Treatment Planning in
Radiation Oncology

THIRD EDITION

Treatment Planning in
Radiation Oncology

EDITORS

Faiz M. Khan, PhD

Professor Emeritus
Department of Radiation Oncology
University of Minnesota Medical School
Minneapolis, Minnesota

Bruce J. Gerbi, PhD

Professor
Department of Radiation Oncology
University of Minnesota Medical School
Minneapolis, Minnesota

Wolters Kluwer | Lippincott Williams & Wilkins
Health

Philadelphia · Baltimore · New York · London
Buenos Aires · Hong Kong · Sydney · Tokyo

Senior Executive Editor: Jonathan W. Pine, Jr.
Senior Product Manager: Emilie Moyer
Vendor Manager: Alicia Jackson
Senior Manufacturing Manager: Benjamin Rivera
Senior Marketing Manager: Angela Panetta
Designer: Joan Wendt
Production Service: Aptara, Inc.

© 2012 by LIPPINCOTT WILLIAMS & WILKINS, a WOLTERS KLUWER business
Two Commerce Square
2001 Market Street
Philadelphia, PA 19103 USA
LWW.com

Printed in China

Library of Congress Cataloging-in-Publication Data
Treatment planning in radiation oncology / editors, Faiz M. Khan, Bruce J. Gerbi – 3rd ed.
    p. ; cm.
  Includes bibliographical references and index.
  Summary: "With the advent of computer technology and medical imaging, treatment planning in radiation oncology has evolved from a way of devising beam arrangements to a sophisticated process whereby imaging scanners are used to define target volume, simulators are used to outline treatment volume, and computers are used to select optimal beam arrangements for treatment. As such, this book is designed to provide a comprehensive discussion of the clinical, physical, and technical aspects of treatment planning. The intent of Treatment Planning in Radiation Oncology is to review these methodologies and present a contemporary version of the treatment planning process"–Provided by publisher.
  ISBN 978-1-60831-431-7 (hardback)
  I. Khan, Faiz M. II. Gerbi, Bruce John.
  [DNLM: 1. Neoplasms–radiotherapy. 2. Radiotherapy Planning, Computer-Assisted.
3. Radiation Oncology–methods. QZ 269]
  LC-classification not assigned
  616.99'40642–dc23

                                                                    2011030518

To purchase additional copies of this book, call our customer service department at (800) 638-3030 or fax orders to (301) 223-2320. International customers should call (301) 223-2300.

Visit Lippincott Williams & Wilkins on the Internet: at LWW.com. Lippincott Williams & Wilkins customer service representatives are available from 8:30 am to 6 pm, EST.

                                                        10 9 8 7 6 5 4 3 2 1

CCS1011

This third edition is dedicated to the contributing authors, whose expertise and efforts are greatly appreciated.

CONTRIBUTORS

Judy A. Adams, CMD
Director of Dosimetry
Department of Radiation Oncology
Massachusetts General Hospital
Boston, Massachusetts

Robert J. Amdur, MD
Professor
Department of Radiation Oncology
University of Florida
Gainesville, Florida

Jonathan B. Ashman, MD, PhD
Assistant Professor
Department of Radiation Oncology
Mayo College of Medicine
Senior Associate Consultant
Department of Radiation Oncology
Mayo Clinic
Scottsdale, Arizona

James M. Balter, PhD
Professor
Department of Radiation Oncology
University of Michigan
Ann Arbor, Michigan

Jonathan J. Beitler, MD, MBA, FACR
Professor of Radiation Oncology, Otolaryngology, Medical
    Oncology and Hematology
Winship Cancer Institute
Distinguished Scholar, Georgia Cancer Coalition
Emory University School of Medicine
Atlanta, Georgia

Thomas P. Boike, MD
Assistant Professor
Radiation Oncology
University of Texas Southwestern
Dallas, Texas

Frank J. Bova, PhD
Professor
Neurological Surgery
University of Florida
Medical Physicist
Neurological Surgery
Shands Hospital
Gainesville, Florida

Arthur L. Boyer, PhD
Professor of Radiology
Texas A&M University School of Medicine
Director Physics Division Radiology
Scott & White Healthcare
Temple, Texas

Jeffrey D. Bradley, MD
Associate Professor
Department of Radiation Oncology
Washington University School of Medicine
St. Louis, Missouri

Jeffrey C. Buchsbaum, MD, PhD, AM
Associate Professor
Radiation Oncology and Pediatrics
Indiana University School of Medicine
Indianapolis, Indiana
Attending Physician
Radiation Oncology
Indiana University Health Proton Therapy Center
Bloomington, Indiana

Matthew D. Callister, MD
Assistant Professor
Radiation Oncology
Mayo Clinic Arizona
Scottsdale, Arizona

George T. Y. Chen, PhD
Professor
Department of Radiation Oncology
Massachusetts General Hospital
Boston, Massachusetts

Kevin S. Choe, MD, PhD
Assistant Professor
Radiation Oncology
University of Texas Southwestern Medical Center
Dallas, Texas

Benjamin M. Clasie, MD
Resident Physician
Radiation Oncology
Rush University Medical Center
Chicago, Illinois

Adam Dickler, MD
Attending Physician
Department of Radiation Oncology
Little Company of Mary Hospital
Evergreen Park, Illinois

Lei Dong, PhD
Professor
Department of Radiation Physics
The University of Texas MD Anderson Cancer Center
Houston, Texas

Bahman Emami, MD
Professor and Chairman
Radiation Oncology
Loyola University Chicago—Stritch School of Medicine
Professor and Chairman
Radiation Oncology
Loyola University Medical Center
Maywood, Illinois

Gary A. Ezzell, PhD
Associate Professor
Department of Radiation Oncology
Mayo Medical School
Rochester, Minnesota
Consultant
Department of Radiation Oncology
Mayo Clinic
Phoenix, Arizona

Bruce J. Gerbi, PhD
Professor
Department of Radiation Oncology
University of Minnesota Medical School
Minneapolis, Minnesota

Benjamin T. Gielda, MD
Resident Physician
Radiation Oncology
Rush University Medical Center
Chicago, Illinois

Glenn P. Glasgow, PhD
Professor
Radiation Oncology
Loyola University Medical Center
Maywood, Illinois

Katherine L. Griem, MD
Professor
Radiation Oncology
Rush University Medical Center
Attending Physician
Radiation Oncology
Rush University Medical Center
Chicago, Illinois

Daniel A. Hamstra, MD, PhD
Assistant Professor
Radiation Oncology
University of Michigan
Director of Genitourinary Radiation Oncology
The University of Michigan Medical Center
Ann Arbor, Michigan

Andrew Jackson, PhD
Associate Attending Physicist
Medical Physics Computer Service
Memorial Sloan-Kettering Cancer Center
New York, New York

Sheena Jain, MD
Resident
Radiation Oncology
University of Texas Southwestern Medical Center
Dallas, Texas

Jian-Yue Jin, PhD
Senior Staff Physicist
Radiation Oncology
Henry Ford Hospital
Detroit, Michigan

Eric Kielhorn, MD
Resident
Radiation Oncology
Loyola University Chicago—Stritch School of Medicine
Resident
Radiation Oncology
Loyola University Medical Center
Maywood, Illinois

Faiz M. Khan, PhD
Professor Emeritus
Department of Radiation Oncology
University of Minnesota Medical School
Minneapolis, Minnesota

Feng-Ming Kong, MD, PhD
Associate Professor
Radiation Oncology
University of Michigan Medical School
Associate Professor
Radiation Oncology
University of Michigan Hospitals and Health Centers
Ann Arbor, Michigan

Hanne M. Kooy, PhD
Associate Professor
Department of Radiation Oncology
Massachusetts General Hospital
Boston, Massachusetts

Gerald J. Kutcher, PhD
Professor
Department of History
State University of New York at Binghamton
Binghamton, New York

Guang Li, PhD
Assistant Member
Memorial Sloan-Kettering Cancer Center
Assistant Attending Physicist
Department of Medical Physics
Memorial Hospital for Cancer & Allied Diseases
New York, New York

Hui Helen Liu, PhD
Professor
Department of Radiation Physics
The University of Texas MD Anderson Cancer Center
Houston, Texas

Thomas R. Mackie, PhD
Professor Medical Physics
University of Wisconsin
Madison, Wisconsin

Gig S. Mageras, PhD
Member, Memorial Hospital
Memorial Sloan-Kettering Cancer Center
Chief Attending Physicist
Medical Physics
Memorial Hospital for Cancer & Allied Diseases
New York, New York

Mary K. Martel, PhD
Radiation Physics
University of Texas MD Anderson Cancer Center
Houston, Texas

Edwin C. McCullough, PhD
Professor Emeritus
Division of Radiation Oncology
Mayo Clinic and Mayo Foundation
Rochester, Minnesota

Loren K. Mell, MD
Assistant Professor
Radiation Oncology
University of California San Diego
La Jolla, California

William M. Mendenhall, MD
Professor
Department of Radiation Oncology
University of Florida
Physician
Department of Radiation Oncology
Shands Hospital at University of Florida
Gainesville, Florida

Dimitris N. Mihailidis, PhD
Chief of Medical Physics Radiation Oncology
Charleston Radiation Therapy Consultants
Charleston, West Virginia

Radhe Mohan, PhD
Professor
Department of Radiation Physics
University of Texas MD Anderson Cancer Center
Houston, Texas

Arno J. Mundt, MD
Professor and Chair
Department of Radiation Oncology
University of California, San Diego
Chair
Department of Radiation Oncology
UC San Diego Moores Cancer Center
La Jolla, California

Lee T. Myers, PhD, DABMP
Senior Clinical Physicist
Radiation Oncology and Molecular Radiation Sciences
Johns Hopkins University
Senior Clinical Physicist
Radiation Oncology and Molecular Radiation Sciences
Sidney Kimmel Comprehensive Cancer Center
Baltimore, Maryland

Lucien A. Nedzi, MD
Assistant Professor
Radiation Oncology
University of Texas Southwestern Medical Center
Dallas, Texas

Colin G. Orton, PhD
Professor Emeritus
Wayne State University
Detroit, Michigan

Niko Papanikolaou, PhD
Medical Physics
University of Texas Health Science Center at San Antonio
San Antonio, Texas

Matthew B. Podgorsak, PhD, FAAPM
Associate Professor and Chief Physicist
Division of Radiation Oncology
Roswell Park Cancer Institute
Buffalo, New York

Arnold Pompos, PhD
Assistant Professor
Radiation Oncology
Medical Physicist
University of Texas Southwestern Medical Center
Dallas, Texas

Karl L. Prado, PhD
Associate Professor Radiation Physics
University of Texas MD Anderson Cancer Center
Houston, Texas

Ezequiel Ramirez, MSRS
Assistant Professor
Radiation Oncology
Medical Dosimetrist
University of Texas Southwestern Medical Center
Dallas, Texas

Michael E. Ray, MD, PhD
Radiation Oncologist
Martha Siekman Cancer Center
Appleton Medical Center
Appleton, Wisconsin

Lawrence E. Reinstein, PhD, FAAPM
Chief Medical Physicist
Department of Radiation Oncology
St. Peter's Cancer Care Center
Albany, New York

William G. Rule, MD
Resident Physician
Radiation Oncology
University of Texas Southwestern Medical Center
Dallas, Texas

Michael T. Selch, MD
Professor
Department of Radiation Oncology
David Geffen School of Medicine
University of California–Los Angeles
Los Angeles, California

Gregory C. Sharp, PhD
Assistant Professor
Radiation Oncology
Harvard Medical School
Assistant Radiation Physicist
Radiation Oncology
Massachusetts General Hospital
Boston Massachusetts

George Starkschall, PhD
University of Texas MD Anderson Cancer Center
Houston, Texas

Kenneth R. Stevens Jr., MD
Professor Emeritus
Department of Radiation Medicine
Oregon Health & Science University
Sherwood, Oregon

Bruce R. Thomadsen, PhD
Professor
Medical Physics
University of Wisconsin
Madison, Wisconsin

Jacob Van Dyk, MSc
Professor Emeritus
Oncology, Medical Biophysics, Medical Imaging, Physics and
    Astronomy University of Western Ontario
Former Manager/Head Physics and Engineering
London Regional Cancer Program
London Health Sciences Centre
London, Ontario, Canada

Kenneth J. Weeks, PhD
Chief Physicist Radiation Oncology
Radiation Oncology
Rex Hospital
Raleigh, North Carolina

John A. Wolfgang, PhD
Instructor
Department of Radiation Oncology
Harvard Medical School
Physicist
Department of Radiation Oncology
Massachusetts General Hospital
Boston, Massachusetts

Joachim Yahalom, MD
Member
Department of Radiation Oncology
Memorial Sloan-Kettering Cancer Center
New York, New York

Catheryn Yashar, MD
Associate Professor
Department of Radiation Oncology
University of California San Diego
Chief of Breast and Gynecologic Radiation Services
Radiation Oncology
UC San Diego Moores Cancer Center
La Jolla, California

Cedric X. Yu, DSc
Radiation Oncology
University of Maryland School of Medicine
Baltimore, Maryland

PREFACE

This edition is an update of the last edition, which was published in 2007. The contributing authors have made revisions and additions wherever necessary to cover new advances and refinements in the field. Several new chapters were added to bring this edition to the current state of the art. These include chapters on normal tissue tolerances, treatment simulation, electron beam therapy, proton beam therapy, image-guided radiation therapy, and stereotactic body radiation therapy.

This book emphasizes modern treatment planning as it involves physics, biology, and clinical radiation oncology. Because of its primary focus on treatment planning, this book presents this topic at a much greater depth than in the books on general topics of medical physics or radiation oncology. Another unique feature of this book is that it is written for the benefit of the entire treatment planning team, namely, radiation oncologist, medical physicist, therapist, and dosimetrist, instead of one group of specialists. It is intended to be useful for both the student and the practitioner of radiation oncology.

We acknowledge Jonathan W. Pine Jr., senior executive editor; Emilie Moyer, senior product manager; and Franny Murphy, development editor, for their valuable contribution in making this publication possible.

Faiz M. Khan

Traditionally, treatment planning has been thought of as a way of devising beam arrangements that will result in an acceptable isodose pattern within a patient's external contour. With the advent of computer technology and medical imaging, treatment planning has developed into a sophisticated process whereby imaging scanners are used to define target volume, simulators are used to outline treatment volume, and computers are used to select optimal beam arrangements for treatment. The results are displayed as isodose curves overlaid on multiple body cross sections or as isodose surfaces in three dimensions. The intent of the book is to review these methodologies and present a modern version of the treatment planning process. The emphasis is not on what is new and glamorous, but rather on techniques and procedures that are considered to be state of the art in providing the best possible care for cancer patients.

Treatment Planning In Radiation Oncology provides a comprehensive discussion of the clinical, physical, and technical aspects of treatment planning. We focus on the application of physical and clinical concepts of treatment planning to solve treatment planning problems routinely encountered in the clinic. Since basic physics and basic radiation oncology are covered adequately in other textbooks, they are not included in this book.

This book is written for radiation oncologists, physicists, and dosimetrists and will be useful to both the novice and those experienced in the practice of radiation oncology. Ample references are provided for those who would like to explore the subject in greater detail.

We greatly appreciate the assistance of Sally Humphreys in managing this lengthy project. She has been responsible for keeping the communication channels open among the editors, the contributors, and the publisher.

Faiz M. Khan

Roger A. Potish

CONTENTS

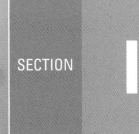

SECTION I

Physics and Biology of Treatment Planning

CHAPTER 1

Introduction: Process, Equipment, and Personnel

Faiz M. Khan

Every patient with cancer must have access to the best possible care regardless of constraints such as geographic separation from adequate facilities and professional competence, economic restrictions, cultural barriers, or methods of health care delivery. Suboptimal care is likely to result in an unfavorable outcome for the patient, at greater expense for the patient and for society.

—BLUE BOOK

Radiotherapy procedure in itself does not guarantee any favorable outcome. It is through meticulous planning and careful implementation of the needed treatment that the potential benefits of radiotherapy can be realized. The ideas presented in this book pertain to the clinical, physical, and technical procedures in radiotherapy treatment planning. Optimal planning and attention to details will make it possible to fulfill the goal of the Blue Book (1), namely, to provide the best possible care for every patient with cancer.

TREATMENT PLANNING PROCESS

Treatment planning is a process that involves the determination of treatment parameters considered optimal in the management of a patient's disease. In radiotherapy, these parameters include target volume, dose-limiting structures, treatment volume, dose prescription, dose fractionation, dose distribution, positioning of the patient, treatment machine settings, and adjuvant therapies. The final part of this activity is a blueprint for the treatment, to be followed meticulously and precisely over several weeks.

Target Volume Assessment

Treatment planning starts right after the therapy decision is made and radiotherapy is chosen as the treatment modality. The first step is to determine the tumor location and its extent. The *target volume*, as it is called, consists of a volume that includes the tumor (demonstrated through imaging or other means) and its occult spread to the surrounding tissues or lymphatics. The determination of this volume and its precise location is of paramount importance. Considering that radiotherapy is basically an agent for local or regional tumor control, it is logical to believe that errors in target volume assessment or its localization will cause radiotherapy failures.

Modern imaging modalities such as computed tomography (CT), magnetic resonance imaging (MRI), ultrasound, single photon emission computed tomography (SPECT), and positron emission tomography (PET) assist the radiation oncologist in the localization of target volume. However, what is discernible in an image may not be the entire extent of the tumor. Sufficient margins must be added to the demonstrable tumor to allow for the uncertainty in the imaging as well as the microscopic spread, depending upon the invasive characteristics of the tumor.

Next in importance to localization of the target volume is the localization of critical structures. Again, modern imaging is greatly helpful in providing detailed anatomic information. Although such information is available from standard anatomy atlases, its extrapolation to a given patient is fraught with errors that are unacceptable in precision radiotherapy.

Assessment of the target volume for radiotherapy is not as easy as it may sound. The first and foremost difficulty is the fact that no imaging modality at the present time is capable of revealing the entire extent of the tumor with its microscopic spread. The visible tumor, usually seen through imaging, represents only a part of the tumor, called the *gross tumor volume* (GTV). The volume that includes the entire tumor, namely, GTV and the invisible microscopic disease can be estimated only clinically and is therefore called the *clinical target volume* (CTV).

The estimate of CTV is usually made by giving a suitable margin around the GTV to include the occult disease. This process of assessing CTV is not precise because it is subjective and depends entirely on one's clinical judgment. Because it is an educated guess at best, one should not be overly tight in assigning these margins around the GTV. The assigned margins must be wide enough to ensure that the CTV thus designed includes the entire tumor, including both the gross and the microscopic disease. If in doubt, it is better to be more generous than too tight because missing a part of the disease, however tiny, would certainly result in treatment failure.

Added to the inherent uncertainty of CTV are the uncertainties of target volume localization in space and time. An image-based GTV, or the inferred CTV, does not have static boundaries or shape. Its extent and location can change as a function of time because of variations in patient setup, physiologic motion of internal organs, patient breathing, and positioning instability. A planning target volume (PTV) is therefore required, which should include the CTV plus suitable margins to account for the above uncertainties. PTV, therefore, is the ultimate target volume—the primary focus of the treatment planning and delivery. Adequate dose delivered to PTV at each treatment session, presumably, assures adequate treatment of the entire disease-bearing volume, the CTV.

Because of the importance of accurate determination of PTV and its localization, the International Commission on Radiation Units and Measurements (ICRU) has come up with a systematic approach to the whole process, as illustrated in Figures 1.1 and 1.2. The reader is referred to ICRU Reports 50, 62, and 71 for the underlying concepts and details of the system (2–4).

Although sophisticated treatment techniques such as intensity-modulated radiation therapy (IMRT) and image-guided radiation therapy (IGRT) are now available, which account for organ motion and positional uncertainties as a function of time, the basic problem still remains: How accurate is the CTV? Unless the CTV can be relied upon with a high degree of certainty, various protocols to design PTV from it and the technical advances to localize it precisely in space and time would seem rather arbitrary, illusory, or even make-believe. Therefore, the need for technological sophistication (with its added cost and complexity) must be balanced with the inherent uncertainty of CTV for a given disease.

The above seemingly pessimistic view of the process, however, should not discourage the development or the use of these technologies. It should rather be taken as a cautionary note for those who may pursue such technologies with a blind eye to their limitations. Technological advances must ultimately be evaluated in the context of biological advances. "Smart bombs" are not smart if they miss the target or, worse yet, produce unacceptable collateral damage.

Treating the right target volume conformally with the right dose distribution and fractionation is the primary goal of radiotherapy. It does not matter if this objective is achieved with open beams or uniform-intensity wedged beams, compensators, IMRT, or IGRT. As will be discussed in the following chapters, various technologies and methodologies are currently available, which should be selected on the basis of their ability to achieve the above radiotherapy goal for the given disease to be treated. In some cases, simple arrangements such as a single beam, parallel-opposed beams, or multiple beams, with or without wedges, are adequate, while in others IMRT or IGRT is the treatment of choice.

Treatment Volume

Armed with knowledge from the clinical evaluation, biological characteristics of the disease, imaging studies, and laboratory tests, the radiation oncologist is in a position to design the PTV, as discussed earlier. The *treatment volume* must be larger than the PTV to allow for limitation of the treatment technique. The treatment volume is defined by an isodose surface that adequately covers the PTV, and its value represents the minimum required target dose. The margin between the treatment volume and the PTV is dictated by the particular treatment technique and equipment. Strictly speaking, the treatment volume cannot be optimally designed without an accurate knowledge of PTV and isodose distribution, both in three dimensions.

Traditionally, the first attempt at designing the treatment volume is made in the simulator room. By this time, all the diagnostic information about the disease must be available. Although diagnostic CT or MRI is usually obtained with the patient positioning differing from that to be used for radiotherapy treatment, the information provided by these images can still be used to design a rough outline of the treatment volume. Treatment fields, possible beam directions, patient positioning, patient immobilization, and surface contours are initially planned using simulator radiographs to visualize the treatment volume. Since a detailed dose distribution in the volume to be irradiated is not available at this stage, the setting up of accurate margins between the target volume and the treatment volume is not possible. However, approximate field boundaries can be marked on the simulator film to include, with suitable margins, the target volume. Modification or fine-tuning of the plan should be possible after dose distribution has been obtained.

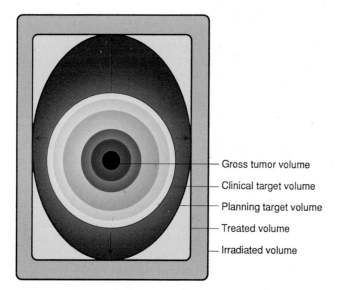

Gross tumor volume

Clinical target volume

Planning target volume

Treated volume

Irradiated volume

Figure 1.1. Schematic illustration of ICRU volumes. (From ICRU. Prescribing, recording, and reporting photon beam therapy. ICRU Report 50. Bethesda, MD: International Commission of Radiation Units and Measurements, 1993.)

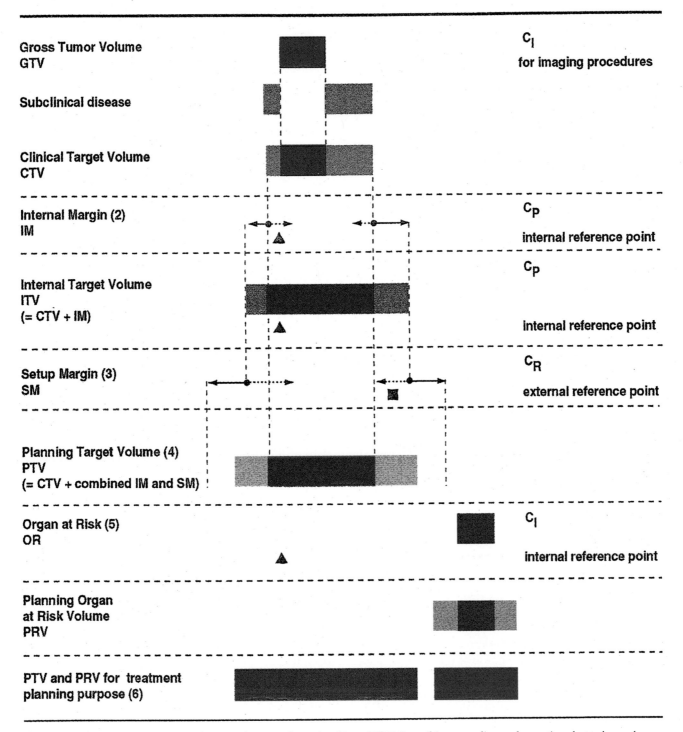

Figure 1.2. Schematic representation of ICRU volumes and margins. (From ICRU. Prescribing, recording, and reporting photon beam therapy [supplement to ICRU Report 50]. ICRU Report 62. Bethesda, MD: International Commission on Radiation Units and Measurements, 1999.)

A more modern simulation procedure involves the acquisition of CT images every few millimeters in the region of interest, with the patient in the treatment position. Immobilization devices and fiducial markers are used to make patient positioning reproducible, as well as to allow registration of positioning landmarks. These closely spaced CT slices provide all the volumetric data one needs to perform a *virtual simulation.* Computer software allows pro-

cessing of CT data to create images in any plane. Radiographs simulating any field orientation with appropriate beam divergence can be reconstructed. These digitally reconstructed radiographs (DRRs) form the basis of *CT simulation.* If PTV and critical structures (organs at risk) are outlined on each slice, the DRRs can incorporate these structures in radiographs reconstructed in any plane. Treatment planning tools allow treatment fields to be shaped and directed for an optimally determined direction to provide appropriate coverage of the PTV and to minimize the dose to critical structures.

In defining field boundaries, one takes into account the physical penumbra of the beam (e.g., lateral distance between the field edge and the 90% or 95% isodose curve). Therefore, the initial outline of the field includes the PTV plus estimated margins to allow for beam penumbra in order to provide adequate dosimetric coverage of the PTV. The final confirmation of the fields drawn must await the isodose plan.

Isodose Distribution

The objective of isodose planning is to optimize the irradiation technique and provide the best possible dose distribution. Ideally, one would like to deliver the necessary dose to the tumor-bearing areas and spare all the normal tissues. However, because of particular beam characteristics and limitations of the radiotherapy equipment, a certain amount of normal tissue irradiation is unavoidable. Moreover, the greatest problem continues to be the determination of CTV, as discussed earlier. Because of the uncertainty of microscopic tumor spread, targets have to be drawn more generously, at the risk of irradiating additional normal tissue.

Optimization of beam placement, beam modifiers, beam weights, and beam energy is traditionally done by iterative techniques. Numerous treatment techniques and field arrangements for different tumors and body sites have been developed over the years. Most treatment planners start with the well-established techniques and make modifications as needed to optimize dose distribution for a given patient. Since the process is essentially iterative and interactive, it is important to have computer software that is reasonably fast and user-friendly. Of course, as the system becomes more sophisticated, such as for three-dimensional (3D) planning, it can become slow and unfriendly.

Treatment planning for modern techniques such as IMRT and IGRT is best accomplished using *inverse planning*. These sophisticated algorithms allow planners to specify the desired dose distribution from the very start and let the computer program the machine settings, and the dynamic multileaf collimators (MLCs) achieve a treatment plan as close to the desired distribution as possible. These techniques will be discussed in the following chapters.

Treatment Fields

Next to target volume delineation, the most important task of treatment planning (non-IMRT) is treatment field delineation. Treatment fields initially set by simulation (conventional or CT scan) may require adjustments in shape, size, and orientation, depending on the isodose plan and other practical considerations. The final delinea-

tion of fields must be made after evaluating the isodose plan. For example, if a simulated field is not large enough to provide adequate isodose coverage of the target volume in three dimensions, it has to be suitably enlarged. The isodose plan can be used as a guide to make the final adjustments in field dimensions, shape, and other relevant treatment parameters. If these adjustments are major, such as beam orientation or beam location, it may be necessary to resimulate the patient. If it is simply a question of field margins around the target, these may be adjusted without resimulation or a repeat isodose plan. Nevertheless, any changes made in the isodose plan or the simulation films must be carefully and explicitly documented. One advantage of CT simulation is that once the volumetric data set is available, field modifications and other changes in the treatment plan can be made without resimulation. The DRRs can be obtained to document the final field arrangement.

Field Shaping

In designing fields, it is important to ensure that the appropriate margins are provided among the field, the target, and the critical structures, three-dimensionally. Although this can be ascertained more conveniently and completely by 3D planning systems, the adequacy of a treatment field can be evaluated slice by slice by measurement of field margins around the target, on which the target and isodose distribution have been displayed. As discussed earlier, field margins are established by examining 3D isodose plans or individually on representative CT scans.

Custom blocking with cerrobend (non-IMRT) has freed the radiotherapist from having to use rectangular or square fields irrespective of target shape. Fields can be designed in any shape by drawing on to a beam's-eye-view (field outlined on a plane perpendicular to beam's central axis) simulator film or DRR. With the use of hot-wire Styrofoam cutters, custom blocks can be designed to provide the desired field.

Availability of computer-controlled MLC has almost completely replaced the cutting of custom cerrobend blocks. These and other related developments, such as conformational radiation therapy, will be discussed later in this book.

Intensity Modulation

Traditional radiotherapy uses beams of a uniform-intensity profile. The uniformity criteria for individual beams are specified by flatness and symmetry. In some cases, the intensity profiles are intentionally modified, as in wedges, so that by combining beams of modified profiles, a conformal and uniform composite dose distribution is obtained. Compensators are another class of beam modifiers that are designed to make the beam profile uniform when it has been skewed or modified by the patient's surface contour or tissue heterogeneity. Wedges and compensators can be called *intensity modulators*. Their use for what we call IMRT is possible but not practical.

Intensity modulation for modern techniques of IMRT and IGRT (to be discussed later in the book) is best accomplished by computer-controlled MLCs as in *sliding window* or *step and shoot* techniques of IMRT or special collimators using dynamic apertures as in *tomotherapy* machines. The required intensity modulation of beams in IMRT, IGRT, or tomotherapy is obtained through the use of inverse planning algorithms, which are designed to produce dose distributions with preset criteria of dose uniformity and conformity for the PTV and tolerance dose for the organs at risk.

Brachytherapy

The treatment planning process for brachytherapy is very similar to that for the external beam except that the treatment indications and treatment parameters are uniquely determined for each procedure. In most brachytherapy applications, the goal is to provide a boost dose to the clinically or radiographically demonstrable tumor or tumor bed (after surgical excision) using interstitial or intracavitary implantation of radioactive sources. Therefore, one of the most important parts of treatment planning, as in external beam therapy, is the target volume localization. This is accomplished by clinical examination, radiologic imaging, and/or CT scanning.

A number of systems have been established for low-dose-rate (LDR) brachytherapy implants: The Manchester, Quimby, Paris, Memorial, and Computer. These systems are characterized by their own rules of implantation and dose specification. Some of them require the use of elaborate patterns of source distribution and precalculated dosage tables. Current treatment planning techniques, however, use computerized treatment planning systems in which dosages are specified according to isodose distribution in relation to the implanted target volume. The evaluation of implants is aided by computer displays of dose distribution in three dimensions or in multiple planes of interest.

While LDR using manual after-loading or remote after-loading techniques is still popular, there is a definite trend toward high-dose-rate (HDR) brachytherapy because of its many advantages over LDR such as treatments on an outpatient basis, higher throughput for institutions with high patient loads, greater capability and flexibility of optimizing dose distribution, and greater personnel protection against radiation exposure. Although the clinical advantages or disadvantages of HDR versus LDR are not well established, HDR technology is fast gaining acceptance and may well replace LDR altogether in the not-too-distant future.

Several chapters in this book are dedicated to brachytherapy techniques and treatment planning. Brachytherapy is a well-established treatment modality in radiation therapy and, in some cases, is considered indispensable.

Facility Organization

Many radiotherapy facilities in the United States have only a single megavoltage unit and a large number of them are staffed by a single physician or with no full-time medical physicist. Such facilities are often not equipped or staffed to do adequate treatment planning. Realizing this nationwide problem, the authors of the Blue Book (1) wrote: "Treatment planning skills, a computer-based treatment planning system, simulation, direct medical radiation physicist involvement, high energy photon and electron beams, skilled brachytherapy and the capability to fabricate treatment aids must be available to the patients in small facilities, either on-site or through arrangements with nearby centers."

Each patient undergoing radiotherapy requires careful treatment planning. Clinical evaluation, therapeutic plan, imaging, simulation, and isodose planning are all part of this process. The quality of the final treatment plan and of the treatment itself depends on how the facility is organized to carry out these tasks. As demonstrated by the Patterns of Care Study (5), the outcome of radiotherapy process depends critically on the facility structure, principally equipment and staffing.

EQUIPMENT

Treatment planning is a process essentially of optimization of therapeutic choices and treatment techniques. This is all done in the context of available equipment. In the absence of adequate or versatile equipment, optimization of treatment plans is difficult, if not impossible. For example, if the best equipment in an institution is a cobalt unit or a traditional low-energy (4–6 MV) linear accelerator, the choice of beam energy for different patients and tumor sites cannot be optimized. If a good-quality simulator (conventional or CT) is not available, accurate design of treatment fields, beam positioning, and portal localization are not possible. Without modern imaging equipment, high accuracy is not possible in the determination of target volumes and critical structures, so that techniques that require conformal dose distributions in three dimensions cannot be optimized. Accessibility to a reasonably sophisticated computerized treatment planning system is essential to plan isodose distributions for different techniques so as to select the one that is best suited for a given patient. Therefore, the quality of treatment planning and the treatment itself depend on how well equipped the facility is with regard to treatment units, imaging equipment, and treatment planning computers.

External Beam Units

Low-Energy Megavoltage X-ray Beams

Low-energy megavoltage beams without IMRT capability (e.g., cobalt-60 and/or 4–6-MV x-rays) are principally used for relatively shallow or moderately deep tumors such as in the head and neck, breast, and extremities. For treatments using parallel-opposed beams, the body thickness in the path of these beams should not exceed approximately 17 cm. This is dictated by the ratio of maximum peripheral dose to the midline dose (6).

In addition to the beam energy, it is also important to have machine specifications that improve beam characteristics as well as accuracy of treatment delivery. Some of the major specifications, for example, are isocentric capability with source-to-axis distance of 100 cm (not <80 cm for cobalt-60), field size of at least 40 × 40 cm, versatile and rigid treatment couch, asymmetrical or MLCs, and other features that allow optimization of treatment techniques.

For IMRT or IGRT techniques, a 6-MV x-ray beam is sufficient so far as the energy is concerned. However, the unit must be equipped with a special collimator having dynamic MLC or apertures suitable for these techniques. Its operation must be computer controlled to allow for intensity-modulated beam delivery in accordance with the IMRT or IGRT treatment plans.

Medium- or High-Energy Megavoltage X-ray Beams

X-ray beams in the energy range of 10 to 25 MV allow optimal treatment techniques for deep-seated tumors in the thorax, abdomen, or pelvis. For parallel-opposed beam techniques, the deeper the tumor, the higher the energy required to maximize the dose to the tumor, relative to the normal tissue. Again, the ratio of the maximum peripheral dose to the midline dose is an important consideration (6). In addition, the dose buildup characteristics of these beams allow substantial sparing of normal subcutaneous tissue in the path of the beams.

One may argue that the degree of normal tissue sparing achieved by x-ray beams of energy >10 MV can also be achieved by lower megavoltage beams using more than two beam directions, as in multiple isocentric fields, rotation therapy, or IMRT. However, for certain cases in which anteroposterior and posteroanterior (AP/PA) parallel-opposed beam techniques are preferred because of simplicity, accuracy, and reproducibility, higher energy beams offer significant tissue-sparing advantages. Also, critical structures may preclude the use of beam arrangements other than the AP/PA parallel-opposed or allow only a limited number of fields, for which high-energy beams are best suited. It is therefore important to have a high-energy-beam capability for optimizing the energy parameter for certain techniques. For deep-seated tumors, high-energy beams offer greater tissue sparing for all techniques, including IMRT.

Charged-Particle Beams

1. Electrons. Electron beams in the range of 6 to 20 MeV are useful for treating superficial tumors at depths of ~5 cm. They are often used in conjunction with x-ray beams, either as a boost or a mixed-beam treatment, to provide a particular isodose distribution. The principal clinical applications include the treatment of skin and lip cancers, chest wall irradiation, boost therapy for lymph nodes, and the treatment of head and neck cancers.

Depth–dose characteristics of electron beams have unique features that allow effective irradiation of relatively superficial cancers and almost complete sparing of normal tissues beyond them. The availability of this modality is essential for optimizing treatments of approximately 20% to 30% of cancers managed with radiotherapy. The indispensability of electron beams for certain clinical situations is best stated by Gilbert Fletcher: "There is no alternative to electron beam therapy" (7).

2. Protons. Proton beam therapy has been used to treat almost all tumors that are traditionally treated with x-rays and electrons (e.g., tumors of the brain, spine, head and neck, breast, lung, gastrointestinal malignancies, prostate, and gynecological cancers). Because of the ability to obtain a high degree of conformity of dose distribution to the target volume with practically no exit dose to the normal tissues, the proton radiotherapy is an excellent option for tumors in close proximity of critical structures such as tumors of the brain, eye, and spine. Also, protons give significantly less integral dose than photons and, therefore, should be a preferred modality in the treatment of pediatric tumors where there is always a concern for a possible development of secondary malignancies during the lifetime of the patient. As of 2009, about 30 facilities worldwide are using proton beams for radiotherapy.

3. Carbon ions. Efficacy of charged particles heavier than protons such as nuclei of helium, carbon, nitrogen, neon, silicon, and argon has also been explored. Currently, there are about three facilities (two in Japan and one in Germany) using carbon ion therapy. Although, carbon ions or heavier charged particles have the potential to be just as good as protons, if not better, it is debatable whether the benefits justify the high cost of such machines (>$200 million). As it stands, even the acquisition of protons is hard to justify over the far less expensive but very versatile megavoltage x-ray and electron accelerators.

Protons and heavier charged particles no doubt have unique biological and physical properties, but "Are they clinically superior to x-rays and electrons with IMRT and IGRT capabilities?" The answer awaits more experience. Clinical superiority of heavy charged particles needs to be demonstrated by carefully conducted clinical trials.

Patient Load Versus Treatment Units

The number of patients treated on a given unit can be an important determinant of the quality of care. Overloaded machines and overworked staff often give rise to suboptimal techniques, inadequate care in patient setup, and a greater possibility of treatment errors. As in any other human activity, rushed jobs do not yield the best results. In radiotherapy, in which the name of the game is accuracy and precision, there is simply no room for sloppiness, which can easily creep in if the technologist's primary concern is to keep up with the treatment schedule. An assembly line type of atmosphere should never be allowed in a radiotherapy facility because it deprives the patients of their right to receive the best possible care that radiotherapy has to offer.

A report like the Blue Book is the best forum for setting up guidelines for equipment use. The recommendation of this document is that the load for a given megavoltage unit should not exceed 6,000 standard treatments (single patient visit equivalent) per year. Depending upon the complexity of procedures performed on a machine, its calibration checks, and quality assurance, the patient load per megavoltage machine for full use can vary from 20 to 30 patients treated per day. Details of calculating realistic load for a megavoltage unit and criteria for replacing or acquiring additional equipment are given in the Blue Book.

Brachytherapy Equipment

Brachytherapy is an important integral part of a radiotherapy program. Some tumors are best treated with brachytherapy, alone or in conjunction with an external beam. It is therefore important to have this modality available if optimal treatment planning is the goal. Although electrons are sometimes used as an alternative, brachytherapy continues to have an important role in treating certain tumors such as gynecologic malignancies, oral cancers, sarcomas, prostate cancer, and brain tumors.

Currently, the sources most often being used are cesium-137 tubes, iridium-192 seeds contained in ribbons, iodine-125 seeds, and palladium-103 seeds. These isotopes can be used in after-loading techniques for interstitial as well as intracavitary implantation. Numerous applicators and templates have been designed for conventional LDR brachytherapy. The institution must follow a particular system consistently with all its hardware, rules of implantation, and dose specification schemes. Remote after-loading units, LDR as well as HDR, are becoming increasingly popular, especially among institutions with large patient loads for brachytherapy. Brachytherapy hardware, software, and techniques are discussed in later chapters.

Imaging Equipment

Modern treatment planning is intimately tied to imaging. Although all diagnostic imaging equipments have some role in defining and localizing target volumes, the most useful modalities currently are the CT, MRI, and PET.

Most radiotherapy institutions have access to these machines through diagnostic departments. The only problem with this kind of arrangement is that the fidelity of imaging data obtained under diagnostic conditions is quite poor when used for treatment planning. This is caused primarily by the lack of reproducibility in patient positioning. Besides appropriate modifications in the scanner equipment (e.g., flat tabletop, patient positioning aids), the patient setup should be supervised by a member of the treatment planning staff. With the growing demand for CT, 4D CT (respiration-correlated) and MRI in radiotherapy and the large number of scans that 3D treatment planning requires, dedicated scanners in radiotherapy departments are becoming the norm.

Simulator

There is still a role for conventional simulators in a radiation therapy department although their presence is becoming less common. As the Patterns of Care Study (5) revealed, there is a correlation between simulation and treatment outcome. Obviously, this correlation is not due to the simulation procedure being therapeutic in any way; it is rather a measuring stick for the treatment planning activity.

Detailed specifications of a conventional treatment simulator are discussed elsewhere (6,8). It is important that the simulator has the same geometric accuracy as the treatment machine. In addition, it should allow simulation of various treatment techniques that is possible with the treatment machines, with the exception of some overly large source-to-surface distances (>200 cm).

A good-quality imaging system, including fluoroscopy, enhances the treatment planning capability. Tomographic scanning available with simulators can be useful if the images are good enough to identify important internal structures. They may be used to verify the localization accuracy of CT scans. However, they are not a substitute for the complete CT scan data set needed for 3D treatment planning.

According to the Blue Book, one simulator can accommodate approximately seven patients per day for "standard" simulations. More complex techniques modify this estimate downward. With increasing sophistication of the treatment planning process and a trend toward repeat simulations to verify the final treatment plan, there appears to be a steady growth in simulator use.

Computed Tomography Simulator

With the advent of 3D treatment planning, conformal field shaping, MLCs, 4D CTs, and electronic portal imaging, it is logical to move into CT simulation. A conventional simulator may be useful for final verification of the field placement, but with the availability of good-quality DRRs and special software for CT simulation, this need no longer exists. Final field verification before treatment can be obtained with the portal imaging system available on modern linacs.

CT scanners have been used for treatment planning for many years because of their ability to image patient anatomy and gross tumor, slice by slice. These data can be processed to view images in any plane or in three dimensions. In addition, CT numbers can be correlated with tissue density, pixel by pixel, thereby allowing heterogeneity corrections in treatment planning. The only drawback of diagnostic CT scans is that of geometric accuracy of localization needed in radiotherapy. Diagnostic CT units, with typically narrow apertures and curved tabletops, cannot reproduce patient positions that would be used for treatment. Although variations due to positioning can be minimized by using flat tabletops and units with wide aperture (e.g., ≥70 cm diameter), the personnel operating diagnostic equipment are not trained to set up patients accurately to reproduce radiation therapy conditions. In addition, diagnostic simulation units are usually too busy to allow sufficient time for therapy simulations. Because of these technical and logistic problems, a dedicated CT scanner for radiation therapy has gained wide acceptance.

A dedicated radiation therapy CT scanner, with accessories (e.g., flat table identical with those of the treatment units, lasers for positioning, immobilization, and image registration devices, etc.) to accurately reproduce treatment conditions, is called a *CT simulator*. Many types of such units are commercially available. Some of them are designed specifically for radiation therapy with wide apertures (e.g., 85 cm diameter) to provide flexibility in patient positioning for a variety of treatment setups. The CT image data set thereby obtained, with precise localization of patient anatomy and tissue density information, is useful not only in generating an accurate treatment plan, but also in providing a reference for setting up treatment plan parameters. This process is sometimes called *virtual simulation*.

PET/CT

The physics of PET is based on the positron–electron annihilation into photons. For example, a radiolabeled compound such as fluorodeoxyglucose (FDG) incorporates ^{18}F as the positron-emitting isotope. FDG is an analog of glucose that accumulates in metabolically active cells. Because tumor cells are generally more active metabolically than normal cells, an increased uptake of FDG is positively correlated with the presence of tumor cells and their metabolic activity. When the positron is emitted by ^{18}F, it annihilates a nearby electron, with the emission of two 0.511-MeV photons in opposite directions. These photons are detected by ring detectors placed in a circular gantry surrounding the patient. From the detection of these photons, a computer software (e.g., filtered back projection algorithm) reconstructs the site of the annihilation events and the intervening anatomy. The site of increased FDG accumulation, with the surrounding anatomy, is thereby imaged with a resolution of ~4 mm.

Combining PET with CT scanning has several advantages:

1. Superior quality CT images with their geometric accuracy in defining anatomy and tissue density differences are combined with PET images to provide physiologic imaging, thereby differentiating malignant tumors from the normal tissue on the basis of their metabolic differences.
2. PET images may allow differentiation between benign and malignant lesions well enough in some cases to permit tumor staging.
3. PET scanning may be used to follow changes in tumors that occur over time and with therapy.
4. By using the same treatment table for a PET/CT scan, the patient is scanned by both modalities without moving (only the table is moved between scanners). This minimizes positioning errors in the scanned data sets from both units.
5. By fusing PET and CT images, the two modalities become complementary.

Although PET provides physiologic information about the tumor, it lacks correlative anatomy and is inherently limited in resolution. CT, on the other hand, lacks physiologic information but provides superior images of anatomy and localization. Therefore, PET/CT provides combined images that are superior to either PET or CT images alone.

Accelerator-Mounted Imaging Systems

After the treatment planning and simulation comes the critical step of accurate treatment delivery of the planned treatment. Traditionally, patients are set up on the treatment couch with the help of localization lasers and various identification marks on the patient, for example, ink marks, tattoos, or palpable bony landmarks. Sometimes identification marks are drawn on the body casts worn by the patient for immobilization. These procedures would be considered reasonable, if only the patient would not move within the cast and the ink or tattoo marks did not shift with the stretch of the skin. Bony landmarks are relatively more reliable, but their location by palpitation cannot be pinpointed to better than a few millimeters. Good immobilization devices are critical in minimizing setup variations and are discussed later in the book.

With the advent of 3D conformal radiation therapy (CRT), including IMRT and IGRT, it has become increasingly apparent that the benefit of these technologies cannot be fully realized if the patient setup and anatomy do not match the precision of the treatment plan within acceptable limits at every treatment session. As the treatment fields are made more conformal, the accuracy requirements of patient setup and the PTV coverage during each treatment have to be made more stringent accordingly. These requirements have propelled advances in the area of patient immobilization and dynamic targeting of PTV through imaging systems mounted on the accelerators themselves. Thus began the era of IGRT.

Each of the three major linear accelerator manufacturers, Varian, Elekta, and Siemens, provide accelerator-mounted imaging systems allowing online treatment plan verification and correction (adaptive radiation therapy) and dynamic targeting, synchronized with the patient's respiratory cycles (gating). The commercial names for the systems are Trilogy (www.varian.com), Synergy (www.elekta.com), and ONCOR (www.siemens.com). These products come with various options, some of which may be works in progress or currently not FDA approved. The reader can get the updated information by visiting the corresponding Web sites.

The important consideration in acquiring any of these systems is dictated by the desire to provide state-of-the-art radiation therapy. Such a system is expected to have the following capabilities:

1. 3D CRT with linac-based megavoltage photon beam(s) of appropriate energy (e.g., 6–18 MV)
2. Electron beam therapy with five or six different energies in the range of 6 to 20 MeV
3. IMRT, IGRT, and gated radiation therapy capabilities
4. Accelerator-mounted imaging equipment to allow the treatment techniques mentioned earlier (such as IMRT and IGRT)

Typically, such a system consists of an electronic portal imaging device (EPID), a kVp source for radiographic verification of setup, an online fluoroscopic mode to permit overlaying of treatment field aperture on to the fluoroscopy image, and cone-beam CT capability for treatment plan verification. Many of these devices and their use in modern radiotherapy such as IGRT are discussed in the following chapters.

Treatment Planning Computers

Commercial treatment planning computers became available in the early 1970s. Some of the early ones such as the Spear PC, the Artronix PC-12, Rad-8, Theratronics Theraplan, and ADAC were instant hits and provided a quantum jump from manual to computerized treatment planning. They served their purpose well in providing fast and reasonably accurate 2D treatment plans. Typically, they allowed the input (through the digitizer) of external patient contours, anatomic landmarks, and outlines of the target volume and of the critical structures in a specified plane (usually central). Beams were modeled semi-empirically from the stored beam data obtained in a water phantom. Various corrections were used to apply the water phantom data to the patient situation, presenting irregular surfaces, tissue inhomogeneities, and multiple beam angles. From today's standards, however, the old systems would be considered very limited in capability and rudimentary in the context of modern 3D treatment planning.

With the explosion of computer and imaging technologies in the last 20 years or so, the treatment planning computers and their algorithms have accordingly become more powerful and sophisticated. Systems that are currently available allow 3D treatment planning in which patient data obtained from CT scanning, MRI, PET, and so on, are to be input electronically. Beams are modeled with sophisticated computational algorithms, for example, pencil beam, convolution–superposition, semi Monte Carlo, or full Monte Carlo. These algorithms for photons, electrons, and brachytherapy sources are discussed in later chapters.

Besides major improvements in dose computational methods, there have been revolutionary advances in software, which allow planning of complex treatments such as 3D CRT, IMRT, IGRT, and HDR brachytherapy. One of the most powerful treatment planning algorithms is called *inverse planning*, which allows the planner to specify the desired dose distribution and let the computer generate a plan as close to the input specifications as possible. Again, these techniques and algorithms are topics of discussion later in the book.

Major 3D treatment planning systems that are commercially available are Pinnacle (www.medical.philips.com), Eclipse (www.varian.com), and CMS (Computerized Medical Systems) (www.cms.stl.com). As these systems are constantly evolving and undergoing revisions, the reader should be mindful of the fact that an older version of any given system may not carry much resemblance to the newest version. Therefore, anyone in the market for such a system needs to do some researching and check out each system with its most current version. Also, because these systems and their software are frequently revised and updated, the user is advised to carry a service contract for maintenance as well as the option of receiving future updates as they come along.

STAFFING

The American College of Radiology (ACR) (9) standards require staffing in accordance with the recommendations of the Blue Book (1). The basis for these recommendations is the fundamental principle that radiation oncology practice requires a team of personnel with appropriate educational and training background. Besides the physician specialists, the radiation oncologists, radiotherapy requires the services of medical physicists, dosimetrists, therapists, and nurses. The minimum level of staffing recommended to meet the ACR standards is shown in Table 1.1.

In the specific areas of treatment planning, the key personnel are radiation oncologists, medical physicists, and dosimetrists. The quality of treatment planning largely depends on the strength of this team.

Radiation Oncologist

The radiation oncologist, who has the ultimate responsibility for the care of the patient, heads the treatment

TABLE 1.1	Minimum[a] Personnel Requirements for Clinical Radiation Therapy
Category	**Staffing**
Radiation oncologist-in-chief	One per program
Staff radiation oncologist	One additional for each 200–250 patients treated annually; no more than 25–30 patients under treatment by a single physician
Radiation physicist	1 per center for up to 400 patients annually; additional in ratio of 1 per 400 patients treated annually
Treatment planning staff	
Dosimetrist or physics assistant	One per 300 patients treated annually
Physics technologist (mold room)	One per 600 patients treated annually
Radiation therapy technologist	
Supervisor	One per center
Staff (treatment)	Two per megavoltage unit up to 25 patients treated daily per unit; four per megavoltage unit up to 50 patients treated daily per unit
Staff (simulation)	2 for every 500 patients simulated annually
Staff (brachytherapy)	As needed
Treatment aid	As needed, usually 1 per 300–400 patients treated annually
Nurse[b]	1 per center for up to 300 patients treated annually
Social worker	As needed to provide service
Dietitian	As needed to provide service
Physical therapist	As needed to provide service
Maintenance engineer/electronics technician	1 per 2 megavoltage units or 1 megavoltage unit and a simulator if equipment serviced in-house

[a]Additional personnel will be required for research, education, and administration. For example, if 800 patients are treated annually with three accelerators, one Co teletherapy unit, a superficial x-ray machine, and one treatment planning computer, the clinical allotment for physicists is two to three. A training program with eight residents, two technology students, and a graduate student would require another 1 to 1.5 full-time equivalent. Administration of this group would require 0.5 full-time equivalent. If the faculty had 20% time for research, a total of five to six physicists would be required.
[b]For direct patient care. Other activities supported by licensed vocational nurses and nurses aides.
ACR recommendations are updated from time to time. The reader should consult the most recent publication on the subject by visiting www.acr.org.
Reprinted with permission from ISCRO. Radiation oncology in integrated cancer management. Reston, VA: American College of Radiology, 1991.

planning team. It is his or her responsibility to formulate the overall plan for the treatment, including dose prescription to tumor-bearing sites of the body. Details of the actual treatment technique, beam energies, beam directions, and other specific details of the treatment are finalized after a number of isodose plans have been calculated and an optimal plan has been selected. The final plan must meet the approval of the radiation oncologist in charge of the patient.

The ACR standards require that the radiation oncologist be board-certified to practice radiation oncology. In addition, the number of radiation oncologists in a given institution must be in proportion to the patient load (Table 1.1). No more than 25 to 30 patients should be treated by a single physician. It is important to ensure that each patient receives adequate care and attention from the physician and that the treatments are not compromised because of the physician's lack of time.

Medical Physicist

No other medical specialty draws as much from physics as radiation oncology. The science of ionizing radiation is the province of physics, and its application to medicine requires the services of a physics specialist, the medical physicist. It is the collaboration between the radiation oncologist and the medical physicist that makes radiotherapy an effective treatment modality for cancer. Ralston Paterson (10), emphasizing this relationship, stated in 1963: "In radiotherapy the physicist who has given special study to this field is full partner with the therapist, not only in the development of the science, but in the day-to-day treatment of patients. The unit team, therefore, even for the smallest department, consists of a radiotherapist and a physicist."

The unit team of radiation oncologist and medical physicist must have a supporting cast to provide radiotherapy service effectively to all patients referred to the department. Dosimetrists, radiation therapists (previously called technologists), nurses, and service engineers are the other members of the team. It must be recognized by all concerned that without this infrastructure and adequate staffing in each area of responsibility, radiotherapy is reduced to an ineffective, if not unsafe, modality of treatment.

The adequacy of the support of physics has been spelled out in the Blue Book (Table 1.1). These are only rough guidelines and radiation therapy practices have expanded greatly since its publication. The number of physicists required in a radiotherapy institution depends not only on the number of patients treated per year but also on the complexity of the radiotherapy services offered. For example, special procedures such as stereotactic radiotherapy, HDR brachytherapy, total-body irradiation for bone marrow transplantation, 3D CRT, IMRT, IGRT, respiratory gating, TomoTherapy, CyberKnife treatments, and intraoperative radiotherapy are physics-intensive procedures and therefore require more physicists than the number recommended by the Blue Book.

According to the American Association of Physicists in Medicine (AAPM), a medical physicist involved with clinical services must have a PhD or MS degree and be board certified in the relevant specialty, in this case radiation oncology physics. Also, most physicists in an academic setting teach and do research, and therefore a doctorate degree is more desirable for them. Such research plays a key role in the development of new techniques and in bringing about new advances to radiation oncology. Paterson (10) emphasized this role by stating "While the

physicist has a day-to-day routine task in this working out or checking of cases, it is important that he has time for study of special problems. These may include the development of new x-ray techniques, the devising of special applicators to simplify or assist treatment, the critical analysis of existing techniques, or research work of a more fundamental nature."

A medical physicist's role in radiotherapy is summarized in Table 1.2. Specifically in treatment planning, the physicist has the overall responsibility of ensuring that the treatment plan is accurate and scientifically valid. That means that the physicist is responsible for testing the computer software and commissioning it for clinical use. He or she is also responsible for proper interpretation of the treatment plan as it relates to the dose distribution and calculation of treatment duration or monitor units.

One important role of a medical physicist that is often overlooked is that of a consultant to radiation oncologists in the design of the treatment plan. Physicians working directly with the dosimetrists to generate a treatment plan without any significant input from the physicist can often be seen. This process may be operationally smooth and less costly but can be risky if serious errors go undetected and the final plan is not optimal. It must be recognized that a qualified medical physicist, by virtue of education and training, is the only professional on the radiotherapy team who is familiar with the treatment planning algorithm and can authenticate the scientific validity of a computer treatment plan. It is important that he or she be actively involved

TABLE 1.2	**Roles and Responsibilities of Physicists**			
Equipment (teletherapy, brachytherapy, simulator)	**Treatment planning (teletherapy and brachytherapy)**	**Dosimetry**	**Radiation protection**	**Academic, administrative**
Selection, specifications	Management, QA of treatment planning computer	Dose calculation formalism	Regulatory	Teaching
Acceptance testing	Beam data management	Special treatment techniques	Radiation survey	Research
Commissioning, beam data measurement	Simulation consultation	Special dosimetry	Personnel monitoring	Developmental
Calibration	Patient data for treatment planning	*In vivo* dosimetry	Facility design	Administrative
Quality assurance	Technique optimization, iso-dose planning; plan analysis, evaluation; treatment aids; beam modifiers			

QA, quality assurance.
Reprinted with permission from Khan FM. Residency training for medical physicists. *Int J Radiat Oncol Biol Phys* 1992;24:853.

with the treatment planning process and that the final plan receives his or her careful review. Because of the tendency of some physicians to bypass the physicist, some institutions have developed the policy of having the physicist present during simulation and doing the treatment planning either personally or closely working with the dosimetrist in the generation and optimization of the treatment plan.

Dosimetrist

Historically, dosimetrists were classified as physics personnel with a Bachelor of Science degree in the physical sciences. They assisted physicists in routine clinical work such as treatment planning, exposure time calculations, dosimetry, and quality assurance. They could be called a *physicist assistant*, analogous to physician assistant.

Today the dosimetrist's role is not much different, but the basic educational requirements have been lowered to a high school diploma. However, more emphasis has been placed on specialized training. A qualified dosimetrist is now a high school graduate with certification in medical dosimetry (CMD). Most medical dosimetrists are also certified radiation therapy technologists (RTTs).

The number of dosimetrists recommended by the Blue Book is 1 for 300 patients treated annually (Table 1.1). However, the number of dosimetrists versus physicists varies from institution to institution according to the total physics support, special procedures, and physicist's involvement in treatment planning. As discussed earlier, the role of a dosimetrist is traditionally to assist the physicist in all aspects of physics service. However, in some institutions, dosimetrists substitute for physicists, and/or the treatment planning procedure is made the sole responsibility of the dosimetrist with no supervision from the physicist. Whether it is done for economic or practical reasons, leaving out the physicists from the treatment planning process is not appropriate and definitely not in the best interest of the patient. The dosimetrist's role is to assist the physicist,

not to replace him or her. The radiation oncologists must understand that a computer treatment plan necessitates the physicist's input and review just as much as it necessitates consultation of other medical specialists in the diagnosis and treatment of a patient.

REFERENCES

1. ISCRO. Radiation oncology in integrated cancer management: report of the Inter-Society Council for Radiation Oncology (Blue book). Reston, VA: American College of Radiology, 1991.
2. ICRU. Prescribing, recording, and reporting photon beam therapy. ICRU Report 50. Bethesda: International Commission on Radiation Units and Measurements, 1993.
3. ICRU. Prescribing, recording, and reporting photon beam therapy (supplement to ICRU Report 50). ICRU Report 62. Bethesda: International Commission on Radiation Units and Measurements, 1999.
4. ICRU. Prescribing, recording, and reporting electron beam therapy. ICRU Report 71. Bethesda: International Commission on Radiation Units and Measurements, 2004.
5. Hank GE, Herring DF, Kramer S. The need for complex technology in radiation oncology: correlation of facility characteristics and structure with outcome. *Cancer* 1985;55:2198.
6. Khan FM. The physics of radiation therapy, 4th ed. Baltimore: Lippincott Williams & Wilkins, 2010:185–188.
7. Fletcher GH. Introduction. In: Tapley N, ed. Clinical applications of the electron beam. New York: Wiley, 1976:1.
8. British Institute of Radiology. Treatment simulators. *Br J Radiol* 1989;(Suppl 23):1–49.
9. ACR. ACR standards for radiation oncology. Reston, VA: American College of Radiology, 1995.
10. Paterson R. The treatment of malignant disease by radiotherapy, 2nd ed. Baltimore: Williams & Wilkins, 1963:527.

2 Imaging in Radiotherapy

George T.Y. Chen ■ Gregory C. Sharp ■ John A. Wolfgang

INTRODUCTION

Imaging is the basis of modern radiotherapy. Imaging plays a major role in localizing the extent of disease, improving treatment planning, guiding treatment delivery, and therapy response assessment.

One of the key advances has been the capability of visualizing patient anatomy in tomographic planes. Malignancies often alter the spatial relationships of normal organs (1) and imaging is essential in defining the volumetric extent, shape, and location of the tumor and adjacent normal organs. Four-dimensional computed tomography (4D CT) additionally provides trajectory information of organs relevant to treatment of moving tumors. Dose calculations utilize electron density data extracted from computed tomography (CT) scans. Serial imaging can also be used to visualize and quantify changes in tumor size and tissue densities for adaptive radiotherapy.

With advances in radiation delivery such as intensity modulated or charged-particle-beam radiotherapy (2–6), radiation therapy is now capable of delivering highly conformal doses. These delivery advances have increased the interest in the development of more accurate methods to image and treat moving targets. Complementary advances in treatment-room imaging have further provided the capability of image-guided radiotherapy (IGRT), in which images obtained on a daily basis before or during treatment are used to correct for variations in setup and organ motion. This chapter surveys the imaging modalities and image processing techniques relevant to achieving accurate radiotherapy.

Examining sources of uncertainties in the radiation process (7) provides insights into ways in which imaging can be used to improve treatment. Uncertainties in the process begin with those associated with target delineation. Early studies on the use of CT scan in treatment planning documented that tumor coverage without a CT scan was inadequate in 20% of the patients, marginal in another 27%, and adequate in 53% of the studied population (8). Defining the extent of the target volume in an accurate, consistent, and efficient manner is clearly important (9). With target positional uncertainties due to physiologic processes (10) (e.g., breathing, variable bladder filling), attention must be paid to adequate coverage of a dynamic target.

Another uncertainty is prescribing the appropriate dose sufficient for local tumor control. The dose prescribed may be limited by concern for nearby dose-limiting normal tissues. Imaging provides anatomic and functional localization of normal structures. A more accurate knowledge of the location of normal structural and functional regions may, in conjunction with sophisticated delivery techniques, lead to delivery of higher tumor doses while sparing normal structures, in order to achieve greater local control without increasing treatment-induced morbidity.

Even if the tumor is precisely contoured and an adequate dose is prescribed, uncertainties in dose delivery exist. The root causes of these uncertainties include (a) random and systematic patient setup error, (b) variations in organ physiologic states, which may cause interfractional target motion, and (c) intrafractional organ motion. Imaging can be used to monitor, quantify, correct, and adapt for these variations prior to treatment delivery. IGRT is addressed in detail in Chapter 12.

The image data sets used in treatment may be broadly categorized into acquired and processed images. Acquired anatomical images include volumetric data, most commonly CT scan, magnetic resonance imaging (MRI), emission tomography (PET, SPECT), and ultrasound (US). Radiographic projection images remain an important component of radiotherapy imaging and include film and electronic portal images acquired during simulation and treatment. Processed images in this chapter are defined as images derived from acquired image data. Examples include digitally reconstructed radiographs (DRRs) and volume-rendered images, both of which can be generated from CT studies.

The general principles of medical image formation are described in textbooks on diagnostic radiology and selected oncology texts (7,11). A clinical review of oncologic imaging is found in "Oncologic Imaging" edited by Bragg Rubin Hricak (12). For a historical perspective of imaging, the observance of the centennial anniversary of the discovery of x-rays by Roentgen has resulted in several excellent historical reviews (13–15).

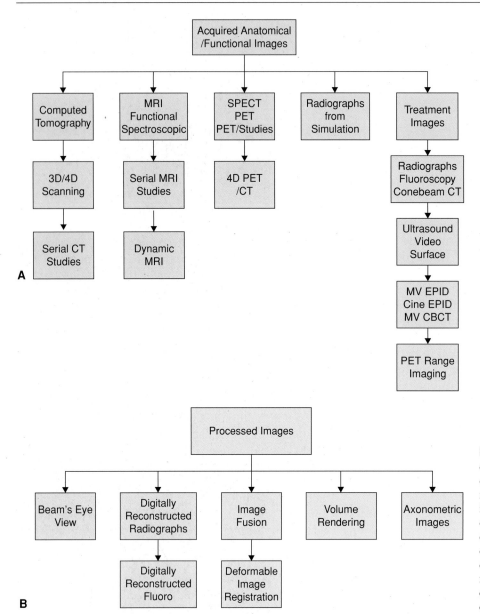

Figure 2.1. Schematic diagram of image data types, (**A**) acquired and (**B**) processed images, used in the course of radiotherapy. MRI, magnetic resonance imaging; SPECT, single photon emission computed tomography; PET, positron-emission tomography; 3D, three-dimensional; 4D, four-dimensional; CT, computed tomography; MV EPID, megavolt electronic portal imaging device; MV CBCT, megavolt core-beam computed tomography.

ACQUIRED IMAGES

Volumetric Imaging

Figure 2.1 diagrammatically summarizes the diverse imaging modalities used in radiotherapy. Volumetric images are used principally to define the geometric shape and location of targets and the location of organs or functional areas at risk. The volumes of interest in treatment planning are defined interactively though a digitizing device such as a computer mouse or trackball.

The terminology and definitions associated with volumes of interest have evolved over time (ICRU 50,62,71). Table 2.1 (16) defines terminology commonly in use (17). Target volume delineation is subjective, and there are uncertainties introduced by interobserver and modality-specific variability (18,19). More advanced computer

automated techniques to aid in image segmentation are under development (20).

Volumetric images are also acquired for target localization pretreatment to improve treatment accuracy (IGRT, typically with cone-beam CT). Serial volumetric studies are frequently acquired during the course of treatment and followup to monitor anatomical changes.

In this chapter, we group acquisition of volumetric images according to the imaging modality, beginning with x-ray computed tomography, followed by MRI and emission tomography. We conclude with a brief overview of projection radiography.

Computed Tomography

Excellent overviews of the history, theory, and basics of CT image formation are covered in texts and articles (21,22).

Abbreviation	Description	Definition
TABLE 2.1 **Target and Normal Organ Volume Definitions**		
GTV	Gross tumor volume	Visible tumor volume
CTV	Clinical target volume	Region of subclinical disease
ITV	Internal target volume	CTV plus motion margin
PTV	Planning target volume	ITV plus setup margin
PRV	Planning organ at risk volume	

Briefly, CT measures the relative linear attenuation coefficient of each pixel (picture element) in the transverse imaging plane. A fan beam of x-rays passes through the patient, and the transmitted radiation is measured. Multiple projection views are acquired as the x-ray source system rotates around the patient. From these projections, image reconstruction algorithms generate an image matrix, typically 512×512 pixels, in which each pixel is a measure of μ_x, the linear attenuation coefficient (relative to water μ_w) at diagnostic x-ray energies. The pixel values are quantified in Hounsfield units (HU):

$$CT \text{ pixel value (HU)} = 1,000 \, (\mu_x - \mu_w)/\mu_w$$

The linear attenuation coefficient is a function of both electron density and atomic number of the tissue within a pixel. Tissue characterization to unfold the relative components of atomic composition and electron density can be achieved with dual energy scanning, although most radiotherapy planning scans are performed at a single x-ray tube potential. For a planning scan (typically 120 kVP), the HUs associated with various tissues and materials are as follows: air, −1000 HU; water, 0 HU; fat, approximately −100 HU; and bone variable up to 1000 HU. HUs of different tissues at diagnostic energies can be approximately extrapolated to electron density (23,24) values that are used for dose calculations.

The anatomic detail imaged with CT is compared with a photograph of the corresponding anatomy in Figure 2.2. The left image is a color photograph of the male pelvis, while the right image is the corresponding CT image (Visible Human Project of the National Library of Medicine) (25). Delineation of an organ (e.g., prostate) on CT may not precisely correspond to ground truth, defined as segmentation of the organs on the visible human cadaver photograph (18,26).

CT acquisition modes include step and shoot as well as helical mode. In step and shoot, a scan in the axial plane is acquired, the x-ray source is gated off, and the couch is advanced to the next longitudinal position. In helical mode, the couch is continuously advanced while the x-ray tube continuously rotates, leading to faster volumetric scan acquisitions. CT simulators currently use multislice detector rings (MDCT), which permit acquisition of multiple slices (from 4 to 64 slices) in one tube rotation. Tube rotation time is ~0.5 second.

The spatial resolution of a CT image is quantified by the modulation transfer function and is a function of scanner geometry (focal spot size, detector size, field of view [FOV], slice thickness) and algorithm characteristics (27). Modern scanners with multiple detector rows can have isotropic submillimeter resolution. Contrast resolution is a measure of the ability to detect objects that have a small difference in HU from the background. CT is capable of detecting

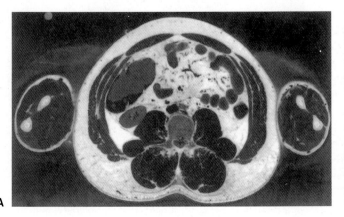
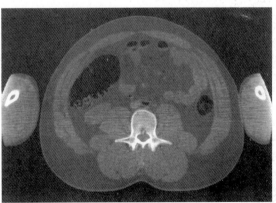

Figure 2.2. A: Photographic section of a human abdomen. **B:** The corresponding CT scan. Visible Human Project.

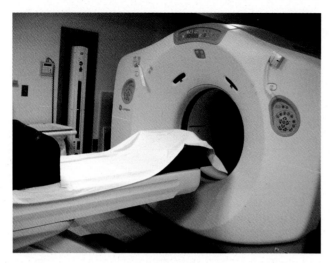

Figure 2.3. A CT simulator providing volumetric images of the gross tumor volume and normal tissues on a patient specific basis. A wide aperture facilitating scanning with immobilization accessories.

and quantifying differences on the order of 0.5% relative to water. Image quality and its relation to scan parameters is reviewed by Judy (28) and Hu (29).

CT Scan Acquisition for Treatment Planning

Scans are most frequently obtained for treatment planning in the radiation therapy department on a dedicated CT simulator as shown in Figure 2.3. Multidetector CT (MDCT) scanners with a wide bore (80 cm) are used for treatment planning scan acquisition because they accommodate treatment positioning accessories during scanning. MDCT scanning is three to five times faster depending on the number of detector rings (4–64). High-speed scanning can capture a bolus of contrast before dissipation, potentially reduces motion artifacts, and minimize issues related to x-ray tube heating.

The scan FOV is selected to permit visualization of the external skin contour, which is required for dose calculations. Longitudinal scan limits are chosen to capture the tumor extent and complete volume of organs at risk (for dose volume histogram analysis). Slice thickness of 3 mm and a total of 200 slices per scanning study (for a helical scan) are typical in planning scans. Convention dictates that cross-sectional images are displayed as viewed from below; for a patient in the supine position on the table, head first into the scan gantry, the image's left is the patient's right. Icons and alphanumeric information imprinted on the scan image provide details of pixel size, slice thickness, and radiographic parameters used during imaging.

Artifacts may degrade CT planning studies. Beam hardening causes streaks when the photon beam crosses particularly opaque regions, such as the bone in the posterior fossa of the brain, or metallic fillings in teeth (27). Physiologic motion can also cause streak artifacts. These artifacts perturb the calculation of radiographic path length. Such perturbations can affect an intensity-modulated

fluence calculation or the calculated penetration of a charged particle beam.

Partial volume sampling is another imaging artifact present in transaxial scanning. Selection of slice thickness influences the detectability of small lesions if the dimensions are not well matched. Temporal aliasing can also result in artifacts (30).

Imaging Moving Anatomy

Respiratory motion artifacts during CT scans have been recognized for many years (31,32). A common observation in a thoracic CT scan of a patient breathing lightly during helical scanning is the presence of discontinuities at the diaphragm/lung interface. Figure 2.4 is an example of such an artifact, where the diaphragm/lung interface is unrealistically visualized due to motion.

These temporal aliasing artifacts have been studied in phantom and simulation (30,33) experiments to elucidate both their source and magnitude. In Figure 2.5, the first column is a photograph of test objects embedded in a foam block, scanned on a moving stage to simulate respiratory motion. Surface rendering of the scan with the phantom in a static state shows life-like realism, as seen in the second column. When the phantom is set into respiration-like motion and scans are acquired in conventional helical scan mode, the resulting images of the spherical objects are significantly distorted, as shown in the next three columns. If a sphere of 6 cm in diameter is imaged during motion with an amplitude of 1 cm (2 cm peak to peak), it may be observed with a longitudinal axis dimension of 4 cm, 2 cm smaller than its actual physical size. The distortion visualized is highly dependent on both scan and object motion parameters, as well as the respiratory phase at the instant the imaging planes intersects the test object (34), which is why the distortions can vary in magnitude. The presence of significant motion artifacts led investigators toward the development of imaging

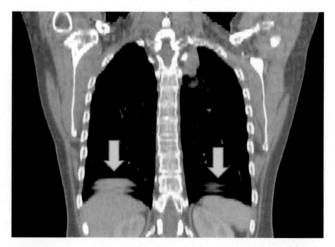

Figure 2.4. Artifacts from helical CT scanning during light breathing. Note discontinuities at the lung/diaphragm interface, indicated by blue arrows.

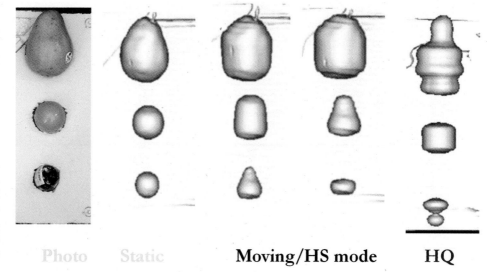

Figure 2.5. Images of phantom, surface renderings of the phantom during static and respiration simulated motion. Note the geometric distortions of the pear and spherical balls. These artifacts arise from temporal aliasing. HS, high speed mode; HQ, high quality mode.

algorithms that imaged object motion as a function of time or 4D imaging.

Four-dimensional CT Scanning

In its broadest sense, 4D scanning includes scans taken at very different time scales and technically includes 3D scans spaced weeks or months apart. 4D CT scanning in this chapter is defined as CT acquisition in the respiratory time scale. The objective of 4D CT scanning is to capture the shape and trajectory of moving organs during breathing. Proof of principle of 4D scanning was initially done on single-slice scanners (35–37) in 2003 and became commercially available shortly thereafter. Respiration-correlated CT uses either a surrogate signal, such as the motion of the abdominal surface, volume of air measured by spirometry, or internal anatomy, to provide a signal needed to re-sort the approximately 1,500 slices of reconstructed image data to coherent spatiotemporal CT data sets at specific instances of the respiratory phase. Scan times for a 4D CT scan with multidetector scanners are of the order of a few minutes, and the end result is typically 10 CT volumes, each with a temporal spacing of approximately one-tenth of the respiratory period (~0.4 s). Details of the 4D CT acquisition methods are described elsewhere (38). Dose during a 4D CT scan is approximately five times that of a conventional treatment planning scan, but may be reduced by altering the radiographic technique without significant reduction of motion information (39,40).

A 4D CT scan provides an imaging method that quantifies and characterizes tumor and normal tissue shape and motion as a function of time. This enables the radiation planning team to design an aperture that adequately covers the internal target volume (ITV) (assuming respiration during treatment is reproducible to that during CT simulation). The 4D CT data can also be used to decide if a motion mitigation strategy is needed (e.g., gating).

Figure 2.6 A and B show images from a 4D CT scan at two specific respiratory instants; the lung lesion is seen in extreme lateral positions, corresponding to inhale and exhale. In this patient, the tumor motion is lateral rather than craniocaudal. Figure 2.6 C shows the difference image, where dark and light areas identify the regions of greatest organ motion. Note that there is relatively little motion of the bony anatomy, and only a slight shift of the trachea between respiratory extremes. The value of 4D CT scan is that it provides a patient-specific estimate of organ trajectories, which can be used to customize treatment apertures and other parameters.

A 4D scan is suitable for assessing organ motion at the ~1-second time scale, but does not have temporal resolution adequate to accurately study motion associated with the heart. Ultrafast scanners, initially designed for cardiac imaging, have been used to study the motion of structures in the radiation field near the heart. A scanned electron beam scanner has been used to acquire CT images near the heart within 50 milliseconds. Scanners of this speed have shown that vessels and tumors near the heart can move by >1 cm (41).

While 4D CT allows for visualization of anatomical displacement and deformation as the result of respiratory motion, the acquisition can still have residual artifacts. Phase-based 4D CT reconstruction, the predominant method used in commercially available 4D CT systems, models the patient respiration as cyclical, assigning a physiological phase (0–2π) to fixed points (inhale → exhale → inhale) during a single period of the respiratory cycle. Images reconstructed at common phase points are used to form a single static CT reflecting a fixed phase point in the patient's respiratory cycle. While this method best reflects the physiological mechanisms occurring during respiration, it neglects the potential variability of lung tidal volume during a free breathing 4D CT exam.

Figure 2.7 demonstrates a characteristic artifact from phase-based 4D CT resorting if breathing amplitude is variable. The target volume splits at the boundary of sequential couch positions during axial cine mode

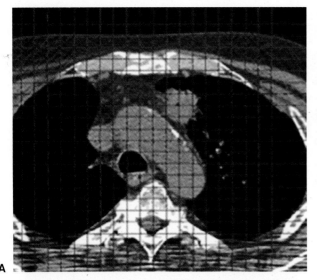

A

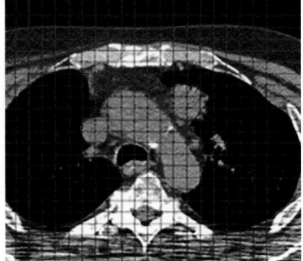

B

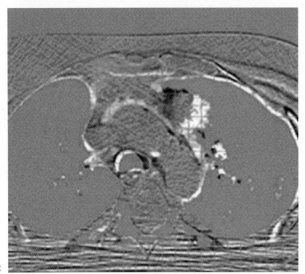

C

Figure 2.6. Images of a lung tumor that moves laterally during respiration. **A,B:** At the lateral extrema of the 4D CT scan. **C:** The subtraction image, where dark and light areas show the greatest internal organ shifts.

acquisition. In this study the patient experienced a relatively large variation in respiratory amplitude between the two couch positions, as shown by the signal from the external abdominal surrogate (RPM) (lower Fig. 2.7). This presents an amplitude mismatch, where points of common phase map to different lung volumes, introducing a distorted target volume.

Variation of tidal volume creates similar artifacts independent of 4D acquisition mode (prospective, retrospective, axial, or helical), due to irreproducibility of respiratory motion. 4D scans require several minutes of data acquisition, during which patients can breathe with variations in amplitude, periodicity, and trajectory. Strategies to coach breathing during 4D scanning have included voice prompts, visual feedback but with variable success. Physical breathing control has been attempted through abdominal compression or active breathing control, where the patient breathes through a regulated valve and is forced to hold his breath at a specific respiratory phase.

Cone-Beam Computed Tomography

X-ray tomography may be acquired at treatment using a flat panel radiation detector available on linear accelerators for IGRT. Imagers of this type are known as cone-beam computed tomography (CBCT). Projection images are acquired at multiple angles, with the x-ray source and detector rotating around the patient in ~1 minute. Reconstruction algorithms suited for this projection geometry are applied to generate volumetric information (42). The value of CBCT lies in its ability to localize soft tissue organs just prior to therapy to enable more accurate targetry.

Current CBCTs have a limited FOV of ~25 cm diameter; by offsetting the detector; the FOV can be enlarged to ~50 cm. Figure 2.8 shows cone-beam images of a lung tumor case. Note that a characteristic of CBCT is the cubic isotropic pixel; the spatial resolution along the longitudinal axis is comparable to that in the transaxial plane. Performance of CBCT data acquisition has been reported, for

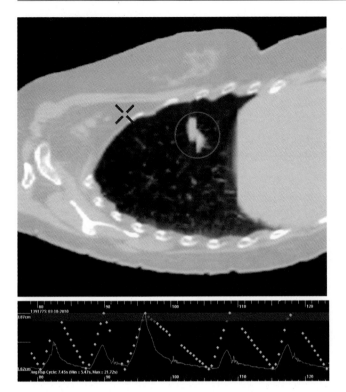

Figure 2.7. 4D residual scan artifacts. Irregularities in the breathing amplitude (RPM trace) below the sagittal image are the cause of these artifacts.

example, by Jaffray and Siewerdsen (43). CBCT can also be implemented at therapeutic energies (MV) to provide volumetric images on a linear accelerator. The therapeutic beam can be used in combination with an electronic portal imaging device (EPID) to acquire image projections (44,45).

Figure 2.9 shows a comparison between conventional CT data and MV CT data acquired by Tomotherapy Inc. (46). Although soft tissue contrast is reduced in the megavoltage CBCT images, there is adequate information for patient positioning. MV CT has potential advantages over kV imaging: (a) attenuation coefficients need not be extrapolated from diagnostic to therapeutic energies and (b) megavoltage tomography is less susceptible to imaging artifacts due to high density objects such as metallic hip implants or dental fillings. As with other tomography imaging, CBCT is affected by motion during data acquisition. Blurred edges of moving structures are clearly visible in the 3D CBCT data. In contrast to conventional CT imaging, where slice-by-slice data acquisition results in distinct artifacts, motion artifacts in CBCT result in blurring. Time-resolved data can be obtained by sorting the acquired projection data into different bins according to motion phases before reconstruction (47).

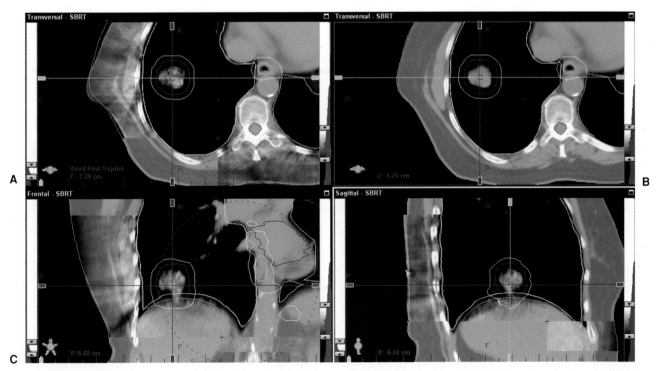

Figure 2.8. Cone-beam computed tomography (CBCT)-guided lung treatment. **A–C:** Checkerboard axial, coronal, and sagittal images of CBCT compared to the planning CT. In a checkerboard image, the image is divided into quadrants as indicated by light blue lines. Upper left and lower right quadrants are portions of the CBCT scan; upper right and lower left quadrants are from the planning CT scan. Boundaries of normal anatomy (outline of the lung, ribs) are interactively aligned. Red and white contours of target contours from the planning scan are seen to enclose the target on treatment day. The upper right panel image is an axial slice from the planning scan.

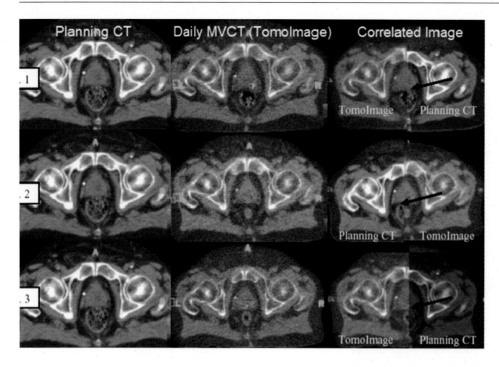

Figure 2.9. CT scan and megavoltage computed tomography (MVCT) scan images of a pelvis showing differences in imaging with MV and kilovoltage radiation. (Courtesy of Tomotherapy Inc.)

Magnetic Resonance Imaging

MRI provides complementary information to CT for target delineation, particularly for treatment sites involving the central nervous system (CNS). It is of growing importance, and some major radiation oncology departments have installed MRI scanners within the department. MRI is used most frequently in combination with CT scans after image registration of the image data sets to a common coordinate system. Figure 2.10 shows CT and MRI scans of the abdomen of a patient at the same anatomical level.

Basics of MR Imaging

MR imaging involves determination of the bulk magnetization of nuclei within a given voxel through the use of radio frequency (RF) radiation and magnetic fields. A stationary magnetic field orients spins of nuclei in the region of interest (ROI), most prominently hydrogen. Orthogonal pulses of radio frequency radiation are applied to perturb these magnetization states, and the nuclei acquire discrete amounts of energy. After each pulse, the relaxation times of the spins to return to the orientation forced by the stationary magnetic field can be measured. During

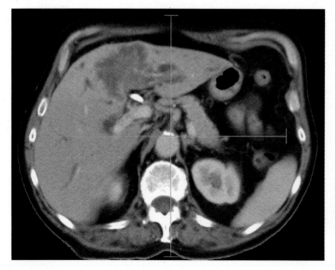 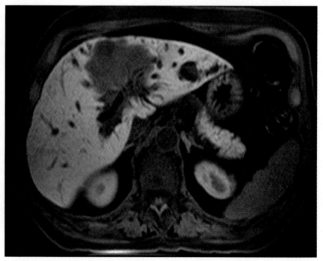

Figure 2.10. CT and MRI scans of patient with liver tumor, acquired at different times, but approximately at the same anatomical level. Lesion is well visualized in the MRI due to superior soft tissue contrast. Bone in CT (white) appears dark on MRI. Fat, due to hydrogen content, appears bright on MRI.

relaxation, electromagnetic radiation is emitted and measured. The quality of MRI depends strongly on variables used in the acquisition. Factors that influence image appearance include the proton density within the voxel, relaxation times, blood flow, and magnetic susceptibility (21). Spatial resolution, contrast, and acquisition time are interdependent. Spin density and relaxation times of soft tissues vary considerably, leading to images with superior contrast resolution in comparison to CT.

Unlike CT, MRI is not constrained to axial acquisition of image data. A 2D imaging plane can be arbitrarily chosen by applying appropriate field gradients during RF excitation. Only spins resonant with the RF will be observed (48). This permits the direct visualization of sagittal, coronal, and arbitrarily oriented imaging planes from MR images. Dynamic MRI is also feasible (49) and has been used to image anatomy continuously in cine mode for organ motion studies relevant to radiotherapy (50–52).

The most commonly acquired MRI scans are hydrogen images. Generally two images are acquired: a T1-weighted image and a T2-weighted image. T1/T2 refer to the spin-lattice relaxation and spin-spin relaxation times, respectively. Paramagnetic materials, such as gadolinium, have unpaired electrons, which result in magnetic susceptibility. The effect of these materials on imaging with MRI is to alter T1 and T2 relaxation rates. Gadolinium chelates are used as contrast media for brain imaging when a breakdown of the blood–brain barrier is suspected.

Magnetic field inhomogeneity, RF field spatial distribution, and effects associated with rapidly changing magnetic field gradients cause artifacts in MR images. Artifacts due to magnetic field inhomogeneity can result in geometric distortion, such as pincushion or barrel distortions, which lead to slight differences in scale along the image axes. Foreign materials may also result in a local geometric distortion. Surgical clips are known to cause problems. On MRI, these materials can cause artifacts characterized by loss of signal and spatial distortion, even when the metallic fragments are too small to be seen on plain x-ray film. If the patient moves, multiple ghosts may appear in the image. Planning scans using this modality therefore must pay particular attention to geometric distortions (53). Phantoms may be used to calibrate MR scanners, but *in vivo* variations are difficult to correct. Typically, a CT scan is also available, and direct comparison provides some measure of establishing geometric integrity. Insensitivity to calcifications, lack of visualization of cortical bony detail (important in assessment of tumor invasion of bone), and degradation of the images caused by motion artifacts are also problems in treatment planning.

MRI in Radiation Therapy

The primary advantage of MR imaging over CT imaging is superior soft tissue discrimination, especially for CNS structures. In general, MRI is more sensitive than CT in detecting abnormalities in the brain. This is particularly true in the posterior fossa, where the CT image is degraded by beam-hardening artifacts, and for low-grade astrocytomas with indistinct CT margins. Under such circumstances, investigators have analyzed and contoured both CT-defined and MRI-defined lesions and combined the corresponding targets (53,54) through image registration (discussed later). In the abdomen and pelvis, multiplanar imaging and improved contrast enable more accurate delineation of the extent of the malignancy.

Dynamic Studies

Cine MRI has been used to study organ motion (50,51). In these studies, the patient is scanned every few seconds in the desired anatomical plane for up to 1 hour. During that time, physiologic motion in the bowel and bladder filling are visualized. Advantages of MRI over CT in documenting organ motion include no dose from ionizing radiation and imaging in the plane of interest.

Lymph Node Visualization

A novel technique in MR imaging is visualization of lymph nodes with iron nanoparticles. Lymphotropic nanoparticle-enhanced magnetic resonance imaging (LNMRI) has been shown to identify the location and extent of the lymphatic system involved with cancer. LNMRI employs a magnetic lymphotropic nanoparticle (e.g., Combidex; Advanced Magnetics Inc., Cambridge, MA; Sinerem; Guerbet, Paris, France) that effectively increases contrast of the lymphatic system during optimized MRI pulse sequences (dual echo gradient sequences). Figure 2.11 presents the results of an LNMRI study for prostate cancer (55). In this case, LNMRI labeled lymph nodes were mapped from 18 prostate patients to a model subject's anatomy, delineating the distribution of lymph nodes. Node positions were registered to the iliac vessels, generating an ideal, generalized treatment margin expansion (purple) of the iliac vessels that encompasses the identified nodes.

Functional Magnetic Resonance Imaging

Functional MRI (fMRI) reveals physiologic and neurologic activity in contrast to structural information (56). fMRI techniques detect changes in blood flow associated with activation of specific regions of the brain. When a task is performed, oxygen demands in that region rise, resulting in a net increase in oxyhemoglobin due to overcompensation. Since deoxyhemoglobin is paramagnetic, changes from increased blood flow result in changes in the signal. Functional imaging of the brain is feasible at magnetic field strengths of clinically available scanners (1.5 T) and is capable of mapping the human visual system during visual stimulation (57), language processing areas; and sensory and motor cortex (58). These areas identified by fMRI can be useful in planning the dose distribution to avoid organs at risk for the specific patient. With conventional imaging

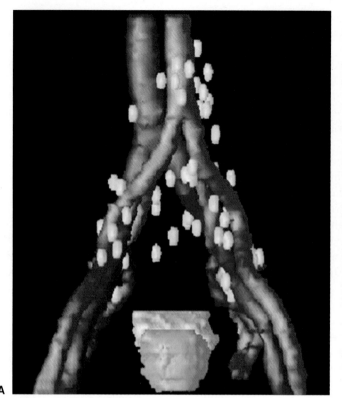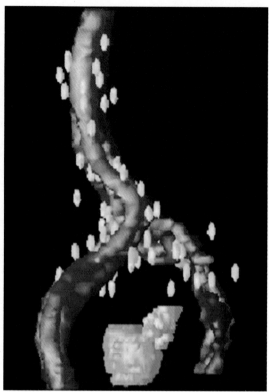

Figure 2.11. Metastatic lymph nodes (yellow) from several patients studied are mapped on to pelvic vessels of a reference patient. The prostate (green) and seminal vesicles (gold) are also shown (**A**) anterior to posterior view (**B**) left lateral view.

of intracranial lesions, only a few brain structures are segmented. Tolerance doses for the optic chiasm, brainstem, optic nerves, and area postrema are known with some confidence and can be defined from anatomical scans (CT or MRI). Although functional regions tend to be generally found in the same anatomic regions of the brain, individual variations can be significant. Furthermore, functional volumes may be displaced from their expected locations by mass effect or functional reorganization caused by an intracranial lesion. If the neuropsychologic activation sites of a specific patient are localized before treatment planning, it may be possible to avoid irradiating these eloquent areas during focal radiotherapy.

Magnetic Resonance Spectroscopy Imaging

The dominant MR signals result from the ^1H nuclei of water. Suppression of signals from water permits the measurement and analysis of properties of other compounds. Spectroscopy was initially limited to small regions of interest but has evolved to imaging multiple voxels. Water-suppressed ^1H spectroscopy techniques are commercially available. For each voxel, the MR spectrum reveals the chemical composition. Differences in metabolite concentrations – either observed by peak heights, peak ratios of different peaks, or the integral of the spectrum – can be used to characterize the tissue. Application of MRS imaging in radiation therapy includes applications to characterize brain and prostate tumors (54,59).

Emission Tomography

Biological imaging can provide important information on the biochemical activity of tumors. Specific biological characteristics of tumors being developed and validated using positron emission tomography (PET) include imaging hypoxia, the degree of cell proliferation, angiogenesis, apoptosis, and response to therapy. Nuclear imaging by emission tomography is of increasing importance in oncologic imaging, and therefore of use to radiation oncology.

Tomographic imaging based on the detection of γ-rays emitted from administered radionuclides includes single photon emission computed tomography (SPECT) and PET. Images are acquired with a γ-camera that consists of a scintillator crystal in front of a camera. The crystal absorbs γ-rays and emits flashes of visible light (scintillations) that are amplified by photomultiplier tubes. Reconstruction of these signals provides volumetric information on the 3D and 4D biodistribution of the radionuclide.

Radionuclides are typically administered to the patient intravenously. The radionuclides are conjugated with biological molecules chosen to bind to selected tissue, producing images that measure biochemical distributions. In SPECT imaging, γ-emitting isotopes are administered, while for PET, positron emitters are used. The positrons annihilate nearby electrons with emission of opposed γ-rays. PET scanners consist of a full ring of detectors to allow simultaneous detection of the emitted γ-rays in all

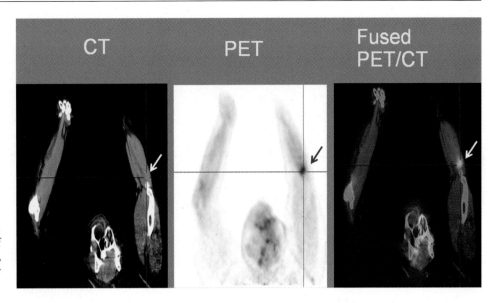

Figure 2.12. PET and CT images of a metastatic lesion of the left elbow, from a PET CT scanner. (Courtesy of G. El-Fakhri, MGH Radiology.)

directions. Volumetric data sets are acquired at several couch positions, requiring several minutes at each position.

PET can be useful in staging the extent of disease. In a study of the impact of FDG-PET on GTV and PTV definitions for planning, Grosu et al. (60) cite numerous uses, including upstaging of disease due to detection of lymph node involvement, increase in size of GTV or PTV to treat regions previously thought to be uninvolved, decrease of the target by excluding atelectasis in lung or lymph nodes.

Increased metabolic uptake can indicate metastases not visible in CT. For example, Figure 2.12 shows planar images of a patient with a metastatic lesion in the left elbow as seen by the enhanced uptake in the PET scan. The tumor is not visible in the corresponding radiograph.

Positron Emission Tomography in Treatment Planning

The role of PET in oncology has increased in importance as a result of the development of PET/CT scanners (60,61). A PET CT scanner is a union of a conventional multislice CT scanner with a PET scanner (62–64). By mechanical integration of these imaging devices, many image registration issues are resolved, although data acquisition times for the modalities are still very different. This significant difference can result in ambiguities in distributions that arise from different patient positioning during scanning (64).

Assessing the extent of cancer with metabolic imaging is one of the potential advantages (60). PET is more sensitive in detection of small masses that take up tracers. In lung cancer, PET is helpful in differentiating between malignancy and atelectasis. In principle, PET is helpful in head and neck cancer in localizing unknown primary tumors as well as detecting lymph node involvement. Data are still being acquired, and the impact of PET in the planning process still requires further analysis.

As with other tomographic imaging techniques, respiratory motion poses a challenging problem to PET imaging. During the ~20 minutes of data acquisition time, periodic motion leads to blurring of the reconstructed

isotope distributions (65). 4D PET acquisition has been reported (61,66). Data acquisition is performed in temporal correlation to respiratory motion by labeling each detected event with the actual motion state. Following encoded temporal data acquisition, reconstructions are performed using temporal bins of detected events.

Ultrasound

The most common application of ultrasound (US) in external beam therapy is localization of the prostate for image guided therapy. High-frequency sound waves, in the range of 1 to 10 MHz, are generated by a piezoelectric crystal. A hand-held US probe is positioned manually over the region of interest. To image the prostate, the probe is placed superior to the pubic bone. When US waves are sent into the body, they are reflected at tissue interfaces, resulting in reflected sound waves. These reflected waves are detected and used to generate an anatomic image that can have high spatial resolution and tissue characterization capabilities after image texture analysis (67).

US imaging immediately before each treatment can be used to determine the location of the prostate (68). After localization, the spatial transformation required to bring the target to the planned position is determined. The target is then positioned to isocenter. A typical radiotherapy US image for prostate alignment during external beam conformal therapy is shown in Figure 2.13.

3D Video Imaging

Surface Imaging

Video imaging to aid patient repositioning was proposed as early as 1970s (69). With current digital video imaging, a 3D map of the patient at simulation can be captured. A corresponding 3D surface image can be acquired on the treatment machine. In 3D video guided setup, the patient surface *du jour* is brought into congruence with the 3D

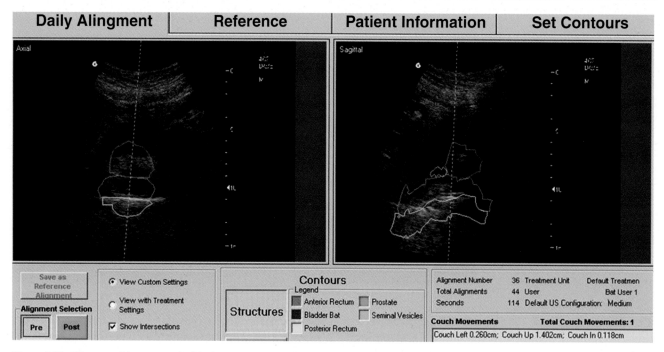

Daily Alingment	Reference	Patient Information	Set Contours

Axial

Sagittal

Save as Reference Alignment

Alignment Selection

Pre | Post

◉ View Custom Settings
○ View with Treatment Settings
☑ Show Intersections

Structures

Contours
Legend
☐ Anterior Rectum ☐ Prostate
■ Bladder Bat ☐ Seminal Vesicles
☐ Posterior Rectum

Alignment Number 36 Treatment Unit Default Treatmen
Total Alignments 44 User Bat User 1
Seconds 114 Default US Configuration: Medium

Couch Movements **Total Couch Movements: 1**

Couch Left 0.260cm; Couch Up 1.402cm; Couch In 0.118cm

Figure 2.13. Ultrasound image acquired before treatment to align prostate to isocenter. Contours from the planning scan are projected onto daily ultrasound image. The patient is moved to the corrected position. The interface between the bladder, rectum, and prostate are used in the alignment process.

reference image in real time. The key assumption in surface guided target setup is that reproducible repositioning of external surface leads to precise subsurface target alignment.

A 3D video generated image is shown in Figure 2.14. In this technology, stereo camera pods view the patient during the flash exposure of a speckle pattern. The system reconstructs the surface topology to an accuracy of <1 mm. The surface at treatment is fitted to a reference surface to determine the transformation needed to bring the two surfaces into congruence. The system is of particular use in aligning the breast (70,71) or extremities. Accuracy of repositioning using video for internal targets (e.g., lung/prostate) is subject to greater uncertainty because of respiration, varying

physiologic conditions, and soft tissue movement. These uncertainties also affect the current three-point and line laser patient alignment. The system can also perform real-time surface surveillance, and alert the radiation therapist of changes in patient position during treatment.

Fiducial-Based Video

There are alternatives to surface-based video for patient alignment. Video tracking of multiple fiducials can also be used. One fiducial-based technique for patient positioning uses a bite block with video-visible fiducials (white balls attached to the bite block). Video cameras triangulate the coordinates of the point fiducials to establish position relative to the treatment apparatus (72).

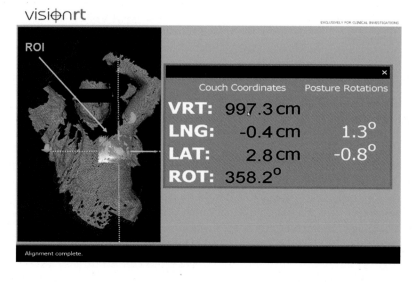

visionrt

EXCLUSIVELY FOR CLINICAL INVESTIGATIONS

ROI

Couch Coordinates	Posture Rotations
VRT: 997.3 cm	
LNG: -0.4 cm	1.3°
LAT: 2.8 cm	-0.8°
ROT: 358.2°	

Alignment complete.

Figure 2.14. Surface imaging by video used to align breast for external beam irradiation. The region of interest (ROI) includes the surface to be aligned to the reference surface. The required moves include the four degrees of freedom of a linac couch (vertical, longitudinal, lateral translations, and couch kick rotation). Posture rotations indicate roll and yaw.

Projection Imaging

Discussion thus far has been on volumetric/3D/4D image acquisition. 2D projection imaging, "films," still have a role in radiotherapy, although diminished. Because projection imaging does not visualize soft tissues well, radioopaque markers (clips) embedded near the tumor are frequently used. Radiographic films are being phased out, increasingly replaced by digital images that can be electronically archived and distributed.

Simulation Images

Many departments still have conventional radiographic simulators capable of radiography and fluoroscopy. Digital radiation detectors have replaced film. 2D projection images are an adequate technique for many palliative setups, such as whole brain irradiation or simulation for bone metastases. In this scenario, the radiation oncologist outlines the region to be treated on a projection image (electronically) and typically uses simple single or AP–PA fields.

An example of a right lateral simulation radiograph for a head and neck cancer is shown in Figure 2.15. The skeletal anatomy and airways are clearly depicted but details of soft tissues are not. In this sim film, a wire has been used to outline a palpable neck lesion. The treatment isocenter is at the intersection of the vertical and horizontal reticule, identified with centimeter tick marks. Solid wires delineate the selected linac jaw settings. Orthogonal radiographs are

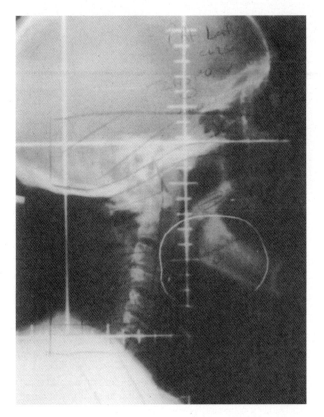

Figure 2.15. Simulator radiograph of a patient with head and neck lesion.

acquired as reference images to establish field placement relative to bony anatomy. If more complex oblique or non-coplanar beam angles are used, reference films still provide data useful for confirming isocenter placement. Fluoroscopic imaging on a digital simulator produces dynamic planar images that can be used to assess tumor motion.

Electronic Portal Images and Image Guidance Radiographs

Projection images are routinely acquired for image guided setup and field placement quality assurance. On current linear accelerators, image guidance is performed at diagnostic energies, with an x-ray tube and amorphous silicon detector mounted orthogonal to the treatment beam. Therapeutic field outlines can be electronically superimposed on the image guidance radiograph. Image quality is good. When high accuracy is required, image guidance radiographs may be taken on a daily basis.

Portal images on the linear accelerator are typically acquired once per week per field to verify radiation port setup. The imaged radiation is the therapeutic megavoltage beam collimated by the treatment portal (e.g., multileaf collimator). Images of the radiation port, superimposed on a larger bony anatomy radiograph, are compared by the radiation oncologist with simulation films or DRRs to determine concurrence of isocenters. Images at megavoltage energies are typically poorer contrast than at diagnostic energy. If the target registration is within the specified accuracy (typically <5 mm), no change is requested by the attending physician. If a field movement relative to anatomy is requested, it is usually a translation in the aperture plane rather than an in-plane or out-of-plane rotation. Six to seven port films per field are acquired during the course of fractionated radiotherapy for quality assurance purposes.

Digital portal images are integrated into the Department's electronic record. Instead of using film, the transmission image is captured by a digital detector. Computer software facilitates the comparison of the simulation film and EPID images. Computer-aided registration of these films quantitates the magnitude and direction of differences and aids the radiation therapist in repositioning.

An EPID can be run in the cine mode, where a continuous sequence of images is captured. Frame rate is determined by the capability of the imaging hardware to read out an image and reinitialize the detector before the next frame. Typical frame rates are of the order of 5 to 15 frames per second. At this rate, it is feasible to visualize the exit therapeutic beam during respiration. When radioopaque clips are visible, cine EPID can be useful in verifying that the motion of the tumor (as represented by the clips) is within the planned range of motion (73).

Image Transfer to Planning Systems

Digital data acquired on volumetric scanners are transferred to treatment planning computers for segmentation, processing, and planning by electronic network. Image format standards such as DICOM transfer between imaging devices and treatment planning computers is the industry standard; DICOM RT, a format that accommodates radiotherapy-specific parameters, is under development (74,75).

PROCESSED IMAGES

Acquired tomographic images may undergo extensive image processing to generate new types of images. The primary data extracted from the acquired studies are those that help determine the size, shape, location, and motion of the target volume relative to adjacent normal tissues likely to receive treatments.

Beam's Eye View and Digitally Reconstructed Radiographs

Beam's eye views (BEVs) and DRRs are processed images that are generated for virtually all patients undergoing conformal radiotherapy (76–78); these two components are complementary. The target and adjacent organs at risk are segmented on the volumetric CT scan and represented as a ring-stack of contours or as outlines. The DRR component generates a projection image principally of the

bony anatomy and low-density anatomy (airways, lung), which provide an internal anatomy coordinate system. The DRR is generated by 3D ray tracing from the radiation source through the volume of CT data, projecting the final image onto a plane. The DRR is the reference image against which the IGRT radiograph is compared to make final adjustments in patient position. The two components are typically fused into one image on the treatment planning workstation display.

Since the viewpoint is from the radiation source, the BEV image accurately portrays the projection of the radiation field as it passes through both target and normal organs. The 3D target projected onto a 2D plane defines the aperture shape, and interactively varying the beam angle permits the choice of a portal entry to avoid or minimize the irradiation of critical structures while encompassing the target (79). A typical BEV display is shown in Figure 2.16.

Image Registration

Image registration, the alignment of two different image data sets, is an important image processing technique used in radiotherapy to improve target delineation, image understanding, and alignment of planning and treatment images. Use of multiple images typically requires that the images be analyzed in a common coordinate system. For

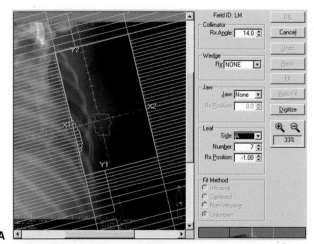
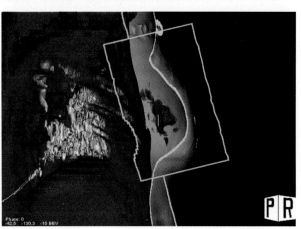
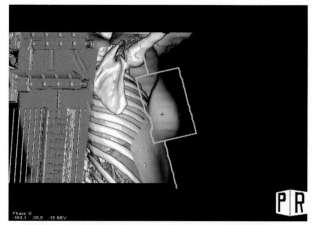

Figure 2.16. Beam's eye view of tangential breast. (**A**) conventional BEV showing DRR of breast with bony anatomy visible. (**B**) Volume rendered surface view showing breast skin surface and radiation field outline. The cut plane is advanced to reveal the scapula and ribs. (**C**) Volume rendered view is windowed and leveled to reveal lesion in breast (red) with part of lung and chest wall visualized. The bright yellow line indicated the intersection of the cut plane with the breast skin surface. Cross hairs indicate planned position of isocenter.

example, the extent of a tumor might be visible on MRI, but must be accurately mapped into the coordinate system of a CT image for treatment planning. The enabling technology for mapping information between different image data is known as image registration. Ideally, image registration defines a one-to-one mapping between the coordinates of a point in one space with a corresponding point in the second space (80). The coordinate systems involved may be image spaces or physical space such as the patient or the treatment room. Therefore, aiming a physical radiation beam at an image-defined target within a patient requires the solution of at least one and possibly multiple registration problems. Such image-to-physical space registration is the essence of virtual simulation. Strategies for daily IGRT, whether adaptive or not, also depend on registration of the daily anatomy as defined by pretreatment images. These images are acquired in (or registered with) the coordinate system of the treatment machine, with the planned radiation beams, and the 3D planning images with respect to which those beams were originally defined.

In radiation oncology, image registration is used for a wide range of applications, including the visualization, delineation of anatomical and function structures, pretreatment patient positioning, and evaluation of treatment response. For example, a preoperative scan can be registered to a postoperative treatment planning scan to define the target volume at risk. Anatomic and functional images from MRI or emission tomography can also be defined and mapped onto CT scans for planning (81,82). Another use of image registration is the correlation of multiple serial scans of the same patient to provide data on the 3D movement of internal organs needed to determine appropriate portal margins. Several groups have reported on the variation of prostate and seminal vesicle position during the course of fractionated external beam therapy (83–85). In these studies, the serial CT data sets must first be aligned relative to each other (bony anatomy alignment). The position of the prostate/seminal vesicles is then measured relative to the common coordinate system. These studies show anisotropic prostate motion with daily variations of a few millimeters in the left–right axis to upward of 1 to 1.5 cm in the anteroposterior (AP) axis.

Several comprehensive reviews of medical image registration have appeared (80,86–88). We will briefly survey some of the most commonly used image registration methods and describe their inner workings. The first distinction we will make is based on the degree of automation. Registration can be performed manually, semiautomatically, or fully automatically. Manual registration is common for routine clinical use, especially when performing translational (3-DOF) or rigid (6-DOF) matching. The operator visually inspects and adjusts the match using interactive tools, such as a custom viewport where the operator can slide the images back and forth or a landmark selection tool to define matching points. As the user adjusts the transformation parameters, the display is updated with blended sections through the newly

transformed second scan. Semiautomatic tools allow for a limited degree of feedback from the user, such as a starting guess or an incomplete set of matching points. Fully automatic methods generate a transformation matrix without operator feedback, but still requires inspection of the final alignment to validate its correctness.

Automatic methods are characterized by their *transform* and *cost function*. The transform defines the nature of the mapping between spaces and is either linear (such as pure translation, rigid, and affine) or nonlinear (such as B-spline or free-form). The cost function is a numeric score that defines the relative quality of a match. Methods are broadly classified into either "intensity-based" or "feature-based," though the distinction is not exact and hybrid methods exist as well. Intensity-based methods find the best image match by computing the cost directly from raw or corrected image intensities. In contrast, feature-based methods perform matching based on a reduced representation, such as point or curve landmarks. In either case, the best transform for a given cost function is selected using an *optimizer*. Intensity-based methods generally require the use of a nonlinear optimizer, which finds a local minimum of the cost function. Some feature-based methods can use geometric optimizers that achieve globally optimal solutions, while others require nonlinear optimizers.

The choice of cost function is usually decided based on the image modalities involved. For registration of CT to CT, one can consider the use of the mean-squared error cost function. This cost function computes the intensity difference between corresponding voxels of both images and sums their squared difference. Another commonly used method is one in which locations of high gradients, that is, edges, are matched in 3D by an automated procedure. This requires defining a measure of how well the two sets of edges match; a popular way of doing this is through the distance transform or "chamfer-matching" approach (89). In this method, each voxel in the first image volume is labeled by its distance to the nearest edge feature. This essentially produces a new image volume in which the brightness at each point is given by how far that point is away from an edge. Points close to edges are dark; points far from edges are bright. Matching the second scan to the first is then reduced to finding the transformation of the set of edges from the second scan, such that the sum of the values of the first scan's distance image over all points on the transformed edges is minimized.

Image registration can be applied to both serial studies of the same modality, for example, a planning and daily setup CT scan, or to image studies from different modalities, CT scan and MRI, or anatomic images with functional images. Identification of homologous features in cross-modality registration may become difficult, and much effort has been spent on the development of methods that are robust in registration of multimodality imaging. In the past decade, a method that has come to be widely utilized for both intra- and intermodality registration is maximization of mutual information (86,90–92), which is now briefly described.

The utility of mutual information as an image matching tool is based on the intuitively reasonable assumption that while corresponding anatomical regions may have different distributions of intensities in two different image modalities, it is generally true that the relationship between those intensities is predictable and consistent. Bony anatomy is bright in a CT scan and dark in MRI, for example, and therefore one could map very bright regions in a CT scan onto very dark regions in MRI. Mutual information implicitly extends this idea to every location in the image through its mathematical definition in terms of the joint probability density function of the matched images.

To illustrate how the joint probability distribution can characterize image matching, consider the artificial situation shown in Figure 2.17 A,B, where a CT scan and MRI scan of the same patient's brain are to be matched. In this example, there are only four tissue regions: air, bone,

brain, and fat. Air is dark on both modalities; bone is bright on CT scan and dark on MRI; brain and fat are intermediate in both modalities but their relative intensities are reversed with brain brighter in CT scan and fat brighter in MRI. Assume further that there is one and only one intensity value associated with each of these classes. If the entire 3D image volumes were perfectly registered, then every bone CT voxel would map onto a bone MR voxel, brain onto brain, and so forth. If a joint histogram of the CT scan and MR intensity is constructed as shown in Figure 2.17 C, where each point on the base plane represents a single combination of CT intensity and MR intensity, we would find that the histogram will contain zeros everywhere except at the four points corresponding to CT bone, MR bone; CT brain, MR brain; CT air, MR air; and CT fat, MR fat. Now if the image volumes were to become slightly misaligned, some CT bone voxels would

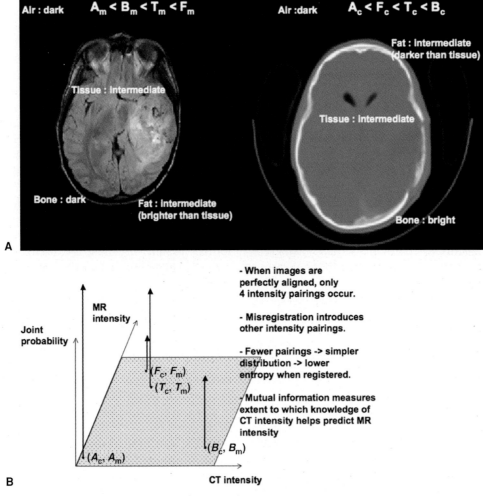

Figure 2.17. **A:** Hypothetical computed tomography and magnetic resonance imaging slices with only four tissue classes to be registered. Relationships between voxel intensities in air, bone, tissue, and fat regions are indicated on the images. **B:** Joint intensity histogram of the hypothetical computed tomographic and magnetic resonance imaging volumes when perfectly registered. All voxels fall into one of only four bins in the histogram, since corresponding tissue types map onto each other perfectly. Misorientation will introduce additional peaks in the distribution, as different tissues map onto each other. CT, computed tomography; MR, magnetic resonance.

map onto MR brain voxels, introducing another peak in the joint histogram. Some MR bone voxels would likewise map onto CT brain voxels, introducing yet another peak, and so forth. In fact, some voxels from each of the four CT tissue classes could map onto all four MR voxel classes, leading to potentially 16 different peaks. Therefore, the effect of misalignment is to reduce the sharpness of the joint histogram. The sharpness of such a distribution can be expressed in terms of its entropy, which is defined in a way analogous to thermodynamic entropy:

$$H(A,B) = -\sum_{a,b} p(a,b) \times \log p(a,b)$$

where $H(A,B)$ is the entropy associated with the distribution of values a and b in images A and B, $p(a,b)$ is the normalized joint intensity distribution, and the sum is the over all image values in each of the two images. The entropies of the individual images A and B are defined analogously:

$$H(A) = -\sum_a p(a) \times \log p(a)$$
$$H(B) = -\sum_b p(b) \times \log p(b)$$

Entropy in this context expresses the lack of order, or the uncertainty, in a distribution, just as in thermodynamics.

One of a number of equivalent definitions of mutual information is

$$I(A,B) = H(B) - H(B|A)$$

where $H(B|A)$ is the entropy of the marginal probability distribution $p(b|a)$, the probability of finding value b in image B, given that the corresponding point in image A has value a. This form shows that $I(A,B)$ represents the reduction in uncertainty in the value of image B, given that the value of image A is known. Referring back to our simple example, when the images are perfectly registered, knowing that a voxel has the bone value in the CT scan means that the corresponding voxel in the MR scan will have the MR bone value, with no uncertainty. In this case, $H(B|A)$ would be small (small uncertainty means low entropy) and $I(A,B)$ would be maximized. Mutual information and its variants have been used to register CT, MRI, PET, SPECT, and various 2D images (anatomic and functional, radiographic, and photographic) with themselves and with each other.

Image registration is an active area of research, and steady improvements in accuracy and reliability are seen each year. In addition to commercial offerings, there are a number of high-quality open source implementations. In addition to general-purpose registration packages such as the Insight Toolkit (http://www.itk.org) or 3D Slicer (http://slicer.org), radiotherapy-specific problems can be solved with applications such as Plastimatch (http://plastimatch.org) or Dirart (DIRART).

A useful application of deformable registration is the propagation of contours of organs from one respiratory phase to another. Figure 2.18 shows such an example. In this case, the liver was segmented by the physician on the T30 phase of respiration. To study organ deformation and perform 4D dose calculations, it is necessary to contour the liver on all 10 phases. This is clearly a tedious and impractical task. Image registration may be used to propagate contours. During the process of deformable registration, the vector mapping of each voxel from one phase to all other phases is calculated. This transformation may then be applied to the voxels that define the contour, to map the organ outline to other phases. There are some small discrepancies, as seen in Figure 2.18, but most contours are acceptable. Editing may be applied to the propagated contours as needed. A full set of 3D contours at each phase permits calculation and quantitative assessment of organ trajectories.

Volume Visualization

An alternative to ring-stack or surface display of anatomy is volume visualization, initially described in computer science literature (93). In volume rendering, the opacity and hue of a voxel of the 3D image data set are set by the operator to be a function of its CT number. Volume-rendered displays have been used in treatment planning for radiotherapy (93–95).

Figure 2.19 is a volumetric display of CT data. The image is of a patient with a lung tumor, and the data rendered are from a high-quality treatment planning scan (0.5-mm slice thickness, 256 slice scanner). The lung parenchyma is rendered transparent, and the tracheobronchial tree is visualized along with bony anatomy. The visualization software used (96,97) displays regions of high gradients in HU that essentially display interfaces. Therefore, the contents of organs (e.g., heart) are not seen.

One advantage of volumetric visualization in radiotherapy planning is that this technique can display anatomic detail not normally segmented. Nerves, vessels, and lymph nodes are difficult to identify and laborious to segment on axial cuts. Yet these structures may be directly seen in a volumetric rendering from a selected BEV. The hypothesis is that visualization of these structures may help in aperture design of the clinical target volume.

The difficulty of volume visualization is that so much anatomy, including overlying tissues, is visualized, and some are not relevant to the planning task. Methods to display only the relevant anatomy from a given beam perspective are needed. Interactive tools capable of selectively peeling away tissues obscuring the volume of interest must be incorporated into these techniques to reveal the volumes of interest.

Imaging Response

Processing serial volumetric images to assess response to therapy is key. For the individual patient, early evidence of

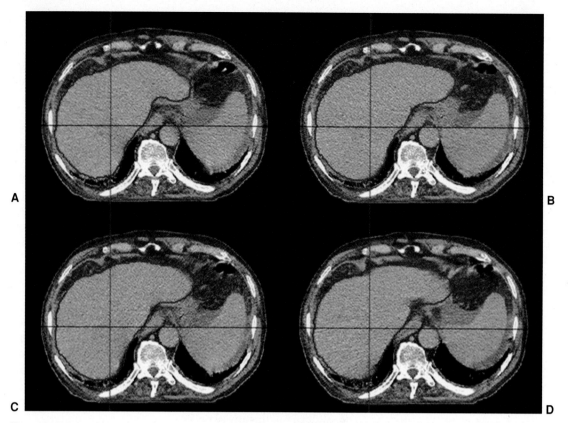

Figure 2.18. Segmentation of liver by deformable registration. Contours are shown at (**A**) T10, (**B**) T30, (**C**) T50, (**D**) T70. The liver was manually contoured volumetrically at T30 respiratory phase; deformable registration was used to map this volume to nine other respiratory phases. Accuracy is best near T30, with a few millimeter inaccuracies at phases farther from reference (T30).

treatment ineffectiveness can prompt adjustments in treatment. In clinical trials, evidence of the effectiveness of a new agent or technique can speed its approval by regulatory bodies. The endpoint of overall survival from a therapeutic modality may take decades to quantify. Biomarkers

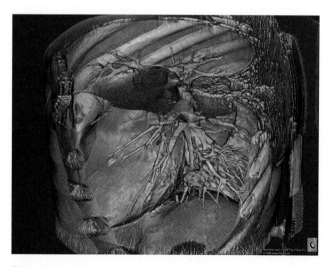

Figure 2.19. Volume visualization of a lung tumor. Lung parenchyma rendered transparent. The tracheobronchial tree is visible as are surface interfaces of bony anatomy and mediastinum. Scan is high resolution 0.5-mm slice thickness 256 slice CT scanner with 14-cm longitudinal coverage. (Courtesy of Fovia.com.)

that indicate response can indicate which therapeutic approaches are most promising. Imaging both anatomical and biologic response to treatment provides a noninvasive method to measure response.

The importance of reliable tumor measurement in the assessment of response to therapy has been long recognized. Grossman and Burch (98) wrote "The ability to compare results of clinical trials depends upon consistent definitions of tumor response and the use of reliable and reproducible methods of tumor measurement." Usually the response of tumors to localized or systemic therapy falls into one of four categories: complete response, partial response, stable disease, or progressive disease. Each of these is associated with an approximate measure of tumor volume changes. Follow-up images may also be useful in correlating complications with delivered dose distributions if there is radiographic visualization of the complications, such as radiation pneumonitis in an irradiated lung.

The two most widely used anatomic tumor response criteria have been the WHO criteria (1980s) and the Response Evaluation Criteria in Solid Tumors (RECIST 1.0 and 1.1) in the past decade. WHO criteria was based on the product of the longest diameter and its perpendicular diameter of a tumor dimension. Its ease of computation and simplicity facilitated response reporting internationally. RECIST was developed to even further simplify measurement and address WHO response criteria limitations. Both WHO and RECIST categorize treatment response into the four categories: complete response, partial response (30% decrease in tumor size from baseline), stable disease, and progressive disease (20% or greater increase in tumor dimension). Limitations in the anatomical approach to measuring response have been discussed in the literature (99).

Advances in molecular and biological imaging are also being actively developed to measure tumor response. Wahl et al. (100) have suggested the use of metabolic imaging to measure tumor response. The biologic signal from 18F-FDG is often more "predictive of histologic and survival outcomes than anatomic imaging." Quantitation of tracer uptake is technically challenging and requires an understanding of the bias and variability of such measurements (101).

REFERENCES

1. Waxman AD. Radionuclide imaging in cancer medicine. In: Holland J et al., eds. *Cancer medicine.* Philadelphia: Lea & Febiger, 1993:483–486.
2. Boyer AL, Butler EB, DiPetrillo TA, et al. Intensity-modulated radiotherapy: current status and issues of interest. *Int J Radiat Oncol Biol Phys* 2001;51(4):880–914.
3. Chen GTY, Castro JR, Quivey JM. Heavy charged-particle radiotherapy. *Ann Rev Biophys Bioeng* 1981;10: 499–529.
4. Loeffler JS, Smith AR, Suit HD. The potential role of proton beams in radiation oncology. *Semin Oncol* 1997;24(6):686–695.
5. Orecchia R, Krengli M, Jereczek-Fossa BA, et al. Clinical and research validity of hadrontherapy with ion beams. *Crit Rev Oncol Hematol* 2004;51(2):81–90.
6. Schulz-Ertner D, Tsujii H. Particle radiation therapy using proton and heavier ion beams. *J Clin Oncol* 2007;25(8):953–964. doi:10.1200/JCO.2006.09.7816.
7. Goitein Michael. *Radiation oncology: a physicist's-eye view.* Heidelberg, Germany: Springer Science. 2008.
8. Munzenrider JE, Pilepich M, Rene-Ferrero JB. Use of a body scanner in radiotherapy treatment planning. *Cancer* 1977;40:170–179.
9. Leunens G, Menten J, Weltens C. Quality assessment of medical decision making in radiation oncology: variability in target volume delineation for brain tumors. *Radiother Oncol* 1993;29:169–175.
10. Langen KM, Jones DT. Organ motion and its management. *Int J Radiat Oncol Biol Phys* 2001;50(1):265–278.
11. Dendy PP, Heaton B. Physics for diagnostic radiology. Second edition. *Medical science series.* Bristol: Institute of Physics, 1999.
12. Bragg DG, Rubin P, Hricak H. Oncologic Imaging. Second edition. Philadelphia: Saunders, 2002.
13. Rosenow UF. Notes on the legacy of the Roentgen rays. *Med Phys* 1995;22:1855–1868.
14. Selgier HH. Wilhelm Conrad Roentgen and the glimmer of light. *Phys Today* 1995;48:25–31.
15. Siebert JA. One hundred years of medical technology. *Health Phys* 1995;69:695–720.
16. Berthelsen Anne Kiil, Dobbs Jane, Kjellén Elisabeth, et al. What's new in target volume definition for radi-

17. Van Den Berge DL, Ridder MD, Storme GA. Imaging in radiotherapy. *Eur J Radiol* 2000;36(1):41–48.
18. Gao Z, Wilkins D, Eapen L, et al. A study of prostate delineation referenced against a gold standard created from the visible human data. *Radiother Oncol* 2007;85(2):239–246. doi:10.1016/j.radonc.2007.08.001.
19. Rasch C, Barillot I, Remeijer P, et al. Definition of the prostate in CT and MRI: a multi-observer study. *Int J Radiat Oncol Biol Phys* 1999;43(1):57–66.
20. Sims R, Isambert A, Grégoire V, et al. A pre-clinical assessment of an atlas-based automatic segmentation tool for the head and neck. *Radiother Oncol* 2009;93(3): 474–478. doi:10.1016/j.radonc.2009.08.013.
21. Bushong SC. *Radiologic science for technologists: physics, biology and protection.* St. Louis: Mosby, 1993.
22. Pan XC, Siewerdsen J, La PJ, et al. Anniversary paper: development of x-ray computed tomography: the role of medical physics and AAPM from the 1970s to present. *Med Phys* 2008;35(8):3728–3739. doi:10.1118/1.2952653.
23. Battista JJ, Bronskill MJ. Compton scatter imaging of transverse sections an overall appraisal and evaluation for radiotherapy planning. *Phys Med Biol* 1981;26: 81–99.
24. Schneider W, Bortfeld T, Schlegel W. Correlation between CT numbers and tissue parameters needed for Monte Carlo simulations of clinical dose distributions. *Phys Med Biol* 2000;45(2):459–478.
25. Spitzer V, Ackerman MJ, Scherzinger AL, et al. The visible human male: a technical report. *J Am Med Inform Assoc* 1996;3(2):118–130.
26. Olsen DR, Thwaites DI. Now you see it... Imaging in radiotherapy treatment planning and delivery. *Radiother Oncol* 2007;85(2):173–175. doi:10.1016/j.radonc.2007.11.001.
27. Gould RG. CT overview and basics. In: Siebert JA, Barnes GT, Gould RG, eds. *Specifications, acceptance testing, and quality control of diagnostic x-ray imaging equipment. American Association of Physicist in Medicine, Summer School.* Woodbury, NY: American Institute of Physics, 1991:801–831.
28. Judy PF. CT image quality and parameters affecting the CT image. In: Goldman LW, ed. *RSNA categorial course in diagnostic radiology physics: CT and US cross-sectional imaging.* Oak Brook, IL: Radiological Society of North America, 2000:117--125.
29. Hu H, He HD, Foley WD, et al. Four multidetector-row helical CT: image quality and volume coverage speed. *Radiology* 2000;215(1):55–62.
30. Chen GT, Kung JH, Beaudette KP. Artifacts in computed tomography scanning of moving objects. *Semin Radiat Oncol* 2004;14(1):19–26. doi:10.1053/j.semradonc.2003.10.004.
31. Balter JM, Ten RK, Haken TS, et al. Uncertainties in CT-based radiation therapy treatment planning associated with patient breathing. *Int J Radiat Oncol Biol Phys* 1996;36(1):167–174.

32. Balter JM, Lam KL, McGinn CJ, et al. Improvement of CT-based treatment-planning models of abdominal targets using static exhale imaging. *Int J Radiat Oncol Biol Phys* 1998;41(4):939–943.

33. Sarker J, Chu A, Mui K, et al. Variations in tumor size and position due to irregular breathing in 4D-CT: a simulation study. *Med Phys* 2010;37(3):1254–1260.

34. Chen GT, Kung JH, Beaudette KP. Artifacts in computed tomography scanning of moving objects. *Semin Radiat Oncol* 2004;14(1):19–26.

35. Ford EC, Mageras GS, Yorke E, et al. Respiration-correlated spiral CT: a method of measuring respiratory-induced anatomic motion for radiation treatment planning. *Med Phys* 2003;30(1):88–97.

36. Low DA, Nystrom M, Kalinin E, et al. A method for the reconstruction of four-dimensional synchronized CT scans acquired during free breathing. *Med Phys* 2003;30(6):1254–1263.

37. Vedam SS, Keall PJ, Kini VR, et al. Acquiring a four-dimensional computed tomography dataset using an external respiratory signal. *Phys Med Biol* 2003;48(1):45–62.

38. Pan T, Lee TY, Rietzel E, et al. 4D-CT imaging of a volume influenced by respiratory motion on multi-slice CT. *Med Phys* 2004;31(2):333–340.

39. Li T, Schreibmann E, Thorndyke B, et al. Radiation dose reduction in four-dimensional computed tomography. *Med Phys* 2005;32(12):3650–3660.

40. Wang J, Li T, Liang Z, et al. Dose reduction for kilovoltage cone-beam computed tomography in radiation therapy. *Phys Med Biol* 2008;53(11):2897–2909. doi:10.1088/0031–9155/53/11/009.

41. Ross CS, Hussy DH, Pennington EC. Analysis of movement in intrathoracic neoplasm using ultrafast computerized tomography. *Int J Radiat Oncol Biol Phys* 1990;18:671–677.

42. Feldkamp LA, Davis LC, Kress JW. Practical cone-beam algorithm. *J Opt Soc Am* 1984;1(6):612–619.

43. Jaffray DA, Siewerdsen H. Conebeam computed tomography with flat panel imager: initial performance characterization. *Med Phys* 2000;27:1311–1323.

44. Morin O, Gillis A, Chen J, et al. Megavoltage cone-beam CT: system description and clinical applications. *Med Dosim* 2006;31(1):51–61.

45. Pouliot J, Bani-Hashemi A, Chen J, et al. Low-dose megavoltage cone-beam CT for radiation therapy. *Int J Radiat Oncol Biol Phys* 2005;61(2):552–560.

46. Mackie TR, Kapatoes J, Ruchala K, et al. Image guidance for precise conformal radiotherapy. *Int J Radiat Oncol Biol Phys* 2003;56(1):89–105.

47. Sonke JJ, Zijp L, Remeijer P, et al. Respiratory correlated cone beam CT. *Med Phys* 2005;32(4):1176–1186.

48. Dixon WT. Physics and instrumentation. In: Sogel S, Lee JKT, eds. *Computed body tomography with MRI correlations.* New York: Raven Press, 1989:23–30.

49. Plathow C, Zimmermann H, Fink C, et al. Influence of different breathing maneuvers on internal and external organ motion: Use of fiducial markers in dynamic MRI. *Int J Radiat Oncol Biol Phys* 2005;62(1):238–245.

50. Feng M, Balter JM, Normolle D, et al. Characterization of pancreatic tumor motion using cine MRI: surrogates for tumor position should be used with caution. *Int J Radiat Oncol Biol Phys* 2009;74(3):884–891. doi:10.1016/j.ijrobp.2009.02.003.

51. Ghilezan MJ, Jaffray DA, Siewerdsen JH, et al. Prostate gland motion assessed with cine-magnetic resonance imaging (cine-MRI). *Int J Radiat Oncol Biol Phys* 2005;62(2):406–417.

52. Padhani AR, Khoo VS, Suckling J, et al. Evaluating the effect of rectal distension and rectal movement on prostate gland position using cine MRI. *Int J Radiat Oncol Biol Phys* 1999;44(3):525–533.

53. Thornton A. F, Sandler HM, Ten Haken RK, et al. The clinical utility of MRI in 3-dimentional treatment planning of brain neoplasms. *Int J Radiat Oncol Biol Phys* 1992;24:767–775.

54. Nelson SJ. Multivoxel magnetic resonance spectroscopy of brain tumors. *Mol Cancer Ther* 2003;2(5):497–507.

55. Shih HA, Harisinghani M, Zietman AL, et al. Mapping of nodal disease in locally advanced prostate cancer: rethinking the clinical target volume for pelvic nodal irradiation based on vascular rather than bony anatomy. *Int J Radiat Oncol Biol Phys* 2005;63(4):1262–1269. doi:10.1016/j.ijrobp.2005.07.952.

56. Orrison WW, Lewine JD, Sanders JA, et al. Functional brain imaging. Chicago: Mosby Year Book, Inc., 1995.

57. Nakajima T, Fujita M, Watanabe H, et al. Functional mapping of the human visual system with near-infrared spectroscopy and BOLD functional MRI. San Francisco: Society of Magnetic Resonance Medicine, 1994.

58. Cao Y, Towel V, Levin D, et al. Functional mapping of human motor cortical activation with conventional MR imaging at 1.5 T. *J Magn Reson Imag* 1993;3:869–871.

59. Hamilton RJ, Sweeney PJ, Pelizzari CA, et al. Functional imaging in treatment planning of brain lesions. *Int J Radiat Oncol Biol Phys* 1997;37(1):181–188.

60. Grosu AL, Piert M, Weber WA, et al. Positron emission tomography for radiation treatment planning. *Strahlenther Onkol* 2005;181(8):483–499. doi:10.1007/s00066–005-1422–7.

61. Nehmeh SA, Erdi YE, Pan T, et al. Four-dimensional PET/CT imaging of the thorax. *Med Phys* 2004; 31(12):3179–3186.

62. Townsend DW. A combined PET/CT scanner: the choices. *J Nucl Med* 2001;42(3):533–534.

63. Townsend DW. Combined positron emission tomography-computed tomography: the historical perspective. *Semin Ultrasound CT MR* 2008;29(4):232–235.

64. Townsend DW, Beyer T, Blodgett TM. PET/CT scanners: a hardware approach to image fusion. *Semin Nucl Med* 2003;33(3):193–204.

65. Marks L. B, Spencer DP, Bentel GC, et al. The utility of SPECT lung perfusion scans in minimizing and assessing the physiologic consequences of thoracic irradiation. *Int J Radiat Oncol Biol Phys* 1993;26:659–668.

66. Caldwell CB, Mah K, Skinner M, et al. Can PET provide the 3D extent of tumor motion for individualized internal target volumes? A phantom study of the limits of CT and the promise of PET. *Int J Radiat Oncol Biol Phys* 2003;55(5):1381–1393.

67. Martinez A, Gonzalez J, Stromberg J, et al. Conformal prostate brachytherapy: initial experience of a phase

I/II dose-escalating trial. *Int J Radiat Oncol Biol Phys* 1995;33:1019–1028.

68. Lattanzi J, McNeeley S, Pinover W, et al. A comparison of daily CT localization to a daily ultrasound-based system in prostate cancer. *Int J Radiat Oncol Biol Phys* 1999;43(4):719–725.

69. Conner WG, Boone MLM, Veomett R, et al. Patient repositioning and motion detection using a video cancellation system. *Int J Radiat Oncol Biol Phys* 1975;1:147–153.

70. Bert C, Metheany KG, Doppke K, et al. A phantom evaluation of a stereo-vision surface imaging system for radiotherapy patient setup. *Med Phys* 2005;32(9):2753–2762.

71. Bert C, Metheany KG, Doppke KP, et al. Clinical experience with a 3D surface patient setup system for alignment of partial-breast irradiation patients. *Int J Radiat Oncol Biol Phys* 2006;64(4):1265–1274.

72. Meeks SL, Bova FJ, Wagner TH, et al. Image localization for frameless stereotactic radiotherapy. *Int J Radiat Oncol Biol Phys* 2000;46(5):1291–1299.

73. Berbeco RI, Neicu T, Rietzel E, et al. A technique for respiratory-gated radiotherapy treatment verification with an EPID in cine mode. *Phys Med Biol* 2005;50(16):3669–3679.

74. Law MY, Liu B. Informatics in radiology: DICOM-RT and its utilization in radiation therapy. *Radiographics* 2009;29(3):655–667. doi:10.1148/rg.293075172.

75. NEMA. 2006. The DICOM Standard, http://dicom.nema.org.

76. Bosch WR. Integrating the management of patient treatment planning and image data. In: Purdy JA, ed. *Categorical course syllabus: 3-dimensional radiation therapy treatment planning*, Chicago: Radiology Society of North America, 1994:151–160.

77. McShan DL, Silverman A, Lanza DN, et al. A computerized three- dimensional treatment planning system utilizing interactive color graphics. *Br J Radiol* 1979;52:478–481.

78. McShan DL, Kessler ML, Fraass BA. Advanced interactive planning techniques for conformal therapy: high level beam descriptions and volumetric mapping techniques. *Int J Radiat Oncol Biol Phys* 1995;33:1061–1072.

79. Goitein M, Abrams M, Rowell D, et al. Multidimensional treatment planning: 2. Beam's eye view, back projection, and projection through CT sections. *Int J Radiat Oncol Biol Phys* 1983;9:789–797.

80. Chen GTY, Pelizzari CA, Levin DN. Image correlation in oncology. In: Hellman S, Devita V, eds. *Important advances in oncology*. Philadelphia: JB Lippincott, 1990:131–142.

81. Chen L, Price RA, Wang L, et al. MRI-based treatment planning for radiotherapy: dosimetric verification for prostate IMRT. *Int J Radiat Oncol Biol Phys* 2004;60(2):636–647.

82. Das IJ. The digitally reconstructed radiograph. In: Schulthesis TE, Coia LR, eds. *A practical guide to CT simulation*. Madison: Advanced Medical Publishing, 1995:39–50.

83. Beard C, Bussiere M, Plunkett M, et al. Analysis of prostate and seminal vesicle motion. *Int J Radiat Oncol Biol Phys* 1993;27(Suppl 1):136.

84. Melian E, Kutcher G, Leibel S, et al. Variation in prostate position: quantitation and implications for three dimensional conformal radiation therapy. *Int J Radiat Oncol Biol Phys* 1993;27(Suppl 1):137.

85. Roeske JC, Forman JD, Messina CF, et al. Evaluation of changes in the size and location of the prostate, seminal vesicle, bladder and rectum during a course of external beam radiation therapy. *Int J Radiat Oncol Biol Phys* 1995;33:1321–1329.

86. Maintz JBA, Viergever MA. A survey of medical image registration. *Med Image Anal* 1998;2:1–36.

87. Maurer CR, Fitzpatrick JM. A review of medical image registration. In: Maciunas RJ, ed. *Interactive image guided neurosurgery*. Park Ridge, IL: AAN, 1993:17–44.

88. Pluim JPW, Maintz JBA, Viergever MA. Mutual information based registration of medical images: a survey. *IEEE Trans Med Imaging* 2003:22(8):968–1003.

89. Van Den Elsen PA, Maintz JB, Viergever MA. Geometry driven multimodality matching of brain images. *Brain Topogr* 1992;5(2):153–157.

90. Collignon A, Maes F, Delaere D, et al. Automated multimodality image registration based on information theory. In: Bizais Y, Barillot C, DiPaola R, eds. *Information processing in medical imaging*. Dordrecht: Kluwer, 1995.

91. van Herk M, Gilhuis K, Holupka E, et al. A new method for automatic three-dimensional image correlation. *Med Phys* 1992:19(4):11–34.

92. Viola P. Alignment by maximization of mutual information. Ph.D. Thesis, Artificial Intelligence Laboratory, Massachusetts Institute of Technology, Cambridge MA, AI Technical Report 1548 (1995).

93. Drebin R, Carpente RL, Hanrahan P. Volume rendering. *Comput Graph* 1988;22:65–74.

94. Kuszyk BS, Ney DR, Fishman EK. The current state of the art in three dimensional oncologic imaging: an overview. *Int J Radiat Oncol Biol Phys* 1995;33:1029–1040.

95. Pelizzari CA, Ryan MJ, Grzeszczuk R, et al. Volumetric visualization of anatomy for treatment planning. *Int J Radiat Oncol Biol Phys* 1995;34:205–212.

96. Computing, Scientific, and Imaging Institute. 2004. The SCIRun Problem Solving Environment, http://software.sci.utah.edu/scirun.html.

97. Gehring M, Mackie T, Kubsad S, et al. Three dimensional volume visualization package applied to stereotactic radiosurgery treatment planning. *Int J Radiat Oncol Biol Phys* 1991;21:491–500.

98. Grossman SA, Burch PA. Quantitation of tumor response to anti-neoplastic therapy. *Semin Oncol* 1988:15:441–454.

99. Jaffe CC. Response assessment in clinical trials: implications for sarcoma clinical trial design. *The Oncologist* 2008;13(Suppl 2):14–18. doi:10.1634/theoncologist.13-S2-14.

100. Wahl RL, Jacene H, Kasamon Y, et al. From RECIST to PERCIST: evolving considerations for PET response criteria in solid tumors. *J Nucl Med* 2009;50(Suppl 1):122S–150S. doi:10.2967/jnumed.108.057307.

101. Kinahan PE, Doot RK, Wanner-Roybal M, et al. PET/CT Assessment of Response to Therapy: Tumor Change Measurement, Truth Data, and Error. *Transl Oncol* 2009;2(4):223–230.

CHAPTER 3

Patient Data Acquisition

Bahman Emami

INTRODUCTION

Radiation oncology is a clinical specialty devoted to the management of patients with malignant neoplasms by using ionizing radiation alone or in combination with other modalities. This endeavor also includes investigation of biological and physical basis of radiotherapy and training of professionals in this field. The aim of radiotherapy is to deliver a precisely measured dose of radiation to a defined target volume with as small as dose as possible to the surrounding healthy tissues. The aim is eradication of cancer, with side effects as few and mild as possible, resulting in improved quality of life and prolongation of survival, at reasonable cost.

Although patients are usually referred to radiation oncologist after the diagnosis has been made or is highly probable from diagnostic studies, it is absolutely essential that radiation oncologist be fully knowledgeable and able to execute the entire process of workup, diagnosis, and staging of patients. They direct any additional medications needed during treatment and are available in any emergency. As emphasized in Perez and Brady (1), it is essential for the radiation oncologist to cooperate closely with specialists in other fields in the management of patient to provide better care.

DIAGNOSIS

Clinical Presentation

Persistent changes in normal body functions, such as alterations in eating habits, loss of appetite, and difficulty in swallowing, demand evaluation and explanation. Other presentations, such as a lump or a nodule at any site, unnatural bleeding of orifices, and fever or infections not responding to antibiotic therapy, also fall into this category. These early signs of cancer have been sketched for different sites in general (Table 3.1). Thorough evaluation of these signs can often lead to detection of cancer at early stages, in which therapy most often proves successful. An important point in all of these presentations is a high index of suspicion. Periodic screening tests are very important to early detection. Annual chest x-ray films for lung cancer, annual mammograms for breast cancer, and annual Pap smears for uterine cancer have shown to help

with early detection and improved cure rate periodic colonoscopy and prostate-specific antigen (PSA; for men) have proven to save many lives.

The role of tumor markers in the diagnosis of cancer has yet to be defined, with the exception of PSA as a most significant indicator of prostate cancer. As yet no simple test with sufficient sensitivity and specificity to detect the presence of cancer is available. Most tumor markers, such as carcinoembryonic antigen (CEA) in colon cancer and human gonadotropin hormones (BHCG) and α-fetal protein (AFP) in nonseminomatous testicular cancers, are more useful for monitoring the patient's response and detecting recurrence than as a definitive diagnostic tool in screening early cancer.

Surgical Biopsy

Once cancer is suspected, a careful workup, including a thorough history and physical examination, a detailed examination of the anatomical site under suspicion, and the appropriate radiological examination, should be undertaken.

Most importantly, clinical leads should be pursued and investigative studies should not be unduly procrastinated. Surgical biopsy (or excision), however, is the single most important procedure in establishing a firm diagnosis of cancer. With rare exceptions a histologic diagnosis is essential before undertaking any radical treatment. Oncological imaging can precede or follow surgical biopsy, depending on the given clinical condition. Once the pathological diagnosis is made, the anatomical extent or stage of the disease should be determined (discussed later in the chapter).

Oncological Imaging

An extended array of radiological studies is available. The aim of these studies is to determine the extent of local disease, involvement of regional nodes by a given cancer, and the presence or absence of distant metastasis. In ordering these radiographic studies, the physician has to be discriminating and cost-effective, obtaining the fewest studies adequate for answering the question. Familiarity with multimodality imaging is essential for practicing modern radiotherapy. Radiographic studies include chest x-ray

TABLE 3.1	**Cancer's Seven Warning Signals**

Change in bowel or bladder habits

A sore that does not heal

Unusual bleeding or discharge

Thickening of lump in breast or elsewhere

Indigestion or difficulty in swallowing

Obvious change in wart or mole

Nagging cough or hoarseness

If you have a warning sign, see your doctor!

Reprinted with permission from American Cancer Society: *CA Cancer J Clin* 1990;40:101–128.

film, mammogram, radionuclide scan, ultrasound, computed tomography (CT), magnetic resonance imaging (MRI), and recently positron emission tomography (PET). Although the use of one or more of these studies depends on the clinical condition at hand and is under the decision of the treating physician, certain radiographic studies are in general use in oncology. For example, CT scan of the chest and upper abdomen is a prerequisite for accurate staging of patients with lung cancer. This study not only evaluates the extent of primary tumor in the chest, status of involved mediastinal nodes, and presence or absence of pleural effusion but also investigates the status of liver and the adrenals, which are frequent sites of metastasis. MRI is the radiographic study of choice for almost all tumors of the central nervous system and possible sarcomas at any site in the body. Patients with head and neck cancer, especially in the advanced stage, almost always require a CT scan of the head and neck area, and mammography is the essential radiographic workup for patients with breast cancer. Nuclear imaging still plays an important role, although it has been replaced by CT scan or MRI for detecting brain metastasis. Gallium scan in Hodgkin's disease, radioactive iodine scan for evaluation of thyroid cancer, and finally bone scan for evaluation of suspected bony metastasis are considered routine procedures.

Ultrasound remains the least expensive and the least hazardous alternative to any of the other studies, but unfortunately, because of the inferior quality of the information, it is less useful in most cases.

CT scan, the most widely used imaging modality, is the essential part of the simulation process in modern radiotherapy planning procedures, as will be discussed below.

During the past 10 years, in almost every field of oncology the impact of PET imaging has been evaluated, leading to current practice with PET or PET/CT contributing widely to oncological patient care by its proven advantages over anatomical imaging in staging and restaging of cancer (2,3). Majority of PET examinations are being performed with glucose analog fluorodeoxyglu-

cose (FDG), which is accumulated in most active tissues including malignant tumors. FDG-PET has shown to have clinical impact on diagnosis, staging and/or restaging of lung cancer, head and neck cancer, colorectal cancer, melanoma, lymphoma, breast cancer, gastroesophageal cancer, pancreatic cancer, testicular cancer, and thyroid cancer. FTG-PET is a routine use in staging of lung cancer (4), malignant lymphomas (5), and colorectal cancer.

Vast experience of the last 10 years with FDG-PET has resulted in significant progress in oncological imaging especially in the era of functional imaging. Modern imaging technologies allow visualization of not only anatomical structures within the body (CT) but also biological markers of relevance for the response to treatment especially radiation therapy (PET and MRI) (6). Tumor images based on PET technology allow visualization of a specific biomarker, whereas advanced MRI gives information about the physiological and metabolic status of the cancer tissue. Ongoing research scientists are studying functional imaging techniques by comparing with the pathologist specimens of various disease sites (7). Progress in functional imaging will allow radiation oncologists for individual treatment adaptation. Imaging of the biology of cancer tissue also makes it possible to identify regions within the patient's tumor that will benefit from higher radiation dose. Combined with modern radiation technologies, such as IMRT/IGRT, this allows selective radiation of particularly important regions within the cancer tissue. By confining the radiation dose according to biological features of cancer tissue, more patients could potentially be cured without compromising healthy tissue (8).

Classification of Cancer

One of the key factors influencing treatment decision making in oncology is accurate classification of cancer based on anatomical and histological consideration. A description such as early, moderate, or advanced cancer, that is, "locally advanced head and neck cancer," is meaningless at best. National and international organizations over the years have attempted to bring some order and a generally agreeable consensus to these classifications. Although many proposed classifications appear in the literature from time to time, not many of them gain widespread applicability and use in clinical practice. A workable classification should have the following characteristics (9): (a) usefulness to the clinician in making therapy decisions, (b) prognostic implications, (c) help in evaluating the results of treatment, (d) ease with the exchange of information, and (e) help with the continuing investigation of cancer. Two of the most important organizations in this regard, whose classifications have been most widely accepted by the oncology community, are UICC (International Union against Cancer) (10) and AJCC (American Joint Committee for Cancer Staging and End Results Reporting) (11).

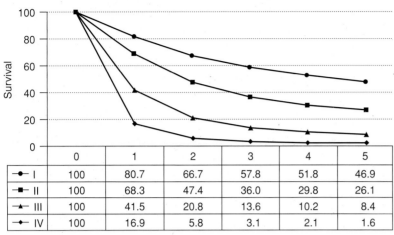

	0	1	2	3	4	5
─●─ I	100	80.7	66.7	57.8	51.8	46.9
─■─ II	100	68.3	47.4	36.0	29.8	26.1
─▲─ III	100	41.5	20.8	13.6	10.2	8.4
─♦─ IV	100	16.9	5.8	3.1	2.1	1.6

Years following diagnosis

Figure 3.1. Relative survival rates for non-small-cell lung cancer diagnosed in the United States in 1992 and 1993. Cases classified by the current staging classification, where pathologic stage group was used to classify each case when available, and clinical stage group was used. Stage I includes 30,260 patients; stage II, 8,893 patients; stage III, 38,498 patients; and stage IV, 44,410 patients. Data from the National Cancer Data Base (Commission on Cancer of the American College of Surgeons and the American Cancer Society).

Histopathological Classification

The importance of knowing the type of cancer needs no further emphasis. In addition to the commonly used morphological characteristics, recent innovations on histochemical, immunochemical, and electromicroscopic information have made this area of histopathological classification more complex and definitely more accurate. Although some intrapathology and interpathology difference of opinion always exist, there is common agreement in the majority of cases. Assistance of a committed, knowledgeable, and oncology-oriented pathologist in this regard is invaluable.

The second important aspect of histopathological classification is the grading of the cancer. Grading means the expression of the degree of malignancy of the cancer. It is usually shown by grade I (well differentiated), grade II (moderately well differentiated), and grade III (poorly differentiated). Grading has significant therapeutic and prognostic implications, and in some cancers, such as sarcomas, is part of the staging.

Staging Classification

Anatomical staging simply means quantifying the extent of the disease. Since the introduction of the Tumor, Node, and Metastasis (TNM) system, numerous variations of this classification have appeared in the literature in the past 45 years. Until 1982 there were two separate anatomical classifications, one by UICC and one by AJCC. In order to have a uniform language, in 1982 the international committees agreed on a uniform staging system, TNM (11). It has three components: T for primary or direct extension, N for secondary or lymphatic involvement, and M for vascular dissemination or distant metastasis. Various subcategories of T, T1, T2, T3, and T4 describe increasing extent of the primary tumor. The advancing nodal disease is classified as N0 (no evidence of clinical involvement of the regional lymph nodes), N1, N2, or N3; again, these are for graduations of nodal disease. The presence or absence of metastasis is depicted by M0

or M+. A combination of T, N, and M has been defined as various stages of disease, depending on the site.

As mentioned earlier, the staging system, as well as having both therapeutic and prognostic implications, plays a major role in the evaluation of the results of therapy and exchange of information. Figure 3.1 reveals the prognostic value of the TNM staging system in non-small cell lung cancer.

TREATMENT DECISION

The basic principle in therapy is to cure the patient with minimal functional and structural impairment. The process of treatment decision making, a very complex one, involves factors related to tumor, such as histopathological type and anatomical extent, and personal factors such as physical, psychological, and emotional status of the patient and sometimes his or her relatives. This process always involves participation from various specialists such as surgeon, radiation oncologist, medical oncologist, pathologist, radiologist, and social worker. Without doubt, this most important phase of management of the patient with cancer is best accomplished by a multidisciplinary effort of these specialists. Because of the importance of the matter, most specialties also have subspecialty areas dealing with cancer patients, such as surgical oncology, gynecological oncology, and pediatric oncology. The team members should be knowledgeable about the potential and capabilities of not only their areas of subspecialty but also to some extent of the others. Through an honest and open dialogue the team should come up with a therapeutic decision consensus in the best interest of the patient. Proper knowledge of natural history of cancer and its patterns of spread and of the effectiveness and potential morbidity of each therapeutic modality (therapeutic ratio) is the basis of the process. One of the first steps in this decision making is to decide, considering all factors, whether the treatment will have curative potential or will be purely palliative. The second step is to decide which modality, surgery, radiotherapy, chemotherapy, or any combination thereof has the best chance to achieve the goals with minimal functional and anatomical deficits. In clinical situations in which surgery and radiotherapy have an equal chance of cure, usually the one with less consequential morbidity is preferred. In many situations, a combined modality approach is most likely to result in a favorable outcome, and therefore a judicious use of each modality mandates thorough teamwork of the multidisciplinary team.

Patient selection criteria for three-dimensional conformal radiotherapy (3D CRT), intensity-modulated radiotherapy (IMRT), image-guided radiotherapy (IGRT), and stereotactic radiotherapy (STS/STR): the radiation oncologist, who has the ultimate responsibility of radiotherapeutic treatment of patients, should have adequate knowledge of the various techniques available to him/her in order to properly oversee the course of treatment process.

3D CRT and IMRT have made a significant improvement in the quality of the practice of radiation oncology. These goals have been accomplished by protocols aimed at increasing tumor dose, reducing dose to uninvolved normal tissue, or both. In general, the published clinical experiences with 3D CRT/IMRT technologies can be divided into two broad categories. The first group has been to better spare uninvolved normal tissues and therefore preserve the function of these organs such as patients with head and neck cancers. In this group of patients the preservation of salivary gland functions has resulted in significant improvement in the quality of life. Similarly, acquired knowledge on the functional tolerance of other organs such as the cochlea and pharyngeal constrictor muscles and limiting the dose to these organs to tolerance level via proper planning has shown to significantly decrease or eliminate these potential complications in radio-chemotherapeutic management of head and neck cancer patients.

In the second group the goal is to improve local control by dose escalation protocols using 3D CRT/IMRT. Patients with localized prostate cancer are an example of this group. Dose escalation in radiotherapeutic management of patients with localized prostate cancer using IMRT technology has significantly improved cure rate in this group of patients.

Dose escalation is impossible in certain sites with serial architecture such as spinal cord or brain because of the potential for higher complication rates. In these tissues destruction of a single functional unit is sufficient to incapacitate organ function and cause complications. Also, organ such as the esophagus, although not considered a tissue with serial architecture, may develop severe complications (stricture or perforation) with doses beyond the tolerance of the organ. Caution should be exercised in considering these tissues and dose escalation 3D CRT/IMRT protocols.

Tumors arising from tissues with parallel architecture such as lung, prostate, head and neck (certain sites), and liver are being treated with 3D CRT/IMRT on dose escalation protocols in various institutions.

Reducing radiation dose to normal tissue structures with 3D CRT/IMRT has shown significant gain in controlling malignancies originating from tissues not suitable for dose escalation studies. Central nervous system tumors are an example of this group. Moreover, a group of patients such as children with malignancies, whose low tolerance to irradiation of normal tissue structures and organs has long been a major challenge to radiation oncologists, can significantly benefit from this new technology.

The limited ability to control a tumor's location compromises the accuracy of radiotherapy. The result is a requirement for larger treatment volumes to account for target uncertainty that restricts the radiation dose because more surrounding normal tissue is exposed. Theoretically with image-guided radiation therapy (IGRT) these volumes can be optimized and eradicable tumor doses can be delivered, achieving maximum tumor control with minimal complications. With high precision dose delivery and presumed real-time knowledge of target location, IGRT has initiated the exploration of new possibilities in radiotherapy. In clinical practice there are two pathways to accomplish the above goal. One is to use various imaging modalities during the period of dose deliveries on a day-to-day basis in order to improve on day-to-day uncertainties (random errors). The second scenario is using imaging modalities on a weekly or biweekly basis in order to detect major changes of the volume of tumor and/or normal tissues and by replanning to assure the correct dose is delivered to the correct volumes. To date, the first scenario still remains theoretical research and there is no solid data to show that this version of IGRT will improve patient care or if it is just so called "gilding the lilies." The second scenario, "adaptive radiotherapy," is a true improvement on radiotherapeutic care of patients but has significant economic ramifications.

By ever increasing use of IMRT in radiotherapy, dose escalation studies have become an important part of clinical research in many institutions. However, to deliver an adequate dose requires a long period with conventional fractionation, which may lead to a significant tumor repopulation. Moreover, acute toxicity and long-term complications of normal tissues have also been of major concern. Based on long-term experience with intracranial stereotactic radiosurgery, and the significant technological advancements with planning and delivery of high precision radiotherapy, utilization of stereotactic radiotherapy (STS/STR) in extracranial sites either in the form of single fraction or so-called stereotactic radiosurgery and/or hypofractionation (three to five fractions) in extracranial cancers such as lung and liver has become a common practice with very impressive results.

Process of Treatment Planning

The process of treatment planning is a very complex procedure that requires the following: (a) thorough knowledge of the natural history of a given tumor pathology; (b) accurate knowledge of the true extent of disease (staging); (c) knowledge of volumetric tolerance of normal tissue organs to radiation, especially tissues harboring cancer and their functional and physiological status; (d) decision as to whether the aim of the therapy is definitive, adjuvant, or palliative and which therapeutic modality or combination thereof will best achieve the above goal with minimal functional and anatomical deficit; (e) physical treatment planning, which includes accurate delineation of the target volume and normal tissue structures as well as designing the radiation portals; (f) computation to determine the distribution of radiation within the volume of interest that will produce volumetric isodoses; (g) reproducible repositioning and immobilization technique for simulation and day-to-day treatment delivery; and (h) verification procedures to ensure quality control throughout the course of therapy. In using IMRT for treatment planning and delivery, physicians, physicists, and dosimetrists are faced with an even more complex process. IMRT is a new paradigm, which shows significant potential for further improvement in the therapeutic ratio and reduction in toxicities. In this process the physicians, physicists, and dosimetrists are faced with an even more complex process, which requires more detailed knowledge of the steps, aforementioned for 3D CRT with added complexities of inverse planning and delivery (12,13).

After determining that radiation will be used, the course of radiotherapy itself is planned. Treatment planning is the first and one of the most important parts of the radiation process. It outlines the course of action for the next several weeks of individual treatment sessions. Unlike pharmaceuticals, radiation is not metabolized. Once the dose of radiation has been delivered, it cannot be removed. Thus it is most important that the initial planning should be done critically, meticulously, and judiciously. There is little chance to rectify a poorly planned course of radiation treatment. Radiation kills cancer cells by depositing energy within the cell. Malignant cells that are not struck by radiation will not be affected by treatment and can regrow, resulting in locoregional recurrence and the death of the patient. Similarly, when a large number of normal tissue cells are hit by radiation, they most likely die, resulting in anatomical and/or functional complications for the patient. Therefore, treatment planning designed to treat all tumor-bearing tissues accurately and avoid unnecessary irradiation of normal tissues has unquestioned importance.

The detailed technical process of treatment planning will be discussed in other chapters in this book. Treatment planning is essential in delivering the optimal course of therapy, and the responsibility for critical judgment rests with the radiation oncologist. As emphasized by Emami and Perez (14), radiation oncologists must (a) have sufficient training to interpret treatment planning information and to guide the technical staff in achieving the best dose distribution, (b) have sufficient knowledge to select the best combination of dose and fractionation for the given tumor type and site, and (c) understand the capabilities and limitations of the staff and the radiation treatment planning systems in order to judge the quality of dose distribution and technical feasibility and accuracy of the proposed plan.

REFERENCES

1. Halperin EC, Schmidt-Ullrich RK, Perez CA, et al. Overview. In: Perez CA, Brady L, eds. *Principles and practice of radiation oncology.* Volume 4. Philadelphia: JB Lippincott, 2004:1–69.
2. Schrevens L, Lorent N, Dooms C, et al. The role of PET scan in diagnosis, staging, and management of non-small cell lung cancer. *Oncologist* 2004;9:633–643.
3. Gambhir SS, Czernin J, Schwimmer J, et al. A tabulated summary of the FDG PET literature. *J Nucl Med* 2001;42:1S–93S.
4. Baum RP, Hellwing D, Mezzetti M. Position of nuclear medicine modalities in the diagnostic workup on cancer patients: lung cancer. *Q J Nucl Med Mol Imaging* 2004;48:119–142.
5. Cheson BD. New response criteria for lymphomas in clinical trials. *Ann Oncol* 2008;19(Suppl 4):IV35–IV38.
6. Nestle V, Weber W, Hentschel M, et al. Biological imaging in radiation therapy: role of positron emission tomography. *Phys Med Biol* 2009;54:R1–R25.
7. Groenendaal G, Moman MR, Korporaal JG, et al. Validation of functional imaging with pathology for tumor delineation in the prostate. *Radiother Oncol* 2010;94:145–150.
8. Deniaud-Alexandre E, Touboul E, Lerouge D, et al. Impact of computed tomography and 18f-deoxyglucose coincidence detection emission tomography image fusion for optimization of conformal radiotherapy in non-small-cell lung cancer. *IJROBP* 2005;63(5):1432–1441.
9. Rubin P, Cooper RA. Statement of the clinical oncologic problem. In: Rubin P, ed. *Clinical oncology: a multidisciplinary approach for physicians and student,* 7th ed. Philadelphia: WB Saunders, 1993:1–21.
10. International Union against Cancer. *TNM classification of malignant tumors.* Geneva: UICC Commission on Clinical Oncology, 1968.
11. American Joint Committee for Cancer Staging and End Results Reporting. *Manual for staging of cancer,* 4th ed. Philadelphia, PA: AJC, 1993.
12. Intensity Modulated Radiation Therapy Collaborative Working Group. Intensity-modulated radiotherapy: current status and issues of interest. *IJROBP* 2001;51:880–914.
13. Galvin JM, Ezzell G, Eisbrauch A, et al. Implementing IMRT in Clinical Practice: A Joint Document of the American Society for Therapeutic Radiology and Oncology and the American Association of Physicists in Medicine. *IJROBP* 2004;58:1616–1634.
14. Emami B, Perez C. Carcinoma of the lung and esophagus. In: Levitt S, ed. *Technological basis of radiation therapy.* New York: Lea & Febiger, 1991:248–262.

CHAPTER 4

Patient and Organ Movement

James M. Balter

INTRODUCTION

The driving tenet of conformal radiotherapy is the precise delivery of focal radiation doses to the target, so that an effective dose can be delivered while limiting concomitant normal tissue irradiation and related toxicity risk. Technical advancements, such as three-dimensional (3D) treatment planning and intensity-modulated radiation therapy (IMRT), have provided significant gains in specifying means to provide such dose distributions. Accurate delivery, so that intended and actual doses agree, is a more complicated matter.

The problems of patient positioning and motion have been studied extensively. Although there are currently areas that need further exploration, it is possible to consider the magnitude of various uncertainties in dose delivery due to patient position variation and organ movement, and to discuss rational strategies for dealing with these uncertainties in the context of precision radiotherapy.

DESCRIPTION OF THE PROBLEM OF GEOMETRIC VARIATION

The International Congress on Radiological Units (ICRU) has addressed the relative problem of geometric variations. In reports 50 and 62, concepts are evolved to attempt to standardize means of reporting doses. Some of the concepts presented in these reports have served as the basis for numerous investigations over the past few years, and have been adopted as standards for clinical trials. A brief discussion of the key concepts as they apply to geometric variation follows.

The key structures that are delineated are the gross tumor volume (GTV) and organs at risk (OARs). The GTV is generally defined as the "visible" target, that is, that can be delineated from imaging or related information. The OARs are tissue structures that are dose limiting due to risk of radiation-induced toxicity.

The next volume of interest is the clinical target volume (CTV). This target volume ideally expands about the GTV to include a reasonable expectation of the true target extent on a (static) patient model. The basis for CTV expansions includes intraobserver and interobserver variations in tumor delineation, as well as a reasonable expectation of

the extent of disease below the sensitive range of the imaging modality.

Geometric uncertainty influences both the target volume and the OARs. To ensure adequate geometric coverage of the target, the CTV is expanded. Internal organ movement is encompassed by an internal margin (IM) about the CTV to make the internal target volume (ITV), and setup error influences a setup margin (SM) about the ITV to yield the planning target volume (PTV).

When the patient is imaged to define the CTV and critical structures, the position is sampled. In general, this sample occurs once, specifically during the computed tomography (CT) scan for treatment planning. To obtain this sample, the patient is immobilized and positioned with typical reference marks placed on the skin and/or immobilization device at the principal axes of the CT scanner for verification of position and orientation. The sample of the patient serves as the model for treatment planning, and all subsequent targeting and density modeling are based on the information obtained during this session.

Suppose the patient has the same treatment planning scan repeated several times over the course of a typical fractionated treatment regimen (4–8 weeks). With no prior reference to positioning (i.e., no attempts to match the reference marker positions from one CT scan to the next), each CT scan will yield a patient model that differs in both position and configuration. These variations may be slight (indicating good reproducibility of patient position) or severe. Let us now suppose that attempts are made to reproduce the position of the patient so that the external reference marks line up relative to the CT scan lasers. This process, which in effect simulates multiple positioning by the "3-point setup" method to external references, will still yield a variety of patient positions and configurations in the CT scans obtained. The variation in these scans determines the extent to which external references properly configure and position the patient.

The magnitude of position variation has been studied by several hospitals over the past two decades. Table 4.1 (1–7) highlights some of these measurements, and indicates a reasonable range of expected variations. Note, however, that these reported values are unique to specific hospitals, immobilization equipment, and procedures. They are also influenced to a lesser extent by the means of

TABLE 4.1	Example Measured Setup Variations

Investigator	Body site	Nature of measured setup variation
Hong et al.	Head/neck	Mean error 6.7 mm, σ 3.63 mm
Michalski et al.	Various	6% of monitored fractions with errors >10 mm
Meijer et al.	Bladder	3 mm (1 σ)
Marsh et al.	Head/neck	Range of up to 4.5 mm (5 w into treatment)
Pisani et al.	Various	Mean error of 6.6 $\pm$ 2.4 mm
Weber et al.	Prostate	1.9–2.2 mm (systematic), 3.6 mm (random)
Van de Steene et al.	Thorax	Random σ 4.5-mm longitudinal and 5.7-mm transverse

measuring position variation. It is critical that a department determines its own position variation distributions, both as a baseline for treatment planning and as a means of improving positioning in an efficient manner.

Multiple samples of patient position (translation only) will form a scatter distribution. If we accept the position from the initial (treatment planning) CT scan as the "true" patient position, then a reasonable method of describing this distribution of subsequent positioning is by the translation necessary to make the patient position match that of the treatment planning CT scan. Conventionally, the average coordinate of this distribution is considered as the "systematic" error, in that it is the effective offset that persists throughout the samples (multiple CT scans in the above example, or multiple patient positions over a course of treatment). The spread of sampled positions about this average coordinate represents the random setup variation. It is important to note that the average coordinate may never be sampled.

Figure 4.1 shows a scatter distribution of patient position over multiple samples (about two axes), relative to the treatment planning CT scan representation of a patient. Note that the treatment planning CT scan does not reflect the average position or configuration of the patient. At best, it is just one of the random samples of position. At worst, due to patient discomfort or unfamiliarity with the immobilization equipment and process, it is a very biased sample of the later position distribution. Nonetheless, the

patient at simulation generally reflects the model that subsequent positioning and localization attempt to match.

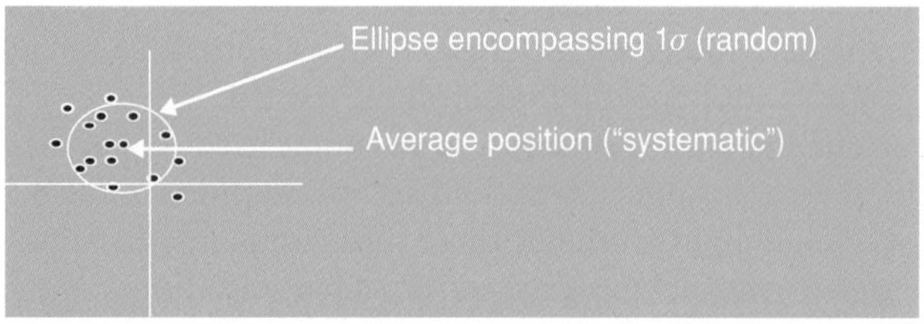

Let us consider positioning to be described by a Gaussian probability density function. By this assumption, the "average" magnitude of error in any sample is of the order of 0.8 σ, or 80% of the magnitude of the standard deviation of the distribution. Extending this model, it can be shown that the typical magnitude of difference between any two samples of the distribution is approximately 1.1 σ.

Table 4.2 shows some sample random variations measured from patients positioned and evaluated through daily imaging.

There are a number of assumptions that are critical to this simple model. One of the most important is that no time trend exists in patient position. This may not be true in all cases, and time trends in position have been investigated for various body sites.

Minimizing the Impact of Setup Variations on Treatment

Obviously, these setup variations require margins to ensure proper target coverage. The expansion of the CTV to ensure adequate coverage includes a SM to yield the PTV. Reducing the SM yields a smaller volume of tissue

Figure 4.1. Scatter distribution of patient position over multiple samples (about two axes), relative to the treatment planning computed tomography representation of a patient.

TABLE 4.2	Random Variations in Position Measured from Daily Imaging of Patients for Various Body Sites

Site	Average σ (mm)	Range of σ (mm)
Pelvis	3	1–7
Head and neck	2	1–5
Chest	4	1–12

irradiated to high doses, and can potentially reduce the toxicity to normal tissues. As such, significant efforts have been made to minimize the range of variations and their resulting impact on treatment.

POSITIONING SYSTEMS

A significant variety of equipment is in use to aid in repeat setup of patients. This equipment attempts to address a dual role: immobilization and localization. These dual roles are not necessarily compatible for any given piece of technology.

Immobilization

Quite simply, the process of immobilization involves limiting or eliminating movement for the time period of imaging or treatment. The primary objective is to limit target movement, although critical normal tissue movement also needs to be considered.

A number of excellent reviews of immobilization equipment have been published recently. As the technology is evolving, however, it is important to consider a number of key aspects in deciding on a technology and strategy for use of an immobilization system.

The advantage of a given immobilization method may be compromised by the complexity of use. If an immobilization system has many degrees of freedom, improper configuration of the device may lead to systematic errors in patient position or shape at treatment. Examples of complex systems are multiuse boards for fixation, in which the angles and positions of arm supports, angle of the upper thorax, shape of neck support, and other components are adjustable. These devices are very cost-effective, and can be used effectively, but special care must be taken to properly verify the per patient configuration, including notation of all configuration parameters and documented photographs of proper setup.

Some systems (e.g., alpha cradle and vacuum loc) form directly to the patient's shape. This can be beneficial in positioning, but it is important to separate comfort from immobilization. Formed immobilization that extends to distal regions from the target has been shown to be beneficial in reproducing position (8).

Localization Technology

A wealth of technology has been applied to localization in radiation therapy. At present, the most prevalent technology includes in-room lasers and electronic portal imaging devices (EPIDS). Improved image quality and ease of use, as well as better software for image review and management have led to EPIDS replacing film as the standard method of setup verification.

Megavoltage radiography is inherently limited by a lack of contrast, and has further been practically limited by the radiation doses involved. Other localization technologies have been introduced to overcome these limitations.

In-room diagnostic radiography is, in fact, a very old concept. Film-based radiographic systems have existed on linear accelerators for over 20 years (9). Room-based digital systems have been used for radiographic (10–13) and fluoroscopic (14) procedures.

STRATEGIES FOR POSITION CORRECTION

Online

Generally, online position correction refers to the processes of measuring and correcting setup error at the start of each treatment fraction. This is the area in which the vast majority of technical developments have focused recently. The process of online correction includes three steps: measurement, decision, and adjustment. A fourth step (verification) may also be used.

Measurement systems include data collection and analysis. Data can be from imaging (e.g., radiographs, CT scan images, ultrasound, and video) or other markers (e.g., electromagnetic and external fiducial). Analysis is the comparison of reference image or position information to that gathered at treatment.

Decision is the process of choosing to act or not on information from measurements. It is valuable to consider that the measurement systems as well as correction technology are not perfect, and therefore the errors in these systems may increase errors in certain circumstances. The use of thresholds for corrections allows a trade-off between the cost (frequency of adjustment) and benefit (actual reduction of errors). Figure 4.2 shows the cost versus threshold for setup adjustment in prostate patients.

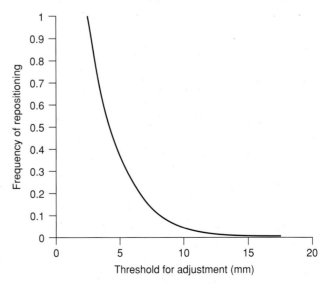

Figure 4.2. Cost (frequency of adjustment) versus threshold for online setup adjustment (based on 6-mm σ for pelvic patients).

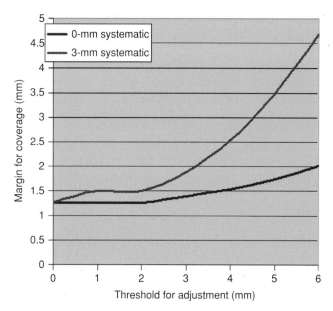

Figure 4.3. Benefit (margin) versus threshold for adjustment (4-mm σ setup, 1.5-mm σ measurement uncertainty, and 1.0 mm σ setup correction uncertainty).

Figure 4.3 shows the impact of positioning strategy on margins under assumptions of systematic error versus none.

Off-line

Studies of the dosimetric impact of setup error (15–18) demonstrate that systematic error has the largest impact on margin needed to adequately dose a target, and that the geometric expansion to account for random error is generally small (less than one standard deviation). Given this observation, it can be seen that, as long as random errors are not exceedingly large, the most significant patient benefit comes from strategies that rapidly reduce the magnitude of systematic setup variation.

A number of strategies have been used to minimize systematic error. Two common strategies are the shrinking action level (SAL) and no action level (NAL) methods (19–21). In the SAL protocol, setup is verified daily for the first few fractions, and adjustments are made with tolerances that reduce in magnitude as the fractions progress. This strategy has shown promising results.

The NAL protocol is also routinely used. In this method, images from setup are acquired for *n* (typically 3–5) fractions. These images are analyzed off-line (thereby minimizing the delay needed to analyze and act on images at the treatment unit), and the best prediction of the systematic error (typically the average position of the fractions analyzed) is corrected before the next fraction treated. This protocol has been tested, and shown to dramatically reduce systematic errors. Table 4.3 shows the average errors found over 4 days of imaging for various body sites. The patients studied had setup adjusted on the first fraction, followed by three fractions of imaging with off-line analysis. The "systematic" errors observed by off-line image analysis would probably have persisted throughout treatment for these patients without the correction adjustment on fraction 5.

Adaptive

Adaptive strategies for position adjustment were first proposed by Yan (22). The adaptive process extends the concept of off-line and online strategies. Essentially, the patient position variability is assumed to follow a population model before patient-specific measurements. As information about that patient's variation is acquired (e.g., through multiple CT scans or daily portal images), the model of variation is refined, and predictions from this refined model can be used to adjust position and margins. The frequency of further measurement can be similarly adjusted as increased confidence in the patient variation is gained, and similarly increased frequency of measurement can be reinstated if, for example, an unexpected outlying measurement occurs during the treatment course. Such strategies form a basis for plan modification, which is a topic of active research and development in radiation therapy.

Organ Movement

Internal organ movement is a further, sometimes significant, factor in dose-limiting geometric uncertainty. The most studied forms of organ movement have been prostate movement and breathing-induced movement in (primarily) the thorax and abdomen. Langen and Jones have published an excellent review of the magnitude of organ movement as studied by several investigators (23).

TABLE 4.3	"Average" Error in Position Seen After Four Fractions		
Site	**Lateral (mm)**	**Anterior–posterior (mm)**	**Cranial–caudal (mm)**
Pelvis	3.1	2.5	2.6
Chest	3.3	3.8	3.7
Abdomen	2.9	2.6	3.9
H/N	2.5	2.5	3.0

Prostate position variability is a combination of pelvic setup variation (mentioned above) with internal movement of the prostate within the pelvis (24–33). The primary factors affecting prostate movement are rectal and bladder filling, with differential influence of these forces in prone versus supine patients. The vast majority of prostate patients are positioned supine, both for patient comfort and owing to observed improvements in setup variation of the pelvis. Prone positioning has been reported advantageous due to a separation of the rectal wall from the prostate, although both setup variation and (breathing-related) internal movement have been observed to increase in these patients.

Internal movement of the prostate has generally been observed in the anterior–posterior (AP) and cranial–caudal directions (CC). Furthermore, a significant component of this movement has been correlated to rotations of the prostate about the left–right (LR) axis, with a pivot at or near the prostatic apex (34) (Fig. 4.4). The magnitude of this movement (of the prostate relative to the pelvic bones) is typically 1 cm or less in the AP and CC directions, and <5 mm in the LR direction.

Although most prostate movement studies have examined interfractional position changes (i.e., on the order of days), some measurements have been made of intrafractional movement. Breathing has been shown to impact prostate movement, most notably during deep breathing and in prone patients (35,36). Peristalsis, gas in the rectum, and bladder filling have a more significant influence on prostate position and potentially short-term movement. A recent study using implanted electromagnetic markers has described high-resolution traces of prostate position over times comparable to a treatment fraction (e.g., Fig. 4.5). Analysis of this data indicates that significant movement can occur during treatment delivery, requiring margins of 6-mm AP and 7.1-mm CC (37).

Prostate movement has been addressed by attempts at reducing motion by diet as well as immobilization through a rectal balloon. Most common attempts at managing pros-

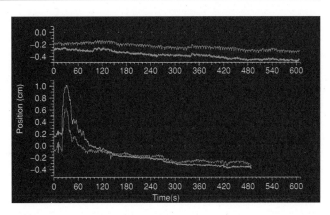

Figure 4.5. Sample traces of intratreatment prostate movement about the left–right (red), anterior–posterior (green), and cranial–caudal (blue) directions, evaluated using implanted electromagnetic transponders. The top figure represents a patient with minimal movement, while the lower graph shows a large transient movement followed by a chronic drift in the posterior and inferior directions.

tate movement, however, have focused on localization. Radiographic localization and tracking of implanted markers, studied by several investigators, is routine practice, with initial localization (before subsequent movement) accuracy of better than 2 mm. Ultrasound and in-room CT scan have also been used for prostate localization before treatment.

Breathing Movement

Vast efforts have recently been focused on the problem of breathing-related movement in radiation therapy. Breathing influences movement and shape change primarily in the thorax and abdomen, although, as noted above, breathing-related movements can also be seen in pelvic structures.

Breathing is a complex process. It is controlled both voluntarily and automatically. Various combinations of thoracic and abdominal muscles (including the diaphragm) can be used to control breathing, and therefore the shape of a patient can vary for the same estimated "phase" of breathing when evaluated sequentially.

A few general observations have been made about breathing in population studies. A typical breathing cycle lasts between 4 and 8 seconds. During normal breathing, patients tend to spend more time to (or near) exhale than inhale. Tumors near the apices of the lungs tend to move less than those near the diaphragm. Although these general observations represent a reasonable population summary, numerous studies have further shown that individual patients may violate any of the above observations. The need for patient-specific motion assessment has been demonstrated (38,39). The advent of four-dimensional (4D) CT techniques (40) provides data that help further elucidate patient-specific movement.

A very thorough summary of the ventilatory movement patterns of intrathoracic tumors was published by

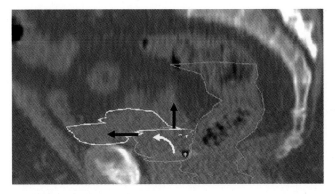

Figure 4.4. Graphic representation of the dominant modes of prostate movement (bladder—yellow, rectum—brown, prostate—pink, intraprostatic implanted markers—white stars). The major translation axes (black arrows) about the left–right and anterior–posterior axes have also been significantly attributed as rotation about the left–right axis (white arrow).

Seppenwoolde (41). In addition to the above observations, this study further showed the influence of heartbeat on some tumors, especially those near the mediastinum. An observation of complex, elliptical movement ("hysteresis") was also noted in this study and further observed by several other investigators. This elliptical movement can be attributed to the complex elastic properties of lung tissue, coupled with the different interactions of muscles and force between the inhale and exhale portions of the breathing cycle.

Motion has been studied in breast cancer as well. In general, the breast and chest wall move <1 cm within a single treatment fraction. Such small movements may not demand significant intrafraction intervention for motion management. Larger interfraction variation of chest wall position has been seen in portal imaging studies. Of note, however, is the potentially significant advantage of deep-inspiration breath hold (42–47), not only for immobilizing the chest wall temporarily, but also, more importantly, for reducing lung density and separating the heart from the medial high-dose region.

The abdomen has demonstrated significant breathing-related movement with typical amplitudes of 1.5 cm or more. The superior region of the liver moves with strong correlation to the diaphragm, while more caudal regions of the liver may move differentially due to deformation (48–51).

A number of technologies have been introduced to manage breathing movement. One common system involves gating (turning on and off) the treatment beam. The feedback for gating has generally been from the monitoring of an externally placed reflective marker on the patient's abdomen, although fluoroscopic tracking systems have also been used with tolerance windows for gating (52). Gating involves a trade-off of residual motion versus efficiency. The narrower the acceptance range for motion, the less frequently the beam is on. The most significant concern with external gating is the relationship between the external marker position and the tumor location. While targets near the skin surface (e.g., breast) may

have significant correlation with external references, other targets, especially those in the thorax, have been shown to vary in location at the same phase (as estimated from external motion) over multiple breathing cycles (53–56).

Another commonly used technology is active breathing control (ABC) (Fig. 4.6). First introduced by Wong (57), this concept involves using a system that monitors breathing, and occludes breath at a given phase of the breathing cycle and/or volume of air relative to exhale. Various studies have shown excellent short-term reproducibility of target position in the thorax and abdomen using this technology (10,58–62). Decreased accuracy in long-term reproducibility suggests the advantage of image-guided localization at the start of a treatment fraction in combination with ABC-aided ventilatory immobilization.

More complex technology for managing breathing movement involves tracking. In this process, an estimate of the target's trajectory is used to adjust the couch, linear accelerator orientation, or field aperture. Such systems are in early developmental and investigational stages, with a working example in robotic-guided stereotactic treatment (63–67).

All breathing management systems rely on the relationship of a surrogate to estimate tumor position at any given time or patient state. Various surrogates have been employed, including implanted fiducial markers, external fiducials (usually tracked in real time by video systems), external surface monitoring, and lung volume and air flow. The relationship between surrogate state/position and tumor position may be variable, and the influence on this variability on geometric accuracy of target position prediction should determine the extent of additional verification needed or residual error expected. One commercial system currently employs a hybrid approach to tracking, in which implanted radiopaque fiducials are periodically localized using biplanar radiographs, and their position is used to update a correlation with the constantly monitored external surface of the patient.

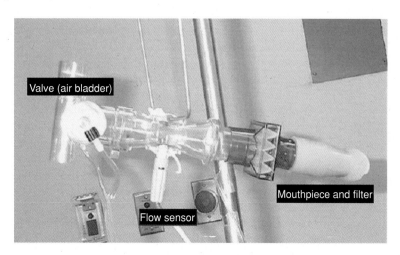

Figure 4.6. Components of an active breathing control (ABC) system.

SUMMARY

The influence of geometric variations in radiation therapy increases in significance with the conformality of the planned treatment. Our understanding of motion and its effects is growing. The most significant geometric variation is systematic positioning error, with interfraction movement, intrafraction movement, and random setup variation.

Interventions to better reduce these movement-related uncertainties are evolving rapidly. A fundamental understanding of the limitations of any given monitoring or tracking system, coupled with the impact of uncertainty in target position on dose, will yield efficient strategies for implementing technology to limit the impact of patient and organ movement on treatment outcome.

REFERENCES

1. Van de Steene J, Van Den Heuvel F, Bel A, et al. Electronic portal imaging with on-line correction of setup error in thoracic irradiation: clinical evaluation. *Int J Radiat Oncol Biol Phys* 1998;40(4):967–976.
2. Hong TS, et al. The impact of daily setup variations on head-and-neck intensity-modulated radiation therapy. *Int J Radiat Oncol Biol Phys* 2005;61(3):779–788.
3. Meijer GJ, et al. Three-dimensional analysis of delineation errors, setup errors, and organ motion during radiotherapy of bladder cancer. *Int J Radiat Oncol Biol Phys* 2003;55(5):1277–1287.
4. Weber DC, et al. Patient positioning in prostate radiotherapy: is prone better than supine? *Int J Radiat Oncol Biol Phys* 2000;47(2):365–371.
5. Pisani L, et al. Setup error in radiotherapy: on-line correction using electronic kilovoltage and megavoltage radiographs. *Int J Radiat Oncol Biol Phys* 2000;47(3):825–839.
6. Michalski JM, et al. Prospective clinical evaluation of an electronic portal imaging device. *Int J Radiat Oncol Biol Phys* 1996;34(4):943–951.
7. Marsh R, et al. Design and analysis of an immobilization and repositioning system for treatment of neck malignancies. *Med Dosim* 1997;22(4):293–297.
8. Bentel GC, et al. The effectiveness of immobilization during prostate irradiation. *Int J Radiat Oncol Biol Phys* 1995;31(1):143–148.
9. Biggs PJ, Goitein M, Russell MD. A diagnostic X ray field verification device for a 10 MV linear accelerator. *Int J Radiat Oncol Biol Phys* 1985;11(3):635–643.
10. Balter JM, et al. Daily targeting of intrahepatic tumors for radiotherapy. *Int J Radiat Oncol Biol Phys* 2002;52(1):266–271.
11. Litzenberg D, et al. Daily prostate targeting using implanted radiopaque markers. *Int J Radiat Oncol Biol Phys* 2002;52(3):699–703.
12. Schewe JE, et al. A room-based diagnostic imaging system for measurement of patient setup. *Med Phys* 1998;25(12):2385–2387.
13. Murphy MJ. An automatic six-degree-of-freedom image registration algorithm for image-guided frameless stereotaxic radiosurgery. *Med Phys* 1997;24(6):857–866.
14. Shirato H, et al. Four-dimensional treatment planning and fluoroscopic real-time tumor tracking radiotherapy for moving tumor. *Int J Radiat Oncol Biol Phys* 2000;48(2):435–442.
15. Bel A, van Herk M, Lebesque JV. Target margins for random geometrical treatment uncertainties in conformal radiotherapy. *Med Phys* 1996;23(9):1537–1545.
16. Remeijer P, et al. Margins for translational and rotational uncertainties: a probability-based approach. *Int J Radiat Oncol Biol Phys* 2002;53(2):464–474.
17. van Herk M, Remeijer P, Lebesque JV. Inclusion of geometric uncertainties in treatment plan evaluation. *Int J Radiat Oncol Biol Phys* 2002;52(5):1407–1422.
18. Balter JM, et al. Evaluating the influence of setup uncertainties on treatment planning for focal liver tumors. *Int J Radiat Oncol Biol Phys* 2005;63(2):610–614.
19. de Boer HC, et al. Electronic portal image assisted reduction of systematic set-up errors in head and neck irradiation. *Radiother Oncol* 2001;61(3):299–308.
20. de Boer HC, Heijmen BJ. A protocol for the reduction of systematic patient setup errors with minimal portal imaging workload. *Int J Radiat Oncol Biol Phys* 2001;50(5):1350–1365.
21. van Lin EN, et al. Effectiveness of couch height-based patient set-up and an off-line correction protocol in prostate cancer radiotherapy. *Int J Radiat Oncol Biol Phys* 2001;50(2):569–577.
22. Yan D, et al. Adaptive radiation therapy. *Phys Med Biol* 1997;42(1):123–132.
23. Langen KM, Jones DT. Organ motion and its management. *Int J Radiat Oncol Biol Phys* 2001;50(1):265–278.
24. Balter JM, et al. Measurement of prostate movement over the course of routine radiotherapy using implanted markers. *Int J Radiat Oncol Biol Phys* 1995;31(1):113–118.
25. Beard CJ, et al. Analysis of prostate and seminal vesicle motion: implications for treatment planning. *Int J Radiat Oncol Biol Phys* 1996;34(2):451–458.
26. Booth JT, Zavgorodni SF. Set-up error & organ motion uncertainty: a review. *Australas Phys Eng Sci Med* 1999;22(2):29–47.
27. Crook JM, et al. Prostate motion during standard radiotherapy as assessed by fiducial markers. *Radiother Oncol* 1995;37(1):35–42.
28. Dawson LA, et al. Target position variability throughout prostate radiotherapy. *Int J Radiat Oncol Biol Phys* 1998;42(5):1155–1161.
29. Melian E, et al. Variation in prostate position quantitation and implications for three-dimensional conformal treatment planning. *Int J Radiat Oncol Biol Phys* 1997;38(1):73–81.
30. Padhani AR, et al. Evaluating the effect of rectal distension and rectal movement on prostate gland position using cine MRI. *Int J Radiat Oncol Biol Phys* 1999;44(3):525–533.
31. Roeske JC, et al. Evaluation of changes in the size and location of the prostate, seminal vesicles, bladder, and rectum during a course of external beam radiation therapy. *Int J Radiat Oncol Biol Phys* 1995;33(5):1321–1329.
32. van Herk M, et al. Quantification of organ motion during conformal radiotherapy of the prostate by three dimensional image registration. *Int J Radiat Oncol Biol Phys* 1995;33(5):1311–1320.

33. Zimmermann FB, Molls M. Influence of organ and patient movements on the target volume in radiotherapy of prostatic carcinoma. *Strahlenther Onkol* 1997;173(3):172–173.

34. Smitsmans MH, et al. Automatic prostate localization on cone-beam CT scans for high precision image-guided radiotherapy. *Int J Radiat Oncol Biol Phys* 2005;63(4):975–984.

35. Dawson LA, et al. A comparison of ventilatory prostate movement in four treatment positions. *Int J Radiat Oncol Biol Phys* 2000;48(2):319–323.

36. Malone S, et al. Respiratory-induced prostate motion: quantification and characterization. *Int J Radiat Oncol Biol Phys* 2000;48(1):105–109.

37. Litzenberg DW, et al. Influence of intrafraction motion on margins for prostate radiotherapy. *Int J Radiat Oncol Biol Phys* 2006;65(2):548–553.

38. Allen AM, et al. Evaluation of the influence of breathing on the movement and modeling of lung tumors. *Int J Radiat Oncol Biol Phys* 2004;58(4):1251–1257.

39. Stevens CW, et al. Respiratory-driven lung tumor motion is independent of tumor size, tumor location, and pulmonary function. *Int J Radiat Oncol Biol Phys* 2001;51(1):62–68.

40. Rietzel E, Pan T, Chen GT. Four-dimensional computed tomography: image formation and clinical protocol. *Med Phys* 2005;32(4):874–889.

41. Seppenwoolde Y, et al. Precise and real-time measurement of 3D tumor motion in lung due to breathing and heartbeat, measured during radiotherapy. *Int J Radiat Oncol Biol Phys* 2002;53(4):822–834.

42. Barnes EA, et al. Dosimetric evaluation of lung tumor immobilization using breath hold at deep inspiration. *Int J Radiat Oncol Biol Phys* 2001;50(4):1091–1098.

43. Chen MH, et al. Respiratory maneuvers decrease irradiated cardiac volume in patients with left-sided breast cancer. *J Cardiovasc Magn Reson* 2002;4(2):265–271.

44. Hanley J, et al. Deep inspiration breath-hold technique for lung tumors: the potential value of target immobilization and reduced lung density in dose escalation. *Int J Radiat Oncol Biol Phys* 1999;45(3):603–611.

45. Rosenzweig KE, et al. The deep inspiration breath-hold technique in the treatment of inoperable non-small-cell lung cancer. *Int J Radiat Oncol Biol Phys* 2000;48(1):81–87.

46. Sixel KE, Aznar MC, Ung YC. Deep inspiration breath hold to reduce irradiated heart volume in breast cancer patients. *Int J Radiat Oncol Biol Phys* 2001;49(1):199–204.

47. Stromberg JS, et al. Active Breathing Control (ABC) for Hodgkin's disease: reduction in normal tissue irradiation with deep inspiration and implications for treatment. *Int J Radiat Oncol Biol Phys* 2000;48(3):797–806.

48. Brock KK, et al. Technical note: creating a four-dimensional model of the liver using finite element analysis. *Med Phys* 2002;29(7):1403–1405.

49. Brock KK, et al. Inclusion of organ deformation in dose calculations. *Med Phys* 2003;30(3):290–295.

50. Brock KK, et al. Accuracy of finite element model-based multi-organ deformable image registration. *Med Phys* 2005;32(6):1647–1659.

51. Brock KM, et al. Automated generation of a four-dimensional model of the liver using warping and mutual information. *Med Phys* 2003;30(6):1128–1133.

52. Shirato H, et al. Physical aspects of a real-time tumor-tracking system for gated radiotherapy. *Int J Radiat Oncol Biol Phys* 2000;48(4):1187–1195.

53. Berbeco RI, et al. Residual motion of lung tumours in gated radiotherapy with external respiratory surrogates. *Phys Med Biol* 2005;50(16):3655–3667.

54. Jin JY, Yin FF. Time delay measurement for linac based treatment delivery in synchronized respiratory gating radiotherapy. *Med Phys* 2005;32(5):1293–1296.

55. Ozhasoglu C, Murphy MJ. Issues in respiratory motion compensation during external-beam radiotherapy. *Int J Radiat Oncol Biol Phys* 2002;52(5):1389–1399.

56. Vedam SS, et al. Determining parameters for respiration-gated radiotherapy. *Med Phys* 2001;28(10):2139–2146.

57. Wong JW, et al. The use of active breathing control (ABC) to reduce margin for breathing motion. *Int J Radiat Oncol Biol Phys* 1999;44(4):911–919.

58. Cheung PC, et al. Reproducibility of lung tumor position and reduction of lung mass within the planning target volume using active breathing control (ABC). *Int J Radiat Oncol Biol Phys* 2003;57(5):1437–1442.

59. Dawson LA, et al. The reproducibility of organ position using active breathing control (ABC) during liver radiotherapy. *Int J Radiat Oncol Biol Phys* 2001;51(5):1410–1421.

60. Dawson LA, et al. Accuracy of daily image guidance for hypofractionated liver radiotherapy with active breathing control. *Int J Radiat Oncol Biol Phys* 2005;62(4):1247–1252.

61. Remouchamps VM, et al. Initial clinical experience with moderate deep-inspiration breath hold using an active breathing control device in the treatment of patients with left-sided breast cancer using external beam radiation therapy. *Int J Radiat Oncol Biol Phys* 2003;56(3):704–715.

62. Sarrut D, et al. Nonrigid registration method to assess reproducibility of breath-holding with ABC in lung cancer. *Int J Radiat Oncol Biol Phys* 2005;61(2):594–607.

63. D'Souza WD, Naqvi SA, Yu CX. Real-time intra-fraction-motion tracking using the treatment couch: a feasibility study. *Phys Med Biol* 2005;50(17):4021–4033.

64. Murphy MJ. Tracking moving organs in real time. *Semin Radiat Oncol* 2004;14(1):91–100.

65. Neicu T, et al. Synchronized moving aperture radiation therapy (SMART): average tumour trajectory for lung patients. *Phys Med Biol* 2003;48(5):587–598.

66. Schweikard A, Shiomi H, Adler J. Respiration tracking in radiosurgery. *Med Phys* 2004;31(10):2738–2741.

67. Sharp GC, et al. Prediction of respiratory tumour motion for real-time image-guided radiotherapy. *Phys Med Biol* 2004;49(3):425–440.

CHAPTER 5

Patient Positioning and Immobilization

Lawrence E. Reinstein ■ Matthew B. Podgorsak

INTRODUCTION

The primary goal of radiotherapy is the delivery of a prescribed radiation dose to a predefined target volume, either to inactivate a tumor or to treat a benign condition that responds to radiation therapy. A frequently conflicting goal is the avoidance of damage to the patient's healthy radiosensitive tissues and organs that may be adjacent to the target volume or are in the path of a radiation beam as it is aimed toward the target volume. For many treatments requiring very high doses of radiation, the determining factor in how well we can achieve both goals is the extent to which we can deliver treatment accurately every day for the entire course of radiotherapy. Inadequate dose to all or part of the target volume may lead to treatment failure and possibly death. On the other hand, excessive dose to all or part of an adjacent organ may cause drastic and intolerable complications such as paraplegia, blindness, kidney failure, and so on, that would result in unacceptable post-treatment quality of life for the patient.

Radiation treatment accuracy can be divided into two separate but highly interrelated concepts: dosimetric accuracy and geometric accuracy. This chapter deals only with the latter. It covers issues related to patient positioning and immobilization that have a strong effect on how well we can accurately cover a specified anatomic volume with a desired radiation dose. It does not deal with issues such as radiation beam calibration and dose calculations but only with patient positioning from the time the target volume and critical organ volumes are defined through the daily treatment setup.

PATIENT SETUP FOR RADIOTHERAPY

Nearly all modern radiotherapy is delivered using a medical linear accelerator. Current medical accelerators provide photon beams in the megavoltage range, typically with a peak energy of 6 MV or greater, and often with dual photon beams and an assortment of electron beams. The photon beam may be controlled by thick tungsten collimators that define a variable field size. These motorized collimators, which can be symmetrical, asymmetrical, or multileaf, are mounted in the head of a gantry that rotates a full 360 degree about an *isocenter* whose position in space is stable

to within 1 mm. A beam *central axis* can be defined as the straight line between the accelerator target (x-ray *source*) and the center of the radiation field defined by the symmetrical collimators. If the accelerator geometry is properly aligned, the central axis passes through the isocenter for all gantry angles, forming a vertical plane. Also, it must continue to pass through the isocenter even when the field-defining collimators are rotated about the central axis. Typical specifications on geometric precision for medical accelerators require that for all possible beam orientations, the central axis must pass through a sphere at the isocenter with a radius of 1 mm (1,2). The newest accelerators equipped with onboard imaging capability through cone-beam computed tomography (CT) reconstruction have even tighter geometrical tolerances (isocenter sphere radius of 0.5 mm) to ensure accurate image reconstruction. The accelerator comes with a light field projecting an optical crosshair that precisely indicates the location of the beam central axis during setup.

As described above, in general, the goal of radiotherapy is to deliver a high dose to the target volume, at the same time keeping the dose to the surrounding tissues and organs to a minimum, or at least within tolerable levels. Once these structures are identified with a variety of different imaging techniques, a treatment plan is created. Usually, the treatment plan necessitates centering the target volume on the isocenter and firing beams of different apertures from several different gantry and/or couch angles toward the target (Fig. 5.1A).

How can we place the patient so as to ensure that the target is at the isocenter? If we make the simplifying but somewhat unrealistic assumption that the patient is a *rigid solid* with a flat posterior surface, and therefore the tumor volume and all surrounding organs are *frozen*, treatment setup is straightforward and well defined. If the patient is supine on a flat, perfectly horizontal treatment couch, a single point (a fiducial mark, often a tattoo or permanent ink) placed on the anterior skin is sufficient to locate the center of the target volume that prior imaging has shown to be at a certain depth, d, beneath the surface. With the gantry angle vertical and central axis pointing downward, the treatment couch can be adjusted in the left-to-right and head-to-toe dimensions until the optical crosshair intersects at this skin mark. Because the accelerator includes a simple tool to indicate the target-to-surface distance (TSD)

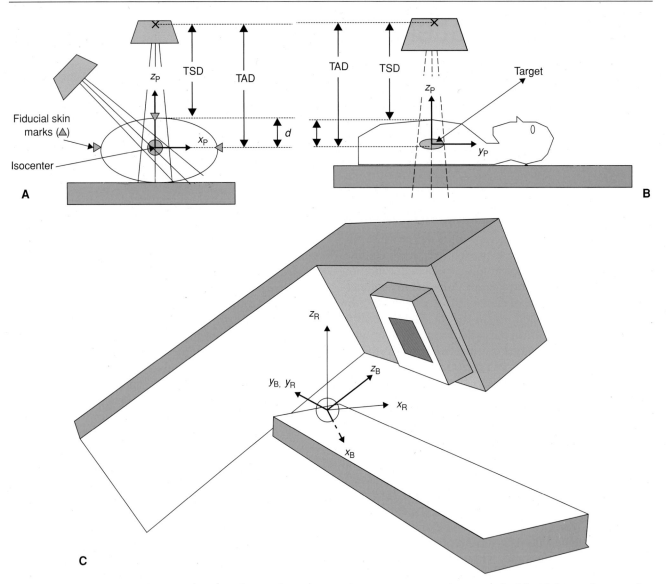

Figure 5.1. **A:** Cross section of patient illustrating the use of two isocentric beams to encompass the target. The fiducial skin marks are used to set up the patient so that the target is at the isocenter at a depth *d*. The target-to-skin distance (TSD) and target-to-axis distance (TAD) satisfy the relationship TSD = TAD − *d*. **B:** The treatment setup parameters and patient coordinate system shown in the sagittal view. **C:** Room coordinate and beam coordinate systems as described in text.

and because the target-to-axis (isocenter) distance (TAD) is fixed (at 100 cm for nearly all therapy accelerators), the treatment couch height is simply adjusted until the TSD indicator, a calibrated *front pointer*, or *optical distance indicator* (ODI), shows TSD = TAD − *d* (i.e., TSD = 100 cm—target depth). This positions the target center at the accelerator isocenter.

Modern medical accelerators come equipped with a precision motorized and often computer-controllable treatment couch, also known as the *patient support assembly*. The movements of the treatment couch are carefully specified so that its translational axes are vertical and horizontal. In addition, the couch rotates about a vertical axis passing through the isocenter to allow for nonaxial (noncoplanar) beams for more complex treatment delivery. The setup procedure just described may not be sufficiently well defined

even for our fictitious rigid patient. Simply superimposing the target center on the accelerator isocenter allows the possibility that the rigid patient is twisted or rotated, and although the target center would still be treated correctly, the full target volume and the surrounding organs might not be treated as planned. By way of analogy, knowing the *x, y, z* center-of-mass coordinates of an airplane on its landing approach does not adequately describe the situation: The pilot also must know its *roll* (lateral tilt), *pitch* (longitudinal tilt), and *yaw* (rotation on vertical axis) to land safely. If the posterior surface of the rigid patient is a flat plane, the treatment couch eliminates any ambiguities with respect to roll and pitch of the patient. The problem of yaw, however, remains. An improved and somewhat more complex approach to patient setup enabling fine-tuning of rigid patient rotation has been recently developed. The system

(HexaPOD evo RT System, Elekta Inc., Norcross, GA) includes a robotic treatment couch top that incorporates 6 degrees of freedom in its movement (three translations and three rotations) and can be used to fine-tune patient rotation as well as the center of mass of the target to ensure accurate orientation of the full target volume relative to the treatment beam.

Modern radiotherapy simulator, virtual simulator, and accelerator rooms are equipped with at least three lasers. Two of these are mounted on the sidewalls to the patient's left and right and are aligned to be horizontal, to pass through the machine isocenter, and to be perpendicular to the isocenter axis. (When these conditions are met, the laser beams are colinear as well.) The third laser is mounted on the ceiling and points straight down through the isocenter. With the patient lying on the couch in the simulator room, the CT room, or any other room similarly equipped, a patient coordinate system can be established, and the points where the laser beams intersect the skin surface can be permanently marked. Although it is typical and convenient to try to place the origin of the patient coordinate system at the target volume center and to align the patient so that his or her longitudinal body axis is parallel to the isocenter axis, it is not altogether necessary. Consistent planning and treatment can be based upon an initial patient origin that is near the target center or even somewhat arbitrary. Optimum choice for the patient coordinate system *setup origin* is often dictated by the location of the associated fiducial skin marks.

The rigid-solid setup procedure consists of establishing an appropriate patient coordinate system on the radiotherapy simulator couch, carefully creating fiducial point surface marks, and then rotating and translating the patient on the accelerator treatment couch so as to achieve congruence between the patient and room coordinate systems. Congruence is demonstrated when the orthogonal lasers in the accelerator treatment room precisely impinge on the three surface fiducials, two side and one top. Other tools to help verify the alignment include the ODI, which, if the treatment setup is perfect, should indicate the correct central axis depth to the target center ($d = $ TAD – TSD), and the sagittal laser, which is mounted on the wall opposite to the accelerator gantry to provide a longitudinal line parallel to and defining a vertical plane with the horizontal isocenter axis.

For implementation of more complex isocentric treatment plans, it is useful to establish three coordinate systems: the patient coordinate system, the room coordinate system, and the beam coordinate system. The patient coordinate system, already described, is usually defined during therapy simulation, CT imaging for therapy planning, or virtual simulation. During this process the patient should be placed in a comfortable and reproducible position that will become the *treatment position*. Typically, in this position the patient is lying flat and level, either supine or prone, on the horizontal table without any obvious bending or twisting. The patient's longitudinal symmetry axis is aligned to the

horizontal to become the y_p axis of the patient coordinate system. A transverse plane orthogonal to the y_p axis contains the z_p (pointing straight upward) and x_p (pointing horizontally to the supine patient's left) coordinate axes (Fig. 5.1B). Treatment planning is often simplified if the origin of the patient coordinate system is placed at the center of the treatment target, but this is not always convenient nor is it absolutely necessary. The patient coordinate system should be more or less permanently delineated through the use of fiducial marks on the patient's skin. It may be advantageous to shift the origin of the patient coordinate system away from the target center to obtain fiducial marks where the skin is taut and relatively immovable and to avoid regions of soft and flabby tissues.

The room coordinate system can be defined with its origin at the isocenter of the medical accelerator. The isocenter plane is defined by the sweep of the beam central axis as the accelerator gantry rotates about the isocenter. The y_r axis is defined as orthogonal to this plane passing through the isocenter, the positive direction being toward the gantry support. The x_r and z_r axes of the room coordinate system are contained in the isocenter plane with positive z_r in the vertical (up) direction and positive z_r in the horizontal (supine patient's left) direction (Fig. 5.1C).

The beam coordinate system is defined by the central ray of the radiation beam (z_b) and the x_b and y_b axes, which are in a plane orthogonal to the central ray and pointing perpendicularly toward the field-defining (symmetrical or asymmetrical) collimators. Note that the origin of the beam coordinate system is also at the isocenter and that the beam coordinate system rotates with respect to the room coordinate system with either accelerator gantry or collimator rotation.

The process of patient treatment setup according to an isocentric radiotherapy treatment plan includes the following steps:

1. The patient is placed on the couch (patient support assembly) in the proper treatment position, supine or prone, with or without wedges, pillows, and immobilization devices.
2. Properly shifting the patient on the treatment couch and raising the couch to the appropriate height (z_r dimension) brings the patient coordinate system into alignment with the room coordinate system, as is verified by precise superpositioning of the orthogonal room lasers with the fiducial skin marks.
3. With the gantry pointing straight down, secondary confirmation checks are made of the TSD using the ODI such that TSD = TAD – d, where d is the depth to the isocenter. This becomes the proper initial treatment setup position.
4. The treatment plan is implemented for each field by proper rotation of the gantry and collimator as well as by choice of field size and beam modifiers. This transforms the beam coordinate system with respect to the room coordinate system and hence, because they are

aligned by the initial setup procedure, to the patient coordinate system as well. Before treatment, a secondary check of TSD should also be made for each field.

5. More complex planning (e.g., noncoplanar, nonaxial, and multiple isocenters) may require further transformation of the patient coordinate system with respect to the room coordinate system and hence with respect to the beam coordinate system. This is achieved by appropriate translation and/or rotation of the treatment couch.

Although the three-point triangulation method is sufficient to prevent the orientation ambiguities (roll, pitch, and yaw) that characterize the single-point method, what about the actual patient, who is far from rigid and who consists of muscle, fat, bone, and so on? It is tempting to suggest that the three-point triangulation method at least ensures that the treatment setup is accurate in the transverse plane defined by this triangle. But even this may not be true. In a *perfectly* accurate setup the treatment fields would correspond exactly to the planned fields with respect to the target volume *and* the surrounding tissues and organs. This can be true only if the interrelationship between these anatomic structures with the surface fiducials remains constant in time, both on the imaging or radiotherapy simulator couch and on the treatment couch. Strictly speaking, this is unlikely to be true for any patient.

As we move away from the central triangulation plane in the cephalad or caudad direction, additional differences may arise between the patient localization data (the CT scan, magnetic resonance imaging (MRI), single photon emission computed tomography (SPECT), positron emission tomography (PET) images, or even external surface contours) and the anatomy of the patient lying on the accelerator couch on the day of treatment. While the patient is lying on a hard flat couch, the arm and leg positions can shift, the spine and the neck can flex differently each time, soft tissues and fat can deform under the force of surface contact or of gravity, muscles can contract or relax, and so on. Depending on the location of the treatment site, we cannot be certain that the patient will lie down on the couch each day in the same way as during the localization procedure. Because organ position can change with respect to the patient coordinate system, this can lead to different areas of target undertreatment and critical organ overtreatment each day, with actual delivered dose-volume histograms (DVH) different from the planned DVH.

Depending on the level of accuracy demanded by a particular treatment protocol, aligning the patient with three triangulation points may not be sufficient. Serious errors can occur, particularly when long (in the cephalocaudal dimension) fields are used. A number of steps can reduce the error associated with the soft and flexible nature of the patient. In general, they all attempt to create a comfortable, relaxed, and stable treatment position for the patient, one that can be reasonably well reproduced each day. The more like a rigid body one can make the patient, the more likely it is that correct setup will be accomplished.

Some straightforward suggestions to improve setup accuracy:

■ Determine a comfortable and relaxed position for the patient. If the position is not comfortable, the patient tends to fidget or move until a more comfortable position is found. Also, if muscles are tense during localization, they may relax as the treatments progress. The use of standard indexed foam wedges, head cups, and Timos can often help.

■ Make use of the modern laser crosshair system that has replaced the older laser dot system. If properly installed and aligned, the sidewall lasers project lines in precisely vertical and horizontal directions, with the intersection of the crosshairs projecting horizontally through the isocenter. The ceiling laser cross-projects lines straight downward in the transverse and sagittal planes, both intersecting the isocenter. It is important to note that the crosshair intersection point for perfectly installed lasers is projected colinearly to each axis of the room coordinate system. Often, similar systems of laser crosses exist in the simulator or imaging rooms, consequently more extensive markings can be made where these lines intersect the patient's surface while in the treatment position. These markings can be used as additional setup guides to help return the patient to the same position each day and to avoid errors that result from the natural twisting and flexing of the body. New developments in technology include HeNe lasers that project a green light providing enhanced contrast on skin tones that are problematic with the traditional red laser. Furthermore, green laser projections are sharper on the patient skin due to reduced light scatter in the fine capillaries beneath the skin surface.

■ Extend the surface markings as far superior and inferior to the central treatment plane as is practical. Rotation of the legs can affect the position of organs within the pelvis. The arms and shoulders can similarly affect the internal anatomy within the thorax. Extending the alignment marks above and below the central plane and even the treatment volume, as discussed in the preceding text, improves reproducibility of target and critical organ placement.

■ Refer to external anatomic landmarks. Additional reassurance in setting up a patient in a reproducible position can be obtained by measuring and recording the distances between several visible anatomic landmarks or between these landmarks and the laser alignment system. For example, proper head tilt can be tested each day by measuring the distance between the bottom of the chin and the suprasternal notch.

■ Make use of immobilization devices. There is a detailed discussion of these devices later in this chapter. Many of the newer devices and materials are based upon modern packaging techniques with which fragile electronic equipment or soft produce is protected by hardened foams and thermoplastics that conform to their external

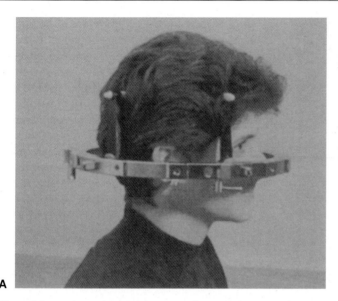
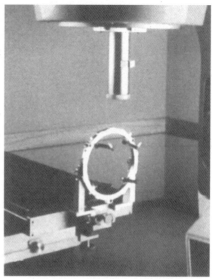

A **B**

Figure 5.2. A: The BRW/CRW (Brown-Roberts-Wells/Cosman-Roberts-Wells) head ring assembly for stereotactic radiosurgery. **B:** Head ring assembly attached to the treatment couch for accelerator-based radiosurgery. (Courtesy of Integra, Burlington, MA.)

surface. In this way, the soft and flexible item becomes a rigid body. Such devices when customized to radiation oncology patients provide comfort, confinement, and stability that assist in achieving an accurate setup. If the customized device is created during patient localization, the appropriate fiducial marks can be permanently applied to its hard outer surface and hopefully establish a more stable patient coordinate system for use during each treatment setup.

Although the surface fiducial three-point triangulation system is commonly used for conventional treatments, there are several specialized systems in use today or under development. One, in particular, is the localization and setup used for stereotactic radiosurgery (3–5). This single-fraction technique uses small-diameter circular fields for the treatment of arteriovascular malformations (AVMs), acoustic neuromas, brain metastases, primary brain tumors, and recently, functional disorders, for which demands for precision may be greater than in any other external beam treatment (<1 mm overall geometric uncertainty). The variety of commercial systems available include a stereotactic head ring such as is used by neurosurgeons for stereotactic biopsy fixed to the patient's skull with head posts and skull screws set into the bone. This is an invasive (although relatively simple and painless) procedure, and the frame remains affixed to the patient's head throughout the localization and treatment (Figs. 5.2A and B).

Specialized localizing devices and fiducial systems attach to the head frame, and allow the positions of the target and critical structures to be determined with a high degree of accuracy within the coordinate system defined by the stereotactic frame. Localizing devices are available for use with CT scan, angiography, and MRI. As with conventional radiotherapy, the planning process includes

digitizing the target center and the relevant anatomic structures, once the stereotactic transformation has been determined. For treatment, the head frame can be *docked* with a base frame mounted either to the treatment couch or the floor. Because the base frames are mechanically aligned to the room coordinate system, it becomes a simple matter to apply a series of spatial translations so that the target is exactly at the isocenter and the head oriented according to the treatment plan. A specialized radiotherapy and neurosurgery tool, known as the *Gamma Knife* (Elekta Inc., Norcross, GA), has also been successfully applied for intracranial radiosurgery treatments.

One of the reasons stereotactic radiosurgery is so accurate is that there are virtually no changes in the positions of the internal anatomy with respect to the bony skull, either during treatment or day to day. Although it is tempting to try to apply this technique to fractionated radiotherapy, there is one major drawback: It is impractical to have the head frame bolted to the patient's skull for an entire course of radiotherapy. To address this objection, several relocatable head frames, invasive and noninvasive, have been developed. These are discussed later in this chapter. Furthermore, several systems for body radiosurgery have also been developed and are based on similar principles to traditional intracranial radiosurgery.

An alternative or supplement to treatment setup using surface fiducial marks is *radiographic setup and alignment.* This approach has been characterized as image-guided radiation therapy (IGRT), and the state of the art in IGRT technology is covered in detail in Chapter 14. A simple example of IGRT is the daily use of portal images before treatment is delivered. To maintain patient flow in a busy clinic, such interventional techniques are practical only if automatic or semiautomatic software tools are available to rapidly compare the portal image taken with an electronic

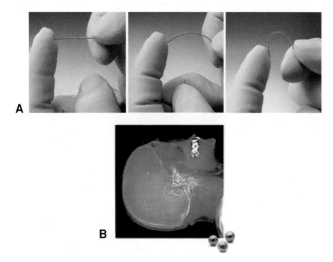

Figure 5.3. **A:** Three implantable radiopaque markers. (Courtesy of CIVCO and IBA-Advanced Radiotherapy, Tyngsboro, MA.) **B:** Radiograph showing implanted fiducial marker in the skull.

portal imaging device (EPID) with the digitally reconstructed radiograph (DRR) previously generated for the radiation field in question. For this method, the DRR, which is based upon CT localization data, should contain the outline of the field aperture designed in the treatment planning process as well as contours of visible anatomic structures. Such software tools have been developed and are readily available from numerous manufacturers (e.g., Visicoil Guided Radiotherapy, IBA-Advanced Radiotherapy, Tyngsboro, MA). Several studies using interventional setup techniques show reasonable success (6,7).

Radiographic alignment of patient anatomy using bony landmarks should be more accurate than surface fiducial methods. Studies of daily radiographic alignment of supine patients treated for intracranial targets (8,9) yield positioning accuracy of 1 mm or better. Reasons for the inaccuracy of surface fiducial methods include the inherent limitations of laser and optical alignment devices (discussed later in this chapter) and the instability of internal organs with respect to the skin surface. However, radiographic alignment has its limitations as well. It is not always possible to find the same point on the bony landmark in the two orthogonal views needed to ensure complete three-dimensional (3D) spatial verification. Also, because this method is based upon imaging and repositioning of the bony landmarks within the treatment volume, it makes the *underlying assumption that the soft tissue organs are fixed with respect to the skeleton.* The reliability of this assumption is highly dependent on the anatomic location and the organs in question, and further study is clearly needed.

The following two forms of radiographic setup *do not* make this important assumption:

■ Localization and alignment using radiopaque markers implanted in the target
■ Setup using daily pretreatment acquisition of patient 3D anatomic information

Implanting radiopaque markers in the target (10,11) make it possible to use, for example, an EPID device to achieve computer-assisted orthogonal localization of the soft tissue target. Several manufacturers currently market implantable fiducial markers (e.g., ACCULOC IGRT fiducial markers [CIVCO], Visicoil [IBA-Advanced Radiotherapy, Tyngsboro, MA]) that are radiographically visible and can be used in conjunction with IGRT techniques for patient setup. Imaging of these radiopaque markers can be done using portal images acquired before treatment delivery. The position of the markers relative to the isocenter is then compared to their position on a DRR obtained from the planning CT scan, and appropriate patient position adjustments can subsequently be made. Figure 5.3A shows two types of implantable fiducial markers and Figure 5.3B shows a radiograph of implanted bone fiducial markers.

Taking this process one step further, the ExacTrac X-ray 6D system (BrainLAB USA, Chicago, IL) is comprised of a pair of kV x-ray tubes recessed into the treatment room floor and aimed at a corresponding pair of amorphous silicon flat panel detectors. These imaging systems, shown in Figure 5.4, provide real-time stereoscopic information regarding the position of bony anatomy or implanted fiducial markers relative to the treatment isocenter. A comparison is then made to the corresponding marker positions on DRRs reconstructed from the planning CT scan, and patient position is robotically modified during treatment to realign the anatomy or markers to their planned positions relative to the isocenter using a treatment couch with 6 degrees of freedom (ExacTrac Robotic Couch, BrainLAB, Chicago, IL).

A different concept in patient setup and positioning involves implanting tiny *beacon transponders*, consisting of small coils encapsulated in a glass enclosure, within a target volume (Calypso 4D Localization System, Calypso Medical,

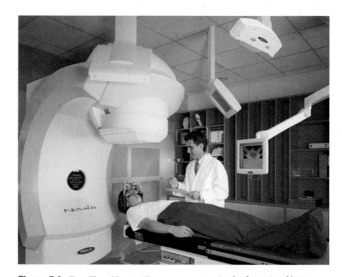

Figure 5.4. ExacTrac X-ray 6D system comprised of a pair of kV x-ray tubes recessed into the treatment room floor and aimed at a corresponding pair of flat panel detectors. (Courtesy of BrainLAB, Chicago, IL.)

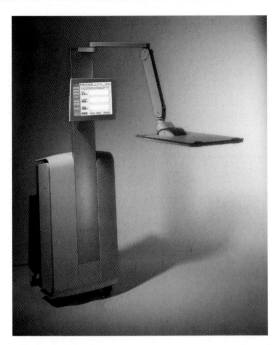

Figure 5.5. Array placed over a patient that activates implanted transponders through a radiofrequency signal and then listens for the signals returned from each transponder. (Courtesy of Calypso Medical, Seattle, WA.)

Seattle, WA). Rather than using radiographic information to localize these markers, an array, shown in Figure 5.5, placed over the patient activates the transponders through a radiofrequency signal and then listens for the signals that are returned from each transponder. The 3D position of each transponder is determined and compared to the baseline geometry, giving shift coordinates that, once implemented, return the implanted transponders, and, presumably, the target volume, to their planned positions relative to isocenter. Multi-institutional clinical trials have shown that this technology can be efficiently applied to improve the accuracy of prostate localization during external beam radiotherapy (12–14). Recently published phantom and animal studies have also documented the potential use of this technology in the treatment of other anatomies (15,16).

The idea of using daily pretreatment CT scans to assist in patient setup on a daily basis may have seemed far-fetched just a few years ago, but several variations of this scheme have been recently developed. The simplest technique is the placement of a commercial diagnostic CT scanner *within* the medical accelerator room (e.g., Primatom [Siemens Medical Solutions, Malvern, PA]). This paradigm includes a medical accelerator coupled with a standard CT scanner mounted on rails that can be positioned around a patient already setup in treatment position on the linac treatment couch. Once imaging of the target volume is complete and the patient has been appropriately shifted, the CT scanner is moved away so that treatment can be delivered. Of course, this approach requires fast and reliable software to determine what translations and rotations of the patient (patient coordinate system) must be

made to best duplicate the dose distribution seen on the approved treatment plan.

A more sophisticated approach involves obtaining tomographic imaging information using the treatment unit itself. One such concept, coined *tomotherapy* (17) and described in detail elsewhere in this textbook, consists of an X-band accelerating waveguide (linac) mounted on a CT gantry. This beam line can be programmed with the appropriate parameters to obtain either a fan beam CT scan or to deliver a treatment. Patient positioning is fine-tuned before treatment based on the CT scan information, therefore in principle making it possible to duplicate on a daily basis the alignment of the planning target volume (PTV) to the isocenter that was captured at the time of planning CT scan. A different approach, covered in detail in Chapter 14, involves the use of cone-beam CT images obtained with an imaging device that is attached to a standard linear accelerator. Two manufacturers (Varian Medical Systems, Palo Alto, CA and Elekta Inc., Norcross, GA) currently have commercial products that are based on this paradigm. Tomographic information is obtained using a complementary beam line oriented perpendicularly to the treatment beam and comprised of a kV x-ray tube coupled with a digital image detector. A third manufacturer (Siemens Medical Solutions, Malvern, PA) has developed a system using the existing treatment beam to produce 3D target imaging with the patient on the treatment table. All three IGRT systems allow an image set to be reconstructed immediately prior to the delivery of each fraction from projections obtained as the system makes a full rotation around the patient. Similar to the tomotherapy concept, patient positioning can be fine-tuned by comparing the treatment CT scan obtained with the patient on the treatment table to the planning CT scan.

Ultrasound-based systems are also used for patient alignment. Although these systems have found their most common applications in patient positioning for pelvic (primarily prostate) radiotherapy, the positioning of any anatomy that lends itself to ultrasound imaging could, in principle, be verified with an ultrasound-based system. The use of these systems (BATCAM [Best Nomos, Pittsburgh, PA], Clarity [Elekta AB, Stockholm], and SonArray [Varian Medical Systems, Palo Alto, CA]) does not appear to significantly affect patient throughput.

All these radiographic setup techniques are interventional and require a means for the interactive correction of patient position, based on the radiographic information. Usually, this can be achieved through motorized couch movements that have recently incorporated motion in six dimensions (three standard translations plus roll, pitch, and yaw). A clinical system that eliminates the need for patient realignment after setup incorporates a miniature accelerator supported by a robotic arm that can accurately point in almost any direction (CyberKnife Robotic Radiosurgery System, Accuray, Sunnyvale, CA). After the patient is securely supported on a conventional treatment couch, stereo radiographs of the patient are taken with two ceiling-mounted x-ray tubes and corresponding amorphous silicon flat panel detectors recessed into the floor. These radiographs are compared with the library of DRRs generated during the planning study. The accelerator position and angle can then be adjusted to compensate for variations between the current and planned anatomic positions. This process is repeated during treatment delivery, and fine adjustments to the accelerator positioning are made to correct for patient motion during treatment.

PATIENT SETUP DURING DELIVERY OF RADIOTHERAPY

Verification of patient setup and interfraction confirmation of PTV alignment with treatment isocenter have been covered in the preceding text. Some PTVs, particularly those in the thorax and upper abdominal areas, have the potential for intrafraction motion, that is, the PTV can move during the delivery of a fraction of radiotherapy. Technologies that account for this motion have been developed (e.g., RPM Respiratory Gating System [Varian Medical Systems, Palo Alto, CA], Active Breathing Coordinator [Elekta Inc., Norcross, GA], ExacTrac Adaptive Gating [BrainLAB USA, Westchester, IL], Anzai Respiratory Gating Hardware [Siemens Medical Solutions, Malvern, PA]). Most of these systems track the position of a surrogate marker, either externally positioned or implanted within the target volume, and rely on reproducible correlation between the positions of the surrogate and the PTV. Delivery using this type of system has been termed *gated radiation therapy* because treatment is delivered through a "gate" defined by surrogate position. At least one manufacturer (Accuray, Sunnyvale, CA) has developed a treatment system (CyberKnife Robotic Radiosurgery System with Synchrony Respiratory Tracking System) that can continuously track patient, and, presumably PTV, position during treatment delivery, thereby obviating the need for

gating techniques. One group has studied the accuracy of a dynamic MLC-defined field moving in synchrony with a PTV that is itself moving due to respiratory motion (18). These approaches have the potential to be superior to gated delivery because they are more efficient and do not rely on a surrogate marker as the position of the PTV itself can be continuously verified.

ACCURACY AND REPRODUCIBILITY

Numerous studies demonstrate (to no one's surprise) geometric uncertainties in the delivery of radiotherapy. Whether these go by the name of patient setup errors, field placement errors (FPEs), field aperture errors, or patient position errors, they generally amount to underirradiating part of the intended target, overirradiating normal critical organs, or both. Byhardt et al. (19) found in a study of 337 patient portal films that setup errors >5 mm occurred in 15% of the setups, and for 10% the error was at least 10 mm. Other studies (20,21) estimate the frequency of setup errors >10 mm to be on the order of 20% across all sites when surface fiducial triangulation methods are used without immobilization devices. Also, a portal film study of mantle fields on nonimmobilized patients with Hodgkin's disease (22) showed block placement errors >10 mm in at least 21% of the patients. Much of the early literature is summarized in a paper by Boyer (23), in which he presents the FPEs as determined by portal film studies of different treatment sites (Table 5.1).

How are we to interpret these studies? What are the causes of these discrepancies? Should they be considered acceptable? Can anything be done to improve the situation? Do these FPEs have a negative clinical effect, and has this been demonstrated?

To answer the last question first, we turn to a theoretical study by Goitein and Buss (24), who found that clinically realistic random setup errors could cause a 12% decrease in tumor control for supraglottic lesions. A clinical study

TABLE 5.1 Field Alignment Discrepancy		
Site	Mean (mm)	Value exceeded by 20% of fields
Brain	7.1	9.2
Head and neck	3.6	5.0
Thorax	9.2	11.7
Abdomen	5.1	8.3
Pelvis	8.4	11.9
Extremities	6.9	8.8
All sites combined	7.7	11.1

Reprinted from Boyer AL. Patient positioning and immobilization devices. Monograph 15. In: Kereiakes JG, Elson HR, Born CG, eds. *Radiation oncology physics.* New York, NY: American Association of Physicists in Medicine, 1986: 438–446, with permission.

by Maruyama and Khan (25) reports a 33% recurrence rate in sites adjacent to the blocked areas in patients treated for Hodgkin's disease with mediastinal involvement, implying that marginal misses have a strong effect on outcome. A more recent report by Kinzie et al. (26), based on Patterns of Care data for 155 patients treated for Hodgkin's disease at several institutions, found that the local recurrence rate increased from 7% for patients with adequate tumor margins to 33% for those with inadequate ones. Similarly, in a retrospective study of 40 patients by Doss (27) head-and-neck recurrences were found to be correlated with blocking errors, defined as 5 mm or greater with respect to the first approved portal film. Only 7% of the patients with correct fields had recurrent disease versus 75% ($p = 0.03$) in those with blocking errors. Another retrospective study of 178 patients treated at a single institution for nasopharyngeal carcinoma showed that patients with adequate coverage of the defined target volume had 20% better local control than those with inadequately covered targets.

Taken as a whole, these and other data suggest what is more or less self-evident: Accurate reproducible treatment of the entire target volume with appropriate margins is important for achievement of the best possible results for the patient with cancer. To understand the individual sources of error that lead to the overall uncertainties, we must more clearly define the parameters involved. Fortunately, this has been made easier by the publication of ICRU *Report 50: Prescribing, recording and reporting photon beam therapy* (28), and the companion publication ICRU *Report 62: Prescribing, recording and reporting photon beam therapy (Supplement to ICRU Report 50)* (29). The ICRU defines a gross tumor volume (GTV) as "gross palpable or visible/demonstrable extent and location of malignant growth." The clinical target volume (CTV) includes the GTV "and/or subclinical microscopic malignant disease which have to be eliminated." It is the CTV that we hope to sterilize or eradicate by the application of radiotherapy.

Another volume introduced and defined by the ICRU is the PTV (Fig. 5.6). This volume is defined in recognition of treatment uncertainties such as organ motion and/or deformation and patient positioning errors and incorporates the concepts of internal margin (IM) and setup margin (SM), respectively, to account for these uncertainties. The PTV therefore includes the CTV and an appropriate margin (IM and SM) to take these treatment uncertainties into account. For any one patient, it is impossible to know exactly what these margins should be. The PTV–CTV margin may be nonuniform in thickness, because the uncertainties are not necessarily the same in every dimension. In principle, however, the CTV is entirely contained by the PTV despite all organ motion and setup uncertainties throughout the entire course of therapy. With this in mind, the task of the treatment planner is to find a combination of beam angles, beam apertures, and beam weights that deliver the prescribed dose to the entire PTV.

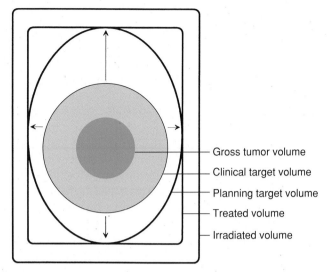

Figure 5.6. Schematic illustration of the different volumes used by Internal Commission on Radiation Units and Measurements (ICRU) for treatment planning. (Reprinted from International Commission on Radiation Units and Measurements. Prescribing, recording and reporting photon beam therapy. Report 50. Bethesda, MD: ICRU, 1993, with permission.)

Of necessity, the plan requires an *aperture margin* that takes into account the beam penumbra, which depends on depth, beam energy, and field size.

Issues of treatment accuracy and reproducibility can be thought of in terms of selection of the appropriate PTV–CTV margin for a particular patient treatment site and setup technique. Local recurrence due to a *marginal miss* in a treatment plan that was otherwise sound ("looked good on paper") means that the PTV–CTV margin may not have been adequate or appropriate. How can these margins be intelligently chosen, because we do not know the extent of organ motion or deformation or how much a particular setup will be off? To do this, it is necessary for the radiation oncology treatment planning team to study and understand the sources of error and uncertainty. Errors that contribute to treatment setup uncertainty include the following:

- Mechanical uncertainties in the medical accelerator. These include, for example, isocenter tolerance with gantry or collimator rotation, misalignment of treatment couch movements, and slack in block tray or couch top positioning.
- Mechanical indicator and readout uncertainties. These include alignment of positioning laser and optical crosshairs, light and radiation field congruence, ODI accuracy, digital readouts of gantry angle, collimator angle and field size accuracy, and so on. Also included in this group are such things as the width of the laser lines and the quality of the visible field light, which can lead to inconsistent interpretations.
- Mechanical uncertainties for all imaging and patient measurement systems with which localization and

treatment planning data were acquired. These include not only the indicators and readouts with which modern radiotherapy simulators, CT scanners, and virtual simulators are equipped, but also external contouring devices, patient calipers, and so on. Other characteristics, such as the difference in how the couch tops flex between the simulator and accelerator, may be considered here.

■ Erratic patient movement during treatment. This includes the extent and likelihood of patient motion caused by lack of cooperation, muscle contractions, discomfort in the treatment position, and its likely effect on the position of the CTV and other organs.

■ Patient repositioning uncertainties from treatment to treatment. This depends on the anatomic site, patient's weight and medical condition, stability and permanence of fiducial skin marks, patient cooperation and *memory* of setup, stability of the treatment position for the individual patient (supine, prone, on side, etc.), training and skill of the radiation therapist, use of ancillary devices such as foam wedges, head cups, and casts, and the clarity and completeness of the setup description in the patient's radiotherapy chart.

■ Intertreatment organ motion uncertainties. These include the extent and likelihood that the CTV will change its position or shape with respect to both the patient coordinate system and the surrounding organs because of such things as weight gain or loss, tumor shrinkage or growth, bladder and rectal filling, and so on. These data can typically be acquired only through *class studies* and can be applied only in a statistical manner. Such studies (30) are usually based upon sequential CT data taken on several days during a course of treatment for a subpopulation of patients.

■ Intratreatment organ motion uncertainties due to rhythmic motion during a treatment. This is the extent to which patient respiration, heartbeat, and peristalsis affect CTV position with respect to the patient coordination system and surrounding organ.

Can anything be done to significantly reduce or eliminate these errors? Obviously errors generated by uncertainties described in the first three categories are far easier to handle than those in the remaining categories. These can be minimized (but not altogether eliminated) by intensive acceptance testing, rigorous maintenance, and regular quality assurance testing. The AAPM TG40 Report (1) and its recent update, AAPM TG142 Report (2), provide complete guidelines that if applied with vigor should reduce these mechanical uncertainties to a well-defined and hopefully insignificant level. For the last four categories we must provide a better understanding of their statistical nature before discussing how their effects can be minimized.

A common way to express setup errors is to divide them into either *systematic* or *random* errors. Random errors are errors whose magnitudes are expected to be distributed as a Gaussian function about a mean with a width that can be

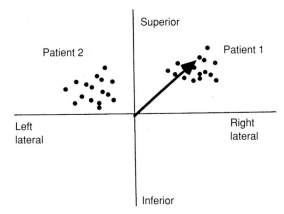

Figure 5.7. The random and systematic errors for two patients. Each dot represents one measurement of the patient's position relative to the planned or prescribed position. The arrow from the origin to the average position (center of gravity) of the dots represents the systematic setup error for the patient; the difference between each of the dots and the average represents the random error distribution for the patient. (Reprinted from Kutcher GJ, Mageras GS, Leibel SA. Control correction and modeling of setup errors and organ motion. Semin Radiat Oncol 1995;5:134–145, with permission.)

used to calculate the probability of being within any given distance from the mean. If we were able to analyze the portal film or EPID image of an individual patient for each treatment field on a daily basis and if we could also determine the error in CTV position with respect to a reference image, either a simulator film or DRR, we would be able to create a *scatter graph* of setup errors similar to that shown in Figure 5.7 (30). As an example, assume that we analyze anteroposterior images only. The vertical axis would represent the superior–inferior dimension and the horizontal would be the right–left lateral dimension. Each daily image comparison would yield a point on this graph that represents the setup error with respect to the reference, which is at the origin of the two-dimensional (2D) coordinate system. A perfect setup would be represented by a point at the origin. After several treatments for an individual patient, the graph contains a cluster of points. A vector from the origin to a single point represents the total error (systematic plus random) in the superior–inferior and left–right lateral directions. Although there is no way to separate the systematic from the random component with a single point, the average position of the cluster of daily setup error points represents the systematic setup error, which can be represented by a vector from the origin to the *center of mass* of the cluster.

The distribution of points about the average (the *ensemble of differences between the setup errors and their mean*) (31) constitutes the random setup error distribution for the patient. After sufficient measurements are made, we would expect to find that the random error distribution is Gaussian, with a standard deviation, σ. The reliability of this method for an individual patient improves with the number of daily measurements, which, unfortunately, are costly and time-consuming. Although an increasing number of institutions have the means to perform electronic daily portal imaging, very few have the manpower or inclination to take the time for this close analysis. An alternative, less costly approach is to look for *class solutions* and derive σ using a *class* of similarly treated patients and appropriate statistical techniques based upon retrospective portal image analysis.

Why are we interested in resolving the total error into its systematic and random components? It helps us decide whether the problem is significant and if so, how we can best deal with it. For example, systematic errors tend to result from errors in or misinterpretations of patient setup instructions; incorrectly cut blocks; discrepancies in mechanical readouts between the simulator, localizer, and medical accelerator; treatment plan transcription errors; and so on. If properly determined early on, these can be addressed and removed for the duration of treatment. Random errors, on the other hand, are usually the result of patient movement, inconsistent repositioning, organ motion, inconsistent interpretation of skin marks, and so on. Many of these will be best addressed by improved patient immobilization, proper training, and better setup procedures.

Numerous advisory groups, including AAPM TG40 (1) recommend taking regular portal images as part of a radiation oncology department's quality assurance program. Most, if not all, clinics are following these recommendations and acquire portal images of treatment fields aligned to patients on a weekly basis. With the advent of the EPID some are even following a policy of daily portal imaging. Given random and systematic errors, however, there is some danger that this increased information about patient treatment accuracy *may not be properly used*. How, for example, should a radiation oncologist respond to an anteroposterior pelvis portal image showing a shift of 8 mm to the patient's right with respect to the reference image? He or she might draw an arrow on the film instructing the radiation therapist to shift the patient setup 8 mm to the left on the following treatment. However, if the error distribution based on this patient's own treatment data (or class data) is dominated by a random error component (e.g., σ = 6 mm), this instruction may not lead to the desired result. If, however, because of careful attention to patient immobilization the random error standard deviation for these patients (σ) is only 2 mm, the physician's instructions make far more sense.

The nature of patient setup errors, organ motion uncertainties, and the effects of respiration are matters of growing interest and concern. A great deal of research and development now under way is intended to allow *automated* evaluation of the plethora of verification image data that results from the increasing availability of EPIDs. An important concern is how best to make use of this new information in an effective and efficient manner. Error correction protocols (32,33) to create an acceptable balance between benefit (improved treatment accuracy) and cost (man-hours for analysis) are being developed and tested.

An obvious question to ask before embarking on costly and labor-intensive patient setup and quality assurance procedures is, "How good is good enough?" Should equal effort be put into improving setup accuracy for all patient treatment sites? Why not design a large enough target margin (i.e., the PTV–CTV margin) that setup errors become unimportant? Clearly, with sufficiently large margins, the CTV will always be within the PTV, so that the hard work of patient immobilization, careful patient setup, and setup error studies is unnecessary. The answer is that accurate treatment of the CTV is not the *sole* aim of radiotherapy; the CTV alone does not fully define the problem. The complete goal is to treat the CTV correctly but keep dose to the surrounding normal tissues and critical organs within tolerable limits. Allowing the PTV–CTV margin to be as large as necessary without attempting to reduce the sources of error increases the volume of irradiated normal tissue, possibly enough to exceed critical organ tolerance.

Nonetheless, the need for large margins to ensure treatment accuracy has been the acceptable conventional assumption for many years and for many treatment situations. Only recently, with increased attention to 3D conformal radiotherapy techniques, has the virtue of this solution been questioned. Still, for low-dose treatments, for a palliative regimen, and for an anatomic site sufficiently far from radiosensitive tissues, large margins indeed may remain the appropriate and most cost-effective way of ensuring that the prescribed dose is properly delivered to the CTV.

Sometimes, the overall cost and effort of reducing treatment margins are not justified by the small clinical gain. At other times, however, when the CTV requires treatment to very high doses and is adjacent to a radiosensitive critical organ, the gain in terms of tumor control may well be worth the effort and increased cost. The goal of 3D conformal radiotherapy is to raise the tumor control probability (34,35) without increasing the normal tissue complication probability (36–38) above acceptable limits. Attempts to achieve this goal are mainly focused on escalating the dose to the CTV. A natural consequence of escalating dose and keeping normal tissue complication probability tolerable is the need to reduce the volume of normal tissue being irradiated by very high doses. Because the high-dose regions are usually adjacent to the CTV, this is tantamount to *requiring a reduction in the PTV–CTV margin*.

We have already seen that reducing the PTV–CTV margin requires an understanding and reduction of all treatment uncertainties, both random and systematic. Attempts to reduce or account for the systematic errors can be made through the following:

- Increased maintenance and quality assurance of treatment and imaging equipment
- Improved training of therapists and better documentation of individual patient setup instructions
- Heightened chart review with added redundancy checks for correct information transfer

It may also be possible to reduce random patient setup errors by implementing state-of-the-art imaging and immobilization techniques such as the use of two-component expanding plastic foams, thermoplastic shells, vacuum bead bags, and so on.

If these attempts at reducing total errors (random plus systematic) are successful, it should be possible to reduce the PTV–CTV margin and even if ICRU 50 definitions (28) are followed, still ensure that the CTV receives the full prescribed treatment dose through the course of therapy.

A striking question remains: Even if we reduce or eliminate most of the geometric setup uncertainties by implementing methods already suggested, can anything be done to reduce errors caused by *organ motion*, both intertreatment and intratreatment? First, as we have already stated, we must study it so as to include these uncertainties in assessing the proper target margins. It may also be possible to incorporate the knowledge of organ motion uncertainty into the computerized isodose and DVH calculation process (30). Although we cannot *stop* the organs from moving, once their motion is properly understood, we may be able to reduce these variations by properly instructing the patient in breathing techniques as well as optimal (consistent) bladder and bowel filling. Pretreatment imaging, as described earlier, can also help to more consistently align a PTV to isocenter, decreasing treatment margins. Radiographic patient setup techniques using implanted radiopaque markers also enable additional reductions in this margin. Finally, methods for *gated radiotherapy and tumor or PTV tracking*, as described earlier, eliminate the problem of rhythmic organ motion altogether.

IMMOBILIZATION AND POSITIONING DEVICES

Accuracy and reproducibility of patient treatment setup are keys to satisfactory radiotherapy. The use of immobilization devices to reduce random setup errors can also reduce the amount of normal tissue irradiated and ensure adequate coverage of the CTV. An *immobilization device* is any device that helps to establish and maintain the patient in a fixed, well-defined position from treatment to treatment over a course of radiotherapy. It is also any device that helps to prevent the patient from moving (ignoring internal motion, of course) during a single treatment session.

A variety of radiotherapy immobilization devices have been used successfully over the past several decades. They vary in construction from the complex to the simple. Some are constructed in-house, and others are manufactured and sold by commercial vendors. The following questions should be considered before implementation of a particular patient immobilization system:

■ Is the patient fully supported in a comfortable and relaxed position? If not, the patient will tend to shift weight and relax muscles if at all possible in order to obtain this comfortable state.

■ Does the device provide a tactile reminder to the patient of how it feels when the setup is consistent with previous treatment? If it does, the patient can assist the therapists in achieving correct setup position.
■ Is the patient secured and is all movement constrained? The ideal device prevents the patient from moving.
■ Does the device conform to the patient's external surface contours? For sites such as head, neck, and extremities the changing surface contours provide the best anchor for reproducing setup.
■ Is the device appropriate to the particular patient and anatomy under treatment? Because of the cylindrical symmetry and surrounding fat, a body cast may not provide adequate positioning and immobilization for an obese patient being treated deep within the abdomen. However, a similar conformal technique (e.g., a thermoplastic mask) may provide excellent support for the same patient in the head-and-neck region, where the surface contours are rapidly changing and the rigid bone is near the skin surface.
■ Can the device be used to position the patient optimally to minimize normal tissue complications? A subcategory of the immobilization device is the ancillary device used to help the patient maintain a special position designed to optimize the relationship between the target (PTV) and the surrounding radiosensitive organs. These *positioning devices,* including arm boards, breast tilt boards, Timos, foam wedges, belly boards, and so on, are discussed further on in this section.
■ Does the device allow an unobstructed path for the radiation beams? The immobilization device must not interfere with the particular treatment plan. High atomic number (Z) materials should not be in or near the beam path, where they can cause unwanted attenuation or scatter. Radio-transparent rigid materials are preferable, and it should be possible to cut away or remove sections if necessary. It is also important to consider whether the immobilization device will become a mechanical obstruction and interfere with the positioning of the accelerator gantry for a particular treatment field or even cause a collision when the beam rotates from one gantry angle to another.
■ Will the device be usable on the radiotherapy simulator, CT scan, MRI, or other treatment planning imaging systems? As discussed earlier, the same patient treatment immobilization device *should* be used during all imaging and localization procedures to establish a consistent patient coordinate system for accurate setup and treatment. In fact, it is common for customized immobilization devices to be designed and constructed in the radiotherapy simulator room while the patient is aligned on the simulator couch in the desired treatment position. If CT scan or MRI will be used in the planning process, the doughnut size, or cylinder diameter, associated with these diagnostic units may limit the overall dimensions of the device. These imaging systems also limit the materials that can be used in the device,

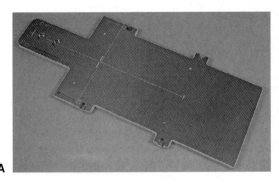 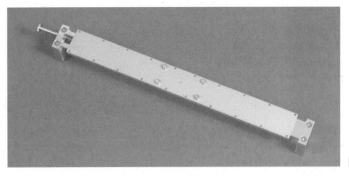

A   B

Figure 5.8. Selection of hardware enabling indexing of older style patient treatment couches. (Courtesy of Orfit Industries N.V., Wijnegem, Belgium.)

because metals, particularly high Z ones, cause artifacts in the CT images, and magnetic materials must be avoided for MRI.

▪ Will the surface dose be adversely affected? If the design of the immobilization device requires the beam to pass through some of its material, its effect on patient surface dose must be determined. The increased surface dose buildup caused by thin thermoplastics and polyurethane foams may be small but should be understood and documented (39).

▪ Does the device provide adequate space for reference marks to fully describe and facilitate reproducibility of the patient setup? The immobilization device helps to define the patient coordinate system. Ultimately, through the setup procedure, this patient coordinate system must be brought into alignment with the room coordinate system using reference marks or indices. A customized device should have space for fiducial marks and other reference indicators to be permanently placed on the surface in an easily visible manner. Noncustomized devices (bite blocks, arm boards, relocatable head frames, and so on) should contain precise indexing to facilitate marking the setup position specific to each patient. All devices should be capable of alignment to the room coordinate system either through the room laser system or careful indexing to the treatment and imaging tables using special adapters (40). Modern radiotherapy treatment couches are designed with precise indexing capabilities that permit the attachment of treatment aids in very reproducible positions on a daily basis. Furthermore, several manufacturers have developed retrofits that can be added to older treatment couches to mimic the indexing capabilities of the newer couches (Fig. 5.8).

▪ Will the immobilization device be rigid and hold its shape over time? It is important for the device to hold its shape over the course of therapy. If over time its fit becomes loose or its walls become flexible, the patient may be able to move within the device, and correct setup cannot be ensured. It would be useful to determine the effects of such factors as temperature, humidity, radiation, and the patient's weight on the materials and construction of any device used for long-term

immobilization. It is also important for the radiation therapists to note the condition and fit of the device before each treatment, whether it is showing signs of wear and tear or even signs of changes in the patient (e.g., loss of weight, tumor shrinkage).

▪ How costly is the immobilization device? Cost is an important consideration in medicine today. The cost of using a complex immobilization device must be evaluated in terms of the potential benefit to the patient for treating a particular tumor. Costs of competing methods must be carefully compared. However, these comparisons should include all cost considerations inherent to the device and its use, including the following:
 ▪ Cost of the materials and the device itself
 ▪ Staff time needed for construction
 ▪ Necessary consumables and supplies
 ▪ Reusability of components
 ▪ Storage space required for devices while in use and for materials that must be kept on hand before use
 ▪ Staff time used for each patient setup (perhaps a *negative cost* if setup time is reduced)

Although the main objective of an immobilizing device is to limit patient movement and to reduce the probability of positioning errors, there may be other incidental benefits, such as these:

▪ Reduction in daily setup time. Some immobilization devices make setup much easier and more efficient, and therefore save time and reduce overall treatment cost.

▪ Reduction in the patient's fear and worry because the patient feels safer and more secure.

▪ No need for patient to be awake, alert, and cooperative.

▪ Conversion of the patient into more of a *rigid body,* diminishing rotation of one part of the patient with respect to another and fixing the relationship between the internal organs and the surface fiducial marks.

There is a wide range of complexity in immobilization devices. I will describe some of the more popular methods by category.

Tapes and Other Daily Reminders to Discourage Movement During Treatment. From the earliest days of radiotherapy, various types of adhesive tapes have been

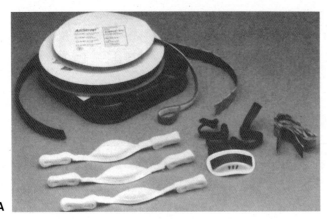 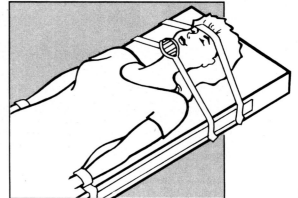

Figure 5.9. A: Velcro restraining straps. (Courtesy of Bionix, Toledo, OH.) **B:** Velcro restraining straps immobilize the patient without the use of sticky adhesives. Typically, straps are padded and reusable. (Reprinted with permission from Smithers Medical Products, Inc., North Canton, OH.)

used to assist patient setup. Paper tapes, cloth tapes, masking tapes, and so on have all been used on a daily basis to discourage movement *once the correct treatment position has been achieved with surface fiducials.* For example, tape across the patient's forehead attached to the couch side rails discourages side-to-side twisting of the head. Leather straps and straps with Velcro backing have been used in a similar way. Strips of adhesive Velcro tape with its hooks facing outward can be permanently affixed to the side rails of the treatment couch. The Velcro strap with its complementary loops can be wrapped around the patient and securely attached to the side rail hooks. The Velcro straps are padded and reusable, and they avoid the pain to the patient associated with removing sticky tapes. They provide a means to help keep the patient's hands at the sides of the body and the feet together. Specialized Velcro-backed chin straps in combination with other head supports can be quite effective in preventing intratreatment head movement (Figs. 5.9A and B).

Generic Body Supports: Nonindexed and Indexed. This category includes foam rubber wedges and other foam rubber supports, one-size-fits-all plastic head cups ("doggie bowls"), neck rolls, knee and lumbar supports, thigh and heel stirrups, prone face holders with cutouts for nose and mouth, and so on (Figs. 5.10A–C). Although they do not, of themselves, offer any guidance for intertreatment setup reproducibility, they do provide added comfort and stability during a single treatment. The plastic head cups and neck rolls can be used in combination with sticky tape to remind the patient to remain motionless during treatment. These simple methods, with proper patient instructions such as "hold still" or "hold your breath," are commonly used today, when reducing the volume of irradiated normal tissue is considered to have critical importance.

A simple improvement in generic body support techniques that provides a means to facilitate intertreatment setup reproducibility is the indexed support. Several manufacturers supply sets of head cups, head and neck supports, foam rubber wedges, and so on, that are carefully indexed by size, shape, elevation above the treatment

couch, and so on. Some of the head and neck supports are molded from clear plastic; others are of opaque foam rubber or polyurethane foam (Figs. 5.11A and B). These devices provide head and neck height and slant information for setup duplication. They can be quite useful for supporting the head during treatment of lung, supraclavicular nodes, esophagus, and generally any supine treatment that necessitates securing the head and neck. The significance of indexing these various devices is in the ability to recreate a given head height or neck slant day after day. Maintaining a complete duplicate set in each treatment room as well as in the radiotherapy simulator makes the patient setup instructions better defined, less ambiguous, and less error prone. Of course, the effectiveness of these methods (and for that matter, all methods) is greatly enhanced by a rigorous quality assurance program that includes regular and careful review of portal images.

Body Cast Techniques. Since the 1960s, the importance of immobilization for complex, definitive isocentric treatment has been appreciated. Techniques and materials for immobilization were borrowed from other specialties such as dentistry and orthopedics. Complete body supports and head helmets were cast from plaster of Paris, often plaster-impregnated tape, and related materials (Fig. 5.12A). Creation of such devices was labor intensive and time-consuming. The creation of a prone body cast, such as was commonly used for craniospinal irradiation, could take almost a full day for a trained technician and demanded the patient's presence for much of the time. Some techniques for creating an immobilization helmet involved several steps, including the creation of a model of the patient's head. Although some clinics were large enough to support full-time shops for creating such ancillary equipment, the smaller departments could not and so would often have to rely on outside consultant orthopedic technicians. When properly made, the resulting plaster immobilization devices conformed exquisitely to the body surface and were initially quite successful in helping to achieve accurate, immobile, reproducible treatment setups. They were particularly useful in stabilizing young children

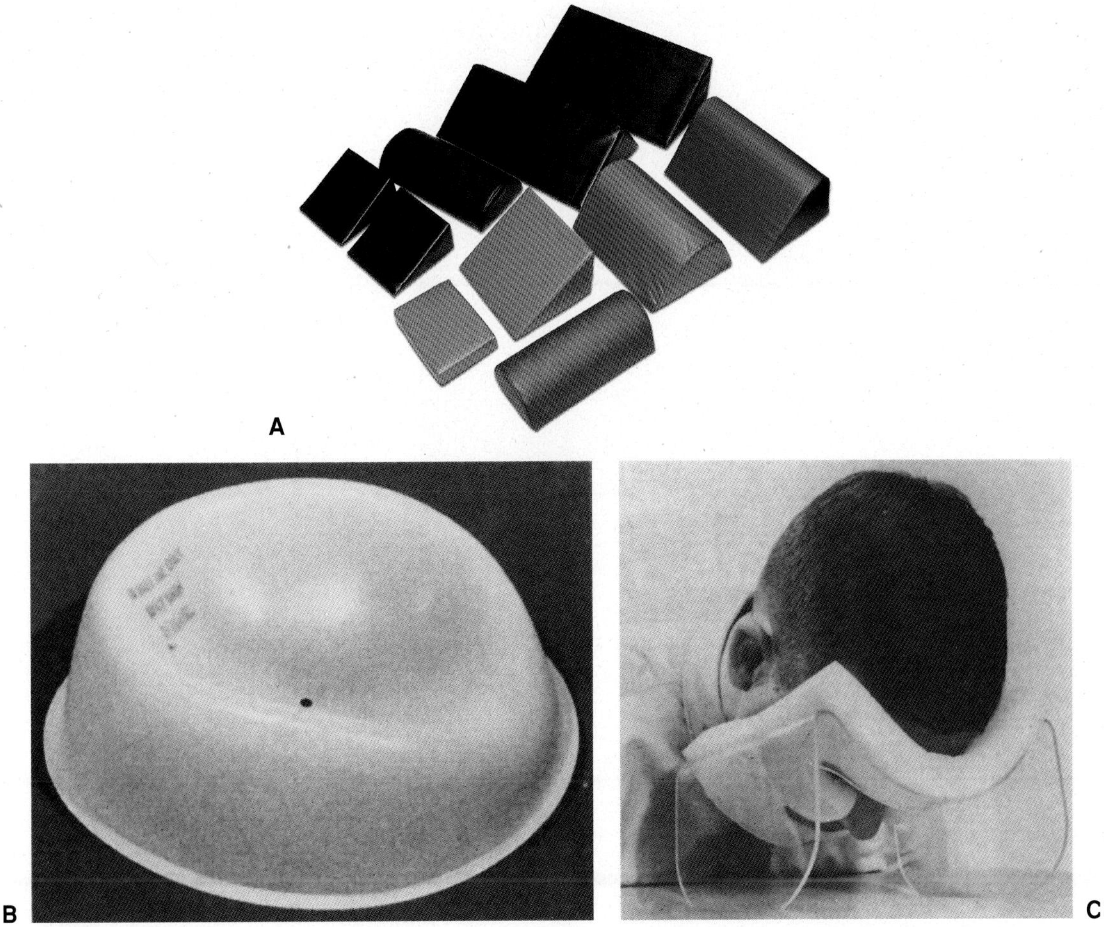

Figure 5.10. **A:** Assorted foam wedges used for patient comfort and support. (Courtesy of Bionix, Toledo, OH.) **B:** Generic head supports. Disposable formed plastic head holder "doggy bowl" provides stability for the head when the patient is supine. **C:** The formed plastic facedown stabilizer has a foam rubber lining with an opening for eyes, nose, and mouth. (**B** and **C** reprinted from Delclos L, Khan FM. Treatment aids for external-beam radiotherapy. In: Levitt S, Khan F, Potish R, eds. Technological basis of radiation therapy. Philadelphia, PA: Lea & Febiger, 1992, with permission.)

for the precise field matching involved in craniospinal radiation used for treatment of pediatric cancers such as medulloblastoma and central nervous system leukemia.

Other than being too labor intensive and time-consuming, the traditional plaster casts tended to become flexible, get damaged, or lose their shape over time. Another technique introduced in the 1970s was based upon a new product packaging method, the bubble pack. A transparent form-fitting plastic shell was fabricated using a special vacuum forming device sometimes called

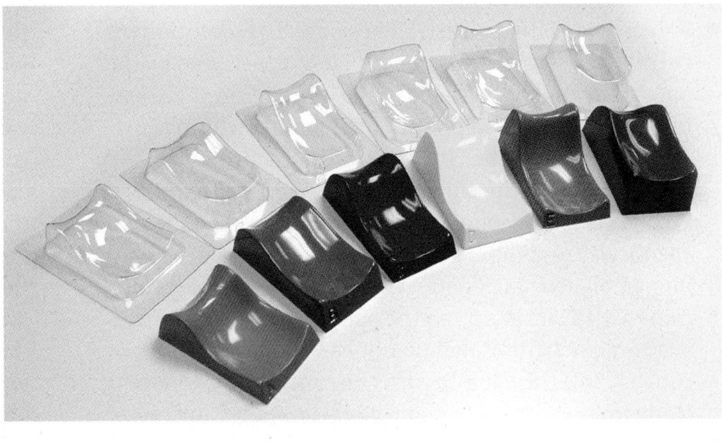

Figure 5.11. A set of Timo head and neck supports indexed to recreate a specific head height or neck slant day after day. Timos are typically either letters or color coded. Hollow clear plastic Timos to reduce scatter and potential skin reaction. (Courtesy of Bionix, Akron, OH.)

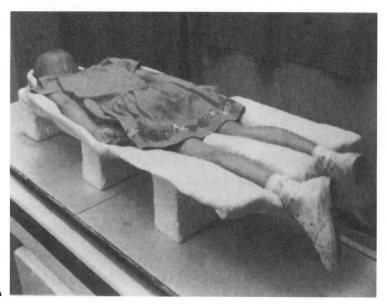

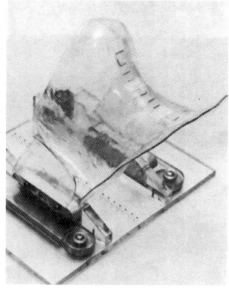

A

B

Figure 5.12. A: Plaster body cast. (Reprinted from Bentel GC. Radiation therapy planning. New York, NY: McGraw-Hill, 1996, with permission.) **B:** Vacu-Former shell for treatment of the larynx. (Reprinted from Watkins OMB. Radiation therapy mold technology. Toronto: Pergamon Press, 1981, with permission.)

a *Vacu-Former*. In this process, the polyvinyl chloride sheet was electrically heated to soften the plastic and then formed over a plaster model of the patient by creating a vacuum between them. Although the material was quite stable and extensively used in Great Britain and Canada, the method did not gain widespread acceptance in the United States, probably because it too was considered labor intensive, because the clear plastic sheet could *not* be stretched directly over the patient but rather required a solid plaster cast of the patient (40) (Fig. 5.12B).

In the late 1970s and early 1980s, there was a general awareness of the need for reducing patient setup errors to allow progress toward 3D conformal therapy, including intensity-modulated radiation therapy (IMRT) at escalated doses. As a result, many new methods and materials based on modern packaging techniques, dentistry, and orthopedics were introduced. Most of these represent the state-of-the-art body cast immobilization. They include the following:

■ Polyurethane foam casts. These are two-component chemical systems, the most popular of which goes by the name Alpha Cradle. The patient is placed in the treatment position atop a plastic bag that rests within a specialized form. The form is usually prefabricated according to the specific anatomy under treatment and is constructed of solid Styrofoam blocks. When the two chemicals are combined in the bag, they begin to expand into a polyurethane foam. As the foam rises, the technician maneuvers it around the patient to offer support to anatomic structures that do not lie flat on the treatment couch. Once the foam hardens, the customized device is ready for use. This technique has been successfully used

for many diseases (often in combination with other patient support systems, e.g., head and neck holders and tilt boards) such as cancers of the breast, prostate, lower extremities, lung, pituitary gland, head and neck region, and Hodgkin's disease (Figs. 5.13A and B). In fact, a prone-patient whole-body cast for treatment of the entire central nervous system can be constructed from these materials (with the special prefabricated styrofoam shell) in a fraction of the time it takes to make a traditional plaster cast. The polyurethane foam casts are rigid, stable, and relatively radiolucent. They form a snug and comfortable patient support device. They do not, however, prevent patient movement and rotation when used by themselves, nor can they conform as completely to the changes in body contour as other methods. For this reason foam cast supports are frequently used in combination with other methods, such as thermoplastics, head supports, and hand grips.

■ Vacuum bags. Radiolucent plastic cushions are filled with tiny polystyrene balls. With the patient lying on it, the semideflated cushion can be molded around the patient's gross body contours. The cushion is then connected to a vacuum pump through a quick-release valve and the air is pumped out, causing the balls to come together and form a firm solid support. The cushion becomes an entirely rigid and comfortable mold of the patient's body (Fig. 5.14). Because of its airtight valve, the vacuum (and therefore the cushion's shape) can be maintained for the entire course of treatment. The cushion is reusable; that is, after the patient's therapy is complete, air can be let back into the cushion and it can be shaped to a new patient. The vacuum bag system provides a comfortable and secure support

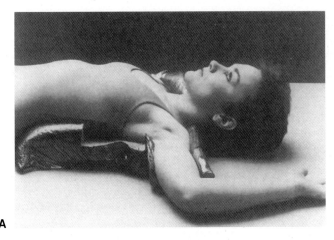

A

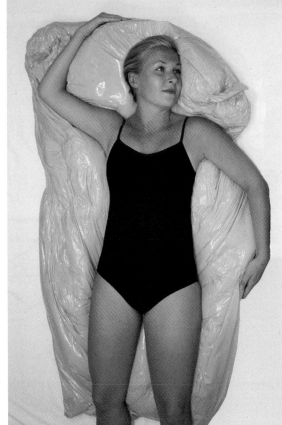

B

Figure 5.13. **A:** Foam repositioning cast. The two-component foam expands to surround external contours and provides for duplication of treatment position. (Reprinted from Levitt S, Khan F, Potish R. Technological basis of radiation therapy. Philadelphia, PA: Lea & Febiger, 1992, with permission.) **B:** A customized foam repositioning system (Alpha Cradle) designed for 3D treatment planning for cancer of the breast. (Courtesy of Smithers Medical Products, North Canton, OH.)

with many precut shapes tailored for support of the head and upper thorax (both prone and supine), the pelvis (with a window for prostate treatment), and the

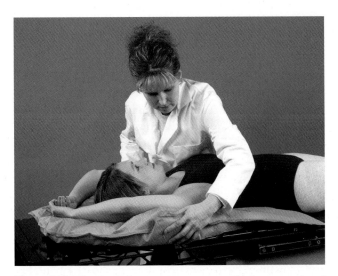

Figure 5.14. The Vac-Lok system creates a cradle for accurate and reproducible patient positioning. After the patient is placed on the inflated cushion, the valve is connected to a vacuum compressor. The cushion is molded to the patient's contours and a complete vacuum is drawn, rendering the cradle rigid. The Vac-Lok can hold its shape for 6 weeks. (Courtesy of CIVCO.)

breast. As with the polyurethane foam system, it conforms well to gross surface changes and less well to the finer details. Therefore patient motion, although discouraged, is still possible, and if strict immobilization is critical, the vacuum bag should be used in combination with one or more other devices (e.g., head holders and thermoplastics).

■ Thermoplastics. Low-temperature orthopedic plastics have become very popular for radiotherapy patient immobilization. A variety of vendors (e.g., CIVCO; Orfit Industries, Wijnegem Belgium; Sinmed, Reeuwijk, Holland) sell different forms of this material under different names. The material itself comes in the form of solid sheets or a flat plastic mesh in a variety of thicknesses. Its useful property is that it becomes soft and flexible, almost like cloth, when soaked in warm water. In its soft and flexible state, the plastic material can be stretched around any part of the patient's anatomy; it is not uncomfortably hot. Once it cools, the plastic becomes rigid again and maintains its new shape indefinitely. (Naturally, the solid sheets are more rigid than the mesh sheets.) Unlike the polyurethane foam and vacuum bag systems, these devices do not have much strength or cushioning properties and so are not used to support the patient's weight. Rather, they are stretched around the topside of a patient who is already in the treatment position (Fig. 5.15A). For example,

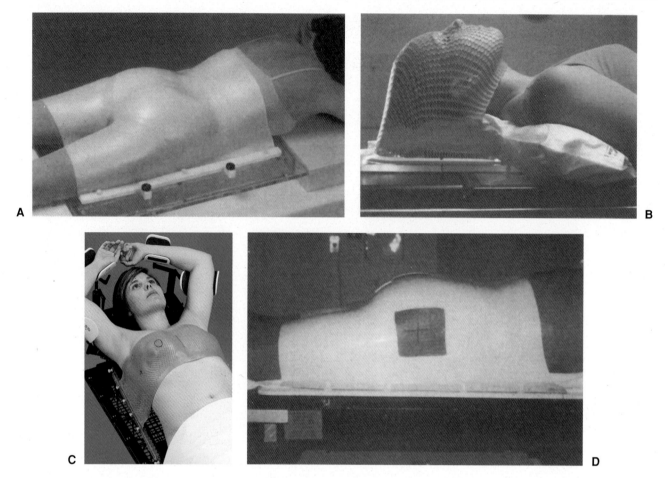

Figure 5.15. **A:** Solid thermoplastic material is used to immobilize pelvis and extremities where rigidity is important. The thermal plastic patient immobilization system (Aquaplast, Wycoff, NJ), in its perforated version, is commonly used for head and neck immobilization and repositioning. The thermoplastic comes ready to use in either a disposable or reusable U-frame, which is easily anchored to the couch-mounted base plate. (Courtesy of Nuclear Associates, Carle Place, NY.) **B:** Perforated thermoplastic material used in combination with a vacuum bag support and a tilt board for comfortable yet secure patient immobilization. **C:** Perforated thermoplastic material used in combination with a breast board to form a brassiere to help stabilize flaccid breasts for tangential breast treatment. (**B** and **C** Courtesy of CIVCO.) **D:** Prostate patient treated prone in custom-designed thermoplastic immobilization device. The cast is attached to a board on the treatment couch and customized cutouts allow beam access without reduction in skin sparing. (**D** reprinted from Leibel SA, Heimann R, Kutcher GJ, et al. 3-dimensional conformal radiation therapy and locally advanced carcinoma of the prostate. *Int J Radiat Oncol Biol Phys* 1994;28:55–65, with permission.)

in treating carcinoma of the prostate, some clinics immobilize prone patients by stretching solid sheets of thermoplastic material around the patient's hips. Sometimes, the plastic material is used over a patient being supported by a polyurethane foam or vacuum bag support or over patients supported by standard head supports, on tilt boards, and so on (Fig. 5.15B). These plastics are even being used to form a brassiere to help stabilize large, flaccid breasts for tangential beam treatment (Fig. 5.15C). The thermoplastics are easy to use in comparison with traditional casting methods. They also allow treatments with few skin marks, because most of the reference lines can be placed on the stretched plastic sheet. However, there may be some loss of skin sparing through the material, so it is important to be careful. When this is critical, the plastic sheet maybe cut out to match the treatment portal, although some rigidity is sacrificed.

Positioning Devices

All *immobilization devices* can, in some sense, be considered *positioning devices*. However, for this discussion we can make the distinction that *positioning devices* are ancillary devices used to help maintain the patient in a *nonstandard* treatment position. One standard radiotherapy treatment position is the patient lying supine on the flat treatment couch with arms at sides, facing the ceiling. Another is the prone, arms at side, straight spine, facedown (in face-holder) position. Oftentimes, however, it is necessary to set the patient up in a special position designed to improve the *therapeutic ratio* and sometimes the patient's comfort for the treatment. For some treatments, the optimal beam access is limited by external anatomic features such as the extremities, a large belly, or a pendulous breast. Other treatment plans are limited by the proximity of the target (PTV) to the surrounding radiosensitive structures. Because the human body is a nonrigid solid,

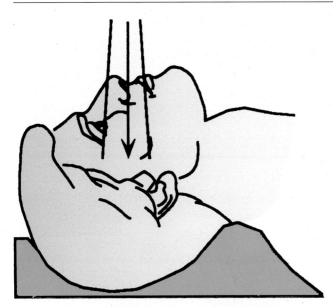

Figure 5.16. To include the apex of the maxillary antrum while excluding the eye, the chin must be hyperextended using a neck roll or Timo device. (Courtesy of Bentel GC. Radiation therapy planning. New York, NY: McGraw-Hill, 1996.)

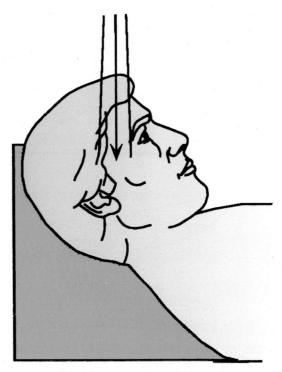

Figure 5.17. A foam head support aids in tilting the head forward for extreme flexing of the neck, which is useful for treatment of pituitary gland and other small brain tumors. (Reprinted from Bentel GC. Radiation therapy planning. New York, NY: McGraw-Hill, 1996, with permission.)

for these cases special accessory supports have been used to manipulate the body features and provide stable and comfortable support in a nonstandard position. Positioning devices include the following:

■ Neck roll, foam wedge, head holder, and Timo. These simple devices are used to maneuver body parts out of the way of the beam or into a better position. For example, in treatment of the maxillary antrum, the patient's head should be positioned with the chin hyperextended so as to include the superior extent of the maxillary antrum in an anterior field without also including the eye (41). Such a position can be achieved and maintained with the use of an appropriate head and neck support (Timo) (Fig. 5.16). Treatment of cancer of the pituitary gland or of small brain tumors often requires the head to be positioned with an extreme flexing of the neck. With the patient in this position, the anterior beam can avoid the dose-limiting structures such as the optic chiasm, the retina, and much of the brain tissue. Again, a foam head support can help hold this position comfortably (42) (Fig. 5.17). In these cases, a customized support such as the vacuum bag or the hardening foam system can be used with even greater comfort. Combined with a thermoplastic mask, this setup provides stability against patient movement as well (Fig. 5.18).
■ Arm board, knee saddle, and thigh stirrups. These ancillary devices, available from vendors of radiotherapy accessories, are specifically designed to position the extremities in a comfortable and reproducible manner. Positioning of the extremities is sometimes useful for treating soft tissue sarcomas in the arms or legs. At other times, it is necessary to remove the arm or leg from the

path of the radiation beam. An arm may be best treated, for example, while it is extended out 90 degrees and with the treatment couch rotated 90 degrees. This allows the axis of the arm to be aligned with the axis of gantry rotation so that precise isocentric treatment can be planned and delivered (42) (Fig. 5.19). The lower extremities

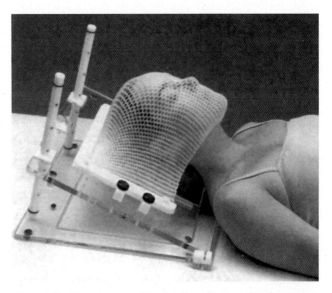

Figure 5.18. Combination of head and neck supporting foam Timo and tilt board provides immobilization and patient positioning. (Courtesy of Nuclear Associates, Carle Place, NY.)

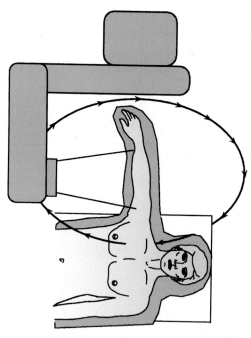

Figure 5.19. An arm board for supporting the patient's arm in an extended position and positioning at an angle of 90 degrees to the couch. (Reprinted from Bentel GC. Radiation therapy planning. New York, NY: McGraw-Hill, 1996, with permission.)

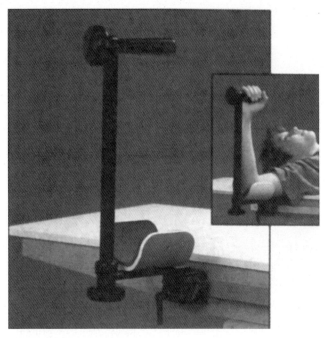

Figure 5.21. Arm positioner can provide comfortable support. (Courtesy of CIVCO.)

cannot be positioned for treatment quite so easily. For treating the leg, the challenge is often to reproducibly position the uninvolved leg sufficiently outside the radiation field. This can be accomplished with knee saddles or stirrups mounted on the couch rail or with a customized solid foam or vacuum bag support (Fig. 5.20).

■ Hand grip, overhead arm positioner, and shoulder retractor. Most often, these devices are used to position the extremities so that they do not interfere with treatment of some other region. Arms can be positioned above the head or at the sides in well-defined and repro-

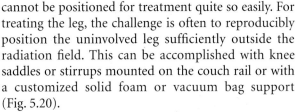

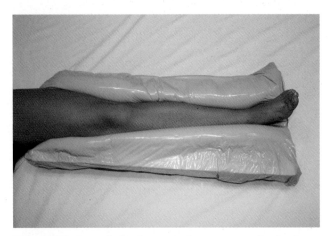

Figure 5.20. Expanded polystyrene foam support for the lower extremity. (Reprinted with permission from Smithers Medical Products, Inc., North Canton, OH.)

ducible locations with either couch rail—mounted or tilt board—mounted hand grips and arm supports (Fig. 5.21) or an overhead arm positioner hand grip device (e.g., the *butterfly* or the *T-bar*) (Fig. 5.22). The T-bar hand grip is mounted on a horizontal plastic board and is used in combination with a head and neck support device. With adjustable hand grip positions (with an engraved scale to allow longitudinal and vertical movement), this device helps to maintain the patient in a reproducible arms-up position, advantageous for treating various lesions in the thorax and abdomen. The couch rail-mounted hand grips and the shoulder retractors are typically used to nudge the patient into a position with arms and shoulders down. The shoulder retractor can consist of a footboard attached to hand grips through nylon ropes with adjustable tension. This device helps pull the shoulders down and out of the way in a reproducible manner, which is very useful for treating head and neck cancers with lateral fields (Fig. 5.23).

■ Patient elevation systems: Tilt board, slant board, and breast board. Positioning supine patients for treatment on tilting or slanting rigid plastic boards has numerous advantages. Some patients, particularly with severe obesity or lung disease, may have a difficult time lying flat on the back. The tilt board typically has built-in hand grips or arm supports that provide comfortable and reproducible arms-up support. Therefore, the tilt board provides an acceptable position for treating lung cancer through lateral fields without the interference of arms or shoulders. It may also help in treatment of patients with severe sloping chests by positioning the patient so that the anteroposterior vertical beam impinges orthogonally on the skin

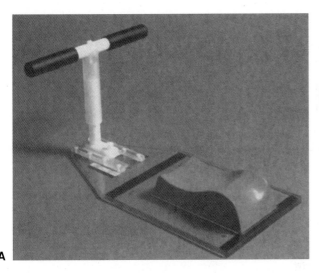

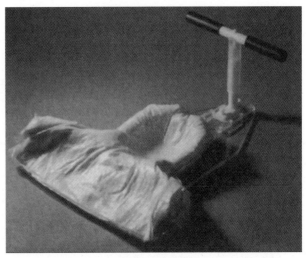

A   **B**

Figure 5.22. **A:** An overhead arm positioner used in combination with Timo head and neck support helps to keep the patient's arms out of the field, which is advantageous for treating lesions in the thorax and abdomen. **B:** It can also be combined with a vacuum bag head support. (Courtesy of CIVCO.)

surface (Fig. 5.24). Probably, the most common use of the tilt board is in the treatment of breast cancer with parallel opposed tangential fields. The *breast board* has been in use for several decades and serves several purposes:

■ Provides arm support to bring the arm above the shoulders and out of the way of the lateral field

■ Provides unobstructed access to the breast by the lateral field

■ Allows the patient to be positioned so that the chest wall is horizontal and therefore avoids angulation of the collimator

■ Takes advantage of gravity to pull the large breast down into a better treatment position

■ Modern breast board. Constructed of rigid plastic, the breast board provides a wide range of indexed tilt angles (Figs. 5.25A and B). The back support includes a head holder and is cut away to prevent interference with the tangential field for steep beam angles. The breast board also contains an arm support system, the simplest being a set of vertical pegs with an assortment of hole posi-

tions and the more complex, a continuously adjustable indexed biaxial support for wrist and forearm. With regard to the treatment of breast cancer, another patient positioning problem arises in the treatment of women with large, flaccid, or pendulous breasts. These women may have severe skin reactions resulting from the skin overlap in the inframammary fold. This problem may be reduced by use of a thin perforated thermoplastic brassiere (Fig. 5.26A) or a breast ring (Fig. 5.26B) to support and position the breast to avoid skin overlap (43).

■ Prone breast platform support. Developed to reduce the potential for skin, lung, and cardiac complications from treating large, pendulous breasts (44) (Fig. 5.26C), this system consists of a rigid trough-like supporting device mounted atop the treatment couch and curved up at

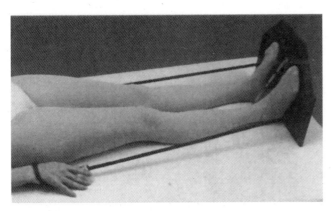

Figure 5.23. A shoulder retractor pulls down patient's shoulders reproducibly to provide improved access for lateral beams. (Courtesy of Nuclear Associates, Carle Place, NY.)

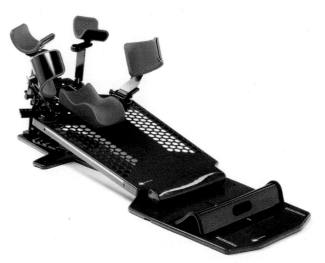

Figure 5.24. Lightweight slant board is designed to facilitate treatments in the thorax, especially when a patient has difficulty lying flat and when a patient's arms must be held overhead, out of the treatment field. (Courtesy of CIVCO.)

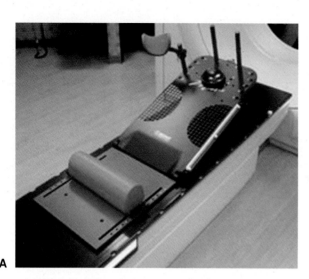

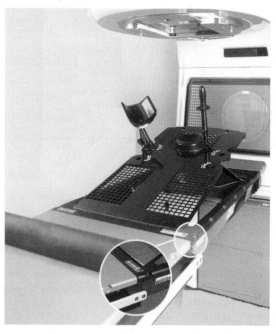

Figure 5.25. A: Adjustable height Plexiglas and aluminum breast board. Tilt angle and arm angle, as well as arm position are indexed for documentation and reproducibility. **B:** Alternative systems provide foam-padded arm and wrist supports as well. Other features to look for in a breast board are adaptability for use with head cups and Timos and beam access; some systems provide cutaway or mesh designs to minimize obstruction to the lateral tangential beam. (Courtesy of Bionix, Toledo, OH.)

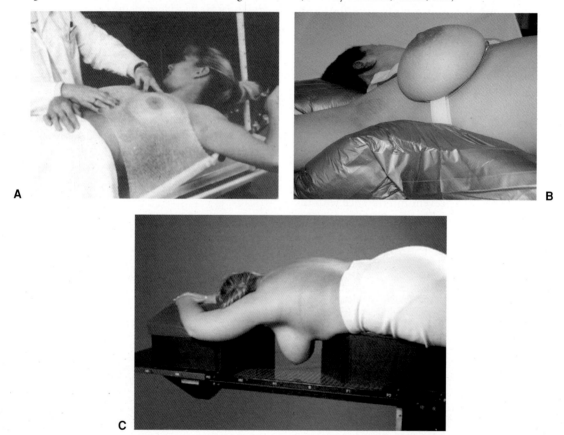

Figure 5.26. A: Perforated thin thermoplastic material (Aquaplast) used as a "brassiere" to stabilize and portion large, flaccid breasts. (Courtesy of Nuclear Associates, Carle Place, NY.) **B:** A supportive ring is placed around the breast and held in place with adjustable foam-lined Velcro chest and shoulder straps. This keeps the breast elevated off the chest wall to allow a wider choice of fields and to reduce the potential for skin reaction in the inframammary fold. (Reprinted with permission from Smithers Medical Products, Inc. North Canton, OH.) **C:** Patient set up for breast irradiation treatment using a prone breast support platform. The treated breast hangs beneath the platform for treatment by lateral beams. (Reprinted from Merchant TE, McCormick B. Prone position breast irradiation. *Int J Radiat Oncol Biol Phys* 1994;30:197–203, with permission.)

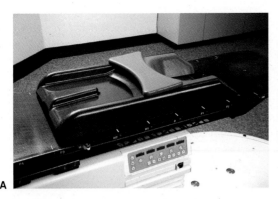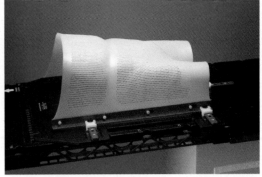

Figure 5.27. **A:** This belly board consists of a 4-in.-thick vinyl-covered foam block with a 30 × 30 cm cutout area and a removable expanded polystyrene block that can be cut to fit the patient's anterior shape. **B:** The belly board can be combined with thermoplastic immobilization to provide additional fixation and reproducible position for prone hip and pelvic treatments. (Courtesy of CIVCO.)

the sides for added security. The patient lies prone on the device, and only the involved breast hangs under its own weight through a window in the bottom of the trough, providing improved separation between the target and the normal tissues. Lateral tangential beams are used for treatment.

■ Belly board. Several specialized and some single-purpose treatment positioning devices have recently been introduced or improved. The belly board is usually a thick mattress for supporting the patient prone with a window cutout for the patient's belly. The purpose of this device is to provide more comfort and stability in the prone position (especially for the obese patient) and to reduce the amount of intestine in the lateral radiation fields. One commercial version of the belly board comes with removable Styrofoam blocks that can be customized to fit each patient's anatomy, whereas another system is based upon an entirely custom-shaped polyurethane foam cast (Figs. 5.27A and B). Both types may be used in combination with a thermoplastic fixation device that, when molded around the patients hips and buttock, provides more rigorous immobilization in addition to the stable support.

■ Treatment chair. Available to the radiotherapy clinic in one form or another for several decades, the treatment chair has never achieved great popularity. Recent use of lighter and stronger modern materials such as carbon fiber grids have led to the development of a more effective and easier-to-use immobilization system. The newer chairs, which can be mounted on the treatment couch, contain head and neck supports as well as arm rests to assist with a variety of arm positions. The treatment chair (Fig. 5.28) can be helpful in treating patients who have trouble breathing and cannot be placed in a recumbent position. It has also been used (45) in the treatment of mediastinal disease, in which the vertical orientation takes advantage of the gravitational effects on the mediastinum and reduces the amount of irradiated normal tissue.

Head Fixation Devices

Stereotactic radiosurgery immobilization requires greater precision and accuracy than any other current treatment. The stereotactic frame is actually bolted to the patient's skull before the target localization procedure and must remain attached until after treatment is complete. Fortunately, because the metal frame is not very comfortable, this is a single-fraction technique. Therefore, it is impractical for fractionated radiotherapy. Several spin-off ideas

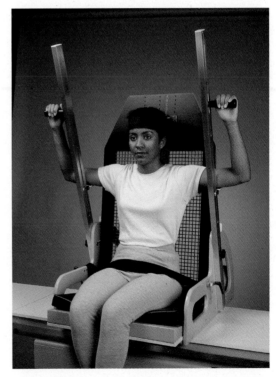

Figure 5.28. Treatment chair facilitates accurate positioning and repositioning for patients who require vertical orientation during radiotherapy. Modern chairs contain rigid, lightweight carbon fiber grid panel to provide radio-translucent treatment window. They also offer adjustable arm and head supports and can be locked to the treatment couch accessory rail. (Courtesy of CIVCO.)

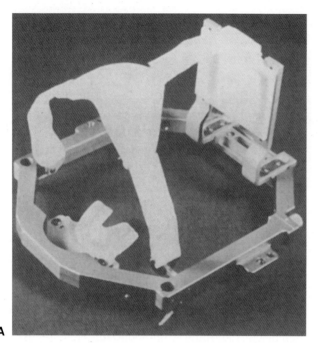
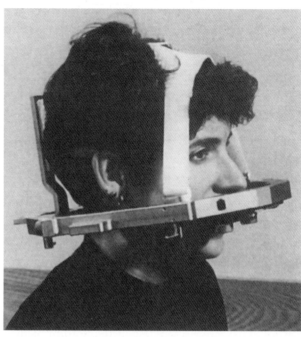

A

B

Figure 5.29. A: Relocatable head immobilization device (Gill-Thomas-Cosman system) for stereotactic radiotherapy. **B:** The same device in place on a patient. This system makes use of a dental mold and an occipital tray with a cast of the occiput for stabilization. (Courtesy of Integra, Burlington, MA.)

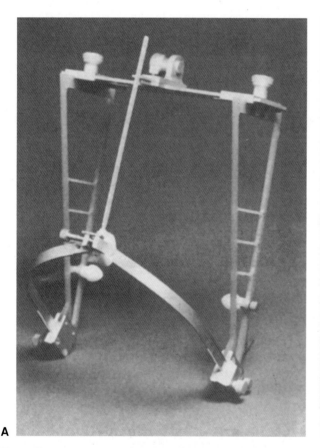
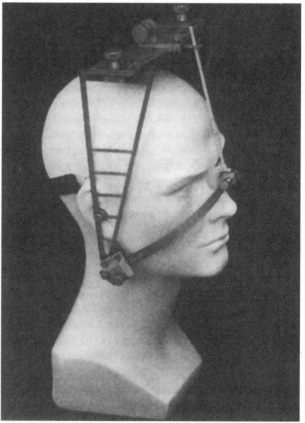

A

B

Figure 5.30. A: Another relocatable head immobilization device for stereotactic radiotherapy. This device relies on a rod in each external auditory canal with a clip molded to the bridge of the nose for repeatable immobilization (**B**). (Courtesy of Sandstrom Trade & Technology, Welland, ON.)

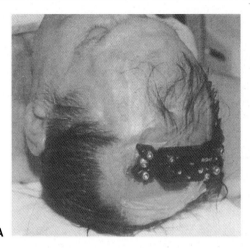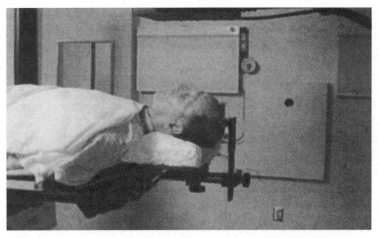

A   B

Figure 5.31. Two views of an invasive yet relocatable head frame. Each day the protruding standoffs, which remain in place during the course of therapy, interlock to the table adapter plate for rapid treatment setup. (Courtesy of Best Nomos, Pittsburgh, PA.)

based upon this technology have been pursued in the development of an effective, noninvasive, relocatable stereotactic localizer–immobilizer frame. One such device, the Gill-Thomas-Cosman system (Fig. 5.29A and B), consists of a frame fixed to the head with a dental mold, an occipital tray with a cast of the occiput, and a strap that holds the device tightly to the head (46,47). Another device immobilizes the head with a rod in each external auditory canal and a clip molded to the bridge of the nose (Fig. 5.30A and B).

A third type of relocatable system is *invasive* yet can be used successfully for fractionated radiotherapy. The system was designed for intensity-modulated radiotherapy of the head and neck. As with radiosurgery procedures, bone screws are set into the inner table of the skull (a relatively painless process). The screws have internal threads and can receive the *standoffs*, which remain in place during the course of therapy and are well tolerated. Each day, the

standoffs interlock to the table adapter plate for a rapid and reproducible treatment setup (Fig. 5.31A and B).

Several other nonstereotactic head immobilization devices based upon the use of *thermoplastic masks* are in common use in the radiotherapy clinic. Most of these systems involve a precut thermoplastic mesh sheet that is either factory bonded or attached by the user to a rigid frame (Fig. 5.32A and B). This unit can be softened by soaking in warm water for a few minutes. The radiotherapist pulls the mask over the patient's face down to a locking base plate. The therapist can mold the soft thermoplastic to the patient's facial contours, and in a few minutes the mask hardens and the rigid head immobilization device is complete. The base plate, which usually has a head cup, can be fastened to the treatment couch. Other face mask immobilization systems make use of different hardening tapes such as fiberglass tape and light-cast tape (a thermoplastic that hardens under ultraviolet light).

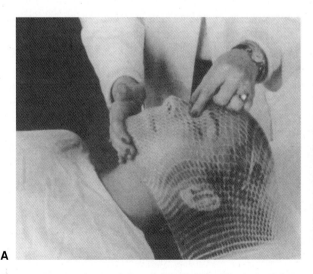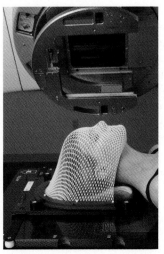

A   B

Figure 5.32. **A:** Perforated thermoplastic (Aquaplast) mask being molded for patient's face. (Courtesy of Nuclear Associates, Carle Place, NY.) **B:** The thermoplastic immobilization mask is shown with its frame locked to the base plate treatment couch mount. (Courtesy of CIVCO.)

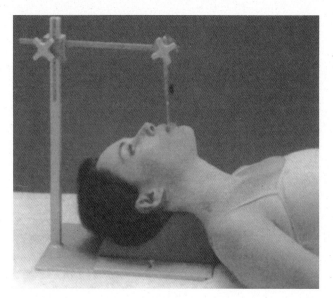

Figure 5.33. Adjustable bite block used in conjunction with a Timo head and neck support. (Courtesy of Nuclear Associates, Carle Place, NY.)

Another head immobilizer is the traditional *bite block*, which usually relies on a dental impression mouthpiece rigidly supported by and referenced to a solid base plate placed under the patient's head and fastened to the treatment couch. The patient's reproducible head position is recorded according to the reference numbers (there is typically at least 3 degrees of freedom) and included in the patient setup instructions in the treatment chart (Fig. 5.33).

Modern bite block systems can incorporate optical tracking systems that verify correct placement of fiducial markers incorporated within the bite block apparatus. Several such systems are commercially available (e.g., nTRAK [Best Nomos, Pittsburgh, PA], RadioCameras [Varian Medical Systems, Palo Alto, CA]). All work by comparing the positions of the fiducial markers relative to the isocenter to their corresponding positions at the time of the acquisition of the planning CT scan. Typically, a graphical user interface suggests shifts in patient position such that the fiducial apparatus, and, presumably, the anatomies of interest, fall back to their planned positions relative to the isocenter. At least one manufacturer has developed an attachment to a standard treatment couch (Radiotherapy Table Adapter [RTA], Best Nomos, Pittsburgh, PA) that permits, in addition to couch rotation and translation along the three cardinal axes, correction for patient tilt and rotation about the patient's long axis.

SUMMARY

Accurate and reproducible treatment has always been an important aspect of high-quality radiotherapy. Its importance today, however, has grown with the increased interest in 3D conformal therapy, static gantry IMRT, and volume-modulated arc therapy (rotational IMRT), along with the associated expectations of dose escalation using these tech-

niques. The success of these new high-dose protocols aimed at improving tumor control may depend on the ability to use tighter target margins and thereby to limit the dose to adjacent normal tissues. The terminology of ICRU Reports 50 and 62 makes it clear that the PTV–CTV margins must be large enough to ensure that the CTV will be included in the PTV for the entire course of therapy, and thereby accurately receive its correct prescribed dose. Therefore, to shrink these margins, we must be prepared to improve our treatment accuracy and daily treatment reproducibility. Because a major cause of nonreproducibility of treatment is random patient setup errors, a reduction of these errors by the implementation of modern patient immobilization systems may let us safely reduce the PTV–CTV margin.

Obviously, absolutely accurate and reproducible treatment delivery according to a complex image-based treatment plan is limited by the extent to which the target and critical organs can be positioned with respect to the external beam reference frame (i.e., the room coordinate system) throughout a single treatment and on a day-to-day basis. In reality, this is most closely achieved with stereotactic radiosurgery because of its very tightly aligned room coordinate system with rigid, invasive patient immobilization and because it is administered to a part of the human anatomy (the cranial cavity) where there can be little or no movement of the internal structures with respect to the patient reference frame (determined by the skull). For more typical radiotherapy, treatment position reproducibility is limited, to a greater or lesser extent depending on anatomical location, by the following:

- Uncertainties in the accelerator, the radiotherapy simulator, and the treatment planning coordinate systems
- Daily organ movement or deformation with respect to soft tissue and bony skeleton
- Organ movement during the treatment caused by rhythmic processes
- The patient moving during treatment
- Flexing and rotation of the skeleton and soft tissues from treatment to treatment
- Treatment setup errors due to changing skin marks, varying interpretations of instructions, and so on

Most, if not all, of these uncertainties can be reduced through the use of quality assurance procedures and the patient positioning and immobilization techniques discussed in this chapter. The quality assurance procedures refer not only to the maintenance of the mechanical specifications of the treatment, imaging, and simulation units, but also to the frequent review of portal images and treatment charts. The immobilization devices include the traditional generic patient supports as well as the more modern hardening foams and thermoplastics to create customized body casts, face masks, and so on.

Will the increased use of immobilization techniques be effective? Two studies (48,49) of the effectiveness of hardened foam casts for prostate treatment show that the average daily positioning errors were 6 to 8 mm in the unimmobilized

TABLE 5.2	Immobilization Capabilities			
Site	Technique	Treatment to treatment	Simulation to treatment	Alignment
Pelvis, abdomen	Alpha Cradle or thermoplastic casts	3–4 mm	—	Laser
	Unimmobilized	6–8 mm	6 mm	Laser
Breast	Alpha Cradle or vacuum bead bags	3 mm	—	Light field
Thorax	Unimmobilized	4 mm	6 mm	Laser
Head, neck	Face mask with neck	2.5–4 mm	—	Laser
	Mechanical	3 mm	2.5 mm	Laser
	Bite block	4 mm	6 mm	Laser
Intracranial	Unimmobilized	3 mm	5 mm	Laser
	Face mask with neck	2.0–2.5 mm	—	Laser
	Cranial fixation (stereotactic)	<1 mm	—	Mechanical
	Noninvasive (stereotactic)	1–1.5 mm	—	Mechanical

Reprinted from Verhey LJ. Immobilizing and positioning patients for radiotherapy. *Semin Radiat Oncol* 1995;5:108, with permission.

patient but only 3 to 4 mm in the immobilized patient. Another retrospective study of 554 head and neck patients (19) showed an error rate of 16% in the unimmobilized patient compared with only 1% using bite block immobilization (errors defined as a localization discrepancy of at least 10 mm). Verhey (50), in an extensive review of the literature, summarizes the reported capabilities of several popular immobilization systems. He estimates the treatment-to-treatment uncertainties to be as shown in Table 5.2.

Many other studies lead to a similar conclusion: Patient immobilization can help to reduce the need for large target margins. New techniques for automated radiographic positioning using either bony anatomy or implanted markers in conjunction with IGRT seem to hold great promise. Verhey (50) estimates the limitation of positioning uncertainty to be plus or minus 1 mm using radiographic alignment of point markers and 1 to 2 mm using radiographic alignment of bony landmarks. He also suggests that laser alignment techniques using skin marks have accuracy limits of 2 to 2.5 mm. The merging of CT localization with radiotherapy in the same room using the treatment machine offers even more possibilities for meeting the challenge.

REFERENCES

1. Kutcher GJ, Coia L, Gillin M, et al. Comprehensive QA for radiation oncology. *Med Phys* 1994;21:581– 618.
2. Klein EE, Hanley J, Bayouth J, et al. Task Group 142 report: quality assurance of medical accelerators. *Med Phys* 2009;36:4197–4212.
3. Lutz W, Winston K, Maleki N. A system for stereotactic radiosurgery with a linear accelerator. *Int J Radiat Oncol Biol Phys* 1988;14:373–381.
4. Siddon RL, Barth NH. Stereotaxic localization of intracranial targets. *Int J Radiat Oncol Biol Phys* 1987;13: 1241–1246.
5. Hamilton AJ, Lulu BA, Fosmiere H, et al. Preliminary clinical experience with linear accelerator—based spinal stereotactic radiosurgery. *Neurosurgery* 1995;36:311–319.
6. De Neve W, Vandan Heuvel F, De Beukeleer M, et al. Routine clinical on-line portal imaging followed by immediate field adjustment using a tele-controlled patient couch. *Radiother Oncol* 1992;24:45–54.
7. Gildersleeve J, Dearnaley DP, Evans PM, et al. A randomized trial of patient repositioning during radiotherapy using an megavoltage imaging system. *Radiother Oncol* 1994;31:161–168.
8. Verhey LJ, Goitein M, McNulty P, et al. Precise positioning of patients for radiotherapy. *Int J Radiat Oncol Biol Phys* 1982;8:289–294.
9. Lyman JT, Phillips MH, Frankel KA, et al. Stereotactic frame for neuro-radiology and charged particle Bragg peak radiosurgery of intra-cranial disorders. *Int J Radiat Oncol Biol Phys* 1989;16:1615–1621.
10. Lam KL, Ten Haken RK, McShan DL, et al. Automated determination of patient setup errors in radiation therapy using spherical radio-opaque markers. *Med Phys* 1993;20:1145–1152.
11. Gall KP, Verhey LJ, Wagner M. Computer assisted positioning of radiotherapy patients using opaque fiducials. *Int J Radiat Oncol Biol Phys* 1993;20:1153–1159.
12. Kupelian P, Willoughby T, Mahadevan A, et al. Multi-institutional clinical experience with the Calypso System in localization and continuous, real-time monitoring of the prostate gland during external radiotherapy. *Int J Radiat Oncol Biol Phys* 2007;67:1088–1098.
13. Willoughby TR, Kupelian PA, Pouliot J, et al. Target localization and real-time tracking using the Calypso 4D localization system in patients with localized prostate cancer. *Int J Radiat Oncol Biol Phys* 2006;65:528–534.
14. Foster RD, Solberg TD, Li HS, et al. Comparison of transabdominal ultrasound and electromagnetic transponders for prostate localization. *J Appl Clin Med Phys* 2010;11:57–67.
15. Smith RL, Lechleiter K, Malinowski K, et al. Evaluation of linear accelerator gating with real-time

electromagnetic tracking. *Int J Radiat Oncol Biol Phys* 2009;74:920–927.

16. Mayse ML, Parikh PJ, Lechleiter KM, et al. Broncho-scopic implantation of a novel wireless electromagnetic transponder in the canine lung: a feasibility study. *Int J Radiat Oncol Biol Phys* 2008;72:93–98.

17. Mackie TR, Holmes T, Swerdloff S, et al. Tomotherapy: a new concept for the delivery of dynamic conformal radiotherapy. *Med Phys* 1993;20:1709–1719.

18. Sawant A, Smith RL, Venkat RB, et al. Toward submil-limeter accuracy in the management of intrafraction motion: the integration of real-time internal position monitoring and multileaf collimator target tracking. *Int J Radiat Oncol Biol Phys* 2009;74:575–582.

19. Byhardt RW, Cox JD, Horngurg A, et al. Weekly localization films and detection of field placement errors. *Int J Radiat Oncol Biol Phys* 1978;4:881–887.

20. Marks JE, Haus AG. The effect of immobilization on localization error in the radiotherapy of head and neck cancer. *Clin Radiol* 1976;27:175–177.

21. Rabinowitz I, Broomberg J, Goitein M, et al. Accuracy of radiation field alignment of clinical practice. *Int J Radiat Oncol Biol Phys* 1985;11:1857–1867.

22. Griffiths SE, Pearcey RG. The daily reproducibility of large complex shaped radiotherapy fields to the thorax and neck. *Clin Radiol* 1986;3:39–41.

23. Boyer AL. Patient positioning and immobilization devic-es. Monograph 15. In: Kereiakes JG, Elson HR, Born CG, eds. *Radiation oncology physics*. New York, NY: American Association of Physicists in Medicine, 1986:438–446.

24. Goitein M, Buss EJ. Immobilization error: some theo-retical considerations. *Radiology* 1975;117:407–412.

25. Maruyama Y, Khan FM. Blocking considerations in mantle therapy. *Radiology* 1971;101:167–171.

26. Kinzie JJ, Hanks GE, MacLean CJ, et al. Patterns of care study: Hodgkin's disease relapse rates and adequacy of portals. *Cancer* 1983;52:2223–2226.

27. Doss LL. *Localization error and local recurrence in upper airway carcinoma: proceedings of the workshop on quality control in the radiotherapy department*. New York, NY: Cancer and Leukemia Group B, 1979.

28. International Commission on Radiation Units and Meas-urements. *Prescribing, recording and reporting photon beam therapy. Report 50*. Bethesda, MD: ICRU, 1993.

29. International Commission on Radiation Units and Meas-urements. *Prescribing, recording and reporting photon beam therapy (Supplement to Report 50). Report 62*. Bethesda, MD: ICRU, 1999.

30. Mageras GS, Kutcher GJ, Liebel SA, et al. A method of incor-porating organ motion uncertainties into 3-dimensional conformal treatment plans. *Int J Radiat Oncol Biol Phys* 1996;35:333–342.

31. Kutcher GJ, Mageras GS, Leibel SA. Control correction and modeling of setup errors and organ motion. *Semin Radiat Oncol* 1995;5:134–145.

32. Bijhold J, Lebesque J, Hart A, et al. Maximizing setup accuracy using portal images as applied to a conformal

boost technique for prostatic cancer. *Radiother Oncol* 1992;24:261–271.

33. Bell A, Bartelink H, Liguad A, et al. Portal imaging and decision rules for correcting patient setups. *Radiother Oncol* 1992;24:S33.

34. Wolbarst AB, Chin LM, Svensson GK. Optimization of radiation therapy: integral response of a model biological system. *Int J Radiat Oncol Biol Phys* 1982;8:1761–1769.

35. Goitein M. Causes and consequences of inhomogene-ous dose distributions in radiation therapy. *Int J Radiat Oncol Biol Phys* 1986;12:701–704.

36. Lyman JT, Wolbarst AB. Optimization of radiation ther-apy: 3. A method of assessing complication probabilities from dose volume histograms. *Int J Radiat Oncol Biol Phys* 1987;13:103–109.

37. Kutcher GJ, Burman C, Brewster L, et al. Histogram reduction method for calculating complication prob-abilities for 3-D treatment planning evaluations. *Int J Radiat Oncol Biol Phys* 1991;21:137–146.

38. Kubo HD, Hill BC. Respiration gated radiotherapy treat-ment: a technical study. *Phys Med Biol* 1996;41:83–91.

39. Fiorino C, Cattaneo GM, del Eecchio A, et al. Skin dose measurements for head and neck radiotherapy. *Med Phys* 1992;19:1263–1266.

40. Purdy JA, Gerber RL, Harms WB. Patient positioning, immobilizing, and treatment verification. AAPM Mono-graph 19. In: Purdy JA, ed. *Advances in radiation oncology physics*. New York, NY: AIP Publishing, 1992:524–534.

41. Watkins DMB. *Radiation therapy mold technology*. Toronto: Pergamon Press, 1981.

42. Bentel GC. *Radiation therapy planning*. New York, NY: McGraw-Hill, 1996.

43. Merchant TE, McCormick B. Prone position breast irra-diation. *Int J Radiat Oncol Biol Phys* 1994;30:197–203.

44. Bentel GC, Marks LB. A simple device to position large/flaccid breasts during tangential breast irradiation. *Int J Radiat Oncol Biol Phys* 1994;29:879–882.

45. Klein EE, Wasserman T, Ermer B. Clinical introduction of a commercial treatment chair to facilitate thorax irra-diation. *Med Dosim* 1995;20:171–176.

46. Gill SS, Thomas DGT, Warrington AP, et al. Relocateable frame for stereotactic external beam radiotherapy. *Int J Radiat Oncol Biol Phys* 1991;20:599.

47. Kooy HM, Dunbar SF, Tarbell NJ, et al. Adaptation and verification of the relocatable Gill-Thomas-Cosman frame in stereotactic radiotherapy. *Int J Radiat Oncol Biol Phys* 1994;30:685.

48. Rosenthal SA, Roche M, Goldsmith BJ, et al. Immobiliza-tion improves the reproducibility of patient positioning during 6-field conformal radiation therapy for prostate carcinoma. *Int J Radiat Oncol Biol Phys* 1993;27:921–926.

49. Soffen EM, Hanks GE, Hwang CC, et al. Conformal static field therapy for low volume, low grade prostate cancer with rigid immobilization. *Int J Radiat Oncol Biol Phys* 1991;20:141–146.

50. Verhey LJ. Immobilizing and positioning patients for radiotherapy. *Semin Radiat Oncol* 1995;5:100–114.

CHAPTER 6

Treatment Simulation

Dimitris N. Mihailidis ■ Niko Papanikolaou

INTRODUCTION

Treatment planning is one of the most crucial processes of radiotherapy, through which the most appropriate way to irradiate the patient is determined. The process is composed by several important steps as follows:

1. Reproducible patient positioning and immobilization
2. Accurate identification of the location and shape of the tumor and neighboring critical organs
3. Selecting the most appropriate beam arrangement
4. Computing the doses to be delivered and evaluation of resulting dose distributions
5. Transfer of the treatment planning information to the treatment delivery system

In today's radiotherapy, three-dimensional (3D) patient anatomy visualization and target definition enable planning to conform the dose to the target volume, delivering as high doses as possible, while avoiding the critical organs. In order to achieve this, a process called *treatment simulation* is necessary to be performed. In essence, treatment simulation is a combination of, or requires that steps 1 to 3 mentioned above have been performed successfully. There are several ways to perform a simulation, each with a different level of complexity. The most common ones are the following:

1. When clinical treatment volume can be determined via simple radiographic and fluoroscopic images from a traditional radiotherapy simulator (1), sometimes called the *anatomical* approach (clinical setup).
2. When only a limited number of transverse computed tomography (CT) images are used for the target delineation along with radiographic planar images (as above) to complete the treatment planning, sometimes called the *traditional* approach.
3. When simulation can be performed on a CT scanner via a special computer software that provides a fully 3D patient representation in the treatment planning position, a process called *CT simulation*. Then, a complete treatment planning strategy can be designed, a process referred to as *virtual simulation* (1,2).

Radiotherapy simulation is a very important process on which treatment planning and delivery depend and are based on. The accuracy of the entire radiotherapy treatment can be influenced by the quality of treatment simulation on patient-per-patient basis.

SIMULATION METHODS

Treatment simulation can also be thought of as a "feasibility study" of the patient treatment strategy. Technological advances of medical imaging and computing have brought great improvement to the simulation process and limitless capabilities.

We will describe the three most common methods of radiotherapy simulation today, which strongly depend on the treatment strategy that will be followed for the patient.

Simple Simulation—Anatomical and Traditional Approach

When the patient is necessary to be prepared for treatment in a short amount of time, or there is a simple treatment to be delivered, a conventional simulation can be performed. In this case, a radiographic simulator, which actually operates in both the radiographic and the fluoroscopic mode, is used (Fig. 6.1A, B). It is an apparatus that uses a diagnostic x-ray tube with an image intensifier (Fig. 6.1C), but duplicates that radiotherapy treatment unit in terms of it geometric, mechanical, and optical properties (3–5).

The patient is setup and immobilized on the simulator the same way that he/she will be treated on the treatment unit. The clinical borders of the treatment area are marked on the patient skin by the physician and radio-opaque markers are placed on skin on these borders. The selection of the treatment isocenter is done via fluoroscopic imaging of the area, typically with two orthogonal reference views: anterior (AP) and lateral (LAT) (Fig. 6.2). Upon selection of the isocenter, two orthogonal radiographic films (or digital images) are produced for further use and comparison with the treatment setup, and documentation purposes. Then, the beams that will be used for treatment are simulated in order to be geographically optimized, depending on the treatment site, by selecting gantry and collimator angles, treatment field sizes, etc.; all in relationship of externally placed markers and internal bony landmarks. A crucial step is the proper marking of the patient: like the isocenter (as a "3-point" marking) and alignment

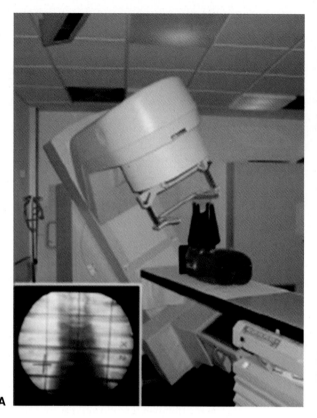

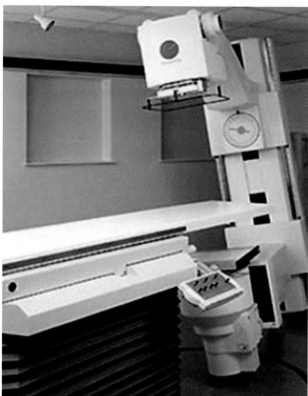

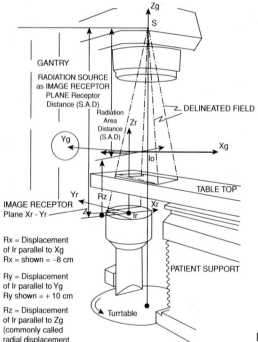

Figure 6.1. Typical radiotherapy simulator. Patient setup represented by a phantom (**A**), room view (**B**), and geometric diagram (**C**).

skin marks using the simulator laser system in all planes. At the same time, other necessary information is collected to be used for setup and dosimetry such as source-to-surface distances of the simulated treatment fields, patient thickness, determination of the time-set or monitor unit calculation point relative to the isocenter (if half-blocked or heavily blocked fields are used, as in Fig. 6.2), simple contours of the patient surface (with contour-makers) through points of dosimetric interest, and evaluation data for bolus or compensator.

Some simulators have a tomographic attachment (simulator-CT) that analyzes and reconstructs the images from the image intensifier using either analog or digital processing (6). However, the quality of the reconstructed

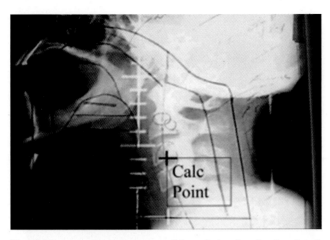

Figure 6.2. Typical simulation portal, lateral view for a head and neck treatment. The blocking is represented by the black marker outlines on the film and the prescription point is denoted as "Calc Point," which is off-axis related to the half-blocked central axis.

image is inferior to the CT-based simulation. In spite of that, it is adequate for acquiring patient contours and identifying bony landmarks. The simulator CT does provide a volumetric reconstruction of the patient's anatomy and, as such, could be used as a basic image data set in treatment planning. The reduced spatial resolution of such volumetric imaging renders this technique unsuitable for high precision conformal radiotherapy planning where a series of many thin slices is required for detail volume reconstruction (7,8).

Interestingly, the concept of simulator CT has recently reemerged and is referred to as cone beam CT (CBCT). Cone beam imaging is currently used in the context of image-guided radiotherapy (IGRT) for daily patient localization and setup verification prior to treatment. Those images could also be used for patient replanning in the context of adaptive radiotherapy, although for the time being this is only a research application. It is expected, however, that once the image quality, imaging dose to the patient, and the speed of replanning improve, CBCT adaptive radiotherapy will become an integral part of advanced radiotherapy.

CBCT imaging can be obtained using the kV imaging system of a linac (Varian, Elekta) or the MV beam itself (Tomotherapy, Siemens). Regardless of the implementation, CBCT is similar to and suffers from the same characteristics as the simulator CT.

Verification Simulation

This is a simulation approach "positioned" between the previous described approach and the virtual simulation that will be described next. This process starts by immobilizing the patient in the treatment planning position with all the necessary devices, this time on the CT scanner flat tabletop. In this case, there is no laser localization system available in the CT room. A standard treatment planning study of the patient will be obtained throughout the

clinical area, after radio-opaque markers are placed by the physician on the patient's skin. The simulation team will need to place "3-point" tattoos or other types of long-lasting markers on the patient's skin. For CT purposes, the "3-point" locations and the treatment area borders will be visible on the CT images. Patient scans are typically obtained in an axial mode, 3- to 5-mm slice thickness. Smaller slice thickness can be used for small areas, when higher resolution and accuracy is necessary.

The CT images are reviewed and then imported to a treatment planning system where a computer simulation will be done off-line. The physician will define the volumes of interest and the isocenter might be adjusted to accommodate the target volume extensions. The coordinates of the treatment isocenter can be referenced to the original "3-point" location marked in the CT room. Next, the remaining treatment planning process is completed and the plan gets finalized. Two orthogonal (AP & LAT), digitally reconstructed radiographs (DRRs) (9,10) at the original CT point and the new isocenter will be produced at this point (Fig. 6.3). DRRs of the treatment fields will also be produced.

A verification simulation is scheduled in the conventional simulator, where the patient is immobilized and setup again in the treatment planning position. The patient then is simulated according to the approved treatment plan. A sample simulation form is shown in Figure 6.4, where all the appropriate shifts from the original CT marks to the final isocenter are implemented. An orthogonal set of setup ports, first at the original CT point ("3-point" mark) and then at the treatment isocenter will assure the proper localization, when compared to the DRRs at the same locations. The patient will be marked appropriately to insure reproducibility of setup during treatment. Further on, additional ports of the treatment fields can be obtained to increase the accuracy of the simulation setup and for documentation purposes. The orthogonal ports and treatment ports will be compared to portal images or portal films in the treatment room, especially at the first day of treatment. A diagram of the verification simulation process is shown in Figure 6.5A.

CT Simulator and Virtual Simulation

This is an exciting development in the area of simulation because it converts a CT (or other scanning modality) scanner into a simulator (1,2,11–13). Both patient and treatment units are virtual, the patient being represented by CT images and the treatment unit by model beam geometry and expected dose distributions. The simulation film is replaced by the DRRs. The DDRs are generated from the CT scan data by mapping average CT values computed along lines drawn from a "virtual source" to the location of the "virtual film." A DRR is essentially a calculated port film that serves as a simulator film, which contains all the useful anatomical information of the patient (Fig. 6.6). A dedicated radiation therapy CT scanner, with

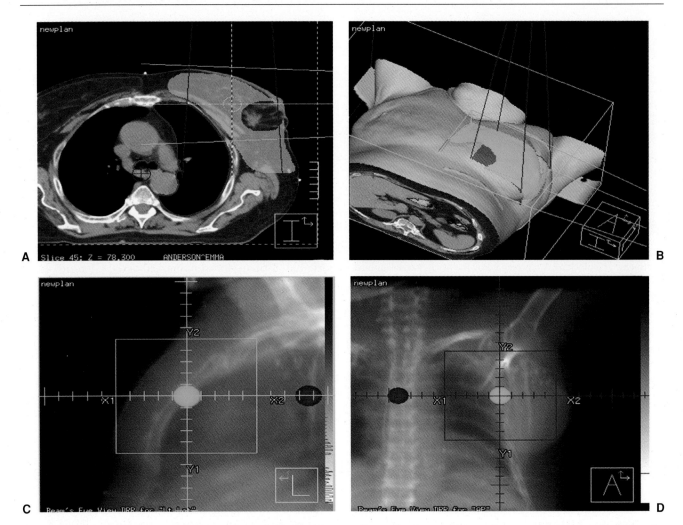

Figure 6.3. Breast patient computed tomography (CT) image with two orthogonal reference fields on the treatment isocenter-GREEN point (**A**), three-dimensional (3D) reconstruction of the patient imaged area with the reference field (**B**), LAT-reference field to the treatment isocenter (**C**), AP-reference filed to the isocenter (**D**). The RED point is the original CT point.

the above described virtual simulation software and simulation accessories (e.g., flat tabletop, immobilization devices, etc.), is called a CT simulator (Fig. 6.7A). In addition, CT simulators are equipped with high precision movable laser systems to mark the isocenter location on the patient during the virtual simulation process. The laser system is mounted on fixed pedestals on the floor and ceiling as shown in Figure 6.7B.

Modern radiotherapy CT simulators are based on the most recent CT scanner technology with multi-slice (multi-detector) detector technology, axial and helical scanning mode capabilities, rapid CT acquisition time, and high image quality performance and wide bore (>75 cm diameter) to accommodate the patient immobilization devices (Fig. 6.8). Further on, an option called *gating* allows the scanner to perform "motion-correlated" scanning, a process called 4DCT (the 4th being the time information), useful for accurate treatment planning on moving anatomy (e.g., respiratory motion in lung). The standard linear accelerator (linac) requirements, for example, large weight capability (up to 450–600 lb load), small sag

(<2 mm), and hard tabletop, apply for CT simulators also.

A diagram that describes the CT simulation and virtual simulation processes is shown in Figure 6.5B.

CT Simulation Process

The patient is immobilized on the CT table and in the treatment planning position. At this initial stage, all special immobilization devices (e.g., head and neck masks, pelvic shells, breast boards, etc.) are required to be constructed and/or utilized, in order to be included in the CT image study of the patient. These devices can be indexed on the CT tabletop, the same way that later on will be indexed on the linac treatment table (Fig. 6.9A–C). Additional planning modifiers, such as skin bolus, are also required to be included. The borders of the clinical area marked by the physician on the patient can be outlined with CT radio-opaque markers (Fig. 6.9C). Sometimes, initial reference skin marks are placed in the middle of the clinical treatment area. The CT movable lasers are used to define and mark the CT reference point on the patient.

Charleston Radiation Therapy Consultants, PLLC   Patient Name:_____

Radiation Oncology   Physicist/Dosimetrist:_____

Plan/Simulation Name:_____

LUNG - VIRTUAL SIMULATION

SPECIAL INSTRUCTIONS: (DRR's: SFD = _____ cm)

SET-UP PARAMETERS:

Set-up Instructions:

1. 3 point set up to CT marks.   Initial [Ant / Post] SSD: _____ cm.

2. Vertical: Shift Isocenter _____cm [Ant / Post].   New SSD: _____ cm.

3. Longitudinal: Shift Isocenter: _____cm towards [Head / Foot].   New SSD: _____ cm.

4. Lateral: Shift Isocenter: _____cm towards patients [Rt / Lt].   New SSD: _____ cm.

Final Couch Coordinates:

Vertical: _____   Lateral: _____   Longitudinal: _____

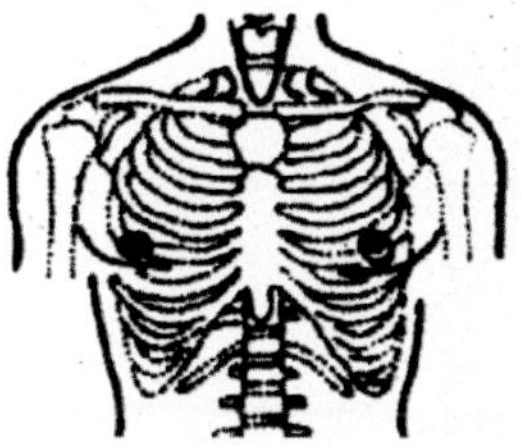

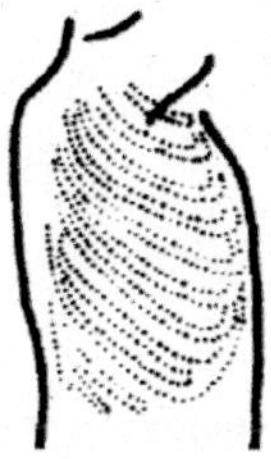

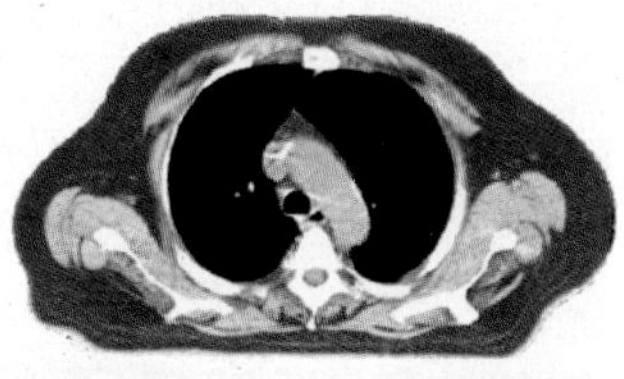

BEAM PARAMETERS:

Field Name / Energy	Gantry Angle	Collim Angle	Table Angle	Field Size						Wedge Angle	SSD Plan	SSD Sim
				X	X1	X2	Y	Y1	Y2			

Created by. D. Mihailidis, PhD/03/15/03

Figure 6.4. Sample in-house simulation form for lung setup. Note the setup instructions and appropriate shift information from the "3-point" computed tomography (CT) mark to the treatment isocenter. Detail information on the treatment fields are entered in the table below. This firm can be used for verification simulation also.

A set of anterior and lateral topograms ("scout views") will assist the patient alignment on the CT table. The patient will be scanned based on a preset protocol according to the disease site and the images will be stored for virtual simulation, while the patient remains on the CT table.

Virtual Simulation Process

There are three tasks that pertain to virtual simulation. First is the treatment isocenter localization, which is typically placed at the geometric center of the treatment volume. The second is the target and critical structures volume delineation. The third is to determine the treatment beam parameters via beam's-eye-view (BEVs) (14) using DRRs, including gantry, collimator and couch angles, field sizes, shielding block, etc. This last part can also be performed at a later time during the treatment planning and isodose computation process.

The CT images will be utilized to render a 3D view of the patient, which will allow the more precise localization of the isocenter, and later on, more efficient placement of the treatment fields (Fig. 6.10). The isocenter will be marked on the reconstructed patient anatomy and two

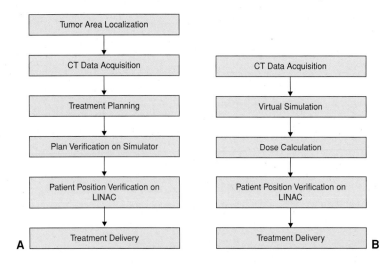

Tumor Area Localization

↓

CT Data Acquisition

↓

Treatment Planning

↓

Plan Verification on Simulator

↓

Patient Position Verification on LINAC

↓

Treatment Delivery

A

CT Data Acquisition

↓

Virtual Simulation

↓

Dose Calculation

↓

Patient Position Verification on LINAC

↓

Treatment Delivery

B

Figure 6.5. Verification simulation process diagram (**A**) and computed tomography (CT) simulation process (**B**).

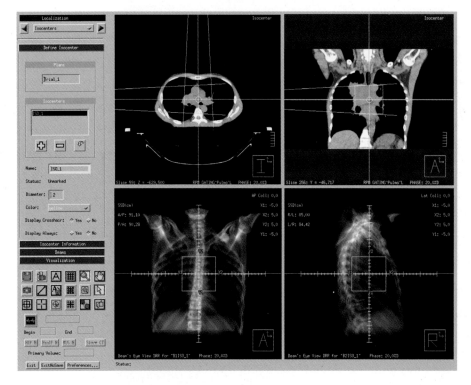

Figure 6.6. Virtual simulation as part of computed tomography (CT) simulation for a lung patient. The user can visualize the anatomical information that will assist appropriate placement of points, such as the treatment isocenter and the fields. In addition, tumor and other critical volumes can be outlined at this stage. This information will be eventually transferred to the treatment planning system.

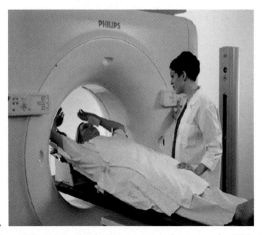

A

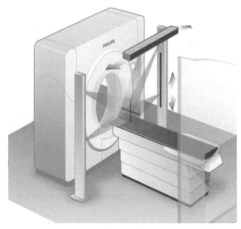

B

Figure 6.7. A large (wide) bore computed tomography (CT) simulator accommodates the majority of immobilization devices to be included in patient setup (**A**). A room view of a CT simulator with the localization laser system (**B**).

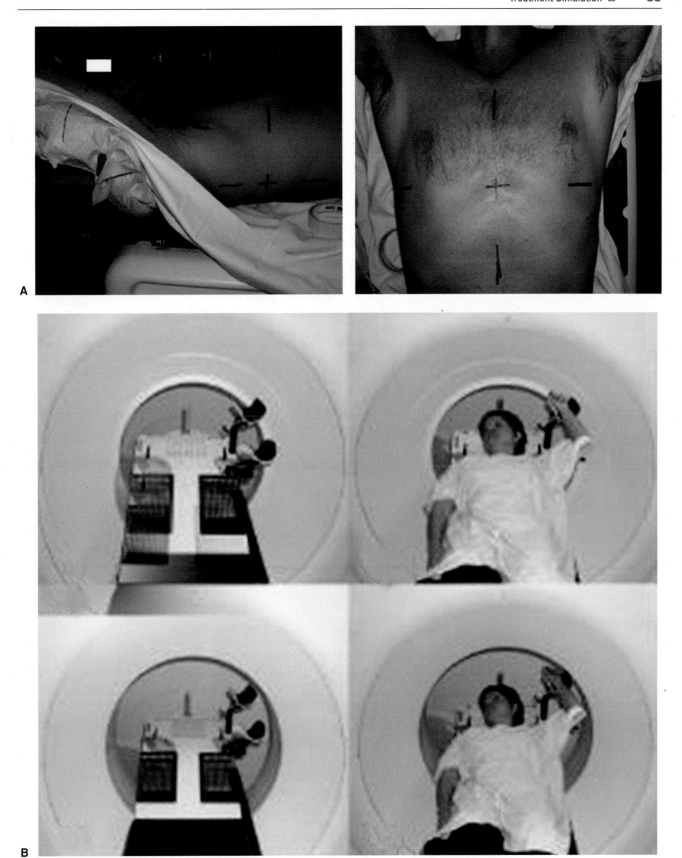

Figure 6.8. Top panel: Patient setup ready to be simulated in a wide bore computed tomography (CT) simulator, with immobilization devices and reference marks ("3-point" mark) (**A**). Bottom panel: Comparison between a standard (UPPER) and wide bore (LOWER) CT simulator when it comes to bulky immobilization devices.

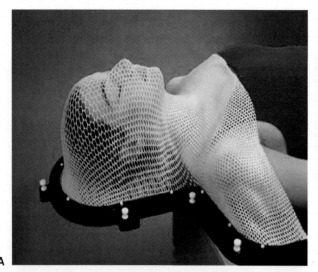

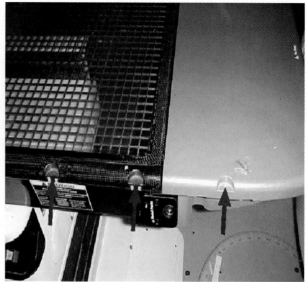

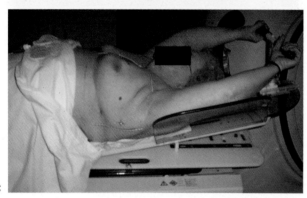

Figure 6.9. Patient immobilization devices as integral part of computed tomography (CT) simulation process for radiotherapy. A head and neck head holder and mask (**A**), indexing grooves for the immobilization devices on the tabletop (**B**) and (**C**) a breast patient on a breast board with reference CT radio-opaque markers ready to be CT simulated.

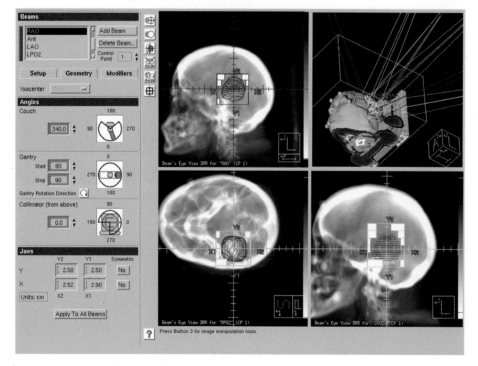

Figure 6.10. Virtual simulation based on three-dimensional (3D) reconstruction allows accurate placement of treatment fields (top-right). In this brain treatment for example, two lateral (top-left and bottom-right) and one vertex (bottom-left) treatment fields shaped by multi-leaf collimators (MLCs) are shown.

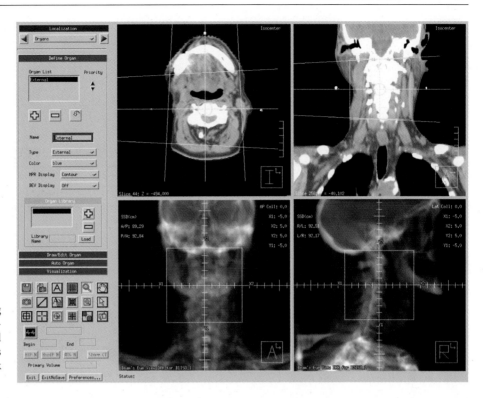

Figure 6.11. Isocenter placement during virtual simulation, based on reconstructed planes (top) and orthogonal digitally reconstructed radiographs (DRRs) (bottom) for a head and neck treatment.

reference fields (typically an AP and an LAT) will be assigned at that point. The DRRs (Fig. 6.11) of the reference fields will be compared with the equivalent ports films later on, the same way simulator films have been used at the past. Having determined the isocenter, the patient is marked with the assistance of the movable lasers, one anterior and two lateral marks on each side of "3-point." Shifts between the original CT reference marks and the isocenter marks should be logged in patient's chart.

At this stage, the patient can be removed from the CT table. The rest of the virtual simulation process can be performed off-line via the special simulation software or the treatment planning system software. Connectivity between the CT scanner's computer system and the treatment planning computer is essential to be evaluated and tested by the physicist on a frequent basis (13). Image format standards such as DICOM (15) and DICOM-RT (16) (developed especially for radiation therapy) transfer protocols between imaging devices and the treatment planning computer are the industry standards. One needs to keep in mind that, DICOM-RT transfer protocol can be highly complex to implement and vary in interpretation from one manufacturer to another.

In the treatment planning system, the patient's CT study and CT simulation information (reference marks, points, reference fields, etc.) should be available for potential registration or fusion with other imaging modalities (other CT studies, MRI, PET, etc.) that the patient might have gone through (Fig. 6.12). The information provided by the multi-imaging studies will allow the physician to outline target and other volumes more accurately.

Starting from the reference marks and setup ports, the treatment isocenter is typically selected at the center of the treatment area. Relative shifts of the isocenter from the reference CT marks are monitored for subsequent patient setup, as described above, and shown in Figure 6.13. The physician will outline the target areas and other critical structures in a slice-by-slice process and will review the 3D representation of these volumes in three major views (axial, sagittal, and coronal). Delineation of target and critical organs is an extremely time-consuming process in most clinical cases. Progress has been made toward computer-assisted automatic contouring, pattern recognition, and auto-segmentation (17). Figure 6.14 compares manually outlined and auto-segmented heart volumes. However, the basic problem remains that target delineation is inherently a manual process, since the extend of target depends on tumor grade, stage, and patterns of spread to adjacent structures. Clinical evaluation of the contouring results by a radiation oncologist provides the final judgment in defining the target volume.

With all the volumes (targets and critical structures) approved by the physician, the treatment planning team can initiate the selection of the appropriate treatment fields via BEVs and 3D reconstruction of internal geometry of the patient (Fig. 6.10). Keeping in mind the clinical and setup margins to the tumor volume, as defined by the International Commission on Radiation Units and Measurements (ICRU) (18,19), appropriate blocks with multi-leaf collimators (MLCs) can be used for 3D conformal treatment planning. It is important to remember that each beam has physical penumbra where the dose varies rapidly and that the dose at the edge of the field is ~50% of the center dose. For this reason, to achieve adequate dose

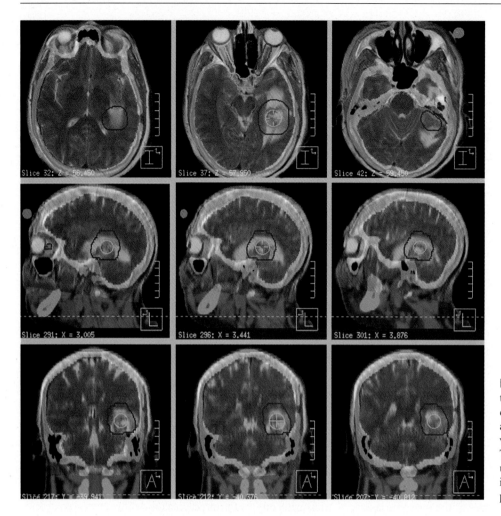

Figure 6.12. Multi-image registration for a brain patient. MRI and computed tomography (CT) are aligned and fused in all three major views: axial, sagittal, and coronal. This allows the user to outline volumes that are visualized in MR images onto the CT images and proceed with treatment planning.

coverage of the target volume, the field penumbra should lie sufficiently beyond the target volume to offset any uncertainties in PTV. Beam apertures can be designed automatically or manually depending on the proximity of the critical structures and the uncertainty involved in the allowed margins to the target volume (Fig. 6.15). Clinical judgment frequently is required between sparing of critical structures and target coverage.

All possible gantry, collimator, and couch angles can be evaluated based on target coverage and critical structures avoidance. Some commercial planning systems provide software-assisted beam geometry parameter optimization (20,21), which is important for highly conformal treatment plans. Beam directions that create greater separation between the target and critical structures are generally preferred unless other constraints such as obstructions in the beam path and gantry collisions with the treatment couch or patient preclude those choices. Alternatively, dose-volume objectives for the target volume and critical structures can be employed to produce an inversely optimized plan, with the majority of commercial planning systems being capable of providing inverse planning optimization algorithms (22). Final dose computations take full advantage of CT electron density information in order to account for tissue inhomogeneities (23). The virtual simulation process smoothly makes a transition into treatment planning and treatment evaluation stage, which is beyond the purpose of this chapter.

A few points of precaution are in order when virtual simulation is performed.

■ Due to precise visualization of internal organ and target volumes, one might be misled to use arbitrary small

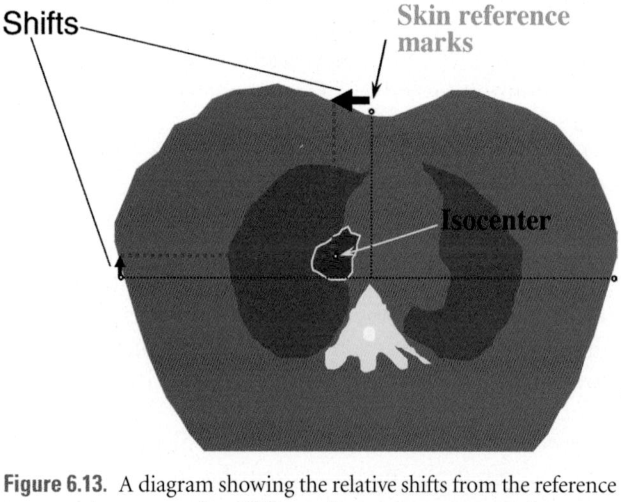

Figure 6.13. A diagram showing the relative shifts from the reference computed tomography (CT) marks to the treatment isocenter. Visualization of internal body structures is essential in this process.

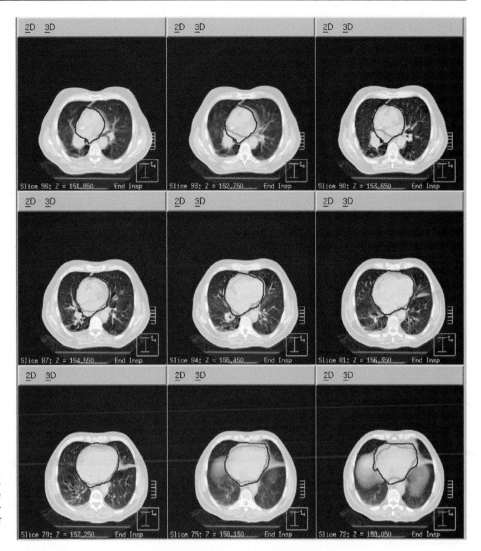

Figure 6.14. Subsequent computed tomography (CT) axial images. Compare the heart volume that has been manually outlined (BLUE line) and the result of auto-segmentation (GREEN line).

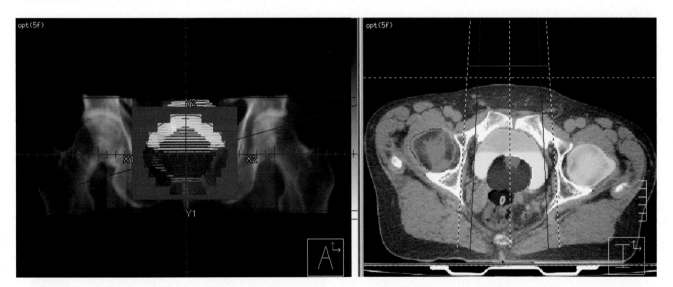

Figure 6.15. A field shaped around the prostate with specific margins using multi-leaf collimators (MLCs). The BEV view (left) and the axial view (right).

margins to the target volume in a feeling of false confidence. Thus, other important effects such as patient setup and target motion might not be taken into account in a proper way, since patient and organ motion are not well visualized by traditional 3D virtual simulation. In absence of 4DCT imaging, an additional fluoroscopic study, in a traditional simulator, might be of great benefit to treatment planning, especially for moving target such as lung.

■ The spatial resolution is generally limited by the spacing of the axial images. Thus, within the target area, it is required that smaller scanning spacing (typically 2–3 mm) is used while a larger spacing (typically 1–2 cm) can be used further from the area of interest. One needs to keep in mind that this will affect the quality of the reconstructed DRRs.

■ Limitation of CT imaging in visualizing all treatment sites can influence the clinical target volume (CTV) design, in other words, CT imaging not always provide the best method to visualize microscopic disease. Most commonly, this is the case for brain tumors that CT imaging cannot provide clear borders of the disease. The clinician needs to keep in mind that combination (image registration process) of the treatment planning CT with other modalities, such as MR or PET, will allow a more accurate delineation of the target volume. It is important to remember that the ability to precisely conform to a target volume has limited value if the target is not determined accurately.

4DCT Simulation Process

Modern CT scanners are capable of providing a high resolution volumetric reconstruction of the patient's anatomy. Each image voxel has a characteristic CT number that is uniquely related to the electron density of that voxel. The density information is used in the computation of dose and accounts for the effects of tissue inhomogeneity in treatment planning. When the anatomy that is imaged is mobile (for tumors and organs that move during the imaging study

due to cardiac or respiratory motion), the image data are subject to motion artifacts. Consequently, the resulting volumetric reconstruction of the patient is a blurred representation of the true patient anatomy. In addition, motion artifacts will result in erroneous CT numbers and correspondingly electron density values in the vicinity of the mobile anatomy. It is therefore important to minimize any motion artifact as it impacts not only the image quality and the specificity by which we can resolve anatomical changes, but also the accuracy of the calculated dose in treatment planning.

There are three different types of motion artifacts that can be observed during a CT acquisition (24):

■ If the CT scanning speed in the superior–inferior direction is much less than the tumor motion speed, then we observe a smeared image of the tumor.

■ If the CT scanning speed is much faster than the tumor motion speed, then the tumor position and shape are captured on the image at an arbitrary phase of the breathing cycle.

■ If the CT scanning speed is similar to the tumor motion speed, then the tumor position and shape can be significantly distorted.

It is therefore evident that patient motion can cause significant artifacts during 3DCT imaging (25,26), which not only degrade the image quality and our ability to delineate anatomical structures (27), but sometimes can even simulate erroneously the presence of disease (28). Figure 6.16 illustrates image artifacts that are caused by superior–inferior motion during conventional CT imaging of a test sphere (29).

Ritchie (30) proposed a high-speed (fast) scan to avoid motion artifacts that was however of limited success with the third-generation CT scanners. The use of multi-slice technology (31) has significantly reduced motion artifacts in CT images when acquired in fast scanning mode. However, fast scans, although less susceptible to motion artifacts, do not portray the full extent of motion of the tumor and are therefore not of clinical use in treatment planning

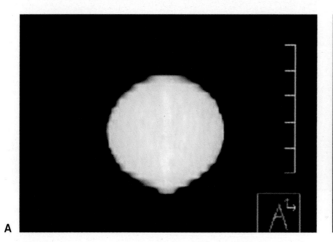
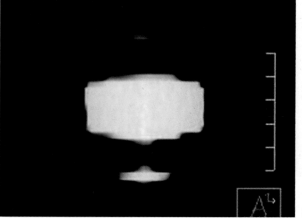

Figure 6.16. Illustration of image artifacts that are caused by superior–inferior (SI) motion during 3DCT imaging. **A:** computed tomography (CT) coronal section of a static sphere. **B:** CT coronal section of the same sphere in oscillatory motion (range = 2 cm, period = 4 s) (29).

of mobile tumors. Multi-slice helical scanning, on the other hand, can be used with a 4DCT scanning protocol to reduce the overall scanning time while achieving the goal of capturing the temporal position of the tumor in the imaging study.

When we consider the organ motion, we have to choose an imaging technique that will minimize motion artifacts during the CT simulation. Several methods have been proposed to address this problem including the following:

■ A breath-hold CT simulation, where the patient is instructed to voluntarily hold their breath while the scanning beam is turned on. A similar result can be achieved using the ABC technique proposed by Wong et al. (32).

■ A slow CT scan, where axial images are acquired at a speed of 4 seconds or slower per slice. A slow scan will ensure that the envelope of motion of any moving organ subject to respiratory motion will be captured in the image (typical respiratory period is 4–6 s).

■ A gated CT scan, where the beam is turned on only when the patient's breathing is at a certain window of the respiratory cycle (typically 30–35% duty cycle). The respiratory-related motion is usually monitored using an external marker. In one of the commercially available implementations, this is accomplished by correlating the respiration-related tumor motion to the displacement of an external marker placed on the patient's chest as measured using an infrared camera. The user can specify which portion of the sinusoidal-shaped signal obtained from the infrared camera is used to trigger the CT scanner using the cardiac gating port. This method of imaging is also known as prospective-gated image acquisition.

■ A 4DCT scan where multiple scans are obtained for each location (oversampling), whereby the organ motion is captured at different sampled phases of the respiratory cycle. At the end of the scan, a very large set of 3D images is produced corresponding to each of the phases in which the breathing cycle was sampled (Fig. 6.17). The collection of those 3DCT scans constitutes the 4DCT study for this patient. This method is also known as retrospective image reconstruction.

Of all the imaging methods that aim to minimize respiration-related motion artifacts, the 4DCT technique is the most comprehensive way to perform such task, because it not only reduces motion artifacts, but also captures the changing topography of the tumor during the respiratory cycle. This information can be used during treatment planning, to optimally delineate treatment volumes and margins, under the assumption that the patient will be breathing the same way during treatment as they did during the 4DCT simulation. Irregular breathing (during imaging or treatment) is not desirable and we often use coaching to help the patient breath regularly and reproducibly. Coaching can be auditory, where a computerized voice instructs the patient to breath in and out, or visual, where, for example, the patient looks at the superposition of their baseline breathing curve and their real-time breathing curve and tries to match them as they control and pace their breathing.

Ultimately, the goal of simulation is to uniquely and reliably identify in the patient's treatment position the exact target shape and location that can be reproducibly localized and treated during the daily treatments. 4DCT simulation allows us to segment the target and organ volumes with high specificity, resulting in more educated decisions on margin selection and improved dose calculation during treatment planning.

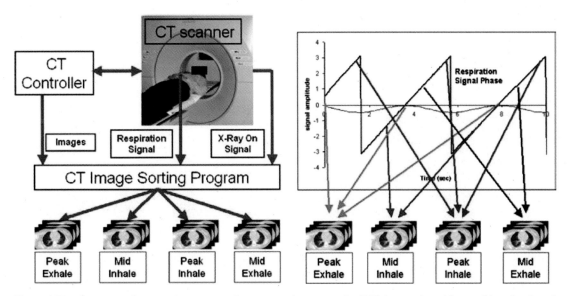

Figure 6.17. The 4DCT phase-sorting process: the computed tomography (CT) images, breathing tracking signal, and 'x-ray ON' signal form the input data stream. The breathing cycle is divided into distinct bins (e.g., peak exhale, mid-inhale, peak inhale, mid-exhale). Images are sorted into those image bins depending on the phase of the breathing cycle in which they were acquired (29).

ACCEPTANCE TESTING AND QUALITY ASSURANCE

When it comes to conventional and CT simulators, the initial acceptance testing is performed to verify that the unit is operating as specified by the manufacturer and to serve as a baseline data pool for future comparisons with periodic quality assurance (QA) testing.

Conventional Simulator

Acceptance testing of a simulator may be divided into two parts: (a) geometric and spatial accuracies verification and (b) performance evaluation of the x-ray generator and the associated imaging system. The first part is similar to the acceptance testing and evaluation of a linear accelerator for mechanical performance. Because the simulators are designed to mimic the treatment accelerators, their geometric accuracies should be comparable with those of the accelerators. To minimize differences between the simulator and the accelerator, it is desired to use the same table design and accessory holders as those on the treatment machine.

The second part is a performance evaluation of a diagnostic radiographic and fluoroscopic unit.

Several authors have discussed the technical specifications of treatment simulators and the required testing procedures and have presented comprehensive reviews on this subject (3,4,33–35). The quality assurance for the x-ray generator and the imaging system has been discussed by various groups (36,37). The most recent recommendations on QA for conventional simulators are coming from AAPM Task Group #40 (Table III in the report) (38). A sample set of monthly QA tests are shown in Figure 6.18. Of course, a well-established QA program requires daily and annual testing for simulators, in addition to the monthly testing.

CT Simulator

Acceptance testing of a CT simulator requires first the acceptance testing of the CT scanner as an imaging device to be done. This process is described in detail by AAPM

Charleston Radiation Therapy Consultants, PLLC

Physicist: ________

Date: ________

Department of Medical Physics

OLDELFT-NUCLETRON SIMULATOR

MONTHLY QUALITY ASSURANCE

I. MECHANICAL CHECKS

A. *Optical Distance Indicator (ODI)*

ODI set @ 100 cm; pointer reads: ________ cm (±2mm) Pass/Fail

ODI set @ 110 cm; pointer reads: ________ cm (±2mm) Pass/Fail

ODI set @ 95 cm; pointer reads: ________ cm (±2mm) Pass/Fail

B. *Field Size Accuracy* *(small, medium and large field sizes)*

Measured Field Size L/R Wires x S/I Wires	Digital Readout L/R Wires x S/I Wires	
____ x ____	____ x ____	
____ x ____	____ x ____	
____ x ____	____ x ____	(±2mm) Pass/Fail

C. *Gantry/Collimator Angle Indicators*

Gantry Angle Measured	Gantry Angle Digital Readout	Collimator Angle Measured	Collimator Angle Digital Readout	
90°	________	90°	________	(C±1°) Pass/Fail
270°	________	270°	________	
360°	________	360°	________	(G±1°) Pass/Fail

D. *Lasers*

Rt. Transverse: ____ mm   Overhead Sagittal: ____

Rt. Coronal: ____ mm   Overhead Transverse: ____

Lt. Transverse: ____ mm   Sagittal: ____

Lt. Coronal: ____ mm   (±2mm) Pass/Fail

E. *Cross-hair Centering* (±2mm diameter) Pass/Fail

F. *Light/Radiation Congruence*

Field Size ________ Collimator Angle ________ (±2mm or ±1%) Pass/Fail

G. *Reviewed Field Service Reports* (through ____________)

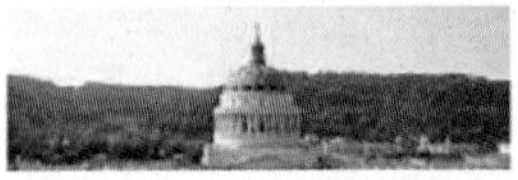

Figure 6.18. Set of monthly QA tests for a conventional simulator. This set of tests is based on AAPM TG-40 (38).

**Monthly CT QA Check Form:
Phillips Big Bore CT**

Date: _____

Charleston Radiation Therapy Consultants   Physicist: _____

Daily Laser QA LAP Laser Phantom Scan: Horz _____ Vert _____ ± 2 mm
                                                              (pass / fail)   (pass / fail)

MedTec CT Simulator Laser QA Device centered at lasers:

Longitudinal distance between LAP lasers and Gantry lasers _____ (500 ± 2 mm)
                                                                              (pass / fail)

Scanned image checks   (pass / fail)

+ Image Definition: Right _____   Center _____   Left _____

Vertical centering _____ ± 2 mm (pass / fail)

Horizontal centering _____ ± 2 mm (pass / fail)

Laser Alignment (± 2 mm)   (pass / fail)

LAP side lasers: Alignment   L _____   R _____

                           Table height   L _____   R _____ (52 ±2 mm)

                           Longitudinal tracking L _____ R _____

                           Vertical tracking   L _____   R _____

Sagittal LAP laser: Longitudinal tracking _____ Vertical tracking _____

                           Alignment (Displacement at center) _____

Gantry lasers: Vertical tracking _____

LAP laser motion (± 1 mm)

Center post _____ (0 ±2 mm) Side post _____ (center ±125 mm ±1 mm)

Table vertical shift (put lasers at top of phantom) _____ (25 ±1 mm) (pass/fail)

Figure 6.19. Set of monthly QA tests for computed tomography (CT) simulator. This set of tests is based on AAPM TG-66 (13).

Report No. 39 (39). For the purpose of CT simulation, additional literature needs to be employed to cover the needs of radiotherapy (see chapter by McGee and Das in Ref. 11). Due to the complexity of the new technology scanners, the manufacturer's acceptance testing procedure (acceptance testing procedure manual [ATP-manual]) provides a great guide to suggested recommendations for testing tolerances for the particular scanner. We recommend that the AAPM Task Group #66 report is followed for all the QA needs of a CT simulator as it applies to radiotherapy procedures (13). Table I in Ref. (13) outlines the electromechanical components testing (e.g., lasers, table, gantry, and scan localization). Table II outlines test specifications for image performance evaluation (e.g., CT number vs. electron density, image noise, contrast, and spatial resolution). A simplified set of tests are shown in Figure 6.19. Keep in mind that the CT simulation process QA should be performed along with the treatment planning process QA, where information and data are transferred between the CT scanner and the treatment planning computers.

When 4DCT scans are used for simulation, the quality assurance is, for the most part, the same as that for the CT

simulator. In addition to the tests described previously, one could include scans of test phantoms that are placed on a moving platform. Such motorized platforms can be programmed to a user-defined moving cycle that is typically 1D or 2D, which is adequate for QA purposes. Since the physical size of the phantom and any objects embedded inside it are known, a 4DCT scan would test the ability of the scanner and the accompanying software to build the 4D model of the phantom and to reproduce the true dimensions of the imaged objects. Although there is not currently much information on QA for 4DCT, such protocols can easily be developed and incorporated in routine quality assurance programs for CT simulation.

CONCLUSIONS

Treatment simulation is a crucial component of the entire treatment planning process and guarantees successful radiotherapy practice. The advancements of today's technology in both hardware and software allow more accurate patient setup and representation with customization of the treatment plans to the specific patient and site. However, stringent QA procedures are necessary to maintain optimum and safe use of such technologies.

REFERENCES

1. Sherouse GW, Bourland JD, Reynolds KL, et al. Virtual simulation in the clinical setting: some practical considerations. *Int J Radiat Oncol Biol Phys* 1990;19:1059–1065.
2. Sherouse GW. Radiotherapy simulation. In: Khan FM, Potish R, eds. *Treatment planning in radiation oncology*, Baltimore, MD: Williams & Wilkins, 1998:39–53.
3. McCullough EC. Radiotherapy treatment simulators. In: AAPM Monograph No. 19, 1990:491–499.
4. McCullough EC, Earl JD. The selection, acceptance testing, and quality control of radiotherapy treatment simulators. *Radiology* 1979;131:221–230.
5. Khan FM. *The physics of radiation therapy*, 4th ed. Baltimore, MD: Lippincott Williams & Wilkins, 2010.
6. Galvin JM. The CT-simulator and the Simulator-CT. In: Smith AR, ed. *Radiation therapy physics.* Berlin: Springer-Verlag, 1995:19–32.
7. Dahl O, Kardamakis D, Lind B, et al. Current status of conformal radiotherapy. *Acta Oncol* 1996;35(Suppl 8):41–57.
8. Rosenwald JC, Gaboriaud G, Pontvert D. Conformal radiotherapy: principles and clarification (in French). *Cancer Radiother* 1999;3:367–377.
9. Siddon RL. Solution to treatment planning problems using coordinate transformations. *Med Phys* 1981;8:766–774.
10. Siddon RL. Fast calculation of the exact radiological path for a three-dimensional CT array. *Med Phys* 1985;12:252–255.
11. Coia LR, Schultheiss TE, Hanks GE, eds. *A practical guide to CT simulation.* Madison, WI: Advanced Medical Publishing, 1995.
12. Aird EG, Conway J. CT simulation for radiotherapy treatment planning. *Br J Radiol* 2002;75:937–949.
13. Mutic S, Palta JR, Butker EK, et al. Quality assurance for computed-tomography-simulation process: Report of the AAPM Radiation Therapy Committee Task Group No. 66. *Med Phys* 2003;30:2762–2792.
14. Goitein M, Abrams M, Rowell D, et al. Multidimensional treatment planning: II Beam's eye-view, back projection through CT sections. *Int J Radiat Oncol Biol Phys* 1983;9:789–797.
15. NEMA, The DICOM Standard, 2006. http://medical.nema.org/dicom/2006.
16. Bosh W. Integrating the management of patient treatment planning and image data. In: Purdy JA, ed. *Categorical course syllabus: 3-dimensional radiation therapy treatment planning.* Chicago: RSNA, 1994;151–160.
17. Ragan D, et al. Semi-automated four-dimensional computed tomography segmentation using deformable models. *Med Phys* 2005;32:2254–2261.
18. ICRU Report No. 50. *Prescribing, recording and reporting photon beam therapy.* Bethesda, MD: ICRU, 1993.
19. ICRU Report No. 62. *Prescribing, recording and reporting photon beam therapy (supplement to ICRU Report 50).* Bethesda, MD: ICRU, 1999.
20. Rowbottom CG, Oldham M, Webb S. Constrained customization of non-coplanar beam orientations in radiotherapy of brain tumors. *Phys Med Biol* 1999;44:383–399.
21. Bedford JL, Webb S. Elimination of importance factors for clinically accurate selection of beam orientations, beam weights and wedge angles in conformal radiation therapy. *Med Phys* 2003;30:1788–1804.
22. Purdy JA, Grant III WH, Palta JR, et al., eds. *3D conformal and intensity modulated radiation therapy: physics and applications.* Madison, WI: Advanced Medical Publishing, Inc., 2001.
23. Papanikolaou N, et al. Tissue inhomogeneity corrections for megavoltage photon beams. AAPM Task Group Report No. 65. 2004. http://www.aapm.org/pubs/reports/RPT_85.pdf.
24. Jiang S. Management of moving targets in radiotherapy: integrating new technologies into the clinic: Monte Carlo and image-guided radiation therapy. AAPM Monograph No. 32, 2006.
25. Mayo JR, Müller NL, Henkelman RM. The double-fissure sign: a motion artifact on thin-section CT scans. *Radiology* 1987;165:580–581.
26. Ritchie CJ, Hseih J, Gard MF, et al. Predictive respiratory gating: a new method to reduce motion artifacts on CT scans. *Radiology* 1994;190:847–852.
27. Keall PJ, Kini VR, Vedam SS, et al. Potential radiotherapy improvements with respiratory gating. *Australas Phys Eng Sci Med* 2002;25:1–6.
28. Tarver RD, Conces DJ, Godwin JD. Motion artifacts on CT simulate bronchiectasis. *Am J Roentgenol* 1998;151:1117–1119.
29. Vedam SS, Keall PJ, Kini VR, et al. Acquiring a four-dimensional computed tomography dataset using an external respiratory signal. *Phys Med Biol* 2003;48:45–62.
30. Ritchie CJ, Godwin JD, Crawford CR, et al. Minimum scan speeds for suppression of motion artifacts in CT. *Radiology* 1992;185(1):37–42.
31. Kachelriess M, Kalender WA. Electrocardiogram-correlated image reconstruction from sub second spiral computed tomography scans of the heart. *Med Phys* 1998;25:2417–2431.
32. Wong JW, Sharpe MB, Jaffray DA, et al. The use of active breathing control (ABC) to reduce margin for breathing motion. *Int J Radiat Oncol Biol Phys* 1999;44(4):911–919.
33. Connors SG, Battista JJ, Bertin RJ. On technical specifications of radiotherapy simulators. *Med Phys* 1984;11:341–343.
34. International Electrotechnical Commission. *Functional performance characteristics of radiotherapy simulators. Draft Report.* Geneva: IEC SubC 62C, 1990.
35. Bomford CK, et al. Treatment simulators. *Br J Radiol* 1989;(Suppl. 23):1–49.
36. National Council on Radiation Protection and Measurements. *Quality assurance for diagnostic imaging equipment.* Report No. 99;1988.
37. Boone JM, et al. AAPM Report No. 74. Quality control in diagnostic radiology. Report of Task Group No. 12;2002.
38. Kuthcer GJ, et al. AAPM Report No. 46. Comprehensive QA for radiation oncology. Report of Task Group No. 40. *Med Phys* 1994;21:581–617.
39. Lin PP-J, et al. AAPM report No. 39. Specification and acceptance testing of computed tomography scanners. Report of Task Group No. 2;1993.

CHAPTER 7

Treatment Planning Algorithms: Model-Based Photon Dose Calculations

Thomas R. Mackie ■ Hui Helen Liu ■ Edwin C. McCullough

INTRODUCTION

This chapter takes a different approach to photon dose calculations in radiotherapy. There are several good books and review articles on radiotherapy dose computation algorithms (1–8). In this chapter, we present the current status of computational approaches to predicting radiotherapy dose distributions.

Computational solutions for complex calculations have a predictable evolution. Computer algorithms in the sciences usually begin by mimicking procedures originally designed for hand calculations. Computers made it possible to gather, organize, and synthesize larger volumes of data to provide input for more complex descriptions of the problem. As computers become faster, new opportunities for increased precision or efficiency present themselves. Procedures that would be undreamed of without computers are described algorithmically. For example, computational meteorology began by storing statistical data of weather patterns so that meteorologists could perform their predictions faster. Soon, satellites were providing enormous quantities of data on cloud cover, rainfall, and wind velocity. These data now fuel meteorologic predictions using fluid and heat transport calculations that involve trillions of operations to model or simulate the global weather. Many sectors of the world economy now rely on accurate predictions for agriculture, air and sea transport, and disaster prediction. Radiotherapy treatment planning (RTP) has entered the modeling or simulation phase of computation.

To generate models, it is necessary to understand the system being modeled. In radiotherapy, the system of interest consists of patients and the equipment that delivers their treatments. With the advent of computed tomography (CT) and magnetic resonance imaging (MRI), reliable representations of an individual patient's anatomy can be obtained at millimeter resolution at reasonable time and cost. Linear accelerators have been routinely used for treating cancer since 1965, but detailed energy spectra about their photon beams were not a high priority. Monte Carlo simulations (MCSs) are routinely used to determine the radiation properties of treatment beams. This information is needed as input data for any model-based treatment planning system. Model-based dose algorithms are used as the basis for the current generation of treatment machines, which will deliver optimized or intensity-modulated radiotherapy (9). Model-based treatment planning demands understanding of the physics of ionizing radiation interactions. Therefore, this chapter provides a short review of the necessary radiologic physics presented in a nontechnical way. Before the background and details of model-based photon dose algorithms can be presented, the history and context of the field must be reviewed.

History of Computation Systems for Radiotherapy

Computerized RTP is more than 40 years old. The first computational techniques applied to radiotherapy are attributed to Tsien (10), who used punched cards to store digitized isodose charts so that the dose distribution from multiple beams could be summed. The dose distribution computed for ~500 points took approximately 10 to 15 minutes per beam. This was still much quicker than doing this work using tracing paper and a slide rule. The 1960s saw development of batch-processing computer planning systems. The first commercial treatment planning systems were introduced in the late 1960s (11). At the outset, commercial treatment planning systems had the following capabilities:

■ To store information on the radiation beams used in the clinic
■ To allow an outline of the patient to be entered
■ To plan the direction of the beam and the beam outline
■ To compute the dose distribution
■ To display the dose distribution with respect to the patient outlines

These features were not very mature in the earliest treatment planning systems. Given the capabilities of the beam and patient representations (e.g., a patient outline), it is not surprising that early dose algorithms were very simple.

The first commercial treatment planning was done on dedicated systems that operated on specialized hardware. The use of dedicated hardware was not isolated to radiotherapy but was the norm for radiology and most small specialized application systems as well. The credit for the use of generic computer systems for radiation treatment planning is attributable to academic institutions. Today, all treatment planning vendors are using generic treatment computer systems controlled by UNIX or Windows-based

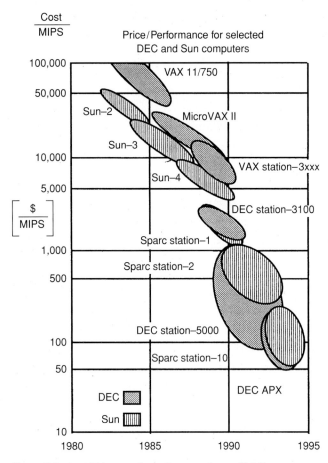

Figure 7.1. A rapid increase in performance is seen if dollars spent per performance (in units of millions of single instructions per second) is plotted for the recent past. The data, which reflect a range of performance characteristics and discounts, are accurate only within a factor of 2.

operating systems. This development allows treatment planning vendors to take advantage of economies of scale and the latest hardware, but most importantly, it lets them devote more time to software development. In addition, software upgrading, as well as hardware maintenance and longevity, is vastly improved.

Progress in RTP is driven by computer technology. The past 20 years have seen an explosive growth in the capabilities of computers. Figure 7.1 illustrates the price–performance ratio since 1980 in units of dollars spent per million instructions per second (MIPS). In 1980, a VAX computer from Digital Equipment Corporation could cost as much as $1 million and would be able to perform ~100,000 operations per second. In 2006, a $2,000 computer with an Intel Pentium 4 can perform approximately a billion operations in a second. Similar performance and price improvements have been achieved with other processors. While it is expected that for single-processor systems this growth will slow down during the next decade, multiple (parallel) processor systems are expected to keep the price–performance curve improving. Computer technology has affected RTP in several ways. Faster computers are enabling more advanced computation algorithms to enter

into clinical use. Three-dimensional (3D) RTP and the use of more sophisticated algorithms began with the advent of CT, which is required for accurate dose computation. CT and 3D RTP allow more complex beam arrangements, which in turn demands more advanced computation algorithms. Fast image manipulation such as volume rendering, has helped to promote and sell 3D treatment planning systems. These processes require fast computers that can in turn be used for more advanced dose computation algorithms.

There is and will continue to be in the near future a trade-off between accuracy and speed of dose computation. It is important to have a good match between the dose planning algorithms and the computer hardware. Since a great deal of time in modern treatment planning is spent segmenting regions of interest, there is no benefit if the dose computation algorithm is fast and not particularly accurate. Fast but relatively inaccurate algorithms do have a role when many beams must be computed and there is a great deal of iteration on the beam parameters. This occurs, for example, in stereotactic radiosurgery planning. At the opposite extreme, it is counterproductive to have an algorithm that is very accurate but takes an inordinate amount of time to compute. From the point of view of software vendors, it is important to keep software accuracy and speed balanced as the performance of computer systems increases. In many instances, it is useful to have quick calculation models for developing the early stages of a treatment plan.

The Representations of the Patient and the Dose Distribution

Patients have been represented in planning systems in a variety of ways. Hand calculations for monitor unit calculations represented the patient as a block of tissue with a surface normal to the beam at a specified source-to-surface distance (SSD). This representation was highly accurate when the field is rectangular, centered on the central axis, and incident normally on the patient, and when the skin contour is flat out to the extent of the field and the field is in a relatively homogeneous region. A moderate-sized treatment to the abdomen is an example. The simplest patient representations used in RTP systems were one or a few contour lines outlining the skin. These could be acquired in a number of ways, from solder wire surface contours to contours acquired from CT. The contours, entered or digitized into the planning system, represented the skin outline in two or three dimensions. Such procedures resulted in the patient being represented as a homogeneous composition (usually water) but do allow surface corrections to be applied. Patient heterogeneities could be represented in simple ways such as using closed contours like the surface representation. Each inhomogeneity had to be outlined individually, with a density assigned. This could usually be done semiautomatically on CT images for tissue such as lung or bone or for air cavities, where the contrast between tissues was sufficiently high. The electron density to assign to the region could be inferred from the CT number (12). The problem with this approach was that tissues such as lung and bone are not themselves homogeneous; there is a variation by ~50% for both bone and lung density. The lung density varies because blood pools from hydrostatic pressure differences.

All modern radiotherapy systems use a fully 3D point-by-point or voxel-by-voxel description of the patient. A CT image set of the treatment region constitutes the most accurate representation of the patient applicable for dose computation. This is because there is a fairly reliable one-to-one relationship between CT number and electron density (12) but this correspondence should be established for each kilovoltage energy setting on each CT scanner separately, and this relationship has to be ensured with ongoing calibrations. Dose algorithms that can use the density representation on a point-by-point basis are easier to use because contouring of the heterogeneities is typically not required. An exception to this is when contrast agents can produce a CT number in the bladder or a brain tumor that mimics bone. Usually, the contrast agent is used to aid in the tissue segmentation, and so only the additional step of providing a more realistic CT number in the segmented region is required to correct for the presence of the contrast agent. The spatial reliability of CT scanners is typically within 2% (which corresponds to ±20 in Hounsfield numbers). For photon beams, this uncertainty leads to dose uncertainties of <1% (12). The information in MRI is not strongly related to electron density. An MRI image set can also be more prone to artifacts during image formation. MRI may not replace reliable electron density information for dose computation, and CT will remain the major imaging modality in radiotherapy for the foreseeable future. The use of MRI as an adjuvant to CT will grow, as it is able to provide superior tissue contrast in many cases.

The resolution of the CT voxels and the spacing of the points at which the dose is computed (the dose grid resolution) should be matched. A CT volume set typically consists of 50 to 200 images with resolutions of $512 \times 512 \times 2$ bytes. The voxel is <1 mm in the transverse directions and 1 to 10 mm in the longitudinal direction. The image set requires 25 to 100 MB of storage. The spacing of the dose computation Cartesian grid points for photon beams is typically 1 to 10 mm on each side. Often, the CT slice thickness is chosen as the voxel size of the dose grid. Presently, a fine-resolution dose grid for photon beam calculations has spacing of $256 \times 256 \times$ the number of CT slices, so there is more resolution in the CT voxels than in the finest grid used to represent the dose computation. To get acceptable times for image manipulation, the entire CT volume has to be in memory at once. If this is not feasible, it may be appropriate to down-sample the CT image set to 256×256. This makes the transverse resolution more closely matched to that of the longitudinal direction and degrades the dose computation little. Degrading the resolution further than 256×256, results in unacceptable loss of detail.

There are five options to obtain quicker dose computations as follows:

1. Use a faster computer
2. Make the algorithm faster
3. Make the grid coarser
4. Restrict the region over which to compute the dose distribution
5. Allow a nonuniform sample spacing and optimize the points at which to do the calculation

The first solution is the industry standard because of the continually decreasing price–performance ratio. Many of the rest of these solutions have associated problems. As already discussed, making an algorithm faster often means making it less accurate. A coarser grid results in a poorer representation in the high-gradient region. Restricting the dose calculation volume may not be possible if the dose to a large organ has to be computed before a plan figure of merit, such as a dose-volume histogram, is assessed. The last option, while the most difficult to implement, is probably the best choice. The use of a nonuniform sample spacing can significantly speed up the dose computation because the dose does not have to be computed at finely spaced intervals in regions where the gradient is low. Therefore, more computations should be performed in high-gradient regions near beam boundaries.

BASIC RADIATION PHYSICS FOR MODEL-BASED DOSE COMPUTATION

Dose computation in external-beam radiotherapy predicts the dose produced by highly specialized linear-accelerator radiation sources. A basic look at important aspects of megavoltage x-ray production and interaction is required to understand the capabilities and limitations of model-based treatment planning algorithms.

The following are the only radiation physics topics absolutely required to understand treatment planning algorithms:

1. The production of megavoltage x-rays
2. The interaction and scattering of photons by the Compton effect
3. The effects of the transport of charged particles near boundaries and tissue heterogeneities

X-rays produced by fluorescence are unimportant. Interactions through the photoelectric effect do occur in materials with a high atomic number in the head of a linear accelerator, and pair production contributes a few percent to the attenuation of photons at the highest beam energies used, but these processes are far less important than the Compton effect.

Megavoltage Photon Production

Bremsstrahlung, or braking radiation, is produced when electrons interact with the strong Coulomb force produced by a nucleus and to a lesser extent by orbital electrons. The broad spectrum of photon beams produced by a linear accelerator typically has a peak of 1 to 2 MeV. The mean energy of the beam is roughly one-third of the nominal accelerating energy. Consequently, there is no dramatic change in the characteristics of megavoltage beams with energy. Megavoltage photon beams become somewhat more penetrating with energy, but the difference between a 10- and a 15-MV beam is much less than between a 100- and 150-kV x-ray beam.

The production of bremsstrahlung occurs when the high-energy electrons produced by the accelerator strike a target, usually consisting of tungsten. The size of the region from which primary photons are produced is one to a few millimeters (13). The finite size of the source results in a small amount of blurring of the edge of the field. The extent of the penumbra also depends on the distance from the collimators to the source.

A primary collimator, fabricated from a tungsten alloy, defines the maximum field diameter that can be used for treatment.

At megavoltage energies, bremsstrahlung is produced mainly in the forward direction. For example, at 10 MV, approximately twice as much photon energy fluence is produced along the central axis as is emitted at approximately 10 degrees from the central axis (14). In a few accelerator models no longer in production, the beam uniformity was obtained by scanning the electron beam before it struck the target. In most C-arm accelerators, to make the beam intensity more uniform, a conical filter positioned in the beam preferentially absorbs the flux along the central axis. In fact, usually the flattening filter slightly overflattens the field so that the intensity increases from the central axis toward the edge of the field. These intensity horns make the dose profile more uniform at depth by compensating for the loss of scatter dose near the edge of the field.

The presence of the field-flattening filter also alters the energy spectrum. The beam passing through the thicker central part of the filter has a higher proportion of high-energy photons and thereby produces a harder beam than does the beam passing through a thinner part of the filter closer to the field edge. Treatment units that are dedicated to IMRT, for example, the Hi-Art™ (TomoTherapy Inc., Madison, WI) helical tomotherapy system, do not have a field-flattening filter because if a uniform field is needed it can be modulated flat (15).

Figure 7.2 illustrates the production of bremsstrahlung photons in a target of a clinical linear accelerator and filtering the beam with a field-flattening filter.

Compton Scatter

Compton scatter influences several aspects of treatment planning with computed dosimetry. There are two general sources of scatter: the treatment head and the patient (or phantom). Production of scatter from either source depends in a complex way on the size and shape of the field. Scatter deep within the patient is mostly generated in the patient.

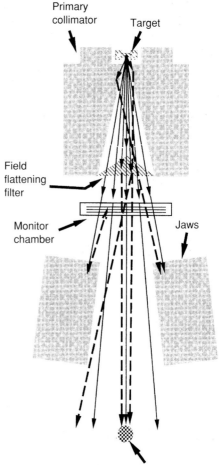

Figure 7.2. The treatment head of a clinical linear accelerator. Primary photons, produced in the target, are shown by the continuous lines. Scattered photons produced in the primary collimator, field-flattening filter, and collimator jaws are shown by dashed lines. These scattered photons have a relatively higher contribution to the photon fluence just outside the field. They are also responsible for the increase in the head-generated output factor as the collimator jaws are opened up.

However, at shallower depths and for higher-energy beams the accelerator-produced scatter contribution can be somewhat higher. Much of the complexity of computation-based treatment planning is due to quantifying the magnitude and spatial distributions of these sources of scatter.

While the primary x-ray beam can be thought of as being emitted at a finite source position, it is subsequently contaminated by electrons and photons scattered (extra-focal radiation) within the head (Fig. 7.2). This has been shown experimentally by several investigators (16–19). The primary collimator and the field-flattening filter produce most of the scatter dose generated by the accelerator head. The primary collimator is close to the target and defines the maximum field radius. More photons interact in this component than in any other in an accelerator, but the vast majority do not escape it. Those that scatter out of the primary collimator do so close to the target and therefore at small radial distances from the central axis. The field-flattening filter intercepts a large fraction of the photons incident on it, mostly by Compton scattering. The photons produced by the accelerator head must be mainly forward-directed to escape the accelerator. The energy spectrum of the accelerator-generated scattered photons overlaps with the primary beam's energy spectrum to a large extent (i.e., has nearly the same penetration characteristics as the primary beam), so the difference must be accounted for only quantitatively, not qualitatively. As the collimator jaws open, more scattered radiation is allowed to leave the treatment head. In addition, increasing the jaw opening decreases by a small amount the number of photons backscattered from the jaws into the monitor chamber. This causes the feedback circuit to increase the accelerator current. Both of these effects are reflected as an increase in the machine-generated output with field size, which is traditionally measured in air with a miniphantom (Fig. 7.2). This has been called *collimator scatter* (5). Even though the collimator jaws themselves contribute little forward scatter, they act as apertures for scatter produced higher in the treatment head. The photons scattered in the primary collimator and field-flattening filter also add to the photon fluence just outside the geometrical field boundary. Helical tomotherapy produces less proportion of scattered photons directed at the patient because of an absence of a field-flattening filter and because the scatter produced by the primary collimator tends to be trapped in downstream collimation.

Scattered photons produced in the patient, while directed mainly forward, contribute to dose in all directions. Like scatter produced by the machine, phantom scatter increases with the size of the field. However, for phantom-generated scatter, the penetration characteristics of the beam are also altered. As the field size increases, the phantom scatter causes the beam to be significantly more penetrating with depth. This effect is significant enough that dose computations, using measured dose distributions directly, must tabulate the penetration characteristics as a function of field size.

The behavior of scatter from beam modifiers such as wedges intermediate between the accelerator head and the patient can mimic the effects of either machine-generated or phantom-generated scatter. When the beam is small, a beam modifier mainly alters the transmission and does not contribute much scatter that arrives at the patient. A multiplicative correction factor (e.g., the wedge factor) that includes both attenuation and the small amount of scatter simply and effectively describes the altered dosimetric properties. However, when the field is large, beam modifiers begin to alter the penetration characteristics of the beam, much as phantom scatter does. For example, the increase in the wedge factor with increasing field size and depth is because of beam characteristics altered largely by scatter from the wedge (20,21).

Electron Transport

Photons are indirectly ionizing radiation. The dose is deposited by charged particles (electrons and positrons)

set in motion from the site of the photon interaction. At megavoltage energies, the range of charged particles can be several centimeters. The charged particles are mainly set in forward motion but are scattered considerably as they slow down and come to rest. The indirect nature of dose deposition results in several features in photon dose distributions.

The dose from an external photon beam builds up from the skin of the patient because of the increased number of charged particles being set in motion distal to the patient's surface. This results in a low skin dose, which spares the patient significant radiation injury. The dose builds up to a maximum at a depth, d_{max}, characteristic of the photon beam energy. At a point in the patient with a depth equal to the penetration distance of charged particles (which is somewhat greater than d_{max}), charged particles coming to rest are being replenished by charged particles set in motion, and charged particle equilibrium (CPE) is said to be reached. (Later, a distinction will be made between CPE and transient charged particle equilibrium [TCPE] that includes consideration for the reduction in the photon fluence with depth.) In this case, the dose at a point is proportional to the energy fluence of photons at the same point. The main criterion for CPE is that the energy fluence of photons must be constant out to the range of electrons set in motion in all directions. This does not occur in general in heterogeneous media, near the beam boundary, or for intensity-modulated beams.

Electrons produced in the head of the accelerator and in air intervening between the accelerator and the patient may be called *contamination electrons*. The interaction of these electrons in and just beyond the buildup region contributes significantly to the dose, especially if the field is large. Figure 7.3 illustrates contamination electron depth–ionization curves for a variety of megavoltage photon beams obtained by magnetically sweeping electrons out of the photon field (22). When the depth axis is normalized to the depth at which the contamination falls to 50% of its maximum value, the curves are nearly energy independent.

CPE does not exist near the field penumbra. In fact, for most linear accelerators most of the field penumbra is due to the fall of equilibrium as electrons that leave the field are not replenished from outside the field. CPE is established only at points farther from the field boundary than the lateral range of electrons.

Perturbation in electron transport can be exaggerated near heterogeneities. For example, the range of electrons is three to five times as long in lung as in water, and so beam boundaries passing through lung have much larger penumbral regions. Bone is the only tissue with an atomic composition significantly different from that of water. This can lead to perturbations in dose of only a few percent (23), and so perturbations in electron scattering or stopping power are rarely taken into account. Bone can therefore be treated as "high-density water."

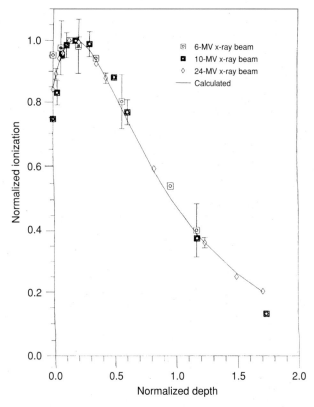

Figure 7.3. The contamination electron ionization as a function of normalized depth in an acrylic phantom. The line is a best fit of data from 6-, 10-, and 24-MV photon beams using the following equation:

$$I(X) = (0.847 + 0.833[1 - exp(-3.725\,X)])\,exp(-1.236X)$$

where $I(X)$ is the normalized ionization curve and X is the normalized depth defined by $X = d/d_{50}$. The d_{50} values in acrylic for the electron contamination components from 6-, 10-, and 24-MV photon beams are 0.89, 1.74, and 2.44 cm, respectively. To scale these d_{50} values to water, multiply by 1.11. (Reprinted from Jursinic PA, Mackie TR. Characteristics of secondary electrons produced by 6-, 10-, and 24-MV x-ray beams. *Phys Med Biol* 1996;41:1499–1509, with permission.)

ALGORITHMS FOR DOSE COMPUTATION

Traditionally, a patient dose distribution was based on correcting dose measurements obtained in a water phantom. Several types of corrections are applied as follows:

- Corrections for beam modifiers, such as wedges, blocks (irregular fields), and compensators, which take into account that a typical field is not the measured open field (i.e., without modifiers)
- Contour corrections, which take into account the irregular surface of the patient as opposed to the flat surface of a water phantom
- Heterogeneity corrections, which take into account that the patient consists of heterogeneous tissue densities instead of a homogeneous tank of water

The magnitude of the correction is much different for each type of correction. Beam modifier corrections are the most important. For example, 60 degrees beam wedges may result in the fluence under the heel (thick end) of the

wedge to be a factor of 3 to 5 less than under the toe of the wedge. Beam intensity in intensity-modulated radiotherapy may vary by a factor of 10. Heterogeneity corrections can result in −10% to +30% change in the dose distal to lung, depending on the size of the field and the lung thickness (24). Under conventional coplanar radiotherapy, contour corrections were the least important, especially if missing tissue compensators were used. Often, these compensators were designed on the basis of missing tissue only, and the errors in this inherent assumption were rarely >3% (25). However, contour corrections are more important than inhomogeneity corrections for relatively homogeneous treatment regions such as the abdomen.

The corrections modify the dose obtained from measurements taken under ideal reproducible conditions. In turn, the corrections are usually based on experiments under ideal conditions. In particular, heterogeneity corrections are based on measurements obtained in slab phantoms (e.g., cork sheets modeling lung) arranged perpendicular to the beam directions and done under open field conditions. Given this, it is somewhat surprising that this method works as well as it does. Noncoplanar radiotherapy with severe contour corrections may be delivered in combination with intensity-modulated beams that have been optimized taking into account internal heterogeneities. There is no reason to be optimistic about the ability of traditional correction-based methods to compute the dose accurately when there are radical corrections from measurements.

A different approach is in common use clinically (8). Instead of correcting measured dose distributions, the dose distributions are modeled from first principles. Measured dose distributions are used to set the parameters for the model and to provide verification of the computed dose. There is no well-defined demarcation between correction- and model-based algorithms, but rather a spectrum of algorithms running from those that only interpolate measured dose distributions to MCS. Correction-based methods usually have models on which to base the corrections, and model-based methods require some measurements to set parameters and verify the model. However, the approaches are operationally quite different. Correction-based algorithms use parameters of dose measured in water phantoms and correct the data to apply to the patient's specific situation. Model-based algorithms directly compute the dose to the patient by modeling the beam and its interactions in the patient representation.

With a model-based approach, there is a possibility to unify the operations inherent in achieving the corrections. Contour corrections can be treated as a special case of heterogeneity corrections by viewing the patient as extending into air. Before the advent of CT the patient contour could be obtained with a variety of devices, and it was possible to gather information to do contour corrections independently of heterogeneity corrections. For example, a Moire fringe device can obtain the whole contour surface. With CT planning it is more convenient to get contour information from the CT image set if the internal anatomy is needed for treatment planning anyway. Model-based algorithms that compute dose using a voxel-by-voxel heterogeneity from the CT values unify contour and heterogeneity calculations, and it can be even more work to perform contour corrections without heterogeneity calculations. In the future, the treatment machine and the in-room imaging system may be modeled as part of the patient. This so-called extended phantom model can take into account the machine-generated scatter (i.e., the head scatter) and compute the signal detected in the imaging system.

MODEL-BASED ALGORITHMS

There are both advantages and disadvantages in the use of a model-based dose algorithm. One disadvantage is that every feature must be explicitly included. For example, the dose buildup, penumbra, and phantom scatter are all present in the measured dose distribution without the need for explicit modeling. However, all these characteristics can be perturbed by patient representations and must be corrected. It is often more efficient and accurate to compute the dose distribution directly with a model that attempts to simulate the radiation transport. Another advantage is that fewer data usually must be acquired to implement the model, but this advantage is traded off because it is more difficult to fit the model parameters to the measurements. It is also more difficult to obtain agreement with the dose measurements than with lookups of parameterization of the measurements. However, this would be a true advantage only if our objectives were to irradiate tanks of water instead of patients.

It is illustrative to describe a simple hypothetical model-based algorithm before more complex models are described.

An Example of a Simple Model-Based Algorithm

3D dose algorithms have to determine the primary and scatter doses arriving at a point from all other points in the field. Assuming CPE, the primary dose D_p and the first-scattered dose from a parallel beam of monoenergetic photons can be computed analytically as follows:

$$D_p(\vec{r}) = (K_c(\vec{r}))_p = \left(\frac{\mu_{en}}{\rho}\right)_p \psi_p(\vec{r})$$

$$= \left(\frac{\mu_{en}}{\rho}\right)_p \phi_p(\vec{r} = 0) h\nu_p e^{-\mu|\vec{r}|} \qquad \text{Equation (7.1)}$$

where $\psi_p(\vec{r})$ and $(K_c(\vec{r}))_p$ are the *primary* energy fluence and collision kerma, respectively, at point $\vec{r}$, $\left(\frac{\mu_{en}}{\rho}\right)_p$ is the mass energy absorption coefficient, $\Phi_p(\vec{r} = 0)$ is the primary photon fluence at the surface of the phantom, $h\nu_p$ is the primary photon energy, and μ is the attenuation coefficient of

primary photons. The total dose is the sum of the primary and scatter components:

$$D_{tot}(\vec{r}) = D_p(\vec{r})$$
$$+ \int D_p(\vec{r}') \frac{(\mu_{en})_{scat}}{(\mu_{en})_p} \frac{(h\nu)_{scat}}{(h\nu)_p} \frac{dP_{scat}(\theta, \vec{r}')}{dV} e^{-\mu_{scat}(\vec{r}'-\vec{r})} dV$$

$$\text{Equation (7.2)}$$

where $dP_{scat}(\theta, \vec{r}')/dV$ is the probability per unit volume of a primary photon being scattered into a solid angle centered about angle θ.

These equations are complicated enough, but they do not take into account any higher-order scatter; they assume that the beam is parallel; they do not take into account heterogeneities; and they are valid only for CPE situations. The primary dose computation is not valid in the buildup region or near the field boundaries, and the scatter dose is perturbed by heterogeneities lying between the scatter site at $\vec{r}'$ and the point $\vec{r}$, where the total dose is being computed.

Convolution–Superposition Method

The convolution–superposition method is actually a class of model-based dose calculation methods that have been under development for a decade and a half by many investigators (4,23,26–38). This method is most commonly used in commercial treatment planning systems, largely because computers have become fast enough to do the calculations required in a reasonable time.

The convolution–superposition method begins by modeling the indirect nature of dose deposition from photon beams. Primary photon interactions are dealt with separately from the transport of scattered photons and electrons set in motion. Before the method is detailed, the roots of the method in classical dosimetry are explained.

Explanation of the Convolution Equation

The convolution method of dose calculation can be understood by considering the dose at a point $\vec{r}$ if there existed CPE. In the case of a monoenergetic beam with a mass energy absorption coefficient μ_{en}/ρ, the dose is given by:

$$D(\vec{r}) = \frac{\mu_{en}}{\rho} \psi(\vec{r}) = K_c(\vec{r}) \qquad \text{Equation (7.3)}$$

where $\psi(\vec{r})$ and $K_c(\vec{r})$ are the *total* energy fluence and collision kerma, respectively, at point $\vec{r}$.

Unfortunately, Equation 7.3 is simplistic because it does not take into account the forward finite range of charged particles. If the mean distance that charged particles travel downstream is $\vec{z}$, the energy fluence that set those charged particles in motion upstream should replace the energy fluence in Equation 7.3:

$$D(\vec{r}) = \frac{\mu_{en}}{\rho} \psi(\vec{r} - \vec{z}) \qquad \text{Equation (7.4)}$$

If it is assumed that the energy fluence increases exponentially as one moves upstream, then the dose can be specified in terms of energy fluence at point $\vec{r}$.

$$D(\vec{r}) = K_c(\vec{r})e^{\mu'|\vec{z}|} = K_c(\vec{r})\beta \qquad \text{EQUATION (7.5)}$$

where μ' is the effective attenuation coefficient and β is the value of the exponential term, which has a value somewhat larger than unity. β is also used in cavity theory to describe the forward transport of charged particles. When Equation 7.5 is true, TCPE is said to exist.

The convolution method can be thought of as a series of extensions of the equations describing TCPE. TCPE supposes that dose at a point arises because of photon interactions elsewhere. A simple extension is to allow multiple sites for the interaction of photons that generate charged particles. Rather than a single effective photon interaction site, this extension requires an integral over the neighborhood of

$$D(\vec{r}) = \int K_c(\vec{r}')A_c(\vec{r} - \vec{r}')d^3\vec{r}' \qquad \text{EQUATION (7.6)}$$

where $A_c(\vec{r} - \vec{r}')$ describes the contribution of charged particle energy that gets absorbed per unit volume at $\vec{r}$ from interactions at $\vec{r}'$ and the integration is over all values of $\vec{r}'$ that make up volume $d^3\vec{r}'$. The charged particle energy absorption kernel has a finite extent because the range of charged particles set in motion is finite and the energy partitioned to positron annihilation in flight, scattered photons, or bremsstrahlung photons by definition is not included.

There is an operational problem with Equation 7.6. It supposes that the collision kerma (or energy fluence) due to both primary and scattered photons is known at all points. Time-consuming transport methods, such as the method of discrete ordinates or the Monte Carlo method would be needed to compute the scattered component accurately. As we have seen, the primary contribution is much more easily computed. The dose that results from interaction of scattered photons can be included in the convolution kernel. Kernels that incorporate scatter partition the primary beam energy that is interacting, not just the energy that gets transferred to charged particles and subsequently absorbed locally. The kernel is now not finite because scatter is included in the kernel. Now only primary photons are explicitly transported. A convolution equation that separates primary photon transport and a kernel that accounts for the scatter photon and electrons set in motion away from the primary photon interaction site is as follows:

$$D(\vec{r}) = \int \frac{\mu}{\rho}\psi_p(\vec{r}')A(\vec{r} - \vec{r}')d^3\vec{r}'$$
$$= \int T_p(\vec{r}')A(\vec{r} - \vec{r}')d^3(\vec{r}') \qquad \text{EQUATION (7.7)}$$

where $\frac{\mu}{\rho}$ is the mass attenuation coefficient, $\psi_p(\vec{r}')$ is the primary energy fluence, and $A(\vec{r} - \vec{r}')$ includes the contribution of scatter. The product of the mass attenuation coefficient and the primary energy fluence is the primary *terma* (total

energy released per unit *mass*) $T_p(\vec{r}')$. Terma, first defined by Ahnesjö, Andreo, and Brahme (39), is analogous to kerma and collision kerma, and has the same units as dose.

The convolution kernels can, in principle, be obtained by analytic computation, deconvolution from dose distributions, or even by direct measurement (40). Most often, the kernels are computed with the Monte Carlo method by interacting a large number of primary photons at one location and determining from where energy is absorbed, that is from primary-generated charged particles, charged particles subsequently set in motion from scattered photons, or both (28,30,39,41). Figure 7.4 illustrates isovalue

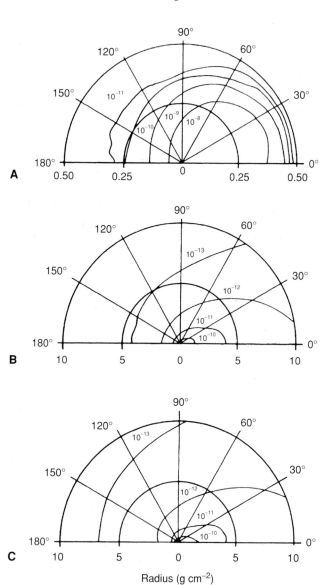

Figure 7.4. Cobalt-60 (more precisely, 1.25-MeV primary photons) kernels for water computed using Monte Carlo simulation (MCS). The isovalue lines are in units of cGy MeV^{-1} photon^{-1}. **A:** The contribution due to electrons set in motion from primary photons (i.e., the primary contribution). **B:** The first scatter contribution. **C:** The sum of the primary and all scatter contributions. (Reprinted from Mackie TR, Bielajew AF, Rogers DWO, et al. Generation of photon energy deposition kernels using the EGS4 Monte Carlo code. *Phys Med Biol* 1988;33:1–20, with permission.)

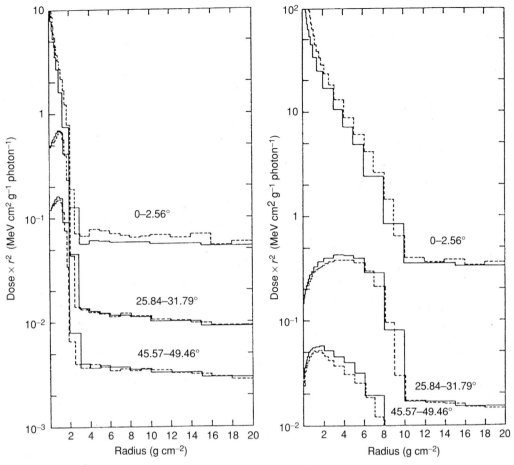

Figure 7.5. Comparison between kernels for water multiplied by r^2 for selected angular intervals. The continuous line is from Mackie et al. and the dashed lines are computed by C. Chui and R. Mohan (personal communication). The left side is for 5-MeV photons and the right side is for 20-MeV photons. (Reprinted from Mackie TR, Bielajew AF, Rogers DWO, et al. Generation of photon energy deposition kernels using the EGS4 Monte Carlo code. *Phys Med Biol* 1988;33:1–20, with permission.)

lines for a 1.25-MeV kernel in water. Even at this low energy, the kernel is mainly forward directed. As the energy increases, the kernel becomes even more forward peaked. Figure 7.5 compares two sets of Monte Carlo kernels along radial lines in several directions. The values have been multiplied by r^2 to eliminate inverse-square fall-off. The finite range of primary-photon-generated charged particles can easily be seen.

Modeling Primary Photons Incident on the Phantom

The convolution equation is restricted to describing monoenergetic parallel beams of primary photons interacting with homogeneous phantoms. The spectrum of a clinical linear accelerator is very difficult to measure. At present, the spectral information is derived from MCS benchmarked by measurement. Using the EGS4 Monte Carlo method, Mohan Chui (42) first quantified the spectrum of clinical accelerators using the Monte Carlo method. These simulations indicated that the spectrum at off-axis points is progressively softer than at the central axis. Chaney and Cullip (43) simulated photon transport

in clinical treatment heads using the Monte Carlo method and qualitatively confirmed the measurements discussed earlier. Lovelock et al. (44) performed simulations describing a scanned photon beam accelerator. Liu et al. (37) used the EGS4-based BEAM Monte Carlo code to model a Varian Clinac 2100 C accelerator (45). Figure 7.6 shows the SSD of photons that arrive at a plane at the isocenter. It is a plot derived by considering the origin along the central axis of all photons from each of the three sources of scatter high in the treatment head. The high narrow peak is from photons produced in the target. The broad peaks are due to scattered photons interacting in the primary collimator and the flattening filter.

Figure 7.7 shows that the mean energy of primary radiation (directly from the target) decreases off-axis, but the extrafocal photons (primary collimator and flattening filter) do not (37). The off-axis decrease of the photons directly from the source is due to hardening of the beam by the field-flattening filter. Since the direct photon component dominates, the model must take into account the change in the energy spectrum across the field.

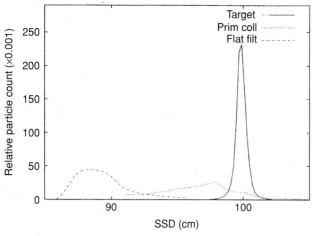

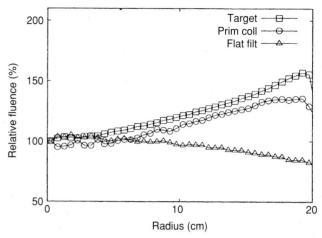

Figure 7.6. The distribution of source positions along the beam central axis generated by the major components of the treatment head; the target, primary collimator, and field-flattening filter. The BEAM Monte Carlo code (42) was used to obtain the results from the simulation of a 10-MV Varian Clinac 2100 C accelerator. The relative particle count is normalized to the total number of particles of the corresponding component that escape the head. For a 40 × 40 cm field, ~84% of the photons are directly from the target, 4% are from the primary collimator, 10% are from the field-flattening filter, and 2% are from all other sources, including the collimator jaws. SSD, source-to-surface distance. (Reprinted from Liu HH, Mackie TR, McCullough EC. A dual source photon beam model used in convolution–superposition dose calculations for clinical megavoltage x-ray beams. *Med Phys* 1997;24:1960–1974, with permission.)

Figure 7.8. The fluence distribution in an open 40 × 40 cm field from a 10-MV photon beam target, primary collimator, and field-flattening filter. The fluence is normalized to each of the component values at the central axis. (Reprinted from Liu HH, Mackie TR, McCullough EC. A dual source photon beam model used in convolution–superposition dose calculations for clinical megavoltage x-ray beams. *Med Phys* 1997;24:1960–1974, with permission.)

The model that describes the primary beam must be simple enough to be tractable, yet general enough to describe a variety of clinical beam conditions, including the influence of beam modifiers and collimator systems. Often, only a single-point source is used to model the photon

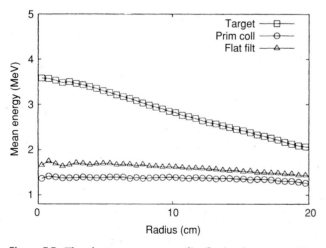

Figure 7.7. The photon mean energy distribution in an open 40 × 40 cm field from a 10-MV photon beam target, primary collimator, and field-flattening filter. Values are for in-air photons arriving at the plane of the isocenter. (Reprinted from Liu HH, Mackie TR, McCullough EC. A dual source photon beam model used in convolution–superposition dose calculations for clinical megavoltage x-ray beams. *Med Phys* 1997;24:1960–1974, with permission.)

beam, although this leads to limited accuracy in the dose distribution in the penumbra and outside the field. As indicated earlier, the three most important components of the clinical treatment head are the target, the primary collimator, and the field-flattening filter. In the Varian Clinac 2100 C, primary photons directly from the target contribute approximately 80% to 90%, the primary collimator contributes approximately 3% to 5%, and the field-flattening filter contributes approximately 8% to 12% of the photons arriving at the isocenter for large field sizes. Figure 7.8 shows the relative fluence at the isocenter as a function of radius from these components (37). Each component has been normalized to its value at the central axis. The target contribution increases off-axis because of overflattening of the beam.

Collimators and block field outlines are usually modeled with a mathematical *mask function*. For a collimator, the mask function inside the field is unity, and underneath the collimator it is equal to the primary collimator transmission. For a block, the mask function inside the field is the primary transmission through the block tray, and underneath the block it is equal to the primary block transmission. The mask function alone would not be able to model the penumbral blurring of the field boundary. This has been modeled by an *aperture function*. The mask function is convolved by a two-dimensional (2D) blurring kernel that represents the finite size of the source. The blurring kernel is usually assumed to be a normal function with a standard deviation equal to the projection of the source spot's width through the collimation system (thereby accounting for magnification of the source at large distances from the collimator system). Finally, the mask function is multiplied by the energy fluence distribution for the largest open field.

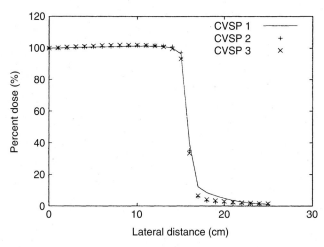

Figure 7.9. Dose profiles 5-cm deep for a 10-MV photon beam at 100-cm source-to-surface distance (SSD) and 30 × 30 cm field from three convolution–superposition calculations of the photon source. CVSP 1 uses both a source at the target and an extrafocal source; CVSP 2 uses only a source located at the target. Both CVSP 1 and CVSP 2 use results from Monte Carlo simulation (MCS). CVSP 3 uses a source position at the target approximated by a Gaussian distribution and a linear increase in energy fluence with radial position. CVSP, convolution–superposition. (Reprinted from Liu HH, Mackie TR, McCullough EC. A dual source photon beam model used in convolution–superposition dose calculations for clinical megavoltage X-ray beams. *Med Phys* 1997;24:1960–1974, with permission.)

The energy fluence outside the field is greater than can be accounted for by collimator transmission of the primary photons generated in the target. It can be modeled by adding short, broad normal distribution to the energy fluence. The source of this component is mainly the extrafocal radiation produced from Compton scattering in the field-flattening filter and to a smaller extent in the primary collimator, and it should be modeled with an upstream displacement. Figure 7.9 illustrates the difficulty in matching the dose outside the field unless the extrafocal radiation is explicitly included (37). The magnitude of the extrafocal radiation source can also be used to account for the variation in the machine-generated output factor, because the scatter outside the field and the increase in machine-generated output are both due to scatter from the primary collimator and the field-flattening filter (19,37).

Conventional wedges and compensators cannot be accurately modeled with primary attenuation only. These components produce scatter and cause differential hardening of the beam. The hardening of the primary beam can be accounted for according to the material of the wedge and the beam spectrum as a function of radial position. Scatter from the wedge is more difficult to account for. The increased scatter results in the wedge factor increasing by a few percent as a function of field size. This can be adequately modeled by a field size-dependent factor that duplicates the effect. Alternatively, the wedge or compensator can be included as part of the patient representation. This extended phantom has a large heterogeneity in it, namely, the air gap between the device and the patient. This

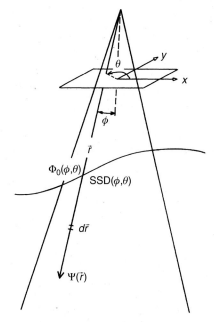

Figure 7.10. The ray-tracing of a two-dimensional (2D) energy fluence distribution through the patient to create a three-dimensional (3D) energy fluence distribution in the patient. SSD, source-to-surface distance.

method can predict the variation in the wedge factor as a function of field size. Another example of an extended phantom will be discussed later.

Ray-Tracing the Incident Energy Fluence Through the Phantom

The incident 2D energy fluence distribution is ray-traced through the patient to create a 3D distribution of energy fluence (Fig. 7.10). The density of the rays followed and the sampling of the rays along their path must be sufficient to represent the attenuation behavior of the phantom. Sufficient sampling density is especially important for head, neck, and breast tangential fields. In general, the sampling density required is higher than the dose resolution desired, so several rays are traversing each calculation voxel. Inverse-square fall-off is accounted for explicitly rather than allowing the sample density to reduce through divergence implicitly.

The operation to determine the terma is not as straightforward as it seems. As the ray traverses the phantom, it is attenuated. The primary ray attenuation coefficient, weighted to the appropriate beam spectrum, is based on the voxel properties (usually CT number is sufficient to determine both density and material composition for the purposes of dose computation). The energy fluence at a sample point is reduced from the previous sample along the ray, and the result multiplied by the mass attenuation coefficient yields the terma sample for the point. Hardening of the primary energy fluence spectrum with depth and off-axis position is accomplished by changing the attenuation coefficient with position. The speed of the ray-tracing operation can be improved significantly by the use of lookup tables to store precomputed results. The terma for the voxel is the average of the samples in the voxel corrected for inverse-square falloff.

Electron Contamination

The electron contamination of the beam is not accounted for in the conventional convolution method. The surface dose from megavoltage photon beams is almost entirely due to the electron contamination component. Studies in which the electron contamination has been removed by magnetically sweeping electrons from the field reveal that dose from the contaminating electrons resembles an electron beam with a practical range somewhat greater than the depth of maximum dose, which is expected from the theoretical grounds discussed earlier (Fig. 7.3). A reasonable agreement with measured depth–dose curves can be obtained by scaling the contamination electron depth–dose curve with the surface dose and adding this component to the convolution-computed dose distribution. Alternatively, the extended phantom concept can be used to merge the entire treatment unit into the patient representation.

Kernel Spatial Variance and Phantom Heterogeneities

The convolution equation assumes that the kernel is spatially invariant in that the kernel value depends only on the relative geometrical relationship between the interaction and dose deposition sites and not on their absolute position in the phantom. When this is true, the convolution calculation can be done in Fourier space, saving much time. Unfortunately, this will not result in an algorithm that is generally useful.

The effects of hardening and divergence of the beam are small and can be calculated in a number of ways. A multiplicative correction to the terma in the patient can be used to correct for hardening of the kernel (36,46). Alternatively, several kernels valid for different depths in the phantom can be used as a basis for interpolation to a specific depth (36,38). Figure 7.11 illustrates a comparison between convolution–superposition calculations with kernel hardening and without it as compared with MCS for a 10-MV beam. It shows that the correction as a function of depth is nearly linear, and not employing any correction results in ~4% discrepancy at 30-cm depth. Explicitly tilting the kernel to match the beam divergence is an expensive computer operation and results in only a few percent improvements in accuracy for the worst-case examples with small SSDs and large field widths (38).

Phantom heterogeneities are a more serious problem. To model the transport of electrons and scattered photons through a heterogeneous phantom would require a unique kernel at each location. Each kernel would be superimposed on the dose grid and weighted with respect to the primary terma. What is required to make the calculation tractable is to modify a kernel, computed in a homogeneous medium, to be reasonably representative in a heterogeneous situation. If most of the energy between the primary interaction site and the dose deposition site is transported on the direct path between these sites, it is possible to have a relatively simple correction to the con-

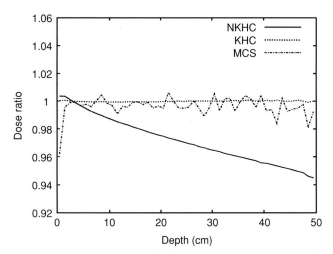

Figure 7.11. The effect of kernel hardening on the central axis for a field 10×10 cm from a parallel 10-MV photon beam. The no-kernel-hardening correction (NKHC) and kernel-hardening correction (KHC) are compared with the Monte Carlo simulation (MCS) result. The result has been normalized to the convolution–superposition method done with a convolution calculation for every spectral bin. One standard deviation of statistical uncertainty of the MCS is ±1%. (Reprinted from Liu HH, Mackie TR, McCullough EC. Correcting kernal tilting and hardening in convolution/superposition dose calculations for clinical divergent and polychromatic photon beams. *Med Phys* 1997;24:1729–1741, with permission.)

volution equation based on ray-tracing between the interaction and dose deposition sites, and on scaling the path length by density to get the radiologic path length between these sites. The convolution equation modified for radiologic path length is called the superposition equation:

$$D(\vec{r}) = \int T_p(\rho_{\vec{r}'} \cdot \vec{r}') A(\rho_{\vec{r}-\vec{r}'} \cdot (\vec{r} - \vec{r}')) d^3\vec{r}' \quad \text{EQUATION (7.8)}$$

where $\rho_{\vec{r}-\vec{r}'} \cdot (\vec{r} - \vec{r}')$ is the radiologic distance from the dose deposition site to the primary photon interaction site and $\rho_{\vec{r}'} \cdot \vec{r}'$ is the radiologic distance from the source to the photon interaction site.

Woo and Cunningham (34) compared the modified kernel using range scaling for a complex heterogeneous phantom with a kernel computed *de novo* for a particular interaction site inside the phantom. The results shown in Figure 7.12 indicate that agreement is not perfect, but the computational trends are clearly in evidence in that isovalue lines contract in high-density regions and expand in low-density regions. Figure 7.13 indicates that the superposition method can compute the absolute dose per unit fluence in a simulated thorax phantom nearly as well as MCS (47). The dose calculation is accurate despite the electronic disequilibrium that is owing to a perturbation in electron transport in the heterogeneous phantom.

The superposition method has been used to predict the dose in even more highly heterogeneous situations. For example, it has been used to predict the dose to an image plane distal to a complex phantom. The method applied to this extended phantom had to account for the scatter

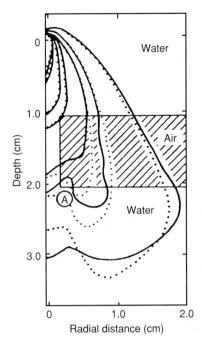

Figure 7.12. Comparison of Monte Carlo–generated 6-MeV primary photon kernel in a water phantom containing a ring of air. The dashed line is a kernel modified for the heterogeneous situation using range scaling from one derived in a homogeneous phantom. The continuous line is a kernel computed expressly for the heterogeneous situation. It is impractical to compute kernels for every possible heterogeneous situation, and there is sufficient similarity to warrant the range scaling approximation. (Reprinted from Woo MK, Cunningham JR. The validity of the density scaling method in primary electron transport for photon and electron beams. *Med Phys* 1990;17:187–194, with permission.)

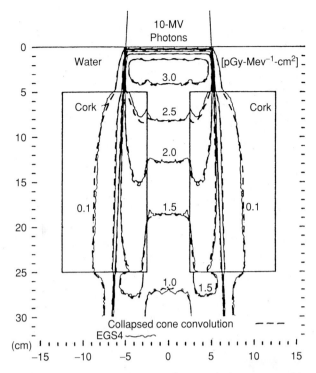

Figure 7.13. Comparison between the convolution–superposition method and EGS4 Monte Carlo simulation (MCS) for a simulated thorax phantom for a 10 × 10 cm 10-MV photon beam. (Reprinted from Ahnesjo A. Collapsed cone convolution of radiant energy for photon dose calculations in heterogeneous media. *Med Phys* 1999;16:577–592, with permission.)

through a large gap to the imaging plane. This method can also be used to invert the problem so as to reconstruct the dose in a phantom on the basis of an electronic image (48). An example using an anthropomorphic thorax phantom is shown in Figure 7.14.

Direct Monte Carlo Treatment Planning

The Monte Carlo technique of radiation transport consists of using well-established probability distributions governing the individual interactions of electrons and photons to simulate their transport through matter. Scoring physical quantities of interest for a large number of simulated particles (*histories*) provides information about average transport properties and the associated distributions, including the deposition of energy (49–53).

MCS is vital for model-based dose computation. It is used to characterize the clinical beam, to produce convolution kernels, and as computation benchmarks. It is possible to use MCS directly to compute photon dose distributions. It is possible to restart histories emerging from MCSs of the heads of clinical accelerator, but the information on the particle states required to do this is prohibitively large. Typical file sizes are several hundred megabytes. More practically, it is possible to use instead the beam characterization models used for the convolu-

tion–superposition, which have, in any case, been set up largely using the results of MCS.

Figure 7.15 shows a fine-resolution dose distribution for a three-field treatment to the sinus produced with the Peregrine Monte Carlo system developed at Lawrence Livermore National Laboratory (50). The dose from a small to a very large number of histories is illustrated. This calculation would take approximately an hour.

More progress has been made for electron beams, because the number of histories required to produce an electron beam dose distribution is about an order or magnitude fewer than for a photon beam. In computational terms, an order of magnitude of reduction in calculation time can be achieved in less than a half decade of performance–price improvements. It is only a matter of time before Monte Carlo treatment planning is commonplace.

The Monte Carlo method reduces the uncertainty from systematic errors at the expense of introducing stochastic or random uncertainties. The greater the number of histories, the smaller is the uncertainty. Ignoring the effects of attenuation and scattering, the number of simulated particles (histories) that has to be directed toward a target volume is approximately given by:

$$N = \frac{A}{\mu \sigma^2 \ell^3} \qquad \text{Equation (7.9)}$$

where A is the exposed beam area, σ is the percent relative error (i.e., the ratio of standard deviation to the mean

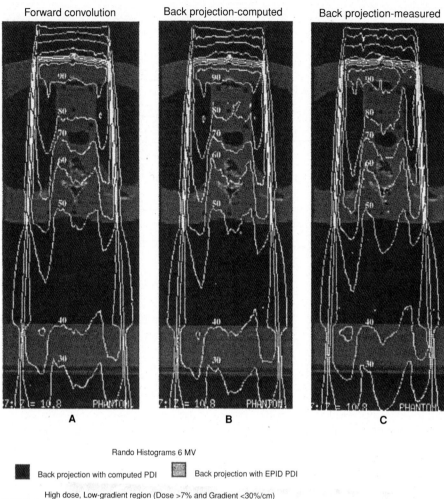

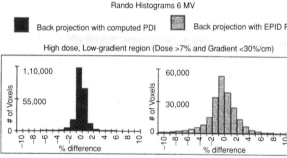

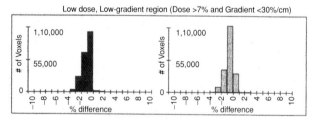

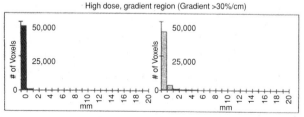

Figure 7.14. The feasibility of modeling dose distributions from portal dose images (PDIs) using the concept of the extended phantom. The upper set of images is isodose lines displayed on computed tomography (CT) data for the Rando thorax phantom on top of a simulated portal dose imaging system. **A:** The forward convolution–superposition method. **B:** Backprojection using the predicted PDI obtained from the forward computation. **C:** Backprojection using the measured PDI from the Varian PortalVision electronic portal imaging system. The lower graphs display error histograms as compared with the forward convolution–superposition calculation. The backprojection, based on the predicted PDI, is a measure of the results if the portal imaging system was noise- and artifact-free. This shows that because the convolution–superposition method is sufficiently accurate, it is possible to reconstruct the dose patients received given an accurate patient representation at the time of treatment and an accurate portal dose imaging system. EPID, electronic portal imaging device. (Reprinted from McNutt TR, Mackie TR, Reckwerdt PJ, et al. Modeling dose distributions from PDIs using the convolution/superposition method. *Med Phys* 1996;23:1381–1392, with permission.)

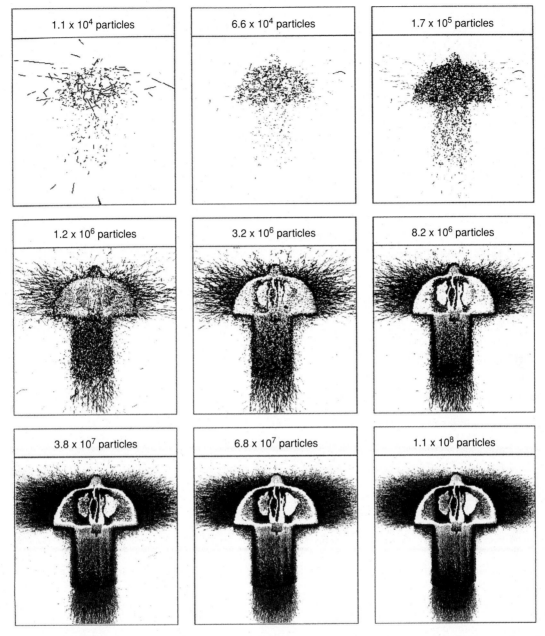

Figure 7.15. Monte Carlo simulation (MCS) of a three-field photon treatment to the sinus using varying number of incident particle histories. (Courtesy of Christine Hartmann-Siantar and William Chandler, Lawrence Livermore National Laboratory.)

expressed as a fraction) being sought, μ is the attenuation coefficient, and l is a typical voxel dimension. To obtain a 0.02 relative error (i.e., 2%) in a 100 cm^2 field for a beam with an attenuation coefficient of 0.05 cm^{-1} (typical for a 6-MV beam) interacting in a phantom with voxel dimensions of 0.5 cm to a side would require 40 million histories. This assumes that there need to be no photons directed outside the field. One advantage is that with the Monte Carlo method it does not matter whether the photons are directed at the target from one direction or many; the same number of histories can be used. The Monte Carlo method, therefore, may take less time than analytic techniques for rotational or multiple-beam techniques.

CONCLUSIONS

RTP was one of the first applications of computation in health care. Its rapid advance is due to the tremendous advances in modern computational performance and improved patient representations obtained from CT and MRI imaging.

RTP has entered the model-building phase of computation. This natural evolution inherent in scientific computation is driven by the need to handle more input data and to increase capabilities. Photon beam techniques such as intensity-modulated radiotherapy have put demands on the traditional dose computation models that they were not designed to deal with. Rather than patch together further corrections of measurement-based dose computations, model-based dose calculations predict the dose distributions from first principles.

Model-based dose calculations require a great deal of attention to the details of the photon transport in the linear accelerator head. The distribution of fluence and energy emerging from the accelerator can be obtained with MCS. This information can be used to set parameters for relatively simple beam characterizations that can be used both for the convolution–superposition method and MCS.

Several examples of model-based photon beam dose computations have been described. The most effort has been spent on the convolution–superposition method, which is capable of computing dose distributions in situations of electronic disequilibrium and is in common use. In the future, the Monte Carlo method will gain acceptance as the price–performance ratio of computers continues to drop.

REFERENCES

1. Cunningham JR. Tissue inhomogeneity corrections in photon-beam treatment planning. In: Orton CG, ed. *Progress in medical physics, Vol. 1.* New York, NY: Plenum Publishing, 1983:103–131.
2. Johns HE, Cunningham JR. *The physics of radiology.* Springfield: Charles C Thomas Publisher, 1983.
3. Wong JW, Purdy JA. On methods of inhomogeneity corrections for photon transport. *Med Phys* 1990;17:807–814.
4. Battista JJ, Sharpe MB. True three-dimensional dose computations for megavoltage x-ray therapy: a role for the superposition principle. *Australas Phys Eng Sci Med* 1992;15:159–178.
5. Khan FM. *The physics of radiation therapy.* Baltimore, MD: Williams & Wilkins, 1994.
6. Mackie TR, Reckwerdt P, Papanikolaou N. 3D photon beam dose algorithms. In: Purdy JA, Emami B, eds. *3D radiation therapy planning and conformal therapy.* Madison: Medical Physics Publishing, 1995.
7. Cunningham JR, Battista JJ. Calculation of dose distributions for x-ray therapy. *Phys Can* 1995;51:190–218.
8. Mackie TR, Reckwerdt P, McNutt T, et al. Photon beam dose computations. In: Mackie TR, Palta JR, eds. *Teletherapy: present and future.* College Park, MD: American Association of Physicists in Medicine, 1996.
9. Webb S. *The physics of three-dimensional radiation therapy.* Bristol, UK: Institute of Physics Publishing, 1993.
10. Tsien KC. The application of automatic computing machines to radiation treatment planning. *Br J Radiol* 1955; 28:432–439.
11. Sontag MR. *Photon beam dose calculations in regions of tissue heterogeneity using computed tomography,* Dissertation. Toronto: University of Toronto, 1979.
12. Sontag MR, Battista JJ, Bronskill MJ, et al. Implications of computed tomography for inhomogeneity corrections in photon beam dose calculations. *Radiology* 1977;124: 143–149.x

13. Jaffray DA, Battista JJ. X-ray sources of medical linear accelerators: focal and extra focal radiation. *Med Phys* 1993;20:1417–1427.
14. Sharf W. *Particle accelerators: applications in technology and research.* New York, NY: John Wiley & Sons, 1989.
15. Mackie TR, Olivera GH, Kapatoes JM. Helical tomotherapy. In: Palta J, Mackie TR, eds. *Intensity-modulated radiation therapy: the state of the art.* Madison, WI: Medical Physics Publishing, 2003.
16. Munro P, Rawlinson J, Fenster A. Therapy imaging: source sizes of radiotherapy beams. *Med Phys* 1988;15:517–524.
17. Lutz WR, Maleki N, Bjarngard B. Evaluation of a beam-spot camera for megavoltage x rays. *Med Phys* 1988;15:614–617.
18. Loewenthal E, Loweinger E, Bar-Avraham E, et al. Measurement of the source size of a 6- and 18-MV radiotherapy linac. *Med Phys* 1992;19:687–690.
19. Sharpe MB, Jaffray DA, Battista JJ, et al. Extrafocal radiation: a unified approach to the prediction of beam penumbra and output factors for megavoltage x-ray beams. *Med Phys* 1995;22:2065–2074.
20. McCullough EC, Cortney J, Blackwell CR. A depth dependence determination of the wedge transmission factor for 4 to 10 MV photon beams. *Med Phys* 1988;15: 621–623.
21. Palta J, Daftari I, Suntharalingham N. Field size dependence of wedge factors. *Med Phys* 1988;15:624–626.
22. Jursinic PA, Mackie TR. Characteristics of secondary electrons produced by 6, 10, and 24 MV x-ray beams. *Phys Med Biol* 1996;41:1499–1509.
23. Sauer OA. Calculation of dose distributions in the vicinity of high-Z interfaces for photon beams. *Med Phys* 1995;22: 1685–1690.
24. Mackie TR, El-Khatib E, Battista JJ, et al. Lung dose corrections for 6 and 15 MV x-rays. *Med Phys* 1985;12:327–332.
25. Jursinic PA, Podgorsak MB, Paliwal BR. Implementation of a three-dimensional compensation system based on computed tomography generated surface contours and tissue inhomogeneities. *Med Phys* 1994;21:357–365.
26. Dean RD. A scattering kernel for use in true three-dimensional dose calculations (Abstract). *Med Phys* 1980; 7:429.
27. Mackie TR, Scrimger JW, Battista JJ. A convolution method of calculating dose for 15 MV x-rays. *Med Phys* 1985;12: 188–196.
28. Boyer AL, Mok EC. A photon dose distribution model employing convolution calculations. *Med Phys* 1985;12: 169–177.
29. Boyer AL, Mok EC. Calculation of photon dose distributions in an inhomogeneous medium using convolutions. *Med Phys* 1986;13:503–509.
30. Mohan R, Chui C, Lidofsky L. Differential pencil beam dose computation model for photons. *Med Phys* 1986;13:64–73.
31. Field GC, Battista JJ. *Photon dose calculations using convolution in real and Fourier space: assumptions and time estimates. Proceedings of the ninth international conference on computers in radiation therapy.* Amsterdam: Elsevier Science, 1987:103–106.
32. Mackie TR, Ahnesjö A, Dickof P, et al. *Development of a convolution/superposition method for photon beams. Proceedings of the ninth international conference on the use of computers in radiation therapy.* Amsterdam: Elsevier Science, 1987:107–110.

33. Kubsad SS, Mackie TR, Gehring MA, et al. Monte Carlo and convolution dosimetry for stereotactic radiosurgery. *Int J Radiat Oncol Biol Phys* 1990;19:1027–1035.
34. Woo MK, Cunningham JR. The validity of the density scaling method in primary electron transport for photon and electron beams. *Med Phys* 1990;17:187–194.
35. Metcalfe PE, Hoban PW, Murray DC, et al. Beam hardening of 10 MV radiotherapy x-rays: analysis using a convolution/superposition method. *Phys Med Biol* 1990;35:1533–1549.
36. Papanikolaou N, Mackie TR, Meger-Wells C, et al. Investigation of the convolution method for polyenergetic spectra. *Med Phys* 1993;20:1327–1336.
37. Liu HH, Mackie TR, McCullough EC. A dual source photon beam model used in convolution/superposition dose calculations for clinical megavoltage x-ray beams. *Med Phys* 1997;24:1960–1974.
38. Liu HH, Mackie TR, McCullough EC. Correcting kernel tilting and hardening in convolution–superposition dose calculations for clinical divergent and polychromatic photon beams. *Med Phys* 1997;24:1729–1741.
39. Ahnesjö A, Andreo P, Brahme A. Calculation and application of point spread functions for treatment planning with high energy photon beams. *Acta Oncol* 1987;26:49–56.
40. O'Connor JE, Malone DE. A cobalt-60 primary dose spread array derived from measurements. *Phys Med Biol* 1989;34:1029–1042.
41. Mackie TR, Bielajew AF, Rogers DWO, et al. Generation of photon energy deposition kernels using the EGS4 Monte Carlo code. *Phys Med Biol* 1988;33:1–20.
42. Mohan R, Chui C. Energy and angular distributions of photons from medical linear accelerators. *Med Phys* 1985;12:592–597.
43. Chaney EL, Cullip TJ. A Monte Carlo study of accelerator head scatter. *Med Phys* 1994;21:1383–1390.
44. Lovelock DMJ, Chui CS, Mohan R. A Monte Carlo model of photon beams used in radiation therapy. *Med Phys* 1995;22:1387–1394.
45. Rogers DWO, Faddegon BA, Ding GX, et al. BEAM: a Monte Carlo code to simulate radiotherapy treatment units. *Med Phys* 1995;22:505–524.
46. Hoban PW, Murray DC, Round WH. Photon beam convolution using polyenergetic energy deposition kernels. *Phys Med Biol* 1994;39:669–685.
47. Ahnesjö A. Collapsed cone convolution of radiant energy for photon dose calculations in heterogeneous media. *Med Phys* 1989;16:577–592.
48. McNutt TR, Mackie TR, Reckwerdt PJ, et al. Modeling dose distributions from portal dose images using the convolution/superposition method. *Med Phys* 1996;23:1381–1392.
49. Mackie TR. Applications of the Monte Carlo method in radiotherapy. In: Kase KR, Bjarngard BE, Attix FH, eds. *The dosimetry of ionizing radiation, Vol. 3.* San Diego: Academic Press, 1990:541–620.
50. Rogers DWO, Bielajew AR. Monte Carlo techniques of electron and photon transport for radiation dosimetry. In: Kase KR, Bjarngard BE, Attix, eds. *The dosimetry of ionizing radiation, Vol. 3.* San Diego: Academic Press, 1990:427–539.
51. Hartmann-Siantar CL, Chandler WP, Weaver KA, et al. Validation and performance assessment of the peregrine all-particle Monte Carlo code for photon beam therapy. *Med Phys* 1996;23:1128.
52. Ma CM, Mok E, Kapur A, et al. Clinical implementation of a Monte Carlo treatment planning system. *Med Phys* 1999;26:2133–2143.
53. Wyatt M, Corredor C, Tamimi M, et al. Comparison of treatment planning dose calculations with measurements and Monte Carlo calculations in a RANDO phantom. *Radiat Prot Dosim* 2005;116:461–465.

Treatment Planning Algorithms: Brachytherapy

Kenneth J. Weeks

INTRODUCTION

Brachytherapy involves the treatment of cancer using the photon, electron, and positron emissions from radioisotopes. Brachytherapy was developed using naturally occurring radioisotopes such as radium 226. The history, applications, and emission details of radioisotopes are described in Chapter 17 and elsewhere (1–4). It is the goal of brachytherapy treatment planning to determine how many sources, their individual strengths, and the location of each source relative to the treatment volume, so as to treat a volume to a given minimum dose while respecting tolerances of normal tissues. It is important to note that the original brachytherapy clinical applications were developed realizing that brachytherapy demanded three-dimensional (3D) planning because the sources were distributed in three dimensions. Because of this fact and the absence of computers, these original treatment systems were all inclusive. They were systems with rules for distributing the sources, rules for picking and arranging source strengths, and given the latter, precalculated dose-rate tables for determining the dose to a point. The Manchester, Paris, Stockholm, Memorial, and Quimby systems (1–4) all specified in alternate ways how to do this for interstitial and intracavitary implants. See Chapter 17 for discussion of these systems. From this history, we can obtain knowledge of the range of the radioactive source applications, which is important in devising dose calculation algorithms. Thus, we summarize guidelines, which include the following. When distributing lines of sources, attempt to keep them spaced no closer than 8 mm (smaller volumes) and no farther than 2 cm (larger volumes) apart. The periphery of the treatment volume is generally not much farther than 5 cm from the center of gravity of the source distribution. The very high doses close (<5 mm) to the sources are not prescribed or evaluated as to clinical significance. At distances >10 cm from the center of the implant, the dose delivered is low and the precise dose is not considered a treatment objective. Therefore, we conclude that dose calculation algorithms that are very accurate from 5 mm to 5 cm and generally accurate to 10 cm are required. The availability of computers and advanced imaging capabilities means that precalculated dose tables for predetermined patterns of multiple sources are no longer required. Calculation of the dose distribution for the individual patient's source distribution is possible.

Radioisotopes decay randomly with a time-independent probability (1,3,5,6). If there are N_0 radioactive atoms at time $t = 0$, then at a later time t, we have $N(t)$ atoms given by

$$N(t) = N_0 e^{-\lambda t} \qquad \text{EQUATION (8.1)}$$

where λ ($= 0.693 / T_{1/2}$) is the radioisotope's decay constant and $T_{1/2}$ is the half-life (time it takes for half of the sample to decay). The activity (A) at time t is proportional to the number of radioactive atoms present and is defined by

$$A(t) = \lambda N(t) = A_0 e^{-\lambda t} \qquad \text{EQUATION (8.2)}$$

where A_0 is the initial activity. Throughout the following, we will consider the calculation of the dose rate, $\dot{D}$ (in cGy/h). The total dose D delivered during an implant, which lasts for time t, is found from the initial dose rate, $\dot{D}_0$, at the start of the implant from

$$D(t) = \dot{D}_0 (1 - e^{-\lambda t}) / \lambda \qquad \text{EQUATION (8.3)}$$

For the case $t \gg T_{1/2}$ (e.g., a permanent implant), the total dose (D) is simply $D = 1.44\, T_{1/2} \dot{D}_0$, whereas if $t \ll T_{1/2}$, then $D = t\dot{D}_0$. Throughout the following, we will calculate the dose rate at the start of the implant ($\dot{D}_0$). The total dose delivered in time t is then found from Equation 8.3.

The isotope emits energy (in the form of photons, electrons, and sometimes positrons) in all directions and that energy is absorbed in the mass (tissue) around the isotope, giving rise to absorbed dose (absorbed energy/mass). The calculation of dose rate depends on the number of radioactive atoms, the types and energies of the emitted particles, the time rate of emission of those particles, and finally the energy absorption and scattering properties of the surrounding media and the radioactive material itself. In this chapter, we will begin with the simplest case of a point source. From there we will use the point source result to determine the dose rate for an ideal line source and then a real clinical cylindrical source. Finally, we will obtain the dose rate distribution for a 3D source/shield/applicator via numerical integration of the point source result. Various intermediate parameterized calculation methods are discussed. This leads inevitably to systems, which explicitly model the flow of energy from the radioactive sources. These include Monte Carlo and Boltzmann transport theory. These latter techniques owe their existence to the extensive computation power now available. The advantages and disadvantages of these methods will be discussed.

CALCULATION OF DOSE RATES AROUND A POINT SOURCE

A point source is the simplest situation to calculate. The first approximation, used in radiation oncology, is to ignore the charged particle emissions and consider only the photons. The significance of this approximation is best understood by reviewing the basic nuclear decay data (7). Consider the well-known ^{192}Ir, which has a half-life of 73.8 days and decays via β decay (95%) or electron capture (5%). The decay of a single ^{192}Ir nucleus produces on average 2.38 photons (there are 44 possible photon energies ranging from 7.8 to 1,378 keV, which can be emitted in a single decay event) and 0.95 β-decay electrons (with the β decay continuous energy spectrum ranging from 0 to 669 keV). In addition, atomic electrons can be emitted with various discrete energies ranging from 11 to 1,378 keV. In a single decay, the average total energy output from photons is 813 keV (note the average energy of the photons is therefore 341 keV from 813 keV/2.38) and the average electron energy output is 216 keV (7). Therefore, the total average energy output per decay is 1,029 keV. Our decision to ignore the emitted electrons means that we are going to ignore around 21% of the total energy output from the source in our dose-rate calculations. Why is this justified? The reason is that practical commercial sources used for radiation oncology will be encapsulated radionuclides and that encapsulation will scatter and slow down the electrons such that most do not leave the source capsule itself and for those that do escape, their range in tissue outside the source is much smaller than 5 mm and thus will not contribute dose at a clinical prescription distance. This encapsulation of the source is essential for the clinical use of most isotopes used in radiation oncology. Historically, in the early days of radiotherapy, in the United States, a clever technique to enclose radon gas in glass capsules was developed. The high energy of the β particles and the light filtration led to unfavorable clinical results (4). We end this discussion with the observation that there can be a major clinical dose distribution difference between an encapsulated and an insufficiently encapsulated radionuclide.

Consider a sample of radioactive material whose largest dimension is much smaller than 0.1 mm. This will be small enough so that all atoms can be approximately considered as located at a single point. Restricting ourselves to the photon emissions from the point source, we will first think about the dose rate produced in a small volume (dV) of tissue located at a distance (r) from the source. For simplicity, consider the source in vacuum (so no scatter)

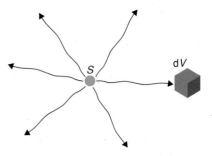

Figure 8.1. Point source (S) emission of photons (wavy lines) in vacuum. Direction is random. Only the photon emitted straight at dV can deposit energy in dV and then only if it randomly interacts with the material in dV.

and that in each decay it emits exactly one photon with energy E. The situation is shown in Figure 8.1. The dose rate must be equal to the product of the following: time rate of emission of the photons (i.e., activity A), the probability of the photon hitting dV (we will abbreviate that as $P[r, dV]$), the probability that the photon of energy E, which hits dV actually interacts with dV as opposed to just passing through ($P[E, dV]$), and the average amount of energy (dE_{abs}) that is absorbed in dV whenever a photon interacts with it, all divided by the mass (m) of dV. The units are energy/mass/time, which is dose rate. Explicitly,

$$\dot{D}(r) = AP(r,dV)P(E,dV)\,dE_{abs}/m \qquad \text{EQUATION (8.4)}$$

The first question is, what happens to the dose rate in dV if we simply change its distance from r to R (Fig. 8.2)? The two things that do not change, at all, are the activity of the source and the mass of the tissue that we move around. $P(E, dV)$ and dE_{abs} should not change if the angles with which the photons hit the volume are similar, that is, the solid angle subtended by dV is small. So, we are left to focus on the probability of a photon hitting dV. When a nucleus decays and gives off a photon, that photon is emitted isotropically, which means the photon is equally likely to go in any direction. Let the cross-sectional entrance area of the mass m be denoted as da (Fig. 8.2). Of course, the total surface area at a distance r is $4\pi r^2$. So, the probability

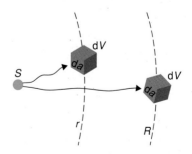

Figure 8.2. Point source (S) emission of photon radiation in vacuum. Cross-sectional area (da) of small material volume dV faces the source. dV is moved from radius r to radius R, causing a reduced probability of being hit by the photons by the factor r^2/R^2.

—

of a photon emitted in a random direction hitting da after it has traveled a distance r is

$$P(r, dV) = \frac{da}{4\pi r^2} \qquad \text{EQUATION (8.5)}$$

If we move to a larger distance R, the probability of hitting da now equals $da/(4\pi R^2)$. Therefore, the probability of hitting da has been reduced by a factor of r^2/R^2 in moving from r to R. This suggests that we can try and approximate Equation 8.4 simply as

$$\dot{D}(r) = \frac{cA}{r^2} \qquad \text{EQUATION (8.6)}$$

where we have defined that $c = P(E, dV)dE_{abs}/m$ and we are hoping that c is a constant, under the assumption that the factors in c do not change much as we move the small volume around in vacuum.

In Equation 8.6 it is understood that we should not move the little volume of tissue someplace where it makes no sense to assume that c remains constant. A counterexample best illustrates why it is not true that c is a constant. Suppose that we had moved the volume dV and centered it on $r = 0$, so that it completely surrounded the radioisotope. The factor $P(r, dV)$, where we got r^2 from the first place, is now $P(r = 0, dV) = 1$, that is, every photon emitted from the radioisotope hits the volume. One can easily see from Equation 8.4 that the dose rate does not become infinite at $r = 0$ (as Equation 8.6 implies). In fact, depending on the photon energy (E) and the size of dV, the dose rate (from the photons emitted) could be extremely small. This example clearly shows the algorithms we devise to calculate dose rate have their regions of validity.

Historically, radioisotope emissions were first measured in air. In particular, the concept of exposure (1,3,6 and Chapter 17) (amount of ionization of air per unit mass) was used extensively because charge collection in air-filled cavities are the easiest measurements to make. The process was, first, measurement of exposure rate in air, second, conversion of that exposure rate in air to dose rate to a small amount of tissue in air, and finally, conversion to dose rate to a point in the patient. The result of this process (1,3) led one to define a dose rate to a small amount of water at a distance r surrounded by air as

$$\dot{D}_{air}(r) = \frac{f_{med} A \Gamma}{r^2} \qquad \text{EQUATION (8.7)}$$

where the single constant c in Equation 8.6 is split into two constants. Γ is the exposure rate constant (in units of R cm²/mCi/h), which represented the conversion of photon energy to ionization of air for the given isotope and f_{med} (in units of cGy/R) is the conversion constant from exposure in air to dose to medium (water) at the average photon energy given off by the radioisotope. Normally, people choose to express dose to water since its radiation properties are similar to tissue and measurements were/are made in water. Values of f

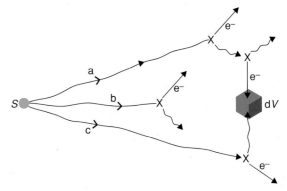

Figure 8.3. Point source (S) emission of photon radiation in homogeneous water medium. Wavy lines are photons, straight lines are electrons, and cross (x) marks are photon interaction points. Three photons are followed. Photon a: Compton scatters above dV, the electron produced misses dV, and the Compton photon scatters again (just above dV). The Compton electron after slowing down deposits its remaining energy in dV. Photon b: It was aimed right at dV coming out of S but halfway it was scattered. Both the Compton photon and electron miss dV. Photon c: Compton scatters below dV and the scattered photon heads right for dV and is photoelectrically captured inside dV; its photoelectron (not shown) is absorbed in dV.

and Γ are given in Tables 17.1 and 17.3 for various radionuclides. The interested reader should refer to Chapter 17 for a further discussion of each quantity.

In Equation 8.7, we have the dose rate to water in air, but what we ultimately want is the dose rate in water (i.e., to the patient). Let us look again at a source radiating photons towards dV but this time in a full water medium. Figure 8.3 shows three examples of photon histories. First, a photon that was going to miss dV ("a" in Fig. 8.3) is scattered several times. Eventually, a secondarily scattered electron deposits a fraction of the original energy into dV. Second, a photon (b), which is emitted from the source aimed right at dV interacts on the way there and no part of its energy reaches dV. Finally, a photon (c), which was going to miss dV, interacts and the scattered photon from that interaction is completely absorbed in dV.

One thing we might guess is that inverse square is not going to be valid anymore because how dV absorbs energy is much more complicated. However, we remember that, inverse square was not a law anyway, and what we want is an approximation in a restricted region of interest. In any event, we could start by describing the dose rate to a point r in water as

$$\dot{D}(r) = \frac{f_{med} A \Gamma}{r^2} e^{-\mu r} + \dot{D}_{scat} \qquad \text{EQUATION (8.8)}$$

In this equation, the major effect of attenuation is represented in the first term where we exponentially attenuate the in-air dose rate of Equation 8.7 with the linear attenuation coefficient (μ) of water for the average energy E emitted by the radionuclide (Table 17.6 for typical values). The exponential attenuation factor takes care of one of these effects above (photon [b] in Fig. 8.3) and scatter out of the path from the radionuclide to dV. D_{scat} now represents the result of all the various scatter possibilities and is far more complicated. Equation 8.8 has merely organized the calculation into a primary part and a secondary scatter part. Now, we note in Figure 8.3 that the attenuation scattering events (b) reduce the dose rate in dV but the scatter events (a and c) increase the dose rate relative to the (Fig. 8.1) in-vacuum case. Maybe, if we get lucky, these will cancel out. It turns out that scatter and attenuation effects do not cancel out at all distances from the source, but close to the source they almost do and their change with distance farther away can be simply parameterized. Meisberger et al. (8) showed that the measured variation in dose rate in water as r changed from 1 to 10 cm was such as to establish Equations 8.9 and 8.10 as a good approximation for the dose rate to water

$$\dot{D}(r) = \frac{f_{\mathrm{med}}A\Gamma}{r^2}T(r) \qquad \text{EQUATION (8.9)}$$

$$T(r) = A + Br + Cr^2 + Dr^3 \qquad \text{EQUATION (8.10)}$$

Application of this algorithm (Equation 8.9) has, in the past, been a popular choice in commercial computerized treatment-planning systems. Technically, f_{med} should now be a function of r to account for the lower energy of the scattered photons with greater distance in water (9,10); however, that detail is usually ignored. Comparing the in-air Equation 8.7 with the in-phantom Equation 8.9, the difference is simply the inclusion of the parameterized factor $T(r)$. $T(r)$, the attenuation and build-up factor, is a polynomial in r (Equation 8.10), which Meisberger et al. (8) used to represent the ratio of the exposure in water to the exposure in air. The free parameters A, B, C, D are determined by least squares fit to the experimental data for each isotope. One sees in Table 17.6 that the value for A is close to 1.0 and that the other coefficients are small. Because of this, the value of $T(r)$ is very close to 1.0 up to a certain distance. Attenuation and in-scatter are balanced at a distance r_A where $T(r_A) = 1.0$. That in-scatter cancels out the attenuation loss was pointed out by Hale (11), and is not obvious. For instance, if we consider ^{137}Cs ($E = 662$ keV), that distance is around 3 cm. If we estimate the reduction in dose from attenuation of 3 cm of water (by using the value for μ in Table 17.6), we would expect a 23% drop-off. Clinically, the fact that a simple dose calculation such as in Equation 8.9 can be used, instead of something as in Equation 8.8, makes calculations easy both by hand and by early computers, and has been extremely useful. The mathematical form, Equation 8.10, which was chosen by Meisberger et al. (8) for $T(r)$ is not a unique parameterization of the attenuation and scatter effects. One could with equal ease use the form proposed by Evans (12)

$$\dot{D}(r) = \frac{f_{\mathrm{med}}A\Gamma}{r^2}e^{-\mu r}[1 + k_a(\mu r)^k_b]$$

$$\text{EQUATION (8.11)}$$

Kornelson and Young (13) fit the coefficients k_a and k_b to Monte Carlo results (14). Venselaar et al. (15) extended the range of the fitted data to 60 cm. The values for various isotopes are given in Table 17.6. Other mathematical expressions (16–18) have also been utilized; there is little difference of clinical significance between them or Equations 8.9 and 8.11. The reader should note that Equation 8.9 or 8.11 can be used with the values in Tables 17.1, 17.3, and 17.6 to perform quick hand-check verifications of clinical implant plans. If one looks at a dose rate at a point 10 cm from the implant center, all the implanted sources can be considered approximately as one point source located at the center of gravity of the implant. Add all the activities together and calculate the cGy/h value expected and compare it to your treatment planning system isodose line. One cannot use this method to determine a small error in the computer plan result, but one can use it to uncover the presence of a major error.

Comparing Equations 8.8 and 8.11, the first term is identical and is the attenuated primary in-air dose rate. Comparing the second terms, one can see that Equation 8.11 assumes that $\dot{D}_{\mathrm{scat}}$ is proportional to the attenuated primary dose rate. This is physically reasonable since scatter comes from the attenuation that occurs in the out-of-path directions and this should be similar to the in-path attenuation. To the extent that this is not true, we make up for that by letting k_a and k_b be completely free parameters for each different isotope. Fitting the parameters can be done in two ways: one is fitting the free parameters to match measured data and the other is fitting (13–15) to match a better calculation such as Monte Carlo. All the parameters (A, B, C, D, and k_i) have no direct physical meaning. They are chosen to allow us to describe the dose rate as accurately as possible. Because of that, it is required to keep track over what range of data the parameters were determined. For example, the best-fit value of D just happens to be negative (Table 17.6) for ^{192}Ir, ^{198}Au, and ^{137}Cs. Hence, at large distances ($r > 25$ cm), where the term r^3 in Equation 8.10 dominates $T(r)$, ($T(r) = 25$ cm) is negative, and therefore Equation 8.9 predicts negative dose rate for those isotopes at large distances. This negative dose result arises because we have applied Equation 8.9 outside the range of the fitted parameters and have obtained a nonphysical (wrong) result.

CALCULATION OF DOSE RATES AROUND A LINE SOURCE

In Equation 8.9, we now have an expression for the dose rate in water due to a simple point source. We can now apply this result (we could have just as easily used Equation 8.11 instead) to help us calculate the dose rate from different source geometries. The next simplest case is a line (length L) of radioactive material (Fig. 8.4). In the point source case, we had spherical symmetry, which meant that the direction from the source did not change the dose, only the distance (r) did. With a line source we need to consider direction and distance relative to the center of the line. There is still symmetry remaining, specifically rotational

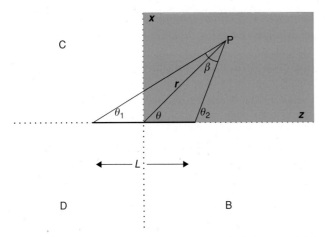

Figure 8.4. Line source geometry. Dose-rate calculation to point P depends on distance and direction (r, θ) of P from the source center. The active length (L) defines angles $(\theta_1$ and $\theta_2)$ from the endpoints of the line source to point P. $\beta = \theta_2 - \theta_1$ is the angle from P to the endpoints of the active source. Results need to be calculated only for the shaded quadrant; dose to points B, C, and D will be identical to point P by symmetry, likewise for all points in 3D space obtained by rotation of the source about the z-axis.

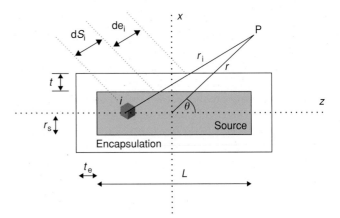

Figure 8.5. Cylindrical encapsulated source geometry, thickness of encapsulation is t, radius of source is r_S, and the end cap thickness is t_e. Radioactive material in the source region is subdivided into N tiny regions. Photons from each of these regions are attenuated by their path length through source material and encapsulation. Dose rate at P (located at r, θ from center of source) involves repeated application of point source calculation for all N cubes. For the ith cube, its distance to P is r_i, the path through the source material is d_{S_i}, and through the encapsulation is d_{e_i}.

and reflection symmetry, so if we can calculate the dose rate to every point in the shaded region, the dose rate anywhere else in the patient volume is determined. For example, the dose rate at P in Figure 8.4 is the same as at point B (reflection of P with respect to Y–Z plane), C (reflection of P with respect to X–Y plane), or D (reflection of B with respect to X–Y plane). Moreover, any point off the plane $(y \neq 0)$ of Figure 8.4 that can be mapped to a point in the plane of Figure 8.4 by a rotation about the z-axis will have the same dose rate as that point in the plane.

The solution can be found in an analytic form by defining an activity per unit length (A/L) of source and integrating the point source expression of Equation 8.9 along the line of the source (dl) to obtain the dose rate at any point $P(r, \theta)$ in the plane (19). The final result is

$$\dot{D}(r,\theta) = \frac{f_{med}\Gamma AT(r)}{L}\int_{-L/2}^{L/2}\frac{dl}{r'^2} = \frac{f_{med}\Gamma AT(r)\beta}{Lr\sin\theta}$$

EQUATION (8.12)

where L is the active length of source and $\beta = \theta_2 - \theta_1$ is the angle subtended by the line source when viewed from point P.

CALCULATION OF DOSE RATES AROUND AN ENCAPSULATED CYLINDRICAL SOURCE

Most applications in radiation oncology entail the use of encapsulated (e.g., stainless steel) cylindrical sources. Consider a cylindrical source S (radioactive source radius r_S, active length L) and enclose it (Fig. 8.5) inside a cylinder of encapsulation material (radial wall thickness t and end cap thickness t_e). Again, we will consider the active source region

to be divided into many small point sources and determine the contribution from each point source separately using Equation 8.9 and add the results. Clearly, the first-order effect of the encapsulation will be to reduce the dose rate by an amount that depends on the path lengths through the encapsulation. As the path length through the encapsulation from every small point source to a given dose point is different, the reduction will be different in different directions. The solution to an encapsulated line source was given by Sievert (20). He presented the equivalent ($T(r)$ was ignored in those days) of the following expression for the dose rate at a point P located at planar coordinates r and θ (measured from the radioactive source center, Fig. 8.5)

$$\dot{D}(r,\theta) = \frac{f_{med}\Gamma AT(r)}{Lr\sin\theta}\int_{\theta_1}^{\theta_2}e^{\frac{-\mu_e t}{\cos\gamma}}d\gamma$$

EQUATION (8.13)

where μ_e is the attenuation coefficient for the radioisotope's photons through the encapsulation material, t is the perpendicular wall thickness of the encapsulation, and θ_1 and θ_2 are the angles from the point P to the ends of the active length of the source. The integral expression in Equation 8.13 is the *Sievert integral*, which can be numerically evaluated with a computer. Young and Batho (21) later provided expressions for an effective wall thickness accounting for source radius. As an aside, Γ would be the unfiltered exposure rate constant (1,3,5,6) in Equation 8.13 because the attenuation of the source's photons by encapsulation is explicitly calculated. The differences between filtered and unfiltered (6,22,23) exposure rate constants are discussed in detail in Chapter 17.

Equation 8.13 is valid for points (such as P in Fig. 8.5) in the patient where path lengths do not go through the ends of the source. Expressions (19,20) that give the dose rate in the other geometrically distinct regions (through ends of the source capsule) will not be presented here, as calculations involving numerical integration (21) can be obtained with computers. We can present a single equation for calculation anywhere in the region by numerical integration. We subdivide the source volume into N equal parts. Each little source volume element i contributes independently to the dose rate at P. The dose rate at a point P located at r, θ, from the center of the source is given by adding all N exponentially attenuated point source contributions

$$\dot{D}(r,\theta) = f_{\text{med}}\,\Gamma\,\frac{A}{N}\sum_{i=1}^{N} e^{-(\mu_s d_{s_i} + \mu_e d_{e_i})}\,\frac{T(r_i)}{r_i^2} \quad \text{EQUATION (8.14)}$$

where d_{s_i} and d_{e_i} (Fig. 8.5) are the individual path length distances through the source (encapsulation) material from tiny source region i to point P. For a clinical ^{137}Cs source, $N = 100$ is a fine enough subdivision. The effect of the attenuation coefficient of the source (μ_s) and its path length (d_{s_i}) is included. The numerical integration method in one form or another has been used often (21,24–28). In Equation 8.14, the coefficients, μ, are either chosen to give the best fit of Equation 8.14 to experimental measurements or directly measured. If the coefficients are directly measured, one sees that measurements (28) of attenuation produced by materials relative to attenuation by water works better than linear attenuation coefficients in Equation 8.14, because the material is a perturbation of the water medium and not a perturbation of air medium.

ENCAPSULATION AND THE LOW ENERGY PROBLEM

In our discussion up to now, we have avoided details such as where do we get the activity (A) of a given source, what is the correct way of calculating the exposure rate constant, how does one calibrate a source and the relationship of the latter procedures to the final step, and calculation of dose rate. To get an idea of the ambiguities, consider a hypothetical encapsulated source where a manufacturer makes the encapsulation container from lead and the radioactive material emits a photon of energy 30 keV half the time the nucleus decays and a photon of energy 1 MeV the other half. If we were to measure the output of this encapsulated source, we would never detect the decays wherein photons of 30 keV are produced because the lead would absorb them. The activity we would infer from measurement would then be less than what it really is because we would only be aware of half the decays. We would be in a dilemma to call that measured activity the activity, because the activity is essentially a measure of the actual number of radioactive atoms (Equation 8.2). This example illustrates why there arose a need for "apparent activity." In short, the source manufacturer would tell you the "apparent activity" under the assumption that you would use the same value

of Γ that he used to derive his apparent activity. Then, when you multiply A and Γ together, you will get the correct result. Look at Equations 8.9 to 8.14; notice that what you need to calculate the dose is the value of $A\Gamma$. You do not need the activity A and do not need Γ. We emphasize that you had to check that the value of Γ, that the source manufacturer quoted, matched the value in your treatment planning system in order to use their reported activity. As an aside, it is no wonder that the use of mg Ra eq (see Chapter 17) for quantifying activity lasted so long after the abandonment of radium implants, because everyone agreed that the value of $\Gamma = 8.25$ (R cm^2/mg Ra eq hour) for radium filtered by 0.5 mm of Pt would be the only number you needed for all isotopes.

The second problem (opposite in nature to the first) comes from the details of calibration of the sources. It is easier to measure the emission output of a radioisotope in air than in water. Suppose a low energy photon is given off by the source and it gets out of the capsule or is scattered from the capsule giving rise to a photon even lower in energy and such a photon travels through air and its ionization is measured by the detector. By everything said above, for determining the activity, that seems like a good thing (a nucleus decayed and its effect was registered). However, suppose that photon is very low in energy that it would be absorbed very quickly by tissue (within an mm or so). Its effect is included in the calibration of the source in air but clinically it is of no significance in delivering a dose at a distance in a patient (29). Therefore, its effects should be excluded.

TWO-DIMENSIONAL DOSE CALCULATION FORMALISM

It should be noted that both these problems were present even from the earliest days of brachytherapy using radium (1–3). The problems were not a great enough danger to warrant rethinking the dose-rate calculation formalism till low energy sources such as ^{125}I and ^{103}Pd came into clinical use. It has been recently decided to define a more consistent method. Task Group 43 (TG43) of the American Association of Physicists in Medicine (AAPM) recommended the adoption of a new system (30–34) for calculating the dose rate to water for low energy sources. This system is designed to be consistent from calibration of the source by the accredited calibration laboratories to the final clinical calculation for the patient. The two-dimensional (2D) dose-rate equation for cylindrically symmetric encapsulated sources in the TG43 formalism (30) is given by

$$\dot{D}(r,\theta) = S_K \Lambda \frac{G_X(r,\theta)}{G_X(r_o,\theta_o)}\,g_X(r)\,F(r,\theta) \quad X = P \text{ or } L$$

EQUATION (8.15)

This dose-rate equation is a 2D calculation as points in the plane with coordinates r and θ are calculated and all other points in 3D space are then found by rotation about the z-axis. Equation 8.15 is really a choice between two equations, where $X = P$ signifies that you will use a point source geometry factor and $X = L$ indicates a line source is used. All quantities in Equation 8.15 are referenced to a single reference position, usually $r_o = 1$ cm and $\theta_o = 90°$ (i.e., 1 cm from the source center in a direction perpendicular to the symmetry axis of the source (e.g., 1 cm along the x-axis in Fig. 8.5). The product $S_K \Lambda$ is the dose rate in water at the reference position, r_o, θ_o.

Two new quantities are defined in Equation 8.15. First, the air kerma strength (1,30,33), S_K, gives a measure of the absolute amount of radionuclide available. Its source calibration unit U equals cGy cm^2/h by definition. The air kerma strength is the air kerma rate in vacuum times d^2 (due to photons of energy greater than a cutoff energy, >5 keV, measured with a free air chamber centered at a distance d); d is usually 1 m. This energy cutoff (5 keV) is chosen so that the calibration effects of low energy photons (which ultimately would not contribute to tissue dose at distances >1 mm from the source) are subtracted from the calibration result. Source manufacturers now provide both the air kerma strength (referenced to the reference position) and apparent activity (for historical comparison). Typical conversions from air kerma strengths to "apparent activity" values (U/mCi) for isotopes used clinically are 1.27, 1.29, 2.86, and 4.12 for ^{125}I, ^{103}Pd, ^{137}Cs, and ^{192}Ir, respectively.

The second new quantity in Equation 8.15 is the radionuclide's dose-rate constant, Λ (units = cGy/h/U). The dose-rate constant is the ratio of a reference dose rate $\dot{D}(r_o, \theta_o)$ in water to S_K. The dose-rate constant is determined once and for all for each manufacturer's source via Monte Carlo modeling plus experimental measurements usually with thermoluminescent dosimeters (TLDs) (30,31,35–38). There are errors in both methods, so results are averaged to produce a "consensus" value for Λ (31,35).

$G(r, \theta)$ is a new symbol for the simple geometry dependence already seen in Equations 8.9 and 8.12, namely, point (P) source and line (L) source (30,31,39). G accounts for the main effects of distance and direction of source from point of measurement. TG43 defines G_P and G_L,

$$\text{Point source } G_P(r,\theta) = r^{-2} \qquad \text{EQUATION (8.16)}$$

$$\text{Line source } G_L(r,\theta) = \frac{\beta}{Lr\sin\theta}, \quad \theta \neq 0$$

$$= \frac{1}{z^2 - (L/2)^2}, \quad \theta = 0 \quad \text{EQUATION (8.17)}$$

The ratio of $G(r,\theta)$ to the reference value $G(r_o,\theta_o)$ is explicitly indicated in Equation 8.15.

In Equation 8.15, the radial dose function $g(r)$ redefines the traditional attenuation and scatter build-up factor. It accounts for photon attenuation and scatter in water in the radial direction to the source symmetry axis ($\theta_o = 90°$).

The radial dose function is essentially $f_{med}(r)T(r)$ renormalized so that $g(r_o) = 1.0$. Since we know that Equation 8.10 is accurate, it is not surprising that a polynomial expansion can be used to represent $g(r)$

$$g_X(r) = a_0 + a_1r + a_2r^2 + a_3r^3 + a_4r^4 + a_5r^5$$

$$\text{EQUATION (8.18)}$$

where $X = P$ or L means that one compares their dose-rate data (at varying positions r with $\theta_o = 90°$) to their calculations using Equation 8.15, and determines the six coefficients a_i in Equation 8.18 using point or line source formula Equations 8.16 or 8.17 for the geometry factor. The dose-rate data required to determine the radial dose functions come from Monte Carlo calculations and are verified by measurements (30,31,40,41). See Table 17.7 for examples of $g(r)$ for several different commercial versions of isotopes.

The anisotropy of source distribution function $F(r, \theta)$ is introduced to account for differences in dose rate as a function of angle from the symmetry axis due to the specific geometry of the encapsulation of the radionuclide source. In other words, it takes into account the different path lengths through the source and encapsulation at various angles. If we have information on the dose rate in all directions, such as from Monte Carlo modeling (42–44) or numerical integration or the Sievert integral, then the anisotropy function can be determined from Equation 8.15. The normalization for F is, $F(r, \theta_o) = 1.0$ (see Table 17.8 for examples).

In high dose-rate afterloader applications using ^{192}Ir (see Chapter 18), there is a single high activity cylindrical source. Optimization techniques (Chapter 18) are used to vary source dwell times at various positions in fixed implanted catheters. Because you must localize the catheters to plan the patient, you have the orientation of the source symmetry axis in the patient at all possible dwell positions and therefore you can determine the angle θ in Figure 8.4 for any position P. Therefore, one uses the 2D dose calculation ($X = L$) of Equation 8.15. Similarly, ^{125}I seed sources loaded into a fixed geometry eye plaque for ocular melanoma treatment can use the line source form.

There is a practical problem in using Equation 8.15 for cylindrical sources that are not constrained to be in a definitive geometric orientation by the applicator, which holds them. That is, it is not always easy to determine orientation. Consider permanent prostate implant that uses ^{125}I seed sources. Computed tomography (CT) scans and/or radiographs cannot easily provide the necessary resolution to determine the line direction in 3D space for all the sources, though methods are being developed to do that (45,46). So, we definitely have line sources but we cannot determine the angle θ (from each and every source to point P). Thus, we are forced to use the point source geometry factor. In this event, there is a better option (31). Although the anisotropy function is a function of r and θ, one can average F over the 4π geometry and F can be approximated by a simple radial function, $\phi_{an}(r)$, called the one-dimensional (1D) anisotropy function (see Table 17.8 for examples). Where a 2D calculation cannot be used for cylindrical sources, the revised TG43 protocol (31) recommends the use of

$$\dot{D}(r,\theta) = S_K \Lambda \frac{G_L(r,\theta_o)}{G_L(r_o,\theta_o)} g_L(r)\phi_{an}(r) \quad \text{EQUATION (8.19)}$$

Compare Equation 8.19 to Equation 8.15 (with $X = L$) with respect to the geometry function. In Equation 8.19, the line source geometry formula is used but regardless of what the angle θ is on the left side of the equation, we evaluate the right-hand side using $\theta = \theta_o = 90°$. The advantage of Equation 8.19 is that it is more accurate for cylindrical sources at distances <1 cm than if we use Equation 8.15 with the point source approximation ($X = P$).

It is important to understand the methodology behind the 2D dose calculation algorithm provided by Equation 8.15. A point or line source approximation for the geometry function is chosen (this choice is determined by practical realities in most cases as almost all clinical sources are cylinders). Experimental measurements and/or Monte Carlo calculations provide the desired 3D dose distribution answer. The radial dose-rate function in point source geometry is then determined by choosing the parameters of Equation 8.18, so that multiplying all the factors together at points where $\theta = \theta_o = 90°$ yields the correct dose rate (which you already know) at those points. Once you have that, you can determine the anisotropy factor in the same way using the already known correct dose distribution. One can either store a table of results (Tables 17.8) or create a fitting function to reproduce the results. Furhang and Anderson (47) proposed the functional form:

$$F(r,\theta) = 1 - (a + b\theta + c\theta^2)\cos(\theta)e^{dr} \quad \text{EQUATION (8.20)}$$

where a, b, c, and d are polynomials in r with a total of 12 free parameters. Sloboda et al. (48) fit those parameters to the results of Monte Carlo calculations. Ling et al. (49) had also used a similar parameterization to fit the dose-rate results for a ^{125}I source.

Equations 8.9, 8.11, 8.12, and 8.14 can be converted to the more modern formalism by substituting $S_K\Lambda g(r)$ for $f_{med}A\Gamma T(r)$. For example, Equation 8.14 for the dose rate about a cylindrical encapsulated source would be

$$\dot{D}(r) = \Lambda \frac{S_K}{N} \sum_{i=1}^{N} e^{-[\mu_s(d_{s_i}-r_s)+\mu_e(de_i-t)]} \frac{g(r_i)}{r_i^2} \quad \text{EQUATION (8.21)}$$

where since ΛS_K would have been determined for the encapsulated source, we subtract the source radius, r_S, and the encapsulation wall thickness, t, from the path differences.

Finally, let us review the rationale of the change in Equation 8.15. In the old system, calibration in air, calculation in air, and then, conversion to dose in medium was the calculation process. The new TG43 system is more akin to external

beam calculations. In Equation 8.15, ΛS_K is the cGy/h calibration in water at a reference position (the analog of linear accelerator calibration at d_{max}). The product of $G(r,\theta_o)$ and $g(r)$ is like a depth dose correction along the x-axis in Figure 8.4, normalized at r_o. Finally, $F(r,\theta)$ is like external beam off-axis ratios. Looked at in this way, the new formalism does not look so foreign.

THREE-DIMENSIONAL DOSE CALCULATIONS— ASYMMETRIC DOSE DISTRIBUTIONS REQUIRED BY APPLICATORS AND SHIELDS

Some treatments involve the use of asymmetric metal applicators to introduce the radioactive sources into the body. In treatment of carcinoma of the uterine cervix (1,2), some of the applicators have tungsten shields attached, which provide a severe asymmetry in the measured dose-rate distribution. The measurement (27,28,50,51) of dose rate in the presence of these asymmetries shows that the effects are to reduce dose rate in particular directions (geometric shadow of the shields) by up to 40%. These applicators clearly have an effect on the dose-rate distribution that is different in different directions, hence the dose-rate algorithm must calculate dose rate over the entire 3D grid centered on the source (25,27,28,52–54). Now, because clinical use involves a source loaded into the same applicator with shields every single time, the calculation can be done once for the source/applicator/shield and the result for that dose distribution stored on the computer. Figure 8.6 shows that the dose point P has paths from the various source volume elements that miss or go through the shield. Numerical integration

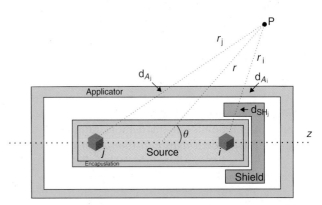

Figure 8.6. Asymmetrical source/applicator/shield geometry. Radioactive material in source region is subdivided into N tiny regions; photons from each of these regions are attenuated by their path length through source material, encapsulation, shield material, and applicator material. Dose rate at P (located at r, θ from center of source) involves repeated application of point source calculation for all N regions. For the ith cube, its distance to P is r_i, the path through the source material is d_{S_i}, through the encapsulation is d_{e_i} (the latter two are not shown here; see Fig. 8.5), the path through the shield material is d_{Sh_i}, and the path through the applicator material is d_{A_i}. For the jth cube, its distance to P is r_j, its path misses the shield and the path through the applicator material is d_{A_j}.

can be extended to this case quite easily, thereby accounting for primary attenuation for path length through source (S), encapsulation (e), shield (Sh), and applicator housing (A). The expression is the following:

$$\dot{D}(x,y,z) = \Lambda S_K / N \sum_{i=1}^{N} e^{-[\mu_S(d_{S_i} - r_S) + \mu_e(d_{e_i} - t) + \mu_{Sh}d_{Sh_i} + \mu_A d_{A_i}]} \frac{g(r_i)}{r_i^2}$$

EQUATION (8.22)

The path length intersection differences (d) have to be evaluated for every direction and the μ are free parameters. The strength of Equation 8.22 is that it is simple and the 3D results can be obtained clinically fast. The 3D calculation for a point P in Equation 8.22 involves numerous ray line (the radial direction from each source subvolume piece to the point P) calculations. The attenuation produced by the metal structure along each path is accounted for, which is the greatest effect. However, the metal structure off the ray line path to point P (secondary effect) is ignored in Equation 8.22. For example, in Figure 8.6, the evaluation of the contribution to dose at P from source subvolume j is the same whether there is a tungsten shield present in the applicator or not. In Equation 8.22, it is $g(r)$ that represents scatter, determined from the case of a homogeneous water medium. We are assuming in Equation 8.22 that $g(r)$ is the same when a nonwater material is lateral to the ray line. Equation 8.22 is a very fast calculation method and comparison to Monte Carlo calculations (53) show that it works very well for ^{137}Cs. Lower photon energies require a method to deal with scatter.

Reasonably fast 3D methods having a scattering component have been developed by Williamson (52) and Russell et al. (55). Monte Carlo calculations of dose results for source/applicator and just source are each separated into primary and scattered components. Monte Carlo calculations are used to create precalculated distance dependent scatter ratios that are a function of distance and mean free path in the patient. Surprisingly, scatter is shown to be fairly isotropic about each applicator, so that scatter dose can be treated as a distance-dependent but angle-independent term. This approximation speeds up the calculations. As Williamson (52) points out, this demonstration of the simple angle independent nature of the scatter also explains why formalisms such as Equation 8.22 work very well for the high-energy photons of ^{137}Cs. At larger distances from the implant or for lower energy isotopes such as ^{125}I, the scatter separation method remains accurate.

Generalization of the TG43 2D dose calculation formalism Equation 8.15, to a form suitable for 3D dose calculation would look something like this:

$$\dot{D}(r,\theta,\varphi) = S_K \Lambda \frac{r_o^2}{r^2} g(r) F(r,\theta,\varphi) \quad \text{EQUATION (8.23)}$$

$F(r,\theta,\varphi)$ is extended to explicitly include the angle φ dependence, $0 < \varphi < 2\pi$ and includes all angular variations. F could be described by a function such as Equation 8.20

with the 12 free parameters themselves a function of φ. This would then involve hundreds of parameters.

At this point, historical review helps us understand that simple equations such as Equations 8.9 or 8.11 among others arose because the developers needed some simple equation to calculate or check treatments by hand. Today, many parameter fits (such as Equation 8.23 would require) can be done on the computer easily. However, it is also true that characterizing the dose-rate calculation directly using Monte Carlo over a full 3D volume $20 \times 20 \times 20$ cm^3 and storing such a 3D matrix would not be a problem either. So one could follow the historical development and precalculate the Monte Carlo result, then fit the parameters of Equation 8.23 to the Monte Carlo, throw away the Monte Carlo result, and use Equation 8.23 with the large number of parameters to calculate the dose distribution. Alternatively, one could just store and use the Monte Carlo results directly (after smoothing to minimize statistical errors). Therefore, it is unlikely that the description of the results of 3D dose calculations will follow TG43 in describing the dose rate as a product of several fitted functions whose parameters were found by comparing to Monte Carlo results. Instead, "consensus" 3D Monte Carlo generated dose-rate matrices normalized to the dose at a reference position could be provided.

3D TREATMENT PLANNING WITH 3D DOSE DISTRIBUTIONS

If we have a precalculated 3D dose-rate distribution, how do we use it clinically? It is necessary to determine the position and orientation of each source's 3D dose distribution in the patient. Figure 8.7 shows a single source, which is arbitrarily angled in the patient. The patient coordinate system (x, y, z) is defined by a 3D imaging device such as a CT scanner. The 3D dose-rate distribution of the source/applicator would have been (pre) calculated in a coordinate system (x', y', z') centered on the source. This is the intrinsic coordinate system of the source/applicator system. If there was cylindrical symmetry about the intrinsic z'-axis,

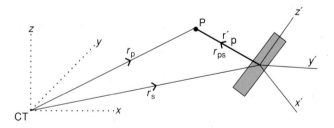

Figure 8.7. Relationship between patient coordinate system (as defined by a computed tomography [CT] scan) and the internal dose-rate calculation coordinate system of a precalculated 3D source, which is rotated relative to the CT system. The center of the source is at r_S (relative to the CT scan). Point P in the patient is located at r_P in the CT scan but at r_P' relative to the internal source coordinate system. r_{PS} and r_P' are physically the same vector, expressed in CT and intrinsic coordinates, respectively.

there would be no need to determine in what direction the x' and y' axes are oriented in the CT scan coordinate system, but here we are assuming that there is no symmetry whatsoever. We define $\dot{D}(\vec{r}_p)$ as the calculated dose-rate distribution in its own intrinsic coordinate system $(\vec{r})$ for a unit air kerma strength source. So in Figure 8.7, the dose rate at point P (located at $\vec{r}_p$ in the CT scan) produced by the source (located at $\vec{r}s$) implies looking up the value for $\dot{D}(\vec{r}_p')$ from the precalculated 3D matrix. We therefore need to determine the vector (distance and direction) $\vec{r}_p$. In practice, this requires that we determine which way the x', y', z' axes point in the CT scanner. Now, $\vec{r}_{PS}$, the vector from S to P, is the same vector as $\vec{r}_P$, only expressed in the coordinates of the CT scanner. These are shown in Figure 8.7 and related via

$$\vec{r}_P = \vec{r}_S + \vec{r}_{PS} = \vec{r}_S + E(\alpha, \beta, \gamma)\vec{r}_P' \quad \text{Equation (8.24)}$$

where $E(\alpha, \beta, \gamma)$ is the rotation matrix (56) for a solid body and α, β, γ are the Euler rotation angles, which rotate the intrinsic coordinate system of the source into correspondence with the CT coordinate system. Our problem is to find the three degrees of rotational freedom, the Euler angles. Finding both ends of the source defines a line in space and decides the z'-axis orientation (equivalent to two degrees of freedom). The last degree of freedom (rotation about that line) is found by identifying a landmark in the CT scan not on the z'-axis. Methods and equations for calculating the Euler angles based on this information have been given for particular 3D source/shield/applicators (57). One last problem is that CT scans do not determine absolute position with a precision better than $\frac{1}{2}$ the scan spacing. A 3D graphic positioning of the entire applicator can make the determination more precise (57).

Continuing on to the case of multiple sources, in Figure 8.8, the dose at point P from two sources requires that the orientations of both sources be determined. In order to look up the value for $\dot{D}(\vec{r}_1')$ and $\dot{D}(\vec{r}_2'')$, we have to determine r_1' and r_2'. So the Euler angles for two coordinate

systems must be found. For N sources, we use Equation 8.24, and the total dose rate $\dot{D}(\vec{r})$ in the patient's 3D coordinate system $(\vec{r})$ for N sources is given by

$$\dot{D}(\vec{r}) = \sum_{i=1}^{N} S_{Ki}\dot{D}_i(\vec{r}_i')$$

$$= \sum_{i=1}^{N} S_{Ki}\dot{D}_i[E_i^{-1}(\alpha_i, \beta_i, \gamma_i)(\vec{r} - \vec{rs}_i)] \quad \text{Equation (8.25)}$$

where S_{Ki} is the source strength and E_i^{-1} is the inverse of the Euler rotation matrix for the ith source. The Euler angles $(\alpha_i, \beta_i, \gamma_i)$ for each source must be determined. It is the latter task, which is the additional work needed to implement 3D dose distributions in a clinical real-time setting (57).

Once a dose-rate calculation algorithm has been implemented, there are two choices in calculating the total 3D dose-rate distribution in the patient from a multitude of sources (enclosed in applicators with or without metal shields). They are (a) dose superposition, that is, addition of individual source/applicator dose distributions independent of the presence of the other sources (Equation 8.25 is dose superposition) and (b) direct dose calculation, that is, using the calculation algorithm with all the sources and applicators accounted for in the calculation. The first is the least computationally taxing because the dose-rate matrices $(\dot{D}_i)$ may be precalculated. The second method is what would be used in real-time clinical Monte Carlo or GBBS applications using CT data.

Commercial treatment-planning systems currently use dose superposition. How important is it to correct for inter-applicator shielding effects, and patient inhomogeneities? The answer depends on the number of sources, shields, or applicators, and their positions relative to one another. At this time, it is not clear how important these effects are to clinical applications. Let us try and estimate this for one particular example where we have a significant amount of metal in the form of tungsten shields in an applicator. Consider, Figure 8.9, which shows just two sources. Let the point P be at a distance of 2 cm from the center of source 2 and 4 cm from source 1 on the left. It is reasonable to assume that the perturbation of having source/applicator 1 to the left of source/applicator 2 cannot affect the contribution that source 2 makes to the dose at P very much. Therefore, that part of the total dose stays the same for dose superposition or direct dose calculation. However, it is obvious that having source/applicator 2 in-between point P and source 1 changes the dose contribution of source 1 to the dose at P. Crudely, we will estimate the error using inverse square considerations alone. In dose superposition, the contribution of source/applicator 1 is roughly $(2/4)^2 = 1/4$ of the contribution that source/applicator 2 makes to the dose rate at point P. So if source/applicator 1's contribution is reduced by 33% (which would only be for points fully in the shadow of the shield), the error in the dose rate (caused by forgetting about

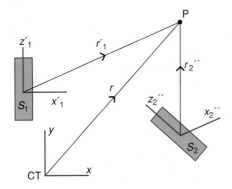

Figure 8.8. Superposition approximation. The dose rate at P is found by adding the contribution from source 1 (assuming source 2 is not present), to the contribution from source 2 (assuming source 1 is not present). The internal coordinate system for each source is shown. Only two out of three axes are shown.

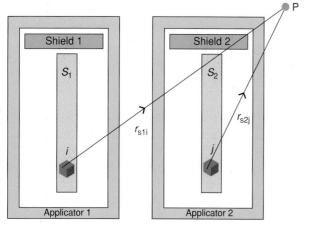

Figure 8.9. Direct calculation of dose from multiple sources. Two radioactive source calculation including attenuation effect of all regions. Sources 1 and 2 are subdivided into N regions each. Dose rate at P involves repeated application of point source calculation for all $2N$ regions and calculation of path lengths through each region from both sources. For the ith cube in source 1, its distance to P is $r_{S_{1i}}$, the path goes through source 1's source material, encapsulation and applicator material, it then enters and leaves source 2 on the way to point P. It passes through source 2, shield 2, and through the second applicator (entering and leaving). For the jth cube in source 2, its distance to P is $r_{S_{2j}}$ and the path does not pass through source 1 and only intersects its own materials.

interapplicator effects, as you do for dose superposition) would be roughly 1/12 or 8% of the total dose. In treatment of carcinoma of the uterine cervix (2) (Fig. 8.9 is an example in a plane through the ovoids to a point lateral to the ovoids) this 8% difference would be reduced even more by the dose-rate contributions from the tandem sources, whose contribution to P would be about the same in superposition or direct calculation.

In low dose-rate permanent implants of the prostate, one may have up to 100 ^{125}I stainless steel clad sources in a 40-cc volume. Surely, the overall inhomogeneity effect caused by seed-to-seed attenuations might be severe, especially since the photon energy is low. Burns and Raeside (58) in a Monte Carlo study of a model two-plane implant showed that the shadowing effect reduces the dose in the interior of the implant but this reduction was not enough to drop the dose below the reference prescription dose. So, the significance is that very high doses here and there inside the implant region are not really as high as one thought. Meigooni et al. (59) also studied inter-seed effects for ^{125}I and found through measurements that variations were dependent on direction but that overall, the dose at the periphery of the implant is reduced by 6%. Chibani et al. (60) used Monte Carlo simulation and found similar results for ^{125}I and [103]Pd. Based on these studies, it is not easy to see the need for any correction other than a 5% reduction of predicted overall dose to the periphery. We emphasize that these studies justify a dose documentation correction, not a 5% boost of the seed activity/strength. The latter is a completely different question, which is beyond the scope of this chapter. At the present time, it is

unclear (61) whether these corrections are needed in permanent seed implants.

Finally, as regards patient heterogeneities, this problem is still harder to evaluate since the variations can be endless. Das et al. (62) found that the dose beyond bone is most affected and that the perturbations of the dose distribution are too complex to be modeled by simple dose calculation algorithms, so Monte Carlo calculations must be used. Meigooni and Nath (63) used measurements plus Monte Carlo simulation and found in their model that lower energy sources such as ^{125}I and [103]Pd have significant changes in dose due to patient heterogeneity, whereas ^{192}Ir does not. Calculation methods to produce simple corrections have been proposed by Williamson et al. (64). They used Monte Carlo-generated primary and scatter components and incorporated empiric parameters into a scatter subtraction method to gain the advantages of Monte Carlo computation but with a large saving in computation time. Agreement with full Monte Carlo simulations was within a few percent in most examples considered. Furstoss et al. (65) studied both inter-seed and breast tissue heterogeneity effects for ^{125}I and [103]Pd seed permanent breast implants using Monte Carlo simulation. At these low energies, they found that breast tissue can change D90 by 10% relative to the homogeneous water case, inter-seed attenuation is not important.

THREE-DIMENSIONAL DOSE CALCULATIONS—MONTE CARLO AND BOLTZMANN TRANSPORT TECHNIQUES

In this section, we move away from macroscopically parameterized calculations and calculate the dose distribution using microscopically parameterized functions. These calculations can handle all inhomogeneities as straightforwardly as the homogeneous case. The techniques require significant computer power, which is available now. The techniques are feasible for brachytherapy applications because the distances and volumes of interest are small. The method of Monte Carlo (66–69) involves the concepts figuratively expressed in Equation 8.4 at the beginning of this chapter. That is, a photon leaves a radioisotope in a random direction and when it hits something, there is a chance of something happening, or not. In Monte Carlo, a photon is randomly created, starts off in a random direction, and each step of the way has a probability (cross section) of photoelectric interaction, Compton interaction, pair production, or coherent scattering. If it spits off an electron at a certain location headed in a certain direction determined by a "roll of the dice," that electron loses energy (6) as it moves through the medium. The medium is split into small volume regions (cells), as electrons lose energy in those cells; that energy loss is tallied as being deposited into that cell. So after the one photon has left and all its scattered photon and electron descendants have ended up as too low in energy to escape any more cells and are absorbed, you say that one history has been completed. After that first history, almost every cell volume around the source has zero dose because most cells were either not geometrically hit by anything or, if hit, no interaction event occurred within them. In order to get useful results, we will have to rerun this "rolling of the dice" process over and over again. The computer is tailor-made to handle this task, many millions of times or more to finally get smooth continuous results close to the source. We note that Monte Carlo simulation tries to mimic what is happening in the patient. Monte Carlo is sometimes thought (67) of as a simulated measurement process carried out on the computer.

The errors in Monte Carlo are of two types: systematic and statistical. The systematic errors arise from the fact that the scattering cross sections are themselves parameterized approximations to the real atomic scattering. When Monte Carlo is used in radiation oncology to predict average macroscopic properties such as dose distributions, these errors are insignificant. The random statistical errors arise because of the need to stop the calculation in some finite time, before statistical variation in each and every volume element of the patient is rendered insignificant. The details can be misleading. Suppose we use 50 million histories in a Monte Carlo modeling of a prostate HDR treatment, this seems like an enormous number. In that case, a 10 Ci source can expose the patient for 300 seconds and therefore, the actual treatment involves around 10^{14} photon histories. So the seemingly huge Monte Carlo computation is actually 2 million times less than the real treatment. Alternatively, one could look at the 50 million history Monte Carlo calculation representing what we would expect from a less than a millisecond HDR treatment. The statistical uncertainty in the dose varies, becoming larger the farther away from the source distribution that one considers. Near the source distribution, that is, in the tumor volume, the 50 million histories modeling is acceptable.

Monte Carlo for brachytherapy investigations has a long history starting with Berger's work (66), which provided analysis and insight into Meisberger et al. results (8). The encapsulated radioactive source can be modeled and the relationship between calibration, measurement, and calculation of 3D distributions determined. An unequaled advantage of Monte Carlo is in handling any case regardless of complexity. All that is required is to determine the radionuclide spatial distribution and the positions of the inhomogeneities, subdivide each into regions, subdivide the entire patient region of interest into small regions, and let the Monte Carlo program run until the results stop changing significantly. This advantage cannot be too highly praised. Consider that the Monte Carlo N-Particle (MCNP) (67) input used for full 3D calculations of a source/shield/applicator (53) required typing only 100 lines of text. Meanwhile, experimental measurements of 3D dose-rate distribution for the same and similar applications (28,50,51) involved machining of positioning devices to allow rotation of applicators with high precision in water tanks. Measurements are made in different orientations and the results have to be merged together. It is obvious which is easier.

Monte Carlo is also useful even when you are not going to use it explicitly. All the approximations for dose-rate calculation in this chapter involve parameters. If one fits the values of the parameters of your algorithm to best match the results of Monte Carlo simulations (53), then one obtains a parameterization that one can have more confidence in than from the traditional method of fitting to experimental results (28). The reasons for this were pointed out by Boyer (70) regarding the limitations of brachytherapy measurement, for example, finite size of detectors, energy response changes of detector with distance, and so on. Monte Carlo does not have these limitations. Monte Carlo does have the limitation or, more precisely, the requirement that the source emission spectrum (7) must be precisely known and that the exact specifications of source/applicator construction are defined correctly. Because of that, there is still a need for measurement but only to spot-check at a few points the results for confidence that the above requirements are correct. In summary, today Monte Carlo simulation is some part of any brachytherapy dose calculation.

Recently, a new method (71–73) has been proposed for brachytherapy dose calculation. Suppose we return to our 50 million history Monte Carlo example and rerun it again on the computer. We would obtain a different (albeit similar) dose distribution result. If we could (we cannot) run the actual 10^{14} histories, get the results, and then rerun that simulation once more and compare, we expect that we would have no difference in results. Therefore, there is an expectation that an exact solution exists, that is, an infinite history solution. To find that solution we turn to methods for solving the linear Boltzmann transport equation (74) that were developed at Los Alamos National Laboratory (75,76). The Boltzmann transport equation governs the motion of a particle in a fluid subject to random collisions. It has no analytic solution. To make the problem computationally feasible, the scattering energies and angles are discretized and the equations are solved on a grid of discrete points. The technique is called lattice or grid-based Boltzmann solvers (GBBS) (77). We can understand this method applied to radiation as having the radioactive source creating the driving flux of photons (see Fig. 8.10). This photon flux flows out, suffers random collisions, and is both modified and creates electron flux. The solution that GBBS finds is the resulting photon and electron final total flux at every grid position throughout the patient. These fluxes are also determined approximately in the Monte Carlo method but far faster in GBBS, that is, thousands of times faster. Error in GBBS is systematic, not statistical. It is said that the solution is exact (77). However, the solutions of the differential equations can be affected by the aforementioned discretization approximations. Hence, there is a danger that the solution could be incorrect. As in Monte Carlo, this is a technique wherein more and more computer-processing power makes the calculations more and more reliable in shorter times.

In Figure 8.10, we show the photon flux in the homogeneous case, assuming a single energy point source emitter.

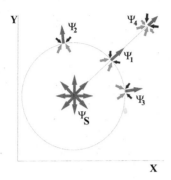

Figure 8.10. Point source S of single energy photons, photon flux Ψ_S in homogeneous medium. Resulting identical photon flux Ψ at positions 1 to 3 and lower energy flux at position 4. Monte Carlo or GBBS can do no better than equal the accuracy of simple parameterized point source dose calculations.

As one goes away from the source, the intensity of the orange photons drops (line gets shorter) and other lower energy photons (shades of blue) appear at different angles. Electron flux is not shown. The assumption with GBBS is that the resulting flux at positions 1 to 4 cannot be random and must be definite and related to each other via the transport equations. Let us compare the use of Equation 8.15 with Monte Carlo and GBBS to illustrate the advantages and disadvantages. In Figure 8.10, if we used Equation 8.15, the dose that we would calculate at equally distant positions 1 to 3 would be exactly equal and correct. Assuming that position 4 is 10 cm away, the dose would be accurate. In contrast, with Monte Carlo the dose would be very close to correct for positions 1 to 3, but the doses would not be exactly equal because of statistical error. With GBBS, the dose would be exactly equal and correct for positions 1 to 3. Both Monte Carlo and GBBS would be more accurate for position 4, especially if it were much greater than 10 cm away. Therefore, for the homogeneous case, really nothing is to be gained over any of the historical methods of dose calculation by using Monte Carlo or GBBS. In Figure 8.11, we show a source distribution S and dose points in the presence of inhomogeneities; gray is bone and blue is air. If we use Equation 8.15 (assume that we can ignore inter-source attenuation effects), the calculated doses at a prescription point such

as D_5 or D_1 are very accurate, while the dose at D_2 is fairly accurate (unless position 2 is very close to the bone), the dose at D_3 is underestimated, and D_4 is overestimated. On the other hand, for Monte Carlo and GBBS, all doses are accurately predicted; moreover, inter-source attenuation effects need not be ignored. There is no question that if inhomogeneity is present, the Monte Carlo and GBBS are superior in dose calculation accuracy throughout the patient.

FUTURE DIRECTIONS IN THREE-DIMENSIONAL DOSE-RATE CALCULATION ALGORITHMS

At the present time, commercial treatment planning systems do not provide 3D calculation of dose and do not allow precalculated 3D dose matrices to be used for planning. TG43 formalism is supported for all sources. It is clear that only Monte Carlo and GBBS can handle all difficulties in brachytherapy dose calculation. One reason is that heterogeneities do not hamper the accuracy of these methods. If the Monte Carlo calculation is deciding whether a photon will randomly scatter as it goes through bone or if it is going through water, it is all the same for the computation procedure. A similar statement applies to GBBS. There is not much extra computation power needed for the inter-applicator/patient heterogeneity calculation relative to a homogeneous calculation. Of course, the calculation time plus time for identification and accurate orientation of all sources, and applicators in the CT scan and definition in the Monte Carlo or GBBS calculation framework are still not a real-time clinical reality except in special cases. However, all these problems will eventually be addressed using increased processing power, both for calculations and for image analysis. In the future, we expect to be able to take all inhomogeneity effects into account, using full clinical Monte Carlo or GBBS calculations.

We now have good reason to expect this. By the time you are reading this, BrachyVision (Varian Medical Systems, Palo Alto, CA) will have introduced a GBBS option for their HDR treatment planning system. The user will generate an optimized plan using Equation 8.15 to calculate dose and thereby determine all dwell times. After completion, they will then have the option to run a GBBS calculation. This will document the dose distribution in the patient accounting for all inhomogeneities. This calculation will take less than 10 minutes. What the user will do with that information is not clear. That the information will now be available is noteworthy. However, it would be a mistake to think that the fact that the inhomogeneity corrected dose is different from the homogeneous dose, justifies changing the integral dose (1) to the patient. That is a more complicated question.

The last paragraph indicates that (unexpectedly) GBBS has leap-frogged Monte Carlo in regards to individual patient-specific clinical utilization. A problem with commercial implementation of Monte Carlo is, "When do you stop

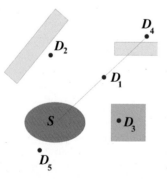

Figure 8.11. Source distribution S and dose at five positions in the presence of bone (gray) and air (blue). Only Monte Carlo or GBBS can accurately predict dose at all positions.

the calculation?" That can be a function of the geometry of the case itself. Since even the homogeneous case takes too long, to design a software system to run more histories than you ever expect to need is not feasible today. So the reasons for GBBS success are increased speed and that GBBS provides an "exact" solution. The former is easy to understand, but the latter should be accepted with caution. Since the solution is exact (and hence when it completes, you are finished), that is a huge software design advantage. There is one potential problem, that is, what happens to the "exact" solution when you have artifact in the CT scan or misinterpretation of the size or density of metal objects or calcifications. Since in GBBS the dose results in all areas of the patient are linked by the differential equations, this could result in the prescription dose result being made inaccurate by other less important regions of the patient being incorrectly specified. This could mean that the "exact" solution is "exactly" wrong. How much wrong is unclear at this time. Having said all that, one has to be excited by this new development as much will be learned from it and in the proposed GBBS implementation for HDR, Equation 8.15 will still control the clinical treatment.

SUMMARY

The history of algorithm development was that extensive use of measurements led to simple calculation algorithms based on a point source. Using numerical integration, these were extended to cylindrical geometries of varying complexity. These developments were then improved by comparison to specialized Monte Carlo studies. The rise in computer power made available more extensive Monte Carlo investigations. These Monte Carlo studies more precisely determined the best parameters of the calculation algorithms to give a better agreement with experiment and later permitted a unification of source calibration and clinical calculation of dose. The ease of these investigations has made extensive 3D measurement projects a thing of the past. In fact, the GBBS literature bypasses experimental measurements and compares to Monte Carlo for justification. The GBBS imminently will be in clinical practice as it is faster than Monte Carlo and gives definite results. As computer power increases in the future, it is obvious that the power and dominance of these two techniques in providing detailed dose distribution results also will increase. It will then seem as if all the simple equations are no longer needed as advanced computer modeling has superseded them. One notes that none of the governing equations for Monte Carlo or GBBS were given in this chapter. There was no need as no one is going to use them to find/check the dose in a patient. The vast computational labor of these methods is such that only the computer can produce a result at even a single point. It is then that the historical methods reappear as the only way to check that the computer results can be believed. One is advised to do exactly that.

Acknowledgments

The author gratefully thanks Glenn Glasgow, PhD, for providing Chapter 17 in advance of publication, Vania Arora, MS, for a careful reading of the manuscript, and Mr. Paul Weeks for producing the figures.

REFERENCES

1. Khan F. *The physics of radiation therapy*. 2nd ed. Baltimore, MD: Williams & Wilkins, 1994.
2. Perez CA, Glasgow GP. Clinical applications of brachytherapy. In: Perez CA, Brady LW, eds. *Principles and practice of radiation oncology*. Philadelphia, PA: JB Lippincott Co, 1987.
3. Johns HE, Cunningham JR. *The physics of radiology*, 4th ed. Springfield, IL: Charles C Thomas Publisher, 1983.
4. Pierquin B, Chassagne DJ, Chahbazian CM, et al. *Brachytherapy*. St. Louis, MO: Warren H. Green, 1978.
5. Glasgow GP, Perez CA. Physics of brachytherapy. In: Perez CA, Brady LW, eds. *Principles and practice of radiation oncology*. Philadelphia, PA: JB Lippincott Co 1987.
6. Attix FA. *Introduction to radiological physics and radiation dosimetry*. New York: John Wiley & Sons, 1986.
7. Brown E, Firestone RB. *Table of radioactive isotopes* (Shirley VS, ed.). New York: John Wiley & Sons, 1986.
8. Meisberger LL, Keller RJ, Shalek RJ. The effective attenuation in water of the gamma rays of gold 198, iridium 192, cesium 137, radium 226, and cobalt 60. *Radiology* 1968;90:953–957.
9. Meli JA, Meigooni AS, Nath R. On the choice of phantom material for the dosimetry of 192Ir sources. *Int J Radiat Oncol Biol Phys* 1988;14:587–594.
10. Dale RG. Some theoretical derivations relating to the tissue dosimetry of brachytherapy nuclides, with particular reference to iodine-125. *Med Phys* 1983;10:176–183.
11. Hale J. The use of interstitial radium dose-rate tables for other radioactive isotopes. *AJR Am J Roentgenol* 1958;79:49–53.
12. Evans RD. *The atomic nucleus*. New York: McGraw Hill, 1955.
13. Kornelson RO, Young MEJ. Brachytherapy buildup factors. *Br J Radiol* 1981;54:136–136.
14. Webb S, Fox RA. The dose in water surrounding point isotropic gamma ray emitters. *Br J Radiol* 1979;52:482–484.
15. Venselaar JL, Van Der Giessen PH, Dries WJ. Measurement and calculation of the dose at large distances from brachytherapy sources: Cs-137, Ir-192, and Co-60. *Med Phys* 1996;23:537–543.
16. van Kleffens HJ, Star WM. Application of stereo X-ray photogrammetry (SRM) in the determination of absorbed dose values during intracavitary radiation therapy. *Int J Radiat Oncol Biol Phys* 1979;5:557–563.
17. Dale RG. A Monte Carlo derivation of parameters for use in the tissue dosimetry of medium and low energy nuclides. *Br J Radiol* 1982;55:748–757.
18. Park HC, Almond PR. Evaluation of the buildup effect of an 192Ir high dose-rate brachytherapy source. *Med Phys* 1992;19:1293–1297.
19. Weaver K. Brachytherapy dose calculations: calculational algorithms. In: Thomadsen B, ed. *Categorical course in brachytherapy physics*. Oak Brook, IL: Radiological Society of North America, 1997:41–49.

20. Sievert RM. Die intensitatatverteilung der primaren-strehlung in der nahe medinizinisher radium-praparate. *Acta Radiol* 1921;1:89–128.

21. Young ME, Batho HF. Dose tables for linear radium sources calculated by an electronic computer. *Br J Radiol* 1964; 37:38–44.

22. Glasgow GP, Dillman LT. Specific γ-ray constant and exposure rate constant of 192Ir. *Med Phys* 1979;6:49–52.

23. Glasgow GP. Exposure rate constants for filtered 192Ir sources. *Med Phys* 1981;8:502–503.

24. Diffey BL, Klevenhagen SC. An experimental and calculated dose distribution in water around CDC K-type Cesium-137 sources. *Phys Med Biol* 1975;20:446–454.

25. Van Der Laarse R, Meertens H. An algorithm for ovoid shielding of a cervix applicator. In: Cunningham JR, Ragan D, Van Dyk J, eds. *The proceedings 8th international conference on the use of computers in radiation therapy, Toronto, Canada, July 9–12.* Los Angeles, CA: IEEE Computer Society, 1984.

26. Williamson JF. Monte Carlo and analytic calculation of absorbed dose near 137Cs intracavitary sources. *Int J Radiat Oncol Biol Phys* 1988;15:227–237.

27. Meertens H, Van Der Laarse R. Screens in ovoids of a selectron cervix applicator. *Radiother Oncol* 1985;3:69–80.

28. Weeks KJ, Dennett JC. Dose calculation and measurements for a CT compatible version of the Fletcher applicator. *Int J Radiat Oncol Biol Phys* 1990;18:1191–1198.

29. Williamson JF. Monte Carlo evaluation of specific dose constants in water for 125I seeds. *Med Phys* 1988;15: 686–694.

30. Nath R, Anderson LL, Luxton G, et al. Dosimetry of interstitial brachytherapy sources: recommendations of the AAPM Radiation Therapy Committee Task Group 43. *Med Phys* 1995;22:209–234.

31. Rivard MJ, Coursey BM, DeWerd LA, et al. Update of AAPM Task Group No. 43 Report: a revised AAPM protocol for brachytherapy dose calculations. *Med Phys* 2004; 31:633–674.

32. Williamson JF, Butler W, DeWerd LA, et al. Recommendations of the American Association of Physicists in medicine regarding the impact of implementing the 2004 Task Group 43 report on dose specification for 103 Pd and 125I interstitial brachytherapy. *Med Phys* 2005;32:1424–1439.

33. DeWerd LA, Huq MS, Das IJ, et al. Procedures for establishing and maintaining consistent air- kerma strength standards for low-energy, photonemitting brachytherapy sources: recommendations of the Calibration Laboratory Accreditation Subcommittee of the American Association of Physics in medicine. *Med Phys* 2004;31:675–681.

34. Rivard MJ, Butler WM, DeWerd LA, et al. Supplement to the 2004 update of AAPM Task Group No. 43 Report. *Med Phys* 2007;34:2187–2205.

35. Chan GH, Nath R, Williamson JF. On the development of consensus values of reference dosimetry parameters for interstitial brachytherapy sources. *Med Phys* 2005;31: 1040–1045.

36. Karaiskos P, Angelopoulos A, Sakellio L, et al. Monte Carlo and TLD dosimetry of an 192Ir high dose-rate brachytherapy source. *Med Phys* 1998;25:1975–1984.

37. Heintz BH, Wallace RE, Hevezi JM. Comparison of I-125 sources used for permanent interstitial implants. *Med Phys* 2001;28:671–682.

38. Mainegra E, Capote R, Lopez E. Dose-rate constants for 125I, 103 Pd, 192Ir and 169Yb brachytherapy sources: An EGS4 Monte Carlo study. *Phys Med Biol* 1998;43: 1557–1566.

39. Williamson JF. The accuracy of the line and point source approximations in 192Ir Dosimetry. *Int J Radiat Oncol Biol Phys* 1990;12:409–414.

40. Thomason C, Mackie TR, Lindstrom MJ, et al. The dose distribution surrounding 192Ir and 137Cs seed sources. *Phys Med Biol* 1991;36:475–493.

41. Mainegra E, Capote R, Lopez E. Radial dose functions for 103 Pd, 125I, 169Yb and 192Ir brachytherapy sources: An EGS4 Monte Carlo study. *Phys Med Biol* 2000;45: 703–717.

42. Kirov AS, Williamson JF, Meigooni AS, et al. TLD, diode, and Monte Carlo dosimetry of an 192Ir source for high dose-rate brachytherapy. *Phys Med Biol* 1995;40: 2015–2035.

43. Nath R, Meigooni AS, Muench P, et al. Anisotropy functions for 103 Pd, 125I, and 192Ir interstitial brachytherapy sources. *Med Phys* 1993;20:1465–1473.

44. Capote R, Mainegra E, Lopez E. Anisotropy functions for low energy interstitial brachytherapy sources: an EGS4 Monte Carlo Study. *Phys Med Biol* 2001;46:135–150.

45. Brunet-Benkhoucha M, Verhaegen F, Lassalle S, et al. Clinical Implementation of a digital tomosynthesis-based seed reconstruction algorithm for intraoperative postimplant dose evaluation in low dose rate prostate brachytherapy. *Med. Phys* 2009;36:5235–5244.

46. Corbett JF, Jezioranski JJ, Crook J, et al. The effect of seed orientation deviations on the quality of 125I prostate implants. *Phys Med Biol* 2001;46:2785–2800.

47. Furhang EE, Anderson LL. Functional fitting of interstitial brachytherapy dosimetry data recommended by the AAPM Radiation Therapy Committee Task Group 43. *Med Phys* 1999;26:153–160.

48. Sloboda RS, Menon GV. Experimental determination of the anisotropy function and anisotropy factor for model 6711 I-125 seeds. *Med Phys* 2000;27:1789–1799.

49. Ling CC, Schell MC, Yorke ED, et al. Two dimensional dose distribution of 125I seeds. *Med Phys* 1985;12:652–655.

50. Ling CC, Spiro IJ, Kubiatowicz DO, et al. Measurement of dose distribution around Fletcher-Suit-Delclos colpostats using a Therados radiation field analyzer (RFA-3). *Med Phys* 1984;11:326–330.

51. Mohan R, Ding IY, Martel MK, et al. Measurements of radiation dose distributions for shielded cervical applicators. *Int J Radiat Oncol Biol Phys* 1985;11:861–868.

52. Williamson JF. Dose calculations about shielded gynecological colpostats. *Int J Radiat Oncol Biol Phys* 1990;19: 167–178.

53. Weeks KJ. Monte Carlo calculations for a new ovoid shield system for carcinoma of the uterine cervix. *Med Phys* 1998;25:2288–2292.

54. Mohan R, Ding IY, Toraskar J, et al. Computation of radiation dose distributions for shielded cervical applicators. *Int J Radiat Oncol Biol Phys* 1985;11:823–830.

55. Russell KR, Ahnesjo A. Dose calculation in brachytherapy for a 192Ir source using a primary and scatter dose separation technique. *Phys Med Biol* 1996;41(6):1007–1024.

56. Rose ME. *Elementary theory of angular momentum.* New York: Wiley, 1957.

57. Weeks KJ. Brachytherapy object oriented treatment planning using three dimensional image guidance. In: Thomadsen B, ed. *Categorical course in brachytherapy physics.* Oak Brook, IL: Radiological Society of North America, 1997:79–86.
58. Burns GS, Raeside DE. The accuracy of single-seed dose superposition for I-125 implants. *Med Phys* 1989;16: 627–631.
59. Meigooni AS, Meli JA, Nath R. Interseed effects on dose for I-125 brachytherapy implants. *Med Phys* 1992;19: 385–390.
60. Chibani O, Williamson JF, Todor D. Dosimetric Effect of seed anisotropy and interseed attenuation for 103 Pd and 125I prostate implants. *Med Phys* 2005;32:2557–2566.
61. Yu Y, Anderson LL, Li Z, et al. Permanent prostate seed implant brachytherapy: Report of the American Association of Physicists in Medicine in Medicine Task Group No. 64. *Med Phys* 1999;26:2054–2076.
62. Das RK, Keleti D, Zhu Y, et al. Validation of Monte Carlo dose calculations near I-125 brachytherapy sources in the presence of bounded tissue heterogeneities. *Int J Radiat Oncol Biol Phys* 1997;38:843–853.
63. Meigooni AS, Nath R. Tissue inhomogeneity correction for brachytherapy sources in a heterogeneous phantom with cylindrical symmetry. *Med Phys* 1992;19:401–407.
64. Williamson JF, Li Z, Wong JW. One-dimensional scatter-subtraction method for brachytherapy dose calculation near bounded heterogeneities. *Med Phys* 1993;20:233–244.
65. Furstoss C, Reniers B. Bertrand MJ, et al. (Monte Carlo study of LDR seed dosimetry with an application in a clinical breast implant. *Med Phys* 2009;36:1848–1858.
66. Berger M. *Energy deposition in water by photons from point isotropic sources. MIRD Pamphlet 2.* Washington, DC: National Bureau of Standards, 1968.
67. Briesmeister JT. MCNP—A general Monte Carlo N-particle transport code. Version 4a: Los Alamos National Laboratory Report, LA-12625, 1993.
68. Nelson W, Hirayama H, Rogers D. *The EGS4 Code System.* SLAC Report 265 Stanford University, 1985.
69. Williamson JF. Monte Carlo evaluation of kerma at a point for photon transport problems. *Med Phys* 1988;14:567–576.
70. Boyer AL. A fundamental accuracy limitation on measurements of brachytherapy sources. *Med Phys* 1979;6: 454–456.
71. Gifford KA, Horton JL, Wareing TA, et al. Comparison of a finite-element multigroup discrete-ordinates code with Monte Carlo for Radiotherapy calculations. *Phys Med Biol* 2006;51:2253–2265.
72. Daskalov GM, Baker RS, Rogers DW, et al. Dosimetric modeling of the microselectron high-dose rate 192Ir source by the multigroup discrete ordinates method. *Med Phys* 2000;27:2307–2319.
73. Zhou C, Inanc F. Integral-transport-based deterministic brachytherapy dose calculations. *Phys Med Biol* 2003; 48(1):73–93.
74. Lewis EE, Miller WF. *Computational methods of neutron transport.* New York, NY: Wiley, 1984.
75. Alcouffe RE, Baker RS, Brinkley FW, et al. DANTSYS: a diffusion accelerated neutral particle transport code system. LA-12969-M, Los Alamos National Laboratory, Los Alamos, NM, 1995.
76. Wareing TA, McGhee JM, Morel JE. ATTILA: A Three Dimensional Unstructured Tetrahedral Mesh Discrete-Ordinates Transport Code. *Trans Am Nucl Soc* 1996;75:146
77. Vassiliev ON, Wareing TA, McGhee J, et al. Validation of a new grid-based Boltzmann equation solver for dose calculation in radiotherapy with photon beams. *Phys Med Biol* 2010;55:581–598.

CHAPTER 9

Treatment Planning Algorithms: Electron Beams

Faiz M. Khan

Most commercial treatment planning systems incorporate electron beam planning programs. However, not all programs have comparable accuracy or limitations. In general, the electron beam algorithms are more complex than those of the photon beams and require more careful testing and commissioning for clinical use.

Early methods of computing dose distribution were based on empiric data or functions that used *ray line geometries* assuming broad-beam depth dose distribution in homogeneous media. Inhomogeneity corrections were determined with transmission data measured with large slabs of heterogeneities. These earlier methods have been reviewed by Sternick (1).

The major problem with the use of broad-beam distributions and slab geometries is that this approach is inadequate in predicting the effects of narrow beams, sudden changes in surface contours, small inhomogeneities, oblique beam incidence, and so on.

An improvement over the empiric methods came about with the development of algorithms based on age-diffusion equation by Kawachi (2) and others in the late 1970s. These models have been reviewed by Andreo (3). A semiempiric pencil beam model developed by Ayyangar and Suntharalingam (4) and based on age-diffusion equation was adopted for the Theraplan treatment planning system (Theratronics, Kanata, Ontario). This semiempiric algorithm, if properly implemented for a given electron accelerator, allows reasonably accurate calculation of dose distribution in a homogeneous medium. Contour irregularity and inhomogeneities are considered only in the plane of calculation, as for example, a computed tomography (CT) slice, without regard to the effects of the third dimension, such as adjacent CT slices. Although pencil beams placed along the surface contour can predict effects of contour irregularity and beam obliquity, inhomogeneity corrections are still based on effective path length between the virtual source and the point of calculations. In these cases, bulk density of the inhomogeneity in the given CT slices is used to determine effective depth. The main limitation of such algorithms is that the effects of the anatomy in three dimensions are not fully accounted for, although empirically derived correction factors may be used in simple geometric situations (5).

PENCIL BEAM MODELS BASED ON MULTIPLE SCATTERING THEORY

In the early 1980s, there was a significant surge in the development of electron beam treatment planning algorithms (6–9). These models were based on Gaussian pencil beam distributions obtained with the application of Fermi–Eyges multiple scattering theory (10). For a review of these algorithms, see Brahme (11) and Hogstrom (12).

Pencil beam algorithms based on multiple scattering theory are the algorithms of choice for electron beam treatment planning. A brief discussion of these algorithms is presented here to familiarize the users of these programs with the basic theory involved.

Assuming small-angle approximation for multiple scattering of electrons, the spatial distribution of electron fluence or dose from an elementary pencil beam penetrating a scattering medium is very nearly Gaussian at all depths. Large-angle scattering events could cause deviations from a pure Gaussian distribution, but their overall effect is considered to be small. The spatial dose distribution for the Gaussian pencil beam can be represented thus:

$$d_p(r,z) = d_p(o,z)e^{-r^2/\sigma_r^2(z)} \qquad \text{EQUATION (9.1)}$$

where $d_p(r,z)$ is the depth dose contributed by the pencil beam at a point at a radial distance r from its central axis and depth z, $d_p(o,z)$ is the axial dose, and $\sigma_r^2(z)$ is the mean square radial displacement of electrons as a result of multiple Coulomb scattering. It can be shown that $\sigma_r^2 = 2\sigma_x^2 = 2\sigma_y^2$, where σ_x^2 and σ_y^2 are the mean square lateral displacements projected into the X, Z and Y, Z planes. The exponential function in Equation 9.1 represents the off-axis ratio for the pencil beam, normalized to unity at $r = o$.

This is another useful form of Equation 9.1.

$$d_p(r,z) = D_\infty(o,z)\frac{e^{-r^2/\sigma_r^2(z)}}{\pi\sigma_r^2(z)} \qquad \text{EQUATION (9.2)}$$

where $D_\infty(o,z)$ is the dose at depth z in an infinitely broad field with the same incident fluence at the surface as the pencil beam. The Gaussian distribution function in Equation 9.2 is normalized so that the area integral of this function over a transverse plane at depth z is unity.

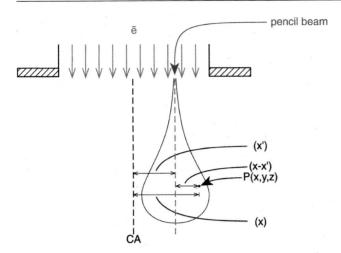

Figure 9.1. A pencil beam coordinate system. Dose at point P is calculated by integrating contributions from individual pencil beams.

In Cartesian coordinates, Equation 9.2 can be written thus:

$$d_p(x, y, z) = D_\infty(0,0,z) \frac{e^{\frac{(x-x')^2+(y-y')^2}{2\sigma^2(x',y',z)}}}{2\pi\sigma^2(x',y',z)} \quad \text{EQUATION (9.3)}$$

where $d_p(x,y,z)$ is the dose contributed to point (x, y, z) from a pencil beam whose central axis passes through (x', y', z) (Fig. 9.1).

The total dose distribution in a field of any shape can be calculated by summing all the pencil beams:

$$D(x,y,z) = \iint d_p(x - x',\ y - y',\ z)dx',dy' \quad \text{EQUATION (9.4)}$$

The integration of a Gaussian function within finite limits cannot be performed analytically. To evaluate it, this function necessitates use of the error function. Thus, convolution calculus shows that for an electron beam of a rectangular cross section $(2a \times 2b)$, the spatial dose distribution is given thus:

$$D(x,y,z) = D_\infty(0,0,z)\cdot\frac{1}{4}\left(\text{erf}\frac{a+x}{\sigma_r(z)} + \text{erf}\frac{a-x}{\sigma_r(z)}\right)$$
$$\times\left(\text{erf}\frac{b+y}{\sigma_r(z)} + \text{erf}\frac{b-y}{\sigma_r(z)}\right)$$
$$\text{EQUATION (9.5)}$$

where the error function is defined thus:

$$\text{erf}(x) = \frac{2}{\sqrt{\pi}}\int_0^x e^{-t^2}\,dt \quad \text{EQUATION (9.6)}$$

The error function is normalized so that $\text{erf}(\infty) = 1$. (It is known that the integral $\int_0^\infty e^{-t^2}\,dt = \frac{\sqrt{\pi}}{2}$.) Error function values for $0 < x < \infty$ can be obtained from tables published in mathematic handbooks (13). Although, $D_\infty(0, 0, z)$ in

Equation 9.5 is given by the area integral of the dose from pencil beams over an infinite transverse plane at depth z, this term is usually determined from measured central axis depth dose data of a broad electron field (e.g., 20×20 cm).

Pencil Beam Characterization

Lateral Spread σ

As discussed earlier, the spatial dose distribution of an elementary pencil electron beam can be represented by a Gaussian function. This function is characterized by its lateral spread parameter σ, which is similar to the standard deviation parameter of the familiar normal frequency distribution function:

$$f(x) = \frac{1}{\sqrt{2\pi}\sigma}e^{\frac{x^2}{2\sigma^2}} \quad \text{EQUATION (9.7)}$$

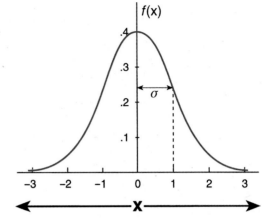

Figure 9.2. Plot of a normal distribution function given by Equation 9.7 for $\sigma = 1$. The function is normalized to unity for limits $-\infty < x < +\infty$.

Figure 9.2 is a plot of the normal distribution function given by Equation 9.7 for $\sigma = 1$. The function is normalized so that its integral between the limits $-\infty < x < +\infty$ is unity.

As a pencil electron beam is incident on a uniform phantom, its isodose distribution looks like a teardrop or onion (Fig. 9.3). The lateral spread (or σ) increases with depth until a maximum spread is achieved. Beyond this depth there is a precipitous loss of electrons as their large lateral excursion causes them to run out of energy.

The lateral spread parameter σ was theoretically predicted by Eyges (10), who extended the small-angle multiple scattering theory of Fermi to the slab geometry of any composition. Considering $\sigma_x(z)$ in the X–Z plane,

$$\sigma_x^2(z) = \frac{1}{2}\int_0^z \left(\frac{\theta^2}{\rho l}(z')\right)\rho(z')(z-z')^2\,dz' \quad \text{EQUATION (9.8)}$$

where $\theta^2/\rho l$ is the mass angular scattering power and ρ is the density of the slab phantom.

There are limitations to the Eyges' equation. As pointed out by Werner et al. (8), σ, given by Equation 9.8, increases

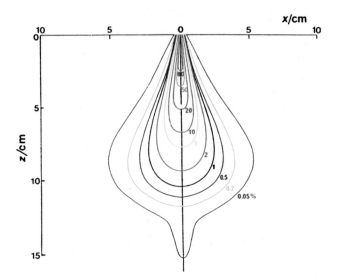

Figure 9.3. Pencil beam isodose distribution measured with a narrow electron beam of 22 MeV energy incident on water phantom. (Reprinted with permission from ICRU Report 35. Radiation dosimetry: Electron beams with energies between 1 and 50 MeV. Bethesda, MD: International Commission on Radiation Units and Measurements, 1984:36.)

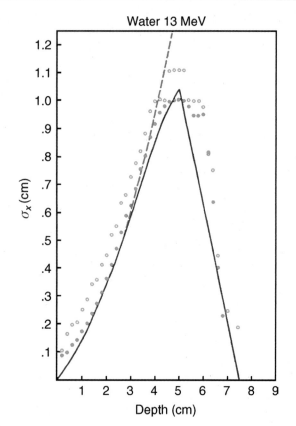

Figure 9.4. Spatial spread parameter, σ_x, plotted as a function of depth in water for a 13 MeV electron beam. Comparison is shown between σ_x's calculated by Eyges' equation (*dashed line*) and Eyges' equation modified for loss of electrons (*solid lines*) with measured data. (Reprinted with permission from Werner BL, Khan FM, Deibel FC. A model for calculating electron beam scattering in treatment planning. *Med Phys* 1982;9:180.)

with depth indefinitely, which is contrary to what is observed experimentally in narrow-beam dose distributions. The theory does not take into account the loss of electrons when lateral excursions exceed the range of the electrons. Also, Equation 9.8 is based on small-angle multiple Coulomb scattering, hence it underestimates the probability of large-angle scatter. This gives rise to an underestimation of σ. Correction factors have been proposed to counteract these problems (8,14,15).

Hogstrom et al. (7) correlated electron collision linear stopping power and linear angular scattering power relative to that of water with CT numbers so that effective depth and σ could be calculated for inhomogeneous media using CT data. Effective depth calculation using CT numbers also allows pixel-by-pixel calculation of heterogeneity correction.

Experimental measurement of $\sigma(z)$ is possible with the use of narrow beams (1–2 mm diameter). The transverse dose distribution in a narrow beam has a Gaussian shape at each depth. The root-mean-square (rms) radial displacement, $\sigma_r(z)$, can be obtained from the profiles by a mathematic deconvolution of the Gaussian distributions.

Several investigators (15–17) used a narrow-beam depth dose distribution to determine σ_r. Some (6) used the edge method, in which a wide beam is blocked off at the center by a lead block; σ is evaluated from the excursion of electrons into the block penumbra.

Werner et al. (8) used strip beams (2 mm wide) to obtain transverse profiles in homogeneous phantoms of various compositions. The strip beam profiles were then fitted by Gaussian distributions at various depths. Figure 9.4 shows the results, comparing σs calculated by Eyges' equation, with and without correction for the loss of electrons.

Central Axis Distribution

As seen in Equation 9.5, the central axis depth dose for a rectangular field of size $(2a \times 2b)$ can be derived from the measured broad-beam central axis distribution. It is given thus:

$$D(o,o,z) = D_\infty(o,o,z)\,\mathrm{erf}\,\frac{a}{\sigma_r(z)}\,\mathrm{erf}\,\frac{b}{\sigma_r(z)} \quad \text{EQUATION (9.9)}$$

The normalization of the dose distribution function against $D_\infty(o,o,z)$ is useful because the central axis dose distribution for a broad beam can be readily measured and includes Bremsstrahlung as well as the inverse square law effect. Multiplication with the error functions provides the required field size dependence factor due to lateral scatter.

SUCCESS AND LIMITATIONS OF PENCIL BEAM ALGORITHMS

Algorithms based on Gaussian pencil beam distribution have solved many of the problems that plagued the previous methods, which used measured broad-beam distributions

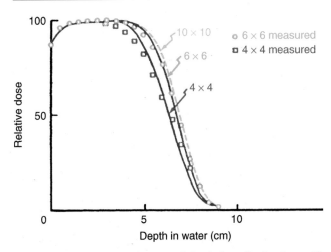

Figure 9.5. Comparison of measured depth dose distributions with those calculated from 10×10 cm field size data. Electron energy, 17 MeV. (Reprinted with permission from Hogstrom KR, Mills MD, Almond PR. Electron beam dose calculations. *Phys Med Biol* 1981; 26:445.)

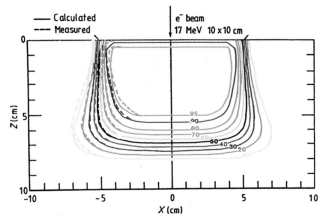

Figure 9.6. Comparison of calculated and measured isodose distribution. (Reprinted with permission from Hogstrom KR, Mills MD, Almond PR. Electron beam dose calculations. *Phys Med Biol* 1981; 26:445.)

or empirically derived best fit functions with separate correction factors for contour irregularity and tissue heterogeneity. Analytic representation of pencil beam allows calculation of dose distribution for fields of any shape and size, irregular or sloping surface contours, and tissue heterogeneities in three dimensions. However, there are limitations to pencil beam algorithms, and they have been discussed by several investigators (12,18–20). Most of the inaccuracies occur at interfaces of different density tissues such as tissue-lung, tissue-bone, and bone edges. Within the homogeneous media of any density, the algorithm has an accuracy of ~5% in the central regions of the field and ~2 mm spatial accuracy in the penumbra.

Central Axis Distribution

One of the essential requirements of a treatment planning algorithm is that it calculates the central axis depth dose distribution in water with acceptable accuracy. For broad beams, there is no problem because measured data are input as part of the formalism (Equation 9.9). So, the critical test of the algorithm is to reproduce depth dose distribution for small and irregularly shaped fields. Figure 9.5 shows such a test of the Hogstrom algorithm.

Isodose Distribution

The next step is to check isodose distributions, especially in the penumbra region. Figure 9.6, from Hogstrom et al. (7), shows a reasonably good agreement. The success of the pencil beam algorithm in this case is in part attributable to the measured broad-beam central axis data, measured off-axis profiles at the surface to provide weighting factors for the pencil beams, and an empirically derived

multiplication factor (1–1.3) to modify calculated values of $\sigma_x(z)$ for a best agreement in the penumbra region. This is true of most algorithms—that some empiric factors are required to obtain a best fit of the algorithm with measured data.

Contour Irregularity

A pencil beam algorithm is ideally suited, at least in principle, to calculate dose distribution in patients with irregular or sloping contour. Pencil beams can be placed along rays emanating from the virtual source, thus entering the patient at points defined by the surface contours. The dose distribution in the X–Z plane from the individual pencil beams depends on the Gaussian spread parameter, $\sigma_x(z)$, which is properly computed as a function of depth along the ray line. The composite dose profile, therefore, reflects the effect of the surface contour shape by virtue of the individual pencil beams entering the contour along ray lines, spreading in accordance with individual depths, and contributing dose laterally. Figure 9.7 shows a schematic representation of the pencil beam algorithm used to calculate dose distribution in a patient correction.

Tissue Heterogeneities

As discussed earlier, the Fermi–Eyges theory is strictly valid for slab geometry. That is, a pencil beam traversing a slab of material is scattered with a Gaussian profile, and the spread, σ, of the transmitted beam depends on the thickness of the slab and its linear angular scattering power (Equation 9.8). Application of this theory to the human body with inhomogeneities of different sizes and shapes becomes tenuous. Not only do many different pencil beams pass through tissues of different composition, but also each pencil with its increasing spread with depth

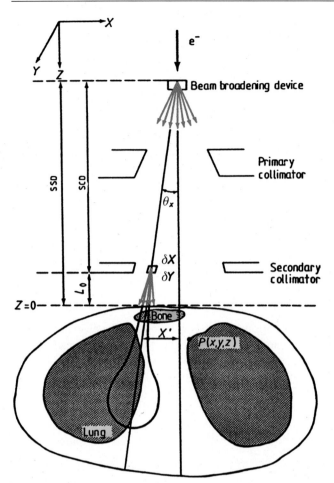

Figure 9.7. Schematic representation of the Hogstrom algorithm for the calculation of dose distribution in a patient cross section. SSD, source-to-surface distance; SCD, source-to-collimator distance. (Reprinted with permission from Hogstrom KR, Mills MD, Almond PR. Electron beam dose calculations. *Phys Med Biol* 1981; 26:445.)

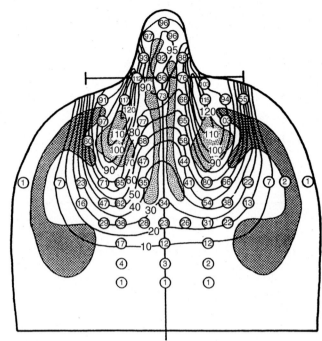

Figure 9.8. Experimental verification of the Hogstrom algorithm. Calculated isodose contours are compared with measured data using TLD in a tissue substitute phantom. Electron energy, 13 MeV; field size, 8 × 8 cm; source-to-source distance (SSD), 100 cm. (Reprinted with permission from Hogstrom KR, Almond PR. Comparison of experimental and calculated dose distributions. *Acta Radiol* 1983; 364(Suppl):89.)

in making therapeutic decisions in the use of electrons when the target or critical structures are encountered in the path of the beam.

may not stay confined to one kind of tissue. Thus, the algorithm is bound to fail where the cross section of the inhomogeneity is smaller than the pencil beam spread or at interfaces where parts of the pencil beam pass through different inhomogeneities. Research in this area continues, but no practical solution to this problem has yet been found.

Figure 9.8 shows an example of how CT-based inhomogeneity corrections have been applied with a pencil beam algorithm. A tissue substitute phantom simulating a nose was irradiated with a 13 MeV electron beam and a detailed thermoluminescent dosimetry was done. The agreement between the measured and calculated distribution was ~13%. This is not an acid test for the algorithm, since many sources of uncertainties can compound the errors in this case. However, if the user understands its limitations of accuracy in complex clinical situations, the pencil beam algorithm is capable of providing clinically useful information about overall dose distribution. These limitations must be considered

COMPUTER ALGORITHM

Implementation of a pencil beam algorithm requires dose distribution equations to be set up so that the dose to a point (x, y, z) in a given field can be calculated as an integral of the doses contributed by Gaussian pencil beams. The points of calculation constitute a beam grid, usually defined by the intersection of fan lines diverging from the virtual point source and equally spaced depth planes perpendicular to the central axis of the beam (X–Y planes). An irregularly shaped field is projected at the depth plane of calculation and is divided into strip beams of width ΔX and length extending from Y^{max} to Y^{min} (Fig. 9.9). The strip is also divided into segments so that σ of the pencil beams and effective depths can be calculated in three dimensions and integration can be carried out over all strips and segments.

Starkschall et al. (18) evaluated the Hogstrom algorithm (7) for one-, two-, and three-dimensional heterogeneity corrections. The general equation that they set up for three-dimensional dose computation is reproduced here

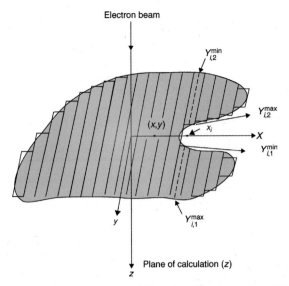

Electron beam

$Y_{i,2}^{min}$

$Y_{i,2}^{max}$

(x,y)

x_i

X

$Y_{i,1}^{min}$

y

$Y_{i,1}^{max}$

Plane of calculation (z)

z

Figure 9.9. Schematic representation of an irregularly shaped field divided into strips projected at the plane of calculation (z). (Reprinted with permission from Starkschall G, Shiu AS, Bujnowski SW, et al. Effect of dimensionality of heterogeneity corrections on the implementation of a three-dimensional electron pencil beam algorithms. *Phys Med Biol* 1991;36:207.)

to illustrate the mathematical formulation of the pencil beam algorithm:

$$
\begin{aligned}
D_e(x,y,z) = \sum_{l=1}^{N_y}\sum_{k=1}^{N_{xy}} W(x_k,y_1)\frac{1}{2}&\left\{ \mathrm{erf}\left[\frac{x_k+\Delta x/2-x}{\sqrt{2a_2(x_k,y_1,z)}}\right]\right.\\
&\left.-\mathrm{erf}\left[\frac{x_k-\Delta x/2-x}{\sqrt{2a_2(x_k,y_1,z)}}\right]\right\}\\
\times\frac{1}{2}&\left\{\mathrm{erf}\left[\frac{y_1+\Delta y-y}{\sqrt{2a_2(x_k,y_1,z)}}\right]\right.\\
&\left.-\mathrm{erf}\left[\frac{y_1+\Delta 2-y}{\sqrt{2a_2(x_k,y_1,z)}}\right]\right\}\\
\times D_e^{meas}&[0,0,d_{eff}(x_k,y_1,z)]\\
\times&\left[\frac{SSD+d_{eff}(x_k,y_1,z)}{SSD+z}\right]^2\\
\times\sum_{i=1}^{N}\frac{1}{2}&\left\{\mathrm{erf}\frac{x_i+\Delta x/2-x_k}{\sqrt{2}\sigma_{air}(z)}\right.\\
&\left.-\mathrm{erf}\left[\frac{x_i-\Delta x/2-x_k}{\sqrt{2}\sigma_{air}(z)}\right]\right\}\\
\times\sum_{j=1}^{M_i}\frac{1}{2}&\left\{\mathrm{erf}\left[\frac{Y_{i,j}^{max}(z)-y_1}{\sqrt{2}\sigma_{air}(z)}\right]\right.\\
&\left.-\mathrm{erf}\left[\frac{Y_{i,j}^{min}(z)-y_1}{\sqrt{2}\sigma_{air}(z)}\right]\right\}
\end{aligned}
$$

EQUATION (9.10)

where $D_e(x,y,z)$ is the electron dose at point (x,y,z); N is the number of strips; M is the number of segments; $W(x_k,y_1)$ is the beam weight along the fan line at point (x_k,y_1); a_2 is the pencil beam spread in the medium at depth z (obtained by integrating linear angular scattering power along a fan line from the surface of the patient to the plane of calculation); σ_{air} is the pencil beam spread in air at the plane of final collimation and projected to the plane of calculation in the absence of the medium; $D_e^{meas}[0,0,d_{eff}(x_k,y_1,z)]$ is the measured broad-beam central axis depth dose; SSD is the effective source-to-surface distance; $Y_{i,j}^{max}$ is the maximum limit of the jth segment of the ith strip; and $Y_{i,j}^{min}$ is the minimum limit of the jth segment of the ith strip.

Equation 9.10 does not include the Bremsstrahlung dose. Assuming that the dose beyond the practical range, R_p, is all due to photons, one can back-calculate the photon dose by using attenuation and inverse square law corrections.

MONTE CARLO METHODS

There is active interest in adopting Monte Carlo methods for treatment planning of photon and electron beams. The Monte Carlo technique consists of simulating transport of millions of particles through matter. It uses the fundamental laws of physics to determine probability distributions of individual particle interactions. Each particle is followed as it travels through the medium and gives rise to energy deposition by interaction with the atoms of the medium. The larger the number of simulated particles (histories), the greater is the statistical accuracy of predicting their distribution. As the number of simulated particles is increased, the accuracy gets better but the computational time becomes prohibitively long. So, the challenge lies in using a relatively small sample of randomly selected particles to predict the average behavior of the particles in the beam. The dose distribution is calculated by accumulating (scoring) ionizing events in bins (voxels) that give rise to energy deposition in the medium. It is estimated that the transport of a few hundred million to a billion histories will be required for radiation therapy treatment planning with adequate precision.

Although Monte Carlo codes require inordinate amount of computational times, they are the most accurate methods of calculating dose distribution. Because of this accuracy, which is not limited by tissue heterogeneity or interfaces, some treatment planning systems have adopted semi-Monte Carlo programs to reduce computational times to retain as much of the accuracy as possible. For example, ADAC Pinnacle uses Monte Carlo-generated kernels in its convolution in superposition algorithm for photons. Eclipse is in the process of implementing what it calls the "fast electron Monte Carlo" or EMC (21), which is based on EGS4 Monte Carlo code but reduces the number of steps in the electron transport. The program requires the input of measured central axis percent depth dose in water and an in-air profile of an open electron beam (without applicator). Clinical tests are in progress to verify that the implementation of EMC in Eclipse would provide a significant improvement in the treatment planning accuracy.

With the continuing advancement in computer technology and computation algorithms, it now seems probable that a full-fledged Monte Carlo code will be implemented for routine treatment planning in the not too distant future.

REFERENCES

1. Sternick E. Algorithms for computerized treatment planning. In: Orton CG, Bagne F, eds. *Practical aspects of electron beam treatment planning.* New York: American Institute of Physics, 1978:52.
2. Kawachi K. Calculation of electron dose distribution for radiotherapy treatment planning. *Phys Med Biol* 1975;20:571.
3. Andreo P. Broad beam approaches to dose computation and their limitations. In: Nahum AE, ed. *The computation of dose distributions in electron beam radiotherapy.* Kungalv, Sweden: Miniab/gotab, 1985:128.
4. Ayyangar K, Suntharalingam N. Electron beam treatment planning incorporating CT data. *Med Phys* 1983;10:525 (abstract).
5. Pohlit W, Manegold KH. Electron beam dose distribution in homogeneous media. In: Kramer S, Suntharalingam N, Zinniger GF, eds. *High energy photons and electrons.* New York: Wiley, 1976:343.
6. Perry DJ, Holt JG. A model for calculating the effects of small inhomogeneities on electron beam dose distributions. *Med Phys* 1980;7:207.
7. Hogstrom KR, Mills MD, Almond PR. Electron beam dose calculations. *Phys Med Biol* 1981;26:445.
8. Werner BL, Khan FM, Deibel FC. A model for calculating electron beam scattering in treatment planning. *Med Phys* 1982;9:180.
9. Jette D. The application of multiple scattering theory to therapeutic electron dosimetry. *Med Phys* 1983;10:141.
10. Eyges L. Multiple scattering with energy loss. *Phys Rev* 1948;74:1534.
11. Brahme A. Brief review of current algorithms for electron beam dose planning. In: Nahum AE, ed. *The computation of dose distributions in electron beam radiotherapy.* Kungalv, Sweden: Miniab/gotab, 1985:271.
12. Hogstrom KR, Starkschall G, Shiu AS. Dose calculation algorithms for electron beams. In: Purdy JA, ed. *Advances in radiation oncology physics. American Institute of Physics Monograph 19.* New York: American Institute of Physics, 1992:900.
13. Beyer WH. *Standard mathematical tables,* 25th edn. Boca Raton, FL: CRC Press, 1978:524.
14. Lax I, Brahme A. Collimation of high energy electron beams. *Acta Radiol Oncol* 1980;19:199.
15. Lax I, Brahme A, Andreo P. Electron beam dose planning using Gaussian beams. *Acta Radiol* 1983;364(Suppl):49.
16. Brahme A. Physics of electron beam penetration: fluence and absorbed dose. In: Paliwal B, ed. *Proceedings of the symposium on electron dosimetry and arc therapy.* New York: American Institute of Physics, 1982:45.
17. Abou Mandour M, Nusslin F, Harder D. Characteristic function of point monodirectional electron beams. *Acta Radiol* 1983;364(Suppl):43.
18. Starkschall G, Shiu AS, Buynowski SW, et al. Effect of dimensionality of heterogeneity corrections on the implementation of a three-dimensional electron pencil-beam algorithm. *Phys Med Biol* 1991;36:207.
19. Hogstrom KR, Steadham RE. Electron beam dose computation. In: Paltra JR, Mackie TR, eds. *Teletherapy: present and future.* Madison, WI: Advanced Medical Publishing, 1996:137–174.
20. Hogstrom KR. Electron-beam therapy: dosimetry, planning and techniques. In: Perez C, Brady L, Halperin E, Schmidt-Ullrich RK, eds. *Principles and practice of radiation oncology.* Baltimore, MD: Lippincott Williams & Wilkins, 2003:252–282.
21. Neuenschwander H, Mackie TR, Reckwerdt PJ. MMC-a high performance Monte Carlo code for electron beam treatment planning. *Phys Med Biol* 1995;40:543–574.

CHAPTER 10

Treatment Planning Algorithms: Proton Therapy

Hanne M. Kooy ■ Benjamin M. Clasie

INTRODUCTION

A clinical dose computation algorithm, a "dose algorithm," must satisfy requirements such as clinical accuracy in the patient, computational performance, representations of patient devices and delivery equipment, and specification of the treatment field in terms of equipment input parameters. A dose algorithm has been invariably imbedded within a larger treatment planning system (TPS) whose requirements and behavior often affect the dose algorithm itself. Current clinical emphasis on the patient workflow and advanced delivery technologies such as adaptive radiotherapy will lead to different dose algorithm implementations and deployments depending on the context. For example, a treatment planner needs highly interactive dose computations in a patient to allow rapid evaluation of a clinical treatment plan. A quality assurance physicist, on the other hand, needs an accurate dose algorithm whose requirements could be simplified considering that QA measurements are typically done in simple homogeneous phantoms.

A dose algorithm has two components: a geometry modeler and a physics modeler. In practice, the choice of a physics model drives the specification of the geometry modeler because the geometry modeler must present the physics modeler with local geometry information to model the local effect on the physics-model calculation. Physics models come in two forms: Monte Carlo and phenomenological. The latter models the transport of radiation in medium with analytical forms and has been the standard in the clinic because of the generally higher computational performance compared to Monte Carlo. Monte Carlo, in general, models the trajectories of a large number of individual radiation particles and scores their randomly generated interactions in medium to yield energy deposited in the medium. Monte Carlo is considered an absolute benchmark and much effort is expanded to produce high-performance implementations. The accuracy of a Monte Carlo model is inversely related to the extent and complexity of the modeled interactions and improved performance can be achieved by limiting the model to meet a particular clinical requirement. We describe, as an example, a basic Monte Carlo, which outperforms a phenomenological implementation because of its simple model and implementation on a graphics processor unit (GPU).

The geometry modeler creates a representation of the patient, which is invariably derived from a CT volumetric data set and the CT voxel coordinates are sometimes chosen as the coordinates for the points for which to compute the dose. Dose points are typically associated to individual organ volumes after the dose calculation proper for the computation of, for example, dose-volume histograms. A more general implementation allows the user to select arbitrary point distributions. The geometry modeler also provides the physical characteristics of the patient including, for example, electron density derived from CT Hounsfield Units and, for protons, the stopping power ratio relative to water also derived from CT Hounsfield Units albeit indirectly. The geometry modeler also implements a model of the treatment field. For a Monte Carlo implementation this is a two-step procedure. First, the treatment field geometry and equipment parameters are used to create a representative phase-space, that is, the distribution of particles in terms of position and energy, and perhaps other parameters, of the radiation particles that impinge on the patient. Second, the particles are transported individually through the patient until they are absorbed in or exit the patient volume. For a phenomenological implementation, the treatment field geometry forms a template whose geometric extents are projected through the patient volume. This projection is typically implemented by a ray tracer where individual rays populate the treatment field to sufficiently sample the features within the patient and where the physics model becomes a function of distance along the ray. Figure 10.1 shows the various computational approaches.

Proton transport in medium has been exhaustively studied and the references in this chapter are but a minimum.

PHYSICS OF PROTON TRANSPORT IN MEDIUM

Interactions

The physics of proton interactions for clinical energies, that is, between 50 and 350 MeV, is well understood. The publication "Passive Beam Spreading in Proton Radiation Therapy" by Bernard Gottschalk (1) provides an in-depth, theoretical and practical, elaboration of this physics and this section relies significantly on that material.

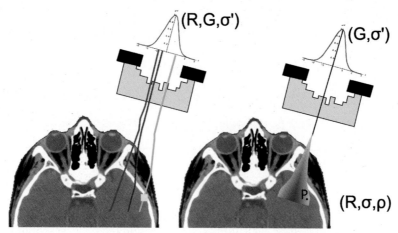

Figure 10.1. The left panel shows a Monte Carlo schematic while the right panel shows a phenomenological schematic. The beam includes an aperture and a range-compensator. The beam for both is assumed subdivided in individual pencil-beam "spots." These spots are physical in the case of pencil-beam scanning (see text) while for a scattered field they are a means for subdividing the field for computational purposes. The initial spot is characterized by a spread σ', an intensity G and an energy R. In the Monte Carlo, the spot properties can be used as a generator of individual protons. Thus, there will be more "red" protons than "blue" protons than "green" protons. The total number of protons is on the order of 10^6 or more. Each proton is transported through the patient and its energy loss is scored in individual voxels (a "yellow" one is shown). In the phenomenological model, the spot defines one or more pencil-beams that are traced through the patient. Each ray-trace models the broadening of the protons in the pencil-beam as a continuous function of density ρ along the ray-trace. Dose is scored to points P, where the deposited dose depends on the geometric location of P with respect to the ray-trace axis and the proton range R and pencil-beam spread σ. The latter may include the initial spot spread σ' if the ray-trace axis represents *all* the protons G in the spot. Otherwise, the spot can be subdivided into multiple sub-spots such that the superposition of those spots equal the initial spot.

Protons loose energy in medium through interactions with orbital electrons, scatter predominantly through electromagnetic Coulomb interactions with the nuclear electric field, and have inelastic interactions with the nucleus itself. Proton–electron interactions produce delta electrons that deposit dose in proximity to the proton geometric track. The mass of the proton is about 2,000 times that of the electron and hence the collision is equivalent to a blue whale moving at near-relativistic speed toward you: the proton emerges unscattered. Proton–nucleus Coulomb interactions result in small angular deviations in the proton direction and produce, to a very good approximation, a Gaussian diffusion profile in a narrow parallel beam of protons. The Gaussian form of this profile is a consequence of the very large number of random scattering events, which, as described by the central limit theorem, approximate to a continuous Gaussian function to describe the underlying discrete random events.

Protons also have inelastic interactions with the nucleus and produce secondary particles including secondary protons, neutrons, and heavier fragments. The secondary protons contribute up to 10% of the dose within a proton depth dose (2). The secondary neutron production is of specific concern because of their long-range effect. These neutrons deposit dose to healthy tissues throughout the patient, far from the target region, and impact on the shielding requirements of a proton therapy facility. The neutron contribution to the dose distribution is only considered implicitly through their contribution in the physics parameters such as a depth-dose distribution. The effect of heavier secondaries is small and can be ignored for dose calculation purposes.

Relative Biological Effectiveness

Dose deposited by protons is considered to be biologically equivalent to Co60 dose. That is, cellular response to proton and photon interactions are considered equivalent. Clinically, though, the proton physical dose (in Gy) is scaled by an RBE factor of 1.1 to yield the proton biological dose with units of Gy (RBE) (3). Thus, a photon fraction prescription of 1.8 Gy (which implicitly has an RBE of 1 as Co60 is the "standard" dose reference) can be delivered with a proton fraction of 1.8 Gy (RBE), which corresponds to 1.64 Gy physical proton dose. The latter is the value one would measure in a radiation detector and to which one would calibrate the field to deliver 1.8 Gy (RBE).

Clinically, the RBE is assumed 1.1 throughout. Of special consideration is the change in RBE at the distal drop-off of the Bragg peak. In this region, the change in RBE has the effect of differentially shifting the distal edge deeper by about 1 mm compared to measurements. That is, the biological dose fall-off is shifted 1 mm deeper compared to the physical dose fall-off. This inherent uncertainty in the distal edge is one reason why the sharp distal edge is not used to achieve, for example, a dose gradient between a target and a critical structure. The other reason (see below) is the uncertainty in the relative stopping power, which is estimated on the order of 2% to 3%. These uncertainties could result in

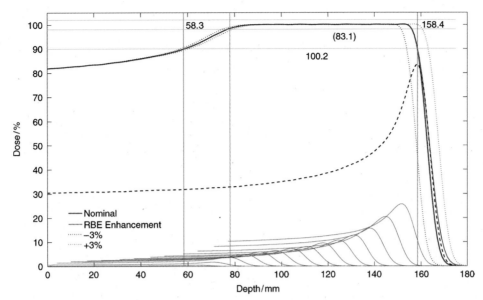

Figure 10.2. An SOBP depth dose distribution with its constituent pristine Bragg peak depth dose distributions scaled relative to their contribution. The deepest pristine peak is at 160 mm, which results in a lower SOBP range of 158.4 mm because of the other peak contributions. The 90-90 modulation width is 100.2 mm while the 90-98 is 83.1 mm. The range uncertainties create a band of uncertainty both distally and proximally (see dashed distal fall-offs). The effect is most pronounced at the distal fall-off and the error must be considered to ensure that the target coverage is respected. The 80% depth, R_{80}, of a pristine peak correlates accurately with the proton energy in MeV. The clinical historical range is in reference to the 90% depth which also depends on the energy spread. The difference in practice is on the order of 1 mm. Care should be practiced especially considering calibration and reference conditions.

overdose to the critical structure or underdose to the target (see Fig. 10.2).

The RBE, in general, depends on other factors such as dose fraction size, number of fractions, clinical end point, and so on. These factors can be ignored for proton radiation computations but are significant for higher LET charged particles such as Carbon. Computation algorithms for such particles are, therefore, much more complicated and must implement a model for the LET distributions in patient to resolve such dependencies.

Stopping Power

The various electromagnetic interactions transfer energy to electrons in the medium and the proton energy is reduced as a consequence. The proton energy loss, transferred to the medium, is quantified as the rate of energy-loss per unit length, dE/dx, where E (MeV) is the energy and x (cm) is the distance along the proton path. The stopping power S is defined in combination with the local material density ρ (g/cm^3):

$$\frac{S}{\rho} = -\frac{1}{\rho}\frac{dE}{dx} \text{ (MeV cm}^2\text{/g)} \qquad \text{EQUATION (10.1)}$$

and is called the mass stopping power.

The mass stopping power in a given medium is a function of the proton energy E and increases significantly when the proton has lost nearly most of its energy. The proton mass stopping power in a given material can be calculated using

the Bethe-Bloch equation (4) or directly from tables (5). For example, the mass stopping power values for protons of energies 100, 10, and 1 MeV, respectively in water are 7.3, 45.7, and 261.1 MeV cm^2/g. Thus, a proton of 1 MeV energy cannot travel more than 0.004 cm in water. It is this rapid increase in energy loss per unit length, and the very localized energy deposition, that leads to the characteristic Bragg peak of the proton depth-dose distribution (Fig. 10.2). Note that a Bragg peak is a characteristic feature of all charged particles, including electrons, of the energy loss along the particle track. The feature disappears for electrons traversing a medium due to their large scattering angle. In effect, the track becomes "tangled-up" and the Bragg peak becomes averaged out over all the entwined tracks. Thus, a mono-energetic electron depth-dose distribution has a broad and flat high-dose region followed by the distal fall-off.

Water-Equivalent Depth and Proton Range, *R*

In a photon algorithm, the computational quantity is the radiological path length, $\tau_{RPL} = \int_0^z \rho(t)\,dt$, that gives the density (ρ in units of g/cm^3 or relative to water) corrected depth along the ray up to the physical depth z in cm. For a proton algorithm, the appropriate quantity is the water-equivalent thickness, τ_{WET} in g/cm^2, which is the thickness in water that produces the same final proton energy as the given thickness in the medium. It is calculated from relative stopping power, S_W^V, defined as the ratio of the

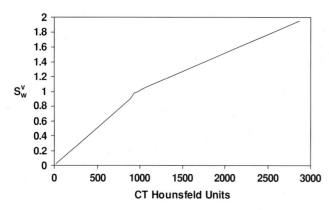

Figure 10.3. Conversion from CT Hounsfeld units of the volume to relative stopping power, S_W^V, for biological tissues. Figure is adapted from Schneider et al. [7].

stopping power of protons in the medium over that in water. In practice, S_W^V is known for the materials such as polyethylene used in range-compensators or derived empirically from CT numbers (see Fig. 10.3). The proton water-equivalent thickness* along a ray trace is given as

$$\tau_{\text{WET}} = \int_0^z \rho_W \cdot S_W^V(t) \cdot dt \, (\text{g/m}^2) \quad \text{EQUATION (10.2)}$$

where ρ_W is the density of water.

The mass stopping power ratio, $\dfrac{\rho_W}{\rho_V} S_W^V$, is almost independent of therapeutic proton energies for biological materials (6). If this ratio is unity, the radiological path length and water-equivalent thickness are mathematically equivalent. In treatment planning, however, the differences between τ_{RPL} and τ_{WET} can be clinically significant.

Range, R, which is often called the mean proton range, is the average water-equivalent depth where protons stop in the medium. This is a very close approximation of the range in the continuous slowing down approximation, R_{CSDA}, and the depth at distal 80% of maximum dose, R_{80}, of a pristine proton Bragg peak (see Fig. 10.2). These definitions of range are often used interchangeably in proton therapy.

Dose to Medium

The dose to a volume element, of thickness t along and area A perpendicular to the proton direction, is given by the energy lost in the voxel divided by the mass of the voxel

$$D \equiv \frac{\text{Energy}}{\text{Mass}} \left[\frac{\text{J}}{\text{kg}} \right] = \frac{dE/dx \times t \times N}{\rho \times A \times t} = \Phi \frac{S}{\rho} \, (\text{Gy})$$

$$\text{EQUATION (10.3)}$$

*Proton pathlength is the thickness of material summed over the track of the proton. Protons at clinical energies, however, undergo little deviation from straight paths and pathlength and thickness can be used interchangeably in proton therapy. Depth is the thickness of material summed along a ray from the entrance of the phantom to a given endpoint.

where $\Phi = N/A$ is the proton fluence in (cm^{-2}). Consider a fluence of 10^9 (1 Gigaproton [Gp]) per cm^2 of 100 MeV protons in water where $S/\rho = 7.3$ MeV cm^2/g. The dose is (Equation 10.3)

$$D = \frac{10^9}{\text{cm}^2} \times \frac{7.3 \text{ MeV cm}^2}{10^{-3} \text{kg}} \times \frac{0.1602 \times 10^{-12} \text{ J}}{\text{MeV}} = 1.17 \, (\text{Gy})$$

$$\text{EQUATION (10.4)}$$

at the entrance of the water (where the proton energy is 100 MeV) and where we used the factor 10^{-3} to convert from gram to kilogram and the conversion factor is 0.1602 $\times 10^{-12}$ J/MeV. Equation 10.4 shows that the number of protons to deliver a clinical dose is on the order of Giga-protons, a number less than 10^{-15} of the number of protons in a gram of water. A convenient rule of thumb is that 1 Gp delivers about 1 cGy to a 1 L (i.e., $10 \times 10 \times 10$ cm^3) volume.

The mass stopping power only measures the energy loss from electromagnetic interactions and does not include the energy deposited from secondary particles. In practice, a measured depth dose is a surrogate for the mass stopping power and thus effectively includes all primary and other interactions in calculational models.

A CT data representation of the patient does not provide the necessary stopping power information; it only provides the electron density on a voxel level. The conversion from this electron density to relative stopping power is empirical and is based on an average for particular organs over all patients (7). Thus, the conversion has inherent uncertainties due to (1) the nonspecificity for a particular patient, and (2) the lack of knowledge of precise stopping powers for particular organs. One, therefore, assumes a 3% uncertainty in the relative stopping power in patients (see Fig. 10.2). This 3% uncertainty must be considered by the treatment planner as is described elsewhere.

A dose algorithm may use longitudinal depth-dose distributions in water for all available proton energies. Dose distributions in the patient are calculated from the dose in water using the local density and relative stopping power, both of which come from CT data. In the presence of heterogeneities, the depth-dose distribution in the medium, $T_M(E, \tau_{\text{WET}})$, is obtained from that in water by (following from Equation 10.3 and assuming constant fluence)

$$T_M^\infty(E, \tau_{\text{WET}}) = T_W^\infty(E, z\rho_W) \times \frac{S_M/\rho_M}{S_W/\rho_W} \quad \text{EQUATION (10.5a)}$$

where E is the incident proton energy, z is the geometric depth in cm, and the superscript ∞ indicates that broad beam depth-dose distributions are at infinite source-to-axis distance (SAD). The effect of inhomogeneities is two-fold. Firstly, the physical depth of the Bragg peak is shifted relative to a water phantom based on the water-equivalent

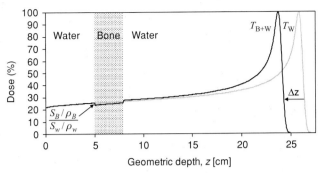

Figure 10.4. T_W is the depth dose distribution in a homogenous water phantom and T_{W+B} is the depth dose distribution in a water phantom with bone at 5 cm depth. The relative mass stopping power, $\dfrac{S_B/\rho_B}{S_W/\rho_W}$, of bone to water gives the ratio of the dose deposited in bone to water in the shaded region. Bone has larger relative stopping power, $\dfrac{S_B}{S_W}$, compared to water and, for 2.9 cm geometric thickness of bone with 1.72 relative stopping power, the Δz is −2.1 cm by Equation (10-5b).

depth in the patient. The shift for material M with geometric thickness z_M and water-equivalent thickness $\tau_{\text{WET,M}}$ is

$$\Delta z = z_M - \frac{\tau_{\text{WET,M}}}{\rho_W}. \qquad \text{Equation (10.5b)}$$

Secondly, the dose in the heterogeneity is scaled by the relative mass stopping powers. The latter ratio of relative mass stopping powers is close to 1 and the scaling of the dose is typically ignored in dose algorithm implementations. These effects are illustrated in Figure 10.4.

It was well recognized early on that protons could be used instead of x-rays for tomography and thus measure the stopping power for a patient directly (8). Such an image measures the energy loss, which is a function of the integrated stopping power, along a particular proton ray instead of an attenuation measurement along an x-ray, which is a function of the integrated electron density. The resultant reconstructed tomographic image is thus a stopping power distribution rather than an electron density distribution. There is considerable interest in this technology to achieve further precision in proton beam dosimetry and to achieve accurate volumetric imaging at very low doses.

Proton Lateral Spread

The numerous multiple elastic scattering events produce, for an initial parallel and infinitesimally narrow beam of protons, a Gaussian lateral distribution profile. The characteristic spread of this Gaussian profile in the Bragg peak region is about 2% of the range (in cm). Thus, a proton beam of 20 cm penetration range in water has a spread of 4 mm in the Bragg peak region. In comparison, an electron beam has a spread of about 20% of its range (Fig. 10.5).

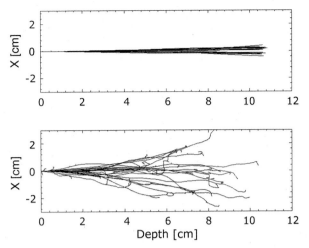

Figure 10.5. Monte Carlo (GEANT4) generated proton and electron tracks in water with comparable penetration range. Protons maintain near constant direction of motion while continuously slowing down by loosing energy in collisions with electrons. An electron track becomes "tangled" up with its collision electron partner and undergoes many wide-angle scattering events. The minimal scatter of the proton makes the dose distribution accurately described by the Gaussian pencil-beam model.

The scattering angle that underlies the widening Gaussian profile was originally described by Molière who investigated single scattering in the Coulomb field of the nucleus and multiple scattering as a consequence of numerous interactions (9). A complete description of scattering theory is beyond the scope of this chapter. In practice, the Highland approximation (10), or similar readily computable variants, are used to compute the lateral beam spread in matter. For dose calculations in thick, heterogeneous matter, the volume is divided into N homogeneous slabs that represent the material along the particle track. The standard deviation of the Gaussian spread $\sigma_{P,i}$ at radiological depth L due to the ith slab is

$$\sigma_{P,i} = \left[1 + \frac{1}{9}\log_{10}\left(\frac{L_i - L_{i-1}}{L_{R,i}} \right) \right]$$

$$\times \left[\int_{L_{i-1}}^{L_i} \left(\frac{14.1\ \text{MeV}}{pv} \times \frac{(L - L')}{\rho_i} \right)^2 \frac{1}{L_{R,i}} dL' \right]^{1/2} \quad \text{(cm)}$$

$$\text{Equation (10.6a)}$$

where pv is the product of the proton momentum and speed (in MeV), L_R is the radiation length (in g/cm²), and the ith slab extends from radiological depth L_{i-1} to L_i. The total Gaussian spread, σ_P, is the quradrature sum of the individual Gaussian spreads from each slab

$$\sigma_P = \left[\sum_{i=1}^{N} \sigma_{P,i}^2 \right]^{1/2} \quad \text{(cm)} \qquad \text{Equation (10.6b)}$$

Solving Equation 10.6b at each dose calculation point is not feasible due to computation time and two simplifications are made: the radiation length in the patient is set to the radiation length of water (36.1 g/cm^2) and the density ρ is set to the density of water (1 g/cm^3) in the integration. The simplified equation for the Gaussian spread

$$\sigma_P(L) = \left[1 + \frac{1}{9}\log_{10}\left(\frac{L}{L_{R,\text{water}}}\right)\right]$$
$$\times \left[\int_0^L \left(\frac{14.1\,\text{MeV}}{pv} \times \frac{(L-L')}{\rho_{\text{water}}}\right)^2 \frac{1}{L_{R,\text{water}}}\,dL'\right]^{1/2} \text{(cm)}$$

EQUATION (10.6c)

is only a function of the radiological depth L in the media. The simplifications are acceptable for most cases. Consider protons with 100 MeV energy incident on a homogeneous water phantom, then σ_P at the maximum water-equivalent depth is 0.179 mm. If the same beam passes through 1 g/cm of compact bone ($L_R = 16.6$ g/cm^2 and $\rho = 1.85$ g/cm^3) followed by water, then σ_P at the maximum water-equivalent depth is 0.169 mm, an acceptable difference compared to the homogeneous phantom. One should, in general, however, give special attention to treatment plans that have materials with properties significantly different than water.

Treatment planning algorithms use tables or parameterizations of σ_P in water to improve the computation time. Numerical solutions of Equation 10.6c are described by Hong et al. (6) and Lee et al. (12). Figure 10.6 shows a similar calculation in water where the momentum and velocity of protons at radiological depth, L, and range, R, are calculated through range-energy tables from J. Janni (5).

MODELS OF DOSE DISTRIBUTIONS

Phenomenological Models

A phenomenological model uses analytical forms to describe the physical processes and, typically, represents the passage of the radiation through the medium as geometric

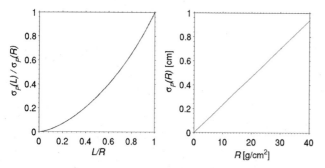

Figure 10.6. Left: The normalized Gaussian spread $\sigma_P(L)/\sigma_P(R)$ vs. normalized radiological depth, L/R. This relation is essentially independent of R; the width of the line gives the variation from 0.1 g/cm^2 < R < 40 g/cm^2. Right: The Gaussian spread at the end of range of the pristine proton beam as a function of range.

rays or pencil beams. Ray tracing, as applied in radiotherapy algorithms, derives primarily from computer graphics techniques to create images of three-dimensional objects as a consequence of light rays interacting with those objects as described by their physical properties. Monte Carlo methods in radiotherapy, in essence, also implement ray tracing methods where individual rays are the particles and their path is, in general, distorted as a consequence of local interactions. We will refer to this technique as particle tracing in distinction from ray tracing.

The performance of ray tracing algorithms through rectilinear volume representations, such as a CT volume, is high and the computation time for this part of an algorithm tends to be small compared to the computation time needed for the physics model calculations. The ray trace along a particular line, typically a line from the radiation source through a point in the isocentric plane, is used to accumulate the volume physical information along the trace.

The main computational burden in a ray-trace algorithm implementation is the association of dose to points surrounding the ray (see Fig. 10.1). In general, at a given depth z, one has to find the points that will receive a relevant contribution from the "particles" modeled by the ray. In the case of a proton algorithm, this means that at a depth z, one has to search an area of radius 3σ as this, for a Gaussian distribution, contains 99% of the laterally distributed profile. To efficiently find these points, as opposed to explicitly checking each point at each depth for the distance from that point to the ray axis, one can resort to sorting and indexing algorithms before commencing the ray-trace calculation. Original implementations of dose calculation algorithms used fan-beam grids where the points on the calculation grid fan out along rays from the source. Such methodologies are impractical when considering requirements such as non-coplanar beams and arbitrary distributions of points. A more general implementation relies on indexing and sorting the dose points, in the beam coordinate system, in the isocentric plane, and along the axis of the beam or ray (see Fig. 10.7).

Gaussian Proton Pencil-Beam Model

The Gaussian behavior of charged particle spread in medium was first used in an electron pencil-beam algorithm described by Hogstrom et al. (13). The use of Gaussian functions has the convenient mathematical property of yielding well-behaved integration and summation results to describe the field profile and lateral penumbrae. In a pencil-beam model, the radiation field is subdivided into narrow subfields, that is, pencil beams. The central axis of the pencil beam, the "ray," is traced through the medium and only density variations along the axis are considered in the calculation of the lateral spread of particles with respect to the pencil-beam axis. The density distribution lateral to the pencil-beam axis is considered to be that encountered on the axis and the calculation is thus insensitive to heterogeneity variations comparable to the width

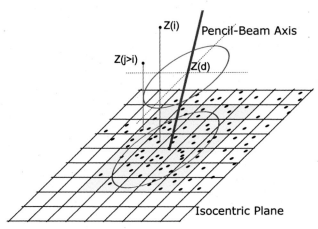

Figure 10.7. A pencil-beam traced through the volume needs to find the points that are within its extent. Consider all dose calculation points Z projected on the isocentric plane ("dots"), binned in rectangles (the grid shown above) in that plane, and sorted along the central axis of the overall field. At a particular depth at Z(d) the pencil-beam has the extent shown above (blue ellipse) which is projected on the isocentric plane (red). The pencil-beam only needs to consider the points in those bins within its extent and only those points Z for which $Z(d)-\Delta < Z < Z(d)+\Delta$ (i.e. those within the thickness of the ray trace step (2Δ). Such an algorithm can improve performance well over 10× compared to a brute force approach.

of the pencil beam. The Gaussian description for electron beams works well in homogeneous medium but less so in heterogeneous media as a consequence of the large scattering angle of electrons (Fig. 10.5). The Gaussian model is a good mathematical and physical representation if the spread is much smaller such as is the case for proton beams.

The Gaussian pencil-beam model was used by Hong et al. (6) to describe a scattered proton field produced by a general delivery device. Such a device contains beam scatterers, an aperture, a range-compensator, an air-gap between the range-compensator and the patient, and the patient itself (Fig. 10.8). A physical narrow pencil beam of protons can be mathematically modeled even in the presence of heterogeneities while retaining good resolution. For example, a pure pencil beam of 15-cm range still has better than 4-mm resolution at depth.

The dose D to a point (x,y,z) from a pencil-beam field is

$$D(x,y,z) = \sum_i \Psi(x_i,y_i)\frac{T_W^\infty(R_i,\tau_{wet})}{2\pi\sigma_T(z)^2}\exp\left(-\frac{(x-x_i)^2-(y-y_i)^2}{2\sigma_T(z)^2}\right)$$

EQUATION (10.7)

where the sum is over all pencil beam i (each of range R_i) whose central axis at a depth at the coordinate z is at (x_i,y_i), $\Psi(x_i,y_i)$ is the number of protons at (x_i,y_i), σ_T is the total spread of the pencil beam, and $T_W^\infty(R_i,\tau_{wet})$ are broad-field depth-dose distributions in water with infinite SAD. $T_W^\infty(R_i,\tau_{wet})$ are determined from measured depth-dose

distributions with finite SAD by correcting for inverse square.

$$T_W^\infty(R_i,\tau_{wet}) = T_W(R_i,\tau_{wet})\times\frac{(SAD+z)^2}{(SAD)^2}$$ EQUATION (10.8)

where z is the longitudinal geometric coordinate of the measurement with axis at $z = 0$.

Equation 10.7 is a general description of proton diffusion through medium as a function of depth. Its basic form is used for describing a scattered proton field, where a proton beam is passively scattered in the lateral dimension and modulated in depth, and a pencil-beam scanning field, where a narrow beam of proton pencils are scanned magnetically in the lateral dimension and modulated in depth.

Scattered Field Implementation

A scattered proton field is not dissimilar from an electron scattered field. The scattered field is characterized by a virtual source from which the protons appear to emanate and diverge and which has a spread σ_S. The source position and size can be determined by measuring the field width and the penumbral width of an aperture as a function of distance from the aperture. The field width projects back to the source position, while the penumbral width is given by the back-projection of the measured penumbra through the aperture, where the penumbra is 0, to that position (as described, e.g., in (13)). The resultant "virtual" source size of the proton beam is large with σ_S between 5 and 10 cm as a consequence of the proton scatter in the scattering system (see Fig. 10.8). This large source size can only be mitigated by placing the aperture as close to the patient as possible (as is the practice for an electron aperture) and to move the source position as far as possible from the patient. The latter is one reason for the size of proton gantries; the other being the bending radius necessary to bend the proton beam toward the patient. The effective source size (the projection of the source to $Z = 0$ through a pinhole at the aperture) thus becomes

$$\sigma_{S,eff} = \sigma_S\frac{SAD-Z_A}{Z_A}$$ EQUATION (10.9)

which for a typical beamline, with an SAD of 300 and an aperture distance Z_A to the patient of 10 cm, reduces the source size by a factor of $(300-10)/10 = 29$ and the contribution of the virtual source is reduced to 3 mm or less.

The proton beam passes through the aperture and subsequently is modified by a range-compensator, which locally shifts the proton range such that the distal surface of the field is beyond the distal target volume surface (with respect to the beam axis). Passage through the range-compensator introduces compensator thickness-dependent scatter, which

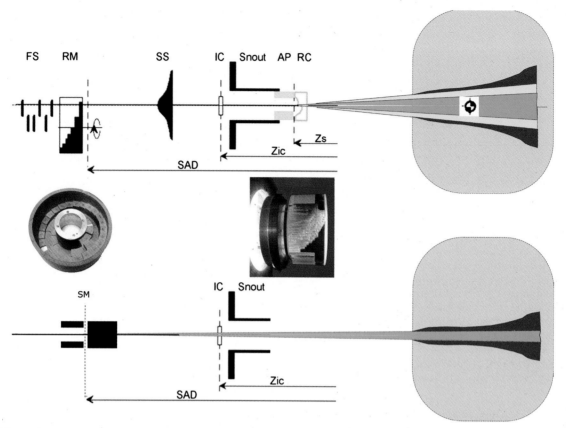

Figure 10.8. A schematic double-scattering nozzle (top) with a range-modulator wheel (RM, insert) and scatterer (SS), ionization chamber IC, and a snout that holds the aperture and range-compensator (insert). The fixed scatterer (FS) inserts thin layers of lead and ensures that the overall mean scattering angle remains constant as a function of energy thus maintaining a flat lateral profile. The protons in the model are assumed to spread as a consequence from the effective source (green profile and eq. 7), from the range-compensator thickness (yellow and eq. 8) and the scatter in patient (red profile and eq. 4b). The bottom shows a scanning nozzle with a pair of scanning magnets (SM). The absence (in general) of an aperture and range-compensator requires that the incoming pencil-beam be as narrow as possible to minimize its contribution (green) to the in-patient spread. The SAD is defined by the bending points in the X and Y magnets (shown here in the center of the magnets). The SAD defines the origin of the proton pencil-beam axis. The relative widths of the pencil-beam are for illustration purposes and do not imply that a scanning beam is, by definition, narrower. The schematics represent the core features of the IBA nozzle (IBA LTD, Louvain la Neuve).

introduces a penumbral spread component in the patient at depth z given by

$$\sigma_R = \theta_0(t(x,y))(z - z_R) \qquad \text{EQUATION (10.10)}$$

where $\theta_0(t)$ is the scattering angle produced by the protons passing through the local thickness t at (x,y) of the range-compensator at position Z_R.

The protons in the patient further scatter and introduce a third spread factor, σ_P, to the total spread of the proton pencil beam. The derivation of σ_P is computed, for example, from the Highland formula (Equation 10.6c). The total spread of the pencil beam is the quadratic sum of the three spread factors in Equations 10.9, 10.10, and 10.6b (Fig. 10.8).

The complete algorithm thus subdivides the scattered field extent circumscribed by the aperture into many small pencil beams, typically spaced in a rectangular grid of 2-mm resolution. This high resolution ensures that heterogeneities within the patient are sufficiently sampled in the lateral extent. Each pencil beam axis is traced through the CT volume from the virtual source through a grid

point and through the CT. The calculation points (x,y,z) are transformed to the beam coordinate system and are sorted in z (Fig. 10.7). The ray trace evaluates the water-equivalent depth (Equation 10.5) for the point whose z is first in this sorted list and whose $(x - x')^2 + (y - y')^2 < 9\sigma_T^2$, that is, those points are close enough to the pencil-beam axis to receive sufficient dose. For those points, the evaluation of Equation 10.7 yields the dose. The ray trace continues and repeats the procedure for the next point z in the list.

Scattered Proton Field Composition

The general framework for the algorithm for scattered fields is the evolution of the proton field in medium described by Equation 10.7 as a composition of individual pencil beams i. The pencil beams for this application should be considered mathematical constructs for the decomposition of the field; the physical field is a laterally uniform flux of protons at different energies. The mathematical decomposition in depth is the weighted superposition of single Bragg peak proton fields, typically uniform in the lateral dimension or weighted according to a measured off-axis ratio profile, to produce a spread-out Bragg peak (SOBP) field. The SOBP is thus a weighted sum of pristine Bragg peaks P_i:

$$\text{SOBP}(z) = \sum_{i=1}^{N} W_i P_i(z) \qquad \text{EQUATION (10.11)}$$

The superposition of Bragg peaks is achieved by mechanically inserting range-shifting material in the monoenergetic proton beam with the insertion time proportional to the required contribution of a peak to the SOBP (Fig. 10.8). The common method is to use a rotating wheel with increasing step thicknesses and where the angular extent of the step is proportional to the weight. A rotating wheel can produce SOBPs of varying modulation by turning the beam off before a full rotation has been completed.

The modulation width traditionally is specified as the distance between the distal and proximal 90%. This definition, however, leads to modulation values larger than the range value for some fields and becomes hard to measure in the shallow entrance dose region. Thus, in our practice at least, we specify the modulation width between the distal 90% and the proximal 98% (see Fig. 10.2).

Absolute dose calculations for SOBP models have, in general, not been implemented and output calculations rely on empirical models (see Kooy et al. (14)). The complexity, specific construction details, and large number of mechanical components in a "modern" scattering nozzle make such a description very difficult. This complexity increases the burden on the physicist to establish a practical quality assurance protocol for output calibrations (Engelsman et al. (15)).

Pencil-Beam Scanning Field Implementation

For pencil-beam scanning fields, we have physical beams of narrow protons whose lateral position, quantified in the isocentric plane, is controlled by the scanning magnets (SMs) and whose penetration depth is quantified by the energy. This energy is nearly uniform with an energy spread dE/E on the order of 0.5% or less. The effect of the energy spread is a broadening of the Bragg peak width.

In principal, one could use the physical pencil beam directly as a representation for the Gaussian form in Equation 10.7. This, however, will lead to an implementation that is insensitive to patient heterogeneities. The physical pencil beam typically has a spread of 4 to 15 mm at the entrance as a consequence of the beam transport system and scatter in air and windows. Thus, considering Equation 10.7, the dose algorithm implementation would be unable to discern inhomogeneities smaller than that spread. Schaffner et al. (16) describe various techniques of modeling dose distributions near lateral heterogeneities and one such model is the Fluence-dose model. The physical pencil beam (PPB) is decomposed at the entrance into constituent mathematical pencil beams (MPB) to retain sufficient resolution of the proton transport inside the patient. This can be represented by considering the spot spread σ_0 separately from the in-patient spread σ_P in the

Gaussian function and modifying Equation 10.7 to the mathematically equivalent form

$$D(\vec{x}) = \sum_S G_S \qquad \text{EQUATION (10.12a)}$$

$$\times \sum_K \left(\oint \frac{1}{2\pi\sigma_O^2(R_S,z)} \exp\left(-\frac{\Delta_{S,K}^2}{2\sigma_O^2(R_S,z)}\right) dA_K \right) \qquad \text{EQUATION (10.12b)}$$

$$\times \frac{T_W^\infty(R_S,\tau_{\text{wet}})}{2\pi\sigma_P^2(R_S,\tau_{\text{wet}})} \exp\left(-\frac{\Delta_K^2(\vec{x})}{2\sigma_P^2(R_S,\tau_{\text{wet}})}\right) \qquad \text{EQUATION (10.12c)}$$

where the first term (Equation 10.12a) is the number of protons G_S (in units of billions or Gigaprotons) in a PPB in the set S, the second term (Equation 10.12b) is the apportionment of these G_S protons, given the intrinsic lateral spread $\sigma_O^2(R_S,z)$ of the PPB, over the set of MPB's K. This set of MPB's K in Equation 10.12c is defined at the highest resolution (~2 mm) necessary to accurately represent the dose in the patient. Equation 10.12c models the diffusion of the number of protons, given by the product of Equations 10.12a and 10.12b, in the patient given the scatter spread $\sigma_P(R_S,\tau_{\text{wet}})$ in the patient due to multiple Coulomb scattering. The intrinsic lateral spread $\sigma_O^2(R_S,z)$ in Equation 10.12b is determined by the scatter in air, magnetic steering, and focusing properties of the PBS system (see Fig. 10.8), and is a function of the spot range R_S and position z along the pencil-beam spot axis. The parameter $\Delta_{S,K}$ denotes the position of a point in the computational pencil beam area A_K with respect to the spot coordinate system. The final term (Equation 10.12c) follows Pedroni et al. (17), where $T_W^\infty(R_S,\tau_{\text{WET}})$ (in units of Gy cm² Gp⁻¹) is the absolute measured depth dose per Gigaproton (see Fig. 10.9) integrated over an infinite plane at water-equivalent depth τ_{wet}, $\sigma_P(R_S,\tau_{\text{WET}})$ is the total pencil-beam spread at τ_{WET} caused by multiple Coulomb scatter in the patient (see Hong et al. (6)), and $\Delta_K(\vec{x})$ is the displacement from the calculation point to the K pencil-beam axis. Equation 10.12 is a phenomenological description of the distribution in the patient of protons delivered by the set of spots S.

A Monte Carlo for Proton Transport in the Patient

The limitation of the Gaussian pencil-beam model is well known: insensitivity to lateral inhomogeneities as only variations along the pencil-beam axis is sampled (Equation 10.2). For clinical purposes, the Gaussian pencil-beam model is a very good representation (18), given the relatively small dispersion of the MPB (Fig. 10.5). Thus, if lateral scatter were accurately modeled, there would be little further improvement necessary. We describe a simple Monte Carlo that only models lateral scatter and is implemented on a GPU, generally available on any personal computer.

The physics of proton transport is well described by considering multiple Coulomb scatter using Molière's theory and energy loss S along the track. Individual

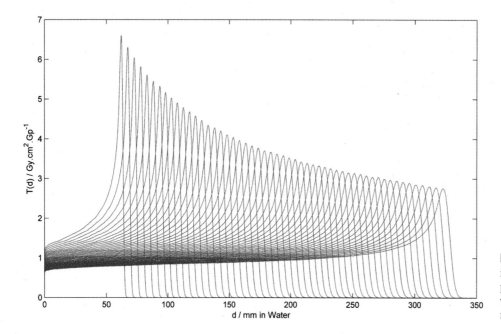

Figure 10.9. A set of pristine peaks in absolute dose (Gy cm²) per giga-proton. Note the change in peak width and height as a function of range.

protons are transported through a volume represented by a rectangular 3D grid of voxels of dimension (dx, dy, dz) and localized by their index (i, j, k). Each voxel has the relative (to water) stopping power S_W^V. The dose to a voxel is the sum of energy depositions along the individual proton tracks that traverse the voxel and divided by the voxel mass.

A proton, of energy E_S, enters a voxel on one of its faces and exits on another. We compute the (unscattered) exit point along the incoming proton direction (u, v, w) and the distance λ between the entrance and this projected exit point. We compute the mean polar scatter angle in the voxel as $\theta = \theta_0(E_S)\sqrt{S_W^V}$ and the azimuthal angle randomly uniform between 0 and 2π. The mean scatter angle $\theta_0(E_s)$ is derived and quantified by Gottschalk (19), analogous to the Highland formula (Equation 10.6c) but more appropriate to traversal through thin layers. The azimuthal angle is the only random variable. The proton direction is

adjusted to (u', v', w'), given the scattering angles and the actual exit point are computed.

The energy loss of the proton along the mean voxel geometric track length $\langle\lambda\rangle$ is derived from either the measured depth-dose distribution, $T_W^\infty(R, \tau_{\text{wet}})$, or from range-stopping power tables as in Fippel et al. (20). The energy loss in a voxel in the former model is

$$\Delta_{\langle\lambda\rangle}(E) = T_W^\infty(R, \tau_{\text{wet}}) \times \frac{S_V/\rho_V}{S_W/\rho_W} \times \rho_V \times \langle\lambda\rangle$$

EQUATION (10.13)

In either model, the depth dose in the Monte Carlo is tuned to match the measured depth dose by adjusting the energy spread at the entrance to the phantom. The use of a mean track length $\langle\lambda\rangle$ solely serves to reduce computational overhead. Figure 10.10 shows the pseudo-code for this simple algorithm and Figure 10.11 shows the ability of the

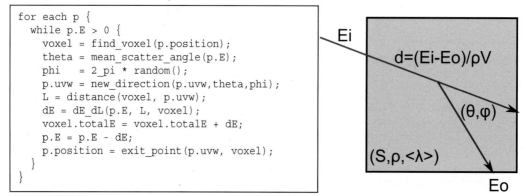

```
for each p {
    while p.E > 0 {
        voxel = find_voxel(p.position);
        theta = mean_scatter_angle(p.E);
        phi   = 2_pi * random();
        p.uvw = new_direction(p.uvw,theta,phi);
        L = distance(voxel, p.uvw);
        dE = dE_dL(p.E, L, voxel);
        voxel.totalE = voxel.totalE + dE;
        p.E = p.E - dE;
        p.position = exit_point(p.uvw, voxel);
    }
}
```

Figure 10.10. Pseudo-code for transporting a single proton through a voxel. The proton enters with energy E_o and scatters by a mean polar angle θ, a random azimuthal (around the proton direction) angle ϕ (green line). The energy loss $(E_i - E_o)$ depends on the energy only and is computed as a function of energy for a mean path length $\langle\lambda\rangle$. The dose d deposited is the deposited energy divided by the mass of the voxel.

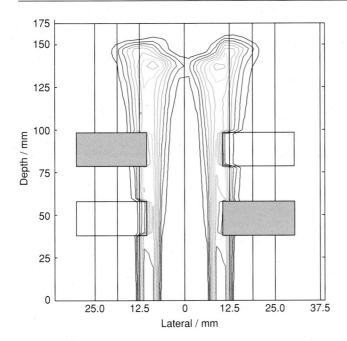

Figure 10.11. Energy loss distribution of 2 physical pencil-beams traversing water with inhomogeneous blocks (gray for "bone" and open for "air." Note the differential lateral scatter as expected.

algorithm to model traversal through heterogeneous medium.

This algorithm is implemented on a GPU, which contains numerous processors and where each processor can execute multiple threads of the code in Figure 10.10. The implementation can transport on the order of 600,000 protons/s on an off-the-shelf graphics card. Such speed is competitive to a "conventional" pencil-beam application and we, therefore, expect that such implementations will replace the conventional implementations.

The clinical proton field is defined by a set of numerous protons ($\sim 10^6$ or 10^7) with a mean energy E, spread $\Delta E / E$, entry point (x, y, z) on the surface of the voxel volume, and direction (u, v, w). This computational set is derived from the properties of the decomposed pencil beams as they are for either scattered or PBS field as described above.

REFERENCES

1. Gottschalk B. Passive beam spreading in proton radiation therapy. Available from huhepl.harvard.edu/~gottschalk/.
2. Paganetti H. Nuclear interactions in proton therapy: dose and relative biological effect distributions originat-ing from primary and secondary particles. *Phys Med Biol* 2002;47:747–764.
3. International Commission on Radiation Units and Measurements. Prescribing, recording, and report-ing proton-beam therapy (ICRU Report 78). *J ICRU* 2007;7(2).
4. Amsler C, et al. (Particle Data Group), *Phys. Lett.* B667 2008;1.
5. Janni J. Proton range-energy tables, 1 keV–10 GeV. *Atom Data Nucl Data Tab* 1982;27:147–339.
6. Hong L, Goitein M, Bucciolini M, et al. A pencil beam algorithm for proton dose calculations. *Phys Med Biol* 1996;41:1305–1330.
7. Schneider U, Pedroni E, Lomax A. The calibration of CT Hounsfield units for radiotherapy treatment planning. *Phys Med Biol* 1996;41:111–124.
8. Cormack AM, Koehler AM. Quantitative proton tomog-raphy: preliminary experiments. *Phys Med Biol* 1976;21:560–569.
9. Molière G. Theorie der Streuung schneller geladener Teilchen II Mehrfach—und Vielfachstreuung-streuung. *Z Naturforsch B* 1948;3A:78–97.
10. Gottschalk B. On the scattering power of radiotherapy protons. *Med Phys* 2010;37:352–367. arXiv:0908.1413v1 (physics.med-ph).
11. Lynch GR, Dahl OI. Approximations to multiple Cou-lomb scattering. *Nucl Instrum Meth* 1991;B58:6–10.
12. Lee M, Nahum A, Webb S. An empirical method to build up a model of proton dose distribution for a radiotherapy treat-ment-planning package. *Phys Med Biol* 1993;38:989–998.
13. Hogstrom KR, Mills MD, Almond PR. Electron beam dose calculations. *Phys Med Biol* 1981;26:445–459.
14. Kooy HM, Schaefer M, Rosenthal S, et al. Monitor unit calculations for range modulated spread-out Bragg peak fields. *Phys Med Biol* 2003;48:2797–2808.
15. Engelsman M, Lu HM, Herrup D, et al. Commissioning a passive scattering proton therapy nozzle for accurate SOBP delivery. *Med Phys* 2009;36:2172–2180.
16. Schaffner B, Pedroni E, Lomax A. Dose calculation mod-els for proton treatment planning using a dynamic beam delivery system: and attempt to include density hetero-geneity effects in the analytical dose calculation. *Phys Med Biol* 1999;44:27–41.
17. Pedroni E, Scheib1 S, Bohringer T, et al. Experimental characterization and physical modelling of the dose dis-tribution of scanned proton pencil beams. *Phys Med Biol* 2005;50:541–561.
18. Jiang H, Paganetti H. Adaptation of GEANT4 to Monte Carlo dose calculations based on CT data. *Med Phys* 2004;31:2811–2818.
19. Gottschalk B. On the scattering power of radiotherapy protons. *Med Phys* 2010;37:352–367.
20. Fippel M, Soukup M. A Monte Carlo dose calculation algo-rithm for proton therapy. *Med Phys* 2004;31:2263–2273.

CHAPTER 11

Commissioning and Quality Assurance

Jacob Van Dyk

INTRODUCTION

Quality assurance (QA) is "all those planned and systematic actions necessary to provide adequate confidence that a product or a service will satisfy given requirements for quality" (1). In radiation therapy, this has been defined by the World Health Organization as "all those procedures that ensure consistency of the medical prescription and the safe fulfillment of that prescription as regards to the target volume, together with minimal dose to normal tissue, minimal exposure of personnel, and adequate patient monitoring aimed at determining the end result of treatment" (2). *Quality control* (QC) is "the regulatory process through which the actual quality performance is measured and, compared to existing standards and finally the actions necessary to keep or regain conformance with the standards" (1). In the context of radiation therapy, *commissioning* means preparing a procedure or a technology for clinical use, whether it be a radiation treatment planning system (TPS), a CT simulator, a radiation treatment machine, a computerized clinical radiation information system, or a new treatment technique such as intensity-modulated radiation therapy (IMRT). *Quality management*, as the words imply, refers to all management issues of the quality process. Quality management must be initiated and continuously encouraged from the top-down and must infiltrate the entire management structure of the organization for it to work successfully.

There are two main considerations for a QA process in radiation therapy. The first is to assure that the radiation treatment is delivered accurately according to the dose-volume prescription provided by the radiation oncologist. The second consideration relates to patient safety and the avoidance of treatment errors.

Figure 11.1 is a block diagram of the many steps in the process of radiation treatment. To ensure accuracy of prescription and the fulfillment of treatment intent, a rigorous program of QA is required at all stages of the radiation treatment process. The shaded region of the figure highlights the stages that relate specifically to treatment planning. Virtual simulation combined with the use of computerized TPS for dose computation and technique optimization is standard practice in the modern radiation therapy department. The extent of their use continues to vary dramatically from simple calculations of dose distributions on two-dimensional (2D) external patient contours to

very complex three-dimensional (3D) treatment planning with the use of various types of patient-specific image data. Recent developments in automated optimization (3), beam intensity modulation (4), the use of a variety of imaging modalities (5), and the inclusion of biological parameters (6) to calculate tumor control probabilities (TCP) and normal tissue complication probabilities (NTCP) have added dramatically to the complexity of the modern TPS. Figure 11.2 is a block diagram adapted from the joint scope of practice document from the American Association of Physicists in Medicine (AAPM) and the American Society for Radiation Oncology (ASTRO) representing the steps of the RT process for modern practice using IMRT (7).

As indicated above, the process of preparing the patient for radiation therapy includes many steps. Uncertainties or errors in any step of the process can have a dramatic effect on outcome, be they related to the control of the disease or to complications as a result of inappropriate treatment. The overall need for QA in radiation therapy is well defined (2,8–10). Although the specific needs for QA of treatment planning computers are described in a number of reports (11–13), the actual implementation of QA procedures is more ambiguous. Very comprehensive reports on treatment planning QA have been developed by the AAPM (14) and, more recently, by the International Atomic Energy Agency (IAEA) (15–17). This chapter addresses issues related to the use of treatment planning computers in the context of purchase, acceptance testing, commissioning, and routine clinical application. Although the emphasis is on commissioning and QC, there is also some discussion on QA of the total treatment planning process. The intent of this chapter is to be as generic as possible so that it applies to both conventional and more sophisticated radiation treatment techniques; however, because of page limitations, details for specialized techniques are confined to references where indicated. The use of IMRT has now become quite routine in a significant number of departments and is no longer considered a special technique. While the general QA and QC principles described here also apply to IMRT, more details can be found in references (3,4,7,18,19).

Historical Perspective

Publications on computer applications in radiation therapy date back to 1951, when Wheatley (20) produced an analog

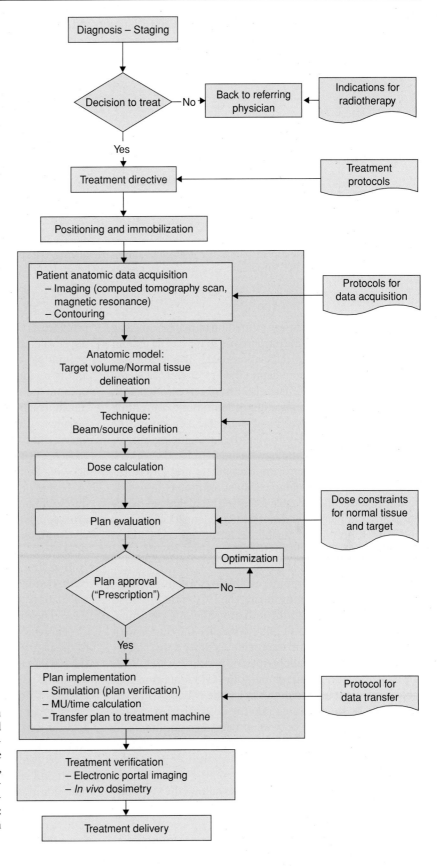

Figure 11.1. Schematic flowchart of the steps in the total radiation therapy process. The shaded region emphasizes those steps specifically associated with treatment planning and the use of the TPS. (Adapted from Van Dyk J, Rosenwald J-C, Fraass B, et al. Commissioning and quality assurance of computerized planning systems for radiation treatment of cancer. IAEA TRS-430. Vienna: International Atomic Energy Agency, 2004, with permission.)

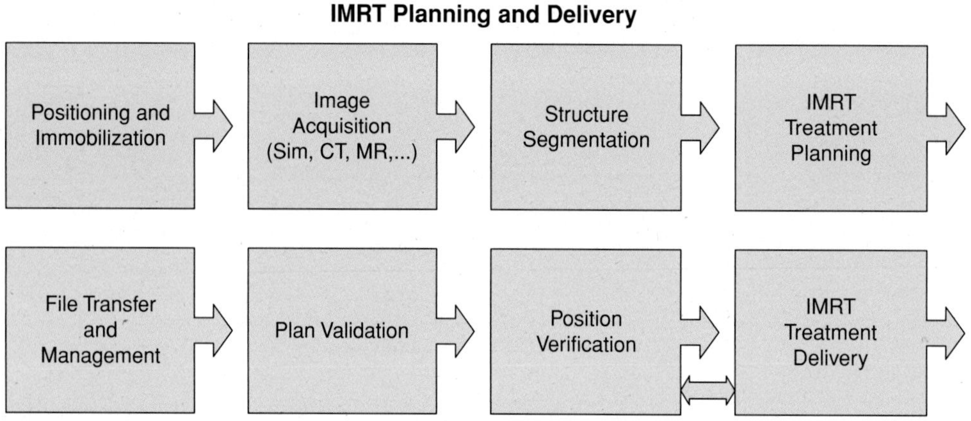

IMRT Planning and Delivery

Figure 11.2. The overall process of IMRT planning and delivery. (Adapted from Ezzell GA, Galvin JM, Low D, et al. Guidance document on delivery, treatment planning, and clinical implementation of IMRT: report of the IMRT Subcommittee of the AAPM Radiation Therapy Committee. *Med Phys* 2003;30:2089–2115, with permission.)

computer to perform "dosage estimation of fields of any size and any shape." The prime purpose was to relieve the tedium associated with dosage calculations (21). It appears that computers were used in radiation therapy as early as in any other field of medicine. Tsien (22) has been credited with being the first in the application of "automatic computing machines to radiation treatment planning." Also, during the past 60 years, there has been an enormous technological evolution of computer technology, including microcomputers, large time-sharing systems, minicomputers, graphics workstations, and today's desktop personal computers, as well as laptops, handhelds, and tablets. During each phase of development, computers provided treatment planners with faster and more sophisticated capabilities for dosage calculations, better image and graphical displays, and improved automated optimization capabilities.

The advances in computer technology led to a revolution of diagnostic imaging during the 1970s that provided a further breakthrough for radiation therapy planning. Until then, it was difficult both to localize the tumor with any kind of accuracy and to provide accurate dose calculations accounting for patient-specific tissue densities. With the advent of computed tomography (CT) it became possible for the first time to derive *in vivo* density information that could be incorporated into the dose calculation process. The combination of developments in computers and in diagnostic imaging resulted in much research, improving dose calculation procedures that accounted for the actual tissue composition of the patient. This, combined with sophisticated display techniques, allows the superposition of dose distributions on any anatomical plane within the human body.

Today, we are able to derive very precise 3D information from a variety of imaging modalities, including CT, magnetic resonance imaging (MRI), single photon emission computed tomography (SPECT), positron emission tomography (PET), digital angiography, and ultrasound (5,23). The superposition of the information from various imaging modalities has

provided a tremendous tool to aid the radiation oncologist in target volume and normal tissue delineation. The routine use of multiple imaging modalities is increasing in availability and is no longer limited to academic institutions. CT has become the standard imaging procedure for therapy planning and is now readily available even in the smaller clinics, usually as CT simulators (24). The modern TPS allows the virtual simulation of the patient by the superposition of radiation beam geometries at any orientation on any image, thus allowing for full 3D treatment planning.

The evolution of these sophisticated technological developments can readily be followed by reviewing the proceedings of a series of international meetings on the use of computers in radiation therapy (25–40). The first of these was held in May 1966 in Cambridge, UK, and the 16th such meeting was held in 2010 in Amsterdam, the Netherlands. While the improvement in accuracy of dose calculations has always been an important component of these meetings, formal discussion on commissioning and QA has received only marginal attention. This is partly due to the nature of QA, which has historically not been considered a major area for high-powered research and partly due to an assumption that QA is something that all medical physicists do but no one really talks about. Admittedly, recent years have seen a formalization of QA activities for TPSs as demonstrated in the national and international reports (14–17,41–44) and textbook chapters (45,46) that have evolved. This chapter summarizes recent developments and recommendations associated with QA issues in radiation treatment planning, especially the implementation and clinical use of computerized radiation TPSs.

Development and Implementation of Treatment Planning Algorithms

The clinical implementation of treatment planning programs involves a number of steps. Some are under the control of the user, and some are not user-controlled

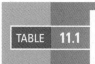

TABLE 11.1	Steps Involved in the Clinical Implementation of Treatment Planning Programs

Development of calculation algorithm (not user controlled)
Based on model of radiation interactions
Physics is complex, incorporates approximations
Model contains inherent uncertainties
Works over limited range of conditions

Development of computer programs implementing algorithm (not user controlled)
Includes input–output routines
Includes image display routines
Includes optimization, evaluation routines
Developer must ensure that programs are correct

Determination of radiation database required by algorithms (user controlled)
Data are limited in range of conditions
Data have uncertainties
Data may be relative or absolute doses

Clinical application (user controlled)
Requires
Patient data (e.g., CT, MRI, contours)
Dose calculations
Optimization, evaluation
Program output on display and hard-copy devices

because they depend on software developed by others. The typical clinical implementation of treatment planning programs usually takes the following steps (Table 11.1).

Development of Calculation Algorithms

Dose calculation algorithms are based on the physics of radiation interactions within tissue. Because of the complexity of the physics of these types of interactions, the algorithms usually involve simplifications allowing the calculations to be completed fast enough to be useful to the treatment planner. These simplifications result in approximations to the complicated physics, and therefore the algorithms have inherent uncertainties and generally work well only over a limited range of conditions. Usually, the more complex algorithms handle the physics in more detail, but also require longer calculation times. The extreme example of this is Monte Carlo calculations, which can take hours to days, depending on the mode of treatment and the complexity of the plan, although recent commercial clinical versions for electron beams can be calculated in minutes (47) and photon beams from minutes to hours (48). To be practical, a clinical algorithm should generate dose distributions nearly in real time but usually in seconds. The details of the algorithm

implemented on a given commercial TPS are not in the control of the user. The user's choice of algorithms is limited to what is provided by the different manufacturers and ultimately to the algorithms supplied with the system purchased.

Development of the Computer Programs Implementing the Algorithms

Once a developer of a TPS has determined the nature of the algorithm, the algorithm must be coded into software. This software must include appropriate input–output routines, image display and manipulation routines, options that allow the user to define the treatment technique, and plan optimization and evaluation routines. The development of the software is not under the control of the user. It is the responsibility of the developer of the software to ensure that the algorithms are properly coded.

It is important for the user to have some knowledge of the nature of the dose calculation algorithms, since a knowledge at some level will help understand their capabilities and limitations. Furthermore, a basic knowledge will also help the user diagnose specific TPS problems and can be of some help in developing a QA process. A detailed description of different dose calculation algorithms can be found in Chapters 7 to 10. A broad overview of dose calculation algorithms has also been given by Van Dyk et al. (45) and a detailed report on external beam tissue inhomogeneity corrections for photon beams has been produced by AAPM Task Group 65 (49). In recognizing that the detailed description of algorithms was also beyond the scope of the IAEA TRS-430 (15), the report provides a series of questions that users may want to address either as part of the search process for a new TPS or in attempting to understand the calculation algorithm(s), currently available on their TPS. Thus, it includes 14 tables addressing different issues related to TPSs. To give an idea as to the subjects covered, the titles of these tables are summarized in Table 11.2. Table 11.3 is an example of one of the tables in IAEA TRS-430 (15) and shows questions related to external beam dose calculation algorithms in a water-like medium without any beam modifiers.

For brachytherapy, an interesting review of the evolution of treatment planning has been provided by Rivard et al. (50).

Determination of the Radiation Database Required by the Algorithms

All algorithms, even sophisticated Monte Carlo procedures, require a basic radiation data set as input. For the standard commercial TPS, these data are determined for each energy on each therapy machine in every radiation therapy department. The quality and accuracy of such data depend on the user of the TPS. Such data are always determined over a limited range of conditions. Thus, calculations that extend beyond the range of the original

TABLE 11.2	**Titles of Tables in IAEA TRS-430 (15) Addressing Questions Associated with TPS Algorithms**

Table number in IAEA report	Table title
2	Automatic extraction of contours or surfaces
3	Building and displaying 3D objects
4	Multiplanar reconstruction and 3D display
5	Expanding objects
6	Digitally reconstructed radiographs
7	Registration of multiple anatomical data sets
8	Automatic design of beam apertures
9	Geometrical reconstruction of sources for brachytherapy
10	Types of external beam calculation algorithm
11	External beam dose calculation algorithm: dose in water-like medium without beam modifier
12	External beam dose calculation algorithm: influence of beam modifier
13	External beam dose calculation algorithm: special collimating systems
14	External beam dose calculation algorithm: influence of patient inhomogeneities and missing tissues
15	Dose normalization and absolute dose calculations

TABLE 11.3	**External Beam Dose Calculation Algorithm: Dose in Water-Like Medium Without Beam Modifier**

	Question
General principle of relative dose calculation.	From interpolation in tables? From analytical functions? By addition of primary and scatter components? By superposition of pencil beam kernels? By superposition of point dose kernels? By Monte Carlo calculation? From a combination of the above possibilities?
If an integration (or super-position, or convolution) algorithm takes place	What are the shape and dimensions of the volume elements? What are the limits of the integration volume? Is it applied differently for each of the dose components (i.e., primary, scatter, etc.)? Is there any correction for spectral modifications with depth?
Influence of flattening filter	Is there a correction for intensity and quality variation across the beam ("horns")? Is there a correction for scatter radiation from head and flattening filter (extra focal)?
Influence of main collimator (photons) and/or applicator (electrons)	What is the model used to describe the profile in the penumbra region? How is it adjusted to match the actual measurements? Is there a difference between the x and the y collimator pairs?
Dose in the build-up region	Is there any specific model to describe the dose in the build-up region? Is it sensitive to patient surface obliquity? How? Is it sensitive to beam modifiers, including block trays? How?

Table 11 in IAEA TRS-430 (15)

measured data may be subject to question, depending on the extrapolation procedures used by the calculation algorithms. Furthermore, measured data have their own inherent uncertainties and depend on the type and size of detectors used and the care taken by the experimentalist to generate the data. The accuracy of the measured data also depends on the stability of the radiation therapy machine and its ability to yield the same kind of radiation characteristics from day to day and hour to hour.

The measured data required by TPSs at minimum are relative, in the form of dose ratios, with the denominator being the dose under some reference condition. Any TPS capable of calculating monitor units (MU) or treatment times also requires absolute information in the form of MUs per gray or grays per minute. These data are all part of the input data set required by the TPS. The quality of the input data depends entirely on the therapy machine reproducibility, the quality of the measurement tools, and the expertise of the individual generating the data.

Clinical Application

Finally, the clinical use of the TPS requires patient-specific information in the form of patient contours, usually generated with the aid of CT and/or MRI. Appropriate parameters must be entered to determine the treatment configuration. Dose calculations are usually performed for each beam independently, with the summed doses displayed on a video monitor or printed on paper. This clinical application of treatment planning depends entirely on the user and his or her knowledge of the capabilities and limitations of the TPS. Admittedly, the newer inverse planning optimization routines (3) used for IMRT are automated and leave little in the control of the user other than entering the dose-volume constraints as required by the objective function for the optimization.

Terminology Associated with QA

Four major topics that are associated with the purchase of any major piece of apparatus are *specifications, acceptance testing, commissioning,* and *QC.* In the context of TPSs, the distinction between some of these terms is not entirely clear, and therefore they warrant special discussion.

System Specifications

According to the dictionary, specification is defined as "a detailed, exact statement of particulars, especially a statement prescribing materials, dimensions, and quality of work for something to be built, installed, or manufactured" (51). In the context of treatment planning computers, specifications are required at two levels at least. First, the user needs specifications to determine what type of TPS to purchase. Second, the specifications determine the standards for acceptance testing and QC. Rigorously speaking, purchasers should develop their own specifications and go through a tendering process to determine

which system best meets those specifications. Practically, manufacturers of TPSs, as well as other therapy equipment, usually provide specifications that define the capabilities of their equipment. For TPSs, the specifications tend to be much more complex than for other equipment because they have so many components. The computer itself can be considered the heart of the system. Attached to the computer are input and output devices, which usually include network connections, possibly some type of magnetic or optical media for backup storage, laser disks, digitizers, film scanners, video displays, and printers. In addition to the hardware, software provides the major capabilities for calculation and display. Software specifications include detailed descriptions of what the software is capable of doing and how accurate the calculations can be made.

Acceptance Testing

Upon the installation of any new device, the user should assess the device to ensure that it behaves according to its specifications. For a TPS, this takes at least two forms: assessment of the hardware and the software. The latter can also be divided into several components, including assessment of the integrity of the operating system, external beam dose calculations, brachytherapy dose calculations, image transfer, and image display.

Commissioning

Commissioning is the process of putting the system into active clinical service. This process includes the production of a basic radiation database, which is entered into the TPS, after which the user tests the system over a range of clinically relevant conditions. Quality evaluations of the programs' outputs are then made. Such a process cannot test all the system's pathways or subroutines; however, it does provide the user with a level of confidence over a wide variety of often-used treatment conditions. In addition, it helps the user understand the degree of uncertainty associated with these specific calculations.

Quality Control

As indicated earlier, QA and QC are closely related. QA is the total process required to ensure that a certain level of quality is maintained for a defined product or service. QC specifically consists of systematic actions necessary to ensure that the product or process performs according to specification. This process contains three components: (a) the measurement of the performance, (b) the comparison of this performance with existing standards or specifications, and (c) the appropriate actions necessary to keep or regain agreement with the standard.

In summary, QA and QC first necessitate defining a series of specifications. Acceptance tests ensure that the system meets the basic requirements as defined by the specifications. Commissioning makes the computer ready for clinical use and provides a series of standards that can be used for ongoing QC to ensure that the system is maintaining the standards. Ongoing QC must be performed at intervals to confirm that there have been no changes in the basic radiation and machine parameter data files, in the input–output hardware, or in the CT, MRI, or other imaging-related software or hardware.

Treatment Planning Process

In its broader sense, treatment planning includes all the steps from therapeutic decision making to target volume and normal tissue delineation, selection of treatment technique, determination of the direction of radiation beams, simulation, fabrication of ancillary devices and treatment aids, MU–time calculations, treatment verification, and finally, first treatment (Fig. 11.1). In its narrower sense, treatment planning includes the outlining of target and critical volumes, the determination of the number and directions of radiation beams, and the corresponding MU calculations. In this narrower definition, treatment planning involves the use of image information and the computer to perform the appropriate virtual simulation and dose calculations. The QA considered in this chapter primarily addresses the use of the TPS to generate appropriate beam arrangements and dose calculations. The following specific issues are associated with that part of the QA process.

Patient Data

Patient data can be derived in various ways, including simple methods of external contour determination and various imaging modalities, most commonly CT. The important issue at this stage of planning is to ensure that the patient is positioned identically to the eventual treatment position and that the derived data represent this position (52). It is important that the data be transferred accurately to the TPS. If a digitizer or film scanner is used, the QA process must ensure the accuracy of the input data. Also, any conversions of digitized data, such as the conversion of CT numbers to electron densities, must be handled accurately by the system.

Display of Patient Data

Once the data have been captured by the TPS, the treatment planner can manipulate the information, look at the data on various slices, and allow the system to perform reconstructions of images. With the patient data on the computer, the radiation oncologist is able to outline target volumes on the appropriate slices as well as the critical structures. While it is well recognized that different physicians can produce large variations in target volume definition for the same patient (53–56), the accuracy of the display of patient data is important for the next step of the planning process, that is, placement of radiation beams.

Display of Beam-Related Information

Beam placement is often performed with the use of a cursor or a mouse, as well as the keyboard to enter some needed parameters such as field size, beam direction, and collimator rotation. At this stage, various options can be used for the definition of the field shape. These include outlining the irregular field shape in its entirety with the mouse, defining the rectangular field and then adding shaped blocks, using the planning target volume and allowing an automatic preset margin, and automated field definition for the multileaf collimator. In each case, the beam edges can be displayed either on a beam's-eye-view perspective or as perspectives of the beam edges intersecting any specified plane. Associated with the beam edge display, information demonstrating gantry angle, collimator angle, beam energy, and collimator size should also be displayed on the screen.

Dose Calculation and Display

Once the beam geometry has been determined, the dose distribution can be calculated and displayed. Displays vary from simple colored isodose lines to color washes to individual point doses. The accuracy of the geometric correctness of isodose lines on the display is very difficult to assess, although very specific phantom geometries, whereby one can assess the position of a specific isodose line can help with this process. Doses calculated at individual points can be correlated to the isodose lines as well as measured data.

Output

Dose-calculation output can be provided on a printer, often in color. Screen dumps allow for a quick copy of everything displayed on the screen. The screen hard copies usually are not on a one-to-one scale, even though this is often preferred by the radiation oncologists for assessing the distribution and making necessary changes.

System Specifications

The system specifications can be divided into various categories, including hardware, system administration software, network and interface software, and planning software. As an example, Table 11.4 gives a summary of the table of contents of one institution's treatment planning computer specifications. Under each section there are many detailed questions as to the system's capabilities. For example, under Section 9.4.3, Program Features, are subsections on anatomy and volume selection, beam definition and display, bolus, and compensators. Each of these subsections has multiple questions as to the programs' capabilities and options.

Sources of Uncertainties

Specifications take various forms. One form is simply a statement of whether the system is capable of doing a particular function or not. Another form is quantitative, for example, speed, number of images it can hold, and so on. A third form is a statement of accuracy. This is

| Table 11.4 | Sample Table of Contents of a Treatment Planning Computer Specifications Document |

1. Document objectives
2. Definitions
   2.1 Base 3D unit
   2.2 Standalone server node
   2.3 Remote 3D node
   2.4 Remote 2D node
   2.5 Remote MU calculation node
   2.6 Remote 3D volume delineation node
3. Summary of essential requirements
4. Regulations, codes, and standards
5. Vendor guarantees
   5.1 Specification guarantee
   5.2 Service guarantees
      5.2.1 Response time
      5.2.2 Hardware support
      5.2.3 Software support
   5.3 Third party products
      5.3.1 Embedded software
      5.3.2 Hardware
   5.4 Performance guarantee
   5.5 Computer protection
   5.6 Upgradeability
   5.7 Indemnity
   5.8 Price guarantee
6. Vendor information
   6.1 Vendor statistics
   6.2 Model statistics
   6.3 Future capabilities
7. Purchase procedure
   7.1 Site preparation
   7.2 Delivery
   7.3 Installation
   7.4 Acceptance testing
8. Payment terms
9. Specifications
   9.1 Hardware
      9.1.1 Host CPUs
      9.1.2 Terminals
      9.1.3 Interactive input devices
      9.1.4 Storage disks
      9.1.5 Networking
      9.1.6 Digitizing tablet
      9.1.7 Backup tape device
      9.1.8 Printer
      9.1.9 Plotter
      9.1.10 Screen dump printer
      9.1.11 Film digitizer
      9.1.12 Nine-track tape drive
      9.1.13 Other peripherals
   9.2 System administration software
      9.2.1 Security
      9.2.2 Backup
      9.2.3 Batch queue support
      9.2.4 Workload
      9.2.5 Other
   9.3 Network and interface software
      9.3.1 Image exchange formats
      9.3.2 X-ray CT images
      9.3.3 Magnetic resonance images
      9.3.4 Simulator digital radiographs
      9.3.5 Film digitizer
      9.3.6 Scanning dosimetry systems
      9.3.7 Portal imagers
      9.3.8 Other peripherals
   9.4 Planning software
      9.4.1 Administration
      9.4.2 General
      9.4.3 Program features
      9.4.4 Installation data requirements
      9.4.5 Calculations
      9.4.6 Calculation speed performance
      9.4.7 Calculated dose accuracy
      9.4.8 Specific phantom tests
   9.5 Documentation and training
      9.5.1 Online help
      9.5.2 Manuals
      9.5.3 Training
   9.6 Service and parts
      9.6.1 Diagnostics
      9.6.2 Preventive maintenance
      9.6.3 Warranty
      9.6.4 Consultant services
      9.6.5 Service contracts
      9.6.6 Parts inventories
   9.7 Environmental requirements
      9.7.1 Power
      9.7.2 Operating conditions
10. Other information
Appendix A. Calculation Tests

Adapted from the treatment planning computer system tender document produced at the Ontario Cancer Institute/Princess Margaret Hospital.

particularly relevant for dose calculations. To assess the accuracy of a system and to define realistic accuracy specifications it is necessary to understand the sources of uncertainties.

The determination of uncertainties in dose calculations is complex because dose calculation algorithms depend on input information, which is usually generated by measurement. Thus, the uncertainty in the calculation output depends on the uncertainties associated with the measurements as well as the limitations of the calculation algorithms. Measurements are of various types, including relative doses in water phantoms, absolute dose calibrations for MU calculations, patient anatomy using imaging techniques or contouring devices, thickness profiles of physical wedges, compensators, or bolus, and distances from x-ray films and optical indicators. Further inaccuracies can be generated by output devices such as printers and screen dumps. Inaccuracies in image display can affect the choice of beam arrangements or field sizes used to cover specified target volumes. Similarly, image distortions can lead to incorrect manual dose optimization procedures.

Suggested Tolerances

Criteria of acceptability for dose calculations have been described by various authors (9,11,57–60). Task Group 53 of the AAPM (14) and IAEA TRS-430 (15) also include discussions on criteria of acceptability and tolerances generally considered achievable. Criteria of acceptability are very dependent on the region of calculation. Greater accuracy can be achieved on the central ray in a homogeneous phantom than in the penumbra region at the beam edge. Generally, four regions can be considered: (a) regions of low dose gradient in the central portion of the beam, (b) regions of large dose gradients such as that occur in the penumbra or in the fall-off region for electron beams, (c) regions of low dose gradients in low-dose areas such as that occur outside the beam or under large shielded areas, and (d) doses in the buildup or build-down regions at the entrance and exit surfaces of the patient. Criteria of acceptability are generally quoted as a percent of the reference dose except in regions of high dose gradients, where a spatial agreement in millimeters is a better descriptor, since the dose uncertainties in such regions can be very large.

Criteria of acceptability should include a statement of confidence. In other words, if we assume that the criterion of acceptability is an accuracy of 2% of the dose calculated on the central ray of the beam for a homogeneous phantom, then the question is whether all the calculated doses on the central ray are within 2%, or does the 2% represent one standard deviation (68% confidence) or two standard deviations (95% confidence)? For one standard deviation, 32% of the results may lie outside the stated criterion of acceptability. This is an important consideration, since ambiguities in these criteria can generate tremendous frustration from the user's perspective as well as some troublesome legal interactions with manufacturers of TPSs. By way of example, Van Dyk et al. (11) produced some tables of criteria of acceptability clearly outlining the system's general capabilities. Tables 11.5 and 11.6 are similar to the Van Dyk data, but some adjustments have been made in the numerical values to indicate a slightly tighter range of acceptability reflecting improvements in dose calculation algorithms available with modern TPSs. These criteria of acceptability represent one standard deviation about the mean. Venselaar et al. (60) have used a somewhat more complex, but more rigorous, definition of a "confidence limit" and this has been discussed in IAEA TRS-430 (15). It should also be noted that calculation accuracies depend not only on the input data and the limitations of the algorithms, but also on the user's performance of the calculation, which includes issues such as the choice of grid spacing. Grid spacing can have a large effect on the accuracy of dose calculations, especially in regions of high dose gradient.

For brachytherapy calculations, uncertainty estimates are more difficult to determine because of the very short treatment distances and the corresponding large dose gradients. Furthermore, brachytherapy calculations usually include absolute dose estimates, which require a detailed understanding of absolute source output specifications. A recent AAPM report suggests that when all uncertainties are combined, the one standard deviation (or one sigma uncertainty, $\kappa = 1$ in the report) of dose rates used in treatment planning can exceed 7% and 5% for low-energy and high-energy photon-emitting brachytherapy sources (61). Table 11.6 gives suggested criteria of acceptability for brachytherapy calculations.

These criteria of acceptability are based on what may be realistically achievable. Ideally, the recommendations of ICRU 42 (59) should be used as a goal for developers of treatment planning computer software. For external beam therapy, ICRU 42 (59) recommends 2% accuracy in low dose gradients and 2 mm accuracy in high dose gradients. For brachytherapy, 3% accuracy in dose at distances of 0.5 cm or more has been suggested (11).

Acceptance Testing

The system specifications determine the acceptance tests that have to be performed. The specifications, as summarized in Table 11.4, provide a broad context to the types of issues that should be considered. As a first step upon completion of the installation of a new system, the user should determine that all the components have been delivered and are consistent with the specifications. This includes a review of each component of the hardware. With rapidly changing technologies, manufacturers often switch one piece of hardware with

TABLE 11.5	Sample Criteria of Acceptability for Photon and Electron Dose Calculations

Descriptor	Criterion
Photon beams	
Homogeneous calculations (no shields)	
Central ray data (excluding buildup region)	2%
High-dose region, low dose gradient	3%
Large dose gradients (>30%/cm)	3 mm
Small dose gradients, low-dose region (<7% or normalization dose)	3%
Inhomogeneity calculations	
Central ray (slab geometry, electron equilibrium)	3%
Composite, anthropomorphic phantom	
Off axis, contour, inhomogeneities, shields, electronic equilibrium, attenuators	
High-dose region, low dose gradient	4%
Large dose gradient (>30%/cm)	3 mm
Small dose gradient, low-dose region (<7% normalization dose)	3%
Electron beams	
Homogeneous calculations (no shields)	
Central ray data (excluding buildup region)	2%
High-dose region, low dose gradient	4%
Large dose gradients (>30%/cm)	4 mm
Small dose gradients, low-dose region (<7% of normalization dose)	4%
Inhomogeneity calculations	
Central ray (slab geometry, electron equilibrium)	5%
Composite, anthropomorphic phantom	
Off axis, contour, inhomogeneities, shields, electronic equilibrium, attenuators	
High-dose region, low dose gradient	7%
Large dose gradient (>30%/cm)	5 mm
Small dose gradient, low-dose region (<7% normalization dose)	5%

Percentages represent one standard deviation and are quoted as a percent of the central ray normalization dose.

an updated version or with a device from another manufacturer. It is up to the user to ensure that the new hardware equals or surpasses the specifications set out in the purchase document.

The next step is to ensure that each component of the hardware functions at a simple level, that is, make a simple assessment of the video monitor, the mouse, the digitizer, the printer, the scanner, the storage media, the network connection, and other such items listed in section 9.1 of Table 11.4. A check that all the relevant manuals and schematics have been delivered is also important.

The next step is to run the system software and to ensure that each component of the software listed in the specifications is actually installed and functional. This includes third-party software (commercial software purchased by the vendor and included in the TPS) in addition to the treatment planning software.

The TPS software acceptance is very complex, primarily because the testing of the software requires measured input data specific to the therapy machines to allow direct comparisons of calculations with measurements. It is possible to use someone else's predetermined package of measurements, such as those produced by Task Group 23 (TG23) of the AAPM (12) for photons or, for electrons, the Electron Collaborative Work Group (ECWG) test set (62). However, this requires much time to enter the basic radiation data set, which is not specific to the purchasing institution, to perform a series of calculations to confirm the accuracy of the system, and then to enter the specific data for the user's machines and to repeat some of the tests. Thus, much added time is required for this type of acceptance.

A more practical approach is to test the system's input–output hardware to ensure that the system is capable of providing the options as defined in the specifications and

TABLE 11.6 — Sample Criteria of Acceptability for Brachytherapy Calculations

Descriptor	Criterion[a]
Single point source	
Distances of 0.5 to 5 cm	5%
Single line source	
Points along lines normal to the central 80% of the active length, distances of 0.5 to 5 cm	5%
Source end effects are difficult to quantify; therefore, no specification is given	

[a]Percent of local dose.

then to assess the accuracy of the calculations as part of the commissioning process. In the signing of the acceptance document, the purchaser should indicate that the software acceptance will be completed as part of the commissioning process. Also, the purchasers of new TPSs should do some prescreening of system capabilities by contacting owners of specific TPSs and asking them for information on the integrity of the software.

It should be noted that acceptance testing for IMRT requires a special emphasis on the system's capability of handling the penumbra region of small radiation fields as well as the leakage radiation outside the field. Small differences between measured and calculated dose in these regions can yield relatively large dose differences when many of these small fields are summed together.

The first level of hardware testing is to use the diagnostic programs provided with the system to ensure that all the hardware components assessed by the diagnostic routines are functioning properly. This provides both a test of the system and a baseline for the user to understand any changes that may be observed in the follow-up QA tests.

A major component of potential error relates to input–output devices such as the digitizer and printers. These devices can be tested by entry of simple shapes with the digitizer or mouse and then printing these shapes using the appropriate print options. The uncertainty in these devices should be <1 mm. Also, the video display should be assessed to ensure that the shapes and dimensions are consistent with the input data. All contours, target volumes, normal tissue structures, CT images, beam outlines, ancillary devices such as wedges and blocks, and isodose lines should be accurate and consistent between screen display and hard-copy output. Scales, distance calipers, and any other measurement routines should be assessed for both function and accuracy. This includes autocontouring, automatic contour expansion for target

volume margins, density assessments, automatic field shaping, and other features used by the planning software.

A more comprehensive process for acceptance testing has been proposed by the IAEA (16). The IAEA process is based on an earlier document specifically made for vendors of TPSs by the International Electrotechnical Commission (IEC) (44), which developed a series of requirements for manufacturers in the design and construction of a TPS. The consultants group for the IAEA has proposed that vendors should perform a series of "type" tests for their system, the results of which should be provided by the vendor to the user as part of the purchase documentation (16). Type tests refer to those tests that are to be done by the manufacturer, normally at the factory, to establish compliance with specified criteria. The type tests proposed by the IAEA are based on data analogous to the AAPM TG23 data (12) but updated and somewhat expanded by Venselaar and Welleweerd (63). In addition to the 6, 10, and 18 MV data in the Venselaar and Welleweerd report, cobalt-60 data have also been added to the IAEA data set. These data are provided by the IAEA to all vendors. The vendors enter the basic radiation beam data as though they were commissioning those beams for their dose calculation algorithms. Then, the vendors should perform all the tests as described in the IAEA document. These test results are to be documented and should be provided by the vendor to the user as part of the purchase documentation (16). Once the TPS is installed at the user's site, a select subset of tests should be performed to demonstrate consistency with the vendor's type tests. The vendors should update the type test results, if necessary, whenever software changes or upgrades are made and again these should be documented and provided to all purchasers of that software. At the time of software updates by the user, another select subset of tests can be made to ensure consistency of results between the vendor's calculations in the factory and the user's calculations in the clinic.

Commissioning

Photon Beams

The clinical implementation of the TPS can be divided into several components. These include entry of basic radiation data, entry of machine-specific parameters, entry of data related to ancillary devices such as wedges, assessment of image transfer capabilities, and assessment of the accuracy of the electron density conversion formula. Each of these components involves data entry and then tests of the algorithms. For each component it is important for the user to understand the capabilities and limitations of the algorithms.

The data entry for dose calculations can have various forms, including a direct entry from data stored in the water phantom computer. These data can be transferred either by some data storage medium or by a network link. The software of both the water phantom systems and TPSs evolves with time and therefore comes in various versions. To ensure version compatibility, it is always important to assess that the data have been read properly by the data entry programs.

Basic radiation data can be entered in various forms, including tissue–air ratios, tissue–phantom ratios, tissue–maximum ratios, percentage depth doses (PDD), and cross-beam profiles. Cross-beam profiles may also have to be measured under a variety of conditions, including profiles for the machine collimators, shielding blocks, wedges, and multileaf collimators. Some older systems also allow the user to enter data with the digitizer tablet. In all situations it is imperative that the user ensures the accuracy of the entered data by looking at the numerical values on the screen or by plotting out the data and comparing directly with what has been entered.

The types of tests that should be used to assess the quality of the algorithms are summarized in earlier reports by Van Dyk et al. (11) and Fraass (46) and more recently through working group reports as seen in references (14,15,43). Table 11.7 provides a summary of the relevant parameters and variables that should be included in the testing process. This is a guide to the kinds of issues that should be considered when assessing the calculation capabilities of the TPS. Further details can be found in relevant references (14,15,43).

Examples of Commissioning Tests

Several examples of the types of tests that can be performed, possible methods of evaluation, and some additional issues to consider will be shown. Figure 11.3 shows an example of simple central axis PDD data. A comparison

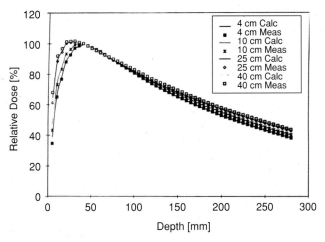

Figure 11.3. Central ray percentage depth doses (PDD) for fields of dimensions 4 × 4 cm, 10 × 10 cm, 25 × 25 cm, and 40 × 40 cm. The data points entered into the treatment planning system are labeled Meas and the calculated data are shown by the lines. The data are for the 25 MV beam from a linear accelerator and are normalized to 100% at a depth of 4 cm.

TABLE 11.7	Initial Dose Calculation Tests: Variables to Consider

Photon beam point calculations
TAR, TPR, PDD, PSF for square fields
TAR, TPR, PDD, PSF for rectangular fields
TAR, TPR, PDD, PSF for complex fields
Inverse square law, distance corrections
Attenuation, tray, wedge, compensator factors
Output or collimator scatter factors

Photon beam dose profiles or distributions
Square fields, normal incidence
Rectangular fields normal incidence
Effects of SAD or SSD
Wedged fields
Contour corrections
Bars or blocks
Multileaf collimators
Asymmetrical fields
Multiple beams
Arcs and rotations
Off-axis calculations
Collimator rotation and/or rotation of plane of calculation
Inhomogeneity corrections
Compensators
Anthropomorphic phantom tests

Electron beam point doses, distributions, or profiles
Square fields PDD and dose profiles
Extended distances
Rectangular fields, normal incidence
Contour corrections
Inhomogeneity corrections
Output factors
Effects of shields and irregular field shapes
Anthropomorphic phantom tests

Machine setting calculations

Clinical examples

Brachytherapy calculations
Entered data
Exposure or air kerma rate constants
Parameters for tissue attenuation and scatter
Half-life and decay calculation
Source wall information
Activity
Anisotropy
Dose calculations
Single and multiple source distributions
Line source calculations
Rotation and translation of plane of calculation
Source trajectories for special applicators
Use of orthogonal and/or stereotactic films
Automatic source identification schemes
Source display routines
Automated optimization, evaluation routines

PDD, percentage depth dose; PSF, peak scatter factor; SAD, source-to-axis distance; SSD, source-to-surface distance; TAR, tissue–air ratio; TPR, tissue–phantom ratio.

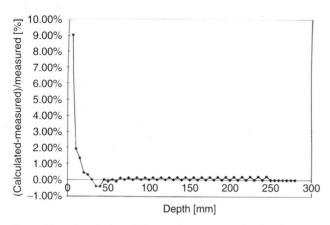

Figure 11.4. The absolute difference between calculated and entered (or measured) percentage depth dose (PDD) data for a 10 × 10 cm field for the 25 MV photon beam from a linear accelerator.

is made between the calculated data (lines) and the entered data (*Meas*). Figure 11.4 shows how the data of Figure 11.3 can be analyzed more critically by taking the absolute difference between the entered and the calculated data for a 10 × 10 cm field size. It is clear that beyond the buildup depth (40 mm) the differences are minimal (<0.2%), but in the buildup region differences can be as large as 9%. The reason for these differences is not clear, but the trends are similar for all field sizes. Figure 11.5 shows another comparison of differences between entered and calculated data but includes a comparison for two different calculation algorithms available in this commercial system, one being a table look-up algorithm and the other a convolution calculation. Figure 11.6 shows a difference comparison for cross-beam profiles, again for the two different algorithms. In these graphs, it is clear that there are sizable differences in dose in the penumbra region, although spatially these differences are quite small (1–2 mm).

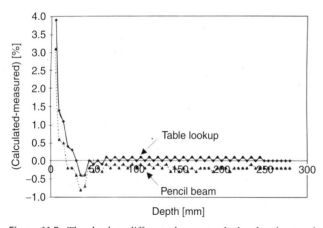

Figure 11.5. The absolute difference between calculated and entered (or measured) percentage depth dose (PDD) data for a 10 cm × 10 cm field for two calculation algorithms available on this commercial treatment planning system (TPS). The data are for the 25 MV beam of a linear accelerator.

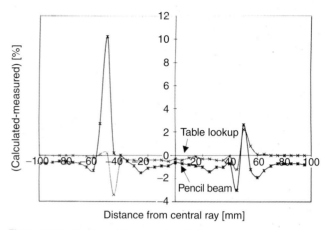

Figure 11.6. Absolute differences in relative doses comparing measurements with calculations for cross-beam dose profiles for two dose calculation algorithms. The beam profiles were measured at a depth of 4 cm for the 25 MV beam of a linear accelerator. The pencil beam (convolution) algorithm shows the largest difference, about 10% in the penumbra region, although this difference represents a spatial uncertainty of only 2 mm.

Figure 11.7 shows a comparison of measured and calculated dose profiles with the gantry angle at 40 degrees incident on a flat water phantom. This comparison tests the integrity of the contour correction algorithm. Figure 11.8 is a demonstration of the accuracy of the wedge calculations for a motorized wedge (a physical wedge that is inserted by motor in the beam for a fraction of the treatment and withdrawn for the remainder). This is a severe test of the algorithms, since the wedge is very thick, with a wedge factor of about 0.25. Figure 11.9 shows different doses for measured and calculated central ray PDD data under the motorized wedge for a number of field sizes.

Figure 11.10 shows cross-beam dose profiles calculated for a multileaf collimator with the three 1-cm leaves covering the central portion of the beam to yield a central beam block. Note that one of the leaves is on one side of the central ray and the other two are on the opposite side. At depths of 4, 10, and 25 cm, the dose profiles agree reasonably well except in the centrally blocked region. A more detailed comparison of this is shown in Figure 11.11, where calculated central ray depth doses are shown first for an open beam and then with the three central leaves covering the beam. Also shown are measured central ray data under the leaves. The differences between calculated and measured data under the leaves are about 5% to 7% except in what is normally the buildup region, where the differences are as large as 28%. These differences are due to this program's inability to handle electron contamination under the leaves or shields. This is a physics problem that occurs in older algorithms but has been improved in some newer commercial treatment planning programs (64,65).

IMRT

There are some unique aspects to commissioning IMRT compared to 3D conformal radiation therapy (CRT).

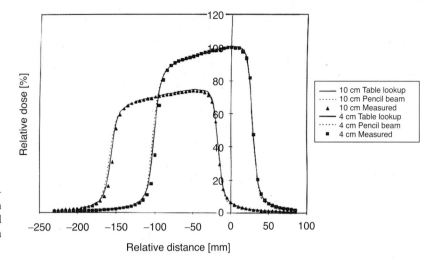

Figure 11.7. Calculated and measured dose profiles with a gantry angle of 40 degrees incident on a flat water phantom for a 10 cm × 10 cm field at depths of 4 and 10 cm for the 25 MV beam of a linear accelerator.

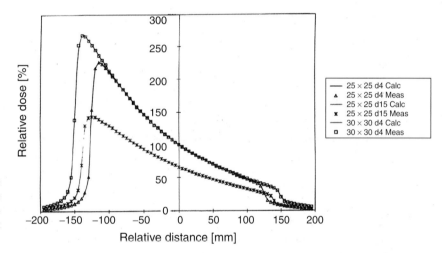

Figure 11.8. Calculated and measured dose profiles under a motorized wedge. Profiles are shown for the 25 cm × 25 cm at depths of 4 and 15 cm as well as a 30 cm × 30 cm field at a depth of 4 cm for a 25 MV beam.

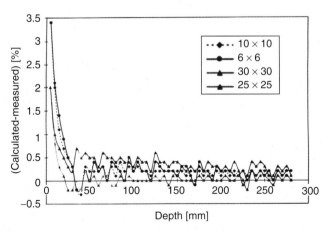

Figure 11.9. Difference profiles comparing measurements with calculations for central ray doses measured under a motorized wedge for 6, 10, 25, and 30 cm square fields for a 25 MV beam. Most differences are within 0.5% except in the buildup region, where differences are as large as 3.5%.

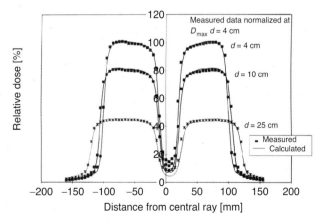

Figure 11.10. Comparison of measured and calculated cross-beam profiles under a multileaf collimator. Three leaves are in the center of the beam, with one leaf on the left side of the central ray and the other two on the right. The largest differences occur under the centrally shielded region of the multileaf collimator.

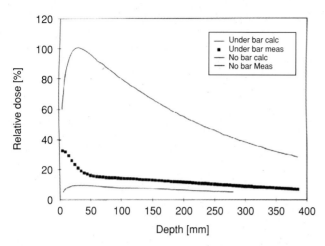

Figure 11.11. Doses along the central ray for the same geometry as Figure 11.9. The upper curve is calculated with no multileaves in the center of the beam. The lower curve is calculated under the leaves, and the individual data points are the measured data under the leaves. The differences between measured and calculated doses in the buildup region under the leaves are due to the inadequacies of the algorithm to handle electron scatter (contamination) under shields.

IMRT uses automated inverse planning routines, which use iterative algorithms to yield acceptable plans based on specified dose-volume constraints. The resulting dose distribution can have steep gradients between the target and the organs at risk. Thus, the commissioning tests need to reflect this added consideration. Because IMRT could involve the summation of very many small fields or multiple field edges, it is extremely important to ensure that the modeling of the penumbra and the low-dose region outside the beam is handled accurately. Furthermore, the accurate calculation of the leakage radiation through the leaves, especially those with curved ends, is very important to yield an accurate penumbra (66,67). Because of these small field considerations, ICRU Report 83 (68) points out that the Van Dyk criteria of acceptability (11) of 3% in the high-dose region and 4% in low-dose regions for 3D CRT may be too restrictive for IMRT in the high-dose region and insufficiently restrictive in the low-dose region.

It should also be noted that the delivered dose distribution is dependent on the leaf sequencing algorithm that is used to convert the TPS-derived intensity maps to a deliverable set of MLC sequences. The results are dependent on leaf width, leaf-travel distance, interdigitization of leaves, and maximum field size. Using smaller MLC steps and a larger number of intensity levels can result in many segments with small field sizes again compounding the need for accuracy in MLC positioning and penumbra modeling. Furthermore, there may be accelerator constraints on the delivery of many segments each with a small number of MUs.

Because of the difficulty in measuring doses in small fields and potential accelerator constraints, the ICRU Report 83 (68) suggests that the use of end-to-end testing, which consists of testing the entire process from data collection, beam modeling, treatment planning and delivery,

and QA of the delivered absorbed dose, is integral to the beam commissioning process.

Electron Beams

Good examples of specific tests for electron beams can be found in papers by Van Dyk et al. (11), Shiu et al. (62), and the recent working group reports (14,15,43). Tests of specific concern to electrons relate to changes in source-to-skin distance (SSD), output factor calculations, contour corrections, and variations in output for shaped fields.

Brachytherapy

Verification of brachytherapy dose calculation should be approached similarly to the external beam tests. In this situation, however, it becomes much more difficult to compare measurements with calculations because of the difficulty in performing measurements over the short distances involved in brachytherapy. The user may have to resort to comparing calculations with previously published source data. Relevant information can be found in various reports (11,14,15,69,70). One unique test for brachytherapy is the assessment of anisotropy calculations if these are provided by the system. A recent report by Rivard et al. (71) provides enhancements to commissioning techniques and QA of brachytherapy TPS that use model-based dose calculation algorithms.

Commissioning of Other Components

Modern TPSs contain many other commissioning aspects than those related to dose calculations. Examples of other types of issues that must be considered and verified are shown in Table 11.8. New phantoms have been developed by us (72–75), and others (75), to specifically address some commissioning and QA issues related to the non-dosimetric components of TPSs.

Special Techniques

Special and individualized techniques require their own unique evaluation. Examples of special techniques that require additional workup and commissioning are summarized in Table 11.9. In addition, there are now a number of new technologies that have specialized TPS specifically made for that technology. Examples include helical tomotherapy (76), robotic radiation therapy (77), and multiple cobalt source, small field radiation therapy, first used mostly for neurological sites (78).

Quality Assurance and Quality Control

QC of a product or process involves three steps: (a) the measurement of the performance, (b) the comparison of the performance with a given standard, and (c) the actions necessary to keep or regain the standard. The commissioning process of the TPS provides the standard for comparison. Once the TPS is fully commissioned, a process to ensure that

TABLE 11.8	Commissioning of Other Components

Image-related issues
Image acquisition
Image transfer
Conversion of CT numbers to electron densities
MRI distortions
Automatic contouring routines
Effects of autocontouring routines with incomplete
   image sets
Effects of unequally spaced slices
Partial volume effects due to slice thickness
Image artifacts
Image registration
Image reconstructions
Image enhancement tools

Display-related issues

Anatomical structures
Contour determination and entry
3D reconstruction of contours
3D surface displays
Bolus generation
Beam display in 3D
Irregular field display
Multileaf collimator display
Wedge display
Display of isodose lines and surfaces
Labeling of relevant parameters and dimensions
Coordinate determination and display
Beam's eye view
Room views
Source display for brachytherapy

Miscellaneous issues
Digitally reconstructed radiographs
Dose-volume histograms
Tumor control and normal tissue complication
   probabilities
Isocenter moves
Data transfer to therapy machine

TABLE 11.9	Techniques Requiring Special Workup

Beam junctions for both photons and electrons
Electron arcs
Stereotactic radiation therapy
Stereotactic brachytherapy
High-dose rate brachytherapy
Automatic optimization routines
Total body irradiation
Total skin irradiation
Intraoperative radiation therapy
Dynamic wedges

the system is able to remain within the standards determined by the commissioning process is necessary. However, the problems associated with maintaining consistency and quality within a TPS are quite different from the problems associated with QA of a CT simulator or accelerator, whose electrical and mechanical components can wear and change with time.

Closely associated with QA is *risk management*. Risk management consists of four components: (a) identifying the possible sources of risk of failure or malfunction, (b) analyzing the frequency of incidents of failure or malfunction, (c) taking corrective action to minimize such failure, and (d) monitoring the outcome of such changes.

Thus, to develop an appropriate QA program for treatment planning computers, an assessment of the likelihood of failure helps focus on the issues of concern rather than performing tasks that are not likely to generate major results in terms of reducing system failures or errors. IAEA TRS-430 (15) provides a good summary of reported errors associated with radiation treatment planning. For the "accidents" (major clinically significant errors) associated with TPSs, they concluded that the key contributory factors include the following:

a. A lack of understanding of the TPS
b. A lack of appropriate commissioning (no comprehensive tests)
c. A lack of independent calculation checks

The major issues related to treatment planning errors were summarized by four key words: (a) education, (b) verification, (c) documentation, and (d) communication.

The development of a thorough QA program is a compromise between cost and benefit. This is shown *schematically* in Figure 11.12, where the vertical axis is benefit, that is, improvements in "quality," and the horizontal axis is increased QA activity or increased cost. While no one knows what this curve really looks like for the QA of TPSs, it can readily be understood that if very little time and effort go into the QA activity, there is likely to be low quality and a high risk of errors. Adding a little time and effort begins to improve the benefit rapidly. However, there comes a point beyond which additional time and effort yield very little improvement in the quality of the process. At that point, it is not worth the cost and effort. Using the schematic of Figure 11.12, we probably should be operating our QA programs in the upper 90% to 96% benefit range. However, the determination of the right amount of QA remains an outstanding issue for which there is no simple answer. The results depend on the requirements of the department, the techniques used, the disease sites treated, and the resources available. Stereotactic radiation

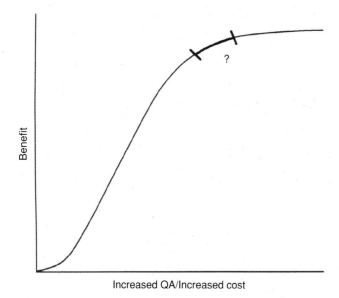

Figure 11.12. Schematic representation of QA cost–benefit relationship.

therapy and total body irradiation have different levels of quality requirements from those of upper-mantle irradiation for Hodgkin's disease, or small-field irradiation for cancer of the larynx, or IMRT.

AAPM Task Group 100 (79) is attempting to deal with the issue of ever-increasing QA activity as new and more complex technologies evolve. They describe a process that has been used in engineering circles and is known as failure mode and effects analysis (FMEA). FMEA focuses on a process, and at each step considers what could possibly go wrong, how that could happen, and what effects would such a failure produce. For each step, there may be many potential failure modes, and each one may have several potential causes and outcomes. For each potential cause of failure, values are assigned in three categories: O, the probability that a specific cause will result in a failure mode; S, the severity of the effects resulting from a specific failure mode should go undetected throughout treatment; and D, the probability that the failure mode resulting from the specific cause will go undetected. Convention uses numbers between 1 and 10. Category O ranges from 1 (unlikely failure, <1 in 10^4) to 10 (highly likely, >5% of the time). Category S ranges from 1 (no appreciable danger) to 10 (catastrophic if persisting through treatment). Category D ranges from 1 (undetected only <0.01% of the time) to 10 (undetected >20% of the time). The product of these three indices forms the risk probability number (RPN = $O \times S \times D$). In industry, RPN values <125 carry little concern. The Task Group is grappling with the values of RPN that should be of concern in radiation therapy. This methodology has been implemented in one radiation oncology center (80) and they identified 127 possible failure modes with *RPN* scores ranging from 2 to 160. Fifteen of the top-ranked failure modes were considered for process improvements, representing RPN scores of 75 and more.

These specific improvement suggestions were incorporated into their practice with a review and implementation by each department team responsible for the process. Thus, the FMEA technique provides a systematic method for finding vulnerabilities in a process before they result in an error. Further experience is required for such an approach to be implemented in every radiation therapy department.

The following section outlines some general considerations for ongoing QA for treatment planning computers.

Program and System Documentation

At the most basic level of QA, the user must be aware of what the programs are doing when any specific option is requested. Even if the programs are perfectly accurate, any error in data entry results in an error in the output. Thus, the user must have adequate information in terms of manuals and online help to aid in the commissioning and operational process of the TPS. The types of documentation that should be available are listed by Van Dyk et al. (11) and in Table A1–1 of AAPM TG53 (14).

User Training

Closely associated with proper manuals and information is user training. The user must be clearly aware of normalization procedures, dose calculation algorithms, image display and reconstruction procedures, and program calculation capabilities and limitations. This training can be carried out at three levels at least: (a) vendor training courses, (b) in-house staff training, and (c) special training courses set up by user groups or third-party software vendors.

Reproducibility Tests

A normally functioning computer is unlikely to generate small changes in output. Computer system hardware malfunctions are likely to be obvious. Changes in digitizer sensitivity, however, have proven to be a concern. Therefore, input and output devices should be checked on a regular basis.

From a risk management perspective, other possible sources of error include intended or unintended changes in software or data files. These can occur within the TPS or in the computers associated with data generation, such as CT scanners and water phantom systems. Software upgrades in these external computer systems can result in changes to the data entered into the TPS.

Another issue of concern is inadvertent access by treatment planners to the basic radiation or machine data files. This can result in changes to accuracy of calculations without the user being aware that changes have taken place.

For inadvertent software or hardware changes, a binary comparison of all the software and data files can test whether any changes have occurred. If changes are found, the details of the changes must be assessed and a partial system recommissioning may have to be implemented. Alternatively, as described in the IAEA report (16), a select subset of the vendor type tests should be performed to demonstrate consistency with previous results.

To aid in the assessment of any software changes, a series of reproducibility tests of the dose calculation algorithms, the image display algorithms, and the plan evaluation tools should be undertaken on a regular basis. Examples of such reproducibility tests can be found in Van Dyk et al. (11) and in the reports from the AAPM (14) and the IAEA (15). Users should develop their own tests based on their particular TPS and what components of the hardware, software, and data files have any likelihood of being changed.

Patient-Specific Tests

Since no system of computer programs is error-free, or are the users of such programs perfect, routine inspection of each treatment plan is a requirement for proper QA. Calculation of the external beam dose usually consists of two components: (a) calculation of a relative dose distribution, and (b) calculation of the machine output in terms of MUs. Both of these components require a check by a participant independent of the first calculation. For relative dose distributions, manual checks can be performed by choosing a specific point, usually on the central ray, and calculating a dose estimate for each of the beams using simplified tables to generate the results. These checks should agree to within about 2% to 3% of the computer-calculated values in regions of uniform dose delivery and relatively simple inhomogeneity corrections. More complicated plans have to be evaluated on an individual basis to assess the trends of the numerical values. Similarly, the machine setting calculation should be checked independently of the first calculation.

With the advent of more complex segmented or dynamic conformal therapy and IMRT, such manual checks become very difficult if not impossible. In these situations, the absolute dose is determined as part of the planning process, with the MUs being defined for each component of the treatment. QC checks for such techniques must be developed for each individual technique. Several commercial software packages are now available that will perform independent MU calculations (81). Georg et al. (81) suggested action levels between ±3% and ±5% dependent on treatment site and treatment technique. They also conclude that independent calculations may be used to replace experimental dose verification once the IMRT program is mature (82). Similarly, ICRU Report 83 (68) describes the use of one or more of the following methods for patient-specific QA:

■ Measurement of the intensity pattern from individual beams for a specific patient
■ Measurement of absorbed dose in phantom of the beam-intensity pattern planned for a specific patient
■ Independent absorbed dose calculations for the patient-specific beam intensity pattern
■ *In vivo* dosimetry

For brachytherapy, manual single-point calculations are more difficult, and therefore a check can be performed with one of the conventional systems of dosage calculations, such as the Manchester system. This approach can be used to make crude checks to an accuracy of about 10%. Again, assessing trends is crucial in evaluating the quality of the calculation.

In vitro *and* In vivo *Dosimetry Checks*

As a final check of the quality of the overall treatment planning process, it is useful to perform measurements using special-purpose or anthropomorphic phantoms (*in vitro* dosimetry) or to perform measurements on or in the patient with the patient in treatment position (*in vivo* dosimetry). *In vitro* dosimetry is an important component of the implementation of any new treatment technique or clinical procedure. Generally, it is performed with thermoluminescent dosimetry (TLD) in a phantom containing humanlike tissue densities and composition, such as the Rando Phantom. More recently, optically stimulated luminescence (OSL) is being used in place of TLD (83). Diodes (84) and metal-oxide semiconductor field-effect transistor (MOSFET) (85–87) dosimetry systems are now readily available and provide instant readout capability. This type of dosimetry ensures that the basic procedures associated with a new treatment technique are in agreement within a predetermined range of accuracy. The level of accuracy achievable depends on the type of treatment technique and the quality of the measurements, although usually the accuracy of dose delivery to a phantom geometry should be better than 3% to 4%, since the dose delivery to the patient should be within 5%. A report by Dunscombe et al. (88) gives a good overview of the use of an anthropomorphic phantom to evaluate the quality of treatment planning computer systems. While providing a good indication of the accuracy of the dose delivery process near the center of the target volume, differences between measurements and calculations away from the central region were difficult to interpret as to whether the calculations were off, the measurements were off, or the beam placement was inaccurate. Thus, *in vitro* dosimetry must be established in such a manner that differences between measurements and calculations can be readily interpreted.

Similar concerns of interpretation also apply to *in vivo* dosimetry (89). There is a general tendency by radiation oncologists to request TLD, OSL, diode, or MOSFET measurements to give them an assurance that the dose delivery process is accurate, especially in regions where there is concern about critical structures such as the eyes, gonads, or a fetus. Sometimes, these regions are close to the edge of the radiation beams. Under such circumstances, small changes in beam alignment can generate large changes in measured dose, leaving ambiguity in the interpretation of the results. These interpretation difficulties should be clearly explained to the radiation oncologist requesting the measurements. Better comparisons of calculations and measurements can be made in regions where doses are not changing as rapidly—either on the entrance or exit surfaces or, if possible, by placing dosimeters in body cavities such as the mouth, trachea, esophagus, vagina, uterus, or rectum. While *in vivo* dosimetry is a recommended check under some treatment conditions and it may provide an opportunity to mitigate treatment errors (90), it is also recognized that it may be inappropriate for some new technologies such as IMRT, where dosimetric checks by phantom irradiations should be done instead (91).

Portal Imaging and Portal Dosimetry—Imaging for Therapy Verification

Port films have been in use for many years as a means of confirmation of the accuracy of beam placement (92–94). The main problems with port films have been their lack of contrast in high-energy photon beams, and therefore an inability to locate relevant critical structures clearly with respect to the actual location of the treatment beam. Furthermore, port films are not very convenient because they require developing, which causes a delay between the time they have taken and the time they are viewed. Often, this is handled by the radiation oncologist viewing the port film after the patient leaves.

Electronic portal imaging devices (EPIDs) provide the possibility of obtaining real-time images of patients while the beam is on. The EPID technology has matured some time ago and is readily available to the average radiation therapy institution (94,95).

Portal images can be obtained in various ways (93). One approach has been the acquisition of the image during treatment and the viewing of the image after treatment. This should provide an indication of the accuracy of the placement of the beam and allow adjustments to be made for subsequent treatments if necessary. Another approach is to make a short exposure at the start of treatment, view the image, and make adjustments as needed prior to the entire treatment being given.

Because of the lack of contrast when using any form of imaging with high-energy photon beams, it is often hard to locate organs or reference structures relative to beam edges. This makes it difficult to evaluate portal images for accuracy. To aid this process, a double exposure is used: one short exposure is made without the blocks and shields and with a larger collimator opening, and another short exposure of the actual treatment field with its ancillary devices in place is made. This helps significantly with the localization of the beam with respect to critical structures or reference organs.

Since EPIDs provide digital images, display contrast can be enhanced by optimizing the windowing and leveling of the image (92). Furthermore, image contrast can be enhanced by image processing using techniques such as adaptive histogram equalization (93). The practical benefit of portal imaging has really evolved with automated image registration techniques. Today, evaluation of the portal image is done either by a direct visual comparison of the portal image with the simulator film or the digitally reconstructed radiograph (DRR) obtained from the TPS or by automated registration techniques. The latter dramatically reduces the tedium and subjectivity of routine evaluation of patient positioning using portal imaging (92,94).

Strategies for intervention and patient adjustment have been described by Balter et al. (96), who indicate that setup adjustments using image registration and setup correction techniques can be made with a reasonable threshold of 3 to 5 mm, depending on treatment site.

As EPID technology has evolved, more effort has been placed on the conversion of the image data to absorbed dose (97). This provides the possibility of obtaining not only beam placement information, but also information on the accuracy of the dose delivery. The process is evolving such that TPSs can generate predicted portal image and portal dose information, which then can be compared directly with the images measured during patient treatment. Criteria of acceptability must be invoked to determine whether the treatment is acceptable and can proceed or whether to terminate the treatment because the beam placement and/or the dose is incorrect. In this context, the portal imaging system is used as a form of *in vivo* dosimetry and provides a 2D dose map of the treatment rather than individual dose points provided by conventional *in vivo* dosimetry methods. Exit dosimetry may prove to be especially useful for 3D dynamic CRT, with which the integrated measured dose can be compared to the planned dose as determined by the TPS. It is also being used for 3D dosimetric evaluation of volumetric arc therapy (97,98).

The use of electronic portal imaging procedures is decreasing as the availability of online cone-beam CT has become more readily available as a tool for daily image-guidance (99) (see Chapter 14). Kilovoltage on-board imaging using planar transmission images is also available as a tool to assess patient setup alignment (100).

Quality Audits

It is always useful to review the QA activities of individual institutions. Recent years have seen the public reporting of various errors or "accidents" in radiation therapy. While such errors can have a devastating effect on individual patients, the actual error rate in radiation therapy is very low. However, it is the responsibility of members of the radiation therapy team to ensure that proper procedures are in place to minimize such errors. As a first approach, an institutional self-auditing process is beneficial. This is best done in the context of a QA committee that should exist in every radiation therapy department (101). External audits have proven to be extremely beneficial for finding inadvertent deviations from acceptable practice. The Radiological Physics Center (RPC) in Houston, Texas, has done this for years for institutions participating in clinical trials involved with the Radiation Therapy Oncology Group (RTOG) (102,103). Dosimetry intercomparisons are also useful especially in the development of new techniques such as IMRT (104). The IAEA has developed an external audit process, which involves a review of the total treatment process (105). They do this through the use of a quality assurance team in radiation oncology (QUATRO), which consists of a radiation oncologist, medical physicist, radiation therapist, and sometimes a specialist in radiation protection.

QA of Total Radiation Therapy Planning Process

As indicated earlier, the total radiation therapy planning process consists of many steps, of which computerized treatment planning is only one component. For the computer plan to be implemented accurately at treatment, it is important that the basic patient data and image information be derived accurately. This requires QC of the imagers generating the data (24,94,95,106). It also requires assurance that the patient is positioned precisely in a manner that will be readily reproducible on subsequent simulation and treatment setups. Ten Haken and Fraass (13) describe various checks that should be considered before planning begins, during planning, after planning, and at treatment.

Geometric accuracy, before planning, begins with proper immobilization and localization of the patient in treatment position. Accuracy during planning includes assessing accuracies associated with image transfer, image registration, target volume and normal tissue localization, beam placement, and dose calculations. To ensure that the plan can be implemented on the therapy unit, the planner must verify that the geometric arrangements are physically achievable. QA after planning may include a verification simulation, the comparison of the radiographs with beam's-eye-view plots or DRRs to verify that the field shapes are correct, as well as confirmation that the internal anatomy is located accurately within the fields. Finally, accuracy can be ensured at treatment by verifying that the treatment setup parameters such as SSDs and depths for each field are consistent, as well as comparing the portal images with the calculated DRRs or verification simulation films. Now available in many institutions, daily online imaging can be used routinely to assure geometric accuracy of the beam positioning and a confirmation of the location of the internal anatomy of the patient, just before each dose fraction is delivered.

QA Administration

A very important component of any QA program is the organization and administration of the program such that it is implemented and carried out according to a predetermined schedule and that ongoing records of the activities and the results are maintained. Proper administration requires that one person, usually a qualified medical physicist, be responsible for the QA program. Although this individual does not necessarily have to carry out all the

tests and their evaluations, he or she must ensure that there is written documentation on the QA process, that the tests are carried out according to their specified frequency, and that appropriate actions are taken as needed.

An important aspect of QA is communication. This is especially important when any changes are made to any component of the TPS, be it hardware or software, or if any changes are made to hardware or software of the imaging or dosimetry devices that feed data into the treatment planning computer.

As TPSs become networked into clusters with various planning and target volume delineation stations, servers, and peripheral devices, system management becomes an integral component of the entire QA of the TPS. This management includes maintaining an adequate check on system security and limiting user access not only to the system, but also to specific software and data file modifications. It is important that the radiation data files should not be inadvertently changed and that patient confidentiality be fully maintained.

To avoid the possibility of any undesired loss of information, a regular schedule for system backup is essential (14). This may include daily backups of the most recent patient additions and changes, weekly backups of all patient information, and monthly backups of the entire TPS. Backups are also warranted immediately after any major changes are made to the software of the system.

In addition to standard backups, it may also be desirable to archive specific patient information, especially if patients are to be grouped for study purposes. In some cases, patient data may have to be forwarded to clinical trial groups such as the RTOG, which accepts such information through the Internet. However, patient data must also be archived in case the patient comes back for retreatment.

Clinical radiation information systems now are becoming a standard component of radiation therapy departments (107). These systems include what used to be called "record and verify" functions on the treatment machine, although they are now much more comprehensive. They may include patient scheduling, the capability to transfer data between the TPS and the therapy machine, as well as provide departmental statistics on the types of patients treated by disease diagnosis (108).

Proper QA of the modern 3D TPS is a time-consuming process. Adequate staff resources must be allocated to ensure that the QA is completed in an appropriate manner. This aspect must be clearly understood as an operational cost of running the TPS and must be incorporated into the purchase plan prior to the purchase of the system.

Summary

QA programs for radiation therapy machines, especially with the clinical implementation of high-energy accelerators have been well defined for many years. Formalized (CT) simulator QA is a more recent phenomenon (24,75,109). While redundant checks for MU and time calculations have also been standard practice, the formalization of a QA program for treatment planning computers occurred more recently. This is partly due to the tremendous variation in TPSs and their algorithms and partly to the complexity of treatment planning QA, since it involves multiple facets, including data measurement, data entry, algorithm verification, image manipulation and verification, assessment of the accuracy of the image display and evaluation tools, and assessment of the quality of the final plan and dose distribution. Because of these complexities, it is clear that a simple unique QA program cannot be defined but that a comprehensive program depends entirely on institutional procedures and the type of planning system in use.

Treatment planning errors can be minimized with a good QA program. As indicated earlier in this chapter, the major issues that relate to treatment planning errors can be summarized by four key words: (a) education, (b) verification, (c) documentation, and (d) communication (15). Education is required not only at the technical and professional level in terms of the use of the TPS, but also at the organizational level with respect to institutional policies and procedures. A very important component of education relates to understanding the software capabilities and limitations. Verification is important since it is recognized that nearly 60% of the reported errors related to the use of TPSs involved a lack of an appropriate independent secondary check of the treatment plan or dose calculation. Clear documentation is required both of each patient's individual treatment plan and of departmental policies and procedures. Finally, communication among staff members is essential for all aspects of treatment, since various people at various professional levels are involved in the treatment process. Poor communication was a key factor in a number of the errors reported that relate to treatment planning.

A carefully executed program of treatment planning computer commissioning and ongoing QA assessment provides users with confidence that their work is being carried out accurately. Furthermore, it gives the user a clear understanding of the TPS's capabilities and limitations. Finally, the quality of the delivery of a radiation dose to the patient depends on the quality of all the steps in the treatment planning process, including patient imaging, simulation, target volume delineation, treatment planning, treatment verification, and quality factors associated with dose delivery and related to the radiation therapy machine. Thus, it is imperative that the medical physicist, as well as all other staff associated with the radiation therapy process, be actively involved in the QA process at all stages. This provides both full awareness of the capabilities and limitations of each step of the process and a mechanism for decision making about any corrective action deemed to be necessary.

Acknowledgments

Dr. Chris Newcomb, formerly of the Princess Margaret Hospital in Toronto, Ontario, Canada, was very much

involved in the measurement of data and the production of Figures 11.3 to 11.11. The data of Table 11.4 were adapted from the tender document produced by a number of members of the Department of Clinical Physics at the Princess Margaret Hospital.

REFERENCES

1. International Organization for Standardization. *Quality management and quality assurance standards—Part 1: guidelines for selection and use. ISO 9000.* International Organization for Standardization, 1994.
2. World Health Organization (WHO). *Quality assurance in radiotherapy.* Geneva: WHO, 1988.
3. Wu Q, Xing L, Ezzell G, et al. Inverse treatment planning. In: Van Dyk J, ed. *The modern technology of radiation oncology: a compendium for medical physicists and radiation oncologists.* Volume 2. Madison: Medical Physics Publishing, 2005:131–183.
4. Xia P, Verhey LJ. Intensity-modulated radiation therapy. In: Van Dyk J, ed. *The modern technology of radiation oncology: a compendium for medical physicists and radiation oncologists.* Volume 2. Madison: Medical Physics Publishing; 2005:221–258.
5. Caldwell C, Mah K. Imaging for radiation therapy planning. In: Van Dyk J, ed. *The modern technology of radiation oncology: a compendium for medical physicists and radiation oncologists.* Volume 2. Madison: Medical Physics Publishing, 2005:31–89.
6. Moiseenko V, Deasy JO, Van Dyk J. Radiobiological modeling for treatment planning. In: Van Dyk J, ed. *The modern technology of radiation oncology: a compendium for medical physicists and radiation oncologists.* Volume 2. Madison: Medical Physics Publishing, 2005:185–220.
7. Ezzell GA, Galvin JM, Low D, et al. Guidance document on delivery, treatment planning, and clinical implementation of IMRT: report of the IMRT Subcommittee of the AAPM Radiation Therapy Committee. *Med Phys* 2003;30:2089–2115.
8. Kutcher GJ, Coia L, Gillin M, et al. Comprehensive QA for radiation oncology: report of AAPM Radiation Therapy Committee Task Group 40. *Med Phys* 1994;21:581–618.
9. Brahme A, ed. Accuracy requirements and quality assurance of external beam therapy with photons and electrons. *Acta Oncol* 1988;27(Suppl. 1):5–76.
10. Williamson JF, Thomadsen BR, eds. Quality assurance for radiation therapy: the challenges of advanced technologies symposium. *Int J Radiat Oncol Biol Phys* 2008;72(Suppl 1):S1–S214.
11. Van Dyk J, Barnett RB, Cygler JE, et al. Commissioning and quality assurance of treatment planning computers. *Int J Radiat Oncol Biol Phys* 1993;26:261–273.
12. Miller DW, Bloch PH, Cunningham JR. *Radiation treatment planning dosimetry verification. AAPM Report Number 55.* New York: American Institute of Physics, 1995.
13. Ten Haken RK, Fraass BA. Quality assurance in 3D treatment planning. In: Meyer JL, Purdy JA, eds. *3D

conformal radiotherapy. Basel: Karger, S., 1996:104–114.

14. Fraass B, Doppke K, Hunt M, et al. American Association of Physicists in Medicine Radiation Therapy Committee Task Group 53: quality assurance for clinical radiotherapy treatment planning. *Med Phys* 1998;25:1773–1829.

15. Van Dyk J, Rosenwald J-C, Fraass B, et al. *Commissioning and quality assurance of computerized planning systems for radiation treatment of cancer. IAEA TRS-430.* Vienna: International Atomic Energy Agency, 2004.

16. International Atomic Energy Agency. *IAEA-TECDOC-1540. Specification and acceptance testing of radiotherapy treatment planning systems.* Vienna, Austria: International Atomic Energy Agency, 2007.

17. International Atomic Energy Agency. *IAEA-TECDOC-1583: commissioning of radiotherapy treatment planning systems: testing for typical external beam treatment techniques.* Vienna, Austria: International Atomic Energy Agency, 2008.

18. Sharpe MB. Commissioning and quality assurance for IMRT treatment planning. In: Palta JR, Mackie TR, eds. *Intensity modulated radiation therapy: state of the art.* Madison, WI: Medical Physics Publishing, 2003:449–473.

19. Galvin JM, Ezzell G, Eisbrauch A, et al. Implementing IMRT in clinical practice: a joint document of the American Society for Therapeutic Radiology and Oncology and the American Association of Physicists in Medicine. *Int J Radiat Oncol Biol Phys* 2004;58:1616–1634.

20. Wheatley BM. An instrument for dosage estimation with fields of any size and any shape. *Brit J Radiol* 1951;24:388–391.

21. Cunningham JR. The Gordon Richards memorial lecture: the stampede to compute: computers in radiotherapy. *J Can Assoc Radiol* 1971;22:242–251.

22. Tsien KC. The application of automatic computing machines to radiation treatment planning. *Brit J Radiol* 1955;28:432–439.

23. Peters TM, Slomka PT, Fenster A. Imaging for radiation therapy planning (MRI, nuclear medicine, ultrasound). In: Van Dyk J, ed. *The modern technology of radiation oncology: a compendium for medical physicists and radiation oncologists.* Madison, WI: Medical Physics Publishing, 1999:192–229.

24. Van Dyk J, Taylor J. CT simulators. In: Van Dyk J, ed. *The modern technology of radiation oncology: a compendium for medical physicists and radiation oncologists.* Madison, WI: Medical Physics Publishing, 1999:131–168.

25. The use of computers in therapeutic radiology. *Special report no. 1. Symposium Proceedings of First International Conference of Computers in Radiotherapy,* Cambridge, UK, 1966. London: British Institute of Radiology, 1967.

26. Cohen M, ed. Computers in radiotherapy. Special report no. 4. Symposium Proceedings of Second International Conference of Computers in Radiotherapy, Chicago. *Br J Radiol* 1970;43:658–663. London: British Institute of Radiology, 1970.

27. Computers in radiotherapy. Special report no. 5. Symposium Proceedings of Third International Conference of Computers in Radiotherapy, Glasgow, 1970. London: British Institute of Radiology, 1971.

28. Computers in radiation therapy. Symposium Proceedings of Fourth International Conference of Computers in Radiotherapy, Uppsala, Sweden, 1972. Uppsala: Radiofysikavdelningen, Akademiska Sjukhuset S-75014, 1972.

29. Sternick ES, ed. *Computer applications in radiation oncology. Symposium Proceedings of Fifth International Conference of Computers in Radiotherapy, Hanover, NH, 1975.* Hanover: University Press of New England, 1976.

30. Rosenow U, ed. *Computers in radiotherapy. Symposium Proceedings of Sixth International Conference of Computers in Radiotherapy, Goettingen, Federal Republic of Germany, 1977.* Goettingen: Strahlenabteilung Universitaets Frauenklinik, D-3400, 1978.

31. Umegaki Y ed. *Computers in radiation therapy. Symposium Proceedings of Seventh International Conference of Computers in Radiotherapy, Kawasaki and Tokyo, 1980.* Tokyo: Japan Radiological Society, 1981.

32. Cunningham JR, Ragan D, Van Dyk J, eds. *Proceedings of the Eighth International Conference on the Use of Computers in Radiation Therapy, Toronto, 1984.* Silver Springs, MD: IEEE Computer Society Press, 1984.

33. Bruinvis IAD, van der Giessen PH, van Kleffens HJ, Wittkämper FW, eds. *The use of computers in radiation therapy. Symposium Proceedings of Ninth International Conference of Computers in Radiotherapy, Scheveningen, Netherlands, 1987.* Amsterdam: Elsevier, 1987.

34. Hukku S, Iyer PS, eds. *The use of computers in radiation therapy. Symposium Proceedings of Tenth International Conference of Computers in Radiotherapy, Lucknow, 1990.* Uttar Pradesh: Department of Electronics, Government of India, Council of Science and Technology, 1990.

35. Hounsell AR, Wilkinson J, Williams PC, eds. *Symposium Proceedings of Eleventh International Conference of Computers in Radiotherapy, Manchester, UK, 1994.* Manchester: North Western Medical Physics Department, 1994.

36. Leavitt DD, Starkschall G, eds. *1997 XIIth International Conference on the use of computers in radiation therapy.* Madison: Medical Physics Publishing, 1997.

37. Schlegel W, Bortfeld T, eds. *The use of computers in radiation therapy.* Heidelberg: Springer-Verlag, 2000.

38. Yi BY, Ahn SD, Choi EK, Ha SW, eds. *The XIVth International Conference on the Use of computers in Radiation Therapy.* Seoul: Jeong Publishing Co., 2004.

39. Bissonnette JP, ed. *Conference Proceedings: XVth International Conference on the Use of Computers in Radiotherapy (ICCR).* Toronto: Department of Radiation Oncology, Faculty of Medicine, University of Toronto, 2007.

40. Sonke JJ, ed. *Proceedings of the XVIth International Conference on the Use of Computers in Radiotherapy (ICCR).* Amsterdam, Netherlands. Het Nederlands Kanker Instituut—Antoni van Leeuwenhoek Ziekenhuis, 2010.

41. Shaw JE. *A guide to commissioning and quality control of treatment planning systems.* New York: The Institution

of Physics and Engineering in Medicine and Biology, 1994.

42. Mijnheer B, Olszewska A, Fiorino C, et al. *Quality assurance of treatment planning systems: practical examples of non-IMRT photon beams.* Brussels: European Society of Therapeutic Radiation Oncology (ESTRO), 2004.

43. Bruinvis IAD, Keus RB, Lenglet WJM, et al. *Quality assurance of 3D treatment planning systems for external photon and electron beams. Report 15 of the Netherlands Commission on Radiation Dosimetry.* Netherlands Commission on Radiation Dosimetry (NCS), 2006.

44. International Electrotechnical Commission (IEC). *Medical electrical equipment—requirements for the safety of radiotherapy treatment planning systems. IEC 62083 (2000–11).* Geneva: International Electrotechnical Commission, 2000.

45. Van Dyk J, Barnett RB, Battista JJ. Computerized radiation treatment planning systems. In: Van Dyk J, ed. *The modern technology of radiation oncology: a compendium for medical physicists and radiation oncologists.* Madison, WI: Medical Physics Publishing, 1999:231–286.

46. Fraass BA. Quality assurance for 3D treatment planning. In: Palta JR, Mackie TR, eds. *Teletherapy: present and future.* Madison, WI: Advanced Medical Publishing, 1996:253–318.

47. Siebers JV, Keall PJ, Kawrakow I. Monte Carlo dose calculations for external beam radiation therapy. In: Van Dyk J, ed. *The modern technology of radiation oncology: a compendium for medical physicists and radiation oncologists.* Volume 2. Madison: Medical Physics Publishing, 2005:91–130.

48. Chetty IJ, Curran B, Cygler JE, et al. Report of the AAPM Task Group No. 105: issues associated with clinical implementation of Monte Carlo-based photon and electron external beam treatment planning. *Med Phys* 2007;34:4818–4853.

49. Papanikolaou N, Battista JJ, Boyer AL, et al. *Tissue inhomogeneity corrections for megavoltage photon beams. Report by Task Group 65 of the Radiation Therapy Committee of the American Association of Physicists in Medicine. AAPM Report 85.* Madison, WI: Medical Physics Publishing, 2004.

50. Rivard MJ, Venselaar JL, Beaulieu L. The evolution of brachytherapy treatment planning. *Med Phys* 2009;36:2136–2153.

51. Houghton Mifflin. *American heritage dictionary of the English language.* 4th ed. Houghton Mifflin, 2006:8–7-2010. http://education.yahoo.com/reference/dictionary/ Last accessed on 2011/05/29.

52. Verhey L, Bentel G. Patient Immobilization. In: Van Dyk J, ed. *The modern technology of radiation oncology: a compendium for medical physicists and radiation oncologists.* Madison, WI: Medical Physics Publishing, 1999:53–94.

53. Leunens G, Menten J, Weltens C, et al. Quality assessment of medical decision making in radiation oncology: variability in target volume delineation for brain tumours. *Radiother Oncol* 1993;29:169–175.

54. Tai P, Van Dyk J, Yu E, et al. Variability of target volume delineation in cervical esophageal cancer. *Int J Radiat Oncol Biol Phys* 1998;42:277–288.

55. Rasch C, Steenbakkers R, van Herk M. Target definition in prostate, head, and neck. *Semin Radiat Oncol* 2005;15:136–145.

56. Hamilton CS, Ebert MA. Volumetric uncertainty in radiotherapy. *Clin Oncol (R Coll Radiol)* 2005;17:456–464.

57. McCullough EC, Krueger AM. Performance evaluation of computerized treatment planning systems for radiotherapy: external photon beams. *Int J Radiat Oncol Biol Phys* 1980;6:1599–1605.

58. Dahlin H, Lamm IL, Landberg T, et al. User requirements on CT-based computed dose planning systems in radiation therapy. *Acta Radiol Oncol* 1983;22:397–415.

59. International Commission on Radiation Units and Measurements. *ICRU Report 42: use of computers in external beam radiotherapy procedures with high-energy photons and electrons.* Bethesda, Maryland: International Commission On Radiation Units and Measurements, 1987.

60. Venselaar J, Welleweerd H, Mijnheer B. Tolerances for the accuracy of photon beam dose calculations of treatment planning systems. *Radiother Oncol* 2001;60:191–201.

61. DeWerd LA, Ibbott GS, Meigooni AS, et al. A prepatient single-source dosimetric uncertainty analysis for photon-emitting brachytherapy sources: report of AAPM Task Group No. 138 and GEC-ESTRO. *Med Phys* 2011;38:782–801.

62. Shiu AS, Tung S, Hogstrom KR, et al. Verification data for electron beam dose algorithms. *Med Phys* 1992;19:623–636.

63. Venselaar J, Welleweerd H. Application of a test package in an intercomparison of the photon dose calculation performance of treatment planning systems used in a clinical setting. *Radiother Oncol* 2001;60:203–213.

64. Zhu TC, Palta JR. Electron contamination in 8 and 18 MV photon beams. *Med Phys* 1998;25:12–19.

65. Bedford JL, Childs PJ, Nordmark H, et al. Commissioning and quality assurance of the Pinnacle(3) radiotherapy treatment planning system for external beam photons. *Br J Radiol* 2003;76:163–176.

66. Cadman P, McNutt T, Bzdusek K. Validation of physics improvements for IMRT with a commercial treatment-planning system. *J Appl Clin Med Phys* 2005;6:74–86.

67. Cadman P, Bassalow R, Sidhu NP, et al. Dosimetric considerations for validation of a sequential IMRT process with a commercial treatment planning system. *Phys Med Biol* 2002;47:3001–3010.

68. International Commission on Radiation Units and Measurements. *ICRU Report 83: Prescribing, Recording, and Reporting Photon-Beam Intensity-Modulated Radiation Therapy (IMRT).* Bethesda, Maryland: International Commission On Radiation Units and Measurements, 2010.

69. Meli JA, Anderson LL, Weaver KA. Dose distribution. In: Anderson LL, Nath R, Weaver KA, et al. eds. *Interstitial brachytherapy: physical, biological, and clinical considerations.* New York: Raven Press, 1990:21–34.

70. Meigooni AS, Chiu-Tsao ST, Smith V. Reference data. In: Anderson LL, Nath R, Weaver KA, et al. eds. *Interstitial*

brachytherapy: physical, biological, and clinical considerations. New York: Raven Press, 1990:261–264.

71. Rivard MJ, Beaulieu L, Mourtada F. Enhancements to commissioning techniques and quality assurance of brachytherapy treatment planning systems that use model-based dose calculation algorithms. *Med Phys* 2010;37:2645–2658.

72. Van Dyk J. Advances in modern radiation therapy. In: Van Dyk J, ed. *The modern technology of radiation oncology: a compendium for medical physicists and radiation oncologists.* Volume 2. Madison, WI: Medical Physics Publishing, 2005:1–29.

73. Craig T, Brochu D, Van Dyk J. A quality assurance phantom for three-dimensional radiation treatment planning. *Int J Radiat Oncol Biol Phys* 1999;44:955–966.

74. McNiven A, Kron T, Van Dyk J. A multileaf collimator phantom for the quality assurance of radiation therapy planning systems and CT simulators. *Int J Radiat Oncol Biol Phys* 2004;60:994–1001.

75. Mutic S, Palta JR, Butker EK, et al. Quality assurance for computed-tomography simulators and the computed-tomography-simulation process: report of the AAPM Radiation Therapy Committee Task Group No. 66. *Med Phys* 2003;30:2762–2792.

76. Mackie TR. History of tomotherapy. *Phys Med Biol* 2006;51:R427–R453.

77. Calcerrada Diaz-Santos N, Blasco Amaro JA, Cardiel GA, et al. The safety and efficacy of robotic image-guided radiosurgery system treatment for intra- and extracranial lesions: a systematic review of the literature. *Radiother Oncol* 2008;89:245–253.

78. Wowra B, Muacevic A, Jess-Hempen A, et al. Safety and efficacy of outpatient gamma knife radiosurgery for multiple cerebral metastases. *Expert Rev Neurother* 2004;4:673–679.

79. Huq MS, Fraass BA, Dunscombe PB, et al. A method for evaluating quality assurance needs in radiation therapy. *Int J Radiat Oncol Biol Phys* 2008;71:S170–S173.

80. Ford EC, Gaudette R, Myers L, et al. Evaluation of safety in a radiation oncology setting using failure mode and effects analysis. *Int J Radiat Oncol Biol Phys* 2009;74:852–858.

81. Georg D, Nyholm T, Olofsson J, et al. Clinical evaluation of monitor unit software and the application of action levels. *Radiother Oncol* 2007;85:306–315.

82. Georg D, Stock M, Kroupa B, et al. Patient-specific IMRT verification using independent fluence-based dose calculation software: experimental benchmarking and initial clinical experience. *Phys Med Biol* 2007;52:4981–4992.

83. Yukihara EG, McKeever SW. Optically stimulated luminescence (OSL) dosimetry in medicine. *Phys Med Biol* 2008;53:R351–R379.

84. Ten Haken R, Fraass B, Lam K. Dosimetry and data acquisition. In: Palta JR, Mackie TR, eds. *Teletherapy: present and future.* Madison: Advanced Medical Publishing, 1996:191–220.

85. Jornet N, Carrasco P, Jurado D, et al. Comparison study of MOSFET detectors and diodes for entrance in vivo dosimetry in 18 MV x-ray beams. *Med Phys* 2004;31:2534–2542.

86. Chuang CF, Verhey LJ, Xia P. Investigation of the use of MOSFET for clinical IMRT dosimetric verification. *Med Phys* 2002;29:1109–1115.

87. Kron T, Rosenfeld A, Lerch M, et al. Measurements in radiotherapy beams using on-line MOSFET detectors. *Radiat Protect Dosim* 2002;101:445–448.

88. Dunscombe P, McGhee P, Lederer E. Anthropomorphic phantom measurements for the validation of a treatment planning system. *Phys Med Biol* 1996;41:399–411.

89. Van Dam J, Marinello G. *Methods for in vivo dosimetry in external radiotherapy.* Brussels, Belgium: ESTRO, 2006.

90. World Health Organization (WHO). *Radiotherapy risk profile: technical manual.* Geneva: World Health Organization, 2008.

91. International Commission on Radiation Protection. ICRP Publication 112—preventing accidental exposures from new external beam radiation therapy technologies. *Ann ICRP* 2009;39:1–86.

92. Munro P. Portal imaging technology: past, present, and future. *Semin Radiat Oncol* 1995;5:115–133.

93. Shalev S. Megavoltage portal imaging. In: Palta JR, Mackie TR, eds. *Teletherapy: present and future.* Madison: Advanced Medical Publishing, 1996;445–470.

94. Munro P. megavoltage radiography for treatment verification. In: Van Dyk J, ed. *The modern technology of radiation oncology: a compendium for medical physicists and radiation oncologists.* Madison, WI: Medical Physics Publishing, 1999:481–508.

95. Jaffray DA, Bissonnette J-P, Craig T. X-ray imaging for verification and localization in radiation therapy. In: Van Dyk J, ed. *The modern technology of radiation oncology: a compendium for medical physicists and radiation oncologists, Volume 2.* Madison, WI: Medical Physics Publishing, 2005:260–284.

96. Balter J, Ten Haken RK, Lam K. Immobilization and setup verification. In: Palta JR, Mackie TR, eds. *Teletherapy: present and future.* Madison: Advanced Medical Publishing, 1996:471–494.

97. Mans A, Remeijer P, Olaciregui-Ruiz I, et al. 3D Dosimetric verification of volumetric-modulated arc therapy by portal dosimetry. *Radiother Oncol* 2010;94:181–187.

98. Mans A, Wendling M, McDermott LN, et al. Catching errors with in vivo EPID dosimetry. *Med Phys* 2010;37:2638–2644.

99. Jaffray DA. Kilovoltage volumetric imaging in the treatment room. *Front Radiat Ther Oncol* 2007;40:116–131.

100. Huntzinger C, Munro P, Johnson S, et al. Dynamic targeting image-guided radiotherapy. *Med Dosim* 2006;31:113–125.

101. Van Dyk J, Purdy JA. Clinical implementation of technology and the quality assurance process. In: Van Dyk J, ed. *The modern technology of radiation oncology: a compendium for medical physicists and radiation oncologists.* Madison, WI: Medical Physics Publishing, 1999:19–51.

102. Ibbott G, Ma CM, Rogers DW, et al. Anniversary paper: fifty years of AAPM involvement in radiation dosimetry. *Med Phys* 2008;35:1418–1427.

103. Ibbott GS, Followill DS, Molineu HA, et al. Challenges in credentialing institutions and participants in advanced technology multi-institutional clinical trials. *Int J Radiat Oncol Biol Phys* 2008;71:S71–S75.

104. Schiefer H, Fogliata A, Nicolini G, et al. The Swiss IMRT dosimetry intercomparison using a thorax phantom. *Med Phys* 2010;37:4424–4431.

105. International Atomic Energy Agency. *Comprehensive audits of radiotherapy practices: a tool for quality improvement, quality assurance team for radiation oncology (QUATRO).* Vienna, Austria: International Atomic Energy Agency, 2007.

106. Ten Haken RK, Kessler ML, Stern RL, et al. Quality assurance of CT and MRI for radiation therapy treatment planning. In: Starkschall GHJ, ed. *Quality assurance of radiotherapy physics: proceedings of an American College Medical Physics Symposium.* Madison, WI: Medical Physics Publishing, 1991:73–103.

107. Brooks K. Radiation Oncology Information Management System. In: Van Dyk J, ed. *The modern technology of radiation oncology: a compendium for medical physicists and radiation oncologists.* Madison, WI: Medical Physics Publishing, 1999:509–520.

108. Siochi RA, Balter P, Bloch CD, et al. Information technology resource management in radiation oncology. *J Appl Clin Med Phys* 2009;10:3116.

109. Van Dyk J, Munro P. Simulators. In: Van Dyk J, ed. *The modern technology of radiation oncology: a compendium for medical physicists and radiation oncologists.* Madison, WI: Medical Physics Publishing, 1999:95–129.

CHAPTER 12

Three-Dimensional Conformal Radiation Therapy

Karl L. Prado ■ George Starkschall ■ Radhe Mohan

INTRODUCTION

The goal of radiation therapy is to irradiate tumor-bearing tissues while sparing normal structures. Specifically, we would like to deliver a dose of radiation to tumor cells that is large enough to produce cell kill at a sufficiently high probability level to control malignant disease, while at the same time limiting the dose to uninvolved surrounding tissues so that the probability of inducing damage to these tissues is kept to a minimum. In external-beam radiation therapy, in which beams of radiation necessarily traverse normal tissues in order to treat tumor-bearing anatomic sites, this goal is often difficult. At dose levels at which tumor control becomes reasonably probable, normal tissue damage becomes a serious consideration.

The primary obstacles to achieving the maximum possible therapeutic advantage in favor of the patient being treated with conventional radiotherapy are the following:

1. The uncertainties in the true spatial extent of the disease
2. Inadequate knowledge of the exact shapes and locations of normal structures
3. The lack of optimal tools for efficient planning and delivery of conformal radiation therapy (CRT)
4. limitations of existing methods of producing desirable radiation dose distributions

These limitations result in the incorporation of large safety margins to reduce the risk of local relapse. However, to ensure that unacceptable normal tissue complications are prevented, the tumor dose often has to be maintained at suboptimal levels, leading to a higher probability of local failures. Therefore, better localization of the extent of the tumor and of normal critical structures and the ability to shape the dose distributions accordingly are essential to reduce the margins, allowing increases in tumor doses and minimizing dose to normal tissues.

Consider a common treatment-planning scenario, in which a tumor lies within a region of uninvolved tissue, and a uniform dose of radiation is delivered to the site. As the dose delivered to this site increases, the probability of tumor control increases, as does the probability of inducing normal tissue damage (Figure 12.1). Depending upon the dose–response characteristics of the tumor and of the surrounding normal tissues, it may not be possible to control the disease at a high enough probability level, without also producing normal tissue damage. Therefore, it very often becomes necessary to deliver higher doses to the tumor than to the surrounding uninvolved tissue. This is accomplished by selectively *targeting* tumor volumes with multiple radiation beams.

Despite considerable progress in improving the accuracy and precision of radiation therapy, many sources of uncertainty remain. These include the limitations of imaging devices to reveal the true extent of the disease, displacement of the internal anatomy at the time of treatment relative to its position at the time of imaging, motion of patient and internal organs during treatment, variation of response to dose from one patient to the next, intratumor variation in response, dosimetric inaccuracies, and so on. These are complex problems, but a reduction in uncertainties is essential for the accumulation of more accurate data and for an improvement of the state of the art of radiotherapy. A considerable amount of effort is being devoted to reducing uncertainties.

TARGETING FOR THREE-DIMENSIONAL CONFORMAL RADIATION THERAPY

The process by which external beams of radiation are designed and used to selectively and exclusively irradiate only tumor-bearing sites is called three-dimensional conformal radiation therapy (3-DCRT). In 3-DCRT, tumor sites are meticulously identified, as are normal structures considered at risk of damage. A treatment plan is created in which radiation beams are carefully designed to include only tumor sites while excluding, as best possible, normal structures considered at risk. The resulting dose distribution is calculated and evaluated in light of dose–response criteria established for the disease and for normal structures at risk. Once approved, the plan can be delivered.

In this chapter, the process of 3-DCRT is reviewed. Initially, necessary terminology is defined. Methods for defining and recognizing tumor-bearing volumes are then described. The rationale for designing radiation-beam portals is explained, emphasizing the concept of margins. The process by which dose distributions are produced and analyzed is then described. Finally, delivery and verification of 3-DCRT are discussed.

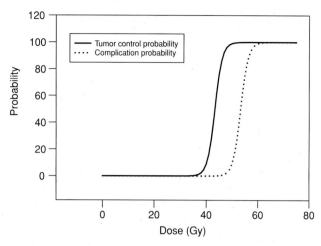

Figure 12.1. Schematic representation of the dependence of tumor control probability (*TCP*) and normal-tissue complication probability on dose. The shape of the curve and its position on the dose axis vary. In the scenario shown here, a relatively high *TCP* can be achieved at dose levels where the probability of normal tissue complications is low. This is very often not the case. In fact, in many instances, normal tissue complications occur at dose levels below those at which tumor control is probable.

International Commission on Radiation Units and Measurements Definitions

3-DCRT has been demonstrated to be a viable method for achieving high precision in radiation therapy. In addition to the geometric precision achievable by 3-DCRT and the dosimetric precision achieved by standardized dosimetry protocols, such as the TG-51 protocol (1), modern radiation oncology needs correspondingly high precision in specifying the radiation dose prescription and the resulting dose distributions. Moreover, when communicating radiation treatment information, for example, in interinstitutional treatment protocols, unambiguous definitions of dose and dose delivery are needed.

The International Commission on Radiation Units and Measurements (ICRU), in a series of reports (2,3), has defined various volumes to support this need for precision and absence of ambiguity in the definition of dose delivery. Two reports have already been written, and it is likely that more may be forthcoming.

The ICRU has defined several regions related to the tumor. The gross tumor volume (GTV) is defined to be the "gross demonstrable extent and location of the malignant growth" (2). The GTV may include primary tumor, involved lymph nodes, and metastatic disease, and is demonstrated using whatever imaging modalities are appropriate, whether it be by visual observation, computed tomography (CT), magnetic resonance imaging (MRI), positron emission tomography (PET), single photon emission computed tomography (SPECT), or by any other method of visualization. Some ambiguity exists in the delineation of the GTV, as different imaging modalities may display different extents of disease. Moreover, differences

in image quality such as spatial resolution, temporal resolution, and contrast-noise ratio may result in differences in the way in which a tumor appears, resulting in differences in the delineation of the GTV. The patient may have several GTVs, depending on the extent of disease, and the treatment goals for each GTV may be different. Furthermore, following surgical intervention, it is possible that the GTV may not necessarily be present.

In addition to the demonstrable disease, the patient is likely to have subclinical disease that is known to be present. The demonstrable tumor plus the microscopic disease constitute the clinical target volume (CTV). The margin surrounding the GTV that defines the CTV is delineated based on clinical experience, or in some cases, pathology studies. In the case where surgical intervention has taken place before radiation treatment and the GTV has been removed, a CTV may exist in the absence of a GTV. The goal of the radiation therapy is to irradiate the CTV to a dose appropriate to control the disease. The GTV and CTV are based on oncologic principles and are not restricted to radiation therapy. For example, the CTV can be the volume defined for surgical resection. Both the GTV and the CTV are defined before any planning for radiation treatment.

In conventional 3-DCRT, the GTV and CTV are based on imaging information acquired several days before treatment. This information is assumed to be an accurate representation of the patient for the entire course of radiation therapy. Patients, however, may change during treatment as a result of factors including gain or loss of weight, bladder, or rectal filling, or changes in the size of the tumor. Intrafractional changes may also occur during an individual radiation treatment due to various physiologic motions such as respiratory motion, cardiac motion, peristalsis, and swallowing. Margins are needed to surround the CTV to ensure that the CTV lies within the treatment field during the entire course of radiation therapy. These internal margins (IMs), in addition to the CTV, constitute the internal target volume (ITV). ITVs can be delineated as a result of IMs implicitly determined based on population studies, or can be explicitly determined by the use of various types of motion studies, often based on acquisition of multiple CT images.

Finally, in order to account for setup uncertainties, one adds a setup margin (SM) to the ITV to generate a planning target volume (PTV). The SM for a specific treatment is generally based on population studies and methods of immobilization. Invasive immobilization techniques such as a stereotactic head frame may result in submillimeter SMs, although other immobilization methods may yield SMs of several millimeters. The PTV is the final volume that must be irradiated to the tumoricidal dose to ensure that the CTV is actually irradiated to the desired dose. If not all the PTV has been irradiated, then the possibility exists that the CTV might not receive the appropriate dose. In the planning of 3-DCRT, beam apertures are designed to ensure complete irradiation of the PTV, whenever

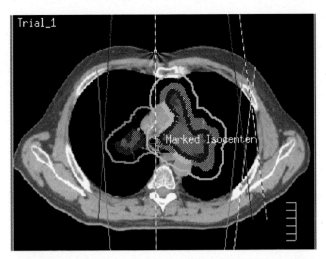

Trial_1

Marked Isocenter

Figure 12.2. The gross tumor volume (GTV), clinical target volume (CTV), and planning target volume (PTV) of patient with lung cancer. The hilar GTV is shown in red color wash surrounded by a thick-line red contour. The CTV extends 8 mm beyond the GTV and is shown in brown color wash. The PTV extends 7 mm beyond the CTV and is represented by the light blue contour. On the patient's right, second CTV and PTV are similarly shown.

possible. Figure 12.2 illustrates an axial CT image with GTV, CTV, and PTV identified and delineated.

In addition to ensuring adequate dose delivery to the PTV, the treatment plan must also account for the presence of uninvolved tissue, which, if given excess radiation, might be damaged, compromising the success of the radiation treatment. The ICRU defines an organ at risk (OAR) to be an organ that, if given an excess radiation dose, would compromise the success of the course of radiation therapy. The identification of the OAR is based on the site to be treated. For example, for thoracic treatments, OARs include each lung, the heart, esophagus, and spinal cord. Organs not likely to be irradiated in the course of radiation treatment are not considered to be an OAR for that treatment.

Just as the CTV must be expanded to account for setup uncertainty and organ motion to generate a PTV, so must the OAR volume be expanded to account for setup uncertainty and organ motion to generate the planning at risk volume (PRV). In some cases, the PTV and PRV might overlap, but often treatment planning is a set of compromises between full irradiation of the PTV and overirradiation of the PRV. Radiation oncologists and treatment planners need to be fully aware when such compromises are being made. It is not correct to make changes in any of the target volumes or the PRVs to make the treatment plan appear better; these volumes must be determined before the plan is developed. If a PTV is to be reduced, some justification needs to be given, such as more precise imaging to reduce the GTV or more precise immobilization to reduce the PTV. Sometimes nonstandard margins may be specified around a PTV or a PRV for the purposes of optimization, but these margins should only be used for the optimization and not be reported in the final assessment of the radiation treatment plan.

Imaging in Three-Dimensional Conformal Radiation Therapy

Accurate methods of imaging play an essential role in the successful implementation of 3-DCRT. Patient images of various types are used in every step of the 3-DCRT procedure. These images may be cross-sectional or projections, and they may come from one or more of various modalities. Before the 3-DCRT era, imaging patients for treatment planning consisted of acquiring one or more cross-sectional images on a CT scanner as well as planar images on a conventional simulator. The conventional simulator was a radiographic/fluoroscopic unit with gantry and collimator motions that simulated those of the radiation treatment machine. Gantry angles were either determined from a plan generated from the CT image or based on class solutions, and then simulated on the conventional simulator. Treatment portals were determined primarily based on two-dimensional (2D) internal anatomy, where known and suspected disease was targeted and critical structures were avoided.

The present state of 3-DCRT practice involves CT-based simulation. Because of the availability of CT scanners capable of high-speed image acquisition and reconstruction, and possessing abundant and inexpensive memory, patient images are now acquired on axial planes with resolutions of 3 mm or less, allowing for accurate volumetric determination of targets and normal anatomy. Treatment planning is then based on 3D anatomy, with design of beam geometries and treatment portals based on the 3D extent of defined targets and normal anatomy. In CT simulation, a 3D CT image set of the patient is obtained in the treatment position. Patients are placed in some form of immobilization device and are appropriately marked to ensure setup reproducibility. Setup reproducibility may vary from submillimeter accuracy in the case of stereotactic and hypofractionated treatments in the head or central nervous system, where critical structures may lie in close proximity to the target volume, to accuracies of 0.5 to 1 cm for some regions of the thorax, abdomen, or extremities.

Various generations of CT scanners have been used to acquire patient information for 3-DCRT. The advent of the third-generation CT scanner, which consists of a single radiation source detected by a single fan-shaped array of radiation detectors, has made image acquisition time sufficiently rapid to make 3-DCRT image acquisition practical. In a third-generation CT scanner, the gantry makes a single (whole or partial) rotation around the patient. The transmission pattern of a single slice is acquired by the array of detectors and is reconstructed. After acquisition of a single slice, the patient table is indexed and another slice is acquired. This procedure continues until the entire 3D CT image has been obtained. The newer technology of helical, or spiral, CT combines gantry rotation with table translation, so that the path of the radiation source makes a spiral trajectory. Coalescing table translation with gantry rotation in this manner significantly speeds up the acquisition of the CT image information. To speed up image acquisition even further, detectors and reconstruction algorithms have been developed that allow acquisition and reconstruction of multiple axial CT slices at one time. This technique of multislice helical CT image acquisition has the potential for scan times as short as 3 to 5 seconds (4). Multislice helical CT scanners used in combination with respiratory monitoring and triggering methods also allow capture of respiratory-induced motion in what is now referred to as "four-dimensional" CT scanning (5,6).

The ability to acquire CT scans with high axial resolution accentuates the question of optimal axial resolution for 3-DCRT planning. Before 3-DCRT, CT image data sets were acquired at axial separations of 10 mm or more. In principle, the axial resolution should be similar to the resolution of a picture element (pixel) in a transverse plane of a CT image, which is somewhat <1 mm. However, such fine axial resolution would result in the production of a very large number of CT images in a data set. Delineating target volumes and normal anatomic structures on such large number of images would significantly increase the time required to develop patient treatment plans, as the contouring process is presently very labor intensive. Effective and efficient contouring tools, as discussed later in this chapter, may be of significant assistance in this process, allowing higher axial resolution image data sets to be incorporated into 3-DCRT planning, but at present, axial resolutions of 2 to 3 mm appear to be the acceptable standard.

Images used in 3-DCRT consist of pixels with a large range of CT-number values. Pixel values in CT images, for example, are normally stored as 12-bit unsigned integers, allowing values from 0 to 4,095. Typically, pixel values are binned into a significantly smaller range of gray-scale values for display. Through appropriate selection of binning methods, one may be able to enhance features of images, possibly enabling better recognition of tumors and anatomic structures. The simplest and most frequently used image enhancement method is that of windowing and leveling. Instead of distributing the entire range of pixel values evenly across the gray-scale spectrum, one selects a window, that is, a limited range of pixel values for display, and a level, which is the location of the window. For example, one could select a range of pixel values between 900 and 1,100 for display. This would be a window of 200 at a level of 1,000. All pixels with values lower than 900 would be displayed as black, and pixels with values greater than 1,100 would be displayed as white. Pixels with intermediate values would then be displayed as shades of gray. Increasing the window width would decrease the contrast of the image; decreasing the window width would increase the contrast of the image. Figure 12.3 illustrates two CT images of an axial slice of a patient's thorax. The figure on the left displays the image using a window typically used to display mediastinal structures, with a window level of 1,060 and a width of 400 (i.e., a range of pixel values from 800 to 1,200), whereas the figure on the right displays the same image using a window typically used to display lungs, with a window level of 500 and a width of 1,600. Note the significantly different contrast in the two images. This may lead to differences in the way tumors are delineated, so it is important that a consistent set of windows and levels be used for tumor delineation in any one site.

In windowing and leveling, the interval of pixel values is divided into equally spaced subintervals, each subinterval being assigned a specific gray-scale value. It is possible, however, that the pixel values in an image may cover a wide range, but the vast majority of pixels may be concentrated in a narrow range and have values less than the average. The details in the darker regions of such images may be difficult to perceive. If the pixel values are divided into bins of equal width and a histogram of the number of pixels in the bins against the pixel value is drawn, it will be sharply peaked, with the peak near the lower end of the intensity range. An alternative method of binning pixel values known as *histogram equalization* allows pixel subintervals of variable width with the requirement that an equal number of pixels are binned into each subinterval. This technique can be of significant utility for images for which there might be a bimodal distribution of pixel

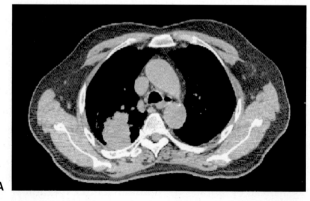
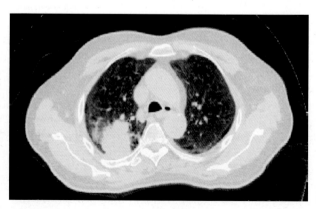

Figure 12.3. An axial computed tomography (CT) image of the thorax, shown in "mediastinal" (**A**) and "lung" (**B**) windows. The pixel values included in the mediastinal window range from 800 to 1,200; those of the lung window range from 300 to 1,300.

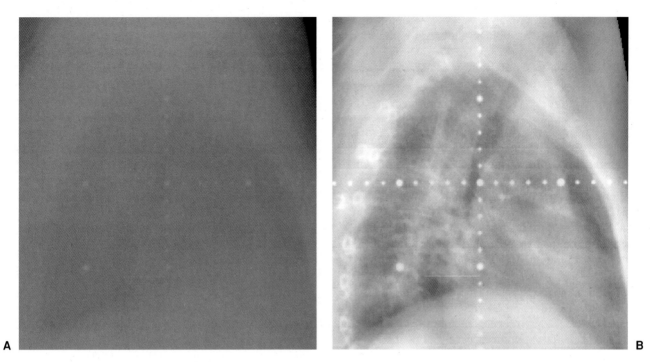

Figure 12.4. Portal image of a lateral chest without image enhancement (**A**) and with histogram equalization (**B**).

values. It is more commonly used to enhance portal images rather than CT images.

An extension of the histogram equalization technique is *adaptive histogram equalization (AHE)*. In AHE, the contrast of each pixel is adjusted according to histograms of pixels in the immediate vicinity of the pixel rather than the histogram of pixels in the entire image. This scheme optimizes the contrast by assigning brightness in the local context. Typically, a 64×64 subimage histogram is selected. Variations of AHE, for example, *clipped,* or contrast-limited AHE (CLAHE), have also been proposed to enhance the images further (7,8). Although AHE and its variants are not yet used extensively in radiation oncology, they have the potential to reveal a great amount of anatomic detail and to aid in the laborious task of manual segmentation as well as in the automatic extraction of anatomy. Histogram equalization techniques are frequently used to evaluate portal images, which tend to be severely lacking in contrast. Figure 12.4 illustrates two portal images of a lateral thoracic field. In the image on the left, only the window and level have been adjusted for clarity, but no other modifications have occurred, whereas in the image on the right, AHE has been applied to improve the clarity of the image. Features that are barely visible on the conventional portal image are quite readily displayed on the histogram-equalized image.

In another form of contrast enhancement, images may be *filtered* to sharpen their edges. A variety of filters are available. Some filtration techniques use Fourier transforms to convert the image into the frequency domain. In the frequency domain, the rapidly changing features (e.g., the edges) are transformed into higher-frequency components.

Reducing the amplitude of lower-frequency components and converting the image back into the spatial domain would enhance the edges of the image. This is called *high-pass filtration.* Other edge enhancement filters, for example, Sobel (9) and Canny (10) filters, use gradient techniques. In some instances, the gradient image showing only the edge information can be obtained.

Gross Tumor Volume Determination

Imaging is used extensively in the definition of 3-DCRT target volumes. Identification of exactly what is to be treated is perhaps the most important component of the 3-DCRT process. To assist in this determination, target and treatment volumes have been clearly defined by the ICRU and have been amply described previously in this chapter. The ICRU definition of the GTV, the ". . . gross demonstrable extent and location of malignant growth . . . ," (2) highlights an important characteristic of this volume, namely that it is "demonstrable," or readily shown or proved. Evidence that a tissue volume contains tumor can be obtained from multiple sources. Among these sources of information are clinical examination, such as palpation, and the use of imaging techniques. Except in circumstances where tissues can be readily observed with the naked eye or palpated directly, imaging is used to define the GTV.

Given the recent advances in imaging technology wherein functional imaging is finding an increasingly significant role in tumor volume definition, the traditional definition of the GTV is undergoing a change (11). The explicit use of ^{18}F fluorodeoxyglucose ([18]FDG) PET imaging, for example, as an aid in defining the GTV, now reveals tumor-bearing tissues that may have been previously occult, excluded from the GTV, and therefore are considered part of the CTV. This issue is discussed in more detail in a later section of this chapter. In this next section, the use of images to define the GTV is explored.

Image Segmentation

Image segmentation is the process by which pixels within an image are identified and classified based on specific properties. Pixels are identified on the basis of their appearance (e.g., density, texture, or pixels bounded by an edge). They can be classified as belonging to a group or class defined as a particular organ system, such as lung, or they can be defined as belonging to a group identified as GTV, or both. For specific applications in radiation treatment planning, the term *image segmentation* is used to describe the task of manually or automatically delineating anatomic regions of interest, including critical normal organs and the target volume, on the 3D patient image. Accurate information about the shapes and locations of anatomic structures is essential for aiming beams at the target volume while minimizing the exposure of normal tissues. Segmented structures are also necessary for the qualitative and quantitative evaluation of treatment plans using dose distribution displays, dose–volume histograms (DVHs), and predicted values of biologic indices. In addition, anatomic structures overlaid on digitally reconstructed radiographs (DRRs) are important for correlating the planning geometry with the treatment geometry using DRRs and portal images.

The process of image segmentation is perhaps the most labor-intensive component of 3-DCRT, as pixels must be individually identified as belonging to one or more groups or classes. The identification process can be either automatic or manual. For many anatomic structures of interest, the contrast near the boundary of the structures is sufficient for automatic edge-detection schemes—often times, it may not be. When automatic edge-detection routines fail to properly identify differences in tissue classification, manual means must be employed. In these instances, outlines must be drawn by guiding the cursor on the image with a mouse, trackball, or light pen. For target volumes, one must delineate a region that includes the gross disease, regions of known extensions, and regions of suspected disease. The latter two are not likely to be discernible on images, and the boundary has to be drawn according to prior knowledge and experience. Considering the arduousness of the task, efficient manual drawing tools are crucial to the success of 3-DCRT.

Many different software tools have become available for accelerating and simplifying the task of manually drawing contours. The choice of the pointing device (e.g., mouse, trackball, light pen) may affect productivity. Tools such as "pencils" and "brushes" of various sizes can also be used to identify individual pixels or groups of pixels and to conform contours to structures (Figure 12.5).

The various image enhancement techniques discussed earlier can be used to maximize the visibility of anatomic detail for manual contouring. The automated selection of the most appropriate enhancement techniques and their parameters for each class of anatomic structure and treatment site can save a significant amount of time and effort. Often anatomic structures, including target volumes, do not vary significantly from one image section to the next. Therefore, a tool to copy contours drawn on the adjacent section and to reshape them can be effective. Another useful capability is the interpolation of contours. Contours drawn on a limited number of widely separated image sections can be interpolated to generate contours on intervening image sections and edited if necessary. The

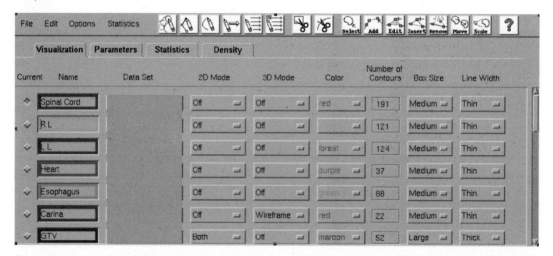

Figure 12.5. Contouring tools that are routinely available in modern treatment-planning and virtual-simulation software are shown in the top toolbar of this contouring panel. Contours can be drawn in a point-by-point or continuous fashion, using "pencils" or "brushes." Contours can be cut, copied, and pasted, as well as edited, moved, and scaled. The resultant regions can then be visualized in multiple colors using various rendering techniques (see text).

efficiency of manual drawing and editing also depends greatly on the user interface and its adaptability to individual user preferences and to individual classes of problems. In general, the best interfaces are those that allow the user to enter and edit the information with a minimum of cursor motion, mouse clicks, and keystrokes.

Although improvements in the manual drawing of contours continue, there is also a need to develop robust techniques to segment anatomic structures automatically. For anatomic structures that appear as high-contrast objects on images, the problem has mostly been solved with the aid of edge detection and edge tracking techniques. Examples of structures that may yield to edge tracking techniques include the boundary of the skin, lungs, bony structures, and cavities in the head and neck. In techniques of this type, the computer automatically tracks the path of a specified pixel value and connects the pixels into a contour outline. To minimize the effect of noise in the image data to obtain a smooth curve, pixel values are averaged over a neighborhood of specified dimensions. In some instances (e.g., for skin and lungs), the computer can be programmed to use some easily definable logic to detect the starting position automatically; in other instances, the starting position may have to be set by the user. Edge tracking may be extended to three dimensions, in which outlines of the specified anatomic structure on all image sections are automatically detected. In one such extension for lung, the position of the centroid of the contour on one image section is used to seek the lung interface on the next image section. Unfortunately, 2D or 3D edge-detection techniques do not always succeed even for such seemingly simple cases as skin and lung, so manual intervention is required. In particular, if the anatomic structure being segmented is not completely surrounded by voxels with a significantly different CT number, edge-detection techniques will fail to generate a reliable contour. Figure 12.6 illustrates this problem. In

Figure 12.6, a right lung is auto segmented using an edge-detection algorithm that detects edges with a CT number of 800. In Figure 12.6A, the right lung is correctly segmented, but in Figure 12.6B, the segmentation also included the left lung. The left lung was included because the tissue separating the right and left lungs was not of sufficiently high density. The failure rate of edge-detection techniques is of the order of a few percent for high-contrast objects but is enough to require review of all automatically drawn contours. Edge detection may be supplemented with edge enhancement and thresholding. Thresholding may be used to highlight pixels in a given range of values. The range is adjusted during visual inspection of all image sections of interest. Any stray pixels and areas of potential problems may be edited away before automatic edge detection is attempted. Even though a modest amount of manual intervention is needed, the process is quite accurate and reliable.

The standard edge-detection techniques may work reasonably well for high-contrast objects; however, they perform poorly for objects with medium contrast and with edges that are diffuse and which are only partially visible. For delineating these objects, considerable attention is being focused on more sophisticated automated and semi-automated methods to fill the gaps in the edge information. It is unlikely that any general solution will be found, and a custom solution for each anatomic structure may have to be developed. A promising approach is the so-called deformable model technique (12,13). In this technique, the image is preprocessed with pixel and texture classification and edge enhancement to identify any edges and clusters of pixels belonging to the object. The edges, pixels, and pixel clusters are used to deform the surface of a model of the anatomic object. The model surface is represented by a series of connected polygons obtained by averaging the manually drawn shape of the organ over a group of patients. Deformation is carried out by forces

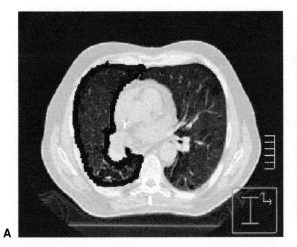 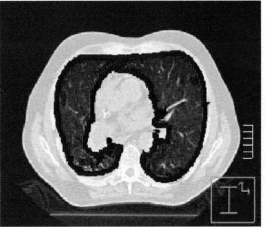

Figure 12.6. Results of autosegmentation of a patient's right lung. **A:** A successful autosegmentation search using edge detection with a threshold computed tomography (CT) value of 800. **B:** An unsuccessful autosegmentation in which the edge detection failed as a result of inadequate separation between the right and left lungs.

applied to each polygon in an attempt to minimize an energy functional. The energy functional consists of two terms, an "internal" term that tends to smooth the surface of the anatomic structure, and an "external" term that tends to fit the surface of the anatomic structure to the intensity edges in the image. Application of the deformable model technique to CT image segmentation in the pelvis has been described by Pekar et al. (14) and that in the thorax by Ragan et al. (15).

The ability to segment an anatomic structure automatically may also depend on the imaging modality. MRI, for instance, provides a much greater contrast in the brain and central nervous system; CT is more appropriate for outlining bony anatomy. Therefore, there is often a need to merge information derived from one imaging modality with that from another. This topic is discussed in detail in the next section.

Image Registration and Correlation

The CT image set comprises the fundamental dataset within which anatomy and targets are defined, dose is computed, and treatment plans are evaluated. This is due to its prevalence as an imaging modality, its high spatial resolution and accuracy, and its necessity for dose computation, as the pixel values can be directly correlated to the interactions of the radiation with tissue. In modern computer systems used for treatment planning, the CT dataset of the patient serves as the basis for the establishment of the spatial coordinate system that will be subsequently used for registration of anatomy and radiation-beam targeting. The CT dataset, therefore, can be thought of as a 3D matrix representing the patient's anatomy. Within this image matrix, volume elements, or voxels, indicate the coordinates of the element, and contain the elements' CT numbers. Additional characteristics can be assigned to these matrix elements as the treatment-planning process progresses. Such characteristics include identification of the element as belonging to a tissue class (such as lung or spinal cord), target group (such as GTV), and dose value (once beams are placed and dose is computed).

As mentioned previously, during the initial phases of the planning process, images are segmented to identify targets and normal tissues. All possible sources of information are used to more accurately define these structures. No single imaging modality may produce all the information needed for the accurate identification and delineation of the target volume and critical organs. Different imaging modalities produce visual renditions of different processes. MRI, for instance, produces images in which the gray scale represents either proton density or proton relaxation times, a characteristic of the chemical environment of the voxel. MRI is well suited for imaging the central nervous system, sarcomas, head and neck cancer, and prostate cancer, as well as for the visualization of lymph nodes. PET with 18 fluorodeoxyglucose (^{18}FDG) produces images in which gray scale is assigned values

proportional to the degree of uptake of FDG by the tissue. The uptake is in turn a function of metabolic activity. Therefore, PET provides metabolic and functional information that may be useful in determining the extent of the tumor, in particular, its microscopic spread. Each unique piece of information needed for the planning and delivery of radiotherapy should ideally be derived from the most suitable source, and then integrated into the CT image set.

Often, the transfer of anatomic and physiologic information is accomplished by manual drawing during visualizations of both sets of images side by side. This process is laborious, approximate, and not particularly well suited for 3-DCRT. Necessary automated methods to assist in image registration are evolving rapidly. Registration of 3D images entails the computation of a transformation function that accurately registers information derived from one 3D image data set to another. The transformation function depends on whether the two sets of images are related through only rigid body transformations, namely, rotations and translations, or whether individual anatomic structures have been deformed or displaced relative to each other. The case of rigid body transformation is much simpler but is accurate in only select circumstances. In essence, a combination of clearly identifiable points, lines, surfaces, and images of anatomic landmarks and external fiducial markers on two data sets are identified and used to match and correlate them. Various techniques, such as cross-correlation (16) or mutual information (17) may be used to obtain the transformation function between the coordinate systems of the two sets. The transformation function is typically a 4 × 4 matrix describing three rotations, three translations, and perhaps simple scaling. This matrix may be used to transform any point or a collection of points (e.g., pixels and contours) on the image correlated to the reference image. Once transformed, the correlated image may be "resliced" to produce image sections in the same coordinate system as the reference image for the side-by-side display and comparison. The outlines and surfaces of anatomic structures abstracted from the correlated image may be transformed to the reference image using the transformation matrix.

For a number of situations, the automatic matching of image data sets may be inadequate or may not be feasible. This may happen, for example, when external fiducial markers are not available, internal landmarks are not easily and accurately identifiable, or when small deformations and relative displacements of anatomic structures are present. In such situations, human judgment may be needed to match two image data sets by interactively manipulating data from both sets of images. Once a satisfactory match has been accomplished, assuming that the rigid body transformation is applicable, the transformation matrix may be computed and used.

If, however, significant deformations and relative organ displacements are present, the problem is considerably more complex. Such distortions are sometimes inherent in the imaging devices, for example, because of inhomogeneities of the magnetic fields in the MRI. Distortions may also be caused by internal organ displacement that occurs naturally, by somewhat different positioning of the patient on different imaging and treatment devices, and by weight loss over the course of treatment. The incorporation of such distortions is a difficult task and a topic of continuing investigations.

A possible limited solution would be to unwarp the distorted image with image metamorphosis techniques. In techniques of this type, also known as *morphing*, surfaces of as many easily identifiable anatomic objects as possible are delineated on both images. A function of the distances of a pixel from various points in the identified objects is used to identify a corresponding pixel on the distorted image bearing the same relationship to the distorted objects. The pixel value at this point in the distorted image becomes the pixel value on the transformed unwarped image (18).

Clinical Target Volume Expansion

Once the GTV has been defined, it then becomes necessary to identify those areas that are *suspect* of containing disease. It is an accepted fact that a cancer cell population extends beyond those areas that can readily be seen or palpated. In the terminology of the ICRU (2), "… in some anatomically definable tissues/organs, there may be cancer cells at some probability level, even though they cannot be detected with present day techniques." The subclinical disease in this extended area is commonly referred to as "microscopic disease" or "microextensions" of the disease, since confirmation of the existence of the disease in this area often requires pathologic validation with a microscope. As defined previously, the anatomic volume that contains both the demonstrable tumor (the GTV) and its associated microscopic extension is called the *CTV*. In the process of defining 3-DCRT target volumes, after the GTV has been identified, a margin is added around the GTV to account for the possible presence of microscopic disease. The volume produced by this extended margin in three dimensions constitutes the CTV. For other anatomic sites, for example, lymph nodes, only the presumed clinical spread of disease is used to define the CTV. These volumes may be also defined as CTVs, even though gross tumor may not be evident in the volume.

The topic of CTV definition is of considerable interest at present. In a recent and relatively comprehensive report that addresses target localization uncertainties, techniques that can be used to quantify GTV-to-CTV expansions are discussed (19,20). The nature and extent of the GTV-to-CTV expansion is based on the particular disease's pathology. It is an area of much needed research, as available data are sparse. Given the definitions of the terms GTV and CTV, the exact extent of malignancy beyond what can be seen or demonstrated has to be determined. This validation can only be accomplished through pathologic examination of tissue specimens after they have been imaged *in vivo*. For example, Giraud et al. report the results of the measurements made of the extent of micro-invasion of non-small-cell adenocarcinoma and squamous cell carcinoma of the lung (21). In their study, the investigators contoured on CT, the lung tumors of patients that subsequently underwent surgical resection. The microscopic extent of the disease was determined by pathologic evaluation, and this extent was then spatially related to the contours previously drawn. They concluded that in 95% of the patients studied, adenocarcinomas extended 6 mm and squamous cell carcinomas extended 8 mm beyond the CT-based contour. In a similar study, Apisarnthanarax et al. (22) measured cervical lymph node extra-capsular extension in 48 patients with squamous cell head and neck cancer. They found that in 96% of nodes sampled, extra-capsular extension was 5 mm or less. Teh et al. (23) published the results of prostatic extra-capsular extension measurements obtained in a series of 712 patients that underwent radical prostatectomies. In the group (26% of patients) where measurable extra-capsular disease was noted, the mean maximum depth of invasion was 3 mm (standard deviation 2.3 mm). Data such as these are essential, if accurate GTV-to-CTV expansions are to be realized in clinical practice.

Methods used to determine the CTV are rapidly, and necessarily, changing as the capabilities of newer functional imaging modalities are explored and validated (24). What may have been considered CTV in the past may now be visualized, therefore leading to a more explicit definition of what has been termed "microscopic extension." The expanding use of multimodality imaging that incorporates some form of functional imaging, such as MR spectroscopy and/or ^{18}FDG PET imaging, appears to be spearheading this effort. Ganslandt et al. (25), for example, have validated the use of metabolic maps obtained from proton magnetic resonance spectroscopic imaging (MRSI) of gliomas *via* histopathologic examination. They conclude that MRSI defines tumor infiltration areas more exactly than does conventional T2 MRI.

Given the current rate of development of techniques that can be used to better define the CTV, methods used clinically at this point in time vary considerably. These methods include explicit definition of anatomic structures (e.g., prostate and seminal vesicles), inclusion of volumes containing external markers (e.g., surgical clips following tumor resection in breast cancer), utilization of functional/molecular imaging modalities to better visualize microscopic disease (26,27), application of published margin expansions or atlases of recommended expansions (28), inclusion of areas of "suspect" image characteristics, and/or use of set margins (e.g., a 1–2 cm margin) defined on the basis of practice "tradition," protocol requirements, and clinical results.

Internal Target Volume Expansion

In the treatment of many disease sites, intrafractional motion, or motion that might occur during beam delivery, requires that the radiation beam treats a volume that is somewhat larger than the CTV, but that accounts for the possible motion of the CTV during a radiation treatment. Internal motion that might affect the CTV may be due to one of several causes, the most common being respiratory motion, cardiac motion, peristalsis, and swallowing. The ICRU (3) recommends that an IM be placed around the CTV to account for intrafractional motion. This margin needs to be sufficiently large to encompass the likely extent of the motion of the CTV during beam delivery. The CTV plus the IM is defined to be the ITV.

Most studies of internal motion at the present time have addressed respiratory motion, and the motion of lung and liver tumors affected by respiratory motion (29–31). For many years, the IM was determined from population studies, based on typical intrafraction motion, and normally consisted of a uniform margin placed around the CTV. With newer imaging methods such as four-dimensional (4D) CT imaging (5,6), in which multiple, phase-specific CT image data sets are acquired, it is possible to track the trajectory of the tumor as it moves during various phases of the respiratory cycle. A GTV is determined for each one of, typically, 10 phases in the respiratory cycle, expanded to generate a CTV, then, the ITV is designed to be the envelope encompassing the CTV over its entire trajectory during a respiratory cycle.

An alternative method for accounting for intrafractional motion during treatment is to restrict the intrafractional motion in some way. To restrict respiratory motion, for example, breath-hold techniques have been used, either voluntary (32) or assisted, using an occlusion spirometer, which restricts the airflow to the patient at a specified point on the respiratory cycle (33). Another technique to reduce the effect of respiratory motion is to gate the delivery of radiation at a specific point in the respiratory cycle (34). In this technique, the respiratory cycle is monitored, either by an external marker, spirometer, strain gauge, or internal marker (35). A region of the respiratory cycle, typically around end expiration, is identified for gating. When the respiratory cycle enters the gate, a signal is sent to the linear accelerator, initiating the beam delivery; when the cycle leaves the gate, radiation is terminated. An implicit assumption in the delivery of gated radiation therapy is that the respiratory monitor is an accurate surrogate for the position of the tumor, and that the position of the monitor accurately and reproducibly represents the position of the tumor. Studies have been undertaken to determine the validity of this assumption.

Planning Target Volume Expansion

Recall that the PTV is that geometric volume in space that, throughout treatment, will always contain the CTV. The PTV, therefore, accounts for all spatial uncertainties associated with the definition and targeting of the CTV. These uncertainties can be classified according to their source (internal organ motion and patient setup uncertainties),

according to when they occur during treatment (interfractional or intrafractional motion), or according to whether they represent errors in treatment plan preparation or execution (systematic or random errors). An example of intrafractional, random, internal motion is peristaltic motion; examples of interfractional, random setup motion are daily setup variation; and examples of systematic uncertainties are those differences that may exist between the patient's condition at planning and at treatment delivery. Some of these errors can be measured and accounted for; others are estimated. A properly defined PTV will take all these uncertainties into account as much as possible.

A review of the targeting procedure up to this point helps illustrate how errors may be accumulated during the process. The GTV has been defined on an image set. Possible errors in this procedure include spatial limitations of the imaging system, variability of observer interpretation of the images (36), and possible motion bias that may be introduced by the use of an initial static (in time) image as representative of average motion over a course of treatment. The GTV is then expanded to a CTV. Here, uncertainties are based mostly on our limited knowledge of microscopic spread of the gross disease. Margins are then established to account for internal motion of organs relative to an immobile patient (the IM), and to account for the motion of the patient relative to a treatment-unit based coordinate system (the SM). Because the topic of *intrafractional* internal organ motion has been discussed in some detail in the previous section, this section will deal mostly with *interfractional* patient setup uncertainties and with systematic differences that may exist between planning and treatment.

To illustrate the challenge, consider the following hypothetical situation in which a series of patients, for example, patients with prostate or head and neck cancer, are imaged on a daily basis during the first week of their treatment. Their daily images are each compared to the corresponding images from their treatment plan, and spatial differences (e.g., differences in anterior–posterior and/or superior–inferior positions) are noted and recorded. For each patient, mean differences are then computed, as also are the standard deviations of these differences. Means and standard deviations are then averaged for the entire group of patients. The statistics obtained from such an evaluation can then be used to determine the systematic and random uncertainties existing in the group of patients studied.

This has been done and reported by van Herk in an excellent review of this topic (37). Using van Herk's terminology, we can define a population-based systematic error, Σ, as the mean spatial difference of all patients, and we can also define a population-based random error, σ, as the root-mean-square spread in spatial differences. Σ describes the mean difference in patient positioning that exists between planning and treatment, and Σ describes the day-to-day uncertainty in patient positioning. The total uncertainty will be a combination of these two types of errors.

As can be expected intuitively, the magnitude of the CTV-to-PTV expansion will depend upon the degree of dosimetric certainty that is desired, that is, the greater the demand for dosimetric certainty, the larger the necessary margin. Recipes for the establishment of population CTV-to-PTV margins have been suggested in order to accomplish given dosimetric goals. Based on what they call coverage probabilities, Stroom et al. (38), for example, have suggested a CTV-to-PTV expansion of $(2 \times \Sigma) + (0.7 \times \sigma)$. Based on this formalism, and using setup-error correction strategies employing electronic portal imaging device (EPID) images and off-line corrections in setup, margins of 6 to 9 mm have been suggested for prostate and head and neck treatments (19). It should be noted that systematic errors dominate the magnitude of the PTV expansion. Recent efforts in image-guided radiation therapy (IGRT) designed to reduce systematic uncertainties should lead to rather significant reductions in PTV margins. This is discussed briefly in a latter section of this chapter and in more detail by other contributing authors.

BEAM DETERMINATION

One of the important features of 3-DCRT is that beam directions are chosen and the beam aperture boundaries are defined according to 3D-based target and anatomic information. The process within which this is accomplished is termed virtual simulation. Noncoplanar beam directions make available many more choices of treatment technique. At present, the beam's-eye-view (BEV) projection (39) is the most prominent mechanism for interactively determining beam directions and defining beam apertures. In a typical implementation of BEV, the 3D information about the target and normal structure may be displayed on the screen as if being viewed from the source of radiation along the central axis of the beam. This graphically conveys exactly which tissues are exposed to radiation. Anatomic structures may be displayed in a variety of surface-rendering techniques, including wire stacks, meshes, and translucent surfaces, and in different colors (Figure 12.7). Color intensity is used to indicate depth (*depth cuing*), and surface shading is employed to indicate surface orientation. Objects are shown in perspective to take into account beam divergence. The scene can be manipulated interactively with a graphic simulator of the treatment machine to view the orientation of the patient's anatomy from different coplanar and noncoplanar beam directions to select a suitable set.

The BEV display may be supplemented with additional visual cues. These may include orthogonal image sections through a reference point with intersections of beams and anatomic structures, the so-called room view or observer view display, in which the viewer can "walk around" a patient's anatomy and beams, and the display of a model of the treatment machine (Figure 12.8). The treatment machine display with the patient's 3D image on the couch may be used to reveal certain beam orientations that may

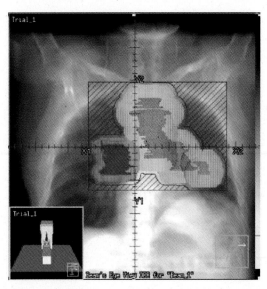

Figure 12.7. A beam's-eye-view (BEV) display of an anterior lung field. Shown within the field are displays of the patient's clinical target volume (CTV) and planning target volume (PTV). (Refer also to the axial computed tomography [CT] slice of Figure 12.2.) Field blocking is designed to cover the PTV with a margin of ~5 mm to account for beam penumbral effects.

be forbidden because of obstructions in the beam path or collision with the machine or the patient. A DRR superimposed on the BEV display has been found useful. Figures 12.9, 12.10, and 12.11 show various components of a typical interactive beam definition system.

For each beam direction, an aperture framing the PTV plus a 5 to 7 mm margin, accounting for lateral transport of radiation (i.e., penumbra), but excluding the normal tissues to the extent desired, is defined. Apertures may be drawn interactively or automatically. In the manual technique, the user draws the outline around the PTV as displayed on the BEV screen, guiding a circular cursor with a pointer. The radius of the cursor may be set to the size of the desired margin and may be adjusted to achieve a variable margin.

Manual techniques are flexible but time consuming, especially when many beams are to be used or explored for treatment or for computer-aided optimization.

Methods for automatically defining the continuous boundary of the aperture enclosing the target volume have been developed by Brewster et al. (40). The automatically drawn aperture may include a margin beyond the PTV but may exclude a critical normal structure if desired. The normal structure may be assigned a negative margin to allow a portion of it to be irradiated to improve target coverage. A typical algorithm may work as follows: The surfaces of 3D target volume and normal anatomic structures to be excluded are tiled (i.e., represented in terms of a set of connected polygon segments) and projected to a plane through the isocenter. The interiors of the projected structures are filled, and an edge-detection process is used to draw their boundaries. These boundaries are extended for a positive margin and contracted for a negative margin.

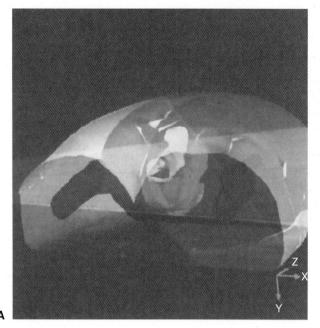
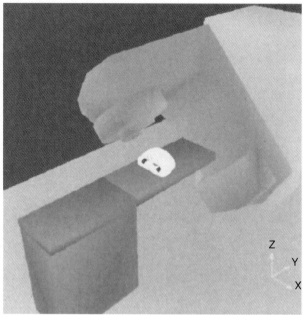

Figure 12.8. **A:** The observer view, a three-dimensional (3D) rendering of the patient's anatomy and beams. The display of previously defined beams is useful for placing the new beam being defined. **B:** The room view, a global view of the patient in the treatment position. The display includes a model of the accelerator and the anatomic surfaces created using the contoured data. The operator may graphically "walk" around in the room looking at the patient and treatment machine from various angles. This display is useful for avoiding directions rendered unfeasible either by the presence of an obstruction such as a couch bar or because of the possibility of collision.

Use of Multileaf Collimation

Three-dimensional conformal treatments are complex and involve many fields. Virtually all of these fields are irregularly shaped, and may also be intensity modulated. Until recently, 3D conformal treatments were delivered manually,

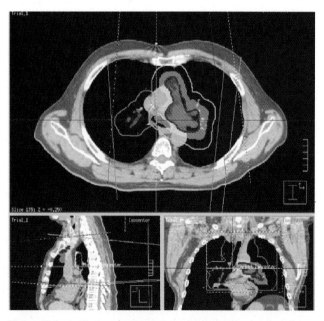

Figure 12.9. A display type that is commonly used in the virtual simulation process. Regions of interest and treatment beams are visualized in the three principal planes: The axial, sagittal, and coronal planes through the isocenter of the beams.

one field at a time, with custom-fabricated blocks, and compensators as intensity modulators. This process is highly labor intensive, time consuming, and prone to mistakes, and it limits the implementation of improved treatment strategies to plans that involve a relatively small number of fields per treatment session. The multileaf collimator (MLC) is essential for making the delivery of these newer treatments practical. The ability of the computer-controlled MLC to set field shapes and produce arbitrary intensity distributions remotely and automatically is ideally suited for delivering complex treatments safely and in times comparable with or even shorter than the manual delivery of conventional treatments.

In addition to lending themselves to the remote and automatic setup of field shapes and the modulation of intensity distributions, MLCs have a number of advantages over conventional field-shaping devices. They save block fabrication costs, storage space, setup time, and the effort of lifting and mounting heavy blocks. They allow on-the-spot modification of the field aperture if the portal image reveals that anatomic landmarks are not at expected locations relative to the boundary. The patient does not have to be sent home while new blocks are fabricated, and there is no danger of injury to the patient or the operator from a falling block. Furthermore, concerns about the toxicity resulting from the handling of blocks made of alloys of lead and cadmium or from inhaling vapors of these metals during fabrication are eliminated.

To realize the efficiency in the delivery of complex treatments possible with MLCs and for greater accuracy, it is important to integrate the MLC into the planning system.

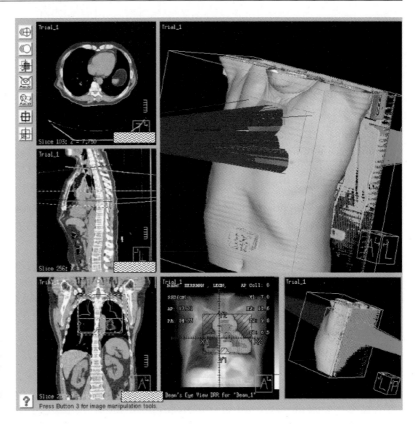

Figure 12.10. Additional views that can be displayed to assist in the processes of virtual simulation and treatment planning. The external surface of the patient can be rendered in a three-dimensional (3D) display that also shows the outline of the treatment fields.

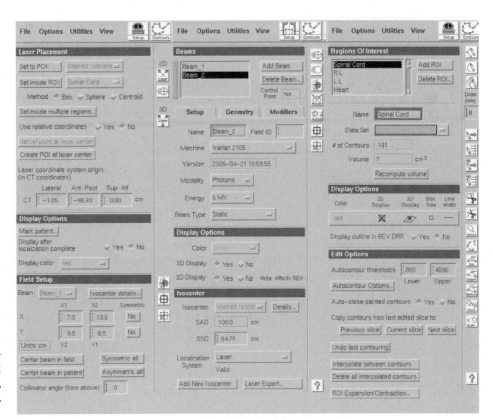

Figure 12.11. Samples of the multiple tool panels that are available for virtual simulation. Shown are tool panels that allow laser placement, beam creation and manipulation, and region of interest management.

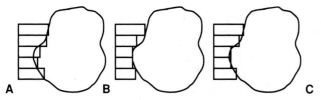

Figure 12.12. Inbound (**A**), outbound (**B**), and cross-bound (**C**) modes of multileaf collimator (MLC) leaf placement. A number of variations of the cross-bound mode are possible. The actual scheme adopted may depend on the treatment site, technique, and the sensitivity of the surrounding normal critical structures. In most instances it is possible to develop a site- and technique-dependent automatic scheme for the placement of leaves.

Toward this objective, certain special features must be explicitly incorporated into the system, in particular, the ability to automatically determine leaf positions and convert the continuous aperture to the corresponding scalloped shape. The leaves can be placed relative to the continuous boundary in different ways. For example, each leaf may touch the continuous boundary but be just outside it, just inside it, or across it. These leaf placement modes have been called *outbound, inbound,* and *cross-bound,* respectively (Figure 12.12). The cross-bound mode allows for several variations. The variation in which the area blocked by each leaf is equalized with the area exposed, shown in Figure 12.13, has been found to be the most suitable (41–44). In this scheme, the total energy fluence incident on the patient is the same as for corresponding cast low-melting point alloy blocks. It is not likely that a universal leaf placement strategy exists. Depending on the treatment site and technique, customization is required to balance the target coverage against the need to spare neighboring normal tissues. Individual leaves may

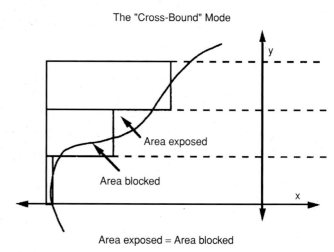

The "Cross-Bound" Mode

Area exposed = Area blocked

Figure 12.13. A specific variation of the cross-bound mode in which the area blocked by the leaf inside the aperture boundary is set equal to the area left exposed outside. In this scheme the energy fluence is the same for the multileaf collimator (MLC)-shaped aperture and the Cerrobend aperture.

have to be adjusted manually if the automated placement method is found to result in dose distributions at variance with the judgment of the planner. With experience, however, it is possible to automate customization of leaf placements for many sites and techniques.

Considerable concern about the jagged edges (*scalloping effect*) of MLC-shaped boundaries has been expressed. The concern is diminishing as experience is gained with these devices. The magnitude of undulations in dose distributions and the width of the 20% to 80% penumbra are functions of the angle between the field boundary and the normal to the direction of leaf travel. Figure 12.14

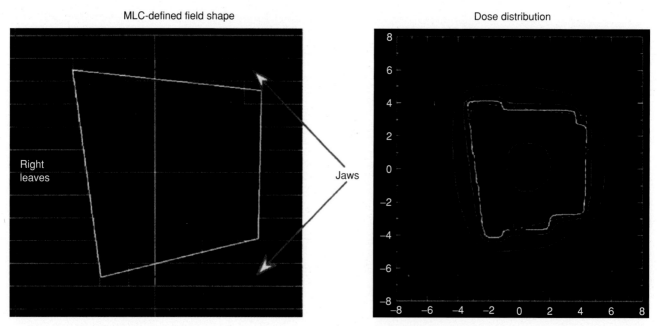

Figure 12.14. Dose distribution for a 15 MV beam in a beam's-eye-view plane at a depth of 10 cm in a phantom for a quadrilateral field defined by a multileaf collimator. It demonstrates the effect of the angle between the field boundary and the normal to the direction of leaf travel on the magnitude of undulations in dose distributions.

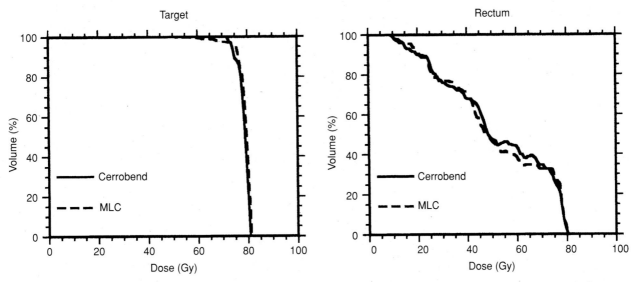

Figure 12.15. Dose–volume histograms for the target and rectum for a typical three-dimensional (3D) conformal treatment of prostate illustrating differences between plans designed with Cerrobend-shaped aperture and multileaf collimator (MLC)-shaped apertures.

demonstrates this fact with a dose distribution in a BEV plane for a quadrilateral field shape defined by an MLC. Measurements by Lo-Sasso et al. (44) and Galvin et al. (45,46) indicate that for a 45-degree angle, the 20% to 80% penumbra for an MLC is 3 to 4 mm wider than the corresponding penumbra for a conventional block. (Note that the penumbra for an MLC-shaped field is defined as the gap between the outer edge of 20% and the inner edge of 80% undulating isodose lines.) The difference between the penumbras for a 15-degree angle was found to be only 1 mm (45,46).

From the point of view of target coverage, the 90% isodose line is considered to be most relevant. It has been demonstrated that even for single fields, the lateral transport of secondary electrons and scattered photons considerably reduces the scalloping effect to an extent that the shape of the 90% isodose line has virtually no undulations and does not shift significantly compared with the corresponding dose distribution for a block-defined field (47). However, the most important contributor to the dilution of the scalloping effect is the smearing effect of multiple fields. Patient motion and variations in daily positioning also play a role. Figure 12.15 shows DVHs for the target and rectum for a six-field conformal prostate treatment designed with both a MLC and a cast block. The differences in dose—volume characteristics are negligible. Furthermore, although the scalloping effect is not a major concern in most instances, the cast block and MLC may not be exactly interchangeable. Minor adjustments in field shape and size and collimator angle may be required. In addition, for some cases, such as treatments with parallel-opposed fields, the residual undulations may not be acceptable.

Whether it is appropriate to substitute cast blocks with multileaf collimated apertures for a particular site and treatment technique depends mainly on whether the

differences in dose distributions at the boundaries significantly alter the target coverage and/or sparing of critical normal tissues. Each class of radiotherapy problems has to be considered case by case. Studies indicate that for a large majority of the cases studied so far, the use of multileaf collimation is appropriate. LoSasso et al. (44) report a quantitative analysis comparing 3D conformal treatment plans for the prostate with blocks and with MLC-shaped apertures and find only insignificant differences. Burman et al. (42,43) examined the use of multileaf collimation for lung and brain patients. For both sites, they compared dose distributions, DVHs, and biologic indices (tumor control probability [*TCP*] and normal tissue complication probability [*NTCP*]) of 3D conformal treatment plans with multileaf collimation against corresponding plans with blocks. For the lung, they reported data for 10 patients and found no clinically significant differences. The change in the irradiated volume of the spinal cord due to the jagged shape of dose distribution near the boundaries was their main concern. They concluded that for some patients it may be necessary to adjust the collimator angle so that the leaf edges are parallel to the cord. For patients with brain cancer, Burman et al. (43) observe that although multileaf-collimator plan dose distributions exhibit undulations, the DVH is virtually indistinguishable from the corresponding DVH for field definition based on shaped blocks. They believe that for most brain plans, the MLC can be used as a substitute for blocks. For some cases in which the PTV is adjacent to the optic chiasm or retina and the dose to these structures is close to the tolerance limit, it may be necessary to adjust the position of the leaves and/or the collimator angle to ensure adequate protection. If such adjustments are deemed inappropriate, blocks should be used. Burman et al. (42,43) also confirm that in general, of the various leaf placement modes, the particular variation of the cross-bound mode in which the area blocked by each leaf is equalized with the area exposed yields the best results.

Another study of 228 blocked treatments of breast, thorax, pelvis, brain, head and neck, spine, bone metastasis, abdomen, and lymphoma conducted at Royal Marsden Hospital was reported by Fernandez et al. (48). It concludes that 6.8% of all cases were found to be unsuitable for treatment with MLC. Lymphomas, brain, and head and neck were the worst offenders. The reasons were varied. For brain, they found that for 4 out of 14 patients acceptable shielding of the back of the eye could not be achieved with a MLC. Of eight lymphoma patients, five were considered to be untreatable with a MLC because of the necessity to create mantle fields with a combination of smaller fields. Also, 3 of a total of 61 thorax cases, 3 of 18 head and neck cases, and 1 of 5 abdomen cases were found to be unsuitable because of difficulties in shielding critical structures or the need to block an isolated organ.

DOSE CALCULATION

Accurate prediction of dose distributions is important for 3-DCRT. However, considerable debate exists about the level of accuracy required for each treatment site and technique and whether that level is achievable with dose computation systems in clinical use. It is commonly believed that accuracy within 5% in delivered dose is required for successful radiotherapy. This belief stems primarily from the information presented in the ICRU Report 24 (49) and references cited therein about the steepness of dose response curves for tumors and normal organs. Because the total uncertainty in delivered dose is composed of several other sources in addition to the uncertainty in predicted dose, the requirements of accuracy in predicted dose should be even higher (2–3%). There may be an erroneous impression on the part of many that the required level of accuracy is achievable in most circumstances of importance. Extensive literature comparing measured dose distributions with the predictions of dose-calculation algorithms implemented in clinical treatment-planning systems shows that under many circumstances this is not the case (50,51). Most of these situations involve tissue interfaces, curvature, inhomogeneities, beam boundaries, and most important, combinations of these.

Van Dyk et al. (52) have specified levels of accuracy in dose calculation in various regions of a dose distribution, distinguishing between high-dose and low-dose regions as well as high-gradient and low-gradient regions. The specific values cited by Van Dyk et al. were repeated in the AAPM Radiation Therapy Committee Task Group 53 report on quality assurance in radiation treatment planning (53) and are explicitly identified as values that are achievable based on the expertise of the authors and do not necessarily represent what is actually desirable. Improvements in the accuracy of dose-calculation algorithms may allow for downward revision of these numbers.

In addition to the inherent accuracy of the dose-calculation algorithm, the size of the dose grid has an effect on the accuracy of the dose calculation, especially in regions of high-dose gradient. Doses are typically calculated on a rectangular grid of evenly spaced dose-calculation points. Isodose lines are then interpolated among the doses at these calculation points. Typical dose grid spacing is in the vicinity of 4 mm. Consequently, in regions of high-dose gradients, isodose lines between these dose grid points may not be appropriately located. If doses in these regions are important, such as in regions where multiple beams are joined with a gap, it may be necessary to reduce the grid spacing to obtain a more accurate realization of the potential hot or cold dose regions. The increase in dose resolution, however, comes with the cost of increased dose computation time.

The precision of 3D dose distributions often requires that the dose be calculated on a fine grid. Depending on dose gradients and the position of points relative to the boundaries of anatomic structures, grid spacing as small as 2 mm may be desired. This means that dose at a million or more points must be computed for each beam, a formidable task, especially when computer-aided optimization is used to explore hundreds or thousands of plans and when more accurate methods of dose computations are employed. The increasing speed of computers may provide some relief. In addition, it is necessary to develop software algorithms to accelerate dose calculations. There is considerable room for improvement. Dose-calculation speed can be accelerated, for example, through the use of variable grid spacing, as suggested by Niemierko and Goitein (54). This technique employs a quadtree or octree approach to reduce the number of points of computations considerably. It takes advantage of the facts that for a single beam the dose is small and dose gradients are small or changes are essentially linear in most regions. The dose at a vast majority of points can therefore be obtained by linear interpolation from dose at the neighboring points. In a typical application of this scheme, dose at a coarse grid of points, say at 16-mm steps, is first calculated. The grid is then subdivided by two along all three axes. The dose values are calculated by linear interpolation if the dose or dose gradient at the neighboring points is small or if the dose gradient is linear, otherwise, by direct calculation. This process is repeated until the desired level of precision is achieved. Depending on the ratio of initial and eventual grid sizes and on the volume of interest, a reduction in number points of a factor of 10 to 100 may be achieved.

Another issue affecting the accuracy of a dose-calculation algorithm involves the commissioning of the beam model and the verification of the accuracy of the model. Commissioning of a beam model is the process of determining those parameters in a beam model that enable the beam to accurately reproduce measured data acquired under a set of well-defined conditions, generally unmodified square fields, normal incidence to the surface, and in a water phantom. Verification of the accuracy of a dose-calculation model is the process of verifying that the commissioned beams accurately calculate dose in configurations that are different from those under which commissioning data was obtained (55). Early dose-calculation algorithms that relied on tables of beam data as measured in a water phantom required little by way of commissioning, but often failed to achieve sufficient accuracy for beam configurations that were different from those of the initial data acquisition, for example, irregularly shaped fields, oblique incidence, or presence of beam modifiers. More sophisticated algorithms, such as those discussed elsewhere in this book, may have large numbers of parameters and require significantly more effort in determining these parameters, although yielding more accurate calculations under a much wider variety of beam configurations. In some cases, the task of beam model commissioning is more of an art than a science (56), although software tools are being developed by vendors of radiation treatment-planning systems and relatively consistent beam characteristics among machines of a single vendor make the commissioning process significantly easier.

Considering the improved precision now possible in the planning and delivery of 3-DCRT, the reduction of margins to reduce normal tissue exposure, and the reduction in other sources (e.g., anatomic structure delineation, motion, and positioning) of uncertainty, it is important that the uncertainty in dose distributions be correspondingly reduced. Improved accuracy of predicted dose may reveal weaknesses in treatment plans in terms of regions of underdose in target volume or overdose in normal structures that could be remedied to improve local control or reduce normal tissue complications. Furthermore, more accurate dose distributions may allow better correlation of dose distributions with outcome, a major weakness in the current practice of radiation oncology.

Specific dose computation algorithms used in radiation treatment planning are described in detail elsewhere in this book. Here, we give only an overview of issues relevant to 3-DCRT. These include accuracy of dose distributions for arbitrarily shaped and intensity-modulated fields and for inhomogeneous patient structure as well as surface irregularities. The important issue of speed of dose computations is also addressed briefly.

Methods of predicting radiation dose range from purely empiric ones to Monte Carlo simulations of radiation transport. The empiric methods, which directly or indirectly use tables of measured dose distribution data, have the advantage that they are simple and fast. However, their accuracy is inadequate when the geometry of dose calculations differs significantly from the conditions under which the dose distributions were measured. Although in principle the Monte Carlo simulations offer the best accuracy, the complexity of implementation and the vast amount of computer resources required make this method somewhat impractical, at least at present, for routine calculation of dose distributions for treatment planning. With improved knowledge of the composition of the incident beam and a better understanding of the mechanism

of radiation transport in patients, new semi-empiric methods of predicting dose have been developed. Examples of such methods are pencil beam convolution, differential pencil beam (DPB), and point-spread array. These methods rely to some extent on basic principles of radiation physics but make simplifying approximations and assumptions. Corrections based on empiric data are often required to improve agreement with measurements. The accuracy of results depends on the nature of the assumptions and approximations. Greater reliance on basic principles often requires smaller corrections and leads to more accurate results for complex geometries that deviate substantially from the conditions of measurements at a cost of increased computation time. As computer technology improves and as more ingenious and efficient algorithms are developed, such methods are likely to become more prevalent.

Since most fields used in 3-DCRT may be shaped and modulated, taking accurate account of the field shape is an important aspect of improving the accuracy of dose distributions. Most conventional systems for predicting dose are inaccurate near the boundaries of fields, especially for irregularly shaped fields. Pencil beam algorithms have been found to be a quite accurate and practical means of predicting dose for irregular and intensity-modulated fields (57,58). In models of this type, pencil beams are convolved with the fluence pattern formed by field-shaping devices and incident on the surface of a flat homogeneous phantom. The results of convolution are corrected for surface curvature and internal inhomogeneities according to the conventional radiologic path length approach. Pencil beams for polyenergetic incident fluence and the energy spectra used for the computation of fluence may be generated with Monte Carlo simulations. Pencil beam algorithms are sufficiently accurate for most treatment sites. Exceptions may be the thorax, and head and neck. Unfortunately, the availability of pencil beam methods is limited. Their widespread implementation will require the generation of accurate energy spectra and pencil beam dose distributions using Monte Carlo simulations for the whole range of treatment machines.

In 3-DCRT, an accurate description of patient's internal anatomy is available in the form of a 3D matrix of CT numbers. To make full use of these data to predict dose more accurately, it is important to consider the effect of the variation in point-by-point densities and the composition of tissue on the lateral transport of scattered photons and electrons. Dose computation models such as the point spread function convolution model (50) and the DPB model (51) have been developed for this purpose. The basic beam data needed for dose calculations with these models is also generated by Monte Carlo simulations. These models can more accurately take into account surface curvature and internal inhomogeneities as well as field-shaping devices but require a large amount of computing resources.

It is noteworthy that both CT and MRI can provide voxel-by-voxel information, but only CT data can be converted into a form suitable for dose calculations. MRI data represent proton densities and nuclear spin relaxation times that are not appropriate for describing the interaction of therapeutic photons and electrons with tissues. These interactions are more closely related to electron densities. Although CT provides effective linear attenuation coefficients for diagnostic energy (~100 kV) photons that do not directly represent radiologic properties of photons of therapeutic energies (1–50 MV), it is possible to convert them to corresponding electron densities empirically. The use of electron densities has been found to yield sufficiently accurate results in most cases. However, the atomic number may be important in making the computed dose more accurate in and around bony structures and in the vicinity of prostheses and dental fillings.

Dose is calculated by tracing rays from the radiation source through the 3D image to the points of computation. Ray tracing is also performed for incorporating the contribution of scattered photons and electrons from all points within the 3D image. The original image set may require 30 MB or more of memory. Furthermore, the 3D CT image is often composed of nonequispaced sections not appropriate for data normally used in ray tracing. Therefore, some preprocessing must be performed to reduce the image to a form suitable for ray tracing. A common technique is to reformat the image into an equispaced 3D matrix of relatively coarse step sizes (typically 4- or 5-mm grid). The values of pixels in the condensed image are averages of the pixels in the original image. In addition, each pixel value may be scaled so that it fits into a single byte. The resulting loss of precision has been found to have only a small effect on computed dose. The 3D image condensed in this manner occupies ~2 MB of memory and lends itself very well to ray-tracing algorithms. However, the precision in calculating path length may be significantly compromised at shallow depths and to some extent at points near the interfaces.

The role of heterogeneities in the calculation of radiation dose distributions has changed over the past several years. In many anatomic sites, the effects of heterogeneities on the dose distribution are relatively small, but in the thorax, these effects may be significant. Clinicians have often refrained from using heterogeneity-corrected dose calculations because their clinical experience has been to correlate radiation effects with doses calculated without making corrections for tissue heterogeneities. Nevertheless, the presence of heterogeneities not only affects the absolute dose delivered to a tumor, but also the relative distribution of dose delivered elsewhere in the patient to the extent that failure to include heterogeneity corrections in the evaluation of a treatment plan may cause changes in the acceptance of a treatment plan. Frank et al. (59) have indicated that by changing the traditional point-dose prescription for lung tumors to a volume dose prescription, previous clinical experience with homogeneous dose calculations can be applied to heterogeneity-corrected dose calculations while preserving the same prescribed dose.

PLAN EVALUATION

Plan Evaluation and Comparison

A crucial component of 3-DCRT is the evaluation of plans, and an accompanying chapter of this book has been devoted to this topic. However, for completeness of the description of 3-DCRT, a brief overview is included here.

In conventional radiotherapy planning, the process of plan evaluation typically consisted of the examination of one or a few cross-sectional isodose distributions, and of a limited amount of quantitative information, such as minimum tumor dose and maximum dose to normal organs. For 3-DCRT, more sophisticated methods are required for the following reasons:

■ 3D dose distributions are voluminous, and their spatial relationship with the tumor volume and critical normal anatomy is complex. The assimilation of this information to draw conclusions about the possible clinical outcome may be a very demanding task. It requires the deployment of advanced display techniques to make the information more easily comprehensible, and schemes to condense the information into a much smaller subset.

■ Dose distributions are often unusual. To evaluate such dose distributions, it is necessary to extrapolate the conventional experience at least to modest degrees, which requires quantitative plan evaluation methods.

■ Many more options can be explored in 3-DCRT. In particular, many more beams, including noncoplanar ones, may be used. These beams may be shaped and intensity modulated to produce conformal dose distributions. The effective evaluation of a sufficient number of plans may be virtually impossible without some special quantitative tools.

■ Quantitative plan evaluation tools are especially important when one considers the need to automate the plan evaluation process. The automation of plan evaluation, and indeed of most aspects of 3-DCRT, is essential if the advantages of this modality are to become widely available. Automated plan evaluation is also a prerequisite for computer-aided optimization when the computer has to generate and compare a large number, perhaps tens of thousands, of plans. Optimization requires condensation of data into a small number of quantities and frequently into a single index that can be considered by physicians to be a reliable overall estimate of clinical consequences.

Dose Distribution Displays

Graphic methods provide the most practical and effective means of evaluating and comparing treatment plans. Properly designed displays supplemented with tools for image enhancement, video attribute control, and rapid navigation, are essential for eliciting satisfactory information. Many ways of displaying dose distributions have been devised, and it is not possible to cover them in their entirety here. Only a few examples are provided.

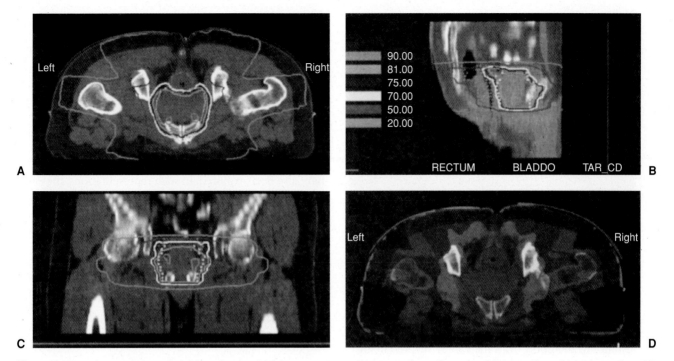

Figure 12.16. Transverse (**A**), sagittal (**B**), and coronal (**C**) image sections of a prostate three-dimensional (3D) conformal treatment plan with overlaid isodose contours. **D:** The same as (**A**) but with color wash. The latter is more quantitative, but the former gives a better global view.

Superimposing dose distributions on a series of transverse, sagittal, or coronal images is the most common method of displaying 2D dose distributions. In some situations, oblique image sections have also been found to be helpful; their usefulness, however, may be limited by the inability to conceptualize their orientation with respect to the patient coordinate system and the lack of experience in comprehending such displays. Figure 12.16, panels A, B, and C, shows three image planes overlaid with isodose contours for a prostate treatment plan: the traditional sagittal, coronal, and transverse cuts. Dose distributions are usually displayed in the form of isodose curves. A somewhat less quantitative but perhaps more easily comprehensible means of examining dose distributions is with the aid of color wash overlays on image sections (Figure 12.16D). In a color wash display, each dose range is assigned a specific color. The CT or MRI is displayed with the various dose range regions flooded with translucent color.

Displays of planar dose distributions are used for evaluation and side-by-side comparison of plans. For the latter, interactive rapid navigation of the whole sequence of parallel image sections has been found to be highly useful in interpreting 3D dose distributions. Color wash dose difference displays may also be used for the comparison of plans. These displays show the difference in dose distributions between two rival plans and highlight their relative merits and demerits. The point-by-point differences in dose values are displayed as color wash regions, with color indicating the magnitude and the sign of the difference (Figure 12.17). This concept has been extended to display the difference between actual and desired dose distribution. In the so-called *images of regret* regions of overdose to normal critical structures and underdose to the target volume may be displayed as color wash overlays on CT images, with color indicating the magnitude of overdose or underdose (Figure 12.18) (60). These displays highlight potential trouble spots without the need to search for them.

Comparing competing plans by displaying 2D image sections side by side can be difficult. A plan may appear to be superior in one plane, but be unacceptable in another. Therefore, a number of additional modes of displaying 3D anatomy and dose distributions have been developed. One example, the surface analog of the color wash, is called the *surface dose display.* The color on the surface of

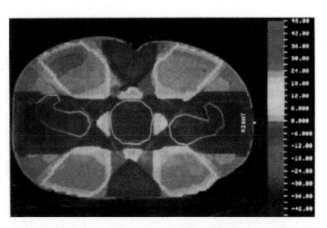

Figure 12.17. A dose difference display. The point-by-point difference of dose values is displayed as color wash regions, with color indicating the magnitude and the sign of the difference.

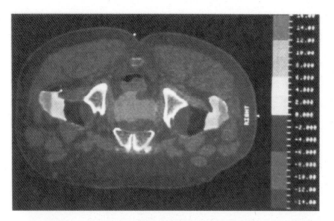

Figure 12.18. An image of regret. Regions of overdose in normal critical structures and underdose in the target volume may be displayed as color wash overlays on computed tomography (CT) images, with color indicating magnitude of overdose or underdose.

a 3D structure indicates the dose level. The color of each point indicates a dose range; the intensity is governed by the distance of the point from the viewer (depth cueing). Several structures may be displayed at the same time. The real-time motion of dose distribution patterns overlaid on the anatomy has been found to aid considerably in the comprehension of displays of 3D data. The concepts of images of regret may also be extended to surfaces of regret in which the color on the surface indicates the degree of deviation from the desired dose.

In another type of surface representation of 3D dose distributions, isodose surfaces may be displayed along with the surface displays of the tumor volume and anatomic structures. For the plan in Figure 12.19A, the target volume is not covered by the prescription dose surface; for the plan in Figure 12.19B, it is. To distinguish anatomy from dose distribution, different surface-rendering techniques are employed. Normally, it is not useful to display more than one isodose surface at a time. Real-time motion enhances the utility of these displays as well.

To enhance the clarity of surface-rendered displays, a combination of surface-rendering schemes may be employed.

Isodose surfaces, for example, may be displayed as wire frames, either as stacks of parallel contours or as tiled polygons, and anatomic structures may be displayed as solids with transparent or opaque surfaces. Alternatively, anatomic structures can be shown as solid surfaces and isodose levels as transparent surfaces or *vice versa*. Interactive control of the opacity of individual structures, rendering method, and other video attributes greatly clarifies whether portions of a structure overlap an isodose surface.

Volumetric displays of the 3D dose distribution data have also been explored. In such representations, the entire volume of image voxel data is shown as semitransparent, much like a radiograph from arbitrary angles. The dose is shown by assigning color and transparency to voxels. The concept of images of regret may be extended to volumes of regret also. The speed of affordable computers does not yet permit the real-time interactive construction of volumetric displays from arbitrary angles. However, a sequence of precomputed rotational views can be used for real-time viewing. Visual cues similar to the ones used for surface-rendered displays can be employed for volume-rendered displays as well. The advantage of volume-rendered over surface is that displays include greater anatomic detail furnished by the 3D image. A more global view of the relationship of dose and anatomy is provided by combining all 2D image planes into a single scene. Conversely, the incorporation of all image and dose data into one view may lead to obfuscation and cluttering, making plan analysis difficult. In addition, the computer resource requirements for generating this type of display are much greater than for surface-rendered displays. Many other possibilities of displaying dose distributions have been investigated (61,62).

Quantitative Plan Evaluation Indices

An advantage of displays of 3D dose distributions is that they can provide dose and position information at every point in the patient. Unfortunately, the information provided may be so overwhelming that in complex situations

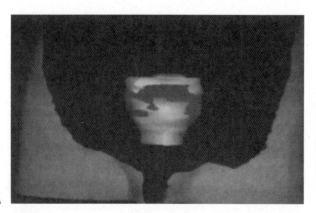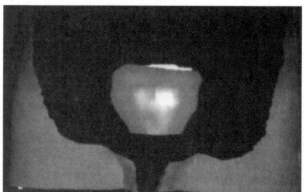

Figure 12.19. Isodose surface displays of two plans of a prostate cancer patient. **A:** A deficient plan in which the prescribed isodose surface does not adequately cover the target volume. **B:** The properly irradiated target.

it may be virtually impossible to absorb a sufficient fraction of it to appreciate the overall clinical effect of the entire dose distribution. Dose distribution displays are essential but not sufficient by themselves for 3D plan evaluation. They must be supplemented with the quantitative indices mentioned earlier. These indices may be either some simple attributes of dose distribution or a condensation of dose distribution into a smaller number of quantities. Next we summarize the quantities that have been found to be useful.

Some features of dose distributions are the same as the ones used conventionally for plan evaluation. These include the minimum tumor dose and the maximum dose to each critical normal organ. Increasingly, other features are being considered useful indicators of the biologic consequences. Examples of these include the mean tumor dose, the standard deviation of tumor dose, the minimum dose to the hottest specified fraction (e.g., 95%) of the target volume, the maximum dose to hottest specified fraction of a normal organ volume, and the fractional volume of an organ receiving a certain specified dose or a higher one.

Dose–Volume Histograms

The DVH is probably the most useful, and certainly the most popular, plan evaluation tool used in 3-DCRT (63). A DVH graphically summarizes 3D dose data into a single curve for each region of interest. An example of a DVH is presented in Figure 12.20. One of its important applications occurs when the DVHs of competing treatment plans are plotted on the same graph for comparison.

Two types of DVH are commonly used. The differential DVH plots volume in each of a set of equal dose bins from the lowest to the highest dose. Therefore, a differential DVH for a totally uniformly irradiated target volume is a

single bar of 100% volume at the prescription dose with all other bars absent. The cumulative DVH is a plot of the volume of the anatomic structure receiving a specific dose or a higher one against the specific dose. In reality, a cumulative DVH is not a histogram at all but simply a continuous curve representing the frequency distribution of volume bins (or points in the anatomic structure) as a function of minimum dose to the volume. The cumulative DVH has been found to be much more useful and more commonly used than its differential counterpart. In fact, the term DVH normally implies cumulative DVH. The precision of the DVH is a topic of interest. This issue is particularly important when dose gradients in the anatomic structure are high and/or the volume is small. The dose distribution in high-gradient regions must be sampled at closely spaced points to ensure that important dose information is not missed. Similarly, the volume must be sampled at closely spaced intervals near the surface or when the shape of the anatomic structure is complex or narrow, as for example, in the rectum or bladder wall. If too coarse a grid is chosen, the resultant DVH has a large uncertainty. On the other hand, too fine a grid requires large computational resources. A relatively coarse grid may be adequate for the prostate target volume, for example, whereas a much finer spacing would be required for an organ like the rectum wall. One method proposed for volume sampling places an adequate number of dose-calculation points in each organ randomly or quasi-randomly, as suggested by Niemierko and Goitein (64). However, the problem as a whole remains unsolved. Similar precision considerations apply when dose distributions are condensed to produce biophysical indices.

DVHs can indicate at a glance the potential for undesired consequences by identifying the existence of hot spots in a critical structure and cold spots in a target volume. Frequently, a clinic will define dose–volume constraints used to evaluate treatment plans. For example, a clinic may establish that for a treatment plan to be acceptable, at least 95% of the PTV be irradiated to the prescription dose. Another such dose–volume constraint might be that no more than 40% of the total lung volume can be irradiated to a dose >20 Gy. The DVH provides a ready display of how the treatment plan meets such dose–volume constraints. However, the DVH provides no information about the precise geometric position of regions that violate these constraints. Consequently, the final judgment about the clinical desirability of a treatment plan is best based on dose distribution displays supplemented with DVHs.

Biophysical Indices

When using DVHs for comparing rival plans, often the DVHs of the plans being compared intersect with each other at one or more points. Under these circumstances it may be difficult to decide which of the two DVHs is better, and further quantitative analysis may be necessary. In

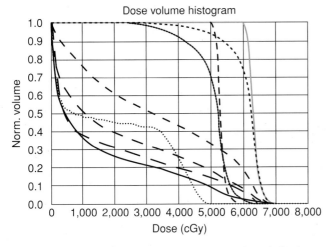

Figure 12.20. A typical dose–volume histogram (DVH) display. A common presentation is normalized volume (*y*-axis) versus absolute dose (*x*-axis). Doses to target volumes and normal structures can be easily and simultaneously evaluated using these displays.

addition, as indicated earlier, it may be necessary to condense dose distribution information further to simplify plan evaluation and comparison and for computer-aided optimization. Further, as Goitein (65) emphasizes, dose is only a surrogate of biologic consequences. Therefore, there is considerable interest in the development and use of models for predicting biophysical indices.

Biophysical indices may simply be "equivalent uniform dose" (*EUD*) and "effective volume" (66,67). The former is the dose, which if delivered uniformly to the whole volume of the anatomic structure, would, in theory, produce the same response as the nonuniform dose in the plan. The latter is the partial volume, which when irradiated to the prescription dose or the maximum dose uniformly, with the remainder of the volume receiving no dose at all, would result in the same response as the nonuniformly irradiated anatomic structure. Other indices, such as the *TCP* and *NTCP*, have been introduced. For predicting the *TCP* of a nonuniformly irradiated tumor, the tumor is divided into voxels, or "tumorlets." The *TCP* of each tumorlet for an individual patient is computed by assuming both a biologic response function and the values of its parameters. The product of the *TCP*s of the tumorlets is the *TCP* of the whole tumor. This *TCP* is averaged over the entire population of patients. The parameters of the model are chosen so that the population-averaged *TCP* for a uniformly irradiated tumor agrees with the observed data (68,69).

Numerous models for computing *NTCP*s of nonuniformly irradiated organs have been proposed. Some are phenomenologic, as for example, the Lyman's model (70,71), and are simple and flexible to use. Others, as for example the models of Jackson et al. (72) and Niemierko and Goitein (73,74), rely on basic biologic principles and attempt to incorporate the underlying architecture of normal tissues. They therefore represent more closely the response to radiation, in particular the volume effect. However, they are more complex and may require significantly greater computational resources.

Unfortunately, the current knowledge of biologic response data for a vast majority of tissues is unreliable and poorly documented. The models for predicting biophysical indices are highly simplistic and subject to criticism. Their computed values cannot be taken seriously in the absolute sense. Even so, they reasonably represent the nonlinear complex shapes of the dose and volume dependence of the response to irradiation. If used judiciously, they can be quite useful for comparing rival plans and for the extrapolation of conventional experience to the unusual dose distributions being observed and anticipated in 3-DCRT.

Treatment Plan Score

Another potentially useful quantity for plan evaluation, comparison, and optimization is a numeric score obtained by combining *TCP*s, *NTCP*s, and other criteria. Often the objective of delivering high and uniform dose to the target volume while keeping the dose to all normal structures below the tolerance limits cannot be met. Different plans yield different radiation burdens to different normal organs. Therefore, compromises have to be made. Each plan evaluation index must be assigned a relative importance. The magnitudes of the relative importance factors depend on the deviation from the desired dose in a complicated nonlinear fashion. There appears to be no source for this information other than the physician's subjective judgment, which is likely to vary from one physician to another. The situation is further confused by such factors as paired organs, for which it may be possible to accept a high degree of complication in one organ in the pair, but not both. Interdependent organs, paired or not, for which the complication of one organ may affect the other, pose another difficult problem. Nevertheless, models for computing plan scores have been proposed. An example is the so-called probability of uncomplicated control (75), defined as:

$$P+ = TCP \prod_i (1 - NTCP_i) \qquad \text{EQUATION (12.1)}$$

This quantity has been used for comparing and optimizing 3D treatment plans. However, as pointed out by Goitein (65), one of the problems with P+ is that it does not assign different weighting to *NTCP*s for different organs and to different end points. Another is that it implicitly assumes that the acceptability of a treatment plan is linearly proportional to the *NTCP* of an organ and that an increase in *NTCP* can be balanced by a corresponding increase in *TCP*. As Goitein (65) observes, "Such a scheme implies that a 6% increase in *TCP* would outweigh a 5% chance of cord transection." In clinical practice, the decision-making process is far too complex. In some cases, a physician may accept a higher probability of complication to save a patient's life, especially if other treatments, such as surgery, are not feasible. In other cases, the effect of complications on the quality of life or life itself may be so severe that the physician chooses to limit the target dose. In general, however, depending on the organ and the end point, a plan's acceptability is often nearly a step function of a clinically relevant parameter, which may be a dose limit, a dose–volume limit, or even a limit on the *NTCP*. That is, below a certain threshold of this parameter little or no penalty is assessed, and the plan is rejected immediately or soon after the limit is reached. Based on such arguments, a score function of the following form has been suggested (76):

$$S = \prod_{k=0}^{N} s_k, \qquad \text{EQUATION (12.2)}$$

where s_k is the anatomic structure-specific subscores. Subscript 0 corresponds to the tumor, and subscore s_0 is the *TCP*. For normal tissues, each subscore is a function of the $NTCP_k$. The choice of the exact functional form of the

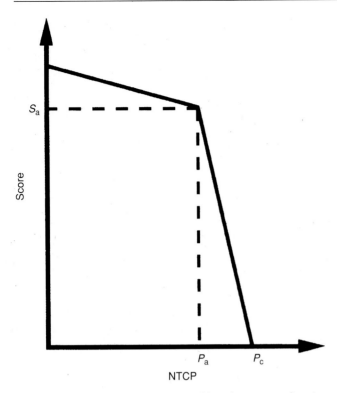

Figure 12.21. Schematic representation of the subscore s_i as a function of computed values of normal tissue complication probability (*NTCP*). For small values of *NTCP* below a physician-specific acceptable level (P_a) the subscore is high and drops slowly and linearly from unity to a value S_a. For values of *NTCP* above P_a the subscore dropped rapidly to a zero, corresponding to a critical level P_c of *NTCP*. *Source:* Reprinted with permission from Mohan R, Wang X, Jackson A. Optimization of three-dimensional radiation treatment plans. In: Meyer JA, Purdy J, eds. Frontiers of radiation therapy and oncology. Proceedings of San Francisco cancer symposium on 3D conformal radiotherapy, 1994. Basel: Karger, 1996:86–103.

subscore function and the values of its parameters are somewhat arbitrary. In order to incorporate the physician's judgment in the score function, a form of the subscore function shown in Figure 12.21 has been suggested by Mohan et al. (66) and Kutcher (77). In this function, the subscore decreases linearly and slowly from unity with increase in the *NTCP*. When the *NTCP* reaches the limit of acceptability, P_a, the subscore begins to drop rapidly, reaching zero when the *NTCP* exceeds a critical limit, P_c. Since the values of *NTCP*s depend partly on the choice of models and parameters, the limits P_a and P_c are relative and are chosen according to the physicians' judgment of dose distributions and DVHs. Other plan evaluation criteria, such as constraints on dose or dose–volume combinations, may be similarly expressed as subscores.

Optimization

The major goal of 3-DCRT treatment planning is to select that set of beam parameters, including beam energies, beam geometries, treatment portals, and beam weights that will generate the best possible treatment plan, or at

least a treatment plan that meets the clinical needs of the radiation oncologist. Although, in theory, this entire procedure can be automated, in practice, not all beam parameters are set automatically. Selection of beam energies is based, to a large extent, on the location, and particularly the depth, of the target volume. Beam geometries are typically set manually so that critical structures are avoided, although some research has been done in automatic beam angle optimization. Treatment portals are generally designed to include the entire PTV along with a margin that accounts for both the geometric and radiation penumbras. Consequently, optimization of treatment plans generally means the automatic selection of beam weights to achieve the clinical goals of the treatment plan. Optimization is much more commonly used in intensity-modulated radiation therapy (IMRT), where the ability to modify the spatial distribution of beam intensities introduces many more degrees of freedom than in 3-DCRT; however, some work has been done to automate the process of selecting beam weights for non-intensity-modulated beams used in 3-DCRT.

The simplest optimization method, and the most commonly used, is trial and error. The treatment planner selects an initial set of beam weights based on class solutions and computes the dose distribution resulting from that set of beam weights. If the plan meets the clinical goals of the dose prescription, the plan is accepted and the planning process ends. If the plan is not acceptable, beam weights or beam geometries are changed to try to improve the quality of the treatment plan. Change is more likely not explicitly algorithmic, but based on the experience and expertise of the treatment planner. In principle, the optimization scheme is finite, that is, after a finite number of iterations, an optimal plan will be found. However, in many cases, the optimal treatment plan may still be unacceptable, so that compromises must be made in the dose prescription so that an acceptable plan can be obtained.

An algorithmic optimization scheme consists of two components. The first component is the identification of a metric, which is a measure of the quality of a treatment plan. This metric is often called an "objective function" or a "cost function." An example of an objective function might be the mean square difference between the calculated dose to the PTV and the prescription dose. Often constraints are also placed on the solution of the optimization scheme. A simple example of such a set of constraints is the obvious requirement that all beam weights be nonnegative. A more complicated example of a constraint might be a dose–volume constraint, such as the requirement that not more than 40% of the total lung volume receives >20 Gy. The second component of the optimization scheme is an algorithm that determines the maximum (or minimum) value of the metric subject to the constraints.

Objective functions can be relatively simple or very complicated. An example of a simple objective function is the mean square difference between the dose calculated to each point in the patient (typically in a rectangular grid) and the dose from an ideal treatment plan. Different ideal doses would apply to different regions in the patient, such as target volume and each OAR. The advantage of this type of objective function is that it is quadratic. If one elected to use a gradient search algorithm for optimization of this cost function, the gradients would be linear, making the optimization problem relatively easy to solve.

A significant disadvantage of this relatively simple objective function is that it does not accurately reflect the clinical desirability of a treatment plan. With this objective function, overdosing of the target volume carries the same weight as an equal underdosing of the target volume. In reality, however, underdosing the target volume is a far more serious failure than the equal overdosing, even though both contributed equally to the objective function. Moreover, even though the most desirable dose to an OAR is zero, a wide range of doses to an OAR would be viewed as acceptable, provided an excessive dose is not delivered to the OAR. Hence the desirability of incorporating dose constraints into the optimization, stating, for example, that any dose up to some maximum dose to an OAR is acceptable, provided the maximum dose is not exceeded. Further refinement can be achieved by incorporating dose–volume constraints. In such constraints, maximum doses are specified to specific volumes of the OAR. Dose–volume constraints are particularly useful in describing the radiation tolerance of parallel organs, such as the lungs, which can function even if a nonnegligible fraction of the organ has been damaged. An example of such a dose–volume constraint would be something like "no more than 40% of the total lung volume may receive more than 20 Gy."

More complicated objective functions might differentiate between target volume and OARs and implicitly incorporate dose–volume constraints. An example of such an objective function would be the squares of the differences between the calculated doses to points in the target volume and the minimum acceptable doses to these points in target volume, or the squares of the differences between the calculated doses to points in OARs and the maximum acceptable doses to these points in the OARs. Objective functions might also incorporate biologic figures of merit such as *NTCP*, *TCP*, or *EUD*.

The second part of optimization involves the development of algorithms to optimize the objective function. If the objective function is quadratic in the beam weights, then gradient search methods can be used. In such cases, the equations used in the gradient search methods are linear in the beam weights and easy to solve. One disadvantage of gradient search methods is that when applied to other forms of objective functions, a gradient search solution might be trapped in a local minimum, whereas a global minimum might be at a significantly lower value of the objective function than that at the local minimum. Stochastic methods, such as simulated annealing or genetic algorithms, can be used if the objective function

might admit local minima. These methods allow one to escape from a local minimum and find a global minimum. The theory of simulated annealing indicates that a global solution can always be found, but no indication is given as to how long it may take to achieve this solution. Consequently, execution times may be prohibitively long.

Another approach to optimization is the class of algorithms known as feasibility search algorithms. Application of these algorithms is based on the idea that an optimal solution may not be needed. Only a feasible solution that meets all the dose–volume constraints is necessary. Provided the space of all feasible solutions forms a convex set in *n*-dimensional beam weight space, algorithms based on the concept of projections onto convex sets (POCS) can be used to either find a feasible solution or demonstrate that no feasible solution exists.

DELIVERY OF THREE-DIMENSIONAL CONFORMAL RADIATION THERAPY

Patient Setup

To implement a 3D treatment plan, it is necessary to spatially register treatment-planning displays with the patient and treatment machine. This requires the placement of alignment marks on the patient at the time of imaging and the determination of the orientation and the position of beams and beam shaping devices relative not only to these markers but more importantly to the internal landmarks of the patient.

The position of the internal anatomy with respect to the beam aperture must be verified before the delivery of treatment. Conventional 2D treatments are verified by comparing port films with simulator films. For 3D treatments, this task may be more difficult and confusing because many beams may be incident obliquely with respect to transverse planes and are arbitrarily shaped. For 3-DCRT, one must digitally reconstruct a simulator-like image, the DRR, from the 3D CT data and compare it with the portal images acquired on film or with EPIDs. In addition to the gray-scale DRR image, the user can display several objects that aid in alignment, the carina for instance. Selected anatomic structure contours can be projected onto the image along with the collimator jaws and aperture outlines, a grid of evenly spaced points as a measurement aid, isocenter crosshairs, and so on. A typical DRR is shown in Figure 12.22.

To ascertain the correctness of the position of the tumor and normal anatomic structures relative to the beam boundary or to estimate the amount of displacement, portal images must be registered with simulator images and/or DRRs. To accomplish this, a common frame of reference between the two images is established by matching either the boundaries or the center of the field. Any of a number of techniques then may be used to determine correlation transformations and to estimate the

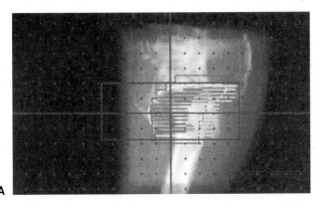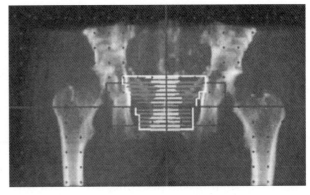

Figure 12.22. Left lateral and posterior digitally reconstructed radiograph (DRR) images of a patient undergoing radiotherapy for cancer of the prostate. The images were constructed using absorption coefficients corresponding to 70 kVp photons. The target volume and rectum contour stacks, jaws, conventional aperture, and the multileaf collimator (MLC)-shaped aperture are superimposed. *Source:* Reprinted with permission from Mohan R, Lovelock M, Mageras G, et al. Computer-controlled radiation therapy and multileaf collimation. In: Meyer JA, Purdy J, eds. Frontiers of radiation therapy and oncology. Proceedings of San Francisco cancer symposium on 3D conformal radiotherapy, 1994. Basel: Karger, 1996:123–128.

error in setup. The simplest of these is the interactive technique, in which drawings of clearly identifiable landmarks and fiducial markers extracted from the simulator image are overlaid on the portal image and interactively translated, rotated, and scaled to obtain the best match. If distortions are minimal, matching can be automated with least-square minimization if well-defined anatomic landmarks can be located on both images (78). Other more sophisticated methods of correlating projection images have been reported by Gilhuijs et al. (79), Jones and Boyer (80), and Chen et al. (81).

Computer-Controlled Radiotherapy

The need for automation of treatment delivery is becoming more apparent as 3-DCRT is implemented into routine clinical practice. The complexity of 3-DCRT is increasing as better planning solutions are developed, and this trend is expected to continue.

Manual delivery of 3-DCRT is inefficient and can benefit only a limited number of patients. The inadequacies of the manual methods will become even more conspicuous as computer-aided optimization improves the design of treatments, resulting in a relatively substantial increase in the number of beams. The use of intensity modulation as an optimization tool requires computer control and monitoring. Computer-controlled treatment machines, in which all moving components as well as dose and dose rate are controlled by computers, are being developed and implemented with the aim of delivering complex 3D conformal treatments rapidly, safely, and more accurately.

A number of issues must be considered when developing and implementing automated radiotherapy. Different models of automation may be adopted, and there are different levels of automation. To take advantage of the efficiency offered by computer-controlled radiotherapy (CCRT), the coupling between the 3D RTP systems and the computer-controlled machine is important. The most important requirement of CCRT is that the automated treatment delivery system be easy to use and safe. While the probability of making mistakes in CCRT is lowered by reducing manual operations, errors in CCRT may have more serious consequences. Therefore, it is important to make CCRT systems even safer than conventional treatment delivery systems.

Over the past decades, the merits of two possible approaches for implementing computer-controlled treatments have been debated. In the early years, the dynamic approach was viewed as essential. In this approach, irradiation continues while various components of the treatment machine are in motion. However, further consideration indicated that the dynamic method offered little if any clinical advantage over the sequential delivery of a set of fixed fields, or segments. In this scheme, called multisegment or step and shoot, a sequence of fixed fields is set up and delivered during each treatment session under computer control, without operator intervention (82). This approach is easier to implement from the engineering point of view, and its safety considerations are somewhat less demanding. Multisegment therapy does not require the synchronization of motions with one another (important for ensuring no collisions) and with the delivered dose. These treatments are also much easier to plan than dynamic treatments. A third mode, the mixed mode, is emerging. In it the treatment session is segmented into fixed fields, but the MLC operates in the dynamic mode to deliver intensity-modulated treatment.

Although treatment machines with full dynamic capability are now available, the multisegment approach to automated treatment delivery has been adopted in the initial phases of CCRT. In the paradigm for the automated treatment delivery adopted in a CCRT system, the computer control functions are divided into those that are carried out by the control computer of the treatment machine and those that are carried out by an external computer. The external computer often consists of a record-and-verify (R&V) system. The external computer imports the treatment plan data of the 3D RTP system. These data consist of treatment machine settings (including MLC leaf positions) for all of the beams (segments) to be employed in the treatment session. Within the external computer, these data and a specified number of monitor units are used to compose a treatment prescription. The prescription and treatment-unit data are downloaded onto the control computer of the treatment unit.

The patient is set up for treatment. For safety and precision, all patients treated with CCRT are immobilized, and the immobilization device is securely attached to the couch. The parameters (couch and gantry positions) for the first segment may be set manually, and portal images are obtained to ensure the correctness of the setup. Any adjustments necessary to the downloaded data are made, and the data in the external computer is modified as necessary so that it can record the corresponding changes in the prescribed values for future treatments. A virtual treatment or "dry run" (all machine motions without irradiation) can be performed to ensure collision-free trajectories.

Treatment is then started. At this point, the external computer verifies that treatment machine components are set to their prescribed positions within tolerances. Tolerances depend on the technique and on the site of treatment. If a discrepancy is discovered, the external computer withholds the permission for the treatment sequence to begin. The user must take a corrective action (change setup or override) and make another attempt to start treatment. The external computer also monitors the treatment delivery process to ensure that machine parameters before the beginning of irradiation of each segment are consistent with their intended values. The external computer records the treatment data on completion of treatment.

In addition to the normal sequence of steps described here, a number of exceptional situations can arise. For example, the treatment may be interrupted and may have to be resumed from the point of interruption. Moreover, the treatment may be terminated prematurely and may have to be resumed later or added to the treatment in another session. The external and control computers manage such situations in conjunction with each other.

VERIFICATION OF DELIVERY

The final step in 3-DCRT is that of verification that the treatment delivered to the patient is consistent with what was planned and approved. All components of the planning and delivery process are reviewed as part of a quality assurance process, including the applicability and correctness of the treatment plan, the accuracy of the treatment unit settings, the validity of the transfer of data from the virtual simulator, through the planning system and R&V system, to the treatment unit. The accuracy of portals for delivery of the radiation beams and the accuracy of the

patient setup is verified as well, as is the accuracy of the actual radiation delivery.

The first steps in corroboration are those of verifying that the treatment plan reflects the radiation dose that has been prescribed for the patient by the attending physician, and of authenticating that the plan accurately reflects the dose designed to be delivered to the patient. This latter requirement is achieved by implementation of a quality assurance program for the treatment-planning system. In such a program, one verifies that the treatment-planning system accurately depicts the patient images, contours, and beams that are provided as input into the dose calculations, and that the beam models are accurate, so that the doses calculated by the treatment-planning system are accurate (83).

The next component of verification is that the machine setting determined by the treatment-planning system will deliver the correct dose to the target. The accuracy of machine settings is verified initially when the beam model is first commissioned and introduced into the treatment-planning system, and is verified for each dose calculation by an independent calculation of radiation doses to individual points within the patient. Software systems generally called "Monitor-Unit (MU) verification systems" are now commonly used as an independent check of MU settings computed by the planning system.

Next, it is necessary to verify that the machine settings, such as beam geometries, and monitor units are accurately transferred from the treatment-planning system to the machine. In many radiation oncology clinics, an R&V system is used to confirm and record the machine settings used to deliver the radiation beams to the patient, ensuring that machine settings lie within clinically accepted tolerances of the values established on the treatment plan. A component of a comprehensive quality assurance program ensures that the machine settings determined by the treatment-planning system are accurately transferred into the R&V system.

Another key step is to verify that the treatment field actually delivered to the patient is identical to the treatment portal as determined on the treatment plan. Commonly, in order to accomplish this task, a radiographic image of the delivered treatment portal is acquired. The portal image is then compared to the DRR of the treatment field extracted from the treatment-planning system. Ideally, the geometric relationship between the target volume and the treatment portal would be compared, but tumors are rarely visible on portal images. Consequently, bony landmarks in the vicinity of the tumors are typically used as surrogates for the target volume locations. Originally, the portal image was recorded on radiographic film, but many radiation oncology clinics are now acquiring this information using an EPID. The use of digital images produced by EPIDs allows for rapid display of the portal images as well as off-site review of the portal images. Figure 12.23 illustrates a DRR and a portal image used to verify the accuracy of the treatment portal.

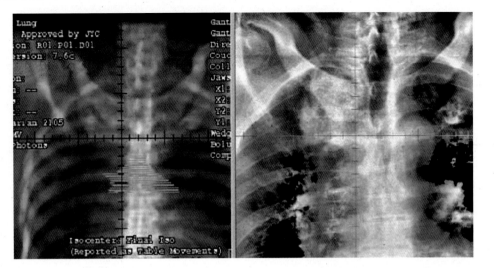

Figure 12.23. Digital portal images can be compared to planning-system digitally reconstructed radiographs (DRRs) for verification of patient positioning. In this figure, the portal image on the right is compared to its corresponding DRR. Note that on the DRR, the carina is shown as a wire contour to aid in its visualization as it is compared to the carina as seen on the portal image.

An important issue regarding the use of portal images for treatment portal verification is the substantial difference in image quality existing between simulation and portal images. Simulation images are typically acquired in the energy range of 50 to 100 keV. In this energy range, the primary interaction between the incident x-rays and the patient results in photoelectric absorption of the incident x-rays. Consequently, the only x-rays that reach the detector are those that are not absorbed in the patient. Moreover, in this energy range, bone absorbs significantly more radiation than soft tissue; hence, the contrast between bony anatomy and the surrounding soft tissue anatomy results in clear, sharp radiographic images. Portal images are acquired at much higher x-ray energies, typically a few MeV, energies that are used in radiation therapy. In this energy range, the difference in absorption of radiation between bone and soft tissue is significantly less, resulting in lower contrast. Moreover, the presence of scattered radiation resulting from x-ray interactions within the patient at these energies results in a significant amount of radiation reaching the detector that gives no indication of the point of origin, resulting in a noisy image. Attempts at overcoming this situation include the application of image enhancement techniques of digital portal images, and generation of DRRs using megavoltage energy spectra.

In addition to verifying the geometry of the treatment portal, the acquisition of a portal image is one of several techniques used to verify that the patient has been set up in a reproducible manner for each treatment. Because the treatment field is often positioned adjacent to critical uninvolved anatomic structures, accurate and reproducible patient positioning is essential so that these uninvolved anatomic structures do not get unnecessarily irradiated. Perhaps the simplest method of position verification is through the use of external markings. Lasers in the walls and ceilings are all directed to a particular point in space, the machine isocenter, where the axis of gantry rotation coincides with the axis of collimator rotation. In 3-DCRT, the patient is often positioned so that the treatment-unit isocenter lies in the approximate center of the target volume. The points at which the lasers intersect the patient surface are marked and used on a daily basis to assist in ensuring that the patient is set up reproducibly. Predicted versus actual source–skin distance verification of treatment portals is an additional means of verifying appropriate patient position.

In conjunction with external markings, patients are often placed in immobilization devices to assist in reproducible positioning. Immobilization devices have many forms. For example, invasive devices, such as stereotactic head frames, which are bolted into the patient's skull, can achieve submillimeter reproducibility and are necessary when the geometric tolerances are very small. When submillimeter tolerance is not as crucial, less invasive devices can be used, including thermoplastic masks, molds, and vacuum bags.

Portal-imaging studies have demonstrated differences between true setup errors and random uncertainties in patient setup, which are a consequence of the degree of patient immobilization, and have indicated guidelines as to when and how to correct for setup inaccuracies. In the treatment of some cancer sites, for example, the prostate, daily variations in patient anatomy have led to the development of more sophisticated methods of setup verification. Differences in bladder and rectal filling on a daily basis combined with the tight treatment margins typical of 3-DCRT may cause one or more radiation beams to miss part of the target volume. One technique that enables correction for daily anatomic variations is to scan the patient just before treatment using an ultrasound technique. Figure 12.24 illustrates an example of a unit used in such an ultrasound process. The outlines of the target volumes and anatomic structures, which are extracted from the radiation treatment plan, are superimposed on the ultrasound scan, and the patient is moved so that the image of the target volume on the scan is superimposed on the outline of the target volume on the treatment plan, therefore ensuring accurate delivery of radiation to the

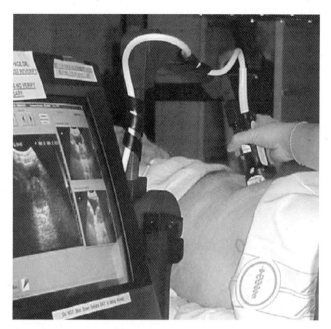

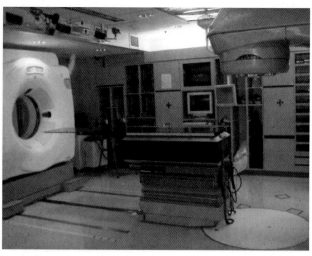

Figure 12.26. A computed tomography (CT)-on-rails image-guided radiation therapy (IGRT) system. Patients can be scanned in treatment position to assess the position of their internal anatomy relative to the position of the treatment unit's isocenter. The patient is aligned using the lasers of the treatment unit. The couch is then rotated so that the CT unit can scan the patient as the unit travels along the rails shown. Image information can then be used to reposition the patient as needed.

Figure 12.24. A B-mode ultrasound unit used to visualize the prostate of a patient undergoing radiation therapy. The position of the ultrasound transducer is registered relative to the treatment unit's isocenter, so that the position of the patient's anatomy at the time of treatment can displayed relative to isocenter (see also Figure 12.25).

target volume. Figure 12.25 illustrates the use of the ultrasound images in realigning a patient.

Another promising technique involves placing a CT scanner in the treatment room in a configuration that allows both imaging and treatment on the same patient

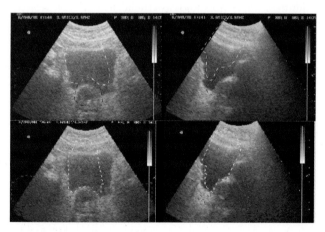

Figure 12.25. Displays of the ultrasound images of a patient undergoing prostate radiotherapy. The images have been registered relative to the treatment unit's isocenter. Also shown are the contours of the patient's prostate and bladder, drawn at the time of treatment planning, which have been transferred to the ultrasound unit's workstation. A spatial relationship also exists between the contours and the treatment unit's isocenter. Shown in the top panel of this figure, is a displacement of the images of the prostate and bladder compared to their respective contours. The images can be moved to achieve better agreement with the planning contours (bottom panel of figure) while specialized software tracks this movement. The treatment couch can then be translated to place the patient in the correct position.

couch. The patient is set up in the treatment position and then scanned. It is then possible to compare the CT image data set, thus, acquired with the data set from which the treatment plan is based, allowing for the patient to be repositioned or even replanned. Rather than allowing the patient table to move through the CT scanner, as is conventionally done, this device moves the CT scanner while the patient remains stationary, hence the device is referred to as *CT-on-Rails/* (Figure 12.26).

The imaging processes previously described are examples of an emerging technology in radiation oncology that is being termed *IGRT.* In IGRT, one tries to reduce the uncertainties introduced into the treatment delivery process by reducing the systematic differences that may exist between simulation and treatment. Recall from our discussion of margins needed to determine the PTV that the SM accounts for systematic and random uncertainties in patient position. A quality assurance system in which information obtained from portal images is used to correct the position of the patient could lead to reduced margins.

In addition to verifying that the radiation beams accurately irradiate the target volume and spare surrounding normal-tissue anatomy, it is necessary to verify that the radiation dose actually delivered to the target is the same as the radiation dose prescribed in the treatment plan. This is achieved by means of a thorough quality assurance system that includes a regular schedule of well-defined daily, monthly, and annual evaluations of the output of the treatment unit, including accurate measurements of the magnitude of the radiation emitted from the linear accelerator as well as the energy of the radiation (83). Additional techniques exist for measurement of doses to accessible parts of the patient during treatment, using small radiation detectors such as thermoluminescent dosimeters (TLD) or diode detectors, which can be placed either on external surfaces of the patient or in accessible cavities within the patient. Current studies are underway to assess the safety and accuracy of radiation detectors that can be implanted inside the patient.

UNCERTAINTIES IN THREE-DIMENSIONAL CONFORMAL RADIATION THERAPY

Although the major objective of 3-DCRT is to improve the accuracy of radiation delivery, this accuracy may be limited by various uncertainties in the planning and delivery process. Although some uncertainties may be controlled, others cannot, and before delivering any sort of radiation treatment, an understanding of what can and cannot be controlled is highly desirable. Because many of these uncertainties are stochastic, they add in quadrature, consequently, a decrease in uncertainty in one variable may not have significant effect on overall uncertainty unless it is accompanied by decreases in uncertainty in several other variables as well. Moreover, the quantitative magnitude of some of the variables may not yet be completely understood.

Uncertainties in radiation therapy are of three main categories: clinical, physical, and dosimetric. Clinical uncertainties include the extent of disease, the delineation of anatomy, and the biologic response of the tumor and normal tissue to radiation. In many respects, the identification of methods for reduction of uncertainties represents a summary of many of the techniques that comprise 3-DCRT. For example, uncertainties in determination of the extent of disease can be reduced by the appropriate selection of imaging modality, as well as by use of multimodality imaging. Uncertainties in delineation of anatomy can be reduced by the use of image segmentation software, which sets standardized criteria for the assignment of image voxels to regions of interest. The incorporation of more sophisticated models for response coupled with additional clinical data is reducing uncertainties in biologic response. Physical uncertainties are somewhat easier to quantify, including intrafractional and interfractional motion as well as setup uncertainties. Various immobilization techniques are used to decrease setup uncertainty, the specific technique selected being appropriate to the level of tolerance of setup uncertainty. Techniques of IGRT such as online kilovoltage imaging and cone-beam CT can reduce setup uncertainty and interfractional motion. Four-dimensional CT, as well as other motion mitigation techniques, can be used to reduce intrafractional motion. Finally, dosimetric uncertainties are perhaps the easiest to quantify, including such components as uncertainties in machine calibration and dose calculation. Uncertainties in machine calibration are based on the relative accuracy with which one can measure radiation output and are well specified in the various calibration protocols (1) and quality assurance reports (83). Uncertainties in the dose calculation depend on the accuracy both of the dose-calculation algorithm (52,53) and of the accuracy by which one determines the various parameters in a beam model (55). It is clearly not possible to eliminate uncertainty altogether. It is important, however, to understand the sources of uncertainty, the magnitude of the various uncertainties in each component of the radiation therapy chain, and to attempt to incorporate these estimates quantitatively into the treatment-planning process (84).

CONCLUSIONS

This chapter has addressed 3-DCRT: Its concepts, processes, characteristics, and issues. The primary goal of 3-DCRT is to provide accurate targeting and delivery of radiation therapy. This is both presently achievable and improving. Techniques currently exist, that permit selective irradiation of tumor-bearing sites, while sparing sensitive normal tissues. Ongoing development in this area is expected to further increase accuracy.

In order to provide accurate targeting and delivery, it is first necessary to accurately define the extent of demonstrable disease and outline normal structures. Clear definitions of target and normal-tissue structures have been proposed and image-based tools have been developed to enable this process. One must properly account for the extent of microscopic disease. Finally, it is necessary to decrease uncertainties due to motion and positioning. Ongoing efforts to achieve these goals include better definition of the CTV through additional pathology studies and molecular imaging, better assessment, and correction of interfraction variation through the use of IGRT, and mitigation of intrafractional motion through the use of various motion-management techniques including explicit delineation of the ITV, gated treatment delivery, and breath-hold treatment delivery. As these techniques are further refined, margins can be adequately and safely reduced, leading perhaps to better tumor control and reduced morbidity.

REFERENCES

1. Almond PR, Biggs PJ, Coursey BM, et al. AAPM'S TG-51 protocol for clinical reference dosimetry of high-energy photon and electron beams. *Med Phys* 1999;26:1847–1870.
2. International Commission on Radiation Units and Measurements (ICRU) Report 50. *Prescribing, recording, and reporting photon beam therapy*. Bethesda, MD: ICRU, 1993.

3. International Commission on Radiation Units and Measurements (ICRU) Report 62. *Prescribing, recording, and reporting photon beam therapy (Supplement to ICRU Report 50)*. Bethesda, MD: ICRU, 1999.

4. Bushberg JT, Seibert JA, Leidholdt EM, et al. *The essential physics of medical imaging, Chap. 13*. Philadelphia, PA: Lippincott Williams & Wilkins, 2003.

5. Pan T, Lee TY, Rietzel E, et al. 4D-CT imaging of a volume influenced by respiratory motion on multi-slice CT. *Med Phys* 2004;31:333–340.

6. Keall PJ, Starkschall G, Shukla H, et al. Acquiring 4D thoracic CT scans using a multislice helical method. *Phys Med Biol* 2004;49:2053–2067.

7. Pizer Sm, Amburn EP, Austin JD, et al. Adaptive histogram equalization and its variations. *Comput Vis Graph Image Process* 1987;39:355–368.

8. Sherouse GW, Rosenman J, McMurry HL, et al. Automatic digital contrast enhancement of radiotherapy films. *Int J Radiat Oncol Biol Phys* 1987;13:801–806.

9. Davis LS. A survey of edge detection techniques. *Comput Graphics Imag Process* 1975;4:248–270.

10. Canny J. A computational approach to edge detection. *Trans Pattern Anal Mach Intell* 1986;8:679–698.

11. Lucignani G, Jereczek-Fossa BA, Orecchia R. The role of molecular imaging in precision radiation therapy for target definition, treatment planning optimization and quality control. *Eur J Nucl Med Mol Imaging* 2004;31:1059–1063.

12. Kass M, Witkin A, Terzopoulos D. Snakes: active contour models. *Int J Comput Vis* 1988;1:321–331.

13. McInerney T, Terzopoulos D. Deformable models in medical image analysis: a survey. *Med Image Anal* 1996;1:91–108.

14. Pekar V, McNutt TR, Kaus MR. Automated model-based organ delineation for radiotherapy planning in prostatic region. *Int J Radiat Oncol Biol Phys* 2004;60:973–980.

15. Ragan D, Starkschall G, McNutt T, et al. Semi-automated four-dimensional computed tomography segmentation using deformable models. *Med Phys* 2005;32:2254–2261.

16. Maintz JB, Viergever MA. A survey of medical image registration. *Med Image Anal* 1998;2:1–36.

17. Wells WM, Viola P, Atsumi H, et al. Multi-modal volume registration by maximization of mutual information. *Med Image Anal* 1996;1:35–51.

18. Baldwin BC, Mohan R. Shape guided image interpolation for radiation treatment planning. *Int J Radiat Oncol Biol Phys* 1993;27(Suppl 1):181–181.

19. Rasch C, Steenbakkers R, van Herk M. Target definition in prostate, head, and neck. *Semin Radiat Oncol* 2005;15:136–145.

20. Giraud P, Kantor G, Loiseau H, et al. Target definition in the thorax and central nervous system. *Semin Radiat Oncol* 2005;15:146–156.

21. Giraud P, Antoine M, Larrouy A, et al. Evaluation of microscopic tumor extension in non-small-cell lung cancer for three-dimensional conformal radiotherapy planning. *Int J Radiat Oncol Biol Phys* 2000;48:1015–1024.

22. Apisarnthanarax S, Elliott DD, El Naggar AK, et al. Determining optimal clinical target volume margins in head-and-neck cancer based on microscopic extracapsular extension of metastatic neck nodes. *Int J Radiat Oncol Biol Phys* 2006;64:678–683.

23. Teh BS, Bastasch MD, Mai WY, et al. Predictors of extracapsular extension and its radial distance in prostate cancer: implications for prostate IMRT, brachytherapy, and surgery. *Cancer J* 2003;9:454–460.

24. Coleman CN. Linking radiation oncology and imaging through molecular biology. *Radiology* 2003;228:29–35.

25. Ganslandt O, Stadlbauer A, Fahlbusch R, et al. Proton magnetic resonance spectroscopic imaging integrated into image-guided surgery: correlation to standard magnetic resonance imaging and tumor cell density. *Neurosurgery* 2005;56(Suppl 2):291–298.

26. Daisne JF, Duprez T, Weynand B, et al. Tumor volume in pharyngolaryngeal squamous cell carcinoma: comparison at CT, MR imaging, and FDG PET and validation with surgical specimen. *Radiology* 2004;233:93–100.

27. Chan R, He Y, Haque A, et al. Computed tomographic–pathologic correlation of gross tumor volume and clinical target volume in non–small cell lung cancer. *Pathol Lab Med* 2001;125:1469–1472.

28. Poon I, Fischbein N, Lee N, et al. A population-based atlas and clinical target volume for the head-and-neck lymph nodes. *Int J Radiat Oncol Biol Phys* 2004;59:1301–1311.

29. Ross CS, Hussey DH, Pennington EC, et al. Analysis of movement of intrathoracic neoplasms using ultrafast computerized tomography. *Int J Radiat Oncol Biol Phys* 1990;18:671–677.

30. Korin HW, Ehman RL, Riederer SJ, et al. Respiratory kinematics of the upper abdominal organs: a quantitative study. *Magn Reson Med* 1992;23:172–178.

31. Davies SC, Hill AL, Holmes RB, et al. Ultrasound quantitation of respiratory organ motion in the upper abdomen. *Br J Radiol* 1994;67:1096–1102.

32. Hanley J, Debois MM, Mah D, et al. Deep inspiration breath-hold technique for lung tumors; the potential value of target immobilization and reduced lung density in dose escalation. *Int J Radiat Oncol Biol Phys* 1999;45:603–611.

33. Wong JW, Sharpe MB, Jaffray DA, et al. The use of active breathing control (ABC) to reduce margin for breathing motion. *Int J Radiat Oncol Biol Phys* 1999;44:911–919.

34. Ohara K, Okumura T, Akisada M, et al. Irradiation synchronized with respiration gate. *Int J Radiat Oncol Biol Phys* 1989;17:853–857.

35. Shirato H, Shimizu S, Kunieda T, et al. Physical aspects of a real-time tumor-tracking system for gated radiotherapy. *Int J Radiat Oncol Biol Phys* 2000;48:1187–1195.

36. Coles CE, Hoole AC, Harden SV, et al. Quantitative assessment of inter-clinician variability of target volume delineation for medulloblastoma; quality assurance for the SIOP PNET 4 trial protocol. *Radiother Oncol* 2003;69:189–194.

37. van Herk M. Errors and margins in radiotherapy. *Semin Radiat Oncol* 2004;14:52–64.

38. Stroom JC, de Boer HC, Huizenga H, et al. Inclusion of geometrical uncertainties in radiotherapy treatment planning by means of coverage probability. *Int J Radiat Oncol Biol Phys* 1999;43:905–919.

39. Goitien M, Abrams M, Rowell DR, et al. Multidimensional treatment planning: II. Beam's eye view, back

projection, and projection through CT sections. *Int J Radiat Oncol Biol Phys* 1983;9:789–797.

40. Brewster L, Mageras GS, Mohan R. Automatic generation of beam apertures. *Med Phys* 1993;20:1337–1342.

41. Mohan R. Field shaping for three-dimensional conformal radiation therapy and multi-leaf collimation. *Semin Radiat Oncol* 1995;5:86–99.

42. Burman C, Armstrong J, Brewster L, et al. Dose distribution comparison for multi-leaf collimator and Cerrobend shaped fields for 3-dimensional lung plans. *Med Phys* 1993;20:925 (abstract).

43. Burman C, Leibel SA, Mohan R, et al. Comparison of dose distributions for 3D brain plans with Cerrobend and multi-leaf collimators. *Med Phys* 1994;21:885 (abstract).

44. LoSasso TJ, Chui CS, Kutcher GJ, et al. The use of a multi-leaf collimator for conformal radiotherapy of carcinomas of the prostate and nasopharynx. *Int J Radiat Oncol Biol Phys* 1993;25:161–170.

45. Galvin JM, Smith AR, Moeller RD, et al. Evaluation of multi-leaf collimator design for a photon beam. *Int J Radiat Oncol Biol Phys* 1992;23:789–801.

46. Galvin JM, Smith AR, Lally B. Characterization of a multi-leaf collimator system. *Int J Radiat Oncol Biol Phys* 1993;25:181–192.

47. Mohan R. *Secondary field shaping, asymmetrical collimators and multileaf collimators. Proceedings of AAPM, summer school.* Woodbury, NY: American Institute of Physics, 1990:307–345.

48. Fernandez EM, Dearnaley DP, Heisig S, et al. Suitability of a multi-leaf collimator as a standard block replacement for different anatomical sites. Proceedings of European Society of Therapeutic Radiology and Oncology second biennial meeting in physics, Prague, 1993.

49. International Commission on Radiation Units and Measurements. *Determination of absorbed dose in a patient by beams of X or gamma rays in radiotherapy procedures, Report 24.* Bethesda, MD: ICRU, 1976.

50. Mackie TR, Scrimger JW, Battista JJ. A convolution method of calculating dose for 15 MV x-rays. *Med Phys* 1985;12:188–196.

51. Mohan R, Chui C, Lidofsky L. Differential pencil beam dose computation model for photons. *Med Phys* 1986;13:64–73.

52. Van Dyk J, Barnett R, Cygler J, et al. Commissioning and quality assurance of treatment planning computers. *Int J Radiat Oncol Biol Phys* 1993;26:261–273.

53. Fraass BA, Doppke KP, Hunt MA, et al. Task Group 53: quality assurance for clinical radiotherapy treatment planning. *Med Phys* 1998;25:1773–1829.

54. Niemierko A, Goitein M. The use of variable grid spacing to accelerate dose calculations. *Med Phys* 1989;16:357–366.

55. Gifford KA, Followill DS, Liu HH, et al. Verification of the accuracy of a photon dose-calculation algorithm. *J Appl Clin Med Phys* 2002;3:26–45.

56. Starkschall G, Steadham RE, Popple RA, et al. Beam commissioning methodology for a 3D convolution/superposition photon dose algorithm. *J Appl Clin Med Phys* 2000;1:8–27.

57. Mohan R, Chui CS. Use of fast Fourier transforms in calculating dose distributions for irregularly shaped fields for three-dimensional treatment planning. *Med Phys* 1987;14:70–77.

58. Zhu Y, Boyer AL, Desobry GE. Dose distributions of x-ray fields as shaped with multi-leaf collimators. *Phys Med Biol* 1992;37:163–174.

59. Frank SJ, Forster KM, Stevens CW, et al. Treatment planning for lung cancer: traditional homogeneous point-dose prescription compared with heterogeneity-corrected dose-volume prescription. *Int J Radiat Oncol Biol Phys* 2003;56:1308–1318.

60. Shaley S, Bartel L, Therrien P, et al. The objective evaluation of alternative treatment plans: 1. Images of regret. *Int J Radiat Oncol Biol Phys* 1988;15:763–767.

61. Kessler ML, McShan DL, Fraass BA. Displays for three-dimensional treatment planning. *Semin Radiat Oncol* 1992;2:226–234.

62. Fraass BA, McShan DL. *3D treatment planning: 1. Overview of a clinical planning system. Proceedings of ninth international conference on the use of computers in radiation therapy,* Scheveningen, the Netherlands, 1987. Amsterdam, North Holland: Elsevier Science Publishers, 1987:273–276.

63. Chen GTY, Austin-Seymour M, Castro JR, et al. *Dose-volume histograms in treatment planning evaluation of carcinoma of the pancreas. Proceedings of the eight international conference on uses of computers in radiation therapy.* Toronto, Canada: Institute of Electrical and Electronic Engineers, 1984:264–268.

64. Niemierko A, Goitein M. Random sampling for evaluating treatment plans. *Med Phys* 1990;17:753–762.

65. Goitein M. The comparison of treatment plans. *Semin Radiat Oncol* 1992;2:246–256.

66. Mohan R, Mageras GS, Baldwin B, et al. Clinically relevant optimization of 3D conformal treatments. *Med Phys* 1992;19:933–944.

67. Kutcher GJ, Burman C. Calculation of complication probability factors for nonuniform normal tissue radiation: the effective volume method. *Int J Radiat Oncol Biol Phys* 1989;16:1623–1630.

68. Goitein M. Probability of controlling an inhomogeneously irradiated tumor. In: Zink S, ed. *Report of the working group on the evaluation of treatment planning for particle beam radiotherapy.* Bethesda, MD: National Cancer Institute, 1987:5.8.1–5.8.17.

69. Niemierko A, Goitein M. Implementation of a model for estimating tumor control probability for an inhomogeneously irradiated tumor. *Radiother Oncol* 1993;29:140–147.

70. Lyman JT. Complication probability as assessed from dose volume histograms. *Radiat Res* 1985;104:S13–S19.

71. Lyman JT, Wolbarst AB. Optimization of radiation therapy: 3. Method of assessing complication probabilities from dose-volume histograms. *Int J Radiat Oncol Biol Phys* 1987;13:103–109.

72. Jackson A, Kutcher GJ, Yorke ED. Probability of radiation induced complications for normal tissues with parallel architecture subject to nonuniform irradiation. *Med Phys* 1993;20:613–625.

73. Niemierko A, Goitein M. Calculation of normal tissue complication probability and dose-volume histogram reduction schemes for tissues with a critical element architecture. *Radiother Oncol* 1991;20:166–176.

74. Niemierko A, Goitein M. Modeling of normal tissue response to radiation: the critical volume model. *Int J Radiat Oncol Biol Phys* 1993;25:135–145.

75. Schultheiss TE, Orto CG. Models in radiotherapy: definition of decision criteria. *Med Phys* 1985;12:183–187.

76. Rubin P. In: Vaeth JM, ed. *Frontiers of radiation therapy and oncology.* Baltimore, MD: University Park, 1972: 489–511.

77. Kutcher GJ. *Quantitative plan evaluation. Proceedings of AAPM summer school.* Woodbury, NY: American Institute of Physics, 1990;998–1021.

78. Munro P. Portal imaging technology: past, present, and future. *Semin Radiat Oncol* 1995;5:115–133.

79. Gilhuijs KGA, van Herk M. Automatic on-line inspection of patient setup in radiation therapy using digital portal images. *Med Phys* 1993;20:667–677.

80. Jones SM, Boyer AL. Investigation of an FFT-based correlation technique for verification of radiation treatment setup. *Med Phys* 1991;18:1116–1125.

81. Chen QS, Defrise M, Deconinck F. Symmetric phase-only matched filtering of Fourier-Mellin transforms for image registration and recognition. *IEEE Trans Pattern Anal Mach Intell* 1994;16:1156–1168.

82. Mageras GS, Podmaniczky K, Mohan R. Model for computer controlled delivery of 3D conformal treatments. *Med Phys* 1992;19:945–954.

83. Kutcher GJ, Coia L, Gillin M, et al. Comprehensive QA for radiation oncology: report of AAPM Radiation Therapy Committee Task Group 40. *Med Phys* 1994;21:581–618.

84. Kutcher GJ, Mageras GS, Leibel SA. Control, correction and modeling of setup errors and organ motion. *Semin Radiat Oncol* 1995;5:134–145.

CHAPTER **13**

Intensity-Modulated Radiation Therapy

Arthur L. Boyer ■ Gary A. Ezzell ■ Cedric X. Yu

INTRODUCTION

The treatment techniques that are collectively known as intensity-modulated radiation therapy (IMRT) compose a broad class in a historical sequence of technical developments for improving local control of cancer by improving the physical delivery of external beam radiation. The mathematically precise geometric information about the patient's anatomy provided by computed tomography (CT) technology enables shaping radiation fields to conform to the projection of the treatment target volume for a radiotherapy beam directed toward a tumor. General deployment of this strategy enabled shaping internally uniform fields with computer-controlled multi-leaf collimators (MLCs) (1–7). This class of external beam treatment techniques has been conventionally known as *three-dimensional conformal radiation therapy* (3-DCRT). The more beams used, the more conformal the cumulative dose in the target. A special variant of this class is the conformal arc therapy method proposed by Takahashi (8). Takahashi envisioned using an MLC to produce a continuous, smoothly connected sequence of aperture shapes that conform to the projection of the target at each gantry angle as a cone beam is continuously rotated around the patient.

3-DCRT reduces the volume of tissue that is irradiated to the prescribed dose outside the target volume, allowing higher prescribed doses to be delivered within the tumor target volume for a given level of normal tissue complications. The magnitude of the normal tissue sparing can be estimated by comparing irradiation of a spherical target volume of diameter D by either four-square, orthogonal fields that enclose the target in a cubic high-dose region of volume D^3 or by many circular-shaped fields from all directions in three dimensions, ideally enclosing the target in a spherical high-dose region having a volume $(4/3)\,\pi\,(D/2)^3 = (\pi/6) \times D^3$. The ratio of these two volumes of tissue irradiated to the prescribed dose is a factor of $\pi/6 = 0.52$. The clinical gain of 3-DCRT is the reduction of tissue irradiated to the prescribed dose by up to a factor of about 2. The full radiobiological advantages of 3-DCRT are a subject of research. Having less damaged normal tissue, especially vasculature, in closer proximity to the tissue stroma within the target volume appears to impart tolerance to higher prescribed tumor doses. However, for more complex tumor shapes, such as target volumes that contain invaginations, internal hollows, and bifurcations, 3-DCRT techniques using internally uniform fluence cannot deliver a complex conforming dose structure. However, one can compute modulations of the internal intensities of shaped fields (9–11) whose sum will produce a relatively uniform dose within a complex target shape while maintaining reduction of dose outside the target in a neighboring organ at risk. One starts with the desired result (a uniform conformal target dose that excludes organs at risk) and works backward toward incident beam intensities, earning the technique the popular name, *inverse treatment planning*. The beam intensities required to deliver the required nonuniform beam intensities can be produced using motion of the MLCs during the irradiation to spatially modulate the intensity, hence the name *intensity-modulated radiation therapy*. This chapter discusses a number of implementations of IMRT that have been put into practice.

Development of IMRT

The development of IMRT was born from the wide adoption of 3DCRT in the 1980s. Brahme et al. demonstrated (9,10) that if the intensities of radiation can be modulated across a radiation field, then the increased freedom would afford a greater ability to shape the volume of high doses, to better conform to the target than 3DCRT. Subsequent to that work, a large number of publications emerged on the use of computer optimization techniques for radiotherapy treatment planning. In 1992, Convery and Rosenbloom derived a mathematical formula for realizing intensity modulation with the dynamic movement of a collimator jaw (11). In 1994–1995, works were published to demonstrate the feasibility of using MLCs for intensity modulation of fixed-gantry fields in either a dynamic mode (continuous movement during radiation) or static mode (alternating motion of leaves with irradiation with motionless leaves) (12–17). The first clinical implementations of the IMRT technique using dynamic MLC leaf motion was at Memorial Sloan Kettering Cancer Center in 1996 using software developed in-house (18). In 1997, IMRT was first planned using commercially available software from the NOMOS Corporation and delivered using a commercially available Varian MLC at Stanford University (19).

In 1993, another form of IMRT using rotational fan beams, called tomotherapy, was proposed by Mackie et al. (20). The idea was quickly commercialized by NOMOS Corporation (21,22) with the trade name Peacock™. The NOMOS Peacock™ was the first commercial IMRT system using a dedicated short-stroke multi-vane intensity modulating collimator (MIMic), as an add-on binary collimator that opens and closes under computer control. The treatment table had to be precisely indexed from one slice to the next. For this reason, the Peacock™ device is often referred to as serial tomotherapy. Serial tomotherapy was first implemented clinically at Baylor College of Medicine in March 1994 (23). Most IMRT treatments delivered in the 1990s employed serial tomotherapy. Helical tomotherapy (HT) was then developed by Tomotherapy, Inc., as a dedicated rotational IMRT system with a slip-ring rotating gantry. It was made commercially available in 2002. More efficient delivery was achieved by continuous gantry rotation and simultaneous treatment couch translation.

In 1995, Yu proposed another form of IMRT called intensity-modulated arc therapy (IMAT) (17). Like tomotherapy, IMAT delivers photon radiation treatment over a continuous arc. Instead of using rotating fan beams as in tomotherapy, IMAT uses rotational cone beams shaped by an MLC to achieve intensity modulation. The strategy was to convert the intensity patterns into segments delivered by a sequence of arcs without table translation. Based on the fact that many beam modulation sequences can yield the same intensity pattern, it is possible to find an MLC aperture at each beam angle such that aperture shapes at successive angles are connected geometrically. The stacks of overlapping beam apertures can then be delivered with multiple overlapping arcs. An initial proof-of-principle study demonstrated that IMAT would be feasible as a treatment delivery technique. The requirement of geometric connectivity of apertures from neighboring angles adds significant complexity to the planning of IMAT treatments. IMRT is not the only way to take advantage of the geometric arrangements of the target and the surrounding avoidance structures. The CyberKnife™ system (Accuray, Sunnyvale, CA), which uses small circular x-ray beams generated by an x-band linear accelerator mounted on a robot (24) to deliver the radiation to the target, does not explicitly modulate the intensity of a beam, but is able to deliver highly conformal treatments.

The rapid adoption of IMRT shortly thereafter was facilitated by additions to the United States Federal funding mechanism for radiation oncology that occurred around the year 2000. In the late 1990s, Medicare began to introduce the hospital outpatient prospective payment system (HOPPS). As part of this system, a payment differential mechanism was included to encourage the introduction of new technology. A Medicare billing code for IMRT treatment was added to the current procedural terminology (CPT) in 2001. The technique-specific payment differential created a financial incentive to purchase treatment planning systems and linear accelerators that included cutting-edge technology for IMRT to improve quality of care, reduce health care costs, and recoup capital costs. Thus, through this explicit federal policy mechanism that encouraged "early adopters," IMRT became available in radiotherapy centers much more rapidly than it would have otherwise (25).

IMRT has been studied extensively for the last two decades. A search on the acronym at the web sites of the major radiation oncology journals yields lists of citations numbering in the thousands. Technical issues and clinical questions are likely to be subjects of research and development for the foreseeable future.

Principles of IMRT Planning and Delivery

Up to a point, treatment planning for IMRT differs little from treatment planning for 3DCRT. The concepts introduced by the International Commission on Radiation Units and Measurements (ICRU) No. 50 are applied to delineate a planning target volume (PTV) as an expansion of a clinical target volume (CTV) that is in turn based on a gross tumor volume (GTV). The expansions are theoretically based on uncertainties in the segmentation, patient positioning, and respiration motion during treatment, and the displacement of structures by physiological processes from one treatment day to the next. An extension of digital imaging and communications in medicine (DICOM) formats, the DICOM-RT format, is the standard for file transfers of imaging studies, structure sets, dose distributions, and treatment sequences. Computer workstations are commercially available for segmenting the target structures and the normal structures using diagnostic studies. Geometric correlation of the disparate studies (CT, MRI, and PET/CT), known as *fusion*, allows the radiation oncologist to take advantage of the imaging advantages peculiar to each type of study. The radiation oncologist can identify the 3D surfaces of these structures by drawing contours along their boundaries in sequential reconstruction planes using a growing suite of artificial-intelligence segmentation tools.

The way IMRT, including IMAT and tomotherapy, spares critical structures is by redistributing the normal tissue dose to less critical regions and by reducing the high-dose volume to just cover the target. For a given case, the geometric arrangement of the target and its surrounding avoidance structures dictates the preferred beam angles, and along each beam angle, the preferred locations at which the radiation is delivered to the tumor. The calculation of fluence required to achieve a desired dose distribution bears certain similarities to the reconstruction of CT scans. How IMRT fluence profiles may be computed has been illustrated by Bortfeld and Webb (26) based on earlier work by Brahme (9) using a simplified two-dimensional (2D) model. This 2D test case contains an OAR of radius r_0 embedded within the side of a PTV of radius r (Fig. 13.1). The OAR is centered on $(x_0, y_0) = (0, -4)$. Using the approximations and methods similar to Brahme (9), an analytic ideal fluence, ϕ, for a continuous arc field

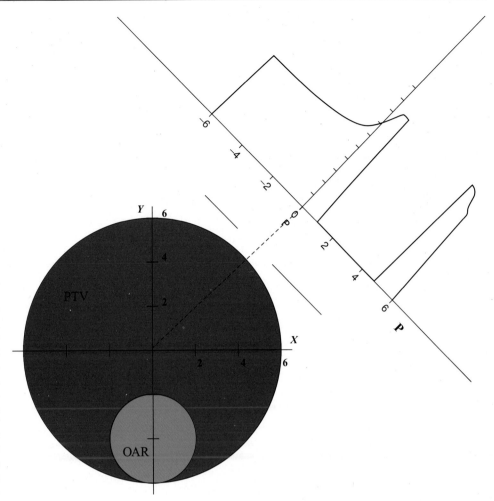

Figure 13.1. Geometry of simple two-dimensional (2D) test case. The planning target volume (PTV) consists of a circle whose radius is $r = 4$ cm. The OAR is a circle whose radius is $r_0 = 2$ cm and is embedded at the bottom side of the PTV. An ideal fluence can be calculated analytically for this case. The fluence in the solution at an angle $\phi = 45$ degrees is depicted as a function of the distance from the center of the treatment beam, p.

as a function of gantry angle ϕ can be calculated based on three conditions on rays passing through the PTV and OAR structures:

$$\Phi(p) = \begin{cases} \dfrac{\left|p - \Delta p_\phi\right|}{\sqrt{(p - \Delta p_\phi)^2 - r_0^2}} & if \ \left|p - \Delta p_\phi\right| > r_0 + w \ and \ |p| \le r \\[3mm] \dfrac{r_0 + w}{\sqrt{(r_0 + w)^2 - r_0^2}} & if \ r_0 \le \left|p - \Delta p_\phi\right| \le r_0 + w \\[3mm] 0 & if \ \left|p - \Delta p_\phi\right| < r_0 \ \ or \ \ |p| > r \end{cases}$$

EQUATION (13.1)

where

$$\Delta p_\phi = x_0 \cos\phi - y_0 \sin\phi$$

Rays that meet the first condition pass through the PTV and are modulated to compensate for rays that are excluded because they pass through the OAR. Rays that meet the second condition pass within a distance w of the OAR. Their amplitudes are cut off at the fixed value given in the equation to avoid a singularity of infinite magnitude that

would otherwise exist at the boundary of the OAR. Rays that meet the third condition are set to zero because they either pass through the OAR or pass outside the PTV. A one-dimensional (1D) beam fluence calculated for an angle $\phi = 45$ degrees at which the beam is directed toward the center of the PTV is shown in Figure 13.1. The entire computed fluence is illustrated as a sinogram plot of fluence across the beam as a function of gantry angle in Figure 13.2. This approach allows no fluence to be directed through the OAR resulting in a zero-fluence valley through the sinogram in Figure 13.2. This simple idealized inverse solution can be modified to apply to tomotherapy and fixed-gantry multiple-field IMRT by using the appropriate parts of the sinogram in Figure 13.2. A search for a generalized 3D analytic inverse solution has not as yet yielded a widely applicable and practical solution (27). The most fruitful approach has been to calculate practical fluence distributions *numerically* using an optimization scheme based on a cost function that reflects some quantitative assessment of the dose distribution that a calculated fluence will deliver. These schemes generally allow some fluence to pass through the OARs to build up a dose in the PTV. Over the last decade, many new methods of treatment delivery using multiple fixed beams or rotating beams have been developed. No matter what form of delivery is

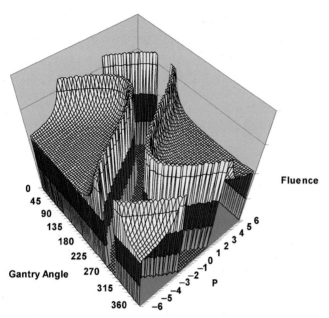

Figure 13.2. The computed fluence (arbitrary units) as a sinogram plot of fluence across the beam as a function of gantry angle. This calculation required that no fluence be delivered to the OAR resulting in the region of zero fluence that winds across the sinogram.

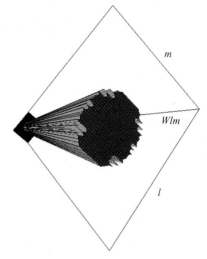

Figure 13.3. A depiction of a beam viewed as a bundle of beamlets. Each beamlet in the bundle can be identified by a row index, l and a column index, m. The fluence within each beamlet is proportional to the beamlet weight or bixel value, $w_{l,m}$.

used, the radiation dose is delivered to the target through multiple radiation fields of varying sizes and shapes. To take full advantage of the geometric arrangements of a specific clinical case, a large number of fields, also referred to as segments, subfields, or apertures, is needed. The number of field segments is case dependent and in general, the more complex the geometric arrangement, the larger the number of field segments required to achieve the optimal plan (28). Where these apertures are placed—within a limited number of beam angles or spaced around the patient as one or more arcs—has been shown to be less important through plan quality comparisons.

Rotational deliveries generally spread the normal tissue dose to a greater volume of normal structures than IMRT methods employing a limited number of fixed gantry beam directions. The key principle is that to deposit a given integral dose to the target, it is necessary to deposit an irreducible integral dose to the surrounding structures (a transit dose), as dictated by the physics of dose deposition. IMRT is appropriate for clinical cases in which delivering a lower dose to a larger volume of normal tissue is better than delivering a larger dose to a smaller volume of normal tissue. Accordingly, volume considerations must be carefully given for parallel organs, such as the lung, and for pediatric applications.

The dose prescription for IMRT is more structured and complex than the single-valued prescription used to guide pre-IMRT therapy. Ideally, one would prescribe some dose value to every voxel in the patient. In practice, blocks of high therapeutic dose and dose limits are prescribed to fractions of the target volume containing many voxels, and dose limits are assigned to fractions of the OAR. A dose calculation is built up within a calculation matrix using

some form of x-ray beam modeling. The dose calculation is based on the beamlets associated with each treatment beam (Fig. 13.3). For a beam directed toward the patient from a given angle, the elements of the 2D array of beamlet weights, $w_{l,m}$ (arranged in rows labeled with an index l, and columns labeled with an index m) are termed *bixel* weights. The beam intensity map will be proportional to the matrix of bixel weights. A set of bixels, $w_{k,l,m}$, is associated with the k beam direction (Fig. 13.4). This 3D set of

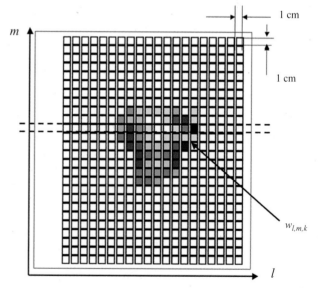

Figure 13.4. An example of a beam intensity map. Each square represents a bixel. The rows are labeled with an index l. The columns are labeled with an index m. This intensity map is associated with a beam direction determined by gantry angle and couch rotation labeled with an index k. Each square represents a bixel with a weight $w_{l,m,k}$. The bixels in which the beam is always blocked by MLC leaves are displayed as white. Shades of gray are used in this figure to indicate levels of beam intensity, $w_{l,m,k}$, black corresponding to the highest intensity.

beamlet weights drives the dose calculation in the 3D voxel matrix, $D_c(x, y, z) = D_c(r)$. The dose calculation that estimates the dose delivered by each beam is based on the values in the beam's bixel matrix. Once the dose is calculated for every beam, the voxels within the patient's skin surface will contain the calculated dose values. The goal of the optimization process is to select those bixel weights that deliver the most favorable dose distribution. The dose distribution is assessed using some mathematical technique for approximating the subjective medical value of the shape and magnitude of the computed dose distribution. This assessment is called *the cost function*, or alternatively, *the objective function*. The simplest cost function simply computes the square of the differences between the computed dose, $D_c(r)$, and doses prescribed for the target volumes and the OARs, $D_p(r)$.

$$F = \sum_i C_i [D_c(r) - D_p(r)]_i^2 \qquad \text{EQUATION (13.2)}$$

where i is the structure index and C_i is the weighting factor used to stress the relative importance of different structures. As the computed dose distribution becomes more similar to the prescribed dose distribution, the value of this cost function decreases. Therefore, the goal of the optimization procedure is to minimize F. What is not shown explicitly in Equation 13.2 is the assignment of dose prescriptions to the planning structures; the target volumes and the OAR. The quadratic cost function given in Equation 13.2 also does not differentiate the target and the OARs. In realistic cost functions, lower doses in the OARs than the prescribed dose limit will be encouraged rather than penalized. Many other measures of the "goodness" of the computed treatment plan have been investigated. Particularly, intriguing are cost functions based on nonlinear tumor response models. Another very general approach is to create a cost function that is itself a summation of many "costlet," functions of relevant parameters such as dose points on the dose–volume histograms (DVH), tissue complication probability, normal tissue complication probability, equivalent uniform dose, and so on. A dose–volume minimum objective is usually applied to a target structure. This objective is met if the dose calculated in all voxels that make up a specified percent of the designated structure volume is greater than or equal to the structure dose objective value.

IMRT is most commonly delivered using the MLC. There are two basic ways to use the MLC (29). One method, called the *step-and-shoot* or *segmented multileaf collimation* (SMLC) approach, alternates between setting MLC apertures without delivering dose and delivering small increments of dose without moving the MLC leaves (30). The dose delivered by SMLC along a beamlet is determined by the amount of time the beamlet remains in an open gap between opposed MLC leaves. The other method, called the *sliding window* or *dynamic multileaf collimation* (DMLC) approach, employs an MLC control

system that can deliver dose while simultaneously moving the leaves by interpolating leaf positions between control points (15). The dose delivered by DMLC along a beamlet is determined by the amount of time the beamlet remains in the gap between continuously moving opposed leaves. There is little, if any, intrinsic difference between the two methods if they are implemented with equivalent fast computer-controlled electromechanical systems.

In both serial and HT implementations, intensity modulation is achieved with a binary MLC, consisting of two opposing banks of tungsten leaves operating in either open or closed states. When all the leaves are open, the binary MLC shapes a fan beam with a width equal to the total leaf travel of the two opposing leaves. Each of the two rows of beamlets is independently controlled to open and close by a computer, and the fraction of time a beamlet is open determines the relative intensity of the beamlet. As this fan beam continuously rotates around the patient, the relative intensities of the beamlets are adjusted with the opening and closing of the corresponding leaf of the binary collimator, allowing the radiation to be delivered to the tumor through the most preferable directions and locations of the patient.

Both serial and HT systems offer a "turn-key" approach to IMRT implementation with the planning system specifically designed for the delivery unit. The Peacock™ system, developed by NOMOS Corporation, optimizes beam intensities for a sequence of 55 radiation beams (every 5 degrees) around the patient based on dose constraints using a simulated annealing optimization algorithm. It encompasses most of the features of current inverse treatment planning systems as described by Carol et al. (22,23). Because the serial tomotherapy uses an add-on device to an existing linac, non-coplanar arcs with the couch at a small angle to its default position are also allowed. HT utilizes a dedicated ring gantry and a computer-controlled couch. The treatment plan is delivered through a 6 MV x-ray fan beam in continuous rotation around the long axis of the patient while the patient is slowly translating through the gantry aperture at a constant speed, which is predetermined by the pitch factor and the gantry period. Each gantry rotation is approximated by 51 equally spaced static beam projections with 64 binary MLC leaves in each projection. Both serial and HT achieve intensity variations of the beamlets with a binary MLC. The degree of modulation by the binary MLC is determined by the gantry period, the modulation factor, and the inherent transit time of leaf motion (<40 ms). Because each MLC is individually controlled and allows full intensity modulation at each projection during dynamic gantry rotation, the degree of intensity modulated is less constrained as compared to MLCs that move continuously to shape extended radiation fields. Therefore, theoretically speaking, tomotherapy provides a planning system with greater freedom to use highly modulated beams than MLC delivery of IMRT employing fixed cone beams.

When a broad photon beam is collimated into a fan beam with the width of only that of two beamlets, most of

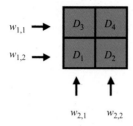

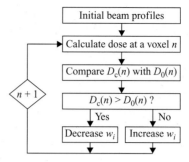

Figure 13.5. A simplified dose calculation matrix used to illustrate inverse treatment planning optimization. In order to make the example easy to calculate, a two-dimensional (2D) matrix consisting of only four voxels is considered. Voxels 1, 3, and 4 are the target structure and voxel 2 is an avoidance structure. In the example shown here, the prescribed dose values (in arbitrary units) in the voxels are set to $D_1 = 1.0$, $D_2 = 0.5$, $D_3 = 1.0$, and $D_4 = 1.0$. Two simplified beams are shown schematically. The bixels in a lateral beam have initial weights $w_{1,1}$ and $w_{1,2}$. The bixels in the vertical beam are indicated to have weights $w_{2,1}$ and $w_{2,2}$. The objective of the optimization is to select weights for the bixels that cause calculated doses in the voxels to be as close as possible to the prescribed doses. For this example, the initial bixel values for Beam 1 will both be set to 0.5 and the initial bixel values for Beam 2 will be set to 0.4.

the x-ray photons generated in the target are blocked, leading to inefficient usage of the monitor units (MUs) and long treatment times for large targets. To compensate for the inefficiency, HT uses a high dose rate of 880 MU/min. The gantry rotation period ranges from 15 to 60 seconds, depending on the fractionation size, the modulation factor, and the pitch. The width of the fan beam can also be preselected in a range of 1.0 to 5.0 cm as a trade-off between the resolution of the intensity pattern and the delivery efficiency.

Treatment Planning for IMRT

The cost function, $F(w_i)$, can be considered to be a function of a space whose dimension is the number of variables, that is, the number of beamlet weights. For IMRT, this is something on the order of 10,000 variables depending on the size of the beamlets, the size of the fields, and the number of beams. A sophisticated computer algorithm is required to minimize the cost function efficiently and effectively. A number of such algorithms have been implemented and are available commercially. To gain an appreciation of how this optimization process works, we

Figure 13.6. A Schematic flow diagram of an iterative process for optimizing the simple example.

will consider a very simple case using a 2D dose matrix containing only four voxels labeled (1) to (4) in Figure 13.5. Three of the voxels, (1) to (3), contain a target for which the dose prescription $D_p = 1$ and one voxel (4) contains an organ at risk for which the prescription will be $D_p = 0.5$. The dose is to be delivered by two beams, one directed horizontally and one delivered vertically. Each beam contains only two beamlets. For example, beamlet 1 of beam 1 irradiates voxels 1 and 2, and beamlet 2 of beam 1 irradiates voxels 3 and 4. A flow diagram of an iterative procedure for optimizing the bixel values is illustrated in Figure 13.6. One starts with an initial guess at the beamlet weights. One calculates the doses delivered by these weights and then compares the dose computed in the voxels with the dose prescribed for the voxels by a const function. Many different cost functions have been employed experimentally and commercially. One cost function computes the average dose difference along the beamlet path through the dose matrix. If the dose averaged over the beamlet voxel path is too large, one reduces the beamlet weight. If the dose in the voxels is too small, one increases the beamlet weight. To carry out this step, one needs a table that maps the beamlets to the voxels and vice versa. One then continues to the next beamlet until all the beamlets have been adjusted for all the voxels. At this point one has computed an entirely new set of beamlet weights. Next, one recomputes the dose distribution with this revised set of beamlet weights (as in Fig. 13.7). Then, one starts at the first beamlet again, and makes adjustments throughout a second iteration. By repeating this cycle many times, one gradually approaches a stable set of beamlet weights (Fig. 13.8). The cost function is used to assess the progress of the

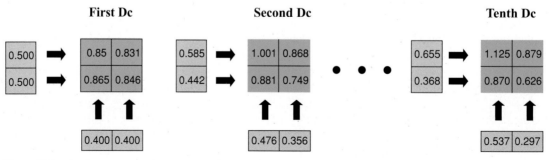

Figure 13.7. The doses computed using bixel values at the first, second, and tenth iteration steps in the simple example.

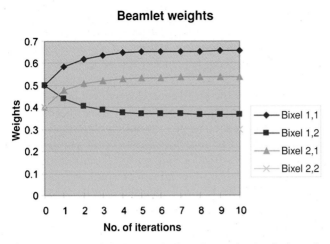

Figure 13.8. Plot of bixel values for beamlets in the simple example as a function of iteration number. After about the fifth iteration, the beamlet weights have converged.

algorithm. For this example, the cost function is given in Figure 13.9. In this example, after 10 iterations, the cost function no longer changes significantly with further iterations. At this point the algorithm has done about as well as it can do. For this example, the dose matrix after 10 iterations is given on the right side of Figure 13.7. The prescribed doses were not achieved. However, the achieved dose is within ~10% of the prescribed dose and a clinically significant difference was achieved between the dose to the target volume and the dose to the organ at risk. The dose to the target volume was not uniform. However, it is uniform within a tolerable range. Similar features are generally exhibited with the inverse planning for clinical cases for which the numbers of voxels, bixels, and beams are considerably greater than this illustrative calculation.

Different algorithms use different search strategies to minimize the cost function. One search strategy changes beamlet weights along the descending gradient of the cost function, $F(w_i)$. One selects an initial set of beamlet weights, $w_i = (w_1, w_2, w_3, \ldots)$, the cost function $F(w_i)$, and the local down-hill gradient, $-grad\ F(w_i)$. On selects a step size Δ_i to compute weights that take a step from w_i to the

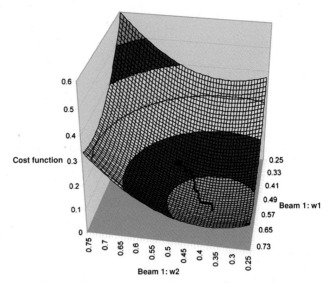

Figure 13.10. A graph of the cost function surface computed in two of the four dimensions of the bixel space for the simple example. The bixel values for Beam 2 were fixed at their optimal values, and the portion of the cost function surface was computed as a function of a range of bixel values for Beam 1 in the vicinity of their optimal values. The locus of the starting values used in the iteration for the bixels of Beam 1 (0.5) is indicated by a small oval. The trajectory of the iterative process is indicated schematically by a red path. The optimal bixel values ($w_{1,1} = 0.655$ and $w_{1,2} = 0.368$) are found at the minimum of the cost function surface where the cost function is slightly over 0.06 in this example.

point $w_i + \Delta_i$ along the down-hill direction of the gradient. After taking this step, one recomputes the dose distribution based on the revised beamlet weights along with a revised value of the cost function and repeats the process. This method will find the minima in the cost function $F(w_i)$ nearest to the starting point. This process is conceptualized in Figure 13.10, a cost function for the simple illustrative case. In this case, the cost function space has four dimensions, but only two dimensions associated with the two beamlet weights of beam 1 are given in Figure 13.10. The minimum found by the iterative procedure is illustrated. Unfortunately, there is no guarantee that there is only one minimum in every case. If the optimization algorithm gets trapped in a local minimum far from the global minimum, the treatment plan may be unsatisfactory. Nevertheless, variants of the down-hill gradient search approach are used widely in commercially available treatment planning systems.

To avoid getting trapped in a local minimum, simulated annealing uses a stochastic strategy, whereby some uphill changes are accepted in addition to the down-hill changes (Fig. 13.11). As long as a change ΔF in the cost function F is negative (e.g., the plan is being improved), the change in a beamlet weight is accepted. When the change in the beamlet weight results in an increase in the cost function, a probability of accepting the change is computed using $P = \exp(-\Delta F/kT)$ where kT is a variable that is used to gradually decrease the probability of accepting an uphill change as long as the search continues. This allows the

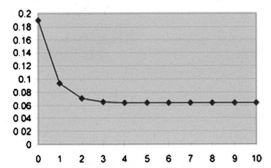

Figure 13.9. Plot of the cost function used for the simple example as a function of iteration number. The cost function has reached a stable value of about 0.06 after 10 iterations, close to an asymptotic limit.

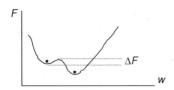

Figure 13.11. A schematic plot illustrating a cost function as a function of a generalized bixel vector, w. The cost function is shown to have two minima. By using simulating annealing, the search for the minimum is given a chance to escape from the higher minimum and enter into the lower minimum.

search to get out of local minima into deeper minima that may be nearby as illustrated schematically in Figure 13.11.

Intensity Modulation

It is fairly obvious that the shape of a 1D beam profile delivered by a static or dynamic leaf sequence is determined by the positions of the leaf ends set at each instance or control point of the sequence. It is also easy to see that there is more than one way to achieve a given profile. This is illustrated in Figure 13.12. The top of the figure depicts a simple 1D ideal fluence pattern having a maximum of three levels near one end. Any completely described profile of finite length must, by definition, start and end at zero intensity. To reach a single maximum of M levels, the profile intensity must increase by M fluence steps (delivered as some fixed number of MUs in each step). Each step up is counted as a setting of a leaf whether the leaf moves or not (assume that it is the left-hand leaf in Figure 13.12, designated the A-leaf). After reaching the maxima, the profile intensity must be decreased by M steps down at positions where the right-hand leaf (designated the B-leaf) has been positioned. The six sequences depicted in the lower portion of Figure 13.12, each consisting of three

instances, all sum up to the profile in the top of the figure. It has been pointed out that any SMLC profile with a single maximum that requires M leaf-end positions could be created by $M!$ unique sequences (31). In Figure 13.12, the first sequence is a "close-in" strategy that starts with the largest extent of the profile and closes down on the maxima. The last instance depicted in Figure 13.12 is the sweeping window strategy that will be described in the subsequent text. In the case illustrated in Figure 13.12 there are $M! = 3! = 6$ unique sequences. The order in which the leaves are set in these sequences is not considered in this calculation. If you consider all permutations of the instances in which the positions are set, there are $(M!)$ (2) possible sequences.

Intuitively, as the profile becomes more structured, the number of possible sequences will increase. Webb considered the more general case in which there are multiple maxima (32). The calculation is illustrated in Figure 13.13. A 1D profile is shown with peak intensities of levels H_1 and H_2. In general, there can be multiple maxima with levels H_1, H_2, H_3, ..., each peak characterized by a change in gradient of the profile from positive to negative. In general, let max be the total number of maxima. Between any two maxima is a minimum that drops to P_1, P_2, ..., each minimum is characterized by a change in slope of the profile from negative to positive. The two potential minima at the beginning and end of the profile are not counted. Therefore, there will be max – 1 such minima. Webb (32) has shown that the number of physically achievable leaf sequences that produce the discrete profile is given by

$$A = \frac{H_1! \cdot H_2! \cdot H_3! \cdot \ldots H_{max}!}{P_1! \cdot P_2! \cdot \ldots P_{max-1}!} \qquad \text{EQUATION (13.3)}$$

This can be a very large number of possible step-and-shoot types of sequences that all create the same discrete

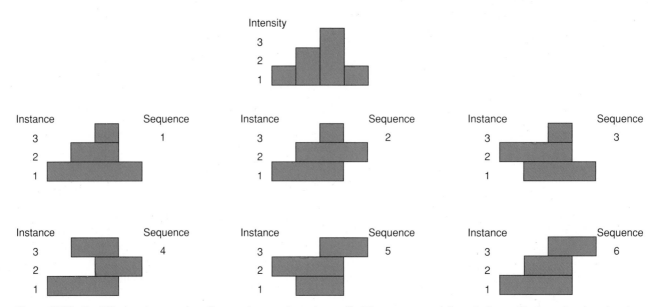

Figure 13.12. Six different sequences that all create the same intensity profile. The top center subfigure is the profile, intensity plotted against positions across the field. The bottom six subfigures show different sequences of three gaps that all lead to the same cumulative intensity profile.

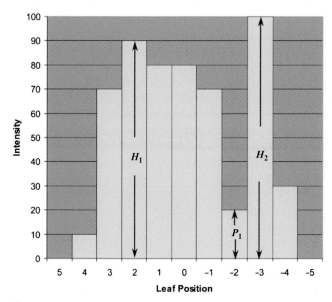

Figure 13.13. A more general one-dimensional (1D) beam profile that contains two maxima separated by a single minima. The total number of different sequences that can produce this profile is 9! X 10!/2! = 6.58 × 10^{11}.

profile. However, for the 1D case, one can still carry out an exhaustive search for a solution that is, in some sense, optimal. For MLC systems that do not allow inter-digitations and leaf-end abutment, the number of physically achievable sequences is smaller. The reduction depends on the details of the MLC system . Webb has calculated a typical value for an Elekta MLC to be ≈10^{94}. In general, an exhaustive search of all possible 2D leaf sequences for an optimal leaf sequence is impractical. Either the delivery sequences must be computed by some specific algorithm or an efficient optimization algorithm must be used to search iteratively for an optimum in this large search space.

Given that one has at hand the technical means to create DMLC and SMLC leaf sequences, and given that there are multiple sequences (in fact, billions) possible for richly structured intensity-modulated beams, what is the best way to determine a leaf sequence to deliver a desired intensity-modulated beam? Methods by which arbitrary x-ray beam intensity profiles may be produced through dynamic jaws or MLCs have been extensively investigated (11,12,15,16,33,34,35,36) considering exhaustive searches, optimization iteration, linear programming, or direct aperture computation to minimize the total beam delivery time.

One commonly used dynamic delivery technique is the so-called sliding window or DMLC technique where both leaves start at one side of the area to be irradiated and move unidirectionally, at different speeds, to the other side (15). The intensity profile to be delivered consists of linear segments of straight lines between closely spaced control points. The delivery is realized by a series of velocity-modulated motions of the leaves with the x-ray beam delivering dose at a constant dose rate.

The required intensity pattern can be expressed as $\Phi_j(x_i) = \mathrm{MU}_{i,j}$ where i (an index locating a point along a leaf trajectory) and j (an index numbering leaves) are indices for the 2D coordinates of finite pencil beams. The leaf sequence trajectory consists of specifications of the positions of the two leaves in each opposing leaf pair as a function of accumulated MUs during the delivery of the field. We will use the convention that the leaves move from left to right and that leaf A will be the trailing leaf on the left and leaf B will be the leading leaf on the right. The sequence of leaf positions along the X-axis can be denoted as $X_A(\mathrm{MU}_n)$ and $X_B(\mathrm{MU}_n)$, where the index n enumerates the sequence of the cumulative meter-set weight (CMW). We will plot the leaf trajectory by placing the independent variable, CMW, on the ordinate axis (Y-axis) and the dependent variables, the A-leaf and B-leaf positions, on the abscissa axis (X-axis). In the practical implementation, the trajectories are ordered pairs of numbers. In each pair, one number is the leaf position and the other is the CMW.

Let $\Phi(x)$ be the fluence down the center of the trajectory of a leaf pair. One way to deliver a prescribed fluence is to determine the arrival "times" at x, $t_A(x)$ for leaf A and $t_B(x)$ for leaf B. The units of the arrival times are expressed in units of CMW. The irradiation "time" interval at x between the opening of a beamlet by leaf B and the shielding of a beamlet by leaf A can be written as

$$\tau(x) = t_A(x) - t_B(x) = \Phi(x)/\Phi_0 \qquad \text{Equation (13.4)}$$

The maximum velocity that the leaves can move is $V_{\max}$. The leaf velocity as a function of the leaf position for the dynamic leaf sequence has been derived independently by several authors:

$$v(x) = V_{\max}/[1 \pm V_{\max} \cdot (d\Phi/dx)] \qquad \text{Equation (13.5)}$$

where the positive sign applies to regions of positive fluence gradient and the negative sign applies to regions of negative fluence gradient. The leaves start the sequence closed at the left side of the field and end the sequence closed together at the right side of the field (e.g., Fig. 13.14). In the initial region and in any subsequent region in which the fluence gradient is positive, the leading leaf, B, moves with the maximum velocity and the trailing leaf A moves along a trajectory with a modulated velocity determined by the fluence profile gradient (see preceding equation). In those regions in which the fluence gradient is negative, the trailing leaf, leaf A, moves with the maximum velocity, while the leading leaf moves along a trajectory determined by the velocity as calculated in Equation 13.5. The DMLC method is a highly efficient delivery technique because the beam does not have to be switched off during the delivery process. However, the quality assurance (QA) procedures for this technique require consideration of the precise location of the effective radiation field edge and the stability

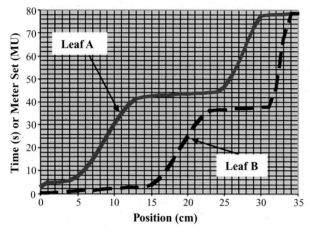

Figure 13.14. An example of the dynamic multileaf collimation (DMLC) continuous leaf position trajectories of a sliding window sequence for one leaf pair. The arrival time of the opposing leaves (leaf A and leaf B) are plotted against leaf position. The arrival time would commonly be replaced by the cumulative meter-set weight (CMW) in units of MU in a practical implementation. A similar trajectory is calculated for each pair of leaves being used to modulate a field at a fixed gantry position.

of leaf speed to ensure that the DMLC performs in accordance with the instruction of the leaf sequence file.

Consider next a strategy that generates an SMLC or step-and-shoot sequence (12). Figure 13.15 depicts a simple example of an intensity pattern. This pattern was computed for the anterior field out of nine fields used to treat a relatively small prostate PTV. This example will be used to illustrate one of the step-and-shoot leaf sequencing methods. The intensity in this 9×5 cm field is expressed using eight nonzero discrete intensity levels, 10 through 80. Five 1-cm wide leaf tracks (numbered 18–22 in Figure 13.15) are to be used to generate the intensity pattern. The delivery sequence is first determined independently for each

profile. We will use the profile determined for leaf pair 19 in Figure 13.15 as an example. The discrete intensity profile for leaf track 19 is shown separately in Figure 13.16. One assumes that one will modulate the intensity along the profile by sweeping the leading leaf, 19B and the following leaf, 19A, from left to right along the X-axis. The first step in this procedure is to divide the total relative beam intensity into a number of equal intervals of width $\Delta\Phi$ as indicated in the illustration. In this case $\Delta\Phi = 10$. The second step in the procedure is to find the x-positions at which the profile passes through the centers of these intensity increment bins as one traces the profile from left to right. Black and white circles in Figure 13.16A indicate these points. The problem has been defined such that the algorithm will find an even number of such points. The third step is to sort the coordinate points into two groups.

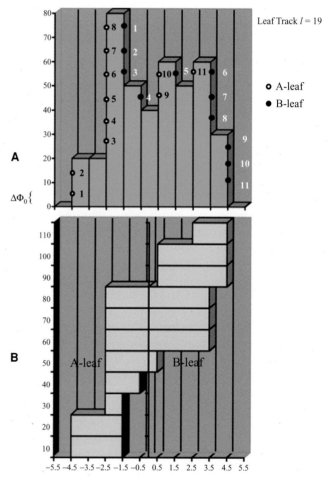

Figure 13.16. In the top half of the figure, (**A**), the cumulative beam profile to be delivered by leaf pair 19 in Figure 13.15. The cumulative meter-set weight (CMW) in units of MU is plotted against position in the field relative to the field center. This illustration is used to explain the logic of the leaf sequence for the segmented multileaf collimation (SMLC) sweeping window algorithm. In the bottom half of the figure, (**B**), the CMW of the SMLC leaf trajectories for the opposing leaves of the pair is plotted against distance across the field relative to the field center. The trajectory for leaf A is on the left border and for leaf B is on the right border.

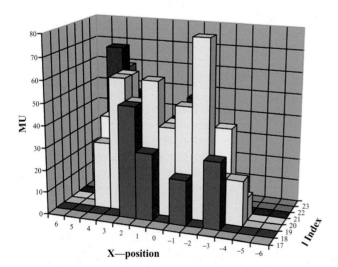

Figure 13.15. An example of an segmented multileaf collimation (SMLC) intensity map. The total cumulative meter-set weight (CMW) in units of MU to be delivered by four leaf pairs (labeled 18, 19, 20, and 21) are plotted against position relative to the field center.

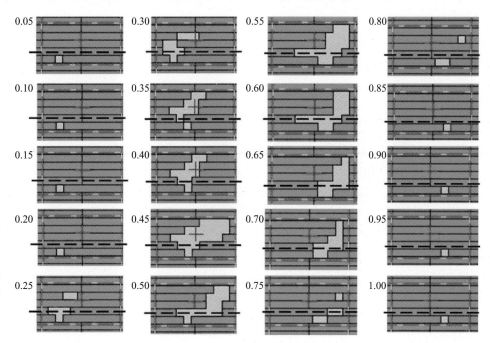

Figure 13.17. The entire leaf sequence for all the leaf pairs plotted as a series of apertures that will deliver the fluence map depicted in Figure 13.15. The numbers to the upper left of each panel are the relative monitor units (MUs) delivered through each aperture.

One group consists of those points lying on an ascending slope of the profile where there is a positive gradient (white circles in Fig. 13.16A), and the other group consists of those points lying on a descending slope of the profile where there is a negative gradient (black circles in Fig. 13.16A). The fourth step is to rank order the points in each group as indicated with the black and white numbers in Figure 13.16A. The numbers indicated are the index numbers for the sequence for the $l = 19$ pair of leaves. Pairing together the coordinates of equal rank order and assigning bin boundary coordinates to the A- and B-leaves produces the desired leaf sequence, $\{x^A_{1,m}, x^B_{1,m}\}$. The number of steps required to create the trajectories will not be the same for all leaf track profiles that make up a field. Steps must be added to the shorter sequences with the leaves abutting beneath a jaw at one side of the treatment field and/or the other so that all sequences for a field will have the same number of step-and-shoot instance pairs. A plot of the sequence derived from Figure 13.16A is given in Figure 13.16B. One can verify that the sequence will produce the desired profile by counting the total CMW in each column of Figure 13.16B. When the sequences for each leaf track are combined, each step instance forms a treatment field consisting of one or more apertures. As the sequence evolves, these apertures form an irregularly shaped window that sweeps across the area to be irradiated. For this example, the calculation produces 20 apertures shown in Figure 13.17 along with the fractional meter set used in each associated shoot instance. This sequence of apertures is displayed for the operator during the delivery process. By examining the apertures in Figure 13.17 one notices that the first four apertures are identical and the last four apertures are identical. These steps could be delivered as one step using four times the fractional meter set in each case. In this example, one can reduce the

total number of steps from 20 to 14 by allowing different numbers of MUs to be delivered at the first and last steps. In general, the step-and-shoot algorithm can be made more efficient by delivering larger increments of MU during certain instances (34). To implement a reduction in the instances one must consider all the leaf tracks at once. This points the way toward leaf sequencing algorithms that consider the entire intensity-modulated aperture at once (37).

The projections of the position of leaves must be accurately encoded for all positions of the leaves across their range of travel. The position encoding mechanisms require calibration at multiple points. Computer look-up tables from which specific values are interpolated during operation are generally used. The curved leaf has its own peculiar issues (38). To discuss this configuration, we will use Figure 13.18, a schematic diagram of an MLC leaf with a rounded end placed at two positions. The distance from the x-ray source to the center of the leaf depth is designated as source to collimator distance (SCD). The tip of the curve on the leaf end is shown as P at the centerline of the leaf depth. The distance from the x-ray source to isocenter is designated as source to axis distance (SAD). The leaf end is shown with an effective radius of curvature R. The projection of W' to the isocenter plane is given by the simple geometric proportion,

$$W = W' \frac{\text{SAD}}{\text{SCD}}$$ EQUATION (13.6)

Equation 13.6 does not describe the position of the light field edge because it refers to the tip of the curved leaf end, point P. The overall light field width, W, will be up to 5 mm smaller than this geometric dimension when curved

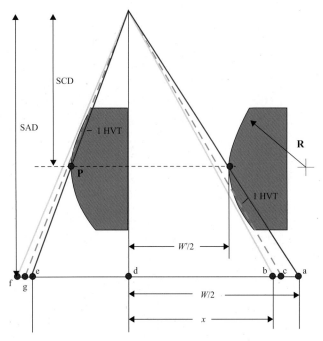

Figure 13.18. Schematic to derive the relation between the leaf positions and the radiation field edge positions. Source to collimator distance (SCD) is from the x-ray source to the center of the leaves. Source to axis distance (SAD) is from the x-ray source to the linac isocenter where the field size is defined. *R* is the effective radius of curvature of the leaf end. The half width of a symmetrical light field is *x*. The physical half width of a symmetrical field is *W′*/2. This distance projected to the plane of the isocenter is *W*/2. The axis of rotation of the collimator passes through isocenter at the point labeled *d*. The rest of the points are described in the text.

leaves define the edge. This light field position *x* is closely approximated by Equation 13.7.

$$ x = \frac{(W/2) \cdot SCD \pm R \cdot SAD \cdot \left(1 - \dfrac{SAD}{\sqrt{SAD^2 + (W/2)^2}} \right)}{SCD \pm R \dfrac{W}{\sqrt{SAD^2 + (W/2)^2}}} $$

EQUATION (13.7)

The relationship is nonlinear with respect to the physical motion of the leaf. The plus sign corresponds to a leaf entering from the right in Figure 13.18 and the minus sign corresponds to a leaf entering from the left.

The edge of the light field is offset from the effective edge of the radiation field. The x-ray fluence is reduced to 50% of the open-field fluence along a ray line that passes through some chord of the arc of the rounded leaf end. The length of this chord is approximately equal to one half-value-thickness (HVT) of the material from which the leaf is fabricated (usually tungsten) at the x-ray energy of the beam. In Figure 13.18, the rays ending at *c* and *e* are depicted passing through such chords. The attenuating chord of arc rolls around the curved leaf end as the leaf is moved from one side of the field to the other. Therefore,

the x-ray field is wider than the light field by a small value that is nearly constant for all leaves and for all positions of the leaves across the field. Calculation of the projection of the 1 HVT chord position in typical curve-ended MLC leaves puts it ≅1 mm outside the light field. For IMRT (and especially for dynamic leaf IMRT), this 1 mm offset has significant dosimetric consequences and should be accounted for in the beam-modeling algorithm. For example, within an SMLC delivery sequence one must abut gaps against each other along each leaf track. When this occurs, it is desirable to minimize the overdose or the underdose that occurs at the junction. This requirement is a more practical criterion for determining the offset value. This parameter should be used in the algorithm that computes the delivery sequence as an offset between the positions for the leaf ends entered into the control file and the positions one needs to place the effective radiation field boundaries. One must be careful with the sign convention used by the algorithm lest one adds a double offset rather than removing the offset.

IMAT

First proposed in 1995 as an alternative to tomotherapy, IMAT is also a rotational IMRT technique. Radiation is delivered with multiple superimposing coplanar or non-coplanar arcs, which can be easily implemented on a conventional linac using a dynamic MLC. In proposing IMAT, Yu predicted that with an increase in the number of gantry angles, the number of intensity levels at each gantry angle can be reduced without degrading the plan quality (31). He argued that the plan quality is a function of the total number of strata, defined as the product of the number of beam angles and the number of intensity levels. In other words, it is the total number of aperture shape variations that determine the plan quality. Assuming this is true, a single arc with a sufficient number of aperture shape variations would be able to create optimal treatment plans. Many subsequent works have attempted to use a single arc for IMAT. Since linacs at the time could not vary the dose rate dynamically during gantry rotation, most previous work on single-arc IMAT was done under the assumption that the machine dose rate had to be constant during arc rotation. To reach the desired plan quality, one must either increase the number of field segments or apertures, or allow the dose rate to vary during gantry rotation, or both.

The feasibility of delivering IMRT with a single arc was first demonstrated by Cameron et al. (39). The technique was termed "sweeping window arc therapy (SWAT)." Shapes of the MLC apertures prior to optimization were initialized so that the MLC leaf positions swept across the PTV during gantry rotation. Optimization of MLC leaf positions was then performed by simulated annealing and arc weight optimization, which assumed a constant or variable angular dose rate.

Tang et al. (40) showed that a multi-arc IMAT could be converted into a single arc by spreading the stacked apertures to neighboring angles with little affect on the plan quality. A 5-arc IMAT plan was created by optimizing the aperture shapes and weights on 36 beam angles. The resulting plan had five apertures stacked at each of the beams spaced every 10 degrees. A new plan was then created by simply rearranging the stacked apertures into neighboring angles by minimizing the movement of the geometric center of the apertures. Dose calculations for the original plan with stacked apertures and for the new plan with spaced apertures showed almost identical results for different plans. This simple exercise elucidated that given the same number of aperture shape variations, single-arc and multi-arc IMATs theoretically have the same degree of freedom for optimizing the dose distributions, if the apertures in the single-arc arrangement could be geometrically connected. It also demonstrated that in rotational delivery, the dose distribution is insensitive to small random errors in the gantry angle.

By assuming that the machine dose rate can vary as needed, Otto (41) developed a single-arc IMAT algorithm that he referred to as volumetric modulated arc therapy (VMAT). In addition to allowing dose-rate variation, the VMAT algorithm used progressive beam angle sampling to optimize a large number (>100) of apertures using direct aperture optimization (DAO). The apertures' shapes and weights were optimized initially for a number of coarsely spaced gantry angles with little consideration of aperture connectivity. Once the solution began to converge, additional gantry angles were inserted. As the angular spacing became smaller, the optimizer considers aperture shape connectivity both in the initialization of aperture shapes and during the optimization. The shapes of the newly inserted apertures were linearly interpolated from their angular neighbors. Such coarse-to-fine sampling is termed progressive sampling, and allows the optimization to converge faster. Because the aperture shape connectivity was ignored initially, the optimizer obtained the freedom to aim for an optimal dose distribution. Since the final plan ensured aperture connectivity, the optimized single arc could be delivered within 2 minutes.

Based on the method developed by Luan et al. for multiple arcs (42), Wang et al. (43) also sequenced the intensity patterns optimized for 36 beams into a single-arc delivery. Other solutions to single-arc IMAT planning were also developed by Cameron (39) and Ulrich et al. (44). These many contributions and their demonstration of superior delivery efficiency led to the present different commercial offerings of single-arc IMAT. A single rotation could theoretically contain hundreds of aperture shape variations, enough to achieve the needed modulation for taking advantage of the angular and positional preferences dictated by the geometric and dosimetric objectives. In reality, however, the apertures cannot be independently shaped because of the physical constraints of MLC leaf motion and gantry rotation. For certain cases, adding a second arc can provide the planning system additional freedom for achieving better treatment plans. This is especially true for MLCs

that cannot (geometrically) cover a large target with one dynamic sequence. For tumors that are not centrally located, and for tumors surrounded by parallel organs, the use of partial arcs is often desirable. For tumors in the brain and in the head-and-neck region, it is often advantageous to use multiple non-coplanar arcs for better tumor targeting and critical structure avoidance.

The general concept and process for IMAT planning is not very different from IMRT planning. The inverse planning principles are almost identical. However, due to the many degrees of freedom in IMAT planning, optimizing an IMAT plan is computationally more difficult. The differences are in the number of beams used to approximate an arc, and the consideration of aperture connectivity. The difficulties in planning IMAT treatment, despite its many advantages, have been the main obstacle in the clinical implementation of IMAT.

Effective planning tools for IMAT have only been developed recently. As with IMRT plan optimization, one may place these methods into two categories: two-step IMAT planning and one-step IMAT planning. Details of these two planning methods are provided in the following sections.

Two-Step Process

The two-step IMAT planning process starts by optimizing the intensity distributions for all beams used for approximating an arc. After the intensity optimization, a leaf-sequencing step is used to convert the optimized beam intensities into deliverable MLC segments to form an arc or arcs. During intensity optimization, no constraint related to delivery is imposed. The conversion of the intensities into segments and the connection of segments into deliverable arcs are both considered in the leaf-sequencing step. In the initial work proving the feasibility of IMAT by Yu (31), the two-step process was used. Recent works also utilize two-step planning. The following summarizes the different approaches.

Optimized intensity distributions on tightly and uniformly spaced beams are first translated into a stack of superimposed irregular fields of uniform beam intensities. Different algorithms can be used for converting the intensity distributions into field segments of different shapes and weights. A leaf-sequencing algorithm attempts to define a sequence of MLC field shapes to create a deliverable intensity distribution that is as close as possible to the distributions obtained from the optimization. The stacks of field segments at all the beam angles must be linked together to form deliverable arcs. These two steps, approximating the intensity distribution using multiple uniform apertures, and connecting the apertures from neighboring angles to form arcs, are normally not separated. In connecting apertures of adjacent beam angles, it may be necessary to alter the shape to force geometric connectivity. The corresponding errors created by such alteration can be compensated by both optimizing new weightings for these apertures, and changing the shapes of other neighboring apertures. The simplest leaf-sequencing algorithm assumes an ideal flat beam with no head scatter, and an ideal MLC with no transmission or leakage. To deliver a predictable dose distribution, a number of other refinements are often added in an accurate dynamic MLC sequence to account for effects such as field flatness, head scatter, penumbra, leaf leakage, rounded leaf ends, and back-scatter into the transmission ion chamber. The under-dosing effects of the tongue-and-groove design of the MLC can also be included. Yu used this two-step process in his initial illustration of using overlapping cone-beam arcs for delivering tomotherapy plans (31). Gladwish et al. (45) developed another work that converted tomotherapy plans for IMAT delivery. By using a "bottom up" segmentation approach and clustering beamlets with similar weightings, the algorithm was able to convert tomotherapy plans to IMAT plans with only minor plan quality degradation. This method would have the potential to improve the plan quality if variable dose rates (VDRs) were allowed within the algorithm. Cao et al. (46) developed a leaf-sequencing method called continuous intensity map optimization (CIMO) for converting the intensity distributions into deliverable segments for step-and-shoot IMRT delivery. They quickly applied the same technique to convert continuous intensity maps optimized for 36 beam angles into deliverable arcs by finding aperture shapes and weights, so that the differences between the intensity created by the overlapping segments and the continuous intensity maps optimized in the plan optimization step were minimized. The algorithm was tested for prostate, brain, head-and-neck, and pancreas cases, and the results showed overall superior plan quality as compared with IMRT using fixed beams.

Luan et al. (42) modeled the interconnectedness of the IMAT beam shapes and MUs using an aperture-based graph algorithm and sequenced continuous intensity maps using the k-link shortest path algorithm. This algorithm was tested for prostate, breast, head-and-neck, and lung, demonstrating that the plans had rivaled HT plans. Based on the method developed by Luan et al. (42), Wang et al. (43) sequenced the intensity patterns optimized for 36 beams into a single-arc delivery. In their approach, the geometric connectivity of all the apertures, designed for approximating the intensity distribution at a given angle, is ensured by using the coupled path-planning algorithm. The geometric connectivity among the apertures derived from intensity distributions from neighboring angles is guaranteed by using the shortest path algorithm over the entire arc. They tested their two-step IMAT planning algorithm for brain, lung, prostate, and head-and-neck cases, and showed that the resulting single-arc IMAT combines the dosimetric advantages of rotational IMRT with speedy deliveries.

One-Step Planning

Realizing that the two-step process may produce a large number of complex field shapes and may lead to inefficient

treatment delivery and increased collimator artifacts, one-step planning was investigated by the research groups in the Ghent University Hospital (47) and University of Maryland (48). De Gersem et al. developed a one-step planning method for step-and-shoot IMRT called leaf position optimization (LPO) (47). Instead of optimizing the fluence distribution with a subsequent MLC leaf segmentation in the two-step planning process, LPO begins an optimization with a set of arbitrary MLC sequences—the MLC shapes are first determined by the beam's eye view (BEV) of the target. Using the simulated annealing approach, the leaf positions are optimized against a dose distribution. LPO also incorporates a segment weight optimization once the leaf sequence is optimized and finalized. In a similar approach, Shepard et al. also developed a one-step planning method for step-and-shoot IMRT delivery called DAO (48). The aperture shapes and weights are simultaneously optimized using a simulated annealing algorithm. Physical constraints of the MLC, such as leaf movement limits, inability to interdigitate, and the minimal gap between opposing leaves and opposing adjacent leaves, can be conveniently considered in the optimization process. Only deliverable MLC shapes are considered and the need for leaf sequencing is eliminated. Without leaf sequencing, the number of apertures can be significantly reduced while maintaining the conformal capabilities of IMRT, considerably reducing the complexity of IMRT. The efficiency advantage of DAO makes it ideal for planning IMAT. Following their successful development of DAO for step-and-shoot IMRT delivery, Earl et al. applied this one-step plan optimization approach to IMAT treatment planning (49). Beams were equally spaced within the range of an arc. The task of DAO algorithm would be to optimize the beam aperture shapes at all the beam angles. To deliver the IMAT plan using a constant dose rate (CDR), a common limitation of treatment machines at the time, all apertures were kept at the same weights. To ensure that the resulting IMAT arcs were deliverable, constraints were placed on the aperture shapes to make sure that they did not differ significantly from one beam angle to the next. As it turned out, these constraints for both the geometry and aperture weights not only reduced the efficiency of optimization, but also limited its potential in terms of plan quality. The possibility of varying dose rates during gantry rotation and irradiation affords greater freedom for DAO. Using a DAO scheme as Earl et al. but employing a more efficient way for selecting the initial aperture shapes, Ulrich et al. showed that IMRT-like dose distributions could be achieved with a single arc (44). When optimizing a large number of beam apertures from a large number of beam angles, the scheme by Ulrich et al. and Earl et al. can take a long time for the optimization to converge. The coarse-to-fine DAO optimization scheme devised by Otto (41) starts with a small number of beams and large angular spacing, and gradually inserts new beam angles to be optimized. Geometric connectivity was facilitated by initializing the shapes of new apertures with shape interpolation between its neighbors and by constraining maximum leaf travel near the end of the optimization process. Both the two-step and one-step optimization methods were successfully applied to planning IMAT treatments employing either multi-arcs or a single arc. The obvious efficiency advantages of single-arc delivery have encouraged linear accelerator vendors to offer different single-arc IMAT solutions. The clinical implementations of single-arc IMAT have shown that beam intensity modulation is not a fundamental requirement for achieving optimal treatment plans, as long as the optimizer is given enough freedom to take advantage of the angular and location preferences intrinsic to a given case (53).

Dose Calculation

Since the doses are calculated beam by beam in IMAT as with other techniques, there is nothing special about dose calculation. On the other hand, due to the large number of beams used to approximate an arc, dose calculation poses new challenges both during the optimization process and in the final dose calculation, offering new opportunities. Tang et al. compared a Monte Carlo-based dose calculation with a collapsed-cone convolution-/superposition-based dose calculation for arc deliveries (50), and it was found that the calculation time for the Monte Carlo-based algorithm is largely independent of the number of beams used, while the calculation time using all the empirical methods linearly increases with the number of beams. If the number of beams is >43, the Monte Carlo-based calculation is faster than a collapsed cone convolution algorithm. Stochastic methods could also offer the opportunity to calculate the doses as with the actual delivery, thereby eliminating the discrepancy between the calculation using the planned static segments and the dynamic delivery.

IMAT Delivery

To understand the delivery of different forms of IMRT, we must first understand how the planning systems handle dynamic delivery and communicates with the linac. In a planning system, a dynamic delivery sequence is approximated with multiple "segments," or "subfields," each defined as the delivery of a fixed number of MUs with a fixed aperture shape at a fixed gantry and collimator angles or spread linearly between two control points. In communicating with the linac for delivery, such segments are defined by a set of control points. How these planned segments are translated to determine the mode of delivery?

In the simplest translation, the first control point always has a cumulative MU of zero, with all other variables, that is, field shape, gantry, and collimator angles, set to that of the first planned segment. For dynamic delivery, the second control point has the cumulative MU of the first planned segment but with the aperture shape, collimator, and gantry angles of the second planned segment. In essence, the first planned static segment is converted into the dynamic transition from the first and the second

control points. The transition from the second to the third control point then delivers the MUs of the second planned segment, and so on. Every pair of neighboring control points defines a dynamic delivery interval and the corresponding planned segment is just a static sample of this delivery interval. The number of control points in a dynamic delivery is always equal to $(N + 1)$, where N is the number of planned segments.

The ability of a single arc to produce dose distributions comparable to tomotherapy is commonly attributed to the freedom provided by dose-rate variation. Palma et al. found that VDR-optimized single-arc plans produced superior dose distributions to those optimized employing a CDR (51). In their study, the treatment plans were generated using a series of evenly spaced static beams, which is the general approach for IMAT planning. VDR delivery not only complicates delivery and QA, but also limits clinical adoption because most of the existing linacs are not equipped with VDR capability.

Based on the observation that the dosimetric error introduced by displacing the beam apertures from the planned angle to a slightly different angular position is minimal, Tang et al. hypothesized (50) that varying the angular spacing of the apertures using CDR delivery is equivalent to varying the weights of evenly spaced beams. They draw the similarity from radio broadcasting, where VDR delivery of evenly spaced beams resembles amplitude modulation (AM) while CDR delivery of unevenly spaced beams resembles frequency modulation (FM). They proved such equivalence by converting Rapid Arc plans, which require VDR delivery, into CDR plans by assigning larger angular intervals to segments with larger MUs and vice versa. The completed CDR plans were delivered and dosimetrically verified using a conventional linac without the capability of dose-rate variation. They found that the plan qualities and the delivery times of the CDR and VDR plans were comparable, and concluded that single-arc IMAT can be delivered using either VDR with even angular spacing or CDR with variable angular spacing. Comparisons between IMRT plans for different delivery methods have been conducted. In a comparison of tomotherapy and MLC delivery, Mavroidis et al. found that linear accelerator delivery with an MLC has slight advantage over tomotherapy for most sites other than head and neck (52). Cao et al. compared the treatment plan quality of IMAT plans and tomotherapy plans for 10 cases including head and neck, lung, brain, and prostate (53). It was found that these two kinds of rotational delivery methods are also equivalent for most cases. For cases where non-coplanar beams are desirable, such as for intracranial tumors and some head and neck cases, the use of partial non-coplanar arcs in IMAT was found to be more advantageous. Shepard et al. compared IMAT plans with IMRT (48) and found that the employment of rotational IMRT is advantageous for most of the cases. Overall, all methods are able to create clinically acceptable and highly conformal treatment plans. Through the initial proof-of-principle

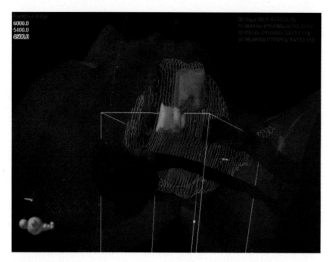

Figure 13.19. Example of an intensity-modulated arc therapy (IMAT) treatment plan. Lymph nodes in the left neck are to be treated down into the clavicular region. Organs at risk include the spinal cord (blue), the cerebellum (red), the larynx and trachea (pink), the right parotid (white), and the oral cavity (orange). They are avoided by the 45 Gy isodose lines (light blue transparency). Multiple planning target volumes (PTVs) are well covered by the 60 Gy isodose lines (yellow wire frame). The treatment was delivered as a single modulated arc.

study, it was shown that IMAT could be a valid alternative to tomotherapy in terms of treatment delivery. However, unlike tomotherapy, IMAT must account for restrictions imposed by the MLC movement as the gantry moves from one beam angle to the next. Because deliverability must take priority, an optimal field shape may have to be altered to produce smooth delivery. As a result, plan quality may be adversely affected. This restriction does not apply to tomotherapy, due to the use of a binary MLC. Therefore, tomotherapy should theoretically have the best plan quality (26). As compared with tomotherapy, IMAT also has a number of advantages: (1) It does not need to move the patient during treatment and avoids abutment issues as seen with serial tomotherapy; (2) it retains the ability of using non-coplanar beams and arcs, which has great value for brain and head/neck tumors; and (3) it uses a conventional linac, thus complex rotational IMRT treatments and simple palliative treatments can be delivered with the same treatment unit.

It is important to note that there are many other issues associated with different delivery techniques besides plan quality. These include the efficiency of planning, delivery, and QA, the complexity and reliability of delivery, and the total MUs required to deliver the prescribed dose. Past attempts in improving treatment efficiency include the use of DAO (49) and the development of single-arc IMAT. By optimizing the aperture shape and aperture weights directly, DAO achieves IMRT plans similar to other planning schemes in quality but with much smaller number of segments, resulting in highly efficient delivery. DAO also provides an efficient method for planning IMAT treatments. Among the different treatment delivery methods,

single-arc IMAT is the most efficient in both MU usage and delivery time with a typical delivery time of about 2 minutes, while tomotherapy is the least efficient.

IMAT has been implemented commercially by the major treatment planning system and medical linear accelerator manufacturers. Given a basic understanding of the underlying principles of planning and delivery, operation of the treatment planning systems can be mastered by persons experienced with IMRT. Figure 13.19 depicts an IMAT treatment computed by the eclipse treatment planning system (Varian Medical Systems, Palo Alto, CA). Lymph nodes in the left neck are to be treated down into the clavicular region. Organs at risk include the spinal cord, the cerebellum, the larynx and trachea, the right parotid, and the oral cavity. The OARs are outside the 45 Gy dose volume. Multiple-shaped PTVs are well covered by the 60 Gy isodose lines (yellow wire frame). The treatment was delivered as a single modulated arc.

COMMISSIONING AND QUALITY ASSURANCE OF IMRT

IMRT and arc-IMRT systems must be thoroughly tested before they can be put into clinical use. This process, known as *commissioning*, is intended to ensure that the IMRT process, as applied in practice, produces dose distributions that can be planned and predicted with sufficient accuracy. The IMRT process is comprised of several complex interacting systems, and the testing must assess the individual systems independently along with end-to-end tests that assess how well they work together. Some of the systems that must be considered include the following:

1. The treatment planning system that predicts the dose distribution and produces the delivery instructions.
2. The delivery system (e.g., linear accelerator, MLC, and control system).
3. The information management system that connects the planning and delivery systems and records the treatments.
4. The QA system (which is discussed later in this section).
5. The process management system, the set of procedures that the clinic uses to control how processes are to be carried out.

This latter point is not always stressed in physicists' publications, but it is a necessary and crucial component for a process such as IMRT that is too complex to test exhaustively all the ways in which it can be used. Standard procedures influence the input to a system and can help prevent it from being used in ways that were not validated. In a complementary way, the QA system can detect variances in the output of the system, perhaps caused by the process being used in an unexpected and untested manner. For example, applying IMRT to a new treatment site with challenging planning goals could push the IMRT planning system into a region in which it was insufficiently accurate. That revelation could come from QA measurements after the plan was computed. However, because QA checks are less exhaustive than commissioning measurements, the problem might escape immediate detection. If, on the other hand, the culture promoted the use of standardized, validated procedures, then the application to a new site would be recognized as a use that needed to be commissioned first. The problem could be recognized, fixed, and the procedures updated. The technical complexity of modern radiation oncology treatments demands such a culture of careful process management.

There are a number of aspects of IMRT that complicate commissioning and QA, which are as follows:

a. IMRT dose distributions are temporally variable (delivered using moving components) and so must be measured using integrating dosimeters.
b. IMRT dose distributions are spatially variable, so must be sampled finely.
c. The evaluation of spatially variant distributions requires assessing, at a given point, the dose agreement and the distance to agreement, which is typically done using the gamma function (54).
d. Differences between planned and measured doses may or may not be clinically important, depending on their location and direction, but assessing that requires correlating measurements in a phantom to location in the patient.

IMRT systems are not only complex, but also continue to evolve rapidly with new capabilities, novel fundamental approaches, and available dosimetry tools. Thus, this text can describe methods that have proved useful to date but must also provide guidance about how to evaluate and deploy new techniques as they develop.

Additional useful recommendations and commentary on the overall aspects of IMRT commissioning and QA can be found in a number of references (55,56,57,58).

Delivery System

IMRT treatments are generally delivered using linear accelerators equipped with MLCs. During the treatment, the MLC leaves move over the area of interest instead of simply defining the outer borders. The number of MUs changes with each MLC shape and can be small. Therefore, the stability of the accelerator for small MU should be determined. Further, the gap between leaf pairs is variable and can also be small, so the gap width must be carefully controlled. For static MLC treatments (SMLC, or "step and shoot"), the MLC leaf position accuracy and reproducibility should be submillimeter (56). For dynamic MLC treatments (DMLC, or "sliding window"), the leaf speed accuracy is also important.

Leaf positioning is often assessed by imaging a series of MLC-defined openings (or dose strips) along an opposing leaf pair track, designed overlap or to abut or to have a 1-mm gap between them. Images of these dose strips may be acquired either with film or with an EPID. Differences from the expected positions can be visualized with a threshold of about 0.5 mm at isocenter. The assessment can be quantified using scans across the images, by positioning the leaf edges over detector arrays, or using an EPID (58,59).

The consistency of the gap width can be monitored by scanning a 0.5-cm slit over a detector and comparing with the output from a static field. Repeating the measurement over time and at different collimator and gantry angles can identify backlash and/or calibration drifts (60).

Some manufacturers employ rounded leaf ends to create consistent penumbra while moving the leaves linearly (60,61). Thus, there is an offset between the leaf edge as determined by the optical field light shadow and edge of the radiation field determined by the 50% transmission ray of about 1 mm. This offset, known as the apparent leaf gap or dosimetric leaf gap, is usually handled by the treatment planning system as an adjustable parameter.

Effective transmission through the MLC leaves includes both primary transmission and scatter, and depends on field size as well as energy. It will also depend on location off-axis because of the spectral changes in the field. Thus, it is useful to measure the transmission over a range of locations and field sizes. It is typically the average MLC leakage, including interleaf and intraleaf transmissions, that is represented in the treatment planning system. Values of 1% to 2% are typical of most MLC systems (60,61,62). The interleaf transmission is reduced by tongue-and-groove construction, but can be about 15% more than mid-leaf transmission. Images of closed leaf banks can check for anomalous leakage patterns.

For the purpose of MLC commissioning, the key point is to establish baseline values for the apparent gap width and MLC transmission that are then used for ongoing QA. Because IMRT MU calculations are highly dependent on the apparent gap width and the effective MLC leaf transmission, it is crucial to create and maintain control over these parameters before moving on to commissioning the planning system. Specific recommendations for MLC systems for the primary vendors have been recently summarized (60,61,62).

Additional factors come into play if the gantry rotates during the IMRT delivery (44,63), as the MLC leaf position, dose rate, and gantry speed can all vary in a mutually dependent manner. By placing a film on a holder such that it remains perpendicular to the axis as the gantry rotates, irradiations can be programmed that produce constant output using different combinations of dose rate and gantry speed or different dose rate and leaf speed (44). Specific recommendations for commissioning and QA of HT have been published (64).

To summarize, accurate IMRT delivery places more demands on the precision of the delivery system compared to 3D conformal delivery. Delivery system commissioning must determine that the accelerator, MLC, and associated components are sufficiently accurate and reproducible at the outset. Furthermore, the baseline values for key parameters, such as leaf gap, are established and maintained going forward with a QA program.

Planning System

Beam modeling for IMRT is more demanding than for 3DCRT. Because the MLCs move through the area of interest, the detailed shape of the penumbra along the leaf end and the sides (tongue and groove) plays a significant role in the calculation accuracy. For example, Yan et al. found (65) that the percent of points in a set of test cases passing gamma criteria of 2 mm/2% increased from 81.6% to 92.6% to 96.8% when a beam model was built based on penumbra measurements made with 6-, 4-, and 0.8-mm diameter detectors, respectively. Another key parameter is the output for small fields, because the MLC leaf sequences in IMRT can have very narrow segments. Inadequate modeling of small field output and depth dose has been shown to degrade the accuracy of IMRT calculations (66). The MLC transmission factor and the offset associated with rounded leaf ends are two other parameters that most planning systems use in their IMRT modeling. Note that although it is possible to derive "true" values for these parameters by direct physical measurements, in practice, the parameters may well need to be modified to best match IMRT calculation to measurement of delivered dose. For example, a recent upgrade to a particular vendor's planning system changed the manner in which tongue-and-groove effect was modeled. Users were advised to check the agreement between calculation and measurement (i.e., recommission) and adjust the modeling of the MLC transmission and the leaf gap if needed. This serves to emphasize that (1) these values are to be treated fitting parameters and (2) a version upgrade to planning system can necessitate revisiting the commissioning process.

Because the planning and delivery systems are so intertwined in IMRT, the natural progression is to first commission the delivery system and establish its baseline performance and then to begin running IMRT plans on a phantom and checking the agreement between calculation and measurement with a suitable dosimeters. Some authors (64,67) have suggested simple geometric shapes with different dose levels as starting points: bands, pyramids, and chair shapes. Although these can indeed be useful beginnings, one should soon move to mock clinical problems that better represent the types of cases that will be seen in practice. AAPM Task Group 119 (68) developed a suite of tests for this purpose, although it is limited and does not, in fact, represent the full range of clinical applications. Even with that limitation, the TG119 approach to commissioning illustrates a reasonable progression.

The first task is to obtain a phantom that is suitable for making ion chamber measurements and integrated planar measurements with a high spatial resolution detector such as radiographic or radiochromic film. The chamber should be small enough so that it can be positioned to avoid high gradient regions: 0.125 cm³ or smaller. The film system should itself be commissioned so that its uncertainties are understood and minimized. Analysis software is needed so that the 2D dose distribution on the film can be compared to predictions with suitable tools such as gamma analysis. Preliminary measurements of simple open-field combinations should be done to ensure that the measured data matches predictions to good precision (<1.5% difference for ion chamber) and the pass rate for gamma analysis on the film is very high (e.g., >97% for 3%/3 mm).

With the dosimetry systems well characterized, the next step is to define a series of IMRT "problems" on the phantom, with targets and avoidance structures that mimic those encountered clinically (see Fig. 13.20), and then test the agreement between calculation and measurement for

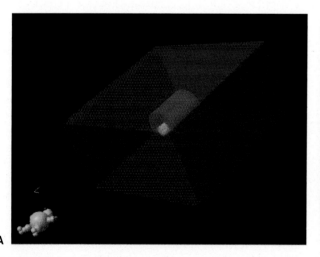
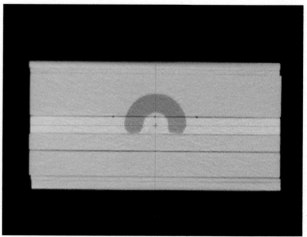

A   B

Figure 13.20. Mock clinical case used for commissioning. **A:** A 3D rendering of a C-shaped target (red) surrounding a structure to be spared (green), drawn on a rectangular phantom. This mimics a perispinal case surrounding the spinal cord. **B:** Transverse view through the center of the phantom.

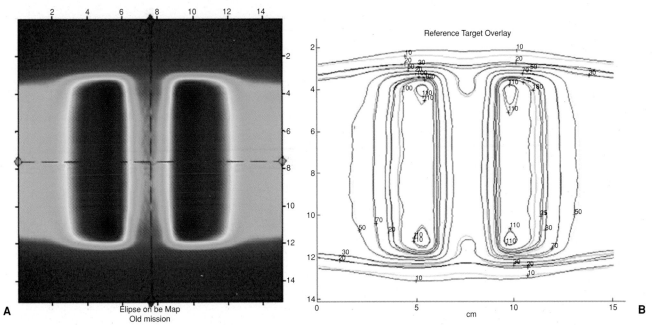

Figure 13.21. Film dosimetry for the C-shape commissioning case. **A:** Shows a scan of the film that was placed in the coronal plane at the phantom center. The density has been converted to dose using standard film dosimetry techniques. **B:** Shows an overlay of the planned isodoses (reference) and the measured isodoses (target).

a variety of situations. To be complete, these studies should include IMRT plans using realistic combinations of beam angles and optimization criteria. Calculations by the treatment planning system are used to predict the mean dose to the chamber volume for locations in low-gradient regions, representative of high-dose targets and low-dose avoidance structures. Treatment planning systems generally provide a means to calculate the 2D planar doses to representative planes that can be measured with film (see Fig. 13.21). It is important to export the irradiation instructions to the delivery system just as they would be for a patient, and to deliver the plan to the phantom using the actual beam angles, etc. Measurements may be compared to the predicted doses, as measured-to-predicted ratios for ion chamber results and as percent of points passing a suitable gamma criterion (see Figure 13.22). If the degree of agreement is not satisfactory, then a parameter in the dose calculation model must be adjusted and the calculations and measurements repeated. If, for example, the measured dose trend were found to be too low, then one might reduce the MLC transmission or the apparent leaf gap parameter. Differentiating which of these two parameters should be adjusted can be difficult; MLC transmission issues may show up more readily as trends with field size.

Despite the widespread application of IMRT clinically, the question of what degree of agreement should be considered satisfactory has not (yet) been resolved. TG119 attempted to address the issue by combining results from a number of institutions that had passed an independent check by the Radiological Physics Center (68). On average, their average ion chamber results agreed with prediction to 0.2% with a standard deviation of 2.2%. Their film

measurements produced an average percentage of points passing gamma criteria of 3%/3 mm of 96.3% with a standard deviation of 4.4%.

The tests so far discussed have been of composite delivery to a phantom. These are very direct measures of the dose as planned, but the sampling of the full distribution is practically limited by the number of points and planes measured. Another type of test is to place a detector perpendicular to each individual beam, measure the dose produced at a standard distance and depth, and compare the measured dose to the predicted dose. This has the advantage of sampling the modulation within each delivery beam over its full range but has the disadvantage of not producing doses directly relevant to the planned distribution. Together, composite and per-beam tests complement each other and both should be used during commissioning. Such per-beam tests have been done with film, detector arrays (69,70,71), and EPIDs (63). The TG119 group, using all three methods but primarily diode arrays, reported an overall gamma pass rate of 97.9% with a standard deviation of 2.5%, again with 3%/3 mm criteria. Other published results (65,72,73) are consistent with these TG119 results for composite and per-field tests.

The commissioning tests described here are end-to-end tests that should treat the phantom as much as possible as the patient is to be treated from the initial CT imaging through the target and structure definition, optimization and planning, communication to the delivery system, and treatment delivery. It is important to realize that *the human planner is part of the system*. The planning for the phantom cases should be done in the same manner as will be done for patients. To have some assurance that this is and will continue to be the case, then part of the commissioning

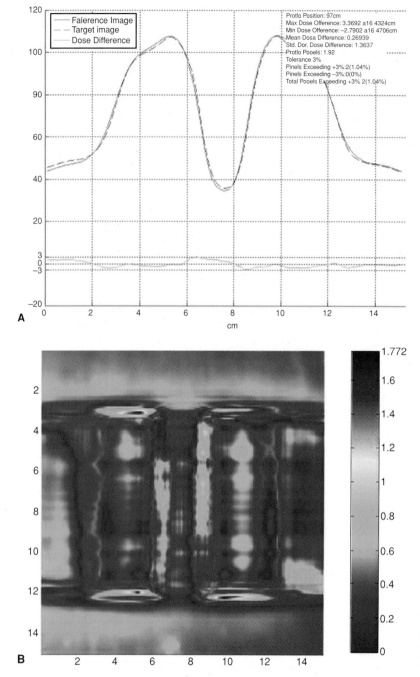

Figure 13.22. **A:** Shows a dose profile through the center of the film, along the horizontal line bounded by green diamonds in Figure 13.21. **B:** Shows a gamma analysis for the film using criteria of 3% dose agreement and 3 mm distance to agreement; 98.6 percent of the points have a gamma of 1.0 or less.

process for each treatment site should be documentation of the manner in which targets and structures will be defined, margins created, treatment goals established, and optimization parameters adjusted. In a department with multiple physicians and planners, it is very instructive to have different people plan the same case and compare results. It is also recommended to include in the commissioning test suite some situations in which the system is pushed very hard and may be expected to fail. Indeed, it is best to push the system until it does fail so that the limits can be determined.

As with the delivery system, one outcome of the planning system commissioning should be a baseline set of tests that can be repeated periodically and whenever the planning software is changed to assure consistency. However, this initial baseline is not likely to be permanently sufficient. As the clinical practice evolves, mock cases that were representative at first will become less so. Periodically, the physicist should reassess whether the practice has changed to the point that testing sample cases in a rigorous fashion is advisable.

Quality Assurance

The QA program for IMRT will include testing of the delivery system combined with a qualitative and quantitative review of each patient's plan. The TG 142 report (74) provides specific guidance on periodic accelerator and MLC QA tests, frequencies, and tolerances for machines used for IMRT. These include weekly, monthly, and annual tests of MLC accuracy. The 2003 Guidance Document (64) discussed the qualitative review of each patient's plan.

"Plan evaluation for IMRT should include an assessment of the potential problems and pitfalls outlined below.

1. Is the dose uniformity in the target acceptable? Are the stated plan goals for hot spots and target coverage satisfied?
2. Are the stated plan goals for normal-tissue sparing satisfied?
3. Were organs contoured in their entirety? Are the plan goals appropriate for the fraction of organ contoured?
4. Are the margins and dose gradients safe given realistic expectations for setup reproducibility? Might geometric miss of the target or overdose to a structure result?
5. Will patient or organ intrafraction motion during the treatment compromise the accuracy?
6. Are there high doses in the buildup region that may be inaccurate or an indication that the inverse planner has struggled to "fix" low doses there?
7. Have inhomogeneity corrections been applied appropriately?
8. How does this plan compare with a conventional alternative? What regions are being treated or spared differently compared with traditional methods?
9. Is the increased whole body dose with IMRT a concern?
10. Are there unusual beam orientations that might involve collision with or shadowing by the treatment table?
11. Are there low-intensity segments that could be removed without compromising plan quality?

This list is not exhaustive but serves to illustrate the caution and skepticism that should be brought to bear."

Patient-specific QA for IMRT includes all the components needed for any patient treatment, such as checking that the information transfer from the planning system to the accelerator control system proceeds correctly via the information management system; checking that the setup information is complete, clear, and correct; and checking via imaging that the treatment isocenter and field shapes are correct. For IMRT, the field shape changes during treatment, so typically the bounding shape is imaged and checked against expectations.

For conventional treatments, a physicist normally checks the MU settings called for by the planning system using some form of independent calculation, perhaps using manual methods. This process is also useful for IMRT, but must be done with dedicated software because of the complexity of the treatment. The treatment data must be imported into the software, and preferably should have been exported from the information system that is used to treat the patient, rather than directly from the planning system, so that any corruption of the data in the treatment control system can be detected.

Independent calculation methods are essentially one computer checking another computer and can detect certain types of problems. However, they cannot verify that the dose delivery will actually occur as planned. Furthermore, such tools usually employ less sophisticated calculation algorithms than the primary planning system, and so one could expect some secondary calculations to fail, that is, differ from the primary by several percent, when in fact the primary calculation is adequately accurate. The prevalence of "false positives" with the independent calculations limits their utility in identifying "true positives," that is, when the primary calculation is not adequately accurate. Therefore, actual measurement of IMRT dose is the norm, and in fact is expected according to the ASTRO practice guidelines for IMRT (62).

Such measurements may be done in a variety of ways with a variety of tools. As with the commissioning process, there are two primary approaches to measurement: (1) delivering the full patient plan to a phantom and sampling the resulting distribution with 1D dosimeters such as ion chambers and/or 2D dosimeters such as film or arrays of discrete detectors (diodes or chambers (see Fig. 13.23), and (2) delivering each field separately to a 2D dosimeter held perpendicular to the beam's central axis. The assumption underlying the first approach is that if the planning system can successfully predict the dose produced by this irradiation plan in a phantom, then the calculation in the patient should be similarly accurate. Of course, the phantom has a different shape and density than the patient, so the actual dose to the phantom will not be the same as the patient. However, the primary concern is that either the primary calculation or the physical delivery is not as expected, and if so, then that would show up in a phantom test.

As noted in the commissioning section, measurements for each field using detectors held perpendicular to the beam have been done using film, arrays of chambers or diodes, and EPIDs. These studies involve using the planning system to predict the dose distribution at some reference distance and depth from each field and then comparing that to the measured using 2D analysis software. This provides no direct data about dose in the patient, but does allow a more complete sampling of the full dose delivery from each beam.

Another approach to per-patient QA is to use accelerator and MLC log files that record the actual MU and MLC position during treatment (75). Although not a direct measurement that is independent of the accelerator system, this has been shown (76) to record accurately the accelerator performance and can be used to verify that the machine performed as expected. This does not, however, check the dose produced.

All these per-field test methods present the problem of correlating any areas of concern within a beam to actual

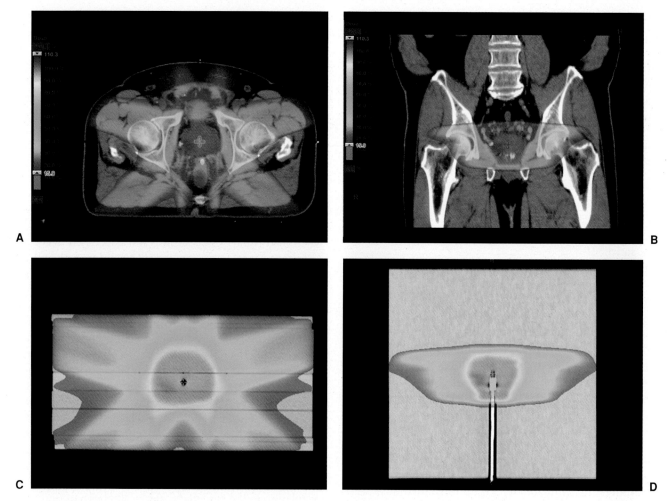

Figure 13.23. Examples of verification measurements for a patient plan: ion chamber measurement in a phantom for composite field delivery. The plan for the patient has been applied to a phantom. Panel *A* shows the patient plan in a transverse plane and panel *B* shows the patient plan in a coronal plane. Panel *C* shows the dose distribution in the phantom in the corresponding transverse plane and panel *C* shows the dose distribution in the phantom in the corresponding coronal plane.

dose and location within a patient. A number of centers and vendors are working on methods to use the measured beam data to adjust the calculated dose to the patient, thereby allowing the clinician to judge the importance of the dose discrepancies. A related approach under development in some centers is to use the EPID as an exit dosimeter and back-project the dose into the model of the patient. This has the potential of allowing ongoing checks of the dose delivery, not just before treatment begins (77).

Although the discussion and references primarily deal with IMRT delivered with stationary gantry beams, these QA processes are applicable or adaptable to rotational techniques as well, and specialized dosimetry tools are currently under development (78).

Action Levels and Process Control

The action levels for per-patient QA should be based on the results of the commissioning studies. TG119, fol-

lowing Palta (79) and Venselaar (80), used the concept of "confidence limit," which is a statistical construct based on the mean and standard deviation of a set of measurements. TG119 used a multiplier of 1.96σ to set a 95% confidence limit for the purpose of comparing commissioning studies between institutions. The action level for routine QA should be set large enough to accommodate this statistical variation without unduly flagging potential problems. The TG119 results support Palta's recommendations for action levels for per-patient QA:

■ Ion chamber measurements: ±5% in a high-dose, low-gradient region and ±7% in a low-dose, low-gradient region
■ Composite irradiations analyzed with radiographic film: 88–90% gamma pass rate at 3%/3 mm
■ Per-field measurements: 90% gamma pass rate at 3%/3 mm

Other authors have published similar results. Both et al. reported (73) per-field results for 747 beams calculated by three planning systems, irradiated on different accelerators, and analyzed with a diode array. They found that the percent of points passing gamma criteria of 3%/3 mm was >95% for prostate treatments and >90% for all treatment sites. Basran and Woo reported (81) that for 115 plans and tested with a diode array, the percent of points passing gamma criteria of 3%/3 mm was >88% for head and neck treatments and >95% for all other treatment sites.

These results could serve as a useful starting point. However, consistently performing patient IMRT measurements provides an excellent data stream for using process control techniques, which are QA concepts that have been developed in industrial engineering. A fairly well-developed industrial QA method is known as *statistical process control* (82). The concept assumes that some initial commissioning of the IMRT procedures has verified the accuracy and integrity of the dose delivery process. One now wishes to set up a QA procedure. Given a QA procedure from which sequential data may be obtained, how can the stream of data be used to draw inductive conclusions about the underlying process? From a measured data set, the physicist needs to know when an anomalous data point is within the limits of random variation in the process or when it is because of a systematic change from the initially verified process. In this method, the average and range charts are used for the location and dispersion statistics. Each chart will have statistically determined upper and lower limits that will serve as action thresholds. The steps to create the charts are as follows:

1. Obtain data from a preliminary application of the IMRT QA process
2. Compute summary statistics of the data
3. Determine process parameters by obtaining limits
4. Use process parameters for clinical QA for patients undergoing IMRT

The data are organized into subgroups. If the subgroups are statistically consistent over time, then the process that created those subgroups is stable, that is, subject to only random variation. If the subgroups are not statistically consistent over time, then the process under consideration is unstable and subject to both random and systematic variations. A process that contains both random and systematic sources of variation is unpredictable, whereas a process that displays only random variation is predictable within the magnitude of random errors in the process. Action thresholds set by process behavior limits will distinguish between these two sources of error. A data point outside the thresholds will very likely have an assignable cause for a systematic error. Data points within the thresholds are within the range of random error and, in most cases, do not have a readily assignable cause.

The IMRT QA process acquires numerical data: x_1, x_2, x_3, ... x_N. Subgroups of this data are then created:

$$x_1 = x_{1,1}$$
$$x_2 = x_{1,2} \qquad \text{average} = \overline{x}_1$$
$$\cdots \qquad \text{range} = R_1$$
$$x_n = x_{1,n}$$
$$x_{n+1} = x_{2,1}$$
$$x_{n+2} = x_{2,2} \qquad \text{average} = \overline{x}_2$$
$$\cdots \qquad \text{range} = R_2$$
$$x_{2n} = x_{2,n}$$
$$\cdots$$
$$x_{N-n+1} = x_{M,1}$$
$$x_{N-n+2} = x_{M,2} \qquad \text{average} = \overline{x}_M$$
$$\cdots \qquad \text{range} = R_M$$
$$x_N = x_{M,n}$$

EQUATION (13.8)

where $n < N$ *and the number of subgroups is* $M = N/n$. The average of a subgroup is $\overline{x}_m$ and the range of values in a subgroup is R_m. When choosing subgroup size n, one seeks to ensure subgroup homogeneity, that is, ensure that the same quantity is being measured in the same way for each subgroup. Using this data, two process behavior charts can be created: An average chart for subgroup averages, $\overline{x}_m$ and a range chart for subgroup ranges, R_m. The centerline for the subgroup average chart is $\overline{\overline{x}}$, which is the average of all the subgroup averages. The centerline for the subgroup range chart is $\overline{R}$, which is the average of all the subgroup ranges. The average chart will have an upper threshold (A_u), centerline (A_c), and lower threshold (A_l) defined as:

$$A_u = \overline{\overline{x}} + 3\frac{\overline{R}}{d_2\sqrt{n}}$$
$$A_c = \overline{\overline{x}}$$
$$A_l = \overline{\overline{x}} - 3\frac{\overline{R}}{d_2\sqrt{n}} \qquad \text{EQUATION (13.9)}$$

where the factor 3 is added as an economical margin for the limits. Similarly, the range chart will have an *upper* threshold (R_u), centerline (R_c), and lower threshold (R_l) defined as:

$$R_U = \left(1 + 3\frac{d_3}{d_2}\right)\overline{R}$$
$$R_C = \overline{R}$$
$$R_L = \left(1 - 3\frac{d_3}{d_2}\right)\overline{R} \qquad \text{EQUATION (13.10)}$$

The quantities d_2 and d_3 depend on the subgroup size n. Values of d_2 and d_3 are given in Table 13.1. An example

TABLE 13.1	Values for the Constants Used to Compute the Centerline and Upper and Lower Thresholds for Control Charts as a Function of Subgroup Size	
n	d_2	d_3
2	1.128	0.8525
3	1.693	0.8884
4	2.059	0.8798
5	2.326	0.8641
6	2.534	0.8480
7	2.704	0.8332
8	2.847	0.8198
9	2.970	0.8078
10	3.078	0.7971
11	3.173	0.7873
12	3.258	0.7785
13	3.336	0.7704
14	3.407	0.7630
15	3.472	0.7562
20	3.735	0.7287
25	3.931	0.7084
30	4.086	0.6927
40	4.322	0.6692
50	4.498	0.6521
100	5.015	0.6052

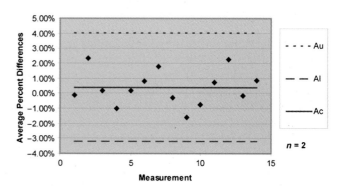

Figure 13.24. An example of a statistical process control chart applied to the quality assurance (QA) measurements for an intensity-modulated radiation therapy (IMRT) treatment. This is the average chart using group sizes of 2.

patient treatments. Any cases for which the average data were to fall outside the calculated limits would be out of statistical process control and should be investigated before the patient treatment proceeded.

Pawlicki et al. have published (83) a control chart analysis for ion chamber tests of IMRT treatments from seven institutions and showed that the variation exceeded the target value of ±5% for sites other than prostate, thus demonstrating the opportunity to improve the system performance. Breen et al. have also published statistical process control results for IMRT dosimetric verification and demonstrated improvements following modeling changes in the treatment planning system (84).

Commissioning and QA Summary

Conventionally, we think of commissioning as work to be done before a technique or apparatus is used clinically and QA as work to be done afterward to monitor performance. For IMRT, at least, it should be expected that this could well be a cyclical process. As IMRT is used in more clinical sites and expected to solve more and more difficult clinical

of a process control average chart for IMRT phantom plan measurements made with an ionization chamber in a ellipsoidal tissue equivalent phantom are given in Figure 13.24. The measured metric was $x_i = (D\text{-}meas_i - D\text{-}calc_i)/D\text{-}pres$ where $D\text{-}meas_i$ was the absolute dose measured with an ionization chamber at a point chosen in the phantom, $D\text{-}calc_i$ was the average dose calculated within a region of interest equal to that of the ionization chamber sensitive volume and centered about the chosen point of measurement, and $D\text{-}pres$ was the dose calculated in the phantom plan equivalent to the prescribed dose. The sample size was $n = 2$. Two measurements acquired by accumulating the dose delivered by all the treatment fields (in this example, seven to nine gantry angles) at two different positions in the phantom were averaged for each datum sample. The accompanying process control range chart is given in Figure 13.25. The upper and lower limits calculated for this entire data set are shown on the charts. Using this data, one can establish a QA procedure to verify

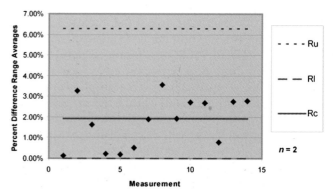

Figure 13.25. A statistical process control range chart applied to the same set of measurements used to generate the SPC average chart in Figure 13.24.

problems, it could well happen that the QA results will show more deviations, indicating that the modeling will need to be revisited. Diligent acquisition and analysis of QA data, especially the use of process control charts, will be needed to identify problems as they develop. Diligent production and conformance to standardized procedures will help prevent problems before they develop, and such should be the culture of any department carrying out advanced therapies such as IMRT. For thoracic tumors treated with conformal therapy, breathing motion can cause the target to move outside the beam aperture, resulting in geometric misses. In breast treatment, breathing motion broadens the beam penumbra at the posterior field boundary, resulting in lower doses to the breast near the posterior field border and higher doses to the underlying lung. To compensate for these effects, large margins are normally assigned around the target volume to ensure proper target coverage. With dynamic intensity modulation, however, the problem is more complicated due to the inter-play of patient motion and the motion of the radiation fields. Yang et al. studied (85) the problem of intra-fraction organ motion for tomotherapy delivery, where the patient is treated by a rotating slit fan beam either in a slice-by-slice or a spiral fashion. They found that ripple-like dose variations occur at the slice boundaries when the target moves in the direction of couch translation. The effect of intra-fraction organ motion on the delivery of intensity modulation with DMLC in a single radiation field was first studied by Yu et al. (86). They simulated the delivery of a sliding window IMRT to a target under cyclic motion with clinically relevant frequency and amplitudes. The simulation revealed that the fundamental mechanism for creating such dosimetric variations in the target is the interplay between the movements of the beam aperture and the target during irradiation. The results showed that, for clinically realistic parameters, the magnitude of intensity variations in the target can be >100% of the desired beam intensity. The magnitude of the photon intensity variations is strongly dependent on the speed of the beam aperture relative to the speed of the target motion, and the width of the scanning beam relative to the amplitude of target motion. In general, the dosimetric effects of target motion increase with narrowing beam aperture. With multiple beams and multiple fractions, the dosimetric errors are averaged and lower. However, the intensity patterns will also be smoothed. Such smoothed beam intensities occurred in all radiation fields will also cause large dose errors in the target.

RADIATION SAFETY CONSIDERATIONS

IMRT treatments require 3 to 10 times more MUs to deliver than conventional treatments. It is important to consider the impact of the increased running of the linear accelerator on personnel radiation safety and the patient whole body dose (87). The increase in the average workload of a linear accelerator being used to treat with IMRT depends on the frac-

tion of patients that receive IMRT treatments. Obviously, if only about a quarter of the patients on a given machine presents with the medical necessity for IMRT treatments, then the workload will only increase proportionately. The increased workload will not, however, cause a requirement for thicker primary barriers. The dose delivered to the target volume within the patient will be, for radiation safety considerations, about the same as for conventional patients. The fraction of the beam blocked by the MLC leaves compensates for the increased number of MUs for primary and scatter considerations. On the other hand, leakage radiation does increase with the total workload. The adequacy of the thickness of secondary barriers around treatment rooms used for IMRT should be reevaluated to consider the increase in overall workload. In addition to the structural barriers in the walls, ceiling (and perhaps floor) of the treatment room, the thickness and composition of the entry door should be evaluated using the increased workload. In addition to the radiation safety of the occupationally exposed personnel and the general public, the radiation safety of the patient is also an issue (88). All patients are subject to some increased risk of induction of secondary malignancies by virtue of the whole body exposure they receive from leakage radiation during the course of their treatment. The increased risk associated with conventional therapy courses is quite low and considered to be reasonable. However, if IMRT is to be delivered by very high x-ray energies and by techniques that require a large increase in MUs, the risk of secondary malignancies may be increased to levels that are not acceptable (89,90). Treatments using x-rays in the 6- to 15-MV range that require increases in MUs of less than a factor of ~5 will be accompanied by acceptable whole body doses to the patient. Higher energy treatments and treatments that require greater numbers of MUs should be carefully evaluated (91).

REFERENCES

1. Boyer AL, Ochran TG, Nyerick CE, et al. Clinical dosimetry for implementation of a multileaf collimator. *Med Phys* 1992;19:1255–1261.
2. Galvin JM, Smith AR, Moeller RD, et al. Evaluation of multileaf collimator design for a photon beam. *Int J Radiat Oncol Biol Phys* 1992;23:789–780.
3. Galvin JM, Smith A, Lally B. Characterization of a multileaf collimator system. *Int J Radiat Oncol Biol Phys* 1993;25: 181–192.
4. Jordan TF, Williams PC. The design and performance characteristics of a multileaf collimator. *Phys Med Biol* 1994;39:231–251.
5. Klein EE, Harms WB, Low DA, et al. Clinical implementation of a commercial multileaf collimator: dosimetry, networking, simulation, and quality assurance. *Int J Radiat Oncol Biol Phys* 1995;33:1195–1208.
6. Frazier A, Du M, Wong J, et al. Dosimetric evaluation of the conformation of the multileaf collimator to irregular shaped fields. *Int J Radiat Oncol Biol Phys* 1995;33:1229–1238.

7. Boyer AL. Basic applications of a multileaf collimator. In: Palta J, Mackie TR, eds. *Teletherapy: present and future.* Madison, WI: Advanced Medical Physics Publishing, 1996: 403–444.

8. Takahashi S. Conformation radiotherapy. Rotation techniques as applied to radiography and radiotherapy of cancer. *Acta Radiol Suppl* 1965;242:1–4.

9. Brahme A, Roos J-E, Lax I. Solution of an integral equation encountered in radiation therapy. *Phys Med Biol* 1982;27: 1221–1229.

10. Brahme A. Optimization of stationary and moving beam radiation therapy techniques. *Radiother Oncol* 1988;12:129–140.

11. Convery DJ, Rosenbloom ME. The generation of intensity-modulated fields for conformal radiotherapy by dynamic collimation. *Phys Med Biol* 1992;37(6):1359–1374.

12. Bortfeld TR, Kahler DL, Waldron TJ, et al. X-ray field compensation with multileaf collimators. *Int J Radiat Oncol Biol Phys* 1994;28(3):723–730.

13. Bortfeld T, Boyer AL, Schlegel W, et al. Realization and verification of three-dimensional conformal radiotherapy with modulated fields. *Int J Radiat Oncol Biol Phys* 1994;30:899–908.

14. Yu CX, Wong JW. Dynamic photon beam intensity modulation. In: Hounsell AR, Wilkinson JM, Williams PC, eds. *Proceedings of the XIth International Conference on the Use of computers in radiation therapy.* Manchester, UK. 1994:182–183.

15. Spirou SV, Chui CS. Generation of arbitrary fluence profiles by dynamic jaws or multileaf collimators. *Med Phys* 1994;2:1031–1041.

16. Stein J, Bortfeld T, Dorschel B, et al. Dynamic x-ray compensation for conformal radiotherapy by means of multileaf collimation. *Radiother Oncol* 1994;32:163–173.

17. Yu CX, Symons MJ, Du MN, et al. A method for implementing dynamic photon beam intensity modulation using independent jaws and multileaf collimator. *Phys Med Biol* 1995;40:769–787.

18. Ling CC, Burman C, Chui CS, et al. Conformal radiation treatment of prostate cancer using inversely-planned intensity-modulated photon beams produced with dynamic multileaf collimation. *Int J Radiat Oncol Biol Phys* 1996;35:721–730.

19. Boyer AL, Li S, Tate D, et al. Potential advantages of modulated therapy in treatment of prostate cancer. *Int J Rad Oncol Biol Phys* 1996;36:388.

20. Mackie TR, Holmes T, Swerdloff S, et al. Toothermapy: a new concept for the delivery of conformal radiotherapy. *Med Phys* 1993;20:1709–1719.

21. Carol MP, Targovnik H, Campbell C, et al. *An automatic 3D treatment planning and implementaion system for optimised conformal therapy.* In: Minet P, ed. Three-dimensional treatment planning. Geneva: WHO, 1993:173–187.

22. Carol MP. Integrated 3D conformal planning/multivane intensity modulating delivery system for radiotherapy. In: Purdy JA, Emami B, eds. *3D Radiation treatment planning and conformal therapy.* Madison, WI: Medical Physics Publishing, 1995:435–445.

23. Butler E, Grant W, Woo S, et al. Prerequisites for the clinical use of the Peacock treatment system. *Radiology* 1994;193(Suppl.):228.

24. Adler JR, Cox RS. Preliminary clinical experience with the Cyberknife: image-guided stereotactic radiosurgery. In: Alexander III E, Kondziolka D, Loeffler JS, eds. *Radiosurgery.* Basel: Karger, 1996:316–326.

25. Szerlag C, Canovas L. Billing and reimbursement issues. In: Mundt AJ, Roeske J, eds. *Intensity modulated radiation therapy: a clinical perspective.* Ontario, Canada: BC Decker Inc., 2005:214–231.

26. Bortfeld T, Webb S. Single-Arc IMRT? *Phys Med Biol* 2009;54:N9–N20.

27. Oelfke U, Bortfeld T. Inverse planning for x-ray rotation therapy: a general solution of the inverse problem. *Phys Med Biol* 1999;44:1089–1104.

28. Bortfeld T. The number of beams in IMRT-theoretical investigations and implications for single-arc IMRT. *Phys Med Biol* 2010;55(1):83–97.

29. Boyer AL, Butler EB, DiPetrillo TA, et al. Intensity-modulated radiotherapy: current status and issues of interest. *Int J Radiat Oncol Biol Phys* 2001;51:890–914.

30. Carol M. An automatic 3D conformal treatment planning system for linear accelerator based beam modulation radiotherapy. In: Hounsell AR, Wilkinson JM, Williams PC, eds. *Proceedings of the XIth international Conference on the Use of computers in radiation therapy.* 1994:172–173.

31. Yu C, Symons M, Du M, et al. A method for implementing dynamic photon beam intensity modulation using independent jaws and a multileaf collimator. *Phys Med Biol* 1995;40:769–787.

32. Webb S. Configuration options for intensity-modulated radiation therapy using multiple static fields shaped by a multileaf collimator. *Phys Med Biol* 1998;43:241–260.

33. Galvin JM, Chen X-G, Smith RM. Combining multileaf fields to modulate fluence distributions. *Int J Radiat Oncol Biol Phys* 1993;27:697–705.

34. Chui CS, LoSasso T, Spirou S. Dose calculation for photon beam with intensity modulation generated by dynamic jaw or multileaf collimation. *Med Phys* 1994;21:1237–1244.

35. Svensson R, Kallman P, Brahme A. An analytical solution for the dynamic control of multileaf collimators. *Phys Med Biol* 1994;39:37–61.

36. Ma L, Boyer A, Ma C-M, et al. Synchronizing dynamic multileaf collimators for producing two-dimensional intensity-modulated fields with minimum beam delivery time. *Int J Radiat Oncol Biol Phys* 1999;44:1147–1154.

37. Ma L, Boyer AL, Xing L, et al. An Optimized leaf-setting algorithm for beam intensity modulation using dynamic multileaf collimators. *Phys Med Biol* 1998;43:1629–1643.

38. Boyer AL, Li S. Geometric analysis of light-field position of a multileaf collimator with curved ends. *Med Phys* 1997;24:757–762.

39. Cameron C. Sweeping-window arc therapy: an implementation of rotational IMRT with automatic beam-weight calculation. *Phys Med Biol* 2005;50:4317–4336.

40. Tang G, Earl M, Luan S, et al. Converting multiple-arc intensity-modulated arc therapy into a single arc for efficient delivery. *Int J Radiat Oncol Biol Phys* 2007;69(3):S673.

41. Karl Otto. Volumetric modulated arc therapy: IMRT in a single gantry arc. *Med Phys* 2008;35:310–317.

42. Luan S, Wang C, Cao D, et al. Leaf-sequencing for intensity-modulated arc therapy using graph algorithms. *Med Phys* 2008;35(1):61–69.

43. Wang C, Luan S, Tang G, et al. Arc-modulated radiation therapy (AMRT): a single-arc form of intensity-modulated arc therapy. *Phys Med Biol* 2008;53(22):6291–6303.

44. Ulrich S, Nill S, Oelfke U. Development of an optimization concept for arc-modulated cone beam therapy. *Phys Med Biol* 2007;52(14):4099–4119.

45. Gladwish A, Oliver M, Craig J, et al. Segmentation and leaf sequencing for intensity modulated arc therapy. *Med Phys* 2007;34:1779–1788.

46. Cao D, Earl M, Luan S, et al. Continuous intensity map optimization (CIMO). A novel approach to leaf sequencing in step and shoot IMRT. *Med Phys* 2006;33:859–867.

47. De Gersem W, Claus F, De Wagter C, et al. Leaf position optimization for step-and-shoot IMRT. *Int J Radiat Oncol Biol Phys* 2001;51:1371–1388.

48. Shepard DM, Earl MA, Li XA, et al. Direct aperture optimization: a turnkey solution for step-and-shoot IMRT. *Med Phys* 2002;29(6):1007–1018.

49. Earl MA, Shepard DM, Naqvi SA, et al. Inverse planning for intensity-modulated arc therapy using direct aperture optimization. *Phys Med Biol* 2003;48:1075–1089.

50. Tang G, Earl MA, Luan S, et al. Stochastic versus deterministic kernel-based superposition approaches for dose calculation of intensity-modulated arcs. *Phys Med Biol* 2008;53:4733–4746.

51. Palma D, Vollans E, James K, et al. Volumetric modulated arc therapy for delivery of prostate radiotherapy: comparison with intensity-modulated radiotherapy and three-dimensional conformal radiotherapy. *Int J Radiat Oncol Biol Phys* 2008;72:996–1001.

52. Mavroidis P, Ferreira BC, Shi C, et al. Treatment plan comparison between helical tomotherapy and MLC-based IMRT using radiobiological measures. *Phys Med Biol* 2007;52(13):3817–3836.

53. Cao D, Holmes TW, Afghan MK, et al. Comparison of plan quality provided by intensity-modulated arc therapy and helical tomotherapy. *Int J Radiat Oncol Biol Phys* 2007;69:240–250.

54. Low DA, Harms WB, Mutic S, et al. A technique for the quantitative evaluation of dose distributions. *Med Phys* 1998;25:656–661.

55. Palta JR, Liu C, Li JG. Quality assurance of intensity-modulated radiation therapy, pages S108–S112. *Int J Radiat Oncol Biol Phys* 2008;71(1):S108–S112.

56. Hartford AC, Palisca MG, Eichler TJ, et al. American society for therapeutic radiology and oncology (ASTRO) and American College of Radiology (ACR) practice guidelines for intensity-modulated radiation therapy (IMRT). *Int J Radiat Oncol Biol Phys* 2009;73(1):9–14.

57. Mijnheer 2008. ESTRO booklet: guidelines for the verification of IMRT (Edited by Mijnheer, Georg), 2008-First edition. ISBN 90–804532-9, ©2008 by ESTRO. Available from http://www.estroeducation.org/publications/Documents/Booklet_n9_P3.pdf.

58. Ezzell GA, Galvin JM, Low D, et al. Guidance document on delivery, treatment planning, and clinical implementation of IMRT: report of the IMRT subcommittee of the AAPM radiation therapy committee. *Med Phys* 2003;30(8):2089–2115.

59. van Elmpt W, McDermott L, Nijsten S, et al. A literature review of electronic portal imaging for radiotherapy dosimetry. *Radiother Oncol* 2008;88(3):289–309.

60. LoSasso T. IMRT delivery performance with a varian multileaf collimator. *Int J Radiat Oncol Biol Phys* 2008;71(1) Supplement 1: S85–S88.

61. Liu C, Simon TA, Fox C, et al. Multileaf collimator characteristics and reliability requirements for IMRT elekta system. *Int J Radiat Oncol Biol Phys* 2008;71(1):S89–S92.

62. Bayouth JE. Siemens multileaf collimator characterization and quality assurance approaches for intensity-modulated radiotherapy. *Int J Radiat Oncol Biol Phys* 2008;71(1):S93–S97.

63. Ling CC, Zhang P, Archambault Y, et al. Commissioning and quality assurance of RapidArc radiotherapy delivery system. *Int J Radiat Oncol Biol Phys* 2008;72(2):575–581.

64. Balog J, Soisson E. Helical tomotherapy quality assurance. *Int J Radiat Oncol Biol Phys* 2008;71(1):S113–S117.

65. Yan G, Fox C, Liu C, et al. The extraction of true profiles for TPS commissioning and its impact on IMRT patient-specific QA. *Med Phys* 2008;35(8):3661–3670.

66. Ibbott GS, Followill DS, Molineu HA, et al. Challenges in credentialing institutions and participants in advanced technology multi-institutional clinical trials. *Int J Radiat Oncol Biol Phys* 2008;71(1):S71–S75.

67. Esch AV, Bohsungb J, Sorvaric P, et al. Acceptance tests and quality control (QC) procedures for the clinical implementation of intensity modulated radiotherapy (IMRT) using inverse planning and the sliding window technique: experience from five radiotherapy departments. *Radiother Oncol* 2002;65(1):53–70.

68. Ezzell GA, Burmeister JW, Dogan N, et al. IMRT commissioning: multiple institution planning and dosimetry comparisons, a report from AAPM Task Group 119. *Med Phys* 2009;36(11):5359–5373.

69. Li JG, Yan G, Liu C. Comparison of two commercial detector arrays for IMRT quality assurance. *J Appl Clin Med Phys* 2009;10(2):2942.

70. Sadagopan R, Bencomo JA, Martin RL, et al. Characterization and clinical evaluation of a novel IMRT quality assurance system. *J Appl Clin Med Phys* 2009;10(2):2928.

71. Buonamici FB, Compagnucci A, Marrazzo L, et al. An intercomparison between film dosimetry and diode matrix for IMRT quality assurance. *Med Phys* 2007;34(4):1372–1379.

72. Gillis S, De Wagter C, Bohsung J, et al. An inter-centre quality assurance network for IMRT verification: results of the ESTRO QUASIMODO project. *Radiother Oncol* 2005;76(3):340–353.

73. Both S, Alecu IM, Stan AR, et al. A study to establish reasonable action limits for patient-specific quality assurance in intensity-modulated radiation therapy. *J Appl Clin Med Phys* 2007;8(2):1–8.

74. Klein EE, Hanley J, Bayouth J, et al. Task Group 142 report: quality assurance of medical accelerators, *Med Phys* 2009;36(9):4197–4212.

75. Litzenberg DW, Moran JM, Fraass BA. Verification of dynamic and segmental IMRT delivery by dynamic log file analysis. *J Appl Clin Med Phys* 2002;3:63–72.

76. Li JG, Dempsey JF, Ding L, et al. Validation of dynamic MLC-controller log files using a two-dimensional diode array. *Med Phys* 2003;30(5):799–805.

77. van Elmpt W, Nijsten S, Petit S, et al. 3D in vivo dosimetry using megavoltage cone-beam CT and EPID dosimetry. *Int J Radiat Oncol Biol Phys* 2009;73(5):1580–1587.

78. Schreibmann E, Dhabaan A, Elder E, et al. Patient-specific quality assurance method for VMAT treatment delivery. *Med Phys* 2009;36(10):4530–4535.

79. Palta J, Kim J, Li J, et al. In: Palta JR, Mackie TR, eds. *Proceedings of the 2003 AAPM summer school, Intensity-modulated radiation therapy: the state of Art.* Madison, WI: Mackie Medical Physics Publishing, 2003: 593–612.

80. Venselaar J, Welleweerd H, Mijnheer B. Tolerances for the accuracy of photon beam dose calculations of treatment planning systems. *Radiother Oncol* 2001;60: 191–201.

81. Basran PS, Woo MK. An analysis of tolerance levels in IMRT quality assurance procedures. *Med Phys* 2008;35(6): 2300–2307.

82. Pawlicki T, Whitaker M, Boyer AL. Statistical process control for radiotherapy quality assurance. *Med Phys* 2005;32: 2777–2786.

83. Pawlicki T, Yoo S, Court LE, et al. Process control analysis of IMRT QA: implications for clinical trials. *Phys Med Biol* 2008;53(18):5193–5205.

84. Breen SL, Moseley DJ, Zhang B, et al. Statistical process control for IMRT dosimetric verification. *Med Phys* 2008;35:4417–4425.

85. Yang JN, Mackie TR, Reckwerdt P, et al. An investigation of tomotherapy beam delivery. *Med Phys* 1997;24(3): 425–436.

86. Yu CX, Jaffray DA, Wong JW. The effects of intra-fraction organ motion on the delivery of dynamic intensity modulation. *Phys Med Biol* 1998;43(1):91–104.

87. Mutic S, Low DA, Klein EE, et al. Room shielding for intensity-modulated radiation therapy treatment facilities. *Int J Radiat Oncol Biol Phys* 2001;50:39–46.

88. Followill D, Geis P, Boyer A. Estimates of whole-body dose equivalent produced by beam intensity modulated conformal therapy. *Int J Radiat Oncol Biol Phys* 1997;38:667–672.

89. Verellen D, Vanhavere F. Risk assessment of radiation-induced malignancies based on whole-body equivalent dose estimates for IMRT treatment in the head and neck region. *Radiother Oncol* 1999;53:199–203.

90. Hall EJ, Wu CS. Radiation-induced second cancers: the impact of 3D-CRT and IMRT. *Int J Radiat Oncol Biol Phys* 2003;56:83–88.

91. Kry S, Salehpour M, Followill D, et al. Out-of-field photon and neutron dose equivalents from step-and-shoot intensity-modulated radiation therapy. *Int J Radiat Oncol Biol Phys* 2005;62:1204–1216.

CHAPTER 14

Image-Guided Radiation Therapy

Guang Li ■ Gig S. Mageras ■ Lei Dong ■ Radhe Mohan

INTRODUCTION

Most modern radiation therapy of cancer involves noninvasive targeting of localized disease and conformal avoidance of nontarget tissues. Radiation dose is delivered to the volume of intended treatment without the benefit of physically seeing the regions being irradiated. Therefore, imaging guidance is crucial in every step of the radiation therapy, including cancer diagnosis, staging, and delineation; treatment simulation and planning; patient setup, tumor localization and motion monitoring; and treatment response assessment, efficacy evaluation and strategy refinement. In fact, most of the significant advances in radiation oncology over the last three decades have been made possible by preceding advances in medical imaging, including computed tomography (CT), magnetic resonance imaging (MRI), magnetic resonance spectroscopic imaging (MRSI), positron emission tomography (PET), single photon emission computed tomography (SPECT), and ultrasound (US). With the aid of CT and MRI, three-dimensional (3D) shapes of treatment regions and critical normal structures are delineated with great precision, thus reducing the chance for marginal misses of the tumor and minimizing the exposure of normal tissues to high radiation dose. MRI, MRSI, PET, and SPECT images provide additional functional and biological information to define and delineate the extent of the disease. Examples of image guidance in various stages of radiation therapy are illustrated in Figure 14.1.

Image-guided radiation therapy (IGRT) is composed of a multitude of major innovations to address some of the problems arising from inter- and intra-fractional anatomic variations. IGRT aims to deliver a radiation treatment as it is planned based on an image acquired at simulated treatment conditions. This simulation image establishes a reference of 3D patient anatomy (with possible inclusion of tumor respiratory motion information) for both image-based treatment planning and image-guided treatment delivery. The former follows the exact 3D anatomy (both the tumor and normal tissues) for dosimetric planning, while the latter focuses mostly on tumor alignment between the reference image and daily images at the treatment unit prior to and during treatment, in reference to the treatment beams. Therefore, the variations of tumor position in the image-guided inter-fractional setup (i.e., variation between treatment fractions) and intra-fractional organ motion (i.e., motion occurring within a treatment fraction) could be corrected for more accurate delivery of the planned treatment dose to the target. As the variation of normal tissues is usually ignored in the current image-guided approach, dosimetric and clinical consequences must be assessed.

Increasing evidence shows that there are substantial inter- and intra-fractional variations in the shapes, volumes, and positions of treatment targets and the intervening and surrounding normal tissues, in contrast to the "snapshot" planning anatomy of a patient. The causes of such variations include body shift, rotation and deformation, respiration-induced organ motion, weight loss, and radiation-induced changes such as tumor shrinkage. These variations could have a significant impact on the outcome of treatments, as they may result in underdosing the target or overdosing the organs at risk (1–3). In the current state of the art of the planning and delivery of radiation therapy, based on the use of CT, PET, and MRI images acquired prior to the course of treatments, it is assumed implicitly that patient's anatomy discerned from initial imaging remains static throughout the course of the radiation therapy. In the current practice, wide treatment margins, derived from population-based studies, are used to ensure coverage of the disease, exposing considerable volumes of normal tissues to unwanted radiation. The use of large margins limits the ability to safely deliver higher tumor doses because of increased risk of normal tissue toxicity, especially for hypo-fractioned stereotactic body radiotherapy (SBRT), in which the high dose per fraction exceeds the normal tissue's capacity for sublethal repair. Furthermore, the margin needed for some patients exhibiting large target variations may exceed the population-based margin, potentially leading to marginal misses, especially with the use of highly conformal modalities, such as 3D conformal radiotherapy (3DCRT), intensity-modulated radiotherapy (IMRT), volumetric-modulated arc therapy (VMAT), and proton therapy (4–6). Treatment planning and delivery techniques that do not correct for such daily volumetric variations adequately may lead to suboptimal treatments. These factors may, in part, be responsible for the poor outcome and high toxicity in radiation therapy for some cancers. IGRT has the potential to target gross and microscopic diseases accurately, to

- **Treatment Planning**
  - Target and normal tissue delineation
    - Gross tumor volume and normal tissue (CT, MRI)
    - Biological tumor volume (PET, SPECT, MRSI, etc.)
    - Internal tumor volume (RCCT or 4DCT)
  - Dosimetric calculation based on patient anatomy
    - Anatomy-based planning (CT, MRI)
    - Biology-based planning (PET, SPECT, MRSI, etc.)
    - 4D planning (RCCT or 4DCT)
- **Treatment Delivery**
  - Image-guided patient setup
    - Radiographs, implanted markers, US, CT, CBCT, MRI, etc.
    - Target alignment: 2D vs. 3D
    - Online vs. offline correction
    - Anatomy-based vs. dose-based
  - Image-guided motion tracking
    - Fluoroscopy, implant markers, optical imaging, MRI, etc.
    - Direct target localization vs. target surrogates
- **Treatment Evaluation**
  - Evaluate patient's setup and dose distributions
    - Repeat CT
  - Follow-up and assessment of treatment outcome
    - Repeat CT, MR, MRSI, PET, MRS, etc.

Figure 14.1. Image guidance at various stages of the radiotherapy process.

individualize treatments to reduce margins, and to allow radiation dose escalation to higher levels with the expectation of improving local control and reducing toxicity (7,8). Although this rationale is supported by increasing evidences, continuing research to further develop IGRT methods for clinical trials is required to determine the true clinical promise of IGRT.

This chapter focuses on IGRT technologies related to treatment planning as well as treatment delivery. The related topics are covered in the following sections: second and third sections introduce various forms of IGRT technologies and their commercial implementations for interfractional and intra-fractional imaging, respectively. Fourth section reviews requirements and considerations for IGRT, including quality assurance (QA). Various possible IGRT strategies, margin assessment and reduction, and clinical implications are described in fifth section. Finally, sixth section attempts to look into the future and speculate on new processes coming into this field.

INTER-FRACTIONAL IGRT IMAGING MODALITIES

In this section, we focus on in-room IGRT imaging modalities for daily patient setup. Images acquired immediately prior to treatment are used to reposition the patient so as to align the target or its surrogate (such as implanted radio-opaque fiducial markers in or near the tumor) with the planned radiation beams. This is the simplest form of image-guided radiotherapy without modification of the original treatment design. A couch positional adjustment is typically used to realign the patient. The inter-fractional imaging modalities may be classified as follows.

2D Radiographic Imaging

Two-dimensional (2D) radiographic (projection) imaging is typically used in treatment rooms to align the patient relative to the radiation beams. Megavoltage (MV) electronic portal imaging (EPI) is the most commonly used form of radiographic imaging (9,10). MV imaging uses therapy x-ray beams and an amorphous-silicon (a-Si) flat-panel imager to verify patient's setup, defined as the position of the skeletal anatomy. Other uses of MV imaging are to verify treatment beam apertures prior to treatment (11,12) and *in vivo* dosimetry during treatment (13). Because the same therapy MV x-ray beam is used for verification, it provides direct in-field verification of treatment delivery, and therefore serves as a "gold standard" for validating new IGRT techniques. Disadvantages of MV imaging include higher radiation dose to the patient from the procedure (typically 1–5 cGy) and poorer image quality due to a large Compton scattering contribution from the higher x-ray energies. Recently, in-line low-energy (~4 MV), with a low atomic number (Z) target (e.g., carbon) without beam flattening filter, has become available, which produces portal images of improved soft-tissue contrast with lower imaging dose (14).

Two general categories of 2D kilovoltage (kV) x-ray imaging are frequently used for IGRT. One is a gantry-mounted kV imaging system on a linear accelerator (linac) that is orthogonal to the therapy MV x-ray beam. The x-ray source and flat-panel imager are mounted on retractable arms. Kilovoltage x-ray imaging provides near-diagnostic quality images. With either kV or MV imaging, determination of the correction to patient position commonly uses orthogonal image pairs that are matched to digitally reconstructed radiographs (DRRs) derived from the planning CT as a reference. The second category of kV imaging is ceiling-mounted systems (15). These systems provide an oblique orthogonal image pair for stereoscopic imaging at a wide range of treatment couch angles. Most kV x-ray radiographic imaging systems have a companion fluoroscopic imaging mode, which is useful for observing motion of the internal anatomy or implanted fiducial markers.

Kilovoltage radiographs are often not sufficient for detecting soft-tissue targets but are more successful in aligning skeletal landmarks or implanted radio-opaque fiducials as target surrogates. In-room kV x-ray imaging represents a major improvement over MV imaging due to its superior image quality and its low imaging dose. The different appearance of kV and MV images, as shown in Figure 14.2 (thorax), results from the higher proportion of Compton scattering and high-energy electrons in MV x-ray beams relative to kV x-rays.

As the kV imaging beam lines are not aligned with MV beam line, the kV-MV isocenter discrepancy must be established within a clinical tolerance through initial and periodic QA processes. The radiation dose from kV imaging is low, typically in the range of 0.01 to 0.1 cGy per

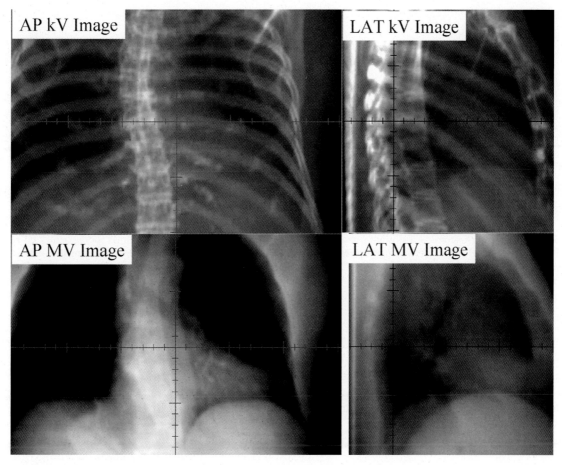

Figure 14.2. The appearance of anatomy kV (top row) and MV (bottom row) radiographs can be quite different. At kV x-ray energies, the bony structures are enhanced; at the therapeutic (MV) energies, the air cavity is enhanced. Direct comparison of kV DRRs with MV portal images can be difficult.

image, which facilitates its use for daily image-guided patient setup.

3D Tomographic Imaging

CT imaging inside the treatment room provides 3D anatomical information and improved soft-tissue visibility, thus providing advantages over radiographic imaging. In-room CT images may potentially be used to reconstruct dose distributions based on anatomy captured at treatment; its application to adaptive radiation therapy, in which a patient's treatment plan is modified in response to changes in anatomy, is an active area of investigation. In the following sections, we describe various forms of in-room CT-based on x-ray systems.

kV Helical CT

Helical single- or multiple-slice CT systems have been widely used in diagnostic imaging and radiation treatment planning for many years. The first integrated clinical system, which combined a linac unit and conventional CT unit in the same room was developed by Uematsu et al. at the National Defense Medical College, Saitama, Japan (16). The system was designed for noninvasive, frameless stereotactic radiotherapy of brain and lung cancers, to reduce the uncertainty in multi-fractional frame-based stereotactic radiotherapy. A combination of single-slice Philips CT scanner and Varian Clinac 2100EX, which used a rail system to transport the patient between treatment and CT couches, was assembled at the Memorial Sloan-Kettering Cancer Center. The system was used for treatment of paraspinal lesions and prostate cancer (17,18).

The first commercial CT-linac system in the United States was installed in 2000 in Morristown Memorial Hospital, New Jersey (19). The system consists of a Siemens medical linac and a moveable Siemens CT scanner that slides along a pair of rails ("CT-on-Rails"). A picture of the system is shown in Figure 14.3A. The CT scan is performed with the patient rotated 180 degrees from the treatment position. The initial clinical experience with this system has been reported by Wong et al. and Fung et al. (19,20). A similar "CT-on-Rails" commercial system is installed at the University of Texas M. D. Anderson Cancer Center (EXaCT™, Varian Oncology Systems, Palo Alto, CA). The mechanical accuracy of the system is found to be within 0.5 mm (21). The system, as shown in Figure 14.3B, has been recently upgraded with a 6-degree-of-freedom couch (HexaPOD™, Medical Intelligence, Germany),

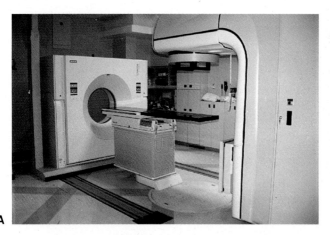
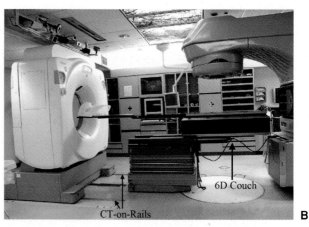

Figure 14.3. A: A Siemens Primatom™ CT-on-rails contains a Primus™ linear accelerator and a Somatom™ sliding-gantry CT scanner. The first Primatom™ was installed at the Morristown Memorial Hospital, New Jersey (Photograph courtesy of Lisa Grimm, PhD). **B:** A CT-on-rails system combining a General Electric Smart Gantry™ CT scanner and a Varian 2100EX linear accelerator. A 6-degree-of-freedom couch (HexaPOD™, Medical Intelligence, Germany) is installed on top of the standard Varian ExaCT™ couch. CT scan of the patient in immobilized treatment position is acquired after rotating the couch 180 degrees.

which allows for more precise couch translations and small rotations. The system has been routinely used for fractionated SBRT, treatment of spinal metastases (22), and lung cancers. The biggest advantage of an in-room CT scanner for IGRT is the similarity of the image quality and fields of view with planning CT images.

kV Cone-Beam CT

Gantry-mounted kV imaging systems are capable of radiography, fluoroscopy, and cone-beam CT (CBCT), providing a versatile solution for IGRT applications (23–25). CBCT imaging involves acquisition of projection images of the patient as the gantry rotates through an arc of at least 180 degrees plus the "cone-beam angle" subtended by the imaging panel (~200 degrees total). A filtered back-projection algorithm is used to reconstruct the volumetric images (26). Geometric calibration of the CBCT system is needed

periodically to maintain image quality and geometric accuracy (27). Corrections on the order of 0.2 cm are required to compensate for the gravity-induced flex in the support arms of the source, detector, and gantry. Sub-millimeter spatial resolution has been demonstrated in phantom. It is possible to reconstruct volumetric images with nearly isotropic spatial resolution, which is useful in cases requiring high resolution, such as stereotactic radiosurgery. Kilovoltage CBCT images demonstrate acceptable soft-tissue contrast for target and organ-at-risk localization.

Since October 2005, all three major manufacturers have offered CBCT capabilities (Elekta Synergy™, Elekta Inc., Sweden; Varian On-board Imager (OBI), Palo Alto, CA; and Siemens Artiste™, Germany). A picture of the commercial implementation of the kV-CBCT system by Elekta (Synergy™) and by Varian (TrueBeam™) is shown in Figure 14.4A and B, respectively. Elekta's system uses a

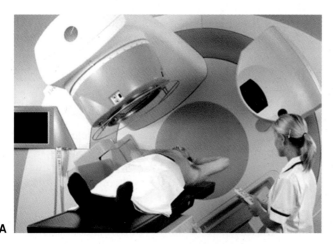
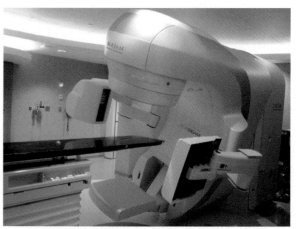

Figure 14.4. A: An Elekta Synergy™ unit (Elekta Inc., Sweden). **B:** A Varian TrueBeam™ unit (Varian Oncology Systems, Palo Alto, CA) (Photograph courtesy of Yingli Yang, PhD). Both linear accelerators have a kV imaging system orthogonal to the therapy beam direction. Both systems provide 2D radiographic, fluoroscopic, and CBCT modes.

slightly larger flat panel detector (41 by 41 cm), compared to Varian's detector (40 cm wide by 30 cm long), which limits the scan length to 15 cm when using the full-fan scanning mode. A "shifted detector" (or half-fan) technique can extend the axial field of view (FOV) to at least 40 cm (28). To further increase the FOV with the existing imager size, Li et al. has recently proposed an "off-axis" ellipse cone-beam scanning method, which shifts the center of rotation during CBCT to increase the sampling outside regular FOV, while sacrificing the sampling in the center (29).

Limitations of CBCT image quality include elevated x-ray scatter, which reduces image contrast and introduces cupping artifacts. Scatter can be reduced by using post-processing methods (Elekta's solution) (30) or anti-scatter grids (Varian's solution). Because of regulations on gantry rotation speed (maximum 1 rpm), CBCT image quality is adversely affected by the breathing motion. The IGRT setup process may add 5 minutes (1–2 min scan time and 1–3 min for image registration and approval) to the regular treatment schedule.

MV Helical CT (Tomotherapy)

Tomotherapy (TomoTherapy Inc., Madison, WI) is an integrated technology that combines a helical megavoltage CT (MVCT) with a linear accelerator, which is specially designed for delivering intensity-modulated radiation in a slit geometry. The concept was originally proposed by Mackie et al. (31,32) and substantially developed by the University of Wisconsin group (33–37). Helical tomotherapy refers to the continuous gantry and couch motion, which, as shown in Figure 14.5A, resembles the motion from a conventional helical CT scanner. Low-dose, typically 1 to 2 cGy, pretreatment MVCT images are obtained from the same treatment beam line but with a nominal energy of 4 MV. The CT detector uses an array of 738 channel xenon ion chambers and an FOV of 40 cm can be reconstructed. There is no limitation in the superior–inferior direction.

Owing to the use of MV beam for imaging, MVCT image quality is not as high as that from a diagnostic CT image: the noise level is higher and low-contrast resolution is less. Nevertheless, the MVCT images provide sufficient contrast to verify patient position (37) and to delineate many anatomic structures (38,39). It is interesting to note that the MVCT numbers are linear with respect to the electron density of material imaged, which yields reliable and accurate dose calculations (40). This capability, together with the strong research effort in treatment plan optimization and image registration by the TomoTherapy group (41–43), makes tomotherapy appealing as an integrated solution for image-guided adaptive radiotherapy.

MV Cone-Beam CT

Megavoltage cone-beam CT (MV CBCT) uses the electronic portal imaging device (EPID) mounted on a linac gantry and the therapy MV x-ray as a basic configuration for CT imaging. The initial attempt was performed by Swindell et al. (44) and subsequently implemented by Mosleh-Shirazi et al. (45). With recent advance in highly sensitive EPIDs, particularly a-Si flat panel detectors (46–48), it has become possible to rapidly acquire multiple, low-dose 2D projection images with current treatment machines. Similar to kV CBCT described in previous sections, a CBCT imaging system uses a large image detector and a single rotation of the x-ray source to complete the image acquisition. In addition to the MV x-ray source, the use of a large-area receptor (EPID) with no effective MV scatter-reduction mechanism limits image quality. The amount of scatter reaching the detector depends on the

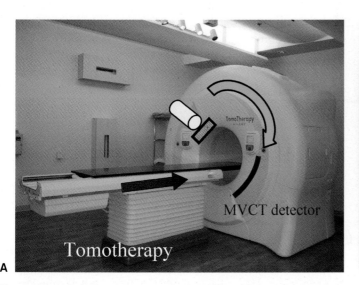
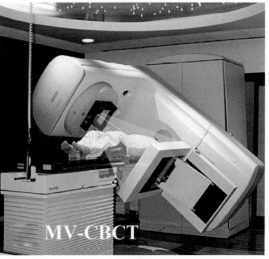

Figure 14.5. A: A picture of tomotherapy unit (TomoTherapy Inc., Madison, WI) (Photograph courtesy of H. Ning, PhD). Tomotherapy is an integrated IGRT system, which combines a linear accelerator with an MVCT image guidance system. **B:** A Siemens MV CBCT imaging system using a conventional linac and a flat-panel EPID. *Source:* Reprinted from Morin O, Gillis A, Chen J, et al. Megavoltage cone-beam CT: system description and clinical applications. *Med Dosim* 2006;31:51–61.

photon energy, field size, and the thickness of the imaged object; however, the imaging system can be optimized by calibrating the system using standard site-specific calibration phantoms (49,50).

Figure 14.5B shows a prototype MV CBCT system from Siemens. The system consists of a standard treatment unit (Primus™, Siemens Medical Solutions, Concord, CA) and an a-Si flat-panel adapted for MV photons on a retractable support. The 41 × 41 cm flat-panel x-ray detector (AG9-ES, PerkinElmer, Optoelectronics) consists of a 1 mm copper plate and a Kodak Lanex fast scintillation plate (Gd2O2 S:Tb) overlaid on a light-sensitive and charge-integrating thin-film transistor (TFT) array. Due to a more stringent requirement for geometric integrity, a calibration procedure is required to correct for mechanical support sag (49,50). The image acquisition lasts ~45 seconds with gantry rotation over a 200-degrees arc, at a rate of one image per degree. Image reconstruction time is less than 2 minutes for a 256 × 256 × 270 image volume (0.7 mm^3 voxel size). Imaging dose ranges from 2 to 8 cGy (51).

The MV CBCT system has good image quality for bony structures and acceptable quality for soft-tissue targets, due to the higher imaging dose. An advantage of both MV CBCT and MVCT systems is the reduced influence of implanted metal objects on image quality, in contrast to kV CT, which exhibits strong artifacts when high-Z material is present. MVCT images thus provide complementary information, which cannot be discerned in conventional CT images (Fig. 14.6). An additional advantage of MV

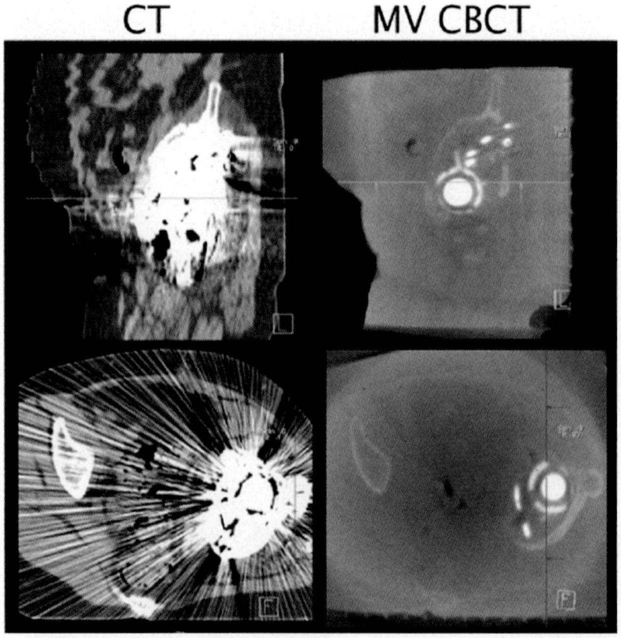

Figure 14.6. Images showing the artifacts due to the presence of metal objects in the conventional kV CT images (left panels). Artifact-free images were obtained with a MV CBCT (right panels). *Source:* Reprinted from Morin O, Gillis A, Chen J, et al. Megavoltage cone-beam CT: system description and clinical applications. *Med Dosim* 2006; 31:51–61.

CBCT is that the physics of absorbed dose from a therapeutic MV beam is well understood, thus enabling accurate calculation of dose from an MV CBCT scan that could be included in the treatment plan (51). Soft-tissue contrast is the principal limiting factor of MV CBCT systems. Investigators at the University of California San Francisco have used a lower-Z target material, which generates more low-energy photons and enhances image contrast (49). One study showed that removal of the flattening filter improved contrast by 200% (14).

Digital Tomosynthesis

Digital tomosynthesis (DTS) is a special situation of tomographic reconstruction, which uses limited arc (20 to 40 degrees) of projection images (53–55). The reconstruction planes are approximately perpendicular to the direction of the x-ray beam at the arc center. They do not have to go through the isocenter, but can be at different depths in the patient. In some methods, reconstruction is followed by a procedure to suppress out-of-plane objects (56,57). The principal advantage of DTS over CBCT is the shorter scan time, which is typically less than 10 seconds. DTS provides soft-tissue image visualization, which can be improved in respiratory disease sites by combining with breath-hold or respiration correlation of the projection images (58).

Depending on the acquisition arc length, spatial resolution is less in the direction perpendicular to the reconstructed planes, which can be addressed by acquisition of a second DTS from a quasi-orthogonal direction to the first. Reference DTS images can be calculated from the planning CT, similar to the calculation of DRRs (59). A comparison of the conventional CT, CBCT, and DTS images of the same patient is shown in Figure 14.7.

Hybrid Cone-Beam CT

Combining kV and MV projection images for CBCT reconstruction has been reported (60). A hybrid CBCT can be achieved by combining orthogonal kV and MV x-ray projection images with a partial arc gantry rotation as little as 90 degrees (61). The resultant projection images span an arc length of 180 degrees. Acquisition requires only 15 seconds, making it optimal for breath-hold imaging.

4D Computed Tomography Imaging

Respiratory motion is one of the important factors in the management of radiation therapy for moving tumors, which can have displacements up to 3 to 4 cm (62). CT scans acquired synchronously with the respiratory signal can be used to reconstruct a set of (3D) CT scans, representing the 3D anatomy at different times (or respiratory phases). This collection of 3D CT data sets is called respiration-correlated CT (RCCT), or 4D CT, which describes the snapshots of patient's 3D anatomy over a periodic respiratory signal. Typically, the breathing cycle is divided

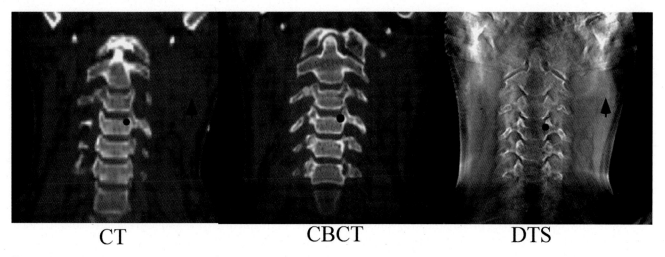

CT   CBCT   DTS

Figure 14.7. A coronal planar image reconstruction based on conventional kV CT (left), CBCT (middle), and digital tomosynthesis (DTS, right) (Photograph courtesy of Fang-Fang Yin, PhD).

into 10 respiratory phases. Four-dimensional medical imaging techniques has been reviewed recently (63).

Respiration-Correlated CT

The approach common to RCCT methods is to acquire sufficient data for generating CT images at all phases of the respiratory cycle while simultaneously recording respiration, then retrospectively correlating the CT projection images with phase. CT acquisition uses either a cine or helical mode. In cine mode, repeat CT projections are acquired over slightly more than one respiratory cycle with the couch stationary while recording patient respiration; the couch is then incremented and the process repeated. Following acquisition, the images are sorted with respect to the respiratory signal, leading to a set of volume images at different respiration points in the cycle (64,65). Helical acquisition uses a low pitch and adjusting the gantry rotation period such that all voxels are viewed by the CT detectors for at least one respiratory cycle (66,67). RCCT images have been widely characterized and applied clinically for estimating the extent of a moving tumor in lung (68–70).

The selection of the type of respiratory signal can vary, which may change the interpretation of the RCCT images; however, a periodic motion is always implied. Deviations from the regular periodic motion will have an impact on the quality of RCCT images and on the accuracy of anatomy discerned from these images. Commercial systems commonly use one of the two types of respiratory monitors. One such monitor (Real-time Position Management, RPM™, Varian Oncology Systems, Palo Alto, CA) captures the up/down motion of a box with infrared reflectors placed on the patient's abdomen or chest using an infrared camera. The other is a "pneumo bellows" system (Phillips Medical Systems, Milpitas, CA) that records the digital voltage signal from a differential pressure sensor wrapped around the patient's abdomen. RCCT scans can be used in so-called 4D treatment planning to explicitly account for tumor motion (63,68,70,72,73).

CT images are sorted based on a respiration phase angle assigned by an algorithm that determines the periodic behavior of the respiratory signal. Phase-based sorting assumes repeatable breathing cycles, that is, that the anatomy is at same position for a given phase in every cycle, which is usually not the case for normal breathing with its varying cycle-to-cycle amplitude variations, and has led to investigations into sorting based on the displacement of the respiratory signal (71,74–76).

Respiration-Correlated CBCT

A limitation of CBCT systems is image degradation caused by patient motion artifacts, which is a consequence of the limited gantry speed and the resultant long (~1 min) acquisition times. Respiratory motion in particular degrades images in the thorax and abdomen. Different methods are under active investigation to reduce motion in CBCT. One approach is respiration-correlated CBCT (RC-CBCT) using retrospective sorting of projection images into different breathing phases (77,78). A slower gantry rotation is required to acquire sufficient projections in each phase bin, resulting in scan times of 3 to 6 minutes. The limited number of projections per phase reduces the contrast resolution and introduces image view artifacts; thus, the method is more suited to detecting high-contrast objects such as tumor in parenchymal lung (77–79).

An alternative approach is to process the CBCT images to correct for motion, using a motion model of the patient (80–84). Most of the methods make use of deformable image registration (DIR) to deform the images to a common motion state.

Non-radiographic Imaging

Ultrasound Imaging

Ultrasound is a noninvasive, non-radiographic, and real-time imaging technique for soft-tissue targeting in radiotherapy, particularly for prostate cancer, but also for upper abdominal malignancies (85–89). Fung et al. have recently reviewed ultrasound guidance for IMRT (90).

The ultrasound transducer, which is made of the piezoelectric crystal, is both a sound source and a sound detector. The ultrasound transducer transmits brief pulses of ultrasound that propagate into the tissues. Whenever there is a change in acoustic impedance, for example, owing to the tissue density or elasticity changes at the interface of two organs, some of the ultrasound will be reflected back to the transducer as echoes. The round-trip time from the pulse transmission to reception of an echo is used to determine the transducer-to-object distances. A scan line converter will construct a 2D image of the patient, in which the amplitude of echoes varies along depth direction. When sweeping the ultrasound through a volume, a 3D ultrasound image can be constructed. The basic principles of this imaging technique limit its use to soft-tissue structures and tumors in pelvic, abdominal, and breast locations.

Although ultrasound has been widely used in patient setup, inherently poor image quality and the unfamiliar appearance of ultrasound images for radiation therapists have limited its potential for more precise image guidance. Figure 14.8 shows a pair of ultrasound images (top row)

and corresponding CT images (bottom row) for a prostate cancer patient undergoing ultrasound-guided setup (91). In this example, the agreement between ultrasound and CT alignments is within 2 mm. It has been shown that the inter- and intra-user variability is large for ultrasound-guided setup, mainly because of the poor image quality, anatomic distortion due to pressure variation and inadequate user training (86,92). When compared with implanted fiducial markers for prostate localization, the ultrasound alignment displayed even more variations (93) and a larger planning margin is recommended (94). Dobler et al. studied the displacement of prostate when acquiring transabdominal ultrasound images (95). X-ray simulations were performed before and during ultrasound image acquisition for 10 patients who had undergone iodine-125 seed implantation. The seeds, which were visible in x-ray images, were used to represent prostate position. A maximum displacement of the prostate of 2.3 mm in anteroposterior and 1.9 mm in craniocaudal direction and a rotational change of up to 2.5 degrees were observed. If the system was not handled correctly and too much pressure was applied, a shift of the prostate of up to 10 mm could be induced. Tome et al. has reported on ultrasound commissioning and QA procedure for radiation therapy (96).

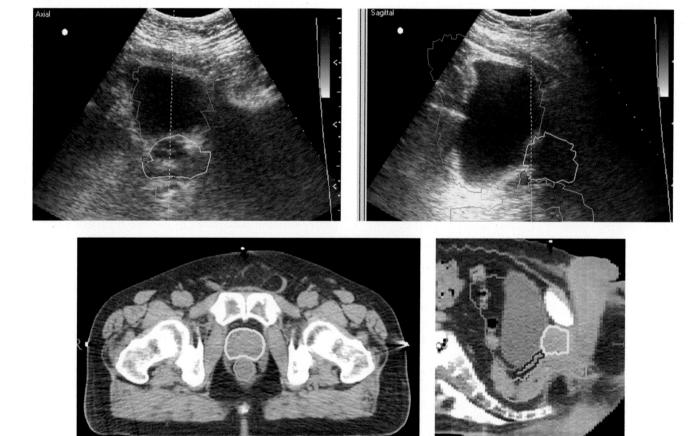

Figure 14.8. A pair of ultrasound images is shown in the top row. The images were acquired from an ultrasound-guided alignment system (BAT™, NOMOS, Chatsworth, CA). A pair of CT images of the same patient is shown in the bottom row. The CT images were acquired using an in-room CT-on-rails scanner within 5 minutes of the ultrasound image acquisition. The alignment relative to the planning CT by these two independent systems was within 2 mm.

Stereoscopic Optical Surface Imaging

Stereoscopic optical surface imaging (OSI) provides real-time imaging capability, primarily used in patient setup for superficial tumors, such as the breasts, or immobile tumors such as in the head. One currently available OSI device (AlignRT™, VisionRT, Ltd., London, UK) is composed of two to three ceiling-mounted stereo-camera pods, each contains two cameras and a speckle pattern projector. The triangulation between the fixed stereo cameras and a skin point identified by the speckle pattern serves to calculate their distances and the location of the point in space. A patient skin surface image is reconstructed from the visible surface points. The accuracy of the surface imaging is within 1.0 mm.

Because OSI does not visualize the tumor, it requires substantial validation against another established image modality, such as radiographic imaging. Early studies of surface imaging in radiotherapy have been reported by Massachusetts General Hospital (97) and Johns Hopkins University (98) in 2005. Validated with x-ray imaging, OSI provides a quick and non-radiologic means for image-guided setup. It has been applied in breast, lung, brain, and head and neck. The common procedure for patient setup is to register the surface image to a reference region of interest (ROI) defined on the delineated patient surface in a simulation CT.

Magnetic Resonance Imaging

MRI is based on the radiofrequency signal from the relaxation process of the dipole moment of an atom with unpaired proton, such as ^1H in tissue, after it is excited with a radiofrequency pulse sequence in the presence of an external magnetic field. The field strength is ~0.2 Tesla (T) for open-field MRI and 1.5 T or 3 T for a regular MRI scanner. The geometric location of the signal is determined using the field gradient, phase and frequency encoding. The soft-tissue heterogeneity provides an environment that alters the relaxation process, thus providing high soft-tissue contrast.

MRI imaging is more versatile than radiologic imaging, as it provides different image appearances when different pulse sequences are applied, such as T1-weighted, T2-weighted, and fast fluid-attenuation inversion recovery (FLAIR) (99). These MRI images are often used in delineating a tumor or postoperation cavity and evaluating local edema, especially for brain cancer. MRI can also produce non-axial scans in any spatial orientation. Like radiologic imaging, MRI can produce 2D planar, 3D volumetric, and 4D volumetric set images (63). Four-dimensional prospective volumetric MRI imaging has been utilized in radiotherapy (100).

MRI may suffer from geometric distortion due to non-uniformity of the external magnetic field strength. This scanner-specific factor can be corrected by measuring the field gradient with a large grid phantom (101). MRI does not produce a visible image in bone due to little relaxation in the solid phase. A limitation for radiotherapy applications is that an MR image cannot be easily converted to electron density, which is essential for dosimetry calculation in a treatment planning system. Recently, MRI-based treatment planning has been reported (102–104).

Several MRI-guided radiotherapy systems are currently under development. Such systems offer not only in-room soft-tissue-based target alignment, but also near real-time MRI volumetric imaging for tumor motion monitoring. The section "MRI Real-Time Volumetric Imaging" discusses these systems in more detail.

INTRA-FRACTIONAL REAL-TIME IMAGING AND MOTION COMPENSATION

The main goal of real-time tracking is to minimize the effect of target motion not only between treatments, but also during a treatment fraction. Real-time tracking usually requires real-time motion monitoring (detection) and the execution of correction with the shortest time delay. In almost all cases, implanted markers are used as surrogates for target position. Therefore, the proximity of the markers to the target and their motion relative to the target are important factors in their reliability for a real-time tracking system. In the following sections, we review different approaches for real-time monitoring and tracking.

Fluoroscopic Imaging with Implant Fiducials

Commercial fluoroscopy-based tracking systems can be categorized into room-mounted and linac gantry-mounted systems. The primary reason for using fluoroscopic imaging is to detect metal fiducials, which are implanted in or near the tumor. The fluoroscopic images can be matched to a reference DRR.

A very interesting, room-mounted system for real-time tracking has been developed by Shirato et al. in collaboration with Mitsubishi at the University of Hokkaido (105,106). It uses a pair of x-ray tubes that rotate on a circular track embedded in the floor, as shown in Figure 14.9A. Each tube has a corresponding x-ray detector that rotates synchronously on a ceiling-mounted track, so as to avoid obstruction of the patient by the treatment gantry. The x-ray tubes allow pulsed imaging interlaced with linac pulses to treat the patient. The radio-opaque marker images are tracked with pulsed fluoroscopy prior to the beginning of the treatment and patient is repositioned so that the end of one of the tracks corresponding to the least mobile portion of the motion is within a predefined gating window. During irradiation, fluoroscopy continues and the beam is automatically switched on when the detected image of the fiducial is within the window; otherwise, it is turned off.

A commercially available room-mounted system, as shown in Figure 14.9B, is developed by BrainLab (ExacTrac® BrainLAB AG, Feldkirchen, Germany). The ExacTrac is an

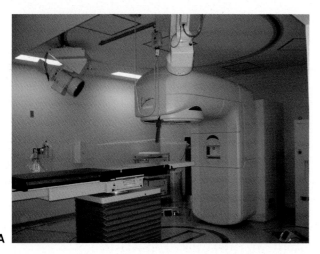
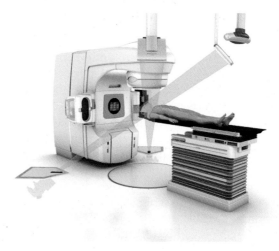

A   **B**

Figure 14.9. Two room-mounted kV image-guided IGRT real-time tracking systems. **A:** A real-time tracking radiation therapy (RTRT) system (Photograph courtesy of Hiroki Shirato, MD, PhD). **B:** ExacTrac system, BrainLAB AG, Feldkirchen, Germany (Photograph courtesy of BrainLAB AG.)

integrated IGRT system for target localization, setup correction, and the delivery of high-precision stereotactic radiotherapy and stereotactic radiosurgery. The image guidance utilizes two distinct imaging subsystems: a real-time infrared (IR) tracking and a kV stereoscopic x-ray imaging subsystem. Two ceiling-mounted IR cameras are used to monitor the movement of infrared-reflecting markers placed on patient's skin or on the reference frame mounted on the treatment couch. The marker images are automatically compared to a stored reference, generating initial couch shift instruction to set up the patient. The x-ray imaging system performs further internal target alignment based on either bony landmarks or implanted fiducial markers. The reference DRRs are provided by the BrainLab treatment planning system. During treatment delivery, the IR tracking system and the fluoroscopic x-ray imaging system work together to monitor target position and to perform treatment interventions. The external fiducial markers can be "tuned" to the internal fiducial markers during a pretreatment verification procedure. Two types of treatment interventions can be performed: adaptive gating of the treatment beam or real-time correction of target offset by using a 6D robotic couch (ExacTrac®, BrainLAB AG, Feldkirchen, Germany). CyberKnife™ system (Accuray Inc., Sunnyvale, CA) has also its own room-mounted stereoscopic x-ray imaging system and 6D robotic couch. Research and clinical experience of using these systems have been reported by various groups (107–110).

Gantry-mounted kV imaging systems usually have only one kV x-ray imager and achieve the orthogonal pair by rotating the gantry. These systems include Varian's Onboard Imager (OBI) and Elekta's Synergy. These kV imaging beam lines are orthogonal to the MV treatment beam line (EPID), sharing the same isocenter of gantry rotation, as shown in Figure 14.4. The gantry-mounted kV imaging system is not blocked by the treatment unit, but it may have limited clearance or the potential for collision with

the immobilization device or the couch. The kV-MV configuration provides a possibility to acquire images during treatment (111). To avoid scatter interference between the two x-ray beams, alternating the beam-on time may be used (112).

A prototype kV-MV dual in-line imaging system is commercially available (Artiste™, Siemens Medical Systems, Germany) (113,114). This is achieved by placing the kV x-ray tube in a retractable lower shelf. The kV image detector is mounted just below the MV collimator. The MV therapy beam must penetrate the kV image detector to treat the patient. This design allows for simultaneous imaging of the beam shaping device (MLC-collimated beams) and patient's anatomy for beam-by-beam verification of treatment delivery or motion compensation.

Optical Fiducial Motion Surrogates

Optical tracking determines an object's position by measuring light either emitted or reflected from the object. The hallmark of optical tracking systems is their high spatial and temporal resolutions (0.1 mm and <0.1 s, respectively) in tracking infrared markers attached to the patient's external surface. The positions of the optical markers relative to the target volume, together with the desired marker positions relative to the treatment isocenter, are determined during CT simulation. In the treatment room, the real marker positions are measured relative to isocenter; a rigid-body transformation determines marker displacements from their desired positions and hence target displacement from the isocenter. Real-time feedback allows one to correct the patient's position continuously during treatment. Meeks et al. have reviewed the technology in several implementations for intracranial and extracranial stereotaxis radiotherapy (115). The first systems used rigid arrays of optical markers that were attached to the patient via a biteplate linkage. Subsequent systems for extracranial radiotherapy tracked external markers to determine the patient position and/or gate the radiation beam based on patient motion.

Video-Based 3D Optical Surface Imaging

Real-time 3D-surface matching has been characterized for clinical use (97,98,116). The reference surface image is either a 3D optical surface image acquired at simulation or a CT/MRI-surface rendering from the treatment plan. The real-time 3D surface images are captured by stereoscopic video cameras mounted on the ceiling of the treatment vault. A fast automatic alignment between the real-time surface and the reference surface using a modified iterative-closest-point method leads to an efficient and robust surface-guided target refixation. Experimental and clinical results demonstrate the excellent efficacy of <2 minutes set-up time and high accuracy and precision of <1 mm in isocenter shifts and <1 degree in rotation (116).

The AlignRT system has been described in a previous section for patient alignment. In addition, it offers capabilities for real-time motion monitoring. Due to processing time required for image reconstruction, it only provides prospective imaging at one to five frames per second (fps), far below its maximum capture rate (~15 fps), (117) depending upon the size and resolution of ROI. Several investigators have shown that this real-time surface imaging capability can be applied to head motion monitoring during frameless stereotactic radiotherapy or radiosurgery (52,118,119). Using a 3D optical surface image acquired at treatment as reference, systematic errors of the imaging system can be cancelled out and achieve a sub-millimeter accuracy for motion detection (52).

Real-Time Electromagnetic Localization and Tracking

Continuous tracking of target position without ionizing radiation is possible with a novel technology utilizing AC electromagnetic fields to induce and detect signals from implanted "wireless" transponder (Calypso Medical Technologies, Inc., Seattle, WA). The system consists of a console, optical tracking system, and a tracking station. The console instrument is situated in the treatment room and includes a display screen and the AC magnetic array (Fig. 14.10). The magnetic array is lightweight and contains source coils that generate signals to excite the transponders, and sensor coils that detect the unique response signals returned by each transponder. Unlike passive fiducial markers, the Calypso system can actively detect the position of transponders without using the radiographic method. The Calypso 4D Localization System can update target position 10 times per second, which is sufficiently fast to track breathing motion of the tumor. Sub-millimeter tracking accuracy and clinical experience in prostate target localization has been reported (120–124).

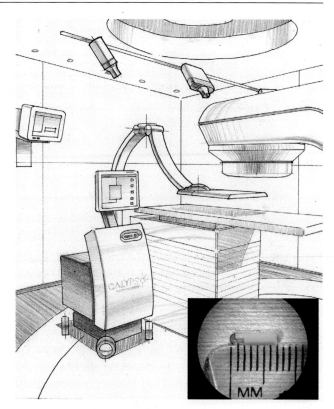

Figure 14.10. A diagram showing the prototype AC electromagnetic field tracking system with the detector array and the infrared cameras (Calypso Medical Technologies, Inc., Seattle, WA) The Beacon™ transponder is shown in the inset.

MRI Real-Time Volumetric Imaging

Another innovative technology being developed for radiation therapy applications is an integrated MRI-guided gamma ray IMRT system (Renaissance System™, ViewRay, Inc., Gainesville, FL). A schematic diagram of the IG-IMRT system is shown in Figure 14.11. The system consists of a low-field open MRI system and three Cobalt irradiation sources; the latter was chosen for its compatibility with the MRI system. The computerized multileaf collimator system provides gamma-ray intensity modulation equivalent to linac-based IMRT systems. The thrust of the technology is the MRI-guided, real-time volumetric imaging system, which can track patient's 3D anatomy every 0.5 to 2.0 seconds without interrupting the treatment delivery. As stated earlier, MRI has superior soft-tissue contrast, which can be used for better definition and tracking of target volumes. As an integrated imaging, adaptive treatment planning and dynamic delivery system, this promising technology is perhaps the only "near" real-time, volumetric soft-tissue targeting system. Because of the known limits of the Cobalt source, such as low energy and large penumbra, the plan quality is compromised.

Recently, there has been development of integrated MRI-linac systems, thus combining the advantages of high soft-tissue discrimination for tracking and linac quality radiation treatment (125–127). There are two designs, with the

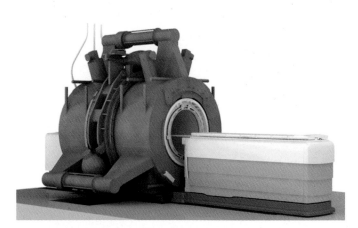
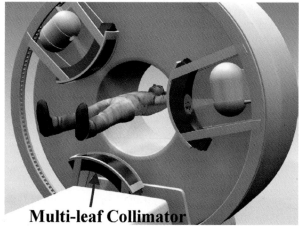

Multi-leaf Collimator

Figure 14.11. A schematic of a prototype MRI-guided real-time volumetric tracking system for IGRT (Renaissance System™, ViewRay, Inc., Gainesville, FL). The system is designed to have a low-field open MRI for real-time imaging and three-headed Cobalt source for intensity-modulated gamma ray irradiation (Photograph courtesy of James Dempsey, PhD).

radiation beam either parallel or perpendicular to the magnetic field. A nontrivial technical task is to shield the magnetic field from the linac in transporting electrons to the target. In addition, the presence of magnetic field affects the motion of the scattered secondary electron scatters, thereby distorting the dose distribution. Nevertheless, integrated MRI-linac systems promise high-precision radiation dose delivery guided by high-quality soft-tissue visualization.

Real-Time Tumor Motion Compensation

Real-time tracking refers to continuous adjustment of the radiation beam or patient position during treatment so as to follow the changing position of the tumor or its surrogate. A means of localizing the target in real time is coupled to the repositioning control system. In principle, real-time tracking provides more efficient treatment than gating, in that the beam duty cycle is at or near 100%, while reducing the margin needed for target motion. In the following sections, we summarize three strategies in various stages of development involving motion tracking of a linac system.

Dynamic Multi-leaf Collimator Approach

Keall et al. have demonstrated motion tracking using dynamic MLC (DMLC) (128). The Calypso electromagnetic system can provide a near real-time signal of prostate motion with <2 mm accuracy and 220 ms system latency (123). One concern of this motion compensation approach is the anisotropic spatial resolution. Depending on whether the motion is along or perpendicular to the leaf motion, the spatial resolution is either <1 mm (the leaf motion accuracy) or 5 mm (the leaf width), respectively. The mechanical motion limitations of MLC pose constraints when DMLC is used simultaneously for motion tracking and IMRT delivery. Investigators have examined different strategies to optimize leaf trajectories for this purpose (129,130).

Mobile Treatment Couch Approach

D'Souza et al. have proposed compensation of the tumor motion using a mobile couch (131). Unlike the DMLC approach, this method compensates for 3D tumor motion with isotropic spatial resolution; however, there may be patient-related physical and medical concerns. For instance, couch motion could induce a counterreaction from the patient, body shift, or tissue deformation when changing motion directions, especially for obese patients. Clinically, a patient may feel dizziness or nausea. Recently, a dynamically adjustable head support was developed for repositioning and for potentially tracking head motion in 6D (translations and rotations) with sub-millimeter accuracy in frameless stereotactic radiotherapy (132,133). As the head is fairly well immobilized with a thermoplastic mask and/or head mold, the motion is slow and the motion range is on the order of 1 to 3 mm. Therefore, the compensating motion for repositioning would be small and slow, posing little or no clinical concerns.

Movable Gantry Approach

The CyberKnife™ (Accuray Inc., Sunnyvale, CA) is an intelligent robotic IGRT system consisting of a small X-band linear accelerator mounted on a 6D robotic arm and a 6D robotic couch for patient alignment. The robotic arm can move at a speed of several centimeters per second, which allows it to keep up with breathing-induced tumor motion. The room-mounted x-ray stereoscopic guidance system provides IGRT setup as well as real-time tracking for image-guided radiosurgery applications, as depicted in Figure 14.12A. An optical tracking system of IR reflectors on a vast worn by the patient provides a real-time target motion signal that is confirmed by periodic x-ray imaging. The CyberKnife is the first clinical radiotherapy system to use real-time motion compensation and has accumulated a wealth of data on the experience of tracking moving targets in a wide variety of treatment scenarios (134–136).

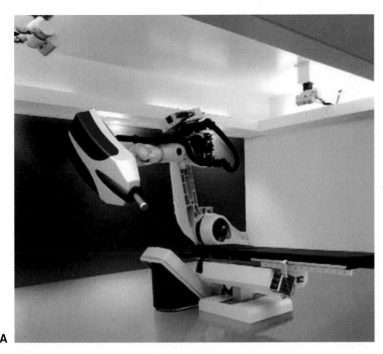 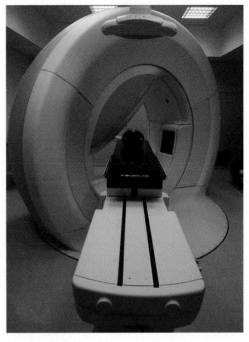

A   B

Figure 14.12. A CyberKnife system (Accuray Inc., Sunnyvale, CA) is shown in (**A**). A VERO system (BrainLAB AG Feldkirchen, Germany and Mitsubishi Heavy Industries, Tokyo, Japan) is shown in (**B**) (Photograph courtesy of Dirk Verellen, PhD). Both systems offer quick gantry movement aiming to a moving tumor, guided by room-mounted or gantry-mounted stereoscopic x-ray imaging systems.

Clinical experience in frameless image-guided cranial (137,138), spinal (139–141), pancreatic (142), and lung radiosurgery (143,144) has been reported.

The VERO™ system is a joint development by BrainLAB AG (Feldkirchen, Germany) and Mitsubishi Heavy Industries (Tokyo, Japan). It is based on a gimbal design, as shown in Figure 14.12B, such that the radiation gantry can rotate quickly to track a moving tumor (145–147). For both panning and tilting rotations, the maximum motion range at treatment isocenter is 4.4 cm (or 2.5 degrees). The response lag time is <50 ms for both panning and tilting rotations. With system lag compensated by using a predicting model, sub-millimeter accuracy of motion tracking has been achieved in initial tests (147). One prototype, installed in UZ Brussels Hospital, the Netherlands, is equipped with an EPID for portal imaging and two orthogonal kV imaging systems that are 45 degrees from the MV beam. CBCT capability is available and patient position corrections are provided by a BrainLAB 5DOF robotic couch that is integrated in the system. Although more characterization studies of the system are needed, initial tests have shown its potential for tumor motion tracking.

IGRT REQUIREMENTS AND CONSIDERATIONS

IGRT Commissioning and Quality Assurance

Commissioning and QA of all IGRT-enabled technologies are essential. In the past few years, the American Association of Physicists in Medicine (AAPM) has issued several task group (TG) reports, covering in-room kV x-ray imaging for patient setup and target localization (TG #104) (148), medical accelerator QA (TG #142) (149), stereotactic body radiation therapy (TG #101) (150), and management of respiratory motion (TG #76) (62). These reports provide guidelines for clinical use and QA of the IGRT imaging systems and procedures. In the following, we summarize three important aspects: geometric accuracy, image quality, and motion detection.

Clinical "Gold Standard" for IGRT

One of most important tasks in commissioning an in-room imaging modality is to compare the imaging isocenter with the treatment isocenter. Traditionally, it is paramount to check the alignment of radiation isocenter, mechanical isocenter, and laser isocenter. When using IGRT imaging modalities, their isocenter coincidence with the treatment radiation isocenter must be initially and periodically checked to assure a clinically acceptable tolerance on their discrepancy. The MV EPID is used as the gold standard as it provides direct reference to the treatment beam line. For stereotactic procedures, the discrepancy should be within 1.0 mm; otherwise, it should be within 2.0 mm (149). Due to the stringent geometric accuracy requirement for the alignment of the OBI and EPID detectors, a calibration procedure is required to correct the mechanical sagging (27,49,50,151). Customized QA phantoms have been developed for different IGRT systems, including kV and MV imaging systems of a linac (149,152) and MVCT imaging system of a helical tomotherapy (153,154).

Imaging Quality QA

Bissonnette and coworkers have established QA program for CBCT imaging quality with the Elekta Synergy and Varian OBI systems. The description includes flat-panel detector stability, performance and image quality of 10 volumetric imaging systems over a period of 3 years (155). Details on correcting background (dark current) and pixel-by-pixel gain uniformity (flood image) of the plat-panel detector are discussed. Similar to diagnostic imaging QA, the CatPhan 500 phantom (The Phantom Laboratory, Salem, NY) is used to quantify image quality (156,157). A comprehensive QA program by Yoo et al. covers safety and functionality, geometric accuracy, and image quality for the Varian OBI system (158). Image quality characterization and QA procedures for EPID (159), MV CBCT (160), and MVCT in helical tomotherapy (154) have also been reported.

Non-gantry mounted x-ray imaging and non-radiological imaging have been reviewed by Bissonnette (155), including the commissioning of image-guided technologies and procedures, QA of geometric accuracy and implementation of a clinical IGRT QA program. A stereotactic head phantom (Model 605 Radiosurgery Head Phantom; CIRS, Norfolk, VA) or equivalent is used for imaging QA of the CyberKnife system (155,161).

Motion-Related QA Processes

In AAPM TG #142 (149), x-ray (MV and kV) 2D radiographic imaging, 3D tomographic (fan-beam and cone-beam) imaging, and 4D imaging are included as part of the QA process for medical accelerators. For 2D fluoroscopic imaging, the temporal resolution should be 100 ms or less, which will produce a uncertainty <2 mm for a moving object at a speed no greater than 2 cm/s. Jiang et al. have laid out major clinical QA challenges in respiratory-related procedures, including respiratory gating, breath holding, and 4D CT imaging (162). As external surrogates are used for most respiratory gating and breath holding, the authors conclude that the biggest challenge is how to ensure treatment accuracy in these cases. Indeed, many reports have discussed the unreliability of the internal–external correlation using external fiducials, such as IR reflectors for motion monitoring. When external respiratory fiducial markers are used, a pretreatment calibration and during-treatment verification against x-ray radiographic imaging is needed. Clinical motion management guideline has been published in AAPM TG #76 (62), covering respiration-induced motions of the target and normal tissue.

Image Registration

Image registration quantitatively aligns the daily 3D or 2D setup images with the planning CT volume or DRR images, respectively. Such image registrations can be suboptimal as the underlying anatomy changes, including daily motion, deformation, or physical changes. Clinically, the focus on

registration of the tumor position is commonly accepted. Visual verification, together with manual adjustment, is necessary for automatic registration. Most visual verification is performed in three orthogonal planar views using color blending, checkerboard, split windows, and difference images. A 3D volumetric visualization to seek most homogeneous color distribution of mono-color images on a volumetric anatomical landmark has been reported with greater spatial accuracy for rigid anatomy (163,164). Image registration method QA should be performed using an appropriate phantom. A QA procedure for image registration and segmentation has been reported (165).

Rigid Image Registration

Most registration tools, which are used for image-guided patient setup, belong to rigid image registration with up to six degrees of freedom (6DOF or 6D). Owing to limitation of the standard treatment couch, three or four DOF are usually employed, unless a 6D robotic couch is available. As patient motion and deformation is inevitable, rigid image registration has limited accuracy. In addition, inter-observer variation for manual image registration is well known. The registration accuracy, couch adjustment accuracy, kV-MV isocenter discrepancy, and couch walk for non-coplanar beams, together with patient immobilization, determine the overall setup accuracy for tumor localization.

Locally focused rigid image registrations are more clinically relevant in the presence of tissue deformation. Zhang et al. (166), Van Kranen et al. (167), and Giske et al. (168) have reported using multiple ROIs for rigid registration and evaluated the local deformation among the three to nine different ROIs in the head and the neck region. Park and coworkers have developed a spatially weighted image registration method to allow users to define the structure of interest, such that a better registration result is achieved with respect to the structure of interest (169). Manual intervention of the semiautomatic registration using visual guidance is always required.

Deformable Image Registration

DIR is not suitable for setup correction with simple couch shifts, as rigid transformation cannot compensate for tissue deformation. Nevertheless, DIR is essential for evaluating cumulative delivered dose distribution, and therefore necessary for adaptive actions to compensate for potential dosimetric deviation from what was planned in the remaining treatment fractions. DIR has been intensively studied (42,170–173) and is an important tool in presenting developments of high-precision radiotherapy. Indeed, many clinical studies using DIR have been reported since 2007, including automatic segmentation and dose distribution mapping for adaptive radiotherapy (174–179).

In the IGRT context, DIR plays a significant role in the following three areas. First, it can track a deformed anatomy voxel by voxel from deformed images to a reference image, producing a deformation transformation matrix,

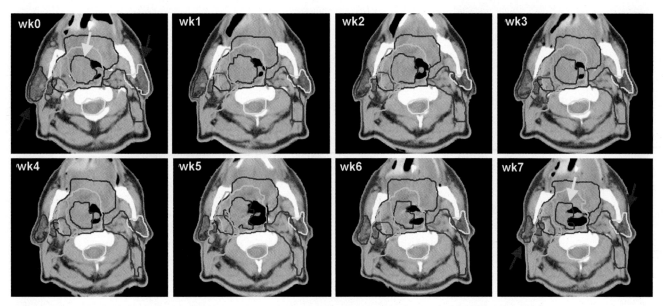

Figure 14.13. Automated image segmentation of multiple repeat CT data sets. In this head-and-neck example, contours drawn manually on the planning CT were deformed to obtain contours for repeat CT scans obtained during the course of radiotherapy. Deformations were carried out using transformation matrices based on deforming planning CT image to match each of the repeat CT images. Such automatic segmentation tools, once validated by clinical studies, would make adaptive replanning practical.

which is useful in studying tumor and organ motion. Zhang et al. have illustrated that the combination of DIR with principal component analysis (PCA) provides a patient-specific motion model (180). Such a DIR-PCA approach has been further developed to predict lung tumor location based on single x-ray projection image (181).

Second, the deformation transformation matrix can be used for mapping segmented anatomic ROIs, such as delineated tumor and organs at risk, from a reference image to other deformed images. Such an auto-contouring technique is essential for 4D and adaptive radiotherapy, as illustrated in Figure 14.13. Wijesooriya et al. have studied the accuracy of the automated segmentation among different phase CT images in 4D CT by comparing 692 pairs of automated and physician-drawn contours. The surface congruence of the gross tumor volume (GTV) and all organs was within 5 mm in >90% of all cases (178). Wang et al. have studied the use of deformable registration to propagate contours in daily CBCT for both lung and head-and-neck cancer patients, and found the volume overlap index to be 83% between the deformed and the physician-drawn contours (175). Physician evaluation of these automated contours is highly recommended, especially in the presence of motion and metal artifacts.

Third, the deformation transformation matrix can be applied to map a dose distribution that is calculated based on static volumetric CT images to a reference volumetric image (70,128). At the end, a cumulative dose distribution can be determined for evaluating delivered radiation dose using daily setup images and for 4D planning based on all phase CTs within a 4D CT image set (183). In IGRT, the principal advantage of DIR is to track radiation doses deposited in a deformed organ over the course of fraction-

ated treatment, which is a basis for image-guided adaptive radiotherapy (184–186).

Information Technology Infrastructure for IGRT

With the increasing use of highly conformal treatment techniques, such as IMRT, VMAT, and SBRT, the need for image guidance is mounting at every stage of the radiotherapy process. Implementation of IGRT into routine clinical workflow requires tighter integration of imaging and treatment systems and more efficient information flow. IGRT represents a shift from a traditionally static treatment planning process to a more dynamic, close-loop practice with multiple feedback check/control points. To meet the technical and logistical needs for this dynamic treatment process, the following infrastructure and software tools are considered important to IGRT applications:

■ IGRT Data Management
  ■ Radiotherapy Picture Archival and Communication System (RT-PACS): Further development is needed to meet the evolving needs of new IGRT workflows and extra data requirements using efficient centralized communication among different imaging and treatment procedures.
  ■ Digital Imaging and Communications in Medicine (DICOM) and its radiotherapy (RT) extension are industrial standards for facilitating connectivity and interoperability of medical image data. Advancements in IGRT have revealed shortcomings in the DICOM-RT standard and the need to address them. The development of new-generation objects is being addressed by a DICOM working group for radiation

therapy objects (187). Compatibility of DICOM and DICOM-RT files among different vendors may need further attention.

- Record and Verify (R&V) server: With the more frequent use of volumetric image acquisition and possible adaptive replanning during the course of treatment, data storage requirements can increase 1 to 2 orders of magnitude. It is also essential to have mirrored servers, robust data backup mechanism, and a disaster recovery strategy for routine, continuous clinical operations (188).
- IGRT Facilitating Tools:
  - DIR: Both rigid and DIR tools are necessary for implementing various IGRT approaches at different levels to correct for geometric and dosimetric variations (171,176,189,190).
  - Fast treatment planning and optimization algorithms: With the increasing need for treatment plan adaptation to the changed anatomy or altered target volumes, it becomes necessary to develop fast treatment planning and optimization strategies (191).
  - Cross-platform planning comparison tools: The computational environment for radiotherapy research (CERR), developed by Deasy and coworkers, provides a common platform for creating multi-institutional IMRT treatment plan database, including adaptive plans. This also provides a platform for data mining in the planning database for clinical outcome research and analysis (192–194).

Selection of IGRT Technology

The selection of an appropriate image-guidance solution is a complex process that is a compromise of clinical objective, product availability, existing infrastructure, and manpower (195,196). The deployment of a new technology requires a thorough understanding of the complete clinical process and the necessary infrastructure to support data collection, analysis, and intervention. The AAPM TG #104 report (148) suggests four aspects of considerations, clinical, technical, resource, and administration, when choosing an IGRT solution. We believe that these considerations will evolve, depending on industry trend and economics. Ten key points are as follows:

i. Clinical objectives (dose escalation/normal tissue sparing)
ii. Structures of interest (target and normal structures)
iii. Strength of surrogates (skin markers, bony landmarks, implanted fiducials, etc.)
iv. Desired level of geometric precision (radiosurgery/hypofractionation)
v. Uncertainties to be managed through the use of margins
vi. Method of intervention/correction (degrees of freedom)
vii. Techniques of managing tumor motion
viii. Magnitude of dose gradients
ix. Available treatment capacity and patient load (treatments/hour)
x. Identification of individuals responsible for maintenance and development

IGRT CORRECTION STRATEGIES AND APPLICATIONS

Online Versus Off-line Corrections

The development of various mechanisms for measuring patient position has created a wealth of valuable data for correction of patient position. The use of these data to stratify treatment decision and to modify the treatment process is referred to as a correction strategy. Strategies are broadly divided into online and off-line approaches. The online approach makes adjustment to the treatment parameters or patient position based upon data acquired during the current treatment session. This may be as simple as adjusting the couch position or as complex as full reoptimization of the treatment parameters based on changes in the shape and relative position of target and normal structures. The off-line approach is one in which the intervention is determined from an accumulation of information that may be drawn from previous treatment sessions or other times of measurement. The online approach is generally categorized as having a greater capacity to increase precision with an associated increase in effort for the same level of accuracy as can be achieved with off-line strategies, but at the cost of a higher workload. In general, clinical implementations typically operate with a hybrid of online and off-line approaches that are invoked under different error thresholds. A familiar example is seen in conventional portal film practice in which the first treatment session is adjusted "online" (at the time of therapy), while subsequent corrections are applied off-line (physician review of portal images). For a detailed review of the numerous strategies in clinical use, the reader is referred to recent reviews in the literature (6,7,146,191,197).

More complex IGRT procedures, which employ increased frequency of imaging, alignment tools, and decision rules, offer potentially increased accuracy compared to conventional practice. The overhead associated with the alignment tools and decision rules can be prohibitive unless properly integrated. The adaptive radiotherapy program at William Beaumont Hospital (184–186,198,199) was made possible only through in-house software integration efforts. Similarly, effort was also required from the procedure and policy perspective to coordinate the actions of the off-line efforts with the radiation therapists operating the machine. Online approaches require elevated levels of software and hardware integration for operation as the analysis and interpretation are performed at the time of therapy.

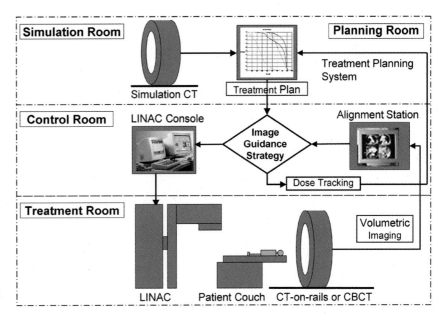

Figure 14.14. An in-room volumetric CT-guided radiotherapy process. CT images of patient's setup and anatomy information are acquired and sent to an alignment workstation where the images are compared and aligned to match with the planning CT. An interventional decision is made based on the magnitude of anatomic variations to assess the need for an online or off-line correction. If necessary, dose tracking may be enabled and used for replanning.

Correction for Inter-fractional Setup Error

Inter-fractional variations are usually larger than intra-fractional ones; therefore, various techniques have been developed for pretreatment setup corrections. Without loss of generality, we consider an in-room CT-guided IGRT system (Fig. 14.14). In the diagram, 3D volumetric CT (CT-on-rails or CBCT) images are acquired after the patient is immobilized and the skin marks aligned with room lasers, then sent to an alignment workstation where the images are registered with the planning CT. The first level of intervention is always the correction of translational shifts. Usually, rotation has smaller effect than the translational shifts of the target, and can be corrected using a 6D couch with isocentric rotation. Depending on the magnitude of the differences observed, an off-line correction protocol may be used to reduce systematic uncertainties while improving operation efficiency (200–202). The second level of intervention may be dose based. In theory, the ultimate treatment goal should be based on the final delivered dose distributions, instead of what was originally planned using the initial planning CT. In-room CT images of the patient's treatment anatomy allows reconstruction of the delivered dose distributions and therefore dose tracking. Cumulative dose distributions can be corrected infrequently using an off-line adaptive correction scheme (191,199,203,204).

Management of Intra-fractional Tumor Motion

In the presence of significant intra-fractional motion, additional geometric and dosimetric variations should also be included. This will set the complexity to another level. There are many different approaches in the management of intra-fractional tumor motion. Not surprisingly, most of these applications are related to the treatment of

lung and liver cancers (62,63,146,191,196). To setup a patient with a moving tumor, marker imaging may be used by aligning the track of the implanted marker, or a portion thereof, with the track discerned from the reference pretreatment 4D CT. Alternatively, bony landmarks may be used for setup alignment. However, the tumor motion trajectory relative to the bony landmark may change, and recent studies have shown that the inter-fractional tumor location has significant variation (205,206).

Real-time monitoring of implanted markers, or of the tumor directly, is needed for accurate "gating" of radiation treatments. Respiratory monitoring and control devices used for imaging may also be used to trigger the beam and the MLC motion on and off during the delivery of gated radiation treatments. The radiation beam is automatically switched on only during a small, generally most reproducible portion of the breathing cycle. In gated IMRT, leaf motion is also correspondingly stopped and resumed, thereby avoiding an interplay effect (207). Similar to imaging, video feedback may be used to improve breathing or breath-hold regularity and reproducibility (208). The same methodology may also be used for "gated breath-hold" treatments in which the patient voluntarily or involuntarily holds his or her breath at the same point in the breathing cycle. In voluntary breath-hold, the beam is turned on only if the breath is held at the same point. Reproducible involuntary breath-hold may be achieved using technology such as active breathing control (ABC) developed by Wong et al. (209,210).

There are considerations regarding implantation of fiducial markers for lung cancers. Implantation is invasive and may cause clinical complications. Marker images do not provide 3D anatomic information on tumor shape changes. Variations of the normal anatomy are ignored altogether. In addition, experience to date shows that markers may get lost and drift appreciably over the course of radiotherapy. Ideally, prospective volumetric imaging would be desirable for both geometric guidance and dosimetric assessment, such as 4D volumetric MRI integrated with a linac (125–127). Nevertheless, implanted markers may be ideal for tracking targets during treatments, and often serve as a gold standard for verification of the target location.

Real-time tumor motion tracking has been implemented with the CyberKnife unit with guidance of both x-ray imaging of implanted fiducial markers and an optical external motion surrogate (211–213). For other types of linacs, such capability is still at the development stage. Zimmerman et al. have demonstrated motion tracking with intensity-modulated arc therapy (214). Depuydt et al. have demonstrated sub-millimeter beam tracking accuracy in a phantom study using a gimbals-based linac unit (147).

Population-Based and Individualized Margins

The relative importance of systematic and random errors in the determination of PTV margins should be considered in the design of the clinical strategy. Geometric errors in radiation field placement are typically characterized by distributions of nonzero mean and variance. The mean describes the systematic discrepancy for an individual patient and the variance for the random component. Several authors have highlighted the relative importance of these two categories of errors in determining appropriate PTV margins (215,216). Their conclusions are not completely general, as the number of fractions is an important factor in determining the relative importance of these two categories of error, especially for SBRT cases with less than five fractions.

A treatment margin depends not only on the imaging modality chosen and tumor surrogate used, but also on the patient immobilization dedicated for a treatment

(217). A proper patient immobilization improves setup reproducibility and reduces voluntary patient motion, therefore decreases systematic and random errors (52). Margin is also dependent on the motion-management technique employed. For involuntary respiratory motion, breath-hold, motion compression, motion gating, or tracking will compensate for tumor motion at different levels. As a consequence, the margin will be reduced, such that it is smaller than a motion-encompassing internal tumor volume (ITV) (184,218–220). The ability to reduce margin by using image guidance will therefore decrease the normal tissue toxicity and increase dose acceleration, particularly important for SBRT.

In prostate cases, image-guided margin reduction is one of most dramatic examples in all anatomic sites. With in-room CT guidance, a 3-mm margin was reported adequate for prostate dose coverage, but may lose some of the seminal vesicles coverage due to daily variation in rectal filling that causes local deformation (221). A comparative study using four different IGRT setup methods, skin marks, 3D bony landmarks, 3D fiducial markers, and Calypso transponders, has shown that the last two methods can achieve 4 mm and 3 mm margin requirement, respectively (222). Another study has compared four setup techniques using skin marks, 2D bony registration, ultrasound guidance, and in-room 3D CT (223). It has proposed a correction for patient-specific systematic shifts after the bony landmark alignment, and provides equivalent dose coverage to ultrasound guidance. A recent Calypso study has shown that a margin of 2 mm would produce sufficient CTV dose coverage based on 1,267 tracking sessions of 35 patients (224). Figure 14.15A demonstrates that the alignment accuracy increases along with the complexity of the alignment technology: from

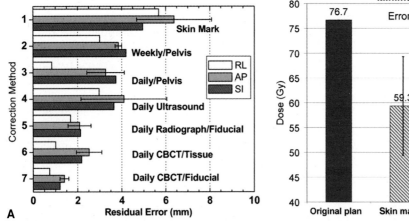

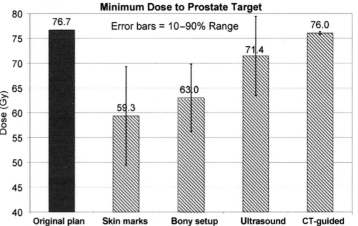

Figure 14.15. **A:** Patient setup accuracy of prostate cancer using different in-room imaging modalities. Generally, the accuracy increases with imaging frequency, dimension, and use of fiducial. The skin mark and ultrasound setup have largest variation, as indicated by the error bars. The margin could be reduced from 8 to 2 mm based on this finding. *Source:* Reprinted with permission from Mageras GS and Mechalakos J, Planning in the IGRT context: Closing the loop, *Semin Radiat Oncol* 2007;17:268–77. **B:** Target coverage based on various types of image-guided setups for treatment. In this example, 24 treatment-time CT scans of a prostate cancer patient were used to compare the effectiveness of four alignment techniques for patient setup using a fixed-margin IMRT plan. The minimum target dose is lowest (59.3 Gy) for skin marks-based setup and highest (76.0 Gy) for the CT-guided setup. The day-to-day variations in the minimum dose (represented by the error bars) are smallest for CT-guided technique and largest for skin-mark and ultrasound-guided techniques.

skin to bone to ultrasound and to CT (6). The dosimetric result (prostate underdose) for one patient exhibiting relatively large organ motion is shown in Figure 14.15B.

In head and neck cases, an IGRT assessment of setup error for 225 patients suggests that 3 mm margin is appropriate (225). The major variation for this anatomical site comes from deformation. Depending on tumor location, locally focused image registration is needed to minimize the setup uncertainty due to deformation (166–168).

In lung cases, both inter- and intra-fractional motion affect setup accuracy, and the overall margin would be the sum of the two terms: regular setup margin plus the ITV. Hugo and coworkers proposed a margin formula that contains both components of population-based and individualized systematic and random errors for lung cancer (217,226). Such a margin formula was applied in clinical cases and 3D CT-guided setup resulted in a 65% to 75% margin reduction. To compensate for the baseline drift, Pepin et al. have reported using a dynamic gating window (227). As the tumor motion is location and patient specific and 4D CT imaging provides the means to measure the patient-specific ITV, individualized tumor motion margin is often applied in lung cancer treatment (217).

Anatomic Variations and Dosimetric Consequences

Inter- and Intra-fractional Variations in Anatomy

Typical inter- and intra-fractional organ variations and setup uncertainties of gynecological tumors, liver, diaphragm, lung tumors, prostate, seminal vesicles, bladder, and rectum have been reviewed by Langen et al. (228) and Booth et al. (229). Both publications have reported significant variations for all organs studied. Even with careful immobilization and alignment of the patient, significant changes occur because of the nonrigidity of anatomy, bowel gas movement, and the variable filling of the bladder (230–233). Li et al. have reported inter-factional anatomic variations for all major sites based on daily CT assessment (234). Target and normal structure variations can also follow certain trends, including volume shrinkage up to 12 months after the initial hormone treatment (235), and soft-tissue changes such as tumor shrinkage and weight loss. Figure 14.16A shows a side-by-side comparison of a head and neck target volume that has shrunk significantly during the course of treatment. The skin contour no longer matches well with the immobilization mask. Changes in target volume and position of normal

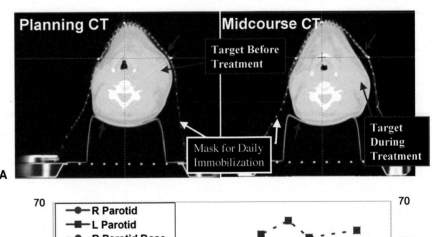

Figure 14.16. A: An example of setup error for a patient immobilized with a thermoplastic facemask due to tumor shrinkage as treatment progresses. Approximately half way through the treatment course (right panel), the lower neck was not centered on the headrest, presumably due to the relatively "roomier" mask. B: Dosimetric impact of inter-fractional variations in head and neck anatomy. The solid lines show the volumes of the parotid glands (left and right) decreased as the treatment progressed. At the same time, the centers of both parotid glands also moved medially due to tumor shrinkage and weight loss. As a result, the percent of parotid volume exceeding 26 Gy increased by least 10% over the course of radiotherapy.

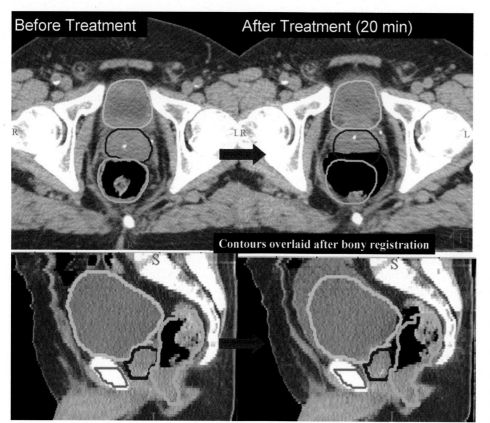

Figure 14.17. Intra-fractional variations of anatomy observed in a prostate patient in the span of 20 minutes. CT images were acquired just prior and immediately after an IMRT treatment fraction. The contours of pelvic anatomy before treatment (left) are overlaid on the CT image of the patient acquired immediately after the treatment (right). Prostate target (red) was displaced anteriorly for >5 mm.

critical organs (such as the spinal cord) could have significant clinical consequences (166,167). In a prostate IMRT treatment, changes in bladder filling can cause prostate and surrounding organs to move away from the planning position, as demonstrated in Figure 14.17. During a 20- to 30-minute IMRT treatment delivery, intrafractional motion may cause significant dose deviation for a session.

Dosimetric Effects due to Inter-fractional Motion

The common approach to evaluating the dosimetric effect of a delivered dose is by applying the treatment plan to the daily setup 3D CT images with the corresponding setup isocenter shift. The actual dynamic leaf sequence can also be retrieved from a treatment log file for synchronized dose reconstruction (236). To generate a cumulative dose distribution over multiple fractions, DIR is applied to map the daily dose distribution to a reference image for final dose evaluation (178).

In prostate cases, it is reported that 25% (8/33) of patients would have geometric or dosimetric miss without daily MVCT improve tumor localization (237). Obese patients and patients with large daily rectal motion would be most subject to such marginal miss. van Herk has pointed out that the systematic uncertainty is more important and should be minimized as much as possible (215). Langen et al. (238) have investigated the dosimetry consequences of prostate motion during helical tomotherapy for 16 patients with 515 daily MVCT scans. The study finds that the mean change in target $D_{95\%}$ is $1 \pm 4\%$ and the average cumulative effect is smeared out after five fractions. In individual fractions, the $D_{95\%}$ may be off by as high as 20%. For normal tissues, such as the rectum, Chen et al. have reported that dose variation is significant due to daily variation of the rectal volume and 27% of actual treatment would benefit from adaptive replanning. The authors recommend an empty rectum for both planning and treatment to avoid such adverse effects (239). Any effort to make patient conditions reproducible is worthwhile so as to treat as planned.

In breast cases, Goddu et al. have demonstrated the potential benefit of daily MVCT setup by simulating the integrated dose distribution without image-guided setup correction. Significant dose reduction in the PTV is observed mostly at the lung interface where steep dose falloff is expected (240). The possible adverse dosimetric effect is anisotropic with regard to the steep dose falloff.

For highly conformal head and neck IMRT treatments, it is desirable to reduce the dose to the parotid glands in order to minimize the incidence of late xerostomia (241). Unfortunately, the parotid glands can decrease in volume and move medially during the course of treatment (242). As a result, parotid dose can increase by 10% and exceed 26 Gy, as illustrated in Figure 14.16B, in which one patient received repeat CT imaging during his course of IMRT treatment. A single mid-course correction to adapt the treatment plan to the anatomical change could help reduce the dose for both parotid glands (243).

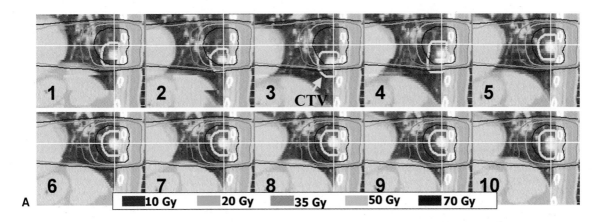

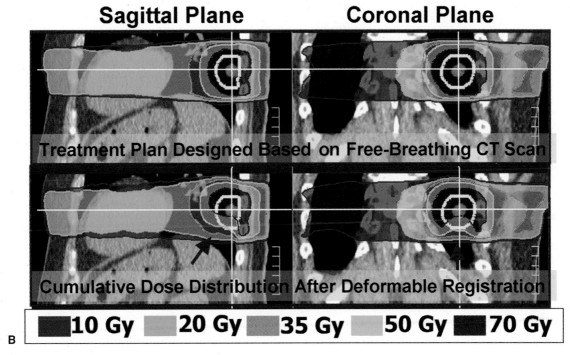

Figure 14.18. **A:** Potential consequence of respiratory motion on target coverage. An IMRT plan, developed using conventional CT, was applied to the patient's 4D CT. Dose distributions were calculated in each of the 10 phases of the breathing cycle. A portion of the CTV, shown in thick yellow line, was not covered by the 70 Gy prescription dose line (red) in phases 1 through 4. **B:** Comparison of a treatment plan as perceived on a free-breathing CT (top row) and as realized after accounting for breathing motion in all 10 phases (bottom row). The latter was obtained by summing dose distributions computed on individual phases of the 4D CT image (**A**), and mapped to a reference CT image using deformable image registration (DIR).

Dosimetric Effects of Intra-fractional Motion

The dosimetric consequence of intra-fractional breathing motion for lung tumors can be demonstrated by 4D CT-based planning. Figure 14.18A shows a case study that used a free-breathing CT image to design a treatment plan with an inadequate 8-mm margin to cover the CTV (shown in yellow). The actual dose distribution does not cover the entire target volume in some of the breathing phases due to respiratory motion, which is not detected in the free-breathing CT. Using DIR, the cumulative dose distribution from the 10 individual phases is calculated and mapped to a free-breathing fast CT scan (near full exhalation, #7). The resultant cumulative dose distribution summed from the entire breathing cycle shows a dose deficiency in the CTV (red arrow), as illustrated in the bottom row of Figure 14.18B. In this case, the cumulative dose distribution when using the internal target volume (ITV) derived from the 10-phase 4D CT does not underdose the target but results in treatment to a larger volume. The ITV method is an example of using an individualized margin to account for target motion in treatment planning. The dosimetric impact of motion in free breathing and gated radiotherapy of lung cancer has been studied using Monte Carlo dose calculation (244). The doses are similar between free breathing and all phases, except for the end-inspiration phase in which the tumor is underdosed by ~10%.

Wu et al. have compared three delivery techniques, 3DCRT, IMAT, and IMRT, in five treatment cases in liver, with tumor motions ranging from 0.5 to 1.75 cm. The variation in $D_{95\%}$ is largest (−8.3%) for IMRT and smallest (<2%) for 3DCRT, with negligible dose–volume histogram variations for normal tissues (177). Kuo et al. have found that with an adequate margin for motion, $D_{95\%}$ variation is <2% in the CTV (72).

Adaptive Approaches for Correcting Dosimetric Deviations

William Beaumont Hospital has pioneered the adaptive radiotherapy strategy by using a purpose-built treatment planning system to facilitate off-line dosimetric evaluation and replanning (185,199). Without the support from a more automated planning system, routine replanning is not feasible under current clinical conditions. Special staff effort may only be reserved for those patients with potentially severe dosimetric consequence (245). Mageras and Mechalakos have discussed treatment planning in the IGRT context and the various challenges to treatment-plan adaptation strategies in various disease sites (6). An alternative treatment planning approach to evaluating a PTV is to simulate motion and other uncertainties directly in the dose calculation. A benefit of this approach is that the resultant dose distributions of not only the CTV, but also organs at risk can be examined.

Recent articles have reviewed clinical applications of adaptive radiotherapy for various treatments (191). The adaptive concept as applied to radiotherapy practice derives from modern informatics and control theory. Offline adaptation has been implemented in various institutions (246–248), and online replanning has been reported, with computation time within 5 to 8 minutes (249). The knowledge gained from geometric and dosimetric variations via clinical IGRT research will be useful for guiding the treatment planning process to be more cautious in certain clinical scenarios.

FUTURE DIRECTIONS

Image-guided radiotherapy is commonly considered in the context of treatment delivery verification, but it is more appropriate to broaden its scope to include imaging at other stages of the radiotherapy process (8). We, therefore, briefly discuss future directions as they apply to this broader definition.

In the application of IGRT to treatment delivery, we have better understanding of various uncertainties, correction strategies, and technical limitations. Geometrically, a large body of evidence has shown the improved accuracy in patient setup and motion management. Dosimetrically, IGRT improves treatment delivery in certain plans that involve sharp dose gradients or a moving target. Clinically, increasing evidence has unveiled the connections of local failure with marginal miss and

high-grade toxicity with organ motion (1–3). Well-designed clinical trials are needed to demonstrate its advantages fully. We believe that further advance in IGRT relies on the innovation and integration of multiple automated technologies to facilitate extra evaluations and additional processes. Parallel computing technologies, such as graphics processing unit (GPU) technology (181), is a solution for increasing real-time performance, especially for intra-fractional motion management and online dosimetric replanning. In motion monitoring, non-radiographic alternatives may be more clinically desirable, such as in-room MRI imaging with near real-time volumetric information (62). In off-line and online dosimetric replanning, automated and integrated systems are necessary to make such actions clinically feasible. The treatment efficacy and benefit of real-time tracking and online adaptation must be evaluated with clinical evidences, such as improved potency of hypo- or single-fractioned SBRT.

In image-based treatment planning, biological imaging with different molecular probes will play an increasing role in reducing the uncertainties in delineation of gross and clinical tumor volumes. Different molecular probes for detecting different biological attributes of cancer may prove useful in accurately defining the biological tumor volume, as shown in Figure 14.19. Various molecular tracers are available for probe tumor metabolism, proliferation, hypoxia, and angiogenesis. The concept of multiplexed imaging used in diagnosis to simultaneously probe different molecular targets may be adopted by the therapeutic clinic as theragnostic imaging (250) to prescribe the distribution of therapeutic dose (8). Microscopic cancerous cells spreading beyond the GTV requires histopathological assessment and accurate registration with 3D anatomic image.

In image-guided treatment evaluation, multi-modality imaging must be applied to assess the complex radiation response. This will remain an intense clinical research arena to improve our fundamental understanding of the radiation response at molecular, cellular, organ functional, and physiological levels. Proper biological attributes, such as DNA double-strand breaks, need to be identified and probed. Ideally, response assessment within the treatment course would be most beneficial for individualized treatments, while the reality is lack of an effective assessment index even after treatment. A response-driven, biologically adaptive radiotherapy is still distant from clinical practice. The dosimetric feedback loop, which is within the reach to ensure that the treatment process goes along the intended course (6,191), can provide more reliable clinical data to tune prediction models of treatment outcome.

Radiation therapy has gone through a series of technological revolutions following several breakthroughs in imaging in the past three decades. We have witnessed the growth of IGRT, which has provided improved geometric and dosimetric accuracy in radiation therapy of localized cancers. We believe that there are more technologic advances to come at all levels of IGRT, closing the physical, biological, and clinical feedback loop for radiation therapy.

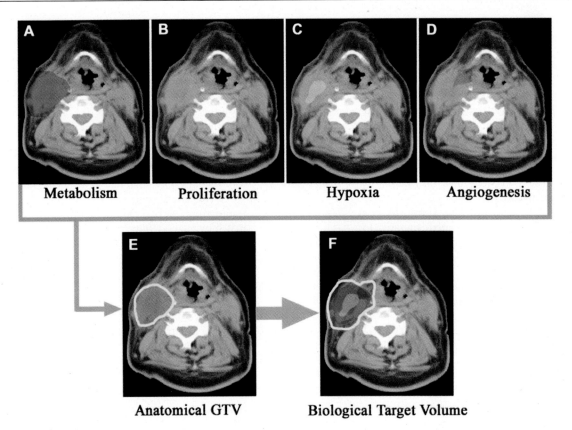

Figure 14.19. Imaging paradigm in radiation oncology hypothetically illustrating the possibility of integrating different functional imaging modalities (panels A–D) with CT-defined gross tumor volume (GTV) (panel E) to obtain a combined biological target volume (BTV) (panel F). Panel A: Metabolism (i.e., FDG); panel B: proliferation (i.e., FLT); panel C: hypoxia (i.e., Cu-ATSM); and panel D: angiogenesis (i.e., MMP). Improved tumor target coverage and/or dose escalation to these physiological sub-regions may be achievable. A region of increased angiogenesis can be seen in panel F that lies outside other biological regions. This may represent a potential area of recurrence that should be included into the overall BTV. Lines (yellow) outlining the anatomical GTV (panel E) and BTV (panel F) accentuate the change in target volume delineation. *Source:* Reprinted with permission from Apisarnthanarax S and Chao KSC, Current imaging paradigms in radiation oncology, Radiation Research, 2005;163:1–25.

REFERENCES

1. Eisbruch A, Harris J, Garden AS, et al. Multi-institutional trial of accelerated hypofractionated intensity-modulated radiation therapy for early-stage oropharyngeal cancer (RTOG 00–22). *Int J Radiat Oncol Biol Phys* 2010;76(5): 1333–1338.
2. de Crevoisier R, Tucker SL, Dong L, et al. Increased risk of biochemical and local failure in patients with distended rectum on the planning CT for prostate cancer radiotherapy. *Int J Radiat Oncol Biol Phys* 2005;62: 965–973.
3. Tucker SL, Jin H, Wei X, et al. Impact of toxicity grade and scoring system on the relationship between mean lung dose and risk of radiation pneumonitis in a large cohort of patients with non-small cell lung cancer. *Int J Radiat Oncol Biol Phys* 2010;77:691–698.
4. Mageras GS, Kutcher GJ, Leibel SA, et al. A method of incorporating organ motion uncertainties into three-dimensional conformal treatment plans. *Int J Radiat Oncol Biol Phys* 1996;35:333–342.
5. Li JG, Xing L. Inverse planning incorporating organ motion. *Med Phys* 2000;27:1573–1578.
6. Mageras GS, Mechalakos J. Planning in the IGRT context: closing the loop. *Semin Radiat Oncol* 2007;17: 268–277.
7. van Herk M. Different styles of image-guided radiotherapy. *Semin Radiat Oncol* 2007;17:258–267.
8. Greco C, Clifton Ling C. Broadening the scope of image-guided radiotherapy (IGRT). *Acta Oncol* 2008;47(7): 1193–1200.
9. van Herk M, Meertens H. A matrix ionisation chamber imaging device for on-line patient setup verification during radiotherapy. *Radiother Oncol* 1988;11:369–378.
10. Boyer AL, Antonuk L, Fenster A, et al. A review of electronic portal imaging devices (EPIDs). *Med Phys* 1992;19: 1–16.
11. Bijhold J, Gilhuijs KG, van Herk M. Automatic verification of radiation field shape using digital portal images. *Med Phys* 1992;19:1007–1014.
12. Dong L, Boyer AL. A portal image alignment and patient setup verification procedure using moments and correlation techniques. *Phys Med Biol* 1996;41:697–723.
13. Van Elmpt W, McDermott, L, Nijsten S, et al. A literature review of electronic portal imaging for radiotherapy dosimetry. *Radiother Oncol* 2008;88:289–309.

14. Faddegon BA, Aubin M, Bani-Hashemi A, et al. Comparison of patient megavoltage cone beam CT images acquired with an unflattened beam from a carbon target and a flattened treatment beam. *Med Phys* 2010;37(4): 1737–1741.

15. Shirato H, Shimizu S, Kunieda T, et al. Physical aspects of a real-time tumor-tracking system for gated radiotherapy. *Int J Radiat Oncol Biol Phys* 2000;48:1187–1195.

16. Uematsu M, Fukui T, Shioda A, et al. A dual computed tomography linear accelerator unit for stereotactic radiation therapy: a new approach without cranially fixated stereotactic frames. *Int J Radiat Oncol Biol Phys* 1996;35:587–592.

17. Yenice KM, Lovelock DM, Hunt MA, et al. CT image-guided intensity-modulated therapy for paraspinal tumors using stereotactic immobilization. *Int J Radiat Oncol Biol Phys* 2003;55:583–593.

18. Hua CH, Lovelock DM, Mageras GS, et al. Development of a semi-automatic alignment tool for accelerated localization of the prostate. *Int J Radiat Oncol Biol Phys* 2003; 55:811–824.

19. Wong JR, Cheng CW, Grimm L, et al. Clinical implementation of the world's first Primatom, a combination of CT scanner and linear accelerator, for precise tumor targeting and treatment. *Phys Med* 2001;17:271–276.

20. Fung AY, Grimm SY, Wong JR, et al. Computed tomography localization of radiation treatment delivery versus conventional localization with bony landmarks. *J Appl Clin Med Phys* 2003;4:112–119.

21. Court L, Rosen I, Mohan R, et al. Evaluation of mechanical precision and alignment uncertainties for an integrated CT/LINAC system. *Med Phys* 2003;30:1198–1210.

22. Shiu AS, Chang EL, Ye JS, et al. Near simultaneous computed tomography image-guided stereotactic spinal radiotherapy: an emerging paradigm for achieving true stereotaxy. *Int J Radiat Oncol Biol Phys* 2003;57: 605–613.

23. Jaffray DA, Drake DG, Moreau M, et al. A radiographic and tomographic imaging system integrated into a medical linear accelerator for localization of bone and soft-tissue targets. *Int J Radiat Oncol Biol Phys* 1999;45: 773–789.

24. Jaffray DA, Siewerdsen JH, Wong JW, et al. Flat-panel cone-beam computed tomography for image-guided radiation therapy. *Int J Radiat Oncol Biol Phys* 2002;53:1337–1349.

25. Siewerdsen JH, Moseley DJ, Jaffray DA, et al. The influence of antiscatter grids on soft-tissue detectability in cone-beam computed tomography with flat-panel detectors. *Med Phys* 2004;31:3506–3520.

26. Feldkamp IA, Davis LC, Kress JW. Practical cone-beam algorithm. *J Opt Soc Am A* 1984;1:612–619.

27. Fahrig R, Holdsworth DW. Three-dimensional computed tomographic reconstruction using a C-arm mounted XRII: image-based correction of gantry motion nonidealities. *Med Phys* 2000;27:30–38.

28. Cho PS, Rudd AD, Johnson RH. Cone-beam CT from width-truncated projections. *Comput Med Imaging Graph* 1996;20:49–57.

29. Li T, Li X, Yang Y, et al. A novel off-axis scanning method for an enlarged ellipse cone-beam computed tomography field of view. *Med Phys* 2010;37:6233–6239.

30. Siewerdsen JH, Daly MJ, Bakhtiar B, et al. A simple, direct method for x-ray scatter estimation and correction in digital radiography and cone-beam CT. *Med Phys* 2006;33:187–197.

31. Mackie TR, Holmes T, Swerdloff S, et al. Tomotherapy: a new concept for the delivery of dynamic conformal radiotherapy. *Med Phys* 1993;20:1709–1719.

32. Mackie TR, Balog J, Ruchala K, et al. Tomotherapy. *Semin Radiat Oncol* 1999;9:108–117.

33. Olivera GH, Shepard DM, Reckwerdt PJ, et al. Maximum likelihood as a common computational framework in tomotherapy. *Phys Med Biol* 1998;43:3277–3294.

34. Lu W, Fitchard EE, Olivera GH, et al. Image/patient registration from (partial) projection data by the Fourier phase matching method. *Phys Med Biol* 1999;44:2029–2048.

35. Ruchala KJ, Olivera GH, Schloesser EA, et al. Megavoltage CT on a tomotherapy system. *Phys Med Biol* 1999;44: 2597–2621.

36. Ruchala KJ, Olivera GH, Schloesser EA, et al. Calibration of a tomotherapeutic MVCT system. *Phys Med Biol* 2000;45:N27–N36.

37. Mackie TR, Jaradat H, Hui S, et al. The utility of megavoltage computed tomography images from a helical tomotherapy system for setup verification purposes. *Int J Radiat Oncol Biol Phys* 2004;60:1639–1644.

38. Meeks SL, Langen KM, Willoughby TR, et al. Performance characterization of megavoltage computed tomography imaging on a helical tomotherapy unit. *Med Phys* 2005;32:2673–2681.

39. Kupelian PA, Meeks SL, Willoughby TR, et al. Serial megavoltage CT imaging during external beam radiotherapy for non-small-cell lung cancer: observations on tumor regression during treatment. *Int J Radiat Oncol Biol Phys* 2005;63:1024–1028.

40. Langen KM, Meeks SL, Poole DO, et al. The use of megavoltage CT (MVCT) images for dose recomputations. *Phys Med Biol* 2005;50:4259–4276.

41. Shepard DM, Olivera GH, Reckwerdt PJ, et al. Iterative approaches to dose optimization in tomotherapy. *Phys Med Biol* 2000;45:69–90.

42. Lu W, Chen ML, Olivera GH, et al. Fast free-form deformable registration via calculus of variations. *Phys Med Biol* 2004;49:3067–3087.

43. Zhang T, Jeraj R, Keller H, et al. Treatment plan optimization incorporating respiratory motion. *Med Phys* 2004;31:1576–1586.

44. Swindell W, Simpson RG, Oleson JR, et al. Computed tomography with a linear accelerator with radiotherapy applications. *Med Phys* 1983;10:416–420.

45. Mosleh-Shirazi MA, Evans PM, Swindell W, et al. A cone-beam megavoltage CT scanner for treatment verification in conformal radiotherapy. *Radiother Oncol* 1998;48: 319–328.

46. Groh BA, Siewerdsen JH, Drake DG, et al. A performance comparison of flat-panel imager-based MV and kV cone-beam CT. *Med Phys* 2002;29:967–975.

47. Ford EC, Chang J, Mueller K, et al. Cone-beam CT with megavoltage beams and an amorphous silicon electronic portal imaging device: potential for verification of radiotherapy of lung cancer. *Med Phys* 2002;29:2913–2924.

48. Sillanpaa J, Chang J, Mageras G, et al. Developments in megavoltage cone beam CT with an amorphous silicon

EPID: reduction of exposure and synchronization with respiratory gating. *Med Phys* 2005;32:819–829.

49. Morin O, Gillis A, Chen J, et al. Megavoltage cone-beam CT: System description and clinical applications. *Med Dosim* 2006;31:51–61.

50. Pouliot J, Bani-Hashemi A, Chen J, et al. Low-dose megavoltage cone-beam CT for radiation therapy. *Int J Radiat Oncol Biol Phys* 2005;61:552–560.

51. Morin O, Gillis A, Descovich M, et al. Patient dose considerations for routine megavoltage cone-beam CT imaging. *Med Phys* 2007;34:1819–1827.

52. Li G, Ballangrud A, Kuo LC, et al. Motion monitoring for cranial frameless stereotactic surgery using video-based three-dimensional optical surface imaging. *Med Phys* 2011;38 (in press).

53. Kolitsi Z, Panayiotakis G, Anastassopoulos V, et al. A multiple projection method for digital tomosynthesis. *Med Phys* 1992;19:1045–1050.

54. Zwicker RD, Atari NA. Transverse tomosynthesis on a digital simulator. *Med Phys* 1997;24:867–871.

55. Godfrey DJ, Yin FF, Oldham M, et al. Digital tomosynthesis with an on-board kilovoltage imaging device. *Int J Radiat Oncol Biol Phys* 2006;65:8–15.

56. Kolitsi Z, Panayiotakis G, Pallikarakis N. A method for selective removal of out-of-plane structures in digital tomosynthesis. *Med Phys* 1992;20:47–50.

57. Badea C, Kolitsi Z, Pallikarakis N. A wavelet-based method for removal of out-of-plane structures in digital tomosynthesis. *Comp Med Img Graph* 1998;22:309–315.

58. Santoro J, Kriminski S, Lovelock DM, et al. Evaluation of respiration-correlated digital tomosynthesis in lung. *Med Phys* 2010;37:1237–1245.

59. Oelfke U, Tucking T, Nill S, et al. Linac-integrated kV-cone beam CT: technical features and first applications. *Med Dosim* 2006;31:62–70.

60. Yin FF, Guan H, Lu W. A technique for on-board CT reconstruction using both kilovoltage and megavoltage beam projections for 3D treatment verification. *Med Phys* 2005;32:2819–2826.

61. Blessing M, Stsepankou D, Wertz H, et al. Breath-hold target localization with simultaneous kilovoltage/megavoltage cone-beam computed tomography and fast reconstruction. *Int J Radiat Oncol Biol Phys* 2010;78:1219–1226.

62. Keall PJ, Mageras GS, Balter JM, et al. The management of respiratory motion in radiation oncology report of AAPM Task Group 76. *Med Phys* 2006;33:3874–900.

63. Li G, Citrin D, Camphausen K, et al. Advances in 4D medical imaging and 4D radiation therapy. *Technol Cancer Res Treat* 2008;7:67–81.

64. Low DA, Nystrom M, Kalinin E, et al. A method for the reconstruction of four-dimensional synchronized CT scans acquired during free breathing. *Med Phy* 2003;30:1254–1263.

65. Pan T, Lee TY, Rietzel E, et al. 4D-CT imaging of a volume influenced by respiratory motion on multi-slice CT. *Med Phys* 2004;31:333–340.

66. Ford EC, Mageras GS, Yorke E, et al. Respiration-correlated spiral CT: a method of measuring respiratory-induced anatomic motion for radiation treatment planning. *Med Phys* 2003;30:88–97.

67. Vedam SS, Keall PJ, Kini VR, et al. Acquiring a four-dimensional computed tomography dataset using an external respiratory signal. *Phys Med Biol* 2003;48:45–62.

68. Keall P. 4-dimensional computed tomography imaging and treatment planning. *Semin Radiat Oncol* 2004;14:81–90.

69. Mageras GS, Pevsner A, Yorke ED, et al. Measurement of lung tumor motion using respiration-correlated CT. *Int J Radiat Oncol Biol Phys* 2004;60:933–941.

70. Rietzel E, Chen GT, Choi NC, et al. Four-dimensional image-based treatment planning: target volume segmentation and dose calculation in the presence of respiratory motion. *Int J Radiat Oncol Biol Phys* 2005;61:1535–1550.

71. Lu W, Parikh PJ, Hubenschmidt JP, et al. A comparison between amplitude sorting and phase-angle sorting using external respiratory measurement for 4D CT. *Med Phys* 2006;33:2964–2974.

72. Kuo HC, Mah D, Chuang KS, et al. A method incorporating 4DCT data for evaluating the dosimetric effects of respiratory motion in single-arc IMAT. *Phys Med Biol* 2010;55:3479–3497.

73. Franks KN, Purdie TG, Dawson LA, et al. Incorporating heterogeneity correction and 4DCT in lung stereotactic body radiation therapy (SBRT): the effect on target coverage, organ-at-risk doses, and dose conformity. *Med Dosim* 2010;35:101–107.

74. Rietzel E, Pan T, Chen GTY. Four-dimensional computed tomography: Image formation and clinical protocol. *Med Phys* 2005;32:874.

75. Fitzpatrick MJ, Starkschall G, Antolak JA, et al. Displacement-based binning of time-dependent computed tomography image data sets. *Med Phys* 2006;33:235–246.

76. Abdelnour AF, Nehmeh SA, Pan T, et al. Phase and amplitude binning for 4D-CT imaging. *Phys Med Biol* 2007;52:3515–3529.

77. Purdie TG, Moseley DJ, Bissonnette JP, et al. Respiration correlated cone-beam computed tomography and 4DCT for evaluating target motion in stereotactic lung radiation therapy. *Acta Oncol* 2006;45:915–922.

78. Sonke JJ, Zijp L, Remeijer P, et al. Respiratory correlated cone beam CT. *Med Phys* 2005;32:1176–1186.

79. Li T, Xing L, Munro P, et al. Four-dimensional cone-beam computed tomography using an on-board imager. *Med Phys* 2006;33:3825–3833.

80. Chang J, Sillanpaa J, Ling CC, et al. Integrating respiratory gating into a megavoltage cone-beam CT system. *Med Phys* 2006;33:2354–2361.

81. Li T, Koong A, Xing L. Enhanced 4D cone-beam CT with inter-phase motion model. *Med Phys* 2007;34:3688–3695.

82. Leng S, Zambelli J, Tolakanahalli R, et al. Streaking artifacts reduction in four-dimensional cone-beam computed tomography. *Med Phys* 2008;35:4649–4659.

83. Rit S, Wolthaus J, Van Herk M, et al. On-the-fly motion-compensated cone-beam CT using an a priori model of the respiratory motion. *Med Phys* 2009;36:2283–2296.

84. Zhang Q, Hu YC, Liu F, et al. Correction of motion artifacts in cone-beam CT using a patient-specific respiratory motion model. *Med Phys* 2010;37:2901–2909.

85. Huang E, Dong L, Chandra A, et al. Intrafraction prostate motion during IMRT for prostate cancer. *Int J Radiat Oncol Biol Phys* 2002;53:261–268.

86. Langen KM, Pouliot J, Anezinos C, et al. Evaluation of ultrasound-based prostate localization for image-guided radiotherapy. *Int J Radiat Oncol Biol Phys* 2003;57:635–644.

87. Kuban DA, Dong L, Cheung R, et al. Ultrasound-based localization. *Semin Radiat Oncol* 2005;15:180–191.

88. Fuss M, Salter BJ, Cavanaugh SX, et al. Daily ultrasound-based image-guided targeting for radiotherapy of upper abdominal malignancies. *Int J Radiat Oncol Biol Phys* 2004;59:1245–1256.

89. Peng C, Kainz K, Lawton C, et al. A comparison of daily megavoltage CT and ultrasound image guided radiation therapy for prostate cancer. *Med Phys* 2008;35:5619–5628.

90. Fung AY, Ayyangar KM, Djajaputra D, et al. Ultrasound-based guidance of intensity-modulated radiation therapy. *Med Dosim* 2006;31:20–29.

91. Dong L, de Crevoisier R, Bonnen M, et al. Evaluation of an ultrasound-based prostate target localization technique with an in-room CT-on-rails. *Int J Radiat Oncol Biol Phys* 2004;60:S332–S333.

92. Fuss M, Cavanaugh SX, Fuss C, et al. Daily stereotactic ultrasound prostate targeting: Inter-user variability. *Technol Cancer Res Treat* 2003;2:161–169.

93. Van Den Heuvel F, Powell T, Seppi E, et al. Independent verification of ultrasound based image-guided radiation treatment, using electronic portal imaging and implanted gold markers. *Med Phys* 2003;30:2878–2887.

94. Scarbrough TJ, Golden NM, Ting JY, et al. Comparison of ultrasound and implanted seed marker prostate localization methods: implications for image-guided radiotherapy. *Int J Radiat Oncol Biol Phys* 2006;65:378–387.

95. Dobler B, Mai S, Ross C, et al. Evaluation of possible prostate displacement induced by pressure applied during transabdominal ultrasound image acquisition. *Strahlenther Onkol* 2006;182:240–246.

96. Tomé WA, Meeks SL, Orton NP, et al. Commissioning and quality assurance of an optically guided three-dimensional ultrasound target localization system for radiotherapy. *Med Phys* 2002;29:1781–1788.

97. Bert C, Metheany KG, Doppke K, et al. A phantom evaluation of a stereo-vision surface imaging system for radiotherapy patient setup. *Med Phys* 2005;32:2753–2762.

98. Djajaputra D, Li S. Real-time 3D surface-image-guided beam setup in radiotherapy of breast cancer. *Med Phys* 2005;32:65–75.

99. Hendee WR, Ritenour ER. *Medical imaging physics*, 4th ed. New York, NY: Wiley-Liss, 2002.

100. Dinkel J, Hintze C, Tetzlaff R, et al. 4D-MRI analysis of lung tumor motion in patients with hemidiaphragmatic paralysis. *Radiother Oncol* 2009;91:449–454.

101. Wang D, Doddrell DM. A proposed scheme for comprehensive characterization of the measured geometric distortion in magnetic resonance imaging using a three-dimensional phantom. *Med Phys* 2004;31:2212–2218.

102. Chen L, Price RA Jr, Wang L, et al. MRI-based treatment planning for radiotherapy: dosimetric verification for prostate IMRT. *Int J Radiat Oncol Biol Phys* 2004;60:636–647.

103. Wang C, Chao M, Lee L, et al. MRI-based treatment planning with electron density information mapped from CT images: a preliminary study. *Technol Cancer Res Treat* 2008;7:341–348.

104. Karlsson M, Karlsson MG, Nyholm T, et al. Dedicated magnetic resonance imaging in the radiotherapy clinic. *Int J Radiat Oncol Biol Phys* 2009;74:644–651.

105. Shirato H, Suzuki K, Sharp GC, et al. Speed and amplitude of lung tumor motion precisely detected in four-dimensional setup and in real-time tumor-tracking radiotherapy. *Int J Radiat Oncol Biol Phys* 2006;64:1229–1236.

106. Onimaru R, Shirato H, Fujino M, et al. The effect of tumor location and respiratory function on tumor movement estimated by real-time tracking radiotherapy (RTRT) system. *Int J Radiat Oncol Biol Phys* 2005;63:164–169.

107. Ding GX, Duggan DM, Coffey CW. Commissioning stereotactic radiosurgery beams using both experimental and theoretical methods. *Phys Med Biol* 2006;51:2549–2566.

108. Verellen D, Soete G, Linthout N, et al. Quality assurance of a system for improved target localization and patient set-up that combines real-time infrared tracking and stereoscopic X-ray imaging. *Radiother Oncol* 2003;67:129–141.

109. Linthout N, Verellen D, Tournel K, et al. Six dimensional analysis with daily stereoscopic x-ray imaging of intrafraction patient motion in head and neck treatments using five points fixation masks. *Med Phys* 2006;33:504–513.

110. Jin JY, Yin FF, Tenn SE, et al. Use of the BrainLAB ExacTrac X-Ray 6D system in image-guided radiotherapy. *Med Dosim* 2008;33:124–134.

111. Nakagawa K, Haga A, Shiraishi K, et al. First clinical cone-beam CT imaging during volumetric modulated arc therapy. *Radiother Oncol* 2009;90:422–423.

112. Wiersma RD, Mao W, Xing L. Combined kV and MV imaging for real-time tracking of implanted fiducial markers. *Med Phys* 2008;35:1191–1198.

113. Amies C, Bani-Hashemi A, Celi JC, et al. A multi-platform approach to image guided radiation therapy (IGRT). *Med Dosim* 2006;31:12–19.

114. Stutzel J, Oelfke U, Nill S. A quantitative image quality comparison of four different image guided radiotherapy devices. *Radiother Oncol* 2008;86:20–24.

115. Meeks SL, Tome WA, Willoughby TR, et al. Optically guided patient positioning techniques. *Semin Radiat Oncol* 2005;15:192–201.

116. Li S, Liu D, Yin G, et al. Real-time 3D-surface-guided head refixation useful for fractionated stereotactic radiotherapy. *Med Phys* 2006;33:492–503.

117. Schoffel PJ, Harms W, Sroka-Perez G, et al. Accuracy of a commercial optical 3D surface imaging system for realignment of patients for radiotherapy of the thorax. *Phys Med Biol* 2007;52:3949–3963.

118. Peng JL, Kahler D, Li JG, et al. Characterization of a real-time surface image-guided stereotactic positioning system. *Med Phys* 2010;37:5421–5433.

119. Cervino LI, Pawlicki T, Lawson JD, et al. Frame-less and mask-less cranial stereotactic radiosurgery: a feasibility study. *Phys Med Biol* 2010;55:1863–1873.

120. Balter JM, Wright JN, Newell LJ, et al. Accuracy of a wireless localization system for radiotherapy. *Int J Radiat Oncol Biol Phys* 2005;61:933–937.

121. Santanam L, Malinowski K, Hubenshmidt J, et al. Fiducial-based translational localization accuracy of electromagnetic tracking system and on-board kilovoltage imaging system. *Int J Radiat Oncol Biol Phys* 2008;70:892–899.

122. Santanam L, Noel C, Willoughby TR, et al. Quality assurance for clinical implementation of an electromagnetic tracking system. *Med Phys* 2009;36:3477–3486.

123. Sawant A, Smith RL, Venkat RB, et al. Toward submillimeter accuracy in the management of intrafraction motion: the integration of real-time internal position monitoring and multileaf collimator target tracking. *Int J Radiat Oncol Biol Phys* 2009;74:575–582.

124. Willoughby TR, Kupelian PA, Pouliot J, et al. Target localization and real-time tracking using the Calypso 4D localization system in patients with localized prostate cancer. *Int J Radiat Oncol Biol Phys* 2006;65:528–534.

125. Raaijmakers AJ, Raaymakers BW, Lagendijk JJ. Integrating a MRI scanner with a 6 MV radiotherapy accelerator: dose increase at tissue-air interfaces in a lateral magnetic field due to returning electrons. *Phys Med Biol* 2005; 50:1363–1376.

126. Fallone BG, Murray B, Rathee S, et al. First MR images obtained during megavoltage photon irradiation from a prototype integrated linac-MR system. *Med Phys* 2009; 36:2084–2088.

127. Kirkby C, Murray B, Rathee S, et al. Lung dosimetry in a linac-MRI radiotherapy unit with a longitudinal magnetic field. *Med Phys* 2010;37:4722–4732.

128. Keall PJ, Joshi S, Vedam SS, et al. Four-dimensional radiotherapy planning for DMLC-based respiratory motion tracking. *Med Phys* 2005;32:942–951.

129. McQuaid D, Webb S. IMRT delivery to a moving target by dynamic MLC tracking: delivery for targets moving in two dimensions in the beam's eye view. *Phys Med Biol* 2006;51:4819–4839.

130. McMahon R, Papiez L, Rangaraj D. Dynamic-MLC leaf control utilizing on-flight intensity calculations: a robust method for real-time IMRT delivery over moving rigid targets. *Med Phys* 2007;34:3211–3223.

131. D'Souza WD, Naqvi SA, Yu CX. Real-time intra-fraction-motion tracking using the treatment couch: a feasibility study. *Phys Med Biol* 2005;50:4021–4033.

132. Wiersma RD, Wen Z, Sadinski M, et al. Development of a frameless stereotactic radiosurgery system based on real-time 6D position monitoring and adaptive head motion compensation. *Phys Med Biol* 2010;55:389–401.

133. Takakura T, Mizowaki T, Nakata M, et al. The geometric accuracy of frameless stereotactic radiosurgery using a 6D robotic couch system. *Phys Med Biol* 2010;55:1–10.

134. Adler JR Jr, Chang SD, Murphy MJ, et al. The Cyberknife: a frameless robotic system for radiosurgery. *Stereotact Funct Neurosurg* 1997;69:124–128.

135. Quinn AM. CyberKnife: a robotic radiosurgery system. *Clin J Oncol Nurs* 2002;6:149, 156.

136. Murphy MJ. Tracking moving organs in real time. *Semin Radiat Oncol* 2004;14:91–100.

137. Chang SD, Adler JR. Robotics and radiosurgery–the cyberknife. *Stereotact Funct Neurosurg* 2001;76:204–208.

138. Chamberlain MC, Blumenthal DT. Intracranial meningiomas: diagnosis and treatment. *Expert Rev Neurother* 2004;4:641–648.

139. Ryu SI, Chang SD, Kim DH, et al. Image-guided hypofractionated stereotactic radiosurgery to spinal lesions. *Neurosurgery* 2001;49:838–846.

140. Gerszten PC, Ozhasoglu C, Burton SA, et al. Evaluation of CyberKnife frameless real-time image-guided stereotactic radiosurgery for spinal lesions. *Stereotact Funct Neurosurg* 2003;81:84–89.

141. Yu C, Main W, Taylor D, et al. An anthropomorphic phantom study of the accuracy of Cyberknife spinal radiosurgery. *Neurosurgery* 2004;55:1138–1149.

142. Murphy MJ, Adler JR Jr, Bodduluri M, et al. Image-guided radiosurgery for the spine and pancreas. *Comput Aided Surg* 2000;5:278–288.

143. Whyte RI, Crownover R, Murphy MJ, et al. Stereotactic radiosurgery for lung tumors: preliminary report of a phase I trial. *Ann Thorac Surg* 2003;75:1097–1101.

144. Silvano G. New radiation techniques for treatment of locally advanced non-small cell lung cancer (NSCLC). *Ann Oncol* 2006;17:34–35.

145. Kamino Y, Takayama K, Kokubo M, et al. Development of a four-dimensional image-guided radiotherapy system with a gimbaled X-ray head. *Int J Radiat Oncol Biol Phys* 2006;66:271–278.

146. Verellen D, Depuydt T, Gevaert T, et al. Gating and tracking, 4D in thoracic tumours. *Cancer Radiother* 2010;14: 446–454.

147. Depuydt T, Verellen D, Haas O, et al. Geometric accuracy of a novel gimbals based radiation therapy tumor tracking system. *Radiother Oncol* 2011;98:365–372.

148. Yin FF, Wong J, Balter J, et al. The role of in-room kV x-ray imaging for patient setup and target localization. December 2009. (ISBN: 9781888340891) http://www.aapm.org/pubs/reports/RPT_104.pdf. Accessed June 6, 2011.

149. Klein FF, Hanley J, Bayouth J, et al. Task Group 142 report: quality assurance of medical accelerators. *Med Phys* 2009;36:4197–4212.

150. Benedict SH, Yenice KM, Followill D, et al. Stereotactic body radiation therapy: the report of AAPM Task Group 101. *Med Phys* 2010;37:4078–4101.

151. Sharpe MB, Moseley DJ, Purdie TG, et al. The stability of mechanical calibration for a kV cone beam computed tomography system integrated with linear accelerator. *Med Phys* 2006;33:136–144.

152. Mao W, Lee L, Xing L. Development of a QA phantom and automated analysis tool for geometric quality assurance of on-board MV and kV x-ray imaging systems. *Med Phys* 2008;35:1497–1506.

153. Goddu SM, Mutic S, Pechenaya OL, et al. Enhanced efficiency in helical tomotherapy quality assurance using a custom-designed water-equivalent phantom. *Phys Med Biol* 2009;54:5663–5674.

154. Langen KM, Papanikolaou N, Balog J, et al. QA for helical tomotherapy: report of the AAPM Task Group 148. *Med Phys* 2010;37:4817–4853.

155. Bissonnette JP. Quality assurance of image-guidance technologies. *Semin Radiat Oncol* 2007;17:278–286.

156. Bissonnette JP, Moseley DJ, Jaffray DA. A quality assurance program for image quality of cone-beam CT guidance in radiation therapy. *Med Phys* 2008;35:1807–1815.

157. Bissonnette JP, Moseley D, White E, et al. Quality assurance for the geometric accuracy of cone-beam CT guidance in radiation therapy. *Int J Radiat Oncol Biol Phys* 2008;71:S57–S61.

158. Yoo S, Yin FF. Dosimetric feasibility of cone-beam CT-based treatment planning compared to CT-based treatment planning. *Int J Radiat Oncol Biol Phys* 2006;66:1553–1561.

159. Gopal A, Samant SS. Use of a line-pair resolution phantom for comprehensive quality assurance of electronic portal imaging devices based on fundamental imaging metrics. *Med Phys* 2009;36:2006–2015.

160. Gayou O, Miften M. Commissioning and clinical implementation of a mega-voltage cone beam CT system for treatment localization. *Med Phys* 2007;34:3183–3192.

161. Antypas C, Pantelis E. Performance evaluation of a CyberKnife G4 image-guided robotic stereotactic radiosurgery system. *Phys Med Biol* 2008;53:4697–4718.

162. Jiang SB, Wolfgang J, Mageras GS. Quality assurance challenges for motion-adaptive radiation therapy: gating, breath holding, and four-dimensional computed tomography. *Int J Radiat Oncol Biol Phys* 2008;71:S103–S107.

163. Li G, Xie H, Ning H, et al. A novel 3D volumetric voxel registration technique for volume-view-guided image registration of multiple imaging modalities. *Int J Radiat Oncol Biol Phys* 2005;63:261–273.

164. Li G, Xie H, Ning H, et al. Accuracy of 3D volumetric image registration based on CT, MR and PET/CT phantom experiments. *J Appl Clin Med Phys* 2008;9:2781.

165. Sharpe M, Brock KK. Quality assurance of serial 3D image registration, fusion, and segmentation. *Int J Radiat Oncol Biol Phys* 2008;71:S33–S37.

166. Zhang L, Garden AS, Lo J, et al. Multiple regions-of-interest analysis of setup uncertainties for head-and-neck cancer radiotherapy. *Int J Radiat Oncol Biol Phys* 2006;64:1559–1569.

167. van Kranen S, van Beek S, Rasch C, et al. Setup uncertainties of anatomical sub-regions in head-and-neck cancer patients after offline CBCT guidance. *Int J Radiat Oncol Biol Phys* 2009;73:1566–1573.

168. Giske K, Stoiber EM, Schwarz M, et al. Local setup errors in image-guided radiotherapy for head and neck cancer patients immobilized with a custom-made device. *Int J Radiat Oncol Biol Phys* 2011;80:582–589.

169. Park SB, Rhee FC, Monroe JI, et al. Spatially weighted mutual information image registration for image guided radiation therapy. *Med Phys* 2010;37:4590–4601.

170. Pluim JP, Maintz JB, Viergever MA. Mutual-information-based registration of medical images: a survey. *IEEE Trans Med Imaging* 2003;22:986–1004.

171. Brock KK, Sharpe MB, Dawson LA, et al. Accuracy of finite element model-based multi-organ deformable image registration. *Med Phys* 2005;32:1647–1659.

172. Wang H, Dong L, O'Daniel J, et al. Validation of an accelerated "demons" algorithm for deformable image registration in radiation therapy. *Phys Med Biol* 2005;50:2887–2905.

173. Liang J, Yan D. Reducing uncertainties in volumetric image based deformable organ registration. *Med Phys* 2003;30:2116–2122.

174. Zhong H, Kim J, Chetty IJ. Analysis of deformable image registration accuracy using computational modeling. *Med Phys* 2010;37:970–979.

175. Wang H, Garden AS, Zhang L, et al. Performance evaluation of automatic anatomy segmentation algorithm on repeat or four-dimensional computed tomography images using deformable image registration method. *Int J Radiat Oncol Biol Phys* 2008;72:210–219.

176. Yue NJ, Kim S, Lewis BE, et al. Optimization of couch translational corrections to compensate for rotational and deformable target deviations in image guided radiotherapy. *Med Phys* 2008;35:4375–4385.

177. Wu QJ, Thongphiew D, Wang Z, et al. The impact of respiratory motion and treatment technique on stereotactic body radiation therapy for liver cancer. *Med Phys* 2008;35:1440–1451.

178. Wijesooriya K, Weiss E, Dill V, et al. Quantifying the accuracy of automated structure segmentation in 4D CT images using a deformable image registration algorithm. *Med Phys* 2008;35:1251–1260.

179. Thongphiew D, Wu QJ, Lee WR, et al. Comparison of online IGRT techniques for prostate IMRT treatment: adaptive vs repositioning correction. *Med Phys* 2009;36:1651–1662.

180. Zhang Q, Pevsner A, Hertanto A, et al. A patient-specific respiratory model of anatomical motion for radiation treatment planning. *Med Phys* 2007;34:4772–4781.

181. Li R, Jia X, Lewis JH, et al. Real-time volumetric image reconstruction and 3D tumor localization based on a single x-ray projection image for lung cancer radiotherapy. *Med Phys* 2010;37:2822–2826.

182. Li G, Xie H, Ning H, et al. A novel analytical approach to the prediction of respiratory diaphragm motion based on external torso volume change. *Phys Med Biol* 2009;54:4113–4130.

183. Hugo GD, Campbell J, Zhang T, et al. Cumulative lung dose for several motion management strategies as a function of pretreatment patient parameters. *Int J Radiat Oncol Biol Phys* 2009;74:593–601.

184. Yan D, Vicini F, Wong J, et al. Adaptive radiation therapy. *Phys Med Biol* 1997;42:123–132.

185. Yan D, Jaffray DA, Wong JW. A model to accumulate fractionated dose in a deforming organ. *Int J Radiat Oncol Biol Phys* 1999;44:665–675.

186. Yan D, Lockman D. Organ/patient geometric variation in external beam radiotherapy and its effects. *Med Phys* 2001;28:593–602.

187. DICOM: Digital Imaging and Communications in Medicine, PS3 Part 3, 2008. NEMA: National Electrical Manufacturers Association. Available from ftp://medical.nema.org/medical/dicom/2008/08_03pu.pdf. Accessed Mar. 25, 2011.

188. Mageras GS, Hu YC, McNamara S, et al. Imaging for radiation treatment planning. In: Curran BH, Starkschall G, eds. *Informatics in radiation oncology*. Boca Raton, FL: CRC Press, 2011 (in press).

189. Lu W, Olivera GH, Chen Q, et al. Automatic re-contouring in 4D radiotherapy. *Phys Med Biol* 2006;51:1077–1099.

190. Söhn M, Birkner M, Alber M, et al. Modelling individual geometric variation based on dominant eigenmodes of

organ deformation: Implementation and evaluation. *Phys Med Biol* 2005;50:5893–5908.

191. Yan D. Adaptive radiotherapy: merging principle into clinical practice. *Semin Radiat Oncol* 2010;20:79–83.

192. Deasy JO, Blanco AI, Clark VH. CERR: a computational environment for radiotherapy research. *Med Phys* 2003; 30:979–985.

193. El Naqa I, Suneja G, Lindsay PE, et al. Dose response explorer: an integrated open-source tool for exploring and modelling radiotherapy dose-volume outcome relationships. *Phys Med Biol* 2006;51:5719–5735.

194. Chow JC, Leung MK, Islam MK, et al. Evaluation of the effect of patient dose from cone beam computed tomography on prostate IMRT using Monte Carlo simulation. *Med Phys* 2008;35:52–60.

195. Jaffray D. Image-guided radiation therapy: from concept to practice. *Semin Radiat Oncol* 2007;17(4):243–244.

196. Mageras GS. Introduction to management of target localization uncertainties in external beam therapy. *Semin Radiat Oncol* 2005;15(3):133–135.

197. Jaffray D, Kupelian P, Djemil T, et al. Review of image-guided radiation therapy. *Expert Rev Anticancer Ther* 2007;7:89–103.

198. Yan D, Ziaja E, Jaffray D, et al. The use of adaptive radiation therapy to reduce setup error: a prospective clinical study. *Int J Radiat Oncol Biol Phys* 1998;41:715–720.

199. Yan D, Lockman D, Brabbins D, et al. An off-line strategy for constructing a patient-specific planning target volume in adaptive treatment process for prostate cancer. *Int J Radiat Oncol Biol Phys* 2000;48:289–302.

200. Keller H, Ritter MA, Mackie TR. Optimal stochastic correction strategies for rigid-body target motion. *Int J Radiat Oncol Biol Phys* 2003;55:261–270.

201. Bortfeld T, Jiang SB, van Herk M. When should systematic patient positioning errors in radiotherapy be corrected? *Phys Med Biol* 2002;47:(23):N297–N302.

202. van Lin EN, Van Der Vight L, Huizenga H, et al. Set-up improvement in head and neck radiotherapy using a 3D off-line EPID-based correction protocol and a customised head and neck support. *Radiother Oncol* 2003;68: 137–148.

203. Wu Q, Liang J, Yan D. Application of dose compensation in image-guided radiotherapy of prostate cancer. *Phys Med Biol* 2006;51:1405–1419.

204. Song W, Schaly B, Bauman G, et al. Image-guided adaptive radiation therapy (IGART): Radiobiological and dose escalation considerations for localized carcinoma of the prostate. *Med Phys* 2005;32:2193–2203.

205. Pepin EW, Wu H, Sandison GA, et al. Site-specific volumetric analysis of lung tumour motion. *Phys Med Biol* 2010;55(12):3325–3337.

206. Riboldi M, Sharp GC, Baroni G, et al. Four-dimensional targeting error analysis in image-guided radiotherapy. *Phys Med Biol* 2009;54(19):5995–6008.

207. Chen H, Wu A, Brandner ED, et al. Dosimetric evaluations of the interplay effect in respiratory-gated intensity-modulated radiation therapy. *Med Phys* 2009;36:893–903.

208. Kini VR, Vedam SS, Keall PJ, et al. Patient training in respiratory-gated radiotherapy. *Med Dosim* 2003;28:7–11.

209. Wong JW, Sharpe MB, Jaffray DA, et al. The use of active breathing control (ABC) to reduce margin for breathing motion. *Int J Radiat Oncol Biol Phys* 1999;44:911–919.

210. Remouchamps VM, Letts N, Vicini FA, et al. Initial clinical experience with moderate deep-inspiration breath hold using an active breathing control device in the treatment of patients with left-sided breast cancer using external beam radiation therapy. *Int J Radiat Oncol Biol Phys* 2003;56:704–715.

211. Schweikard A, Shiomi H, Adler J. Respiration tracking in radiosurgery. *Med Phys* 2004;31:2738–41.

212. Muacevic A, Drexler C, Wowra B et al. Technical description, phantom accuracy, and clinical feasibility for single-session lung radiosurgery using robotic image-guided real-time respiratory tumor tracking. *Technol Cancer Res Treat* 2007;6:321–328.

213. Stintzing S, Hoffmann RT, Heinemann V, et al. Frameless single-session robotic radiosurgery of liver metastases in colorectal cancer patients. *Eur J Cancer* 2010;46: 1026–1032.

214. Zimmerman J, Korreman S, Persson G, et al. DMLC motion tracking of moving targets for intensity modulated arc therapy treatment: a feasibility study. *Acta Oncol* 2009;48:245–250.

215. van Herk M. Errors and margins in radiotherapy. *Semin Radiat Oncol* 2004;14:52–64.

216. van Herk M, Remeijer P, Rasch C, et al. The probability of correct target dosage: dose-population histograms for deriving treatment margins in radiotherapy. *Int J Radiat Oncol Biol Phys* 2000;47:1121–1135.

217. Grills IS, Hugo G, Kestin LL, et al. Image-guided radiotherapy via daily online cone-beam CT substantially reduces margin requirements for stereotactic lung radiotherapy. *Int J Radiat Oncol Biol Phys* 2008;70: 1045–1056.

218. Liu HH, Balter P, Tutt T, et al. Assessing respiration-induced tumor motion and internal target volume using four-dimensional computed tomography for radiotherapy of lung cancer. *Int J Radiat Oncol Biol Phys* 2007;68:531–540.

219. Panakis N, McNair HA, Christian JA, et al. Defining the margins in the radical radiotherapy of non-small cell lung cancer (NSCLC) with active breathing control (ABC) and the effect on physical lung parameters. *Radiother Oncol* 2008;87:65–73.

220. Nelson C, Balter P, Morice RC, et al. Evaluation of tumor position and PTV margins using image guidance and respiratory gating. *Int J Radiat Oncol Biol Phys* 2010;76:1578–1585.

221. Melancon AD, O'Daniel JC, Zhang L, et al. Is a 3-mm intrafractional margin sufficient for daily image-guided intensity-modulated radiation therapy of prostate cancer? *Radiother Oncol* 2007;85:251–259.

222. Tanyi JA, He T, Summers PA, et al. Assessment of planning target volume margins for intensity-modulated radiotherapy of the prostate gland: role of daily inter- and intrafraction motion. *Int J Radiat Oncol Biol Phys* 2010;78: 1579–1585.

223. O'Daniel JC, Dong L, Zhang L, et al. Daily bone alignment with limited repeat CT correction rivals daily ultrasound alignment for prostate radiotherapy. *Int J Radiat Oncol Biol Phys* 2008;71:274–280.

224. Li HS, Chetty IJ, Enke CA, et al. Dosimetric consequences of intrafraction prostate motion. *Int J Radiat Oncol Biol Phys* 2008;71:801–812.

225. Chen AM, Farwell DG, Luu Q, et al. Evaluation of the planning target volume in the treatment of head and neck cancer with intensity-modulated radiotherapy: what is the appropriate expansion margin in the setting of daily image guidance? *Int J Radiat Oncol Biol Phys* 2010.

226. Hugo GD, Yan D, Liang J. Population and patient-specific target margins for 4D adaptive radiotherapy to account for intra- and inter-fraction variation in lung tumour position. *Phys Med Biol* 2007;52:257–274.

227. Pepin EW, Wu H, Shirato H. Dynamic gating window for compensation of baseline shift in respiratory-gated radiation therapy. *Med Phys* 2011;38:1912–1918.

228. Langen KM, Jones DT. Organ motion and its management. *Int J Radiat Oncol Biol Phys* 2001;50:265–278.

229. Booth JT, Zavgorodni SF. Set-up error and organ motion uncertainty: a review. *Australas Phys Eng Sci Med* 1999;22:29–47.

230. Yorke E, Rosenzweig KE, Wagman R, et al. Inter-fractional anatomic variation in patients treated with respiration-gated radiotherapy. *J Appl Clin Med Phys* 2005;6:19–32.

231. Nuyttens JJ, Robertson JM, Yan D, et al. The variability of the clinical target volume for rectal cancer due to internal organ motion during adjuvant treatment. *Int J Radiat Oncol Biol Phys* 2002;53:497–503.

232. Pos FJ, Koedooder K, Hulshof M, et al. Influence of bladder and rectal volume on spatial variability of a bladder tumor during radical radiotherapy. *Int J Radiat Oncol Biol Phys* 2003;55:835–841.

233. Fokdal L, Honore H, Hoyer M, et al. Impact of changes in bladder and rectal filling volume on organ motion and dose distribution of the bladder in radiotherapy for urinary bladder cancer. *Int J Radiat Oncol Biol Phys* 2004;59:436–444.

234. Li XA, Qi XS, Pitterle M, et al. Interfractional variations in patient setup and anatomic change assessed by daily computed tomography. *Int J Radiat Oncol Biol Phys* 2007;68:581–591.

235. Sanguineti G, Marcenaro M, Franzone P, et al. Neoadjuvant androgen deprivation and prostate gland shrinkage during conformal radiotherapy. *Radiother Oncol* 2003;66:151–157.

236. Litzenberg DW, Hadley SW, Tyagi N, et al. Synchronized dynamic dose reconstruction. *Med Phys* 2007;34:91–102.

237. Ramsey CR, Scaperoth D, Seibert R, et al. Image-guided helical tomotherapy for localized prostate cancer: technique and initial clinical observations. *J Appl Clin Med Phys* 2007;8:37–51.

238. Langen KM, Lu W, Willoughby TR, et al. Dosimetric effect of prostate motion during helical tomotherapy. *Int J Radiat Oncol Biol Phys* 2009;74:1134–1142.

239. Chen L, Paskalev K, Xu X, et al. Rectal dose variation during the course of image-guided radiation therapy of prostate cancer. *Radiother Oncol* 2010;95:198–202.

240. Goddu SM, Yaddanapudi S, Pechenaya OL, et al. Dosimetric consequences of uncorrected setup errors in helical tomotherapy treatments of breast-cancer patients. *Radiother Oncol* 2009;93:64–70.

241. Chao KS, Majhail N, Huang CJ, et al. Intensity-modulated radiation therapy reduces late salivary toxicity without compromising tumor control in patients with oropharyngeal carcinoma: a comparison with conventional techniques. *Radiother Oncol* 2001;61:275–280.

242. Barker JL Jr, Garden AS, Ang KK, et al. Quantification of volumetric and geometric changes occurring during fractionated radiotherapy for head-and-neck cancer using an integrated CT/linear accelerator system. *Int J Radiat Oncol Biol Phys* 2004;59:960–970.

243. O'Daniel JC, Garden AS, Schwartz DL, et al. Parotid gland dose in intensity-modulated radiotherapy for head and neck cancer: is what you plan what you get? *Int J Radiat Oncol Biol Phys* 2007;69:1290–1296.

244. Seco J, Sharp GC, Wu Z, et al. Dosimetric impact of motion in free-breathing and gated lung radiotherapy: a 4D Monte Carlo study of intrafraction and interfraction effects. *Med Phys* 2008;35:356–366.

245. Wu QJ, Thongphiew D, Wang Z, et al. On-line re-optimization of prostate IMRT plans for adaptive radiation therapy. *Phys Med Biol* 2008;53:673–691.

246. Sonke JJ, Belderbos J. Adaptive radiotherapy for lung cancer. *Semin Radiat Oncol* 2010;20:94–106.

247. Yang D, Chaudhari SR, Goddu SM, et al. Deformable registration of abdominal kilovoltage treatment planning CT and tomotherapy daily megavoltage CT for treatment adaptation. *Med Phys* 2009;36:329–338.

248. Nijkamp J, Pos FJ, Nuver TT, et al. Adaptive radiotherapy for prostate cancer using kilovoltage cone-beam computed tomography: first clinical results. *Int J Radiat Oncol Biol Phys* 2008;70:75–82.

249. Ahunbay EE, Peng C, Godley A, et al. An on-line replanning method for head and neck adaptive radiotherapy. *Med Phys* 2009;36:4776–4790.

250. Kobayashi H, Longmire MR, Ogawa M, et al. Multiplexed imaging in cancer diagnosis: applications and future advances. *Lancet Oncol* 2010;11:589–595.

CHAPTER 15

Cranial Radiosurgery

Frank J. Bova

DEVELOPMENT

In the mid-twentieth century, the advent of Cobalt tele-therapy units, and subsequently linear accelerators, helped radiation therapy play an increasingly important role in cancer treatment. During this time, external beam radiation therapy relied heavily upon the enhanced ability of normal cells over that of cancer cells to repair sublethal radiation damage. A basic schema was developed where a course of therapy would be divided into small fractions, each delivering a sublethal dose of radiation to a specified target volume. In the time interval between therapeutic fractions, the normal tissues would better repair radiation damage than would the cancerous cells, so that by the end of a course of treatment, the targeted cancer cells would have amassed significantly more radiation damage than would normal cells receiving identical doses (Fig. 15.1).

This delivery technique was necessary for two reasons: the first being that in the mid-twentieth century, neither computed tomography (CT) nor magnetic resonance imaging (MRI) was available, limiting the clinician's ability to map out and plan three-dimensional (3D) conformal radiation distributions. The second, which still exists today, is that the relative ratio of normal tissue cells to cancer cells varies considerably through the volume being targeted by the therapeutic radiation beams. This ratio begins at the site of the primary tumor with a high proportion of cancer cells to normal tissue cells, moves to a more diffuse concentration of cancer cells at the tumor's margin, and finally concludes with the lowest concentration of cancer cells, as regions of suspected microscopic disease are included in the targeted volume. It was necessary to develop a therapeutic tool that resulted in more cancer cell death relative to normal tissue cell death for a given course of therapy across this spectrum of tumor burden.

Radiosurgery, defined as a single-fraction stereotactically targeted radiation therapy, proposed a paradigm shift in the art of radiation delivery. This new approach would not attempt to leverage differential normal cell to cancer cell repair of sublethal damage, but instead deliver a highly concentrated dose of radiation exclusively to the volume of highly concentrated tumor cells. The normal tissue cells would be spared as a result of a very steep dose gradient, significantly reducing the dose to normal tissues.

The term "radiosurgery" was initially conceived by a neurosurgeon, Lars Leksell (1). Leksell's first attempt at a delivery scheme was to provide a concentrated radiation dose by the attachment of an x-ray tube onto an arc-centered stereotactic head-frame system designed to allow a target to be placed at the center of two orthogonal arc systems. The system was provided with a probe holder to point toward the intersection of the two arcing planes. The probe holder could then be moved along either arc while maintaining a trajectory that pointed to the target. Mounting an x-ray tube in place of the probe holder provided a method of delivering a radiation beam that would remain focused on the target. This, in turn, provided delivery of multiple non-coplanar beams, with separate entrance and exit pathways, that all intersected over the target.

In the 1950s, teletherapy was still in its infancy with the transition underway from delivery with x-ray tubes and radium systems to Cobalt-based units. Leksell undoubtedly had a thorough knowledge of state-of-the-art radiation delivery devices. Due to the limited specific activity and the resultant self-shielding, tele-radium sources had a very low dose rate, leading to extended treatment times. Novel approaches at increasing the dose rate were being pursued. One such approach was to develop a device that could simultaneously focus multiple radium sources at a target (Fig. 15.2) (2). These tele-radium beams were focused at a specific depth, converging at a point in space and then diverging as they left the target volume. This geometric-focusing technique is very similar to Leksell's approach used first in his arc-mounted orthovoltage x-ray tube design and then in his 179 Cobalt-60 source Gam-maKnife design (3,4). Leksell's primary contribution to radiation delivery was the realization that the coupling of a multi-focused radiation beam delivery system to a stereotactic reference system could enable a highly focused, high dose of radiation to be delivered to a defined target while providing significant sparing of adjacent normal tissues, a development that preceded isocentric teletherapy designs.

Prior to the development of the GammaKnife unit, in separate efforts, Leksell and Kjellberg had adapted fixed-port proton-beam units for stereotactic radiosurgical applications (Fig. 15.3) (5,6). These pioneering systems treated significant numbers of patients and provided early data on appropriate clinical doses for malignant, as well as

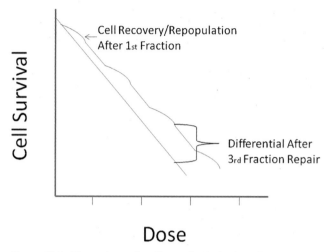

Figure 15.1. Figure shows the effects of a single-dose therapy versus that of a fractionated therapy. After each fraction, cells repair sublethal damage before the next fraction is administered.

benign, targets. The fact that these units were retrofitted for patient application and not readily available to the therapeutic community at large limited their widespread application. Leksell's development of the self-contained GammaKnife provided the first practical, commercial unit to offer dose distributions that rivaled the dose concentration and dose gradient of particle beam therapy (Fig. 15.4). While Leksell's initial intent was to provide a means to produce functional lesion, the anatomic atlases available in the 1950s proved insufficient as the primary image guidance and targeting tools and as mentioned CT and MRI, the tools required for such a target definition, would not be available for several decades.

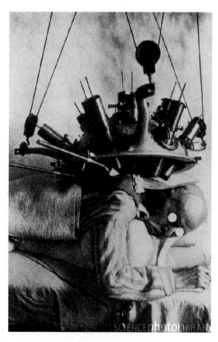

Figure 15.2. Tele-radium device for increasing dose rate over a target volume. Multiple sources are focused at a distance providing unique entry and exit pathways while only overlapping at the target volume.

By the 1980s, techniques for CT-based stereotactic frame localization and subsequent MR–CT image fusion techniques began to provide a novel solution to the problems of 3D target definition (7). Combining these imaging techniques with a new dose computation algorithm allowed a paradigm shift in the treatment of intra-cranial targets. For the first time, the ability to deliver a high dose of radiation that was conformal to a 3D target shape and provide an exceedingly steep dose gradient along the entire target-to-normal tissue interface would become widely available to clinicians.

Over the past two decades, radiosurgery has gone from a novel treatment approach limited to a few academic centers to a treatment modality available in most communities. Systems capable of delivering these precise conformal doses with steep gradients have been developed on multiple platforms. Joining the isotope-based GammaKnife is a multitude of linear accelerator-based systems. These include traditional gantry-based linac approaches as well as robotic arm-mounted systems. These newer devices can provide for not only intra-cranial but also extra-cranial radiosurgical treatments. While each of these delivery platforms presents unique challenges, the underlying principles for targeting and the desired characteristics of the prescribed dose distributions remain the same.

PRIMARY OBJECTIVES

The combination of stereotactic localization and the ability to produce a highly focused dose distribution with exceedingly high gradients provided a radical change from the existing fractionated treatment paradigm. This new imaging/treatment technique could successfully address intracranial targets in a single-fraction therapy, eliminating the dependence upon the ratio of radiation repair in normal tissue cells versus cancerous cells. This paved the way for clinicians to think of radiation as a tool of target elimination, which could be delivered in a single therapeutic event, similar to a surgical approach.

Radiosurgery allowed ionizing radiation to be applied to targets previously resistant to fractionated therapy. Dose distributions with an ever-evolving set of tools for high conformality and with exceedingly steep dose gradients provided new optimization parameters that were effectively leveraged against both benign and malignant targets. Radiosurgery treatment of arterial venous malformations is an example: when differential repair did not provide a sufficient therapeutic advantage relative to normal tissues, single-fraction conformal distributions with high dose gradients provided an effective therapy.

It is difficult to separate the effects of conformality and gradient on the success of radiosurgery treatments. The design of the first dedicated radiosurgery tool, the GammaKnife, allowed the treatment of spherical and irregular targets with a planning/delivery tool, commonly referred to as "sphere packing." This technique uses a class solution

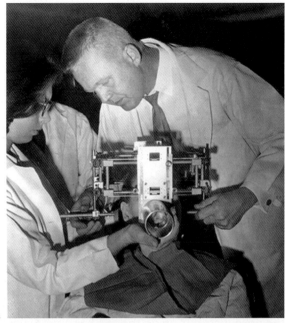

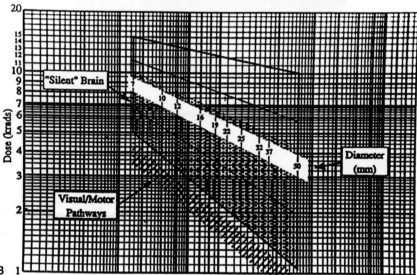

Figure 15.3. A: Image of Dr. Raymond Kjellberg fitting a stereotactic adapter for proto beam treatment. **B:** Adaption of the Kjellberg's proton therapy data relating volume to complication, demonstrating that as the treatment volume increases the safe dose must decrease to remain below the 1% probability of radiation necrosis.

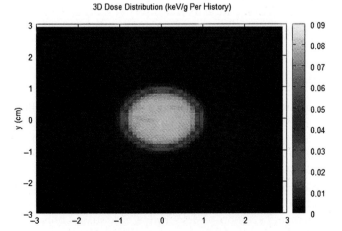

Figure 15.4. GammaKnife with dose distribution for an 18-mm helmet. The distribution and gradient is relatively symmetric about the vertical axis of the displayed dose distribution.

to produce a highly concentrated sphere of dose with very steep dose gradients. For round targets, a sphere is simply fitted to the target volume. For nonspherical targets, the technique fits the largest possible sphere inside the target, removes the volume covered by that sphere, and repeats the process with the remaining volume. The result of this process is an alignment of the target–normal tissue interface with the dose-sphere's steep gradient. The result is a high degree of conformality while maintaining a high dose gradient along the entire target's surface.

Early radiosurgery literature was based on particle beam treatments. For these treatments the Bragg peak provided a delivery tool that allowed both high conformality and little exit dose. The dose distribution provided by such a beam allows a smaller integral dose to be delivered. However, for many targets treated with proton radiosurgery, the effectiveness of the approach has not been shown to out-perform photon beam radiosurgery.

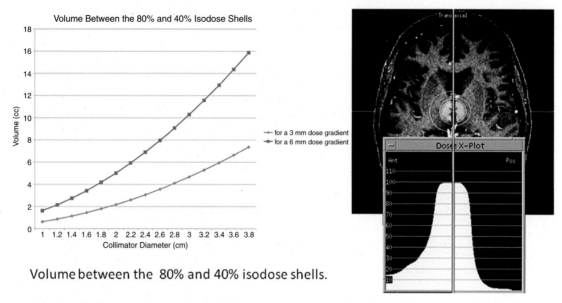

Volume between the 80% and 40% isodose shells.

Dose distribution on the right has a gradient of 3 mm and the dose distribution on the left has a gradient of 6 mm.

Figure 15.5. Volume of steep dose shell for 3- and 6-mm gradients. Figure on the *left* demonstrates the increase in volume encompassed by the 80% to 40% isodose shells for a 3-mm gradient and a 6-mm gradient. The figure on the *right* shows the effect of this change on a metastatic target.

Although eliminating normal tissue from the prescription volume is generally accepted as a necessary parameter for an effective therapy with low complications, a high dose gradient has not been universally recognized as an equally important parameter. When radiosurgery gradients are examined, special attention is paid to the portion of the distribution where the dose decreases from the prescribed target dose to one-half the target dose (6,8–10). As the volume of treated target increases, the volume contained in the rim of normal tissue rapidly expands. Therapies for both malignant and benign diseases have shown limitations on the maximum size of a single fraction's efficacy with targets. As the volume of the target increases, the dose that can be safely delivered decreases. It is thought that this expansion of the high-dose rim is at least partially responsible for the dose volume limit placed on radiosurgery treatments.

The importance of gradient can be appreciated when the volume enclosed in the high dose gradient, a shell defined by the edge of the prescribed isodose volume to one-half the treatment volume, is examined. The first evidence of a volume-limiting normal tissue threshold was the safe dose threshold versus target size published for particle beams (6). This curve demonstrates the relationship between complications and increasing target volume. Many other reports have provided clinical evidence demonstrating the relationship of increasing volumes being associated with increasing complications. Several reports have associated an increase in the 12-Gy volume to correlate with an increase in complications. As can be seen in Figure 15.5, the high-dose shell exposing normal tissue exponentially increases in volume as the target linearly increases. The lower curve in Figure 15.5 demonstrates the increase in this shell's volume if the steep

dose gradient, defined as the volume between the prescribed isodose surface and the isodose surface of one-half the prescribed dose, is maintained at 3 mm. The upper curve is the volume of this shell if the gradient is allowed to degrade from 3 to 6 mm. The net effect of the lower dose gradient is that the limiting dose volume is reached at smaller target volumes. For example, assume that it is safe to expose a rim of normal tissue, 2.0 cc in volume, to a gradient that is decreasing from 20 to 10 Gy. If a plan has a high dose gradient, 3 mm, as described above, this volume will not be reached until targets of ~4 cc (2.0 cm average diameter) are treated. However, if the high dose gradient is allowed to degrade to 6 mm, then the 2.0-cc rim of normal tissue volume is reached when a target of only 0.9 cc (1.2 cm average diameter) is treated. Paying careful attention to the high dose gradient is critical to the delivery of a safe and effective therapy.

IMAGING: ANGIOGRAPHY

To provide a highly conformal treatment with steep dose gradients, the system must be able to provide a spatially accurate description of the tissues to be targeted. While suffering from a lack of true 3D target descriptions, plane film fiducial-based systems can provide the position of a point within a stereotactic reference frame to within a few tenths of a millimeter (Fig. 15.6). The overly defined fiducial system and solution, as described by Siddon, not only provides high-precision spatial accuracy, but also removes the previously required orthogonal geometry (11). In the late 1980s and early 1990s, images used to define intracranial

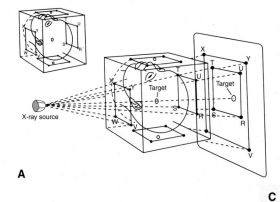

A

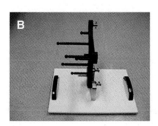

B

C

Coordinates of Test Points Determined from Angiographic Films

AP_m (mm)	Lat_m (mm)	Ax_m (mm)	$|\Delta AP|$ (mm)	$|\Delta Lat|$ (mm)	$|\Delta Ax|$ (mm)
0.04	−0.15	0.08	0.04	0.15	0.08
50.01	−0.22	−0.03	0.01	0.22	0.03
−49.96	−0.05	0.08	0.04	0.05	0.08
0.19	49.65	−0.05	0.19	0.35	0.05
0.17	−50.13	0.02	0.17	0.13	0.02
−0.02	0.1	50.01	0.02	0.1	0.01
0.06	−0.13	−49.91	0.06	0.13	0.09
−0.19	49.73	49.93	0.19	0.27	0.07
50.03	49.74	49.95	0.03	0.26	0.05
−50.17	−49.87	−50.23	0.17	0.13	0.23

Figure 15.6. Stereotactic system for plane films and target localization data. **A:** Angiographic view. **B:** The variable phantom allows targets to be set throughout the entire stereotactic volume. **C:** Table shows the data from nine experiments that examine the results along individual axes and in combinations.

targets, such as arteriovenous malformations (AVMs) were obtained on plane film x-rays. These systems utilized flat-imaging planes that in turn provided the clinician with spatially undistorted projections. The temporal resolution was limited to the speed at which film changers could shuffle film in and out of cassettes, approximately two images per views per second. As x-ray film gave way to the higher speed image intensifiers, these unwarped projections were lost (Fig. 15.7). The image intensifier's distortions were not only complex in any single orientation, but could vary nonlinearly with the orientation of the image intensifier. With the adoption of solid-state detectors, these projections are again presented without spatial distortion.

Simple orthogonal image sets are not capable of providing 3D descriptions of such vascular targets. Figure 15.8 shows a series of objects for which the orthogonal projections do not provide the information required for true 3D reconstructions. Although such views have been utilized for decades to reconstruct implanted radiation sources, the vascular images differ in that unique points in each projection cannot be matched. While these solid-state imaging systems provide clinicians with the perception of the 3D nature of

the vasculature, the systems have not attempted to format and map this data relative to a stereotactic reference system.

Although angiography remains the gold standard for detection of most vascular targets, due to the above limitations, computed tomography angiography (CTA) and magnetic resonance angiography (MRA) have become the stereotactic targeting modalities of choice. This has resulted in many commercial stereotactic systems, abandoning radiographic fiducial frames. Newly introduced imaging platforms capable of rapid rotation during angiographic image acquisition may begin to compete with MRA and CTA as viable stereotactic imaging modalities. However, due to the unavailability of the required fiducial systems, it will be difficult for this mode of targeting to once again gain a clinical foothold.

IMAGING CT

The first significant advance in the ability to define a true 3D intracranial target volume relative to a rigid reference system was the CT fiducial rod system (12,13). The addition

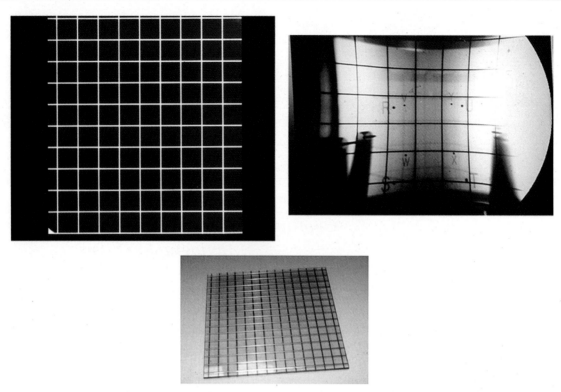

Figure 15.7. *Lower image* shows the lead grid used for imaging. Image in *upper left* shows the result of imaging the grid with a film system. Image on *right* shows the warped images resulting from the imaging with an image intensifying system.

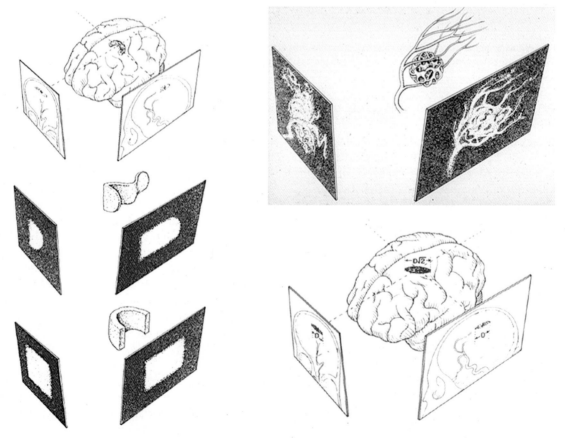

Figure 15.8. Series of objects for which a 2D projection are inadequate for accurate 3D description.

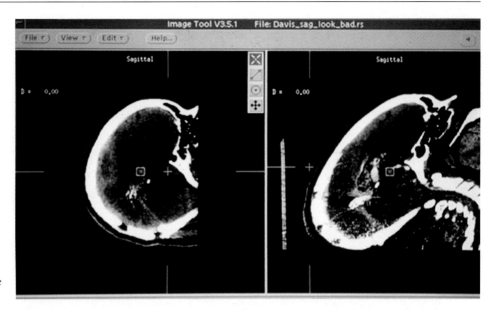

Figure 15.9. Image of effects of severe CT gantry tilt (30 degrees).

of the CT fiducial reference to a stereotactic frame provided a means by which imaged target tissues could be accurately and precisely mapped to a stereotactic reference platform. The stereotactic frame not only provided a method of analyzing each CT slice, providing a method of mapping CT pixels to stereotactic-based voxels (14), but, by analyzing the rods on each image, also provided a framework for image by image quality assessment. These systems removed scanner-dependent parameters from the required image analysis and subsequent mapping. No longer was it necessary to obtain an individual image's relationship based on the CT table's index or the scanner's alignment to the stereotactic frame. All such parameters could now be derived from information contained in each individual CT image.

Not all scanner misalignments are controllable or easily observed during the scanning process. CT tables may not be rigid enough to provide alignment of the patient and reference system to the scan plane. The patient may be rotated along several axes and the scanner gantry may not be perfectly aligned with the axis of table translation.

While a severe gantry tilt (shown in Fig. 15.9) can be readily identified at the time of image acquisition, small tilts may be more difficult to detect by casual visual inspection of the data set. For example, if a patient's stereotactic frame is tilted 0.5 degrees relative to the CT gantry, an error of 2.6 mm in the superior–inferior axis across a 300-mm diameter scan will result. Similar errors will result from misalignments between the reference system and the scanner's imaging plane. If the mapping function is not capable of sorting these misalignments, errors of several millimeters can quickly accumulate. The ability to guarantee such small misalignments during clinical applications is difficult. It is therefore critical for the stereotactic localization system to be rigorously tested for accurate identification and correction of such possibilities.

The ability to perform a local test of stereotactic localization requires the judging of computed-stereotactic coordinates relative to a known standard. It is important not only for the stereotactic coordinates of the test object to be known, but also that the test points are distributed through the defined stereotactic volume. As with the above example, a small tilt may correctly calculate the center of the defined stereotactic space. However, as the stereotactic mapping moves away from the center of the volume to the outer edges, the above-mentioned errors may exist.

A simple test object has been developed initially for frame-based quality assurance (15). This object contains spherical targets spaced throughout the frame's defined stereotactic volume. This allows a series of tests to be performed by the user that verifies the correct computation of these known stereotactic coordinates under varying patient–scanner alignments. Such misalignments that can be individually tested or tested in combination are: (1) gantry tilt, (2) patient frame tilt, and (3) patient frame rotation.

Figure 15.10 shows two types of phantoms: a fixed absolute phantom and a variable phantom. Each phantom can be attached to a fixture that allows the attachment of a CT localizer as well as to a fixture that allows the system to be mounted onto the treatment unit. This provides a system that can examine the alignment of the stereotactic process from imaging through planning and treatment. The fixed phantom has six targets at known stereotactic positions. Figure 15.11 shows the results of a series of tests. In these tests, the phantom was first aligned as precisely as possible to the CT scanner. Then tilts, spins, and gantry tilts were introduced. The CT scans were then processed by the program that automatically found the fiducial rods in each image and then processed the image set, mapping the voxels to the stereotactic ring's reference coordinate system. The results of this test show that the center of each of the known targets was correctly mapped to within one pixel, demonstrating the system's ability to correct for such misalignments during routine scanning. Figure 15.12

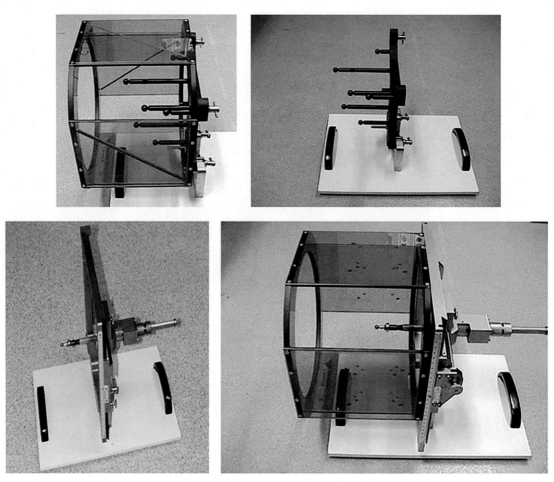

Figure 15.10. *Lower images* show variable Winston–Lutz phantom and angiographic with and without fiducial system. *Upper image* pair shows fixed six target absolute phantoms with CT, and with and without localizer attached.

Scan Descriptor	Calculated Coordinates			Absolute Coordinates			Error				
	AP	Lat	Axial	AP	Lat	Axial	AP	Lat	Axial	Vector Error	Average Vector Error
Ring no Tilt no Spin	24.90	−43.80	50.00	25.00	−43.30	50.00	0.10	0.50	0.00	0.51	0.57
	−50.20	−0.50	29.60	−50.00	0.00	30.00	0.20	0.50	0.40	0.67	
	24.80	43.10	9.50	25.00	43.30	10.00	0.20	0.20	0.50	0.57	
	−100.10	−0.40	−10.40	−100.00	0.00	−10.00	0.10	0.40	0.40	0.57	
	49.80	86.20	−30.50	50.00	86.60	−30.00	0.20	0.40	0.50	0.67	
	49.80	−86.90	−50.20	50.00	−86.60	-50.00	0.20	0.30	0.20	0.41	
Ring Tilt 3 deg	25.00	−43.70	49.80	25 00	−43.30	50.00	0 00	0.40	0.20	0.45	0.56
	−50.40	−0.40	29.80	−50.00	0.00	30.00	0.40	0.40	0.20	0.60	
	24.80	42.80	9.40	25.00	43.30	10.00	0.20	0.50	0.60	0.81	
	−100.40	−0.30	−10.30	−100.00	0.00	−10.00	0.40	0.30	0.30	0.58	
	49.90	86.30	−30.50	50 00	86.60	−30.00	0.10	0.30	0.50	0.59	
	50.00	−86.90	−50.20	50.00	−86.60	-50 00	0.00	0.30	0.20	0.36	
Ring Spin 3 deg	25.30	−43.30	50.10	25.00	−43.30	50.00	−0.30	0.00	−0.10	0.32	0.49
	−49.70	−0.10	29.90	−50.00	0.00	30 00	−0 30	0.10	0.10	0.33	
	25.10	43.30	9.80	25.00	43.30	10.00	−0.10	0.00	0.20	0.22	
	−99.30	0.20	−10.00	−100.00	0.00	−10.00	−0.70	−0.20	0.00	0.73	
	50.20	86.10	−30.30	50 00	86.60	−30.00	−0.20	0.50	0.30	0.62	
	50.20	−86.00	−49.70	50.00	−86.60	−50.00	−0.20	−0.60	−0.30	0.70	
Ring Tilt 3 deg Spin 3 deg	25.30	−43.50	49.80	25 00	−43.30	50.00	−0.30	0.20	0.20	0.41	0.49
	−49.60	−0.10	29.80	-50.00	0.00	30.00	−0.40	0.10	0.20	0.46	
	25.20	43.10	9.70	25 00	43.30	10.00	−0.20	0.20	0.30	0.41	
	−99.40	0.10	−10.10	−100.00	0.00	−10.00	−0.60	−0.10	0.10	0.62	
	50.00	86.20	−30.20	50 00	86.60	−30.00	0.00	0.40	0.20	0.45	
	50.00	−86.00	−50.00	50.00	−86.60	−50.00	0.00	−0.60	0.00	0.60	

Absolute phantom, scan diameter 350 mm 512 × 512 matrix, pixel size 0.67 mm × 0.

Figure 15.11. Table shows results of scanning the absolute phantom with CT localization. Separate runs for phantom spin, tilt and combination spin, and tilt and gantry tilt are shown.

Hidden Targets Test (CT)

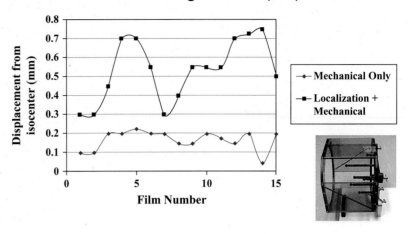

System with average delivery error of 0.2 mm has an overall
A error dominated by the image localization accuracy.

Delivery Testing

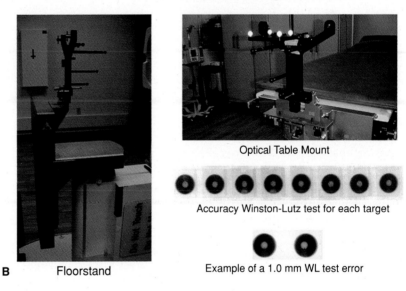

Optical Table Mount

Accuracy Winston-Lutz test for each target

Example of a 1.0 mm WL test error

B Floorstand

Figure 15.12. A: Data shows the results of a hidden target test. Targets are CT-imaged and planned, and Winston–Lutz films are taken and analyzed for total vector error. **B:** Experimental setup for Floorstand and optical guidance systems.

shows the absolute phantom being used with an optical alignment system, again allowing end-to-end testing of the image-planning delivery system.

One important factor in calculating stereotactic coordinates is the ability to account for errors inherent in the pixilation of fiducial systems. With a routine CT image matrix of 512×512 pixels and a scan diameter of ~350 mm to encompass a stereotactic fiducial reference system, the in-plane pixels have dimensions of 0.67×0.67 mm. A fiducial rod of 4-mm diameter that is randomly aligned in the field of view can demonstrate significant sampling errors. Using prior knowledge that the rod is straight and the rod images must therefore fit a straight line, many of the errors introduced by the pixel dimension can be corrected. For the optical system shown in Figure 15.13, the

knowledge that the passive fiducials are round can also be used to help correct for these pixilation effects.

MR IMAGING

Over the past two decades, MRI has become the dominant imaging modality for soft tissue target definition. A host of sequences have been developed that assist in the differentiation between normal and target tissues. Most common are simple T1 and T2 sequences. Most systems heavily rely upon MRI to provide the target-to-normal tissue contrast necessary for targeting definition. While the superior contract of MR scanning for most solid targets is critical for planning, MRI has limitations in providing

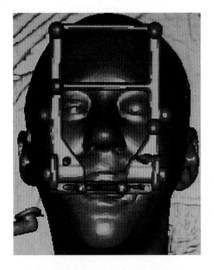
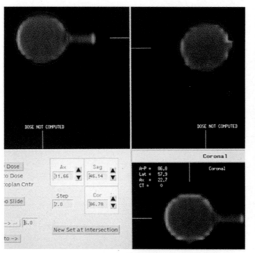
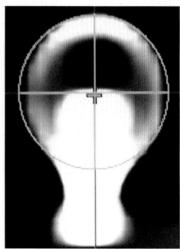

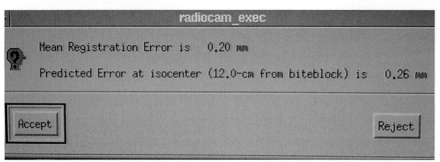

Figure 15.13. Optical target system with known geometry can be used to detect CT scan error or patient inter-scan movement. Image shows an acceptable scan with the reconstructing of the known fiducial system predicting errors less than a pixel in size at 10 cm from the array.

pristine spatial uniformity. The perturbations in the magnetic fields introduced by the patient result in susceptibility errors that warp the MR image. These errors are most dominant at the interface of changes in soft tissue and bone and again at the interface of tissue and air, as well as materials that introduce magnetic perturbations (16). A second set of errors in direct fiducial-based MR stereotactic imaging are introduced by the fiducial systems being at the outer most pixels, an area where magnetic fields are least uniform. A third issue that arises when direct MR stereotactic is attempted is that the size of the fiducial system and the stereotactic ring system often do not fit into head coils that have been optimized to provide the best tissue contrast and image uniformity.

Many systems have adopted MR–CT image registration techniques also referred to as "image fusion techniques." This approach allows the best MR images to be obtained, often requiring head coils that cannot accommodate a stereotactic localizer. Image fusion techniques register these images with the spatially more accurate CT dataset, thereby providing the best of both systems and compensating for each system's limitations. Figure 15.14 shows a typical MR–CT dataset aligned. The structures identified on both scanning systems provide images of common tissue boundaries, thereby allowing clinicians to judge the acceptability of the fusion-alignment process.

Another advantage of nonstereotactic MR scanning is that the imaging of the target tissues can be obtained hours or days before the actual radiosurgical procedure is

to be carried out. For procedures where stereotactic rings are used, this allows consultation and planning without the constraint of a patient waiting on the actual day of procedure.

DOSE PLANNING

Over the past two decades, the area of dose optimization has undergone the most change. As previously mentioned, the criteria of conformality and gradient have been the primary focus for plan optimization. Due to the near uniform sensitivity of intra-cranial tissues, a uniformly steep gradient is, most times, considered optimal. However, one notable exception is for targets near the optic processes, which are considered more sensitive for both single and fractionated treatments. In these cases, gradients can be altered to produce a steeper gradient. For example, gradient alteration is often used in the optimization of treatments involving pituitary targets. In the case of the pituitary, the optic chiasm lies just superior. Producing a steeper gradient in the direction of the optic chiasm, at the sacrifice of more lateral tissues, is often considered beneficial (Fig. 15.15).

As previously mentioned, sphere packing, one of the first radiosurgical planning techniques, was based on the geometric optimization provided by a class solution. In this technique, multiple individual beams are focused at a target providing primary beam overlap over the volume of the target and rapid divergence as the beams both approach

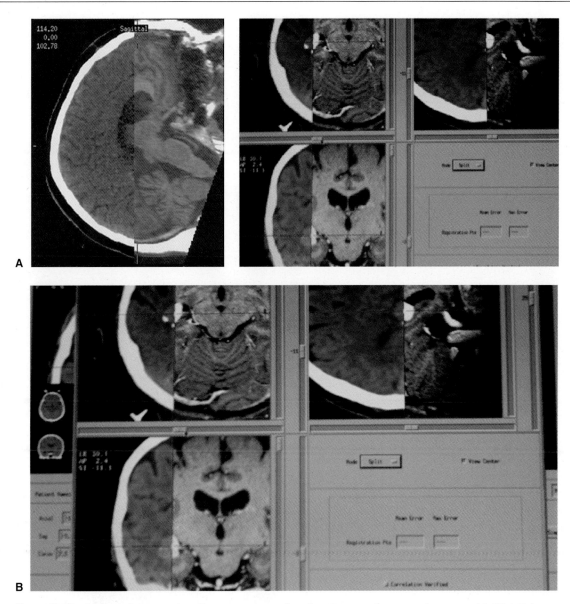

Figure 15.14. A: Image demonstrating alignment at target location. **B:** Image demonstrating successful CT–MR image fusion. Image alignment is inspected in all three anatomic planes.

and move away from the target. When a set of beams uniformly covering 2 pi are used, this solution has the advantages of providing a near-spherical dose distribution, no matter where within the head the stereotactic treatment volume the target lies. This makes the solution simple to program and plan. Where the target shape is not spherical, planning moves to the procedure of filling the target volume with spheres (Fig. 15.16). As previously mentioned, radiosurgery targets have no normal tissue within the targeted volume. Nonuniform intra-target doses have not been shown to be associated with increased complications. This is supported by the GammaKnife system, a targeting system where targets are treated with anywhere from 80% of the maximum dose to 50% of the maximum dose. These same sphere-packing techniques were adopted by early linear accelerator radiosurgery systems.

Many other systems that approach dose planning from other perspectives have been introduced. Dynamic conformal and inverse planning techniques have been applied to radiosurgical treatment. Dynamic conformal planning, a technique using multiple nonconformal arcs and beam's-eye collimation, has difficulty providing a high degree of conformality when addressing very small irregular targets (17,18). The issue of conformality is better addressed by inverse planning and intensity-modulated radiotherapy (IMRT), a technique that generally employs a more limited set of beam paths. While directed gradients against specific adjacent critical tissues can be accommodated, the gradient over 4 pi provides special IMRT challenges that must be carefully evaluated. The gradient over the entire surface of the target volume is particularly critical in cranial radiosurgery.

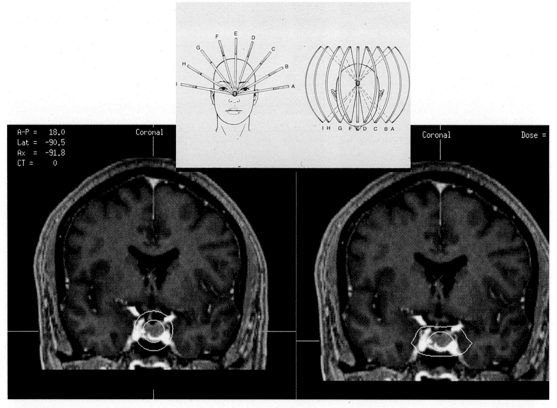

Figure 15.15. *Left image* shows the result of arcing planes distributed symmetrically left to right, *right image* shows the most superior beams (D–F) eliminated, increasing the dose gradient in the anterior–posterior direction, decreasing the dose to the optic chiasm, while decreasing the gradient in the lateral direction.

Because the goal of dose planning is to deliver an effective dose across the target volume while minimizing the dose to normal tissues, the selection of the prescription isodose shell tends to be lower than that used in routine fractionated therapy. Figure 15.17 shows a dose distribution for a metastatic lesion using a conical collimator and five non-coplanar arcs. Cross-plots of the dose along the lateral axis are shown in Figure 15.17A–D. The first plot in Figure 15.16A shows the distance required for the dose

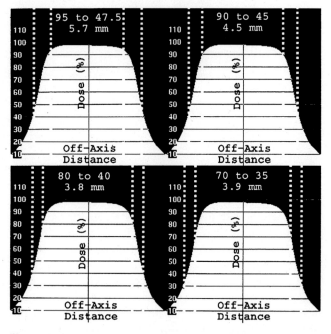

Figure 15.17. Image of metastatic plan on spherical target and the resulting cross plot. The effect of selecting the prescription isodose 95%, 90%, 80%, and 70% of maximum dose, demonstrating that the dose falls most rapidly to one-half the dose when the 80% of maximum dose shell is selected. This provides maximum normal tissue sparing for near-target doses.

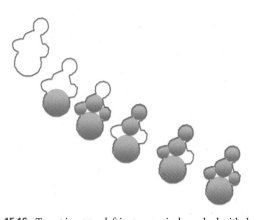

Figure 15.16. Target in *upper left* is progressively packed with decreasing sized spheres until the entire target is covered in *lower right*.

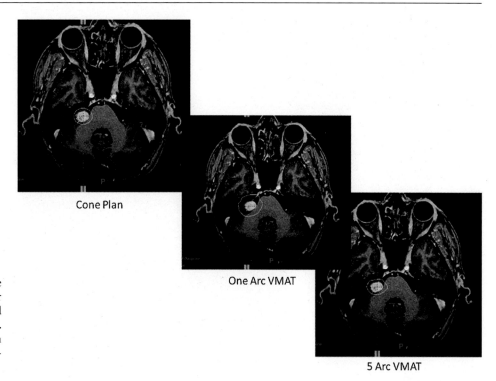

Cone Plan

One Arc VMAT

5 Arc VMAT

Figure 15.18. Plans for a simple acoustic two-isocenter plan for sphere packing and one-arc and five-non-coplanar arc VMAT plans. The cone plan and arc VMAT plan have similar conformality and gradient scores.

to decrease from a target isodose shell of 90% of maximum to 45%, half the target value, is 5.7 mm. Figure 15.17B–D denotes the distance required if the 80%, 70%, and 60% isodose shells are selected as the target isodose. As shown, the minimum distance, 3.8 mm, along with selecting the 80% isodose shell, provides the lowest integral dose to normal tissue (19). This essentially selects a prescription point just past the high-dose shoulder of the dose profile. If a lower prescription isodose shell is selected, then the high dose fall-off in normal tissue encounters a lower plateau of the distribution. If sphere packing is employed, and more than one isocenter is combined over an irregular target volume, a small hot spot is often produced and the resultant normalization can shift the optimized prescription shell down to a lower value. Prescription isodose shells of 70% through 50% are commonly encountered. As previously mentioned, the target volume has no normal tissue, and such hot spots, when confined to the target, have not been correlated with increased complications.

Other planning techniques, such as volume modulation (VMAT), have also been applied to intracranial planning. While these systems show excellent conformality, the ability to maintain exceedingly tight gradients must be carefully evaluated. Figure 15.18 shows the conformality of a simple two-isocenter sphere-packing plan for an acoustic neuroma and one from several VMAT plans. Although both provide excellent conformality, the VMAT plan has, to date, produced a less steep dose gradient for small and mid-size targets, thereby increasing the volume of tissue exposed to near-target dose levels. For larger targets, 2.4 to 3.0 cm average diameters, the ability of sphere packing to rapidly converge and then diverge becomes less

effective, and techniques such as VMAT begin to compare favorably for both conformality and gradient.

Because of the rapid development in treatment planning, the above comparisons are in a constant state of flux. However, the primary objectives of the planning process remain the same: a high degree of conformality and exceedingly steep dose gradients. The evaluation of both conformality and gradient has been suggested by many groups (18,20,21). Wagner introduced a Conformality Gradient Index (CGI) for both conformality (CGIc) and gradient (CGIg) (18). For the gradient score (CGIg), the formulation converts the volume of the prescription isodose and the volume of the isodose that encompasses one-half the treatment isodose into effective spherical volumes and then uses the radii of these effective spheres to compute an average effective radius. Assigning a score of 100 to an average radius of 3 mm, from prescription to one-half the prescription isodose, the score is calculated as

$$\text{CGIc} = 100\left(\frac{\text{Target volume}}{\text{Prescription isodose volume}}\right)$$

$$= (\text{PITV})^{-1} \times 100$$

$$\text{UFIg} = 100 - \left\{100 \cdot [R_{\text{eff, 50\%Rx}} - R_{\text{eff,Rx}}] - 0.3 \text{ cm}\right\}$$

$$R_{\text{eff}} = \sqrt[3]{\frac{3V}{4\pi}}$$

$$CGI = (CGIc + CGIg)/2.$$

Other conformality indexes have also been defined by the ICRU 62 (22) as the volume of the prescription of the

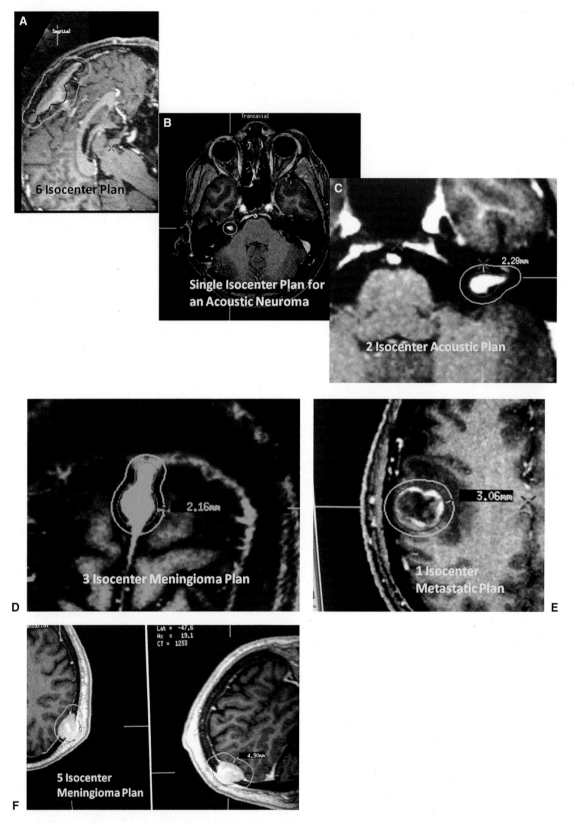

Figure 15.19. (**A**) Six isocenter meningiomas, (**B**) single isocenter for acoustic neuroma, (**C**) two isocenter plans for acoustic neuroma showing gradient (prescription to half prescription) of 2.28 mm, (**D**) two isocenter plans for meningioma showing gradient of 2.16 mm, (**E**) one isocenter 24-mm collimator for metastasis showing gradient of 3.06 mm, and (**F**) five isocenter plans for metastasis showing gradient of 4.9 mm.

isodose volume to that of the planning target volume (PTV).

$$CI_{ICRU} = \frac{V_{Rx}}{V_{PTV}}$$

Another suggested conformality index utilizes the volume that encompasses 95% of the PTV divided by the PTV. Yet, in another version of conformality index formulation, suggested by Paddick, the volume of the treatment isodose that does not include target volume is not counted in the denominator to ensure that the planning volume counted overlaps with the target volume (20).

$$CI_{Inv-Paddick} = \frac{V_{Rx} \times V_{PTV}}{V_{Rx \cap PTV}^2}$$

The goal of radiosurgery is to mimic a surgical resection. The coverage of the PTV is set equal to the imaging target volume. The goal of the planning process is to ensure that the full imaged target is covered. Because of the exceedingly steep dose gradient, the omission of any portion of the target volume is analogous to a subtotal surgical resection. It is therefore common for the prescribed plan to encompass the entire imaged target volume. The sensitivity of the intracranial tissues requires that safe and effective treatments result in conformality indexes between 1.0 and 1.3. With average target volumes in the order of 4 to 5 cc, these plans result in <1 cc of normal tissue being exposed to the prescription dose. The steep dose gradient also minimizes the exposure of normal tissue adjacent to the target volume. Some typical treatment plans with conformality indexes and dose gradients are shown in Figure 15.19.

TREATMENT DELIVERY

The above imaging and highly conformal planning with steep dose gradients requires a highly accurate delivery system. This necessitates that stereotactic targets be aligned with delivery systems, and that delivery systems be able to deliver multiple non-coplanar beams while maintaining accurate alignment.

The early GammaKnife units provided the gold standard for stereotactic delivery. The design of the rigid source alignment with the system's stereotactic reference provided a stereotactic target to isocenter alignment of 0.3 mm (23). Early linear accelerator systems had trouble maintaining such critical alignments (24,25). Winston and Lutz introduced a system that allowed the evaluation of stereotactic target alignment to the delivery system (26). This design provided a means by which non-coplanar delivery accuracy could be measured. In 1989, Friedman and Bova introduced a technique system to correct the linear accelerator's gantry and patient support "wobble" (8). This system was incorporated to provide actions assuring the accuracy and precision of each step of the radiosurgery procedure. Redesigned linear accelerators, capable of maintaining sub-millimeter delivery alignments, were also

introduced in the mid-1990s. For such systems, the Winston–Lutz delivery testing procedure remains the standard for certifying accuracy in delivery.

The phantoms shown in Figure 15.10 can be used with the Winston–Lutz test to provide end-to-end system testing. After evaluation of the CT mapping program, the computer stereotactic coordinates can be used to "treat" the phantom. This provides a process by which the entire image-planning-treatment chain can be evaluated. Figure 15.12 shows the results of such a test. Again, as with previous evaluations, it is critical that targets throughout the volume of the definable stereotactic space be evaluated. Only testing at the center of the defined volume can mask errors in both image mapping and treatment delivery.

The beams used in radiosurgery treatment are often significantly smaller than those used in routine radiation therapy. The complement of beams usually does not exceed 40 mm and usually includes beams as small as 5 mm. The measurement of these small beams poses special problems and requires very small detectors (27). If routine "Farmer style" chambers are employed for such small beams, then significant errors in both beam profiles and output factors can be made. Figure 15.20 shows beam

Effect of Detector Dimension on Penumbra Measurements

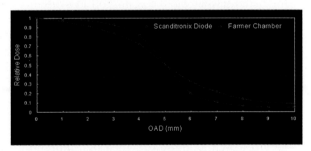

Finite dimensions of larger detectors cause rounding or smoothing of profile

A

Radiosurgery OAR Detectors (AAPM TG 42)

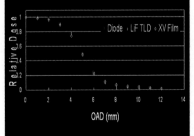

B

- Film is best.
- Diodes, plastic scintillators, TLDs, and ion chambers are all acceptable.
- Detector dimensions must be <2 mm.

Figure 15.20. A: Beam profiles using small diode detector and larger on chamber, demonstrating the errors possible when detectors of large size are used on small radiosurgical beams. **B:** 10-mm circular beam data taken with three high spatial resolution detectors.

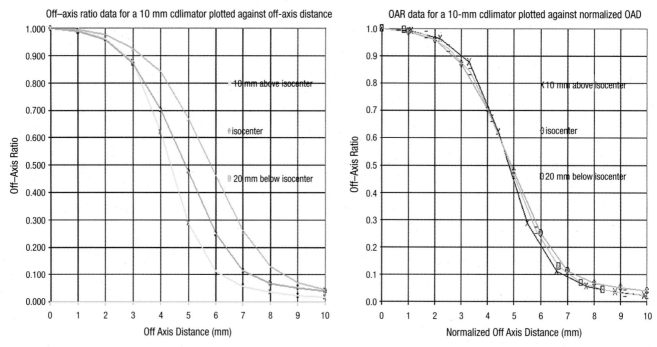

Figure 15.21. Beam cross-plots for absolute distance from central axis and again as percentage of off-axis distance. This can be used to check for effects of detector size.

profiles using numerous high spatial resolution/small cross-section detectors, as well as the effects of a large volume detector. Figure 15.21 shows first how a set of small beams behaves when plotted against off-axis distance and again how they agree when plotted against percent beam diameter. Such cross-tests should be carried out to ensure that detector sizes are not affecting measurement results. Figure 15.22 shows the output factors for a set of circular beams as well as small square fields. Again, cross-checking using multiple detectors is critical in ensuring that errors can be identified as these exceedingly small beams are measured.

Services such as those provided by calibration and quality assurance labs are critical in the commissioning of each radiosurgery system to ensure that all such parameters have been correctly measured and incorporated into

the system's treatment planning and delivery system services. The ability to localize, plan, and treat a test phantom and to have an independent laboratory verify the end result in both accuracy and prescribed dose is critical. Utilizing such services should be part of each new instillation's calibration and certification procedure.

SYSTEM CRITERIA

While it is difficult to define absolute accuracy or precision in stereotactic imaging or treatment delivery, it is possible to examine and provide perspective on the effect of misalignments and errors. Figure 15.23 shows the addition of treatment errors to imaging errors and how these added errors can quickly dominate the overall system accuracy.

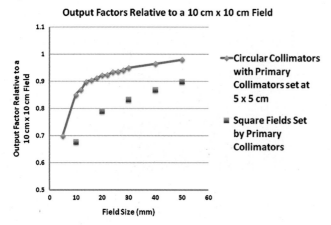

Figure 15.22. Output factors for cones and small square fields.

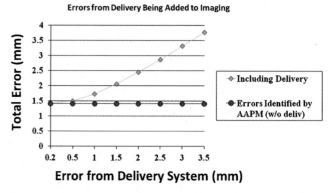

Figure 15.23. Demonstrating the effects of treatment errors when added to imaging errors (AAPM report 42).

Accuracy and precision can be effected by (1) incorrect mapping of stereotactic coordinates during image analysis, (2) planning that does not provide sufficient conformality or gradient, and (3) delivery systems that do not maintain sufficient rigidity and precision during non-coplanar beam delivery. These first two effects have been discussed previously. The third can be simulated in the radiosurgery planning system.

During treatment planning, a simulated radiation source is maneuvered to deliver beams from various directions. The mathematic model is designed to point at a specific stereotactic coordinate without error. During beam delivery, the ability of the actual treatment unit to maintain this accuracy is termed by the isocentric accuracy of the unit. This accuracy is determined by different design and manufacturing parameters that vary with each type of delivery system. In every case, the first critical alignment is the system's ability to place a specific stereotactic coordinate at the unit's nominal isocenter. In the case of the GammaKnife, the unit's delivery accuracy is then determined by how accurately the collimators are aligned within the treatment head. For a linear accelerator delivery system, it is the system's ability to accurately rotate the gantry and patient support unit about this isocenter. For robotic systems, it is the robot's ability to maintain alignment of the beam to a point in space. And for tomographic units, it is the combination of the isocentric rotation of the source and the system's ability to translate the patient through the gantry.

To help understand how isocentric accuracy can affect dose delivery, one can simulate isocentric inaccuracy in the planning system. The resultant dose distributions can then be compared to those derived from perfectly aligned simulations. For an arcing linear accelerator delivery system, dividing the arc into several segments and allowing each segment to aim at a different stereotactic coordinate can accomplish this simulation. Such a simulation was conducted with the gantry and patient support rotation maintaining a ±1 mm isocenter accuracy along each orthogonal axis. For a typical mid-size target of 18-mm diameter, the effects of this degree of inaccuracy result in a shrinking of the 80% prescription isodose shell's volume by 15% and an 80% to 40% isodose fall-off to decrease the sharpness of the gradient by 33%. While it is difficult to translate these effects into treatment failures or treatment complications, they do demonstrate the striking effect of small errors in isocentric accuracy on the delivery of the prescribed dose as well as the maintenance of the steep dose gradient.

THE TREATMENT PROCEDURE

Unlike routine-fractionated radiation delivery, radiosurgery requires more of a surgical mindset. With a single-fraction

Procedure Checklist

Instructions for Staff: Place Initials in the appropriate box indicating complete or enter NA

Step: Process Verification	Radiation Oncology Nurse LPN or RN Complete	Attending Physician Immediately Before any Radioactive Procedure
A. Patient identification: Name and at least one other ☐ MRN ☐ SSN ☐ DOB		
B. Procedure verified with consent for treatment		
C. Procedure verified with history and physical or progress note		
D. Verified availability of materials or treatment unit		
E. "Time Out." The treatment team, led by the attending physician, actively participating in verbal notification of: ☐ Patient Name ☐ Patient MRN ☐ Procedure ☐ Procedure site		

Signature signifies verification of patient ID, intent, correct procedure site

Figure 15.24. Checklist for time-out prior to initiation of the radiosurgical procedure.

therapy all QA and checking must be completed prior to the initiation of the first and only treatment. This places special demands on the radiation oncology department's teletherapy delivery team who are more aligned with an incremental treatment technique.

To assist the procedure, many departments have adopted a rigid checklist to help ensure that each critical step is performed and verified by more than one member of the clinical team. For a ring-based SRS procedure, this checklist would begin when the clinical team meets the patient and continue until the treatment is complete and the ring is removed. The procedure would include:

1. A "time out": Prior to ring placement, a "time out" is used to ensure that the team is focused on the correct radiosurgical target for that individual patient. Figure 15.24 shows a typical "time out" checklist with the accompanying MR image showing the radiosurgical target.
2. Specific written orders to accompany the patient to CT scanning.
3. A sign-off by the treatment team on the quality of image fusion.
4. A sign-off by the treatment team on the final plan.

5. The development of a treatment checklist that includes:
   ■ A check of the plan's transfer to the treatment systems record and verify system.
   ■ The pretreatment QA ensuring that
     ■ The correct patient and prescription has been transferred.
     ■ The unit's accuracy is verified prior to each treatment.
     ■ A step-by-step procedure to ensure that every step is documented and verified, including:
       ■ Verification of the stereotactic coordinate.
       ■ The cone and/or the collimator settings.
       ■ The monitor unit setting for each treatment segment.

An example checklist, automatically generated by the treatment planning system, is shown in Figure 15.25. The use of such a checklist is usually accompanied with a minimum of one double check and often with a second "blind check" to ensure that each parameter is properly set prior to the initiation of each treatment segment.

It is also critical to provide an atmosphere that allows the treatment team to concentrate on delivery and not be distracted by phone calls, scheduling questions or any

```
           STEREOTACTIC RADIOSURGERY TREATMENT CHECKLIST

Date :

Patient Name: Gator, Al E.

Prescribed dose: 1750.0   energy: 6MV Trilogy

Prescription Percent Line: 70.0 % of Maximum Dose
-------------------------------------------------------------
           Setup and Validation Procedure

____ Collinator rotation set to 0 degrees.

____ Field size set to 5 × 5 cm with collinator symmetric.

____ Patient on table in position, table, collinator, and
     jaw movements disabled.

____ Collision avoidance enabled

____ Patient wristband ID checked prior to treatment

____ Patient verified again patient signed picture

____ Prescription validated in Record and Verify System against
     Physician signed prescription

____ Set Winston-Lutz variable phantom to first Isocenter values

Isert collimator and carryout the following test film shots:
          Gantry      PSU
____       270         0
____        0          0
____        0         270
____        90         0

____ Visual approval of test film

____ Second Dosimetry Check compared to Physician signed treatment plan.
-------------------------------------------------------------
____   1.  Verify First isocenter coordinates:
               A-P = -19.3
                    Lat = -29.5
                    Axl = -39.3

____   2.  Install 18nm collimator.

____   3.  Set patient table to 20 degrees.

____   4.  Treat : Start angle = 120
                   End angle   = 30
                   Mon units   = 567
-------------------------------------------------------------
____   5.  Set patient table to 55 degrees.

____   6.  Treat : Start angle = 120
                   End angle   = 30
                   Mon units   = 630
```

```
-------------------------------------------------------------
____   7.  Set patient table to 340 degrees.

____   8.  Treat : Start angle = 240
                   End angle   = 330
                   Mon units   = 704
-------------------------------------------------------------
____   9.  Set patient table to 305 degrees.

____  10.  Treat : Start angle = 240
                   End angle   = 330
                   Mon units   = 744
-------------------------------------------------------------
____  11.  Set patient table to 270 degrees.

____  10.  Treat : Start angle = 240
                   End angle   = 330
                   Mon units   = 718
-------------------------------------------------------------
____  13.  Set Coordinates to A-P = -14.9
                          Lat = -42.7
                          Axl = -41.2

____  14.  Install 10nm collimator.

____  15.  Set patient table to 20 degrees.

____  16.  Treat : Start angle = 120
                   End angle   = 30
                   Mon units   = 315
-------------------------------------------------------------
____  17.  Set patient table to 55 degrees.

____  18.  Treat : Start angle = 120
                   End angle   = 30
                   Mon units   = 348
-------------------------------------------------------------
____  19.  Set patient table to 340 degrees.

____  20.  Treat : Start angle = 240
                   End angle   = 330
                   Mon units   = 449
-------------------------------------------------------------
____  21.  Set patient table to 305 degrees.

____  22.  Treat : Start angle = 240
                   End angle   = 330
                   Mon units   = 461
-------------------------------------------------------------
____  21.  Set patient table to 270 degrees.

____  22.  Treat : Start angle = 240
                   End angle   = 330
                   Mon units   = 418
-------------------------------------------------------------
END OF TREATMENT PROCEDURE
```

Figure 15.25. Checklist for SRS procedures automatically produced by treatment planning system.

other unrelated task. While an awareness of the distraction of cell phones during tasks such as driving a motor vehicle are being realized, similar distractions during complex procedures, such as radiation delivery, are often not appreciated. Providing the proper environment as well as a thoroughly planned procedure and post-procedure reviews are critically important for reducing human errors and identifying general system failures.

REFERENCES

1. Leksell L. The stereotaxic method and radiosurgery of the brain. *Acta Chir Scand* 1951;102(4):316–319.
2. Mould RF. *Mould's medical anecdotes omnibus edition.* CRC Press, 1966:510.
3. Lunsford LD, Flickinger J, Lindner G, et al. Stereotactic radiosurgery of the brain using the first United States 201 cobalt-60 source gamma knife. *Neurosurgery* 1989;24(2):151.
4. Mehta MP. The physical, biologic, and clinical basis of radiosurgery. *Curr Probl Canc* 1995;19(5):265–329.
5. Leksell L. Cerebral radiosurgery. I. Gammathalanotomy in two cases of intractable pain. *Acta Chir Scand* 1968;134(8):585–595.
6. Kjellberg R, Hanamura T, Davis KR, et al. Bragg-peak proton-beam therapy for arteriovenous malformations of the brain. *N Engl J Med* 1983;309(5):269–274.
7. Wu A, Lindner G, Maitz AH, et al. Physics of gamma knife approach on convergent beams in stereotactic radiosurgery. *Int J Radiat Oncol Biol Phys* 1990;18(4):941–949.
8. Friedman WA, Bova FJ. The University of Florida radiosurgery system. *Surg Neurol* 1989;32(5):334–342.
9. Liu R, Wagner TH, Buatti JM, et al. Geometrically based optimization for extracranial radiosurgery. *Phys Med Biol* 2004;49(6):987–96.
10. Pike GB, Podgorsak EB, Peters TM, et al. Three-dimensional isodose distributions in stereotactic radiosurgery. *Stereotact Funct Neurosurg* 1990;54–55:519–524.
11. Siddon RL, Barth NH. Stereotaxic localization of intracranial targets. *Int J Radiat Oncol Biol Phys* 1987;13(8):1241–1246.
12. Heilbrun MP, Roberts TS, Apuzzo ML, et al. Preliminary experience with Brown–Roberts–Wells (BRW) computerized tomography stereotaxic guidance system. *J Neurosurg* 1983;59(2):217–222.
13. Leksell L. Stereotactic radiosurgery. *J Neurol Neurosurg Psychiatry* 1983;46(9):797–803.
14. Saw CB, Ayyangar K, Suntharalingam N. Coordinate transformations and calculation of the angular and depth parameters for a stereotactic system. *Med Phys* 1987;14(6):1042–1044.
15. Phillips MH, Singer K, Miller E, et al. Commissioning an image-guided localization system for radiotherapy. *Int J Radiat Oncol Biol Phys* 2000;48(1):267–276.
16. Li L, Leigh, JS. Quantifying arbitrary magnetic susceptibility distributions with MR. *Magn Reson Med* 2004;51(5):1077–1082.
17. Wagner TH, Yi T, Meeks SL, et al. A geometrically based method for automated radiosurgery planning. *Int J Radiat Oncol Biol Phys* 2000;48(5):1599–1611.
18. Wagner TH, Bova FJ, Friedman WA, et al. A simple and reliable index for scoring rival stereotactic radiosurgery plans. *Int J Radiat Oncol Biol Phys* 2003;57(4):1141–1149.
19. Schell MC, Smith V, Larson DA, et al. Evaluation of radiosurgery techniques with cumulative dose volume histograms in linac-based stereotactic external beam irradiation. *Int J Radiat Oncol Biol Phys* 1991;20(6):1325–1330.
20. Paddick I. A simple scoring ratio to index the conformity of radiosurgical treatment plans. Technical note. *J Neurosurg* 2000;93(Suppl 3):219–222.
21. Bolsi A, Fogliata A, Cozzi L. Radiotherapy of small intracranial tumours with different advanced techniques using photon and proton beams: a treatment planning study. *Radiother Oncol* 2003;68(1):1–14.
22. ICRU Report 62. Prescribing, recording and reporting photon beam therapy (Supplement to ICRU Report 50). Bethesda, MD: International Commission on Radiation Units and Measurements, 1999.
23. Lindquist C. Gamma Knife Radiosurgery. *Semin Radiat Oncol* 1995;5(3):197–202.
24. Betti OO, Galmarini D, Derechinsky V. Radiosurgery with a linear accelerator. Methodological aspects. *Stereotact Funct Neurosurg* 1991;57(1–2):87–98.
25. Colombo F, Benedetti A, Pozza F, et al. Stereotactic radiosurgery utilizing a linear accelerator. *Appl Neurophysiol* 1985;48(1–6):133–145.
26. Lutz W, Winston KR, Maleki N. A system for stereotactic radiosurgery with a linear accelerator. *Int J Radiat Oncol Biol Phys* 1988;14(2):373–381.
27. Rice RK, Hansen JL, Svensson GK, et al. Measurements of dose distributions in small beams of 6 MV X-rays. *Phys Med Biol* 1987;32(9):1087–1099.

CHAPTER 16

Stereotactic Body Radiation Therapy

William G. Rule ■ Sheena Jain ■ Thomas P. Boike

INTRODUCTION

Stereotactic body radiation therapy (SBRT) involves the precise delivery of ablative doses of focused radiation utilizing unique beam arrangements, specialized immobilization, and image guidance equipment. The general principles that guide the optimal delivery of quality SBRT have their roots in cranial stereotactic radiosurgery. Originally described by Lars Leksell in 1951, cranial stereotactic radiosurgery was a novel method of noninvasively treating intracranial pathology (1). In 1967, Leksell and his colleagues developed the Gamma Knife. The Gamma Knife relied upon a stereotactic head-frame coordinate system and multiple cobalt-60 sources to precisely deliver an ablative dose of highly conformal radiation to the target while simultaneously sparing surrounding normal tissues through steep dose gradients. Since that time, numerous investigators have efficiently exploited and confirmed the clinical value of cranial stereotactic radiosurgery (2–7). Although there was significant interest in extending the cranial radiosurgical paradigm to extracranial targets, it was not until technical developments in the linear accelerator, imaging, and immobilization arenas came to fruition that SBRT became feasible. In 1994, Lax and Blomgren, from the Karolinska Institute in Sweden, became the first to publish a system of extracranial stereotactic radiotherapy (8). Since that time, SBRT has grown by leaps and bounds and has found applications in multiple disease sites and clinical scenarios. This chapter will guide the reader through the conceptual and practical framework that surrounds the delivery of SBRT. In addition, published clinical experience in various disease subsites will be presented and summarized.

RATIONALE AND GOALS

The basic radiobiological rationale underlying SBRT is similar to that underlying cranial stereotactic radiosurgery and radiotherapy: A small number, typically 1–5, of high dose fractions delivered over a brief period of time results in a more potent biological effect than what would be expected for the same total dose delivered via conventional fractionation (9). In addition, there is evidence that the high doses utilized in typical SBRT regimens appear to take advantage of microvascular endothelial cell apoptosis to effect tumor cell kill (10,11).

While the argument for the noninvasive and potentially curative nature of SBRT delivery in, for example, a medically inoperable early stage non–small-cell lung cancer patient is relatively easy to make, the delivery of SBRT to sites of metastatic disease requires the examination of several oncologic theories/concepts:

1. Theory of Oligometastases—This theory puts forward the concept that there may be a group of patients with metastatic disease that exists in a discrete number of known sites. Patients with this limited burden of metastatic disease have the potential to be cured if their limited metastatic deposits are eradicated (12–21).

2. Patterns of Failure/Consolidation Concept—Systemic therapy alone may not be sufficient to completely eradicate all clonagens in sites of gross disease. The addition of a potent local consolidative therapy may address the regions of disease that systemic therapy is least likely to successfully address (19–24).

3. The Norton–Simon Hypothesis—Originally utilized in the chemotherapeutic arena, this hypothesis states that tumor response to chemotherapy is proportional to tumor growth rate. In simple terms, the proportion of clonagens killed by a particular chemotherapeutic regimen is greater when the number of clonagens present is low. A potent local therapy such as SBRT, when directed at selected sites of gross disease, may reduce the systemic disease burden and may result in chemosensitization of the remaining clonagens (19–21, 25–27).

4. Immune Mediated Effects—The immune system of the patient receiving ablative SBRT doses may in fact play a role in addressing sites of disease outside of the treatment field (21,28,29).

Regardless of the specific rationale utilized, the delivery of ablative doses of radiation mandates a reduction in the normal tissue volume receiving high-dose exposure. This can only be accomplished with meticulous patient immobilization, respiratory motion management, specialized dosimetric/planning considerations, and image guidance for accurate target localization.

SIMULATION

SBRT simulations consist primarily of three intertwined components. They are: patient immobilization, tumor motion assessment/control, and image acquisition for planning. This process should be directed by the treating radiation oncologist with a physicist either at the simulation or available for consultation. These three aspects set the stage for a safe and successful treatment.

Prior SBRT experiences and trials utilized stereotactic frame-based treatment delivery for daily realignment and patient immobilization. External fiducials within the frame were used to realign patients for treatment. This has been found to be both effective and accurate for a variety of disease sites (8). From that initial experience, SBRT has evolved from an external frame-based approach to one that relies heavily on image guidance. This has made the need for a traditional stereotactic frame obsolete. However, several aspects of the frame should be carried forward for patient immobilization. Patient positioning needs to be comfortable, secure, and reproducible. Typically, patient-specific immobilization consists of a custom-formed pillow that provides ample surface contact with the patient to assure a secure position that will remain consistent during the SBRT treatment. For reproducibility, the patient's arms are typically placed up and out of any fields. This arm position is the major source of discomfort during treatment and the custom-formed pillow must support the arms. Vendors now offer several variations of the body frame with stereotactic localizers and most allow for abdominal compression (30–33).

Frameless approaches that use continuous monitoring of the patient are currently available. These approaches can work well provided that the system can detect and correct for changes in patient positioning. The most widely used and available system is the CyberKnife Image-Guided Radiosurgery System (Accuray, Sunnyvale, CA). This system using a linear accelerator mounted on a robotic arm to deliver treatment while periodic orthogonal kV images are taken to monitor motion. Adjustments for patient positioning and even fiducial/tumor tracking can be made with these images. The system has been shown to have an accuracy of 1.1 ± 0.3 mm for a planning CT slice thickness of 1.25 mm (34). These complex treatments have been very time consuming (35) but an update to the hardware has increased the dose rate and added a resizable collimator that should reduce treatment times.

It is recommended that motion be limited to reduce the target size and thus reduce normal tissue exposed to a high radiation dose. There are several strategies for motion control such as abdominal compression, breath-hold, gating, and tracking which have been described in detail in the Report of AAPM Task Group 76 (36). Abdominal compression is easy to adopt when starting a SBRT program, is tolerated well by patients, and allows for fast treatment delivery. Motion is first assessed using fluoroscopy to visualize the tumor or a surrogate such as the dia-

phragm or fiducials. Compression is applied with a paddle placed on the patient's upper abdomen to limit the excursion of the diaphragm and encourage regular shallower breaths. Patients are coached to expand their chest wall and avoid putting pressure on the compression device. Together, this results in decreased tumor motion for lung and liver targets (37). Pressure is then increased until motion is reduced to less than 1 cm.

Passive and active breath-hold techniques for SBRT have been described with various devices (38–40). Typically, these techniques measure the patient's respiratory cycle and have the patient hold their breath at a moderate deep-inspiration position. These have been shown to be accurate within an average of 2 to 3 mm (38). Patients must be trained for the best results, often at separate visits, and not every patient may be able to tolerate this approach. The length of each breath hold is, on average, 12–16 seconds. This strategy adds time when the treatment beam will be off, thus lengthening the treatment time of an already long radiation treatment visit. This approach may be best applied to patients with liver tumors, other abdominal targets, or metastatic disease to the lung as patients with lung cancer may have difficulty holding their breath due to compromised lung function (Fig. 16.1).

Respiratory gating is another strategy for dealing with diaphragm-related motion. A patient's respiratory cycle is tracked using infra-red cameras and reflectors placed on the patient (41). Alternatively this could be done with stereoscopic video cameras. During treatment planning, a gating window is designed to treat in one or several of the respiratory phases. For treatment delivery, the radiation beam is turned on only when the patient is in the selected part of the respiratory phase. Respiratory gating increases treatment delivery time compared with nongating approaches with published duty cycles (ratio of beam on

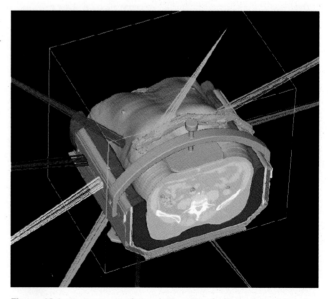

Figure 16.1. Reconstructed simulation CT of a liver patient showing the use of non-coplanar beams and abdominal compression.

time to total beam delivery time) of 30–50% (42,43). The correlation of internal targets to the external surface markers is an area of concern, especially with lung targets (44). An increased dose rate may help shorten treatment delivery. The ideal patient for gated delivery has large amplitude of respiratory motion and a small lung or liver target. It is an area of controversy if the added complexity and time of the treatment outweigh the benefit in other patients.

SBRT necessitates accurate image acquisition for target definition, identification of organs at risk, and treatment planning. This is traditionally accomplished with CT-based images. All organs at risk need to be covered within the scanned volume as well as any potential beam paths. Since noncoplanar beam arrangements are often utilized the volume scanned for treatment planning is often large, extending for 25 cm or greater above and below the target. Slice thickness of <3 mm is recommended for all clinical cases of SBRT. Imaging of moving targets is described in detail in AAPM Task Group 76. This includes slow CT, breath-hold techniques, gated approaches, and 4D CT (36). 4D CT can be reconstructed into maximum, minimum, and average intensity projections. Each of these has their individual strengths and limitations (45,46).

Fused images may aid in identification of targets or organs at risk. For example, prostate and liver targets may be best outlined on MRI. Regarding the spinal cord, it is best seen on T2 MRI images. When images are fused, it is important to make sure that they are acquired in the treatment position with all of the appropriate treatment immobilization devices in place. 18F-fluorodeoxyglucose (18FDG) positron emission tomography (PET) is difficult to use for SBRT but may be helpful in lung and liver targets. However, this should be used with caution as no standardized uptake value (SUV) threshold is standard for tumor definition. In addition, motion artifacts can be created due to the separate acquisition of the CT and PET images. Respiratory-correlated PET-CT may help to minimize artifacts when PET is needed as a fusion dataset for planning (47).

DOSIMETRY

As previously mentioned, minimizing the volume of normal tissue exposed to high dose regions is of primary importance in SBRT. As such, the GTV is typically assumed to be equal to the CTV (48,49). In general, 0.5 cm radial margins and 0.5–1.0 cm superior-inferior margins are added to yield the PTV. These margins may be judiciously modified depending on an individual patient's target motion characteristics as well as individual centers' confidence in their setups.

The two main dosimetric goals in the execution of quality SBRT are a high degree of conformality and dose falloff that is rapid and isotropic (8,48–52). The primary means of achieving a high degree of conformality and rapid and isotropic falloff is the utilization of a relatively large number of nonoverlapping noncoplanar beams (52). Maximal separation of beam intersection (in three dimensions) and avoidance of critical structures must be balanced against the reality of the mechanical constraints and restrictions imposed by modern linear accelerator heads and couches (53). Table 16.1 lists the standard set of beams utilized for right- and left-sided lung lesions at UTSW. Beam weighting should, in general, seek to evenly distribute entrance doses in order to achieve isotropic dose falloff and to limit the possibility of skin toxicity (51,54). In lesions in which isotropic falloff completely surrounding the target may not be ideal (e.g., spinal lesions), beams may be selected to maximize falloff in certain directions in order to minimize

TABLE 16.1 SBRT Couch and Gantry Angles for Right and Left-Sided Lung Lesions

Right lung		Left lung	
Couch angle	Gantry angle	Couch angle	Gantry angle
0	180	0	210
10	220	0	270
345	270	15	315
15	270	90	30
0	315	90	330
90	30	0	50
90	330	15	90
345	45	345	90
0	90	350	160
0	150	0	180

critical structure exposure. Such situations may also benefit from intensity-modulated planning techniques (51,55,56).

Choice of beam energy as well as beam-shaping parameters may also affect dose falloff as SBRT targets are often relatively small. Beam penumbra increases with increasing beam energy (secondary to lateral electron disequilibrium) and this effect becomes more prominent with targets residing within the lungs. Thus, a compromise must be reached between the desire for beam penetration and the desire to control penumbra effects. On most modern linear accelerators 6 MV is the typical photon energy of choice to treat lung targets. Higher energy beams are reserved for targets in other locations (liver, spine, etc.) or in a small number of the total beams for lung targets that must penetrate a significant amount of soft tissue. With regard to beam-shaping parameters, the vast majority of current SBRT treatment delivery is accomplished with multileaf collimators (MLCs). While very fine MLC leaf width (≤3 mm) can theoretically improve dose conformality, 5 mm leaf width appears to be adequate for most SBRT targets (21,56–58).

Another important consideration in planning is the utilization of tissue heterogeneity correction (especially in the setting of lung targets). In a dosimetric analysis of SBRT lung plans with and without heterogeneity corrections from the Radiation Therapy Oncology Group (RTOG) 0236 study, dose modifications were found to be necessary for future protocols utilizing heterogeneity corrections (59). Most modern treatment planning systems utilize algorithms that appropriately account for 3D scatter integration though for specific recommendations, the reader is encouraged to refer to AAPM Task Group 65 (21,60).

SBRT plans must be evaluated carefully, with close attention devoted to target coverage, conformality, normal tissue constraints, as well as the specific locations and falloff characteristics of high and intermediate dose regions. As in intracranial SRS applications, a heterogeneous dose distribution within the target volume is considered acceptable for SBRT (and potentially advantageous as the central portions of tumors often harbor hypoxic cells) (61). In SBRT, this target heterogeneity is achieved by placing the beam block/aperture margins from all beams in close adherence to the outline of the PTV. The resulting prescription lines that conformally cover the PTV are in the 60–90% range (typically ~80%). In general, the prescription isodose line is chosen so that 95% of the PTV is conformally covered by that line and that at least 99% of the PTV is covered by a minimum of 90% of the prescription dose. The plan is normalized so that 100% corresponds to the maximum dose delivered to the patient, with that point ideally located in the center of the PTV (51,59). Conformality can be evaluated by several methods, the simplest of which is by examining the ratio of the prescription isodose volume to the volume of the PTV (59,62).

Table 16.2 lists the normal tissue tolerance doses for single-fraction, three-fraction, and five-fraction SBRT delivery utilized at UTSW. The reader is advised to be cognizant of the fact that normal tissue tolerances for SBRT delivery have been developed relatively recently and are constantly evolving as the peer-reviewed SBRT literature base expands. With regard to the location of high dose regions, every effort should be made to constrain doses greater than 105% of the prescription dose to within the volume of the PTV. Thus, the cumulative volume of tissue outside of the PTV that receives greater than 105% of the prescription dose should equal no more than 15% of the PTV volume (51,59). Intermediate/low-dose spillage is evaluated by examining the maximum dose, 2 cm away from the surface of the PTV ($D_{2\,cm}$) as well as the ratio of the 50% prescription isodose volume to the volume of the PTV ($R_{50\%}$). Tables listing $D_{2\,cm}$ and $R_{50\%}$ values can be found on the RTOG website (www.rtog.org).

QUALITY ASSURANCE

While SBRT may use techniques similar to 3D conformal radiotherapy and IMRT, it is very unique due to the delivery of high doses to small volumes and the amount of technology utilized throughout the patient's treatment course. This physicist plays an important role in quality assurance and should be intimately involved from simulation to treatment delivery with each patient. Accuracy of imaging/fusion, motion assessment/control, treatment planning, patient repositioning/monitoring, and treatment delivery must be confirmed with phantom measurements. This should be done with the commissioning of new equipment to establish a baseline. Ongoing treatment-specific quality assurance should be aimed at reducing systematic errors. Performance of the equipment in the hands of your department should be verified and will aid in developing PTV expansions needed to cover targets reliably. The AAPM Task Group 101 outlines best practice guidelines in SBRT. In addition, suggestions for IGRT/SBRT annual, monthly, and daily QA and tolerances have been published (21) (Fig. 16.2).

While phantom measurements for commissioning and establishing machine tolerances are important, they represent a best-case scenario. Patient-specific departmental QA procedures that ensure consistency for imaging, contouring, normal tissue dose tolerances, target coverage, motion control, treatment verification, and documentation are necessary. Prior to treatment, verification of beam configurations and treatment plans for a given patient should be verified. This can be accomplished with a machine dry run to make sure all angles that are planned are achievable. Also, an absolute point dose and fluence measurement should be made with a small ion chamber and film due to the small fields and steep dose distributions of SBRT. Having well-trained physicist, therapists, and radiation oncologist is necessary because in the end, patient safety and accurate treatment is the responsibility of the entire team.

TABLE 16.2 Normal Tissue Dose Constraints for SBRT Delivery

| Serial tissue | Critical volume | One fraction | | Three fractions | | Five fractions | | Endpoint (≥grade 3) |
		Volume max	Maximum point dose[a]	Volume max	Maximum point dose[a]	Volume max	Maximum point dose[a]	
Optic pathway	<0.2 cc	8 Gy	10 Gy	15.3 Gy (5.1 Gy/fx)	17.4 Gy (5.8 Gy/fx)	23 Gy (4.6 Gy/fx)	25 Gy (5 Gy/fx)	Neuritis
Cochlea			9 Gy		17.1 Gy (5.7 Gy/fx)		25 Gy (5 Gy/fx)	Hearing loss
Brainstem (not medulla)	<0.5 cc	10 Gy	15 Gy	18 Gy (6 Gy/fx)	23.1 Gy (7.7 Gy/fx)	23 Gy (4.6 Gy/fx)	31 Gy (6.2 Gy/fx)	Cranial neuropathy
Spinal cord & medulla	<0.35 cc <1.2 cc	10 Gy 7 Gy	14 Gy	18 Gy (6 Gy/fx) 12.3 Gy (4.1 Gy/fx)	21.9 Gy (7.3 Gy/fx)	23 Gy (4.6 Gy/fx) 14.5 Gy (2.9 Gy/fx)	30 Gy (6 Gy/fx)	Myelitis
Spinal cord subvolume[b]	<10% of sub-volume	10 Gy	14 Gy	18 Gy (6 Gy/fx)	21.9 Gy (7.3 Gy/fx)	23 Gy (4.6 Gy/fx)	30 Gy (6 Gy/fx)	Myelitis
Cauda equina	<5 cc	14 Gy	16 Gy	21.9 Gy (7.3 Gy/fx)	24 Gy (8 Gy/fx)	30 Gy (6 Gy/fx)	32 Gy (6.4 Gy/fx)	Neuritis
Sacral plexus	<5 cc	14.4 Gy	16 Gy	22.5 Gy (7.5 Gy/fx)	24 Gy (8 Gy/fx)	30 Gy (6 Gy/fx)	32 Gy (6.4 Gy/fx)	Neuropathy
Esophagus[c]	<5 cc	11.9 Gy	15.4 Gy	17.7 Gy (5.9 Gy/fx)	25.2 Gy (8.4 Gy/fx)	19.5 Gy (3.9 Gy/fx)	35 Gy (7 Gy/fx)	Stenosis/fistula
Brachial plexus	<3 cc	14 Gy	17.5 Gy	20.4 Gy (6.8 Gy/fx)	24 Gy (8 Gy/fx)	27 Gy (5.4 Gy/fx)	30.5 Gy (6.1 Gy/fx)	Neuropathy
Heart/pericardium	<15 cc	16 Gy	22 Gy	24 Gy (8 Gy/fx)	30 Gy (10 Gy/fx)	32 Gy (6.4 Gy/fx)	38 Gy (7.6 Gy/fx)	Pericarditis
Great vessels	<10 cc	31 Gy	37 Gy	39 Gy (3 Gy/fx)	45 Gy (15 Gy/fx)	47 Gy (9.4 Gy/fx)	53 Gy (10.6 Gy/fx)	Aneurysm
Trachea & large Bronchi[c]	<4 cc	10.5 Gy	20.2 Gy	15 Gy (5 Gy/fx)	30 Gy (10 Gy/fx)	16.5 Gy (3.3 Gy/fx)	40 Gy (8 Gy/fx)	Stenosis/fistula
Bronchi—smaller airways	<0.5 cc	12.4 Gy	13.3 Gy	18.9 Gy (6.3 Gy/fx)	23.1 Gy (7.7 Gy/fx)	21 Gy (4.2 Gy/fx)	33 Gy (6.6 Gy/fx)	Stenosis/atelectasis
Rib	<1 cc	22 Gy	30 Gy	28.8 Gy (9.6 Gy/fx)	36.9 Gy (12.3 Gy/fx)	35 Gy (7 Gy/fx)	43 Gy (8.6 Gy/fx)	Pain/fracture
Skin	<10 cc	23 Gy	26 Gy	30 Gy (10 Gy/fx)	33 Gy (11 Gy/fx)	36.5 Gy (7.3 Gy/fx)	39.5 Gy (7.9 Gy/fx)	Ulceration
Stomach	<10 cc	11.2 Gy	12.4 Gy	16.5 Gy (5.5 Gy/fx)	22.2 Gy (7.4 Gy/fx)	18 Gy (3.6 Gy/fx)	32 Gy (6.4 Gy/fx)	Ulceration/fistula
Duodenum[c]	<5 cc <10 cc	11.2 Gy 9 Gy	12.4 Gy	16.5 Gy (5.5 Gy/fx) 11.4 Gy (3.3 Gy/fx)	22.2 Gy (7.4 Gy/fx)	18 Gy (3.6 Gy/fx) 12.5 Gy (2.5 Gy/fx)	32 Gy (6.4 Gy/fx)	Ulceration

(continued)

TABLE 16.2 Normal Tissue Dose Constraints for SBRT Delivery (Continued)

Serial tissue	Critical volume	One fraction Volume max	One fraction Maximum point dose[a]	Three fractions Volume max	Three fractions Maximum point dose[a]	Five fractions Volume max	Five fractions Maximum point dose[a]	Endpoint (≥grade 3)
Jejunum/ileum[c]	<5 cc	11.9 Gy	15.4 Gy	17.7 Gy (5.9 Gy/fx)	25.2 Gy (8.4 Gy/fx)	19.5 Gy (3.9 Gy/fx)	35 Gy (7 Gy/fx)	Enteritis/obstruction
Colon[c]	<20 cc	14.3 Gy	18.4 Gy	24 Gy (8 Gy/fx)	28.2 Gy (9.4 Gy/fx)	25 Gy (5 Gy/fx)	38 Gy (7.6 Gy/fx)	Colitis/fistula
Rectum[c]	<20 cc	14.3 Gy	18.4 Gy	24 Gy (8 Gy/fx)	28.2 Gy (9.4 Gy/fx)	25 Gy (5 Gy/fx)	38 Gy (7.6 Gy/fx)	Proctitis/fistula
Bladder wall	<15 cc	11.4 Gy	18.4 Gy	16.8 Gy (5.6 Gy/fx)	28.2 Gy (9.4 Gy/fx)	18.3 Gy (3.65 Gy/fx)	38 Gy (7.6 Gy/fx)	Cystitis/fistula
Penile bulb	<3 cc	14 Gy	34 Gy	21.9 Gy (7.3 Gy/fx)	42 Gy (14 Gy/fx)	30 Gy (6 Gy/fx)	50 Gy (10 Gy/fx)	Impotence
Femoral heads (Right & left)	<10 cc	14 Gy		21.9 Gy (7.3 Gy/fx)		30 Gy (6 Gy/fx)		Necrosis
Renal Hilum/vascular trunks	<2/3 volume	10.6 Gy		18.6 Gy (6.2 Gy/fx)		23 Gy (4.6 Gy/fx)		Malignant hypertension
Parallel tissue	**Critical volume**	**Volume max**		**Volume max**		**Volume Max**		**Endpoint (≥grade 3)**
Lung (right & left)	1500 cc	7 Gy		10.5 Gy (3.5 Gy/fx)		12.5 Gy (2.5 Gy/fx)		Basic lung function
Lung (right & left)	1000 cc	7.4 Gy		11.4 Gy (3.8 Gy/fx)		13.5 Gy (2.7 Gy/fx)		Pneumonitis
Liver	700 cc	9.1 Gy		17.1 Gy (5.7 Gy/fx)		21 Gy (4.2 Gy/fx)		Basic liver function
Renal cortex (right & left)	200 cc	8.4 Gy		14.4 Gy (4.8 Gy/fx)		17.5 Gy (3.5 Gy/fx)		Basic renal function

[a]Maximum point dose = 0.035 cc or less.
[b]5–6 mm above and below treated level.
[c]Avoid circumferential irradiation.

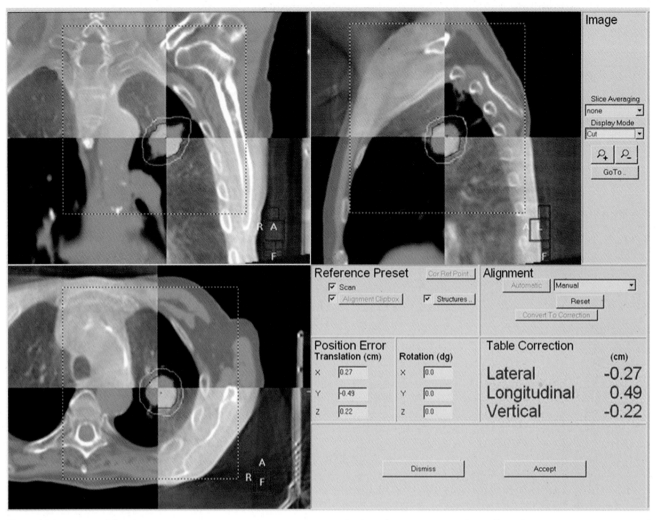

Figure 16.2. Fusion of the planning CT scan to a Cone Beam CT scan acquired on the treatment machine allows for accurate repositioning of lung targets.

EARLY STAGE LUNG CANCER

With an estimated 222,520 new lung cancer cases diagnosed in 2010 and 157,300 deaths, lung cancer remains the leading cause of cancer mortality for men and women (63). Of the new diagnoses, approximately 80% will have NSCLC, and roughly 15–20% of these with have early stage disease. Standard therapy for early stage lung cancer is surgical resection with either a lobectomy or pneumonectomy. Five-year overall survival from surgical resection ranges from 60% to 70% (64,65). However, some patients are not considered candidates for resection given multiple comorbidities, poor cardiac function, or limited pulmonary reserve. In these cases, less extensive surgery with wedge or segmental resections is considered. Limited resections have been associated with higher death rates and increased locoregional recurrence, when compared to lobectomy (66). Primary conventionally fractionated radiotherapy has been utilized in these patients, with 5-year overall survival rates of 10–30% (67,68).

SBRT has been employed in early stage lung cancer with a number of fractionation schemes and doses with

evidence of local control >85% (see Table 16.3). A phase I study performed by Timmerman et al. studied dose escalation in medically inoperable, early stage NSCLC. Dose escalation was started at 24 Gy in 3 fractions and was escalated to 2 Gy per fraction up to a total dose of 66 Gy. Dose was calculated without correction for tissue inhomogeneity. The maximum tolerated dose was found to be 22 Gy × 3 in large T2 tumors (5–7 cm), but was not reached for smaller tumors (32,69). A follow-up phase II study evaluating 70 patients with stage I NSCLC treating patients to 60–66 Gy in three fractions illustrated a 3-year local control of 88% and overall survival of 43%. Increased toxicity was seen in patients with "central" lung tumors, defined as tumors within 2 cm of the proximal bronchial tree (70,71).

A multi-institutional, phase II trial, RTOG 0236 assessed SBRT for peripheral lung tumors. Dose was calculated without correction for tissue inhomogeneity at 60 Gy in three fractions. Results illustrated a 3-year primary tumor local control rate of 98%, tumor plus lobe local control of 91%, and overall survival of 56%. There

TABLE 16.3		Prospective Trials in Lung SBRT			
Study author and year	Number of patients	Median follow-up (months)	Radiation schedule	Local control	Toxicity
Timmerman et al. 2003, McGarry et al. 2005 (7,8)	47	27 for T1, 19 for T2	18–22 Gy × 3	>90%	≥G4 2.1%
Timmerman et al. 2006, Fakiris et al. 2009 (9,10)	70	50	20–22 Gy × 3	88% at 3 y	Peripheral ≥G3 10.4%, Central ≥G3 27.3%
Timmerman et al. 2010 (11)	55	34	18 Gy × 3	98% at 3 y	≥G4 4%
Chang et al. 2008 (12)	27	17	12.5 Gy × 4	100% at 17 m	G2-3 dermatitis/ CW pain 11.1%
Onishi et al. 2007 (13,14)	257	38	3–12 Gy × 1–22	86% at 38 m	≥G3 5.4%
Nagata et al. 2005 (15)	45	30	12 Gy × 4	98% at 30 m	≥G3 0%
Baumann et al. 2009 (16)	57	35	15 Gy × 3	92% at 3 y	≥G4 1.8%

were two grade 4 adverse events and there was no treatment-related mortality (72).

Alternative fractionation schemes have been studied in the United States. Chang et al. at MD Anderson evaluated 27 patients with 50 Gy in four fractions. With a median follow-up of 17 months, local control was 100% with 8% developing mediastinal lymph node metastases and 15% developing distant metastases. One patient developed a brachial plexopathy and three patients (11.1%) developed grade 2 to 3 dermatitis and chest wall pain (73).

In Japan, there is extensive experience with utilizing SBRT in early stage lung cancers. In the largest retrospective series from Japan, published by Onishi et al., 257 patients were treated with SBRT from 14 centers. Doses were delivered at 3–12 Gy in 1–22 fractions and with a 38 month follow-up, local control was 86%. Three- and 5-year overall survival were 57% and 47%, respectively. Patients receiving a BED >100 Gy were found to have higher local control and survival rates (74). A phase I/II study performed by Nagata et al. evaluated 45 patients treated with 12 Gy × 4. No grade 3 toxicities were noted and 3-year overall survival was 83% for stage IA and 72% for stage IB (75).

There are multiple multi-institutional RTOG trials that are further studying the role of SBRT in the treatment of early stage lung cancers. RTOG 0618 is a phase II trial, recently closed to accrual, that is evaluating the role of SBRT in operable stage I/II NSCLC treated to 60 Gy in three fractions. RTOG 0813 is a phase I/II trial evaluating SBRT for early stage, centrally located, NSCLC in medically inoperable patients. In addition, RTOG 0915 is a phase II study comparing 34 Gy in one fraction versus 48 Gy in four fractions for inoperable, peripherally located tumors. The least toxic of these two arms will be compared to 60 Gy in three fractions (utilized in RTOG 0236).

LUNG METASTASES

Since Halsted's initial description of the contiguous spread of cancer, data illustrating long term, disease-free survival in patients with metastases led to Hellman's proposed theory of *oligometastases* (76,77). His theory described a disease state with a limited number of metastases that had not evolved to widespread disease (78). If this is the case, one could implement aggressive local therapy as curative-intent treatment for oligometastases. Surgical resection data for pulmonary metastases have illustrated improvements in survival, with 5- and 10-year overall survival (OS) of 36% and 25%, respectively (79). Based on this improvement in survival with aggressive local control, radiotherapy has also been explored for select patients. In addition, given the success with SBRT in the treatment of primary lung tumors, this technique is now being applied in the oligometastatic setting (32,69–75,80).

Phase II data from Rochester illustrated that 49 patients with 121 metastatic lung lesions had a 3-year actuarial local control rate of 91%. Mean overall survival was 23.4 months and treatment was tolerated well, with 2% grade 3 toxicity (81). Data from Germany showed that 61 patients with lung metastases treated for 71 lesions with SBRT had a 2-year actuarial local control rate and overall survival rate of 74% and 65%, respectively (82). Hoyer et al. published phase II data assessing SBRT in colorectal metastasis with 12 patients with pulmonary metastases treated to 45 Gy in three fractions. Two year actuarial local control was 86% (83).

Recently, a multi-institutional, prospective phase I/II trial evaluating SBRT in patients with 1–3 lung metastases treated to 60 Gy illustrated an actuarial 2-year local control rate of 96%, median survival of 19 months, and grade 3 toxicity rate of 8% (84). In the oligometastatic setting, these studies suggest that SBRT is both well tolerated and effective, with results comparable to metastasectomy, and could be a valuable noninvasive treatment option for patients.

LUNG SBRT SIDE EFFECTS

Side effects from stereotactic radiation treatment can include radiation pneumonitis, bronchial injury, pulmonary function test changes, rib pain, and dermatologic changes. Radiation pneumonitis is an inflammation of the bronchioles and alveoli that can occur weeks to months after treatment. The clinical presentation can be similar to an acute bacterial pneumonia and includes a nonproductive cough, chest pain, shortness of breath,

and fever. Chest X-ray typically illustrates an area of consolidation that can correlate with regions of high dose. Typical treatment includes nonsteroidal anti-inflammatory agents, steroid inhalers, systemic steroids, bronchodilators, and pulmonary toilet. In immunocompromised patients, bactrim can be used to avoid opportunistic infections. It is important to consider GI prophylaxis and monitoring of blood sugar levels in patients receiving steroids.

Bronchial injury can result in downstream atelectasis and can lead to focal collapse of lung. This injury is observed more commonly in central lung tumors and can be more detrimental as a larger portion of subsequent lung collapses. This can result in impaired pulmonary function and can also make it difficult to radiographically evaluate local recurrence from atelectatic tissue. Figure 16.3 shows an example of bronchial injury resulting in lung collapse, in a patient treated with SBRT to a central lung tumor. The patient was treated on protocol, to a total dose of 50 Gy in five fractions. The Indiana experience illustrates that tumor location is a strong predictor of

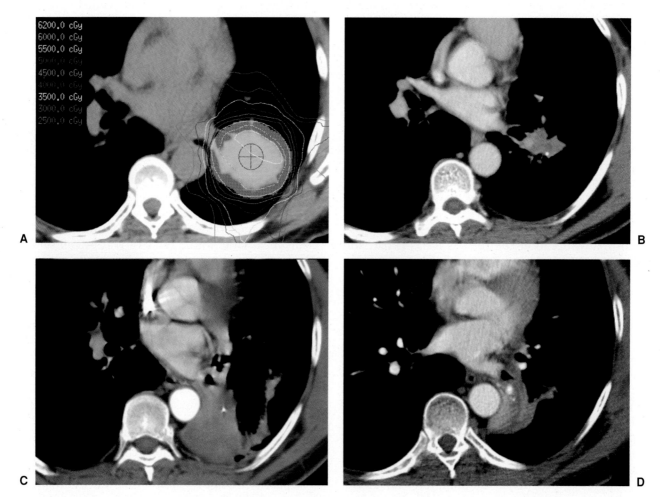

Figure 16.3. Stereotactic body radiation therapy (SBRT) of a central lung tumor treated on protocol. Panel A shows the isodose plan. While follow-up scans are shown at 3 months, 6 months, and 1 year in panel B, C, and D respectively. There was an excellent initial response with eventual collapse of the downstream lung.

toxicity with central tumors, and illustrated a 11-fold increase in grade 3–5 toxicity compared to peripheral tumors (70,71).

Changes in pulmonary function tests can be observed in patients after SBRT treatment and are typically seen in forced expiratory volume in 1 second (FEV1), forced vital capacity (FVC), and diffusion capacity for carbon monoxide (DLCO). These toxicities are graded based on a proportional decline from baseline. The grading scale is rated as follows: grade 1 if the value is 0.9–0.75 times the patient's baseline value, grade 2 if its 0.74–0.5 times the baseline value, grade 3 if its 0.49–0.25 times the baseline value, and grade 4 if its <0.25 times the baseline value and grade 5 if death occurs.

One of the more common side effects seen with patients treated with SBRT to the lung is chest wall pain and rib fractures. The incidence of spontaneous rib fracture has been reported in 3–14% of patients receiving SBRT to the lung, with 17–23% reporting chest wall pain (85–87). Recent data from Dunlap et al. illustrated that the chest wall volume receiving 30 Gy predicted for the risk of severe chest wall pain and/or rib fracture, and should be limited to <30 cm^3 (88). A study performed by Pettersson et al. illustrated a relationship between radiation-induced rib fracture and the dose to 2 cm^3 of the rib (89). Other potential side effects depend on tumor location, and include skin toxicity, brachial plexopathy, cardiac toxicity, and esophageal toxicity. As we continue to study the treatment of lung cancer with stereotactic techniques, the potential risks of therapy will be better elucidated.

LIVER SBRT

In the past, the results of the delivery of fractionated radiation therapy to patients with liver malignancies (primary or metastatic) were largely disappointing secondary to the whole liver's relatively low radiation tolerance (90–92). However, given the fact that the liver is an organ with parallel architecture, ablative does can potentially be delivered as long the volume of irradiation is limited (see Table 16.2) (93). One of the most significant complications that can occur after radiation delivery to the liver is radiation-induced liver disease (RILD). RILD is a clinical syndrome of ascites, anicteric hepatomegaly, and elevated liver enzymes typically occurring 1 to 2 months after completion of radiotherapy. Most patients recover completely within several months, with liver failure and death being quite uncommon (94). While it has been reported in several series, RILD is distinctly rare after SBRT for liver metastases (50,95). Patients with hepatocellular carcinoma (HCC) tend to have baseline hepatic dysfunction, potentially complicating the safe delivery of SBRT. In HCC patients, other liver toxicities, including reactivation of viral hepatitis, a transient increase in liver enzymes, and a general decline in liver function have been reported after SBRT (20) (Table 16.4).

LIVER METASTASES

Blomgren et al. published the first experience of stereotactic radiotherapy for liver tumors (50,96). This exciting work was quickly expanded upon by other investigators (16,97–104). Wulf et al. utilized fractionated stereotactic radiotherapy in 24 patients with 24 hepatic tumors (23 metastatic and 1 primary) (103). The majority of the patients were treated over 1 to 2 weeks with three fractions of 10 Gy prescribed to the PTV enclosing the 65% isodose line. Median follow-up was 9 months and actuarial local control at 1 and 2 years was 76% and 61%, respectively. No acute or late grade 3–5 toxicity was noted in these patients. Wulf et al. updated their experience in 2006 and demonstrated an actuarial local control at 1 and 2 years of 92% and 66%, respectively (102). They noted a borderline significant correlation between dose and local control. The actuarial control at 1 and 2 years in their "high dose" group (3 × 12–12.5 Gy $n = 19$, 1 × 26 Gy $n = 9$) was 100% and 82% compared to 86% and 58% in their "low dose" group (3 × 10 Gy $n = 27$, 4 × 7 Gy $n = 1$, $p = 0.077$). Again, no acute or late grade 3–5 toxicity was observed. Another European phase I/II study treated 17 patients with 34 liver metastases. Fourteen patients received 37.5 Gy in three fractions and three patients received 30 Gy in three fractions. The 2-year actuarial local control rate was 86% (101).

In 2009, Rusthoven et al. published the results of a multi-institutional phase I/II study exploring the safety and efficacy of a three-fraction SBRT regimen for patients with up to three hepatic metastases. Patient eligibility required a Karnofsky performance status (KPS) ≥ 60, ≤3 lesions, a maximum lesion diameter of less than 6 cm, life expectancy >3 months, no concomitant systemic therapy, and adequate liver function. Dose was prescribed to the isodose line covering the PTV (generally the 80–90% isodose line). In the phase I portion, the three-fraction total dose was safely escalated from 36 to 60 Gy in 6 Gy increments (97). Actuarial local control for the combined phase I/II portions (13 patients received <60 Gy, 36 patients received 60 Gy) at 2 years after SBRT was 92%, with 100% 2-year local control in lesions with a maximal diameter of 3 cm or less. The actuarial rate of any grade 3 toxicity was 2% at the time of last follow-up. Median and 2-year overall survival rates were 20.5 months and 30%, respectively. Patients with tumors from unfavorable sites (lung, ovary, noncolorectal gastrointestinal) were associated with worse survival compared to patients with tumors originating in other sites (105).

Further expanding the prospective literature base on SBRT fractionation schemes for liver metastases, investigators at UTSW recently reported the results of a 5-fraction dose-escalation study. Originally conceived as a three-fraction dose-escalation study, the publication of the multi-institutional three-fraction data (97) led to a modification of the study to explore a five-fraction regimen which could be potentially useful for tumors adjacent to critical structures such as bowel, or the larger, more central bile ducts.

TABLE 16.4 **Selected Prospective Trials of SBRT for Liver Metastases**

Study and type	Number of patients	Median follow-up (months)	Radiation schedule	Local control at 2 years	Overall survival	Toxicity
Herfarth et al. (2001) [98, 99] Phase I/II	33	15.1[a]	14–26 Gy in 1 fx -Prescribed to isocenter	68% (81% in phase II portion)	Median Survival: 25 months (27 months in phase II portion)	≥Grade 3: 0%
Mendez-Romero et al. (2006) [101] Phase I/II	14	12.9	37.5 Gy in 3 fxs -Prescribed to 65% isodose	86%	62% at 2 years	Grade 3 Acute: 17.6% Grade 4–5: 0%
Lee et al. (2009) [104] Phase I	70	10.8	27.7–60 Gy (median 41.8 Gy) in 6 fxs -Prescribed to isodose encompassing PTV	71% at 1 year	Median Survival: 17.6 months 47% at 1.5 years	Grade 3 Acute: 10% Grade 4–5: 4.3%
Rusthoven et al. (2009) [105] Phase I/II	47	16.0	36–60 Gy in 3 fxs -Prescribed to isodose encompassing PTV	92%	Median Survival: 20.5 months 30% at 2 years	Grade 3: 2% Grade 4–5: 0%
Goodman et al. (2010) [107] Phase I	26	17.0	18–30 Gy in 1 fx -Prescribed to isodose encompassing PTV	Probability of local failure by 12 months: 23%	Median Survival: 28.6 months 50.4% at 2 years	≥Grade 3: 0%
Rule et al. (2010) [106] Phase I	27	20.0	30 Gy in 3 fxs 50 Gy in 5 fxs 60 Gy in 5 fxs -Prescribed to isodose encompassing PTV	100% in 60 Gy cohort	Median Survival: 37 months 58% at 2 years	≥Grade 3: 0%

[a]Mean follow-up.
SBRT, stereotactic body radiation therapy; fx, fraction; fxs, fractions.

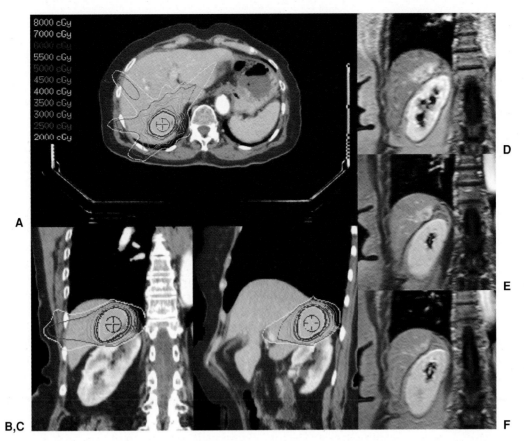

Figure 16.4. Axial, coronal, and sagittal isodoses from liver stereotactic body radiation therapy (SBRT) treated to 60 Gy are show in panel **A–C**, respectively. Panels **D–F** show 3 month, 6 month, and 1 year follow-up.

In this trial, doses were safely escalated to 60 Gy in five fractions of 12 Gy, with no grade 4 to 5 toxicity or treatment-related grade 3 toxicity. Actuarial local control at 2 years for the 60 Gy patient cohort was 100% (106). Figure 16.4 shows a SBRT liver treatment plan from a patient treated on this protocol with control by MRI follow-up.

Herfarth et al., exploring the utility of single-fraction SBRT, escalated the single fraction dose from 14 to 26 Gy in a phase I/II study. Entry criteria required a KPS ≥80, ≤3 lesions, a maximum lesion diameter of 6 cm, and adequate liver function. Sixty lesions (56 metastatic lesions and 4 primary liver lesions) in 37 patients were treated. Dose was prescribed to the isocenter with the 80% isodose line encompassing the PTV. Liver enzymes showed no statistically significant changes during the follow-up after treatment delivery and there was no toxicity greater than grade 2. The actuarial local control rate at 18 months was 68%. It was 81% for the patients treated in the phase II portion, after the initial dose escalation and refinement of patient positioning (98,99).

Goodman et al. recently published the results of a phase I single-fraction dose-escalation study. Twenty-six patients (19 with metastatic disease and 7 with primary liver malignancies) with 40 lesions were treated. Patient eligibility required Eastern Oncology Group (ECOG) performance status ≤2, ≤5 lesions, a maximum lesion diameter of 5 cm,

life expectancy ≥ 6 months, and adequate liver function. The single fraction dose was escalated from 18 Gy to the maximum-planned dose of 30 Gy in 4 Gy increments. Dose was prescribed to the isodose line encompassing the PTV. Dose-limiting toxicity (DLT) was not seen, with no toxic events greater than grade 2 noted. The probability of a patient suffering a local failure by 12 months was 23% (107).

HEPATOCELLULAR CARCINOMA

SBRT is emerging as an important tool in HCC patients with unresectable disease and is being explored in the bridge-to-transplant setting (108). As mentioned previously, patients with HCC tend to have baseline hepatic dysfunction, further elevating the caution that must be exercised when delivering hepatic SBRT. There are currently a limited number of reports describing the utilization of SBRT in patients with HCC, though toxicity and local control outcomes appear promising (96,101,102,107,109–111).

Tse et al. reported a phase I dose-escalation study using an individualized SBRT radiation dose prescription based on the volume of liver irradiated as well as the estimated risk of liver toxicity based on a normal tissue complication model. Thirty-one patients with Child-Pugh Class (CPC)

A HCC were treated, with a median dose of 36 Gy (range 24–54 Gy) delivered over six fractions. No RILD or treatment-related grade 4/5 toxicity was seen within 3 months after SBRT delivery. Five of the thirty-one HCC patients experienced a decline in liver function from CPC-A to CPC-B within 3 months after SBRT delivery. The 1-year in-field local control rate was 65% for all treated patients, with the most frequent site of first progression occurring outside the SBRT treatment volume (109).

A phase I three-fraction dose-escalation study by Cárdenes et al. enrolled 17 unresectable CPC-A and B patients with 1–3 lesions and a cumulative tumor diameter ≤6 cm. The starting dose was 36 Gy in three fractions. Dose in CPC-A patients was successfully escalated to 48 Gy in three fractions without DLT. Two patients with CPC-B developed grade 3 hepatic toxicity at 42 Gy in three fractions and the protocol was subsequently amended to treat CPC-B patients at 40 Gy in five fractions. One CPC-B patient on the 40 Gy/five-fraction regimen experienced a decline to CPC-C, while the remaining CBC-B patients treated with that regimen experienced no DLT. Six patients underwent a subsequent liver transplant. The only factor that was associated with more than one grade 3 (or greater) liver toxicity or death within 6 months was a CPC score ≥8. At the time of publication, 10 patients were alive without progression of disease (111). Given the often medically tenuous nature of the HCC patient population, as well as the general paucity of SBRT HCC data, every effort should be made to treat these patients in the setting of a clinical trial.

SPINE

Each year, more than 100,000 patients in the United States develop bone metastases from spread of their primary cancer (112). While all bones can be affected, the most common site of disease spread is the spine. Complica-

tions from this metastatic spread include pain, pathologic fracture, and spinal cord compression, which are associated with considerable morbidity. RTOG 97-14 found a single dose of 8 Gy to be equally effective to a conventional dose of 30 Gy in 10 fractions for palliation of pain related to skeletal metastases (113). However, lesions frequently recur and require retreatment twice as much as higher dose conventional fractionated treatment (113,114). If the single fraction dose of radiation could be safely escalated, improved rates of pain response and local control may be achieved. Even when employing stereotactic techniques with motion control, IMRT, and IGRT, the spinal cord is in such close proximity that it is the dose limiting structure. Figure 16.5 shows an isodose plan treated with spinal SBRT that spares the spinal cord well. However, this patient did develop asymptomatic radiation pneumonitis as seen on the follow-up PET scan. Henry Ford Hospital treated 49 patients with spine metastases on a dose-escalation protocol allowing a maximum of 10 Gy in a single fraction to 10% of the cord defined 6 mm above and below the vertebral body (115). This dose was found to be a well tolerated and represents a safe constraint. Sahgal has compiled data on patients treated with SBRT with and without prior conventional radiation for spinal neoplasms that have experienced radiation myopathy (116). A conservative recommendation of 10 Gy to a point was made for patients without prior radiation. A range of tolerances is recommended for patients that have prior radiation taking into consideration the dose of prior radiation and time between radiation and SBRT (117).

The primary indication for spinal SBRT has been for pain related to vertebral metastasis. A radiation dose–response relationship for pain control has not been clearly established. In the dose escalation experience from Henry Ford Hospital, a trend toward improved pain control was

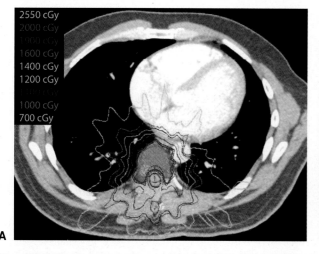
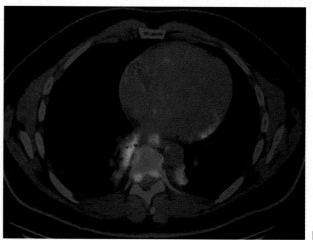

Figure 16.5. Panel a shows a stereotactic body radiation therapy (SBRT) isodose plan of a patient treated to 20 Gy in a single fraction with IMRT used create a sharp dose gradient toward the spinal cord. Panel B shows follow-up at 6 weeks with radiation pneumonitis corresponding to the 10 Gy line.

seen with doses above 16 Gy in a single fraction. Higher doses may lead to improved pain response and improved local control. Gerszten et al. published results of 393 patients treated with single fraction stereotactic radiotherapy for 500 separate spinal metastasis with local control rates of 88% and long-term pain improvement rates of 86% (118). Yamada et al. treated 103 spinal lesions in 93 patients in a single fraction and had 90% freedom from progression at 15 months (119). Amdur et al. treated 25 spinal tumors in 21 patients and found pain control in 43% of patients with 96% local control (120). Doses for these single fraction treatments varied from 15 to 24 Gy. However, the literature has variation in target definition, dose reporting, as well as a lack of target coverage reporting.

Increasing the number of fractions to 3 or 5 may allow for better post-operative treatment or increased safety in the case of re-irradiation. Bilsky et al. has reported safely giving 20 Gy separated over four to five treatments (121). Chang et al. treated 63 patients with either 30 Gy in five fractions or 27 Gy in three fractions (122). Thirty-five of the patients were retreatments and several of them were treated in the post-op setting. Narcotic use dropped by half and 1 year freedom from progression was 84%. Sahgal et al treated 38 patients and 60 different tumors to a median of 24 Gy in three fractions of which 37 of these tumors had prior radiation (123). Pain control was 67% and local control at 1 year was 92% in patients with prior radiation and 78% in patients without prior radiation. The RTOG has begun the first large randomized trial of spinal SBRT comparing 8–16 Gy in a single fraction with a primary endpoint of pain control. Further trials are needed to define the outcomes of SBRT in the post-operative and retreatment settings.

PROSTATE

Prostate cancer is the most common cancer in men in the United States and is often detected when it is localized to the prostate with current screening programs (63). Prostate cancer is divided into risk groups based on PSA, T-Stage, and Gleason score. For low risk patients with a PSA <10, Gleason score ≤6, and T-Stage ≤ T2a there are many treatment options including active surveillance, prostatectomy, brachytherapy, and external beam radiation with IMRT or proton therapy. All of these have high cause-specific survival rates with the differences being primarily in side effect profiles, convenience, and cost. SBRT is an emerging treatment modality in this group of patients and trials are aimed at determining its toxicity and efficacy.

However, this extreme hypofractionation is not a new idea. In the 1960s, patients in the United Kingdom were treated with a total dose of 36 Gy in five fractions over 3 weeks (124). The current rational for prostate SBRT not only builds on this clinical experience but also is rooted in

radiation biology and improved treatment delivery. Evidence supports a low α/β for prostate cancer around 1.5 (125) that is less than the estimated rectal α/β for of 2.3–5.4 (126). IMRT and IGRT currently allow for sculpting of high doses with precise targeting that corrects for inter fraction motion and monitoring intra fraction motion. SBRT is the next logical treatment step for low risk prostate cancer but needs confirmation in carefully executed clinical trials.

Four prospective clinical trials and one large experience have currently been published (127–131). All treatment was delivered in five fractions with total doses ranging from 33.5 to 50 Gy. Characteristics of each trial are outlined in Table 16.5. Out of 460 patients, 345 have been treated on a CyberKnife with total doses ranging from 35 to 36.25 Gy (127,128). The observed grade 3 toxicity in these papers compares favorably to standard dose escalation (132,133). At UT Southwestern, a dose escalation trial was completed of 9, 9.5, and 10 Gy per fraction in groups of 15 patients. For this trial, doses were escalated beyond the previously published ranges. Patients were treated with a rectal balloon in an effort to spare most of the rectum from high doses of radiation (131). Table six shows acute and late toxicity for the various reports. Finally, Freeman et al. performed a pooled analysis of patients from two centers that had a median follow-up of 5 years to access biochemical control (134). For these patients, biochemical progression-free survival was 93% at 5 years. Other clinical trials with SBRT for prostate cancer are underway or in development comparing this treatment modality to conventional IMRT and moderate hypofractionation. Data regarding late toxicity and biochemical control continues to mature.

PANCREAS

Approximately 42,470 people were estimated to be diagnosed with pancreatic cancer in the United States in 2009, with 35,240 expected deaths, resulting in it being the fourth largest cause of cancer mortality (63). Although aggressive multimodality treatments have been utilized, the overall 5-year survival remains less than 5% (2), with surgery being the only potentially curative option. However, only 5–25% of patients present with resectable tumors. For locally advanced disease, chemoradiation remains the standard of care, with a median survival of 9–13 months. SBRT has been studied in phase I and phase II trials in pancreatic cancer. Potential advantages of SBRT for pancreatic cancer include decreasing treatment time, improvements in local control that could potentially lead to decreased tumor seeding and distant metastasis, and earlier initiation of chemotherapy which could result in a decrease in distant spread.

A phase I study performed by Koong, et al. studied the feasibility and toxicity of single fraction SBRT in

TABLE 16.5	Characteristics of Selected Prostate SBRT Trials					
Author	Number of patients	Risk group	Total dose (per fraction)	Schedule	PTV margin	Technique
Madsen et al. (129)	40	Low	33.5 Gy (6.7 Gy)	Consecutive days	4–5 mm	3D with 6 Non-coplanar beams
Tang et al. (130)	30	Low	35 Gy (7 Gy)	Once weekly	4 mm	IMRT with 7 fields
King et al. (128)	41	Low and inter-mediate	36.25 Gy (7.25 Gy)	Consecutive days 21 patients Every other day 20 patients	5 mm and 3 mm pos-teriorly	CyberKnife
Katz et al. (127)	304	Low, interme-diate and high	35 Gy (7 Gy) 50 patients 36.25 Gy (7.25 Gy) 254 patients	Consecutive days	5 mm and 3 mm poste-riorly[a]	CyberKnife
Boike et al. (131)	45	Low and inter-mediate	45 Gy (9 Gy) 15 Patients 47.5 Gy (9.5 Gy) 15 Patients 50 Gy (10 Gy) 15 Patients	Two treatments per week	3 mm	IMRT on linac or tomotherapy

[a]For intermediate and high risk patient the proximal half of the seminal vesicles was added. For high risk patients the PTV was expanded 8 mm on the involved sides.

locally advanced pancreatic patients. Fifteen patients with an ECOG of ≤2 and tumors <7.5 cm were enrolled on the study. Dose escalation was performed at 15, 20, and 25 Gy in single fraction. No dose limiting toxicities were observed, with no grade 3/4 toxicity (135). A follow-up phase II study performed by Koong, et al. assessed the role of a SBRT boost after conventionally fractionated chemoradiation in locally advanced patients. 19 patients were treated with combined 5-FU or capecitabine and 45 Gy at 1.8 Gy/fraction with IMRT followed by a 25 Gy SBRT boost to the primary tumor. Two patients developed a grade 3 gastroparesis (one prior to SBRT and one after). Although excellent local control was achieved, this did not translate to have overall survival (OS) advantage with a median OS of 33 weeks (136).

A Danish study performed by Hoyer et al. evaluated SBRT in locally advanced pancreatic cancer patients. Twenty-two patients with inoperable or recurrent stage I–II disease were treated with SBRT to 45 Gy in three fractions. Only one patient had an isolated local failure, with five patients developing local failure and distant metasta-

ses at the same time. Two weeks after treatment there was a significant decrease in performance status, nausea, and pain compared to baseline. Four patients developed severe mucositis/ulceration of the stomach and one patient had a nonfatal perforation of the stomach. Based on these results, it was recommended that SBRT had unacceptable toxicity and poor outcome for unresectable pancreatic carcinoma patients (137).

A recent phase II study assessing SBRT delivered between cycle 1 and 2 of gemcitabine was assessed by Schellenberg et al. Sixteen patients with locally advanced pancreatic cancer received gemcitabine 1,000 mg/m² weekly on days 1, 8, and 15 with 25 Gy SBRT in a single fraction on day 29. This was followed with gemcitabine 2 weeks later, which was continued until disease progression. Three patients (19%) developed local progression > 1 year after treatment, none of which were in regional lymph nodes. Two patients (13%) developed grade 2 acute toxicity, and one patient (6%) developed acute grade 3 toxicity. There was a increased rate of late toxicity with five patients developing grade 2 ulceration and one patient developing grade 3 duodenal stenosis. Median

| TABLE 16.6 | Toxicity Results From Selected Prostate SBRT Trials |

Author	Median follow-up (Range)	Toxicity scale	Grade 2 GI		Grade 2 GU		≥ Grade 3 GI		≥ Grade 3 GU	
			Acute	Late[a]	Acute	Late	Acute	Late	Acute	Late
Madsen et al. (129)	41 months (12–60)	RTOG	13%	7.5%	20.5%	20%	0%	0%	2%	0%
Tang et al. (130)	12 months (NA)	CTCv3	50%	13%	23%	13%	0%	0%	0%	0%
King et al. (128)	33 months (6–45)	RTOG	NA	15%	NA	24%	NA	0%	NA	5%
Katz et al. (127)	30 months (26–37) Low dose 17 months (8–27) High dose	RTOG	2.9% 3.6%	0% 4%	5.8% 4.7%	2% 4%	0% 0%	0% 0%	0.5% 0%	0% 0%
Boike et al. (131)	30 months (45 Gy) 18 months (47.5 Gy) 12 months (50 Gy)	CTCv3	0% 27% 7%	7% 7% 0%	27% 7% 33%	13% 13% 0%	0% 0% 0%	0% 0% 7%	0% 0% 0%	0% 7% 7%

[a]Toxicity greater than one month post treatment was considered late.

survival was 11.4 months with 50% of patients alive at 1 year. Further analysis was performed to assess if there was a correlation between the volume of duodenum irradiated and toxicity. Although not significant, there was a trend for increased toxicity for the duodenal volume encompassed by the 12.5 Gy (50%) isodose line ($p = 0.13$) (138).

REFERENCES

1. Leksell L. The stereotaxic method and radiosurgery of the brain. *Acta Chir Scand* 1951;102(4):316–319.
2. Flickinger JC, Kondziolka D, Niranjan A, et al. Results of acoustic neuroma radiosurgery: an analysis of 5 years' experience using current methods. *J Neurosurg* 2001; 94(1):1–6.
3. Lunsford LD, Niranjan A, Kondziolka D, et al. Arteriovenous malformation radiosurgery: a twenty year perspective. *Clin Neurosurg* 2008;55:108–119.
4. Andrews DW, Scott CB, Sperduto PW, et al. Whole brain radiation therapy with or without stereotactic radiosurgery boost for patients with one to three brain metastases: phase III results of the RTOG 9508 randomised trial. *Lancet* 2004;363(9422):1665–1672.
5. Izawa M, Hayashi M, Nakaya K, et al. Gamma knife radiosurgery for pituitary adenomas. *J Neurosurg* 2000; 93(Suppl 3):19–22.
6. Pollock BE, Phuong LK, Gorman DA, et al. Stereotactic radiosurgery for idiopathic trigeminal neuralgia. *J Neurosurg* 2002;97(2):347–353.
7. Stafford SL, Pollock BE, Foote RL, et al. Meningioma radiosurgery: tumor control, outcomes, and complications among 190 consecutive patients. *Neurosurgery* 2001; 49(5):1029–1037; discussion 1037–1038.
8. Lax I, Blomgren H, Näslund I, et al. Stereotactic radiotherapy of malignancies in the abdomen. Methodological aspects. *Acta Oncol* 1994;33(6):677–683.
9. Timmerman RD. An overview of hypofractionation and introduction to this issue of seminars in radiation oncology. *Semin Radiat Oncol* 2008;18(4):215–222.
10. Garcia-Barros M, Paris F, Cordon-Cardo C, et al. Tumor response to radiotherapy regulated by endothelial cell apoptosis. *Science* 2003;300(5622):1155–1159.
11. Fuks Z, Kolesnick R. Engaging the vascular component of the tumor response. *Cancer Cell* 2005;8(2):89–91.
12. Hellman S, Weichselbaum R.R. Importance of local control in an era of systemic therapy. *Nat Clin Pract Oncol* 2005;2(2):60–61.
13. Hellman S, Weichselbaum R.R. Oligometastases. *J Clin Oncol* 1995;13(1):8–10.
14. Yang JC, Abad J, Sherry R. Treatment of oligometastases after successful immunotherapy. *Semin Radiat Oncol* 2006;16(2):131–135.
15. Salama JK, Chmura SJ, Mehta N, et al. An initial report of a radiation dose-escalation trial in patients with one to five sites of metastatic disease. *Clin Cancer Res* 2008;14(16):5255–5259.
16. Milano MT, Katz AW, Muhs AG, et al. A prospective pilot study of curative-intent stereotactic body radiation therapy in patients with 5 or fewer oligometastatic lesions. *Cancer* 2008;112(3):650–658.
17. Weber SM, Jarnagin WR, DeMatteo RP, et al. Survival after resection of multiple hepatic colorectal metastases. *Ann Surg Oncol* 2000;7(9):643–650.
18. D'Angelica M, Brennan MF, Fortner JG, et al. Ninety-six five-year survivors after liver resection for metastatic colorectal cancer. *J Am Coll Surg* 1997;185(6):554–559.
19. Kavanagh BD, Bradley J.D, Timmerman R.D. Stereotactic irradiation of tumors outside the central nervous system. In: Halperin EC, Perez CA, Bray LW, eds. *Perez*

and Brady's principles and practice of radiation oncology, 5th ed. Baltimore: Lippincott Williams & Wilkins, 2008: 389–390.

20. Timmerman RD, Bizekis CS, Pass HI, et al. Local surgical, ablative, and radiation treatment of metastases. *CA Cancer J Clin* 2009;59(3):145–170.

21. Benedict S, Yenice KM, Followill D, et al. Stereotactic body radiation therapy: the report of AAPM Task Group 101. *Med Phys* 2010;37(8):4078–4101.

22. Rusthoven KE, Hammerman SF, Kavanagh BD, et al. Is there a role for consolidative stereotactic body radiation therapy following first-line systemic therapy for metastatic lung cancer? A patterns-of-failure analysis. *Acta Oncol* 2009;48(4):578–583.

23. Horning SJ, Weller E, Kim K, et al. Chemotherapy with or without radiotherapy in limited-stage diffuse aggressive non-Hodgkin's lymphoma: Eastern Cooperative Oncology Group study 1484. *J Clin Oncol* 2004;22(15):3032–3038.

24. Miller TP, Dahlberg S, Cassady JR, et al. Chemotherapy alone compared with chemotherapy plus radiotherapy for localized intermediate- and high-grade non-Hodgkin's lymphoma. *N Engl J Med* 1998;339(1):21–26.

25. Norton L. Evolving concepts in the systemic drug therapy of breast cancer. *Semin Oncol* 1997;24(4 Suppl 10): S10-3–S10-10.

26. Norton L, Simon R. The Norton-Simon hypothesis revisited. *Cancer Treat Rep* 1986;70(1):163–169.

27. Simon R, Norton L. The Norton-Simon hypothesis: designing more effective and less toxic chemotherapeutic regimens. *Nat Clin Pract Oncol* 2006;3(8):406–407.

28. Demaria S, Ng B, Devitt ML, et al. Ionizing radiation inhibition of distant untreated tumors (abscopal effect) is immune mediated. *Int J Radiat Oncol Biol Phys* 2004;58(3):862–870.

29. Lee Y, Auh SL, Wang Y, et al. Therapeutic effects of ablative radiation on local tumor require CD8+ T cells: changing strategies for cancer treatment. *Blood* 2009; 114(3):589–595.

30. Chang EL, Shiu AS, Lii MF, et al. Phase I clinical evaluation of near-simultaneous computed tomographic image-guided stereotactic body radiotherapy for spinal metastases. *Int J Radiat Oncol Biol Phys* 2004;59(5): 1288–1294.

31. Fuss M, Salter BJ, Rassiah P, et al. Repositioning accuracy of a commercially available double-vacuum whole body immobilization system for stereotactic body radiation therapy. *Technol Cancer Res Treat* 2004;3(1):59–67.

32. Timmerman R, Papiez L, McGarry R, et al. Extracranial stereotactic radioablation: results of a phase I study in medically inoperable stage I non-small cell lung cancer. *Chest* 2003;124(5):1946–1955.

33. Wulf J, Hädinger U, Oppitz U, et al. Stereotactic radiotherapy of extracranial targets: CT-simulation and accuracy of treatment in the stereotactic body frame. *Radiother Oncol* 2000; 57(2):225–236.

34. Chang SD, Main W, Martin DP, et al. An analysis of the accuracy of the CyberKnife: a robotic frameless stereotactic radiosurgical system. *Neurosurgery* 2003;52(1):140–146; discussion 146–147.

35. Koong AC, Le QT, Ho A, et al. Phase I study of stereotactic radiosurgery in patients with locally advanced pancreatic cancer. *Int J Radiat Oncol Biol Phys* 2004;58(4): 1017–1021.

36. Keall PJ, Mageras GS, Balter JM, et al. The management of respiratory motion in radiation oncology report of AAPM Task Group 76. *Med Phys* 2006;33(10):3874–3900.

37. Heinzerling JH, Anderson JF, Papiez L, et al. Four-dimensional computed tomography scan analysis of tumor and organ motion at varying levels of abdominal compression during stereotactic treatment of lung and liver. *Int J Radiat Oncol Biol Phys* 2008;70(5): 1571–1578.

38. Onishi H, Kuriyama K, Komiyama T, et al. CT evaluation of patient deep inspiration self-breath-holding: how precisely can patients reproduce the tumor position in the absence of respiratory monitoring devices? *Med Phys* 2003;30(6):1183–1187.

39. Wong JW, Sharpe MB, Jaffray DA, et al. The use of active breathing control (ABC) to reduce margin for breathing motion. *Int J Radiat Oncol Biol Phys* 1999; 44(4):911–919.

40. Dawson LA, Brock KK, Kazanjian S, et al. The reproducibility of organ position using active breathing control (ABC) during liver radiotherapy. *Int J Radiat Oncol Biol Phys* 2001;51(5):1410–1421.

41. Meeks SL, Tomé WA, Willoughby TR, et al. Optically guided patient positioning techniques. *Semin Radiat Oncol* 2005;15(3):192–201.

42. Kubo HD, Wang L. Introduction of audio gating to further reduce organ motion in breathing synchronized radiotherapy. *Med Phys* 2002;29(3):345–350.

43. Mageras GS, Yorke E, Rosenzweig K, et al. Fluoroscopic evaluation of diaphragmatic motion reduction with a respiratory gated radiotherapy system. *J App Clin Med Phys* 2001;2(4):191–200.

44. Korreman SS, Juhler-Nottrup T, Boyer AL. Respiratory gated beam delivery cannot facilitate margin reduction, unless combined with respiratory correlated image guidance. *Radiother Oncol* 2008;86(1):61–68.

45. Slotman BJ, Lagerwaard FJ, Senan S. 4D imaging for target definition in stereotactic radiotherapy for lung cancer. *Acta oncologica* 2006;45(7):966–972.

46. Underberg RW, Lagerwaard FJ, Slotman BJ, et al. Use of maximum intensity projections (MIP) for target volume generation in 4DCT scans for lung cancer. *Int J Radiat Oncol Biol Phys* 2005;63(1):253–260.

47. Caldwell CB, Mah K, Skinner M, et al. Can PET provide the 3D extent of tumor motion for individualized internal target volumes? A phantom study of the limitations of CT and the promise of PET. *Int J Radiat Oncol Biol Phys* 2003;55(5):1381–1393.

48. Timmerman R, Papiez L, Suntharalingam M. Extracranial stereotactic radiation delivery: expansion of technology beyond the brain. *Technol Cancer Res Treat* 2003;2(2):153–160.

49. Timmerman RD, Forster K.M, Chinsoo Cho L. Extracranial stereotactic radiation delivery. *Semin Radiat Oncol* 2005;15(3):202–207.

50. Blomgren H, Lax I, Näslund I, et al. Stereotactic high dose fraction radiation therapy of extracranial tumors using an accelerator. Clinical experience of the first thirty-one patients. *Acta Oncol* 1995;34(6):861–870.

51. Kavanagh BD, Timmerman R, eds. *Stereotactic body radiation therapy.* Philadelphia, PA: Lippincott Williams & Wilkins, 2004:57–76.

52. Papiez L, Timmerman R, DesRosiers C, et al. Extracranial stereotactic radioablation: physical principles. *Acta Oncol* 2003;42(8):882–894.

53. Ryu SI, Chang SD, Kim DH, et al. Image-guided hypofractionated stereotactic radiosurgery to spinal lesions. *Neurosurgery* 2001;49(4):838–846.

54. Kavanagh BD, Schefter TE, Cardenes HR, et al. Interim analysis of a prospective phase I/II trial of SBRT for liver metastases. *Acta Oncol* 2006;45(7):848–855.

55. Ryu S, Fang Yin F, Rock J, et al. Image-guided and intensity-modulated radiosurgery for patients with spinal metastasis. *Cancer* 2003;97(8):2013–2018.

56. Wu QJ, Wang Z, Kirkpatrick JP, et al. Impact of collimator leaf width and treatment technique on stereotactic radiosurgery and radiotherapy plans for intra- and extracranial lesions. *Radiat Oncol* 2009;4:3.

57. Monk JE, Perks JR, Doughty D, et al. Comparison of a micro-multileaf collimator with a 5-mm-leaf-width collimator for intracranial stereotactic radiotherapy. *Int J Radiat Oncol Biol Phys* 2003;57(5):1443–1449.

58. Jin JY, Yin FF, Ryu S, et al. Dosimetric study using different leaf-width MLCs for treatment planning of dynamic conformal arcs and intensity-modulated radiosurgery. *Med Phys* 2005;32(2):405–411.

59. Xiao Y, Papiez L, Paulus R, et al. Dosimetric evaluation of heterogeneity corrections for RTOG 0236: stereotactic body radiotherapy of inoperable stage I-II non-small-cell lung cancer. *Int J Radiat Oncol Biol Phys* 2009;73(4):1235–1242.

60. Papanikolaou N, Battista JJ, Boyer AL, et al. Tissue inhomogeneity corrections for megavoltage photon Beams. *AAPM Task Group* 2004.

61. Fowler JF, Tomé WA, Fenwick JD, et al. A challenge to traditional radiation oncology. *Int J Radiat Oncol Biol Phys* 2004;60(4):1241–1256.

62. Hazard LJ, Wang B, Skidmore TB, et al. Conformity of LINAC-based stereotactic radiosurgery using dynamic conformal arcs and micro-multileaf collimator. *Int J Radiat Oncol Biol Phys* 2009;73(2):562–570.

63. Jemal A, Siegel R, Xu J, et al. Cancer statistics, 2010. *CA Cancer J Clin* 2010;60(5):277–300.

64. Mountain CF. A new international staging system for lung cancer. *Chest* 1986;89(4 Suppl):225S–233S.

65. Naruke T, Goya T, Tsuchiya R, et al. Prognosis and survival in resected lung carcinoma based on the new international staging system. *J Thorac Cardiovasc Surg* 1988;96(3):440–447.

66. Ginsberg RJ, Rubinstein LV. Randomized trial of lobectomy versus limited resection for T1 N0 non-small cell lung cancer. Lung Cancer Study Group. *Ann Thorac Surg* 1995;60(3):615–622; discussion 622–623.

67. Dosoretz DE, Katin MJ, Blitzer PH, et al. Radiation therapy in the management of medically inoperable carcinoma of the lung: results and implications for future treatment strategies. *Int J Radiat Oncol Biol Phys* 1992;24(1):3–9.

68. Haffty BG, Goldberg NB, Gerstley J, et al. Results of radical radiation therapy in clinical stage I, technically operable non-small cell lung cancer. *Int J Radiat Oncol Biol Phys* 1988;15(1):69–73.

69. McGarry RC, Papiez L, Williams M, et al. Stereotactic body radiation therapy of early-stage non-small-cell lung carcinoma: phase I study. *Int J Radiat Oncol Biol Phys* 2005;63(4):1010–1015.

70. Fakiris AJ, McGarry RC, Yiannoutsos CT, et al. Stereotactic body radiation therapy for early-stage non-small-cell lung carcinoma: four-year results of a prospective phase II study. *Int J Radiat Oncol Biol Phys* 2009;75(3):677–682.

71. Timmerman R, McGarry R, Yiannoutsos C, et al. Excessive toxicity when treating central tumors in a phase II study of stereotactic body radiation therapy for medically inoperable early-stage lung cancer. *J Clin Oncol* 2006;24(30):4833–4839.

72. Timmerman R, Paulus R, Galvin J, et al. Stereotactic body radiation therapy for inoperable early stage lung cancer. *JAMA* 2010;303(11):1070–1076.

73. Chang JY, Balter PA, Dong L, et al. Stereotactic body radiation therapy in centrally and superiorly located stage I or isolated recurrent non-small-cell lung cancer. *Int J Radiat Oncol Biol Phys* 2008;72(4):967–971.

74. Onishi H, Araki T, Shirato H, et al. Stereotactic hypofractionated high-dose irradiation for stage I nonsmall cell lung carcinoma: clinical outcomes in 245 subjects in a Japanese multiinstitutional study. *Cancer* 2004; 101(7):1623–1631.

75. Nagata Y, Takayama K, Matsuo Y, et al. Clinical outcomes of a phase I/II study of 48 Gy of stereotactic body radiotherapy in 4 fractions for primary lung cancer using a stereotactic body frame. *Int J Radiat Oncol Biol Phys* 2005;63(5):1427–1431.

76. Fong Y, Cohen AM, Fortner JG, et al. Liver resection for colorectal metastases. *J Clin Oncol* 1997;15(3):938–946.

77. Billingsley KG, Burt ME, Jara E, et al. Pulmonary metastases from soft tissue sarcoma: analysis of patterns of diseases and postmetastasis survival. *Ann Surg* 1999;229(5):602–610; discussion 610–62.

78. Hellman P, Ahlström H, Bergström M, et al. Positron emission tomography with 11 C-methionine in hyperparathyroidism. *Surg* 1994;116(6):974–981.

79. Pastorino U, Buyse M, Friedel G, et al. Long-term results of lung metastasectomy: prognostic analyses based on 5206 cases. The International Registry of Lung Metastases. *J Thoracic Cardiovasc Surg* 1997;113(1):37–49.

80. Baumann P, Nyman J, Hoyer M, et al. Outcome in a prospective phase II trial of medically inoperable stage I non-small-cell lung cancer patients treated with stereotactic body radiotherapy. *J Clin Oncol* 2009; 27(20):3290–3296.

81. Okunieff P, Petersen AL, Philip A, et al. Stereotactic Body Radiation Therapy (SBRT) for lung metastases. *Acta Oncol* 2006;45(7):808–817.

82. Hof H, Hoess A, Oetzel D, et al. Stereotactic single-dose radiotherapy of lung metastases. *Strahlenther Onkol* 2007;183(12):673–678.

83. Hoyer M, Roed H, Traberg Hansen A, et al. Phase II study on stereotactic body radiotherapy of colorectal metastases. *Acta Oncol* 2006;45(7):823–830.

84. Rusthoven KE, Kavanagh BD, Burri SH, et al. Multi-institutional phase I/II trial of stereotactic body radiation therapy for lung metastases. *J Clin Oncol* 2009; 27(10):1579–1584.

85. Collins BT, Erickson K, Reichner CA, et al. Radical stereotactic radiosurgery with real-time tumor motion tracking in the treatment of small peripheral lung tumors. *Radiat Oncol* 2007;2:39.

86. Fritz P, Kraus HJ, Blaschke T, et al. Stereotactic, high single-dose irradiation of stage I non-small cell lung cancer (NSCLC) using four-dimensional CT scans for treatment planning. *Lung Cancer* 2008;60(2):193–199.

87. Norihisa Y, Nagata Y, Takayama K, et al. Stereotactic body radiotherapy for oligometastatic lung tumors. *Int J Radiat Oncol Biol Phys* 2008;72(2):398–403.

88. Dunlap NE, Cai J, Biedermann GB, et al. Chest wall volume receiving >30 Gy predicts risk of severe pain and/or rib fracture after lung stereotactic body radiotherapy. *Int J Radiat Oncol Biol Phys* 2010;76(3):796–801.

89. Pettersson N, Nyman J, Johansson KA. Radiation-induced rib fractures after hypofractionated stereotactic body radiation therapy of non-small cell lung cancer: a dose- and volume-response analysis. *Radiother Oncol* 2009;91(3):360–368.

90. Emami B, Lyman J, Brown A, et al. Tolerance of normal tissue to therapeutic irradiation. *Int J Radiat Oncol Biol Phys* 1991;21(1):109–122.

91. Russell AH, Clyde C, Wasserman TH, et al. Accelerated hyperfractionated hepatic irradiation in the management of patients with liver metastases: results of the RTOG dose escalating protocol. *Int J Radiat Oncol Biol Phys* 1993;27(1):117–123.

92. Borgelt BB, Gelber R, Brady LW, et al. The palliation of hepatic metastases: results of the Radiation Therapy Oncology Group pilot study. *Int J Radiat Oncol Biol Phys* 1981;7(5):587–591.

93. Dawson LA, Ten Haken RK. Lawrence TS, Partial irradiation of the liver. *Semin Radiat Oncol* 2001;11(3):240–246.

94. Khozouz RF, Huq SZ, Perry MC. Radiation-induced liver disease. *J Clin Oncol* 2008;26(29):4844–4845.

95. Hoyer M, Roed H, Traberg Hansen A, et al. Phase II study on stereotactic body radiotherapy of colorectal metastases. *Acta Oncol* 2006;45(7):823–830.

96. Blomgren H, L.I., Goranson H, et al. Radiosurgery for tumors in the body: clinical experience using a new method. *J Radiosurgery* 1998;1(1):63–74.

97. Schefter TE, Kavanagh BD, Timmerman RD, et al. A phase I trial of stereotactic body radiation therapy (SBRT) for liver metastases. *Int J Radiat Oncol Biol Phys* 2005;62(5):1371–1378.

98. Herfarth KK, Debus J, Lohr F, et al. Stereotactic single-dose radiation therapy of liver tumors: results of a phase I/II trial. *J Clin Oncol* 2001;19(1):164–170.

99. Herfarth KK, Debus J, Wannenmacher M. Stereotactic radiation therapy of liver metastases: update of the initial phase-I/II trial. *Front Radiat Ther Oncol* 2004;38:100–105.

100. Katz AW, Carey-Sampson M, Muhs AG, et al. Hypofractionated stereotactic body radiation therapy (SBRT) for limited hepatic metastases. *Int J Radiat Oncol Biol Phys* 2007;67(3):793–798.

101. Mendez Romero A, Wunderink W, Hussain SM, et al. Stereotactic body radiation therapy for primary and metastatic liver tumors: A single institution phase i-ii study. *Acta Oncol* 2006;45(7):831–837.

102. Wulf J, Guckenberger M, Haedinger U, et al. Stereotactic radiotherapy of primary liver cancer and hepatic metastases. *Acta Oncol* 2006;45(7):838–847.

103. Wulf J, Hädinger U, Oppitz U, et al. Stereotactic radiotherapy of targets in the lung and liver. *Strahlenther Onkol* 2001;177(12):645–655.

104. Lee MT, Kim JJ, Dinniwell R, et al. Phase I study of individualized stereotactic body radiotherapy of liver metastases. *J Clin Oncol* 2009;27(10):1585–1591.

105. Rusthoven KE, Kavanagh BD, Cardenes H, et al. Multi-institutional phase I/II trial of stereotactic body radiation therapy for liver metastases. *J Clin Oncol* 2009;27(10):1572–1578.

106. Rule W, Timmerman R, Tong L, et al. A phase I dose escalation of stereotactic body radiation therapy in patients with hepatic metastases. *Ann Surg Oncol* 2010. Pending Publication.

107. Goodman KA, Wiegner EA, Maturen KE, et al. Dose-escalation study of single-fraction stereotactic body radiotherapy for liver malignancies. *Int J Radiat Oncol Biol Phys* 2010;78(2):486–493.

108. Lo SS, Dawson LA, Kim EY, et al. Stereotactic body radiation therapy for hepatocellular carcinoma. *Discov Med* 2010;9(48):404–410.

109. Tse RV, Hawkins M, Lockwood G, et al. Phase I study of individualized stereotactic body radiotherapy for hepatocellular carcinoma and intrahepatic cholangiocarcinoma. *J Clin Oncol* 2008;26(4):657–664.

110. Choi BO, Jang HS, Kang KM, et al. Fractionated stereotactic radiotherapy in patients with primary hepatocellular carcinoma. *Jpn J Clin Oncol* 2006;36(3):154–158.

111. Cardenes HR, Price TR, Perkins SM, et al. Phase I feasibility trial of stereotactic body radiation therapy for primary hepatocellular carcinoma. *Clin Transl Oncol* 2010;12(3):218–225.

112. Capanna R, Campanacci DA. The treatment of metastases in the appendicular skeleton. *J Bone Joint Surg Br* 2001;83(4):471–481.

113. Hartsell WF, Scott CB, Bruner DW, et al. Randomized trial of short- versus long-course radiotherapy for palliation of painful bone metastases. *J Natl Cancer Inst* 2005;97(11):798–804.

114. Mizumoto M, Harada H, Asakura H, et al. Radiotherapy for patients with metastases to the spinal column: a review of 603 patients at Shizuoka Cancer Center Hospital. *Int J Radiat Oncol Biol Phys* 2011;79(1):208–213.

115. Ryu S, Jin JY, Jin R, et al. Partial volume tolerance of the spinal cord and complications of single-dose radiosurgery. *Cancer* 2007;109(3):628–636.

116. Sahgal A, Ma L, Gibbs I, et al. Spinal cord tolerance for stereotactic body radiotherapy. *Int J Radiat Oncol Biol Phys* 2010;77(2):548–553.

117. Sahgal A, Ma L, Weinberg V, et al. Reirradiation HUMAN Spinal Cord Tolerance for Stereotactic Body Radiotherapy. *Int J Radiat Oncol Biol Phys* 2010;77:548–553.

118. Gerszten PC, Burton SA, Ozhasoglu C, et al. Radiosurgery for spinal metastases: clinical experience in 500 cases from a single institution. *Spine* 2007;32(2):193–199.

119. Yamada Y, Bilsky MH, Lovelock DM, et al. High-dose, single-fraction image-guided intensity-modulated

radiotherapy for metastatic spinal lesions. *Int J Radiat Oncol Biol Phys* 2008;71(2):484–490.

120. Amdur RJ, Bennett J, Olivier K, et al. A Prospective, Phase II Study Demonstrating the Potential Value and Limitation of Radiosurgery for Spine Metastases. *Am J Clin Oncol* 2009;32(5):515–520.

121. Bilsky MH, Yamada Y, Yenice KM, et al. Intensity-modulated stereotactic radiotherapy of paraspinal tumors: a preliminary report. *Neurosurgery* 2004;54(4):823–830; discussion 830–831.

122. Chang EL, Shiu AS, Mendel E, et al. Phase I/II study of stereotactic body radiotherapy for spinal metastasis and its pattern of failure. *J Neurosurg Spine* 2007;7(2):151–160.

123. Sahgal A, Ames C, Chou D, et al. Stereotactic body radiotherapy is effective salvage therapy for patients with prior radiation of spinal metastases. *Int J Radiat Oncol Biol Phys* 2009;74(3):723–731.

124. Lloyd-Davies RW, Collins CD, Swan AV. Carcinoma of prostate treated by radical external beam radiotherapy using hypofractionation. Twenty-two years' experience (1962–1984). *Urology* 1990;36(2):107–111.

125. Brenner DJ, Hall EJ. Fractionation and protraction for radiotherapy of prostate carcinoma. *Int J Radiat Oncol Biol Phys* 1999 43(5):1095–1101.

126. Brenner DJ. Fractionation and late rectal toxicity. *Int J Radiat Oncol Biol Phys* 2004;60(4):1013–1015.

127. Katz AJ, Santoro M, Ashley R, et al. Stereotactic body radiotherapy for organ-confined prostate cancer. *BMC Urol* 2010;10:1.

128. King CR, Brooks JD, Gill H, et al. Stereotactic Body Radiotherapy for Localized Prostate Cancer: Interim Results of a Prospective Phase II Clinical Trial. *Int J Radiat Oncol Biol Phys* 2009;73(4):1043–1048.

129. Madsen BL, Hsi RA, Pham HT, et al. Stereotactic hypofractionated accurate radiotherapy of the prostate (SHARP), 33.5 Gy in five fractions for localized disease: first clinical trial results. *Int J Radiat Oncol Biol Phys* 2007;67(4):1099–1105.

130. Tang CI, Loblaw DA, Cheung P, et al. Phase I/II study of a five-fraction hypofractionated accelerated radiotherapy treatment for low-risk localised prostate cancer: early results of pHART3. *Clin Oncol (R Coll Radiol)* 2008;20(10):729–737.

131. Boike TP, Lotan Y, Cho LC, et al. Phase I dose-escalation study of stereotactic body radiation therapy for low- and intermediate-risk prostate cancer. *J Clin Oncol* 2011;29(15):2020–2026.

132. Kuban DA, Tucker SL, Dong L, et al. Long-term results of the M. D. Anderson randomized dose-escalation trial for prostate cancer. *Int J Radiat Oncol Biol Phys* 2008;70(1):67–74.

133. Zietman AL, Bae K, Slater JD, et al. Randomized trial comparing conventional-dose with high-dose conformal radiation therapy in early-stage adenocarcinoma of the prostate: long-term results from Proton Radiation Oncology Group/American College of Radiology 95-09. *J Clin Oncol* 2010;28(7):1106–1111.

134. Freeman DE, King CR. Stereotactic body radiotherapy for low-risk prostate cancer: five-year outcomes. *Radiat Oncol* 2011;6:3.

135. Koong AC, Le QT, Ho A, et al. Phase I study of stereotactic radiosurgery in patients with locally advanced pancreatic cancer. *Int J Radiat Oncol Biol Phys* 2004;58(4):1017–1021.

136. Koong AC, Christofferson E, Le QT, et al. Phase II study to assess the efficacy of conventionally fractionated radiotherapy followed by a stereotactic radiosurgery boost in patients with locally advanced pancreatic cancer. *Int J Radiat Oncol Biol Phys* 2005;63(2):320–323.

137. Hoyer M, Roed H, Sengelov L, et al. Phase-II study on stereotactic radiotherapy of locally advanced pancreatic carcinoma. *Radiother Oncol* 2005;76(1):48–53.

138. Schellenberg D, Goodman KA, Lee F, et al. Gemcitabine chemotherapy and single-fraction stereotactic body radiotherapy for locally advanced pancreatic cancer. *Int J Radiat Oncol Biol Phys* 2008;72(3):678–686.

CHAPTER 17

Low-Dose-Rate Brachytherapy

Glenn P. Glasgow

Brachytherapy still prospers! The prior (2nd edition) chapter focused on historical and basic concepts and developments between 1997 and 2005. This revision, best viewed as a supplement to the prior (2nd edition) chapter, deletes some topics, now covered in Chapter 8 (Treatment Planning Algorithms: Brachytherapy), deletes certain historical topics, but adds information published since 2006. Space limitations exclude inclusion of intravascular, liquid I-125 sources, microspheres, nanoparticles, and electronic brachytherapy.

Significant developments include three journal anniversary papers (1–3), a task group report on dose prescriptions for prostate permanent seed implants (4), American Association of Physicists in Medicine (AAPM) and European Society for Therapeutic Radiology and Oncology (ESTRO) recommendations for clinical use of sources with energies higher than 50 keV (5), a Supplement TG-43U1S1 (6) to Task Group 43 (TG-43) absorbed dose formalism (7,8), numerous dosimetry reports on existing and new designs of ^{125}I (9–12) and ^{103}Pd sources (13), and use of photon spectrometry to determine dose-rate constants (14) and numerous dosimetry reports (15–19) and recommendations for use (20) for radionuclide ^{131}Cs for permanent implants. Mixed species radionuclides implants are reported (21–23), as well as imaging with magnetic resonance (MR) (24,25). Improving radionuclide source calibrations is a major interest (26–28). The 2005 AAPM Summer School on brachytherapy physics continues to reflect low-dose-rate (LDR) brachytherapy as practiced today (29). A new monograph considers the radiobiology models for continuous irradiation and brachytherapy (30), and a new book features *The Physics of Modern Brachytherapy for Oncology* (31), and a prospective article looks at the future of brachytherapy treatment planning (32).

This chapter, focusing on treatment planning, offers only an *aperçu* of LDR brachytherapy. Growth brings complexity. Older sources, models, and nomenclature sufficient to approximate the dosimetry of higher energy radium substitute ^{137}Cs linear sources insufficiently describe the dosimetry of currently low energy (e.g., ^{103}Pd, ^{125}I, ^{131}Cs) interstitial sources used in permanent implants. Their dosimetry is more accurately described with nomenclature and modern source models that continue to evolve. However, this chapter retains selected older nomenclature

still of value in understanding basic concepts. Reviews of older dosimetry systems are referenced, as original literature is not always readily available. Together, the old and new concepts, nomenclature, and models, offer the best understanding of LDR brachytherapy—an exciting and continuingly evolving discipline.

INTRODUCTION

Brachytherapy—the placement of radioactive sources in or near cancerous tissue—is over 110 years old. Brachytherapy can be characterized by the physical proximity of the radioactive sources to the tissue, by the duration of treatment, by source strength, by absorbed dose rate, by methods of physical placement of sources in or near the cancer, by dosimetry systems used to prescribe, describe, or determine the absorbed dose, and by the degree of dose uniformity. The radioactive source—a radionuclide safely contained—usually doubly encapsulated, as a needle, tube, seed, wire, sphere, or source train, can be inserted directly (interstitially) into the tissue, into an anatomical lumen (intraluminally) or cavity (intracavitary), or placed (molded) over the tissue.

LDR implants, often defined by absorbed dose rates between 0.4 and 2 Gy/h (0.0067–0.033 Gy/min), usually are temporary and removed after several days. Usually the LDR sources' positions are static. Permanent implants exhibit even lower absorbed dose rates. Procedures with medium dose rates (MDR) >2 Gy/h (0.033 Gy/min) but <12 Gy/h (0.2 Gy/min) and high dose rate (HDR) >12 Gy/h, lasting only for a few minutes, are described in Chapter 18. The discussion is limited to conventional (intracavitary, interstitial) LDR brachytherapy focusing on the use of isodose computation computers, their dosimetry models, and the data required for their correct use. Dynamic LDR with remote afterloading, Selectron LDR (Nucletron Trading BV, Veenendaal, The Netherlands) had limited commercial success in the United States, and units are no longer marketed, but still used (University of Texas MD Anderson Cancer Center, Houston, TX). The radiation oncologist faces five primary tasks: Defining the extent of anatomy to be treated, establishing desired therapeutic goals, identifying methods to achieve them, placing the applicators and/or sources in a desired manner relative to the anatomy to achieve the desired therapeutic goals and (except for permanent implants) then removing applicators and/or sources, and reporting the dosimetry in a meaningful and consistent method.

Brachytherapy is characterized by a progressive knowledge of the spatial dosimetry of individual radioactive sources and the composite spatial dosimetry of source arrays. The earliest methods of planning intracavitary implants, the Paris technique (1920s) and the Manchester system's (1930) point dose specifications (points A and B), used simple calculations and concepts (32,33). For interstitial implants the widely described Manchester and Quimby (1930s and 1940s) systems (32,33), and the later systems, Memorial and Paris Interstitial (1960s and 1970s) developed for ^{125}I and ^{192}Ir sources (32,33), used parametric tables, nomograms, minimum calculations, and strict adherence to system rules to report implant dosimetry and achieve desired therapeutic goals. While historical concepts still offering clinical guidance, most have abandoned these older systems for image-based planning using computer calculations.

Since the 1950s, knowledge of single-source dosimetry has continually improved (1–3). Computer algorithms now display in three dimensions the dosimetry of individual sources (point and line), accounting for source end effects, applicator shield effects, medium scatter, attenuation, and tissue heterogeneities. Methods of target localization and source localization have evolved from two-film techniques to computed tomography (CT) imaging and magnetic resonance imaging (MRI), allowing 3D displays of source arrays and increasingly accurate dose distribution data. Modern physics parameters (7,8) describing source strengths and models increasingly are used.

However, many clinical computer software packages still offer the option of older models, nomenclature, and methods used in the 1980s and 1990s. In a review of semiempirical dose-calculation models, Williamson observes that "For high-energy photon-emitting seeds and linear ^{137}Cs sources, properly implemented semi-empirical dose-calculation algorithms have a predictive accuracy comparable to Monte Carlo simulation . . . and will continue to play an important role in LDR ^{137}Cs based brachytherapy . . ." He further notes, "Classical methodologies will continue to play important roles" (34). However, modern source models and nomenclature to describe permanent seed dosimetry are commonly available on isodose computation computers (35). This chapter presents a limited review of basic and modern brachytherapy concepts in each of these major areas as used today in brachytherapy isodose planning.

BASIC PHYSICS CONCEPTS

We begin with a fundamental review of concepts. Complementary discussions are available (33,36,37). With the exception of ^{103}Pd, ^{125}I, ^{131}Cs, and ^{169}Yb which decay by

electron captures, radionuclides in sealed sources decay through β-decay, producing undesired β-rays (usually with energies <3 MeV) and usually a spectrum of desirable γ-rays (usually with energies <1 MeV). Absorption of the β-rays in the capsule prevents undesired high-absorbed doses to the tissue in contact with the capsule. The average γ-ray energy, $\overline{E}_\gamma$—a useful parameter for comparing radionuclides—is usually much less than the maximum γ-ray energy. When atoms transform, or decay, the change (decrease) in the number of atoms, ΔN, occurs in a period Δt. The activity, A—the rate at which atoms decay—is proportional to the number of atoms, N, with the potential to decay. The fractional decay rate, $\Delta N/N$ per unit time, is a constant, λ, the decay constant (transformation constant), defined by $\lambda = -(\Delta N/N/\Delta t)$ with units of reciprocal time (per second, per day, per year). Hence, $A = \Delta N/\Delta t = \lambda N$. In a half-life, $T_{1/2}$ (seconds, hours, days, or years) some initial number of atoms, N, decay to one-half, $N/2$. Hence, $T_{1/2} = 0.693/\lambda$. The mean life, T_m, equal to $1.44 \cdot T_{1/2}$, is a useful concept for describing decay processes for very short half-life radionuclides. The total number of transformations (decays), ΔN_{total}, which is directly proportional to the total absorbed dose, equals the product of the mean life, T_m, and the initial activity, A_0. (Chapter 8 offers the mathematical relationships of the quantities.)

Exposure, denoted by the symbol, X, is the measure of the ability of x-rays and γ-rays of energies 10 keV to <3 MeV to ionize air and is the quotient of $\Delta Q/\Delta m$ where ΔQ is the sum of all charges of one sign produced in air when all of the electrons liberated by photons in a mass Δm of air are completely stopped. Exposure is expressed in a special unit, the roentgen (R), equal to 258 μC of charge per kilogram of air at standard temperature and pressure. The continued use of exposure is not recommended in the System International d' Unites (SI); however, because of its historical use in science and medicine, exposure remains a widely used term (38). Kinetic energy released per unit mass of material, denoted in lower case, by the acronym, kerma, is a measure for indirectly ionizing radiations (photon, neutron) interacting in a material of the total kinetic energy of all charged particles released per unit mass of material. Kerma possesses a collision component from the kinetic energy imparted by inelastic collisions with electrons and a radiation component (usually much smaller) from interactions with nuclei. For x-rays absorbed in air, collision kerma in air is the product of exposure and the average energy, $\overline{W}$ required to produce an ion pair per unit of electrical charge. Kerma is measured in gray (Gy)—one joule (J) of energy released per kilogram (kg) of the medium. Khan offers a complete description of kerma and its relationship to other quantities (36).

The penetrability of radionuclides, historically, is expressed by HVL—the thickness of material (for comparisons, usually lead) that reduces the exposure rate by half in a specified (good [narrow-beam]) or bad [broadbeam]) geometry and tenth-value layer (TVL), a similar measure where the exposure rate is reduced one tenth. The

		HVLe (lead; cm)[a]	TVLe (lead; cm)[a]	Physical density[b] (g/cm³)	Specific activity[c] (Ci/g)	$f_{water/air}$ (cGy/R)
Isotope	$T_{1/2}$					
¹³⁷Cs	30 y	0.62	2.0	1.93	87	0.973
¹⁹²Ir	73.83 d	0.58	1.9	22.47	9200	0.970
¹⁹⁸Au	2.695 d	0.33	1.1	19.40	244800	0.971
¹⁶⁹Yb	32.02 d	0.17	0.55	6.81	24100	0.96
¹²⁵I	59.4 d	0.002[c]	N/A	4.85	17600	0.910
¹⁰³Pd	16.991 d	0.0008[b]	N/A	11.62	74700	0.886
¹³¹Cs	9.69 d	0.002[b]	N/A	1.91	103000	0.879

TABLE 17.1 Physical Properties of Radionuclides Currently Used in Brachytherapy

[a]HVLe,TVLe per P. Papagiannnis et al. *Med Phys* 2008;35:4898–4906; Assumes broad-beam geometry, a condition not found around brachytherapy applicators.
[b]Approximate value.
[c]For pure radionuclides; sources likely exhibit lower specific activities.
N/A, Data not available.

historical HVL and TVL are being replaced with the refined concepts of first HVL_1 and TVL_1 and equilibrium HVL_e and TVL_e that account for spectral changes with depth. The "equilibrium" notation (e) denotes the reduction achieved at greater depths (after 1/100th reduction in intensity) where dosimetry equilibrium is achieved; the notation "first" denotes reduction in the first layers of material (before 1/100th reduction in intensity) before equilibrium dosimetry is established. Shielding data for several brachytherapy radionuclides are available (39). ¹³⁷Cs, ¹⁹⁸Au, ¹⁹²Ir, and ¹⁶⁹Yb emit higher energy γ-rays with greater penetrability and present more radiation protection challenges than ¹⁰³Pd, ¹²⁵I, and ¹³¹Cs, that emit less penetrating lower-energy x-rays. Table 17.1 shows that TVL_e is about three times HVL_e for ¹³⁷Cs, ¹⁹²Ir, ¹⁹⁸Au, and ¹⁶⁹Yb; but this is not true for the less penetrating ¹⁰³Pd, ¹²⁵I, and ¹³¹Cs. The large separation in air between the source and attenuating material positions inherent in the shielding definitions of either "equilibrium" or "first" HVL and TVL do not occur in brachytherapy applicator treatment geometries. In applicators, the source beam is wide and shields are very close to the source. The degree of attenuation actually achieved when a lead shield is placed very close to a brachytherapy source can differ markedly from that expected from the application of shielding definitions of either "equilibrium" or "first" HVL and TVL.

The curie (Ci), the historical measure of radioactivity, was originally defined as the number of α-particles per unit time emitted by radon in secular equilibrium with 1 g of ²²⁶Ra; it is now defined as 3.7×10^{10} disintegrations per second. The becquerel (Bq)—one disintegration per second (1 Ci = 3.7×10^{10} Bq)—is the SI unit of activity (38).

The curie and becquerel are used in nuclear medicine and health physics to describe amounts or quantities of unencapsulated radionuclides. The curie and becquerel are used in brachytherapy physics only as shorthand notations to specify approximate content quantities of encapsulated radioactive materials, for example, 10 mCi or 37 MBq, or to describe quantities of radioactive materials possessed under a regulatory license. For example, a license may list the maximum possession limit of a radionuclide, for example, ¹²⁵I, in either curies or becquerels. For brachytherapy physics of encapsulated sources, encapsulated content quantities, in curie and becquerel, used historically to describe and identify sources have been replaced by other parameters, discussed later, that more accurately describe strengths of encapsulated sources.

The specific activity of pure radionuclides is the activity per unit mass (Ci/g) and is the product of Avogadro's number, N_0 (6.023×10^{23} atoms per gram atomic weight), and the decay constant, λ, divided by atomic weight, M. Radionuclides such as ¹⁹²Ir, exhibiting high specific activity (low atomic weight and short high-life) and high physical density, permit construction of encapsulated small (0.59 × 10 mm) dimension, high activity (12 Ci [444 GBq]) HDR sources.

The apparent activity, A_{app}, of an encapsulated source is the activity of an unencapsulated source that produces the same exposure rate in air, $\dot{X}$, at a known distance in the same geometry as that produced by the encapsulated source. The content activity, A, in the encapsulated source exceeds A_{app}, because the capsule attenuates not only most of the β-rays, but also some of the γ-rays emitted from the radioactive material inside the capsule. As a *concept*, A_{app}, is still useful in describing how encapsulation of a known activity of a radionuclide in a capsule of particular design decreases the exposure rate or reference air kerma rate at locations around the capsule to give an exposure rate equivalent to that of another source. However, use of A_{app} as a method of source strength specification and in computational quantities in brachytherapy is discouraged (40).

An important parameter of any radionuclide is the quantity of radiation (γ-rays, characteristic x-rays, β-rays, bremsstrahlung) emitted per unit time per amount of radioactive material. The concept has a long history that has suffered from notational confusion and inconsistent application. In early literature the concept was generally called the *k factor*; its value for each radionuclide was not known well. In 1962, the term *specific γ-ray constant*, Γ, was defined (41). The specific γ-ray constant, Γ (which by definition applied to sources of *specific* encapsulation because of photons of energy greater than δ), was usually expressed in roentgen square centimeter per hour per millicurie (R cm^2/h/mCi). The definition notes, "[I]t is assumed that the attenuation in the source and along its length is negligible" (41).

The specific γ-ray constant definition did not include the exposure rate of the lower-energy-emitted x-rays, and a new term, the *exposure rate constant*, was adopted in 1971 (42). The exposure rate constant, $(\Gamma_\delta)_X$ (in R cm^2/h/mCi), which measures the ability of photons from the radionuclide to transfer energy to air, is given by the quotient of l^2 $(dX/dt)_\delta$ by A (in millicuries), where $(dX/dt)_\delta$ is the exposure rate because of photons of energy greater than δ at a distance l (in centimeters) from a point source of activity A. In its *original definition*, for radionuclides *other than* ^{226}Ra, it was defined for an ideal *unencapsulated* point source; it includes all photon radiation, both nuclear and nonnuclear (characteristic x-rays and bremsstrahlung radiation arising from conversion electrons), with energies greater than δ, where δ often is 11.3 keV, and depends on the application. The *original definition* applied filtration only for ^{226}Ra for a 0.5-mm thick (10% iridium, 90% platinum) wall, $(\Gamma_\delta)_X = 8.25$ R cm^2/h/mg. For ^{226}Ra tubes with 1-mm iridioplatinum walls, the constant is 7.71 R cm^2/h/mg. Note that the same mathematical symbol, Γ, is used for these two differing concepts: *specific γ-ray constant* and *exposure rate constant*. Reports on the *specific γ-ray constant, exposure rate constant, and filtered exposure rate constant* of ^{192}Ir contain calculations that clarify the concepts (43,44). Contrary to its original definition, in current popular usage, the exposure rate constant $(\Gamma_\delta)_X$ is frequently stated for sources of certain design and specific encapsulation. The popular use assumes that in a source of finite size, attenuation and scattering occur and annihilation radiation and external bremsstrahlung may be produced, requiring significant corrections. When used in this manner, the source model or specific encapsulation must be stated but, unfortunately, often is not.

Since 1980 the air kerma rate, $\dot{K}_{air}$, has been recommended to replace exposure rate in air as the fundamental concept for brachytherapy absorbed dose calculations (45). The air kerma rate is:

$$\dot{K} = \dot{X}(\overline{W}/e) \qquad \text{EQUATION (17.1)}$$

An exposure of 114.5 R, when multiplied by the ratio $\overline{W}/e$ (0.876 cGy/R) is equivalent to an air kerma of 1 Gy. $\dot{K}_{air}$ is commonly expressed in units of μGy/h or cGy/h.

The air kerma rate constant, $(\Gamma_\delta)_K$, as originally defined, is a fundamental property of the *unencapsulated* idealized point source and neglects activity distribution, self-absorption, and filtrations in encapsulated sources. Hence, it was defined with the same restrictions as the exposure rate constant (46). For ^{226}Ra, the air kerma rate constant, $(\Gamma_\delta)_K$, for 0.5-mm iridioplatinum filtration is 7.227 cGy cm^2/h/mg or 7.227 μGy m^2/h/MBq. In SI units, this is 2.0075 fGy m^2/s Bq. The *reference* air kerma rate, $\dot{K}_1$, measured in μGy m^2/h, at a known reference distance (1 m), on the perpendicular bisector of a source is the SI recommended measure of source strength (45). $\dot{K}_1$ can be expressed for the *entire* source (μGy m^2/h) at 1 m or per unit source length (per cm; in μGy m^2/h/cm). In the United States a related concept recommended by the AAPM (47), air kerma strength, S_K, in μGy m^2/h at 1 m, is the product of the air kerma rate in free space, $\dot{K}_{air}$, at distances l, and the distance squared, l^2, is given by:

$$S_K = (\dot{K}_{air}) \cdot l^2 \qquad \text{EQUATION (17.2)}$$

The air kerma strength, S_K, is numerically equal to the reference air kerma rate, $\dot{K}_1$, but its unit (μGy m^2/h), includes distance squared (m^2). By definition, 1 μGy m^2/h at 1 m (or 1 cGy cm^2/h at 1 cm) is 1 U, a unit of convenience. However, air kerma strength, S_K, is not a recommended SI term, and its unit, U, is not a recommended SI unit (38). Nevertheless, S_K is now *the recognized parameter for encapsulated source strength specification* and subsequent absorbed dose calculations in the United States.

The original parameter of interest in brachytherapy, from which one extracted the absorbed dose rate in the tissue medium, was the exposure rate in air, $X/\Delta t$, in R/h, at some distance, l, from a point source encapsulated radionuclide. This is given by:

$$\Delta X/\Delta t = (\Gamma_\delta)_X \cdot A_{app} l^{-2} \qquad \text{EQUATION (17.3)}$$

where $(\Gamma_\delta)_X$, for a specific source filtration, is the specific γ-ray constant or exposure rate constant in R cm^2/h/mCi. A_{app} is its apparent activity in millicuries, and l is the distance in centimeters from the source to the point where the exposure rate is stated. For radium substitute sources, it was common practice to express apparent activity in millicuries of the source as being equivalent to milligrams of radium (mg Ra eq), for example, $A_{app,equivalent}$ (mg Ra eq). For example, the milligram radium equivalent of an equivalent radionuclide such as ^{137}Cs is the mass in milligrams of ^{226}Ra in equilibrium with its decay products screened by 0.5-mm thick iridioplatinum wall that would yield the same exposure rate in air in scatter-free conditions as produced by an encapsulated ^{137}Cs source at the same distance and in the same geometry. It follows that:

$$A_{\text{app,equivalent}}(\text{mg Ra eq}) \cdot (\Gamma_\delta)_{X,\text{equivalent}}$$
$$= A_{226\text{Ra}}(\text{mg}) \cdot [8.25(\text{R cm}^2/\text{h/mg})]$$

EQUATION (17.4)

Depending on the design and encapsulation (doubly encapsulated in iridioplatinum or stainless steel), and, hence, an appropriate choice of $(\Gamma_\delta)_{X,\text{equivalent}}$, for example, 3.226 R cm^2/h/mCi, a ^{137}Cs source containing ~25.57 mCi (946.2 MBq) yields an exposure rate equivalent to a 10 mg ^{226}Ra source with 0.5-mm iridioplatinum walls. For exposure and absorbed dose calculations, if the $A_{\text{app,equivalent}}$ of the equivalent radium substitute source is expressed in milligram radium equivalents, the specific γ-ray constant or exposure rate constant to be used is that of ^{226}Ra, $\Gamma = 8.25$ R cm^2/h/mg, for a 0.5-mm thick wall of iridioplatinum (10% iridium, 90% platinum), from which the equivalency was drawn, *not* that of the radionuclide actually used (e.g., ^{137}Cs) for the treatment. Misunderstanding of this point has led to the mistreatment of numerous patients. While physicists have abandoned the use of milligram radium equivalency for source strength specifications, the concept of milligram hours, mgh, is still used clinically by some radiation oncologists because it is a simple clinical concept with a long clinical history. Indeed, the *current* American Brachytherapy Society Cervical Cancer Brachytherapy Task Group still retains LDR prescriptions in milligram-hours (48).

The fundamental parameter of interest in brachytherapy is neither source activity nor exposure rate; it is the absorbed dose rate to the medium $\dot{D}_{\text{med}}$—commonly water or muscle. Simplistically, neglecting the perturbing influences of source and medium, one obtains the absorbed dose rate to the medium by first calculating the exposure rate in air, $\dot{X}$, and then multiplying by an appropriate factor, f_{med}, that converts the exposure in air to absorbed dose in the medium. The f_{med} factor is the product of $\overline{W}/e$ (the average energy required to produce an ion pair in dry air divided by the charge of an electron; the quotient is 33.97 J/C [joules per coulomb] or 0.876 cGy/R), and the ratio of mean mass energy transfer coefficients $(\mu_{\text{tr}}/\rho)^{\text{med}}$ $(1-g)/(\mu_{\text{tr}}/\rho)^{\text{air}}(1-g)$, where g is the very small fraction of the energy transferred that leads to bremsstrahlung radiation. Generally, for the brachytherapy radionuclides, g is <0.3% for both water and air and is usually neglected; hence, the ratio can be expressed as $(\mu_{\text{en}}/\rho)^{\text{med}}/(\mu_{\text{en}}/\rho)^{\text{air}}$. For most radionuclides with photon energies between 180 keV and 4 MeV, this ratio of mean mass energy absorption coefficients for water to air is almost constant at 1.11. For ^{125}I, it is 1.02. Hence, f_{med} equals 0.876 $(\mu_{\text{en}}/\rho)^{\text{med}}/(\mu_{\text{en}}/\rho)^{\text{air}}$ cGy/R. As shown in Table 17.1, values range from approximately 0.879 for ^{131}Cs to 0.973 for ^{137}Cs.

A more complete expression reflecting the perturbing influence of source and medium in the radial dimension is:

$$D(r) = [A_{\text{app}}(\Gamma_\delta)_X/r^2]f_{\text{med}}T(r)\overline{\phi}_{\text{an}}(r) \quad \text{EQUATION (17.5)}$$

where $T(r)$ represents radial attenuation and radial multiple scattering effects in the medium and $\overline{\phi}_{\text{an}}(r)$ is an anisotropy constant to account for any source radial anisotropy—both topics are discussed later.

Similar expressions exist using the air kerma rate. The air kerma rate in air is multiplied by the ratio of the mean mass-energy absorption coefficients of water or muscle and air, previously described, to yield the absorbed dose rate in the medium:

$$\dot{D}(r) = \dot{K}(r)(\mu_{\text{en}}/\rho)^{\text{med}}/(\mu_{\text{en}}/\rho)^{\text{air}} \quad \text{EQUATION (17.6)}$$

Including the radial attenuation and multiple scattering in the medium and possible source radial anisotropy, the dose rate in a medium is expressed thus:

$$\dot{D}(r) = \dot{K}[(\mu_{\text{en}}/\rho)^{\text{med}}/(\mu_{\text{en}}/\rho)^{\text{air}}]T(r)\overline{\phi}_{\text{an}}(r)$$

EQUATION (17.7)

This simple model or its analog (Equation 17.5) was widely used in computer algorithms for dose calculations in brachytherapy in the 1980s.

In 1990, a new dose formulation that describes two-dimensional (r,θ) (Fig. 17.1) dose distribution for ^{192}Ir and ^{125}I was introduced (49). TG-43 adopted and recommended this formulation and expanded it in 1995 to include ^{103}Pd seed sources. The methodology, generally called the TG-43 formalism (50), its update (7), erratum

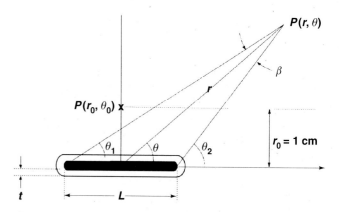

Figure 17.1. TG-43 schema for calculating the dose at point $P(r,\theta)$ from a line source of length L with wall thickness t. The point $P(r_0,\theta_0)$ is the normalization point ($r_0 = 1$ cm) on the bisector for normalization of the radial dose function $g(r)$, the geometry factor $G(r, \theta_{\text{TG-43}})$, and the anisotropy function $F(r, \theta_{\text{TG-43}})$. Note that in TG-43 formalism, $\theta_{\text{TG-43}}$ is the angle of the radius, r, with respect to the axis, z. (Historically, θ is the angle of the radius, r, with respect to h, the bisector of the source; see Fig. 17.4 for comparison). (Reprinted with permission from *Medical Physics* (Copyright 2004); Rivard et al. Update of AAPM Task Group Report No.43 Report: a revised AAPM protocol for brachytherapy dose calculations. *Med Phys.* 2004;31:633–674.)

(8), and supplement (6) are widely used for brachytherapy seed dose calculations. Using the formulation of TG-43, the dose rate in a medium is:

$$\dot{D}(r,\theta) = S_K \Lambda [G(r,\theta)/G(1,\pi/2)]g(r)F(r,\theta)$$

EQUATION (17.8)

where S_K is the air kerma strength in cGy cm²/h, Λ is the dose-rate constant, in cGy/h/U, $G(r,\theta)/G(1,\pi/2)$ is the geometry factor, without units, $g(r)$ is the radial dose function, without units, and $F(r,\theta)$ is the anisotropy function, without units.

The dose-rate constant, Λ, is defined as the absorbed dose rate to water, $\dot{D}(r_0,\Theta_0)$, at a distance of 1 cm on the transverse axis of a unit air kerma strength source, S_K, in a water phantom. It includes the effects of source self-attenuation and filtration, analogous to the prior discussion on exposure rate constants for specifically encapsulated sources. Mathematically,

$$\Lambda = \dot{D}(r_0,\Theta_0)/S_K$$

EQUATION (17.9)

The geometry factor, $G(r,\theta)$, accounts for the variation of relative dose only because of the spatial distribution of activity within the source, ignoring absorption, and scattering in the source. Two models, a point source, $G(r,\theta) = r^{-2}$, and a line source, $G(r,\theta) = \beta \cdot (L\,r\sin\theta)^{-1}$, where L is the source active length and β is the angle subtended by the active source with respect to the point (r,θ). Table V of TG-43 offers values of $G(r,\theta)\cdot r^2$ for a 3-mm line source (50). For $r = 1$ cm, typical values range from 1.023 for $\theta = 0$ degree to 0.9926 for $\theta = 90$ degrees (50).

The radial dose function, $g(r)$, accounts for the absorption and scatter in the medium along the transverse axis of the source. Specific to each source and its design, values range from 1.29 at 0.5 cm to 0.0893 at 5 cm for a certain design of ¹⁰³Pd source to 0.994 at 0.5 cm to 0.891 at 9 cm for an ¹⁹²Ir source. TG-43 (7,8) offers explicit equations that are given for numerous sources of different designs, and new source design dosimetry reports (11,17) usually include $g(r)$ values. Taylor and Rogers (51) report an improved fitting function for $g(r)$ for 18 ¹²⁵I seed models and 9 ¹⁰³Pd seed models.

The anisotropy function, $F(r,\theta)$ accounts for the anisotropy (nonuniformity) of the dose distribution around the source. TG-43 offers tabular values for specific source designs. For example, for an ¹⁹²Ir source, values range from 0.806 (at 1 cm, 0 degree) to 1.00 (at 9 cm, 90 degree).

If one applies a point source approximation, the two-dimensional anisotropy function $F(r,\theta)$ is replaced by the one-dimensional anisotropy factor $\phi_{an}(r)$. This factor is the ratio of the absorbed dose rate at distance r, averaged with respect to solid angle, to the absorbed dose rate on the transverse axis at the same distance r. For example, for a Model 6711 ¹²⁵I seed, values range from 0.944 at 1 cm to 0.901 at 7 cm. A simpler approximate concept, independent of distance, is the anisotropy constant, $\bar{\phi}_{an}(r)$. For the same seed described, the value is 0.93. Commercial isodose computation systems now support the TG-43 dosimetry model (35). There is no way this limited discussion of TG-43 can do justice to the volumes of literature that TG-43 and its revisions has evoked—it is the second most cited article in Medical Physics literature (52). Readers are encouraged to consult the original document (50), its update (7), erratum (8), and supplement (6) for a thorough discussion of concepts.

As noted, the TG-43 formalism was revised (and the revision subsequently corrected) in 2004 (7,8). The revision was prompted for several reasons, including improved source calibrations at NIST and a dramatic increase in the number of seeds with different designs marketed and for which dosimetry studies were performed. This revised formalism, TG-43U1, is now on commercial isodose computers. With some trepidation of committing sins of omission, a most *limited* comparison of the two protocols is offered.

First, TG-43U1 contains *no new* ¹⁹²*Ir seed data*—data in the original TG-43 report is valid.

TG-43U1 expands the three permanent seed recommended data sets (two models of ¹²⁵I seeds, one model of ¹⁰³Pd seed) to eight (six models of ¹²⁵I seeds, two models of ¹⁰³Pd seed) (7,8). Some changes are notational, adding subscripts (e.g., "P" for point, "L" for line) to the geometry factor, $G(r,\theta)$, now $G_P(r,\theta)$ or $G_L(r,\theta)$, as required. Other changes are minor, such as clarifying that S_K is *in vacuo*, meaning that during its measurement corrections are made for air attenuation. Unchanged are definitions of the dose-rate constant, Λ, and the anisotropy function $\phi_{an}(r)$ (but continued use of the anisotropy constant $\bar{\phi}_{an}(r)$ is *not recommended*). The most significant changes are the inclusion of the radial dose function $g(r)$ for both a point source and a line source, changes in the consensus data set for the three original permanent seed models in TG-43, and the inclusion of five more consensus data sets for new permanent seeds (7,8). Table 17.2 offers examples of the TG-43U1 data for the two original permanent seed models 6711 and 200. This table is included to stress that the dosimetry for the two original permanent seeds models 6711 and 200 was changed and that the 2007 supplement (6), TG-43U1S1, contains new data for an additional seven ¹²⁵I and one new ¹⁰³Pd source. Readers must study TG-43 (50), TG-43U1 (7,8), and the supplement (6) to fully appreciate all source dosimetry.

In summary, four methods have been used to specify the strength of a brachytherapy source. The two historical methods, apparent activity, A_{app} (mCi), and $A_{app,equivalent}$ (mg Ra eq) are conceptually valid, and useful in understanding the historical development of brachytherapy, but are no longer recommended for source strength specification. The reference air kerma rate, $\dot{K}_{air}$ (μGy m²/h at 1 m or μGy/h at 1 m per unit source length), is the recommended SI methodology, and is used in Europe (38). The alternate air kerma strength, S_K (U, μGy m²/h or cGy cm²/h) is used

TABLE 17.2	Example Data from Task Group 43U1 and Task Group 43U1S1; Partial Data Sets for Models 6711, 6733 and Models 200, 2355			
Seed	6711	6733	200	2355
Parameter	TG-43U1	TG-43U1S1	TG-43U1	TG-43U1S1
Dose-Rate Constant Λ (cGy/h/U)	0.965	0.980	0.686	0.685
Radial Dose Function $g(r)$ for r(cm)				
0.5	1.048	1.069	1.248	1.307
1.0	1.00	1.00	1.00	1.00
2.0	0.819	0.821	0.561	0.533
3.0	0.636	0.656	0.306	0.296
4.0	0.499	0.495	0.165	0.158
5.0	0.367	0.379	0.090	0.092
Anisotropy Function $F(r,\theta)$				
(1,0)	0.370	0.305	0.541	0.797
(2,0)	0.422	0.397	0.549	0.690
(3,0)	0.488	0.451	0.534	0.674
(4,0)	0.520	0.502	0.538	0.672
(5,0)	0.550	0.533	0.510	0.663
Anisotropy Factor $\phi_{an}(r)$				
1.0	0.944	0.967	0.855	0.879
2.0	0.941	0.964	0.870	0.872
3.0	0.942	0.953	0.884	0.881
4.0	0.943	0.966	0.845	0.881
5.0	0.944	0.953	0.897	0.890

in the United States. Commercial source "strengths" may be stated by any or all of these methods. Expressing source "strength" as absorbed dose rate at a reference distance (1 m), $\dot{K}_{air}$ (μGy m^2/h or μGy/h per unit length) (Europe) or air kerma strength, S_K (μGy m^2/h or U) (United States), for a specified filtration, avoids any confusion associated with apparent or equivalent activities and the associated constants.

Users must apply great caution when using any source strength for absorbed dose calculations either manually or from parameters entered into computers, as *incorrect use of one of the four parameters of strength* (A_{app} [mCi], $A_{app,equivalent}$ [mg Ra eq], A_{app} [MBq], S_K [U, μGy m^2/h, or cGy cm^2/h]) *with incorrect use of one of the four corresponding constants* (exposure rate constant, $(\Gamma_\delta)_X$, in R cm^2/h/mCi, for specific filtration; exposure rate constant of ^{226}Ra, with 0.5-mm iridioplatinum wall, $(\Gamma_\delta)_{X,226Ra}$, 8.25 R cm^2/h/mg; air kerma rate constant, $(\Gamma_\delta)_K$, in μGy/h/MBq, for a specific filtration; and finally, dose-rate constant, Λ, in cGy/h/U), *yields an incorrect absorbed dose calculation.*

The correct products of these two key parameters are: (a) A_{app}, (mCi) $\cdot$ $(\Gamma_\delta)_X$ (R cm^2/h/mCi) for specific filtration; (b) $A_{app,equivalent}$ (mg Ra eq) $\cdot$ 8.25 R cm^2/h/mg, exposure rate constant of ^{226}Ra filtered by 0.5-mm iridioplatinum; (c) A_{app},(MBq), $\cdot$ $(\Gamma_\delta)_K$ (μGy m^2/h/MBq), for a specific filtration; and (d) S_K (U) $\cdot$ Λ (cGy/h/U) for a specific filtration. Other products, for example, A_{app} (mCi) $\cdot$ Λ (cGy/h/U) or S_K (U) $\cdot$ $(\Gamma_\delta)_{X,equivalent}$ (R cm^2/h/mg) are *incorrect* and will yield incorrect absorbed dose calculations. All four correct products must be appropriately multiplied by other terms, previously described, to determine the absorbed dose rate at a point (r,θ) near the source.

Source activity stated in air kerma strength, S_K, in μGy m^2/h or U, for a specified filtration, mathematically, is the product of an air kerma rate constant (in μGy m^2/h/MBq) for a specific filtration and the corresponding apparent activity (in MBq). Use of S_K, however, requires no knowledge of either term, and separation of S_K into two pseudo terms is discouraged. However, some computer algorithms require separate values of the two parameters, and dummy values may be used as long as they yield the proper product for S_K. It is important to determine whether the algorithm makes a correction for source filtration (53). If it does, the dummy values must be selected so that *after the source filtration correction*, the product of the two terms yields the correct value of S_K.

RADIONUCLIDES

Numerous radionuclides (e.g., phosphorus 32, cobalt 60, selenium 75, strontium 90, yttrium 90, palladium 103, ruthenium 106, iodine 125, cesium 131, cesium 137, samarium 145, ytterbium 169, thulium 170, tantalum 182, gold 198, iridium 192, radon 222, radium 226, americium 241, californium 252) have either been commercially marketed or proposed, investigated (and in some instances, abandoned) for various forms (LDR, HDR, intravascular, infusion, or eye plaques) of brachytherapy. The historical significance of ^{226}Ra and radon 222 (^{222}Rn) is briefly reviewed but attention is concentrated on ^{137}Cs, ^{192}Ir, ^{198}Au, ^{125}I, ^{103}Pd, ^{131}Cs, and ^{169}Yb use for conventional LDR intracavitary or interstitial brachytherapy. Tables 17.1 and 17.3 list useful physical parameters of these seven radionuclides.

TABLE 17.3 Properties of Some[a] Radionuclides Used in Brachytherapy

Isotope	β-Ray energies	Prominent photon energies	Average photon energies	Exposure rate constant[b]	Air kerma rate constant[c]	Manufacturer and model	Dose-rate constant[d]
	E_β (MeV)	E_γ (MeV)	$\overline{E}_\gamma$ (MeV)	$(\Gamma_\delta)_X$ (R cm²/h/ mCi)	$(\Gamma_\delta)_K$ (μGym²/h/ MBq)		Λ (μGy/h/U) at 1 m
^{137}Cs	0.514, 1.17	0.662	0.662	3.275	0.0773	CIS CSM11	1.096
						Amersham CDC-1	1.113
						Amersham CDC-3	1.103
						Rad'n Th'py Res. 67800[e]	0.932
						3M 6500/6D6 C	0.960
						3M 6500	0.973
						Amersham CDCS. J	0.979
						IPL 67–6520	0.948
^{198}Au	0.96	0.412–1.088	0.416	2.376	0.0561	Best Industries	1.11
^{192}Ir	0.24–0.67	0.136–1.062	0.38	4.69	0.1110	Best Industries	1.12
^{169}Yb	None	0.063, 0.198	0.143	1.80	0.043	X1267	1.191
^{125}I	None	0.027–0.0355	0.028 (includes x-rays)	1.51[f] (1.45)	0.0355	Amersham 6702	1.036
						Amersham 6711	0.965
						Best Industries 2301	1.018
						NASI MED 3631-A/M	1.036
						Bebig/Th'genics I25.506[e]	1.012
						Imagyn IS-12501	0.940
						Amersham 6733	0.980
						Draximage LS-1	0.972
						Implant Sciences 3500	1.014
						IBt 1251 L	1.038
						IsoAid IAI-125 A	0.981
						MBI AL-125/SH-125	0.953
						SourceTechMedSTM125I	1.018
^{103}Pd	None	0.02–0.48	0.021	1.48	0.0361	Theragenics 200	0.686
						NASI MED 3633	0.688
						Best 2335	0.685
^{131}Cs	None	0.029–0.034	0.030			IsoRay Medical CS-1	1.059[g]
						CS-1 Rev 2	1.046

[a]Amersham 6702 not currently used; ^{131}Cs data not TG-43 approved; ^{169}Yb, used in Europe; other models available.
[b]For an unfiltered point source with δ from 1 to 11.3 keV, depending on isotope.
[c]Air kerma rate constant in μGy m²/h/MBq at 1 m; 1 R cm²/h/Ci = 1.937×10^{-19} C m²/kg/s Bq = 0.0236 μGy m²/h/MBq.
[d]Includes filtration inherent in commercially available seeds.
[e]Rad'n Th'py Res. = Radiation Therapy Resources; Bebig/Th'genics = Bebig/Theragenics.
[f]See Reference (50), Table II; 1.45 R cm²/h/mCi used by convention.
[g]Literature data shows wide variations; 1.059 is recommended; See Reference (20).

[226]Ra is excluded from Tables 17.1 and 17.3 but deserves limited mention because of its historical importance. Details of [226]Ra and [222]Rn sources were previously described (33). The key [226]Ra parameter to remember is the well-known constant, $\Gamma = 8.25$ R cm²/h/mg, for a 0.5-mm thick wall of iridioplatinum (10% iridium, 90% platinum).

The relatively long half-life (30 years) and medium energy (0.66 MeV) of the nearly monoenergetic ^{137}Cs made it a popular substitute for [226]Ra. Most facilities have disposed of their ^{137}Cs needles but a few facilities still perform LDR gynecological brachytherapy from a permanent inventory of ^{137}Cs tubes. The dosimetry of source models Amersham CDCS-J and 3M 6500/6D6 C (53,54), Radiation Therapy Resources 67–800 (55), CDC miniatures (56), CIS CSM11 (57), and Amersham CDCS-M (58) are reviewed by Liu et al. (59) with useful TG-43 data (effective attenuation coefficients, radial dose functions, and anisotropy functions) for the dosimetry of certain models. Melhus and Rivard report new Monte Carlo dosimetry for ^{137}Cs sources (60), whereas Vianello and de Almedia investigated photon fluence nonuniformity near linear ^{137}Cs sources (61). Interest in conventional LDR brachytherapy with ^{137}Cs sources is sufficient to support the market for a new model 67–6520 ^{137}Cs source (Manufacturer: Eckert & Zigler Isotope Products, Valencia, CA; Vendor: Radiation Products Design, Albertville, MN) (62). Each source tube (Fig. 17.2) contains a labeled ceramic rod as the active element surrounded by two stainless steel encapsulations—each of which is of welded construction. The standard size tube is 20 mm long by 3.05 mm diameter, and the inner ceramic active element is 14.8 mm long by 1.52 mm diameter.

[192]Ir, with a modest half-life (73.83 days) and a complex spectrum of γ-ray energies (average energy 0.38 MeV) exhibits a high specific activity (450 Ci per g) suitable for 10 Ci (370 GBq) sources for HDR remote afterloaders (see Chapter 18). A wire coil is popular in Europe, and its dosimetry has been reported (63–65). A new method of modeling wires has been reported (64). In the United States, seeds with activities of tenths of millicuries to several millicuries, in nylon ribbons, are widely used for interstitial implants (66–68). Seed design varies by manufacturer but generally consists of a 0.3-mm diameter core of a mixture of 10% to 25% iridium and the rest platinum, coated with an additional 0.1-mm thickness of either pure platinum or stainless steel to form a 0.5-mm diameter seed ~3 mm long. The sources are not considered sealed or encapsulated, as are other brachytherapy sources, and are subject to wipe test requirements different from encapsulated sources. Integrity of the coating must be maintained during any source manipulations to prevent removing the coating and releasing any undesired β-ray irradiation during use. Recommended dosimetry values are in TG-43 (50). Recent investigations have studied the effects of phantom material composition and size on ^{192}Ir dosimetry (69,70). Glasgow et al. (71) investigated the feasibility of a low-cost permanent ^{192}Ir seed.

[198]Au is the least popular of the seven radionuclides. A few universities with cyclotrons capable of producing [198]Au have used it as an interstitial source for prostate, bladder, or brain

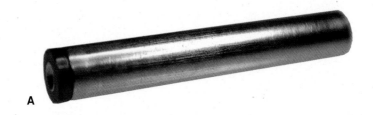

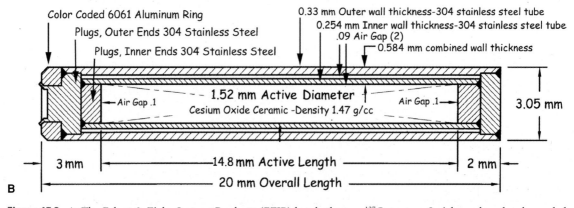

Figure 17.2. A: The Eckert & Zigler Isotope Products (EZIP) brachytherapy ^{137}Cs source. Serial numbered, color-coded sources are available from 5 mg Ra equivalent to 40 mg Ra equivalent, in 5 mg Ra equivalent increments. (Reprinted with permission from Radiation Products Design, Inc., Albertville, MN 55301.) **B:** Construction details of the tube source. It contains a cesium labeled ceramic rod as the active element surrounded by two stainless steel encapsulations, each of which is of welded construction. (Reprinted with permission from Radiation Products Design, Inc., Albertville, MN 55301.)

implants and it is commercially available. ^{198}Au, with a short half-life (2.7 days) suitable for permanent implants, releases a dominant 0.412-MeV γ-ray that produces issues regarding personnel radiation exposure. The short half-life makes source production and distribution by commercial carriers more difficult; moreover, there is no NIST national calibration standard for ^{198}Au. Hence these sources are not popular in the United States, but they do enjoy some popularity in Europe. The seeds or grains are approximately 2.5 mm long and 0.15 mm in diameter; the outer casing is 0.15-mm platinum capsule with the ^{198}Au radioactive matrix inside. The dosimetry of ^{198}Au has been reported (72,73).

^{125}I seeds have had limited use in temporary implants (breast) and eye plaques, but are popular for permanent implants in the prostate and lung. With a modest half-life (59.40 d), they emit a low-energy 35.5-keV γ-ray and x-rays with lower energies, 31.7 to 27.2 keV. The low energy allows local shielding with metal foils only a few tenths of a millimeter thick and allows numerous applications not available with other radionuclides. The original seed design, model 6702 (Medi-Physics, Arlington Heights, IL)—no longer sold—exhibited a highly anisotropic dose distribution. A subsequent design, model 6711 (also from Medi-Physics), exhibited a somewhat less anisotropic dose distribution. The popularity of prostate permanent seed implants led many manufacturers to enter the commercial market with seed designs with alleged improved dose distribution. The AAPM TG-43U1 update (7) includes the recommended dosimetry of six ^{125}I sources: American Health models 6702 and 6711, Best Industries model 2301, North American Scientific Inc. model MED3631-A/M, Bebig/Theragenics Model I25.S06, and Imagyn Medical Technologies Inc. *isotar* IS-12501 (now discontinued). The TG-43U1 supplement (6) provides data for seven more seed designs: Amersham model 6733, Draximage model LS-1, Implant Science model 3500, IBt model 1251 L, IsoAid model IAI-125 A, Mentor model SL-125/SH-125, and SourceTech Medical STM125I. Dosimetry has been reported for four other models: SelectSeed (9), IsoSeed model I25.S17 (10), Bacon Co. (Buenos Aires, Argentina)

model Braquibac (11), and Oncure/GE Healthcare (Arlington Heights, IL) model 9011 (12).

The history of the dosimetry of ^{125}I seeds requires careful study and is beyond the scope of this chapter (50). The dosimetry of specific seed designs and their activities varies, and an absolutely thorough literature review with subsequent testing of applicable computer models is required before attempting to replicate the dosimetry (and clinical results) of the original ^{125}I seeds. Moreover, over the years, and among different groups, there have been changes in clinical prescriptions. Hence, application of computer models for permanent seed implants requires very careful work and *cross-comparison of dosimetry results among those using the same seed designs and the same isodose planning systems is strongly encouraged*!

^{103}Pd, a substitute for ^{125}I, exhibits higher seed activity, correspondingly higher absorbed dose rate, and shorter half-life, all considered *theoretically* more radiobiologically advantageous for permanent implants in more rapidly growing cancers. ^{103}Pd sources, with a short half-life (16.991 days), release characteristic x-rays with energies of 20.07 to 23.18 keV, with a few very weak photons with higher energies. Seeds typically have activities of up to 5 mCi, which produce higher dose rates than those achieved with conventional ^{125}I seeds. The update of AAPM TG-43 included recommended dosimetry of two ^{103}Pd sources: Theragenics Corporation model 200 and North American Scientific Inc. model MED3633 (7). The recent TG-43 supplement, TG-43U1SI, includes data for the Best Medical Model 2335 (5). Source designs (^{103}Pd adsorbed onto silver beads, a coiled wire, and seeds without markers) have been described (74–78).

A ^{131}Cs seed, Model CS-1 (IsoRay Medical, Inc., Richland, WA) for permanent implants was introduced in 2004. With the exception of its short half-life—9.69 days—it is similar to ^{125}I, as its most prominent x-ray peaks are from 29 to 34 keV. Descriptions of its dosimetry and proposed therapeutic absorbed doses equivalent relative to ^{125}I and ^{103}Pd and dose-rate constants were reported (79–81). The modified seed design, Model CS-1 Rev. 2 (Fig. 17.3), was

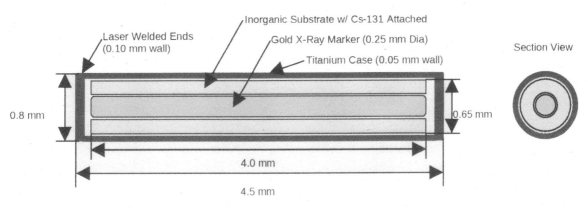

Current Proxcelan Cesium-131 Brachytherapy Seed

Figure 17.3. Model CS-1, Rev 2 Proxcelan ^{131}Cs Brachytherapy Seed. (Reprinted with permission from IsoRay Medical. Inc. Richland, WA 99354–5411.)

introduced later and there are four dosimetry reports (15–19). However, TG-43 consensus dosimetry is not yet available. Originally used to treat prostate cancer and ocular melanoma, seeds are also available in flexible, bio-absorbable braided strands that can be attached to a bio-absorbable mesh that can be implanted to provide radiotherapy to surgical margins after resection of primary lung tumors. These strands have been used to treat head and neck tumors, chest wall tumors, and colorectal cancer.

Ytterbium 169 (^{169}Yb) emits 0.063 and 0.198 MeV photons (average energy 0.143 MeV) and has a half-life of 32.02 days. It has been investigated as a potential HDR source (82,83), and several models of seeds for permanent implants have been used in Italy (84), but not in the United States.

SOURCES AND SOURCE MODELS IN VACUO

Two source models—static point and static line—are widely used to approximate the LDR dosimetry of sources. Karaiskos et al. offer a useful review of the limitations of each model as applied to commercial sources (85).

The point source model is the simplest. Lacking a perturbing surrounding medium (air, tissue, applicators, other sources), the radiation intensity around a point source decreases inversely with the square of the radial distance, as described in Equation 17.3, and is isotropic, equal in all directions. There are, of course, no treatments *in vacuo* and few truly spherical sources. However, sources (e.g., ^{198}Au grains, ^{192}Ir, ^{125}I, ^{103}Pd, and ^{131}Cs seeds) are often modeled as point sources, as the physical orientation of their long (<0.5 cm) axis cannot always be discerned on radiographs or electronic images. TG-43U1 provides data sets for their representation as point sources (7,8). Radiation intensity near their welded or enclosed ends is less than the radiation intensity along the perpendicular bisector of the source. The radiation intensity at points at equal distance around the source, normalized to the radiation intensity at a reference distance on the radius bisecting the source, is called the *anisotropy function* $F(r,\theta)$ of the source. In the point source approximation, the two-dimensional anisotropy function $F(r,\theta)$ is replaced by the one-dimensional anisotropy factor $\phi_{an}(r)$. This anisotropy factor, $\phi_{an}(r)$, is the ratio of the absorbed dose rate at distance r—averaged with respect to solid angle—to the absorbed dose rate on the transverse axis at the same distance r. For example, for a Model 6711 ^{125}I seed, values range from 0.944 at 1 cm to 0.901 at 7 cm. A simpler approximate concept, independent of distance averaged and over 4π geometry, is anisotropy constant, $\bar{\phi}_{an}(r)$. TG-43 values of $\bar{\phi}_{an}(r)$ are 0.93 for ^{125}I seed model 6711, 0.98 for ^{192}Ir stainless steel-clad seeds, and 0.9 for ^{103}Pd seed model 200 (Theragentics, Norcross, GA) (50). The point source model with use of an average anisotropy constant is reasonably accurate when large numbers of seeds are regularly distributed but randomly oriented in volume implants. However, if the seeds are in linear arrays, this simple expression of their anisotropy is inappropriate. Moreover,

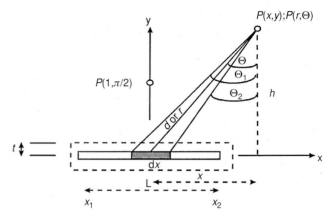

Figure 17.4. The historical schema for calculating the dose at point $P(x,y)$ or $P(r,\theta)$ from either an unfiltered (*center dark line*) line source of length L or a filtered (*outer dashed line*) line source of half-thickness t. Note that θ is the angle of the radius, r, with respect to h, perpendicular to the axis, x. (see Fig. 17.1 for comparison). (Reprinted with permission from *Oxford University Press* (Copyright 1993); Modified from Arid EG, Williams JR. Brachytherapy. In: Williams JR, Thwaites DI, eds. *Radiotherapy physics*. Oxford: Oxford University Press, 1993:187–226, 192.)

TG-43U1 no longer retains the anisotropy constant $\bar{\phi}_{an}(r)$ as a concept (7).

Most commercial computers with algorithms for seed implants offer a simple point source model for computer isodose calculations for seed arrays. The dosimetry at a point from an array of point sources is a straightforward summation—manually or by computer—of the radiation contribution at that point from each individual source.

An unfiltered line source model closely approximates the geometry of the early ^{226}Ra sources, ^{137}Cs tubes and needles, and segments of ^{192}Ir wire. This simple geometry (Fig. 17.4) has been widely described in many mathematical notations. The description is offered in air kerma. For a source with air kerma rate constant $(\Gamma_\delta)_K$, an activity, A, and length L, the air kerma rate $\dot{K}_{air}$, at a point, $P(x,y)$, and a distance, d, from the center of a source segment, dx, is given thus:

$$\dot{K}_{air}(x,y) = \int_{x_1}^{x_2} [(\Gamma_\delta)_K A/(d^2 L)] dx \quad \text{EQUATION (17.10)}$$

Expressing the point location $P(x,y)$ in polar coordinates $P(r, \theta)$ where h is the perpendicular distance of point P from the source axis, it follows that as $d = h/\cos\theta$ and $x = h\tan\theta$, in polar coordinates the integral becomes:

$$\dot{K}_{air}(r,\theta) = \int_{\theta_1}^{\theta_2} [(\Gamma_\delta)_K A/(hL)] d\theta \quad \text{EQUATION (17.11)}$$

Following integration of the length of the source, the air kerma rate from all source segments is given by this well-known expression:

$$\dot{K}_{air}(r,\theta) = (\Gamma_\delta)_K [A/L][\{\theta_2 - \theta_1\}/h] \quad \text{EQUATION (17.12)}$$

The air kerma rate $\dot{K}_{air}$ at point $P(r,\theta)$ is the product of the linear activity (A/L), the air kerma rate constant, $(\Gamma_\delta)_K$, and the angle $(\theta_2 - \theta_1)$ (in radian) subtended by the source, divided by the perpendicular distance, h, from point P to the source axis. It should be noted that in Figure 17.4 θ is the angle between radius r and the perpendicular distance, h, to the x-axis. In the TG-43 formalism (Fig. 17.1), the angle, β, subtended by the source is the *complementary angle* (90 degrees − θ), that is, the angle between the radius, r, and the x-axis. The component $(\theta_2 - \theta_1)/hL$ is identical to the line source geometry factor $G(r,\theta) = \beta/(Lr \cdot \sin\theta)$ in the TG-43 formalism. As expressed, this is for an unfiltered line source. However, while each segment of a line source contributes air kerma rate to a point following the basic inverse square law, near the line source the summation of the air kerma rates from each point source yields a variation that depends on the ratio of the angle subtended to the distance—not to the distance squared. When properly applied with other concepts, this equation is highly useful for dose estimates from line sources or pseudo-line sources (a linear string of point sources).

What is the dosimetry of a "point" versus a "line"? Figure 17.5 shows the variation in dose rate as a function of distance, on a log–log graph, for a 7.227 cGy/h/U (1 mg radium equivalent) point source, a 12-mm line source of the same activity, and a hypothetical source with an inverse (not inverse square) dependency on distance. Far from a line source, at distances beyond three times the length (36 mm in this example) of the source, the dose rates in air begin to approximate, to within ~7%, those calculated from point source geometry. As the distance from the source increases, the line source more nearly approximates a point source. In the lower right corner, the two curves nearly coincide. The dosimetry of some implants requires knowledge of the doses within dimensions similar to the source lengths. Close to such sources, the inverse square law poorly estimates the dose. At close distances, 6 to 10 mm, the dosimetry exhibits a dependency that is similar to that of a source dependent on the inverse of the distance $(1/r)$. Numerous patients have been mistreated because of

misapplication of the inverse square law to estimate doses within 1 to 2 cm of line sources of these same lengths. Of course, the inverse square concepts correctly apply to *each element* of a line source; the true dependency of dose with distance is in the ratio $\dot{K}_{air}(r,\theta) = (\Gamma_\delta)_K[A/L][\{\theta_2 - \theta_1\}/h]$, which changes as h changes. At very close distances, that is, from approximately 0.5 to 0.1 cm from the sources the dosimetry is complex (86,87). Ballester et al. (88) report that 99% of electronic equilibrium is achieved at 3 mm for ^{137}Cs, 2 mm for ^{192}Ir, and 1 mm for ^{169}Yb, and that electronic emissions become important (>0.5%) within 1.7 mm for ^{192}Ir. Nath and Chen (89) reported on the silver florescent yield and its influence on the dose-rate constants of nine low-energy brachytherapy sources.

Radiations from brachytherapy sources are filtered by the radioactive matrix and the encapsulation materials around the matrix. Simply expressed (Fig. 17.4), the source's half-thickness and encapsulating walls are represented by thickness t, and the attenuation of the radiation by the source and wall is characterized by the linear attenuation coefficient μ. As the thickness of source and wall transversed by radiation is a function of angle, the air kerma rate at point P must now be expressed thus:

$$\dot{K}_{air}(r,\theta) = \int_{\theta_1}^{\theta_2} [(\Gamma_\delta)_K A/(hL)] \exp(-\mu t/\cos\theta)\,d\theta$$

EQUATION (17.13)

This is the Sievert integral, which requires evaluation by numerical methods. For a filtered line source, the appropriate product of an air kerma rate constant for some filtration and apparent activity is required. The actual thickness used depends on the source design and is usually an effective or equivalent thickness, t_{eff}, that represents the attenuation in the composite wall material and radioactive matrix. Similarly, the spectrum of γ-ray energies may require the use of an average or effective linear attenuation coefficient, μ_{eff}, often more than one, to represent attenuation in the radioactive matrix and wall with an effective thickness, t_{eff}.

The accuracy of Sievert integral calculations has been widely investigated, and the model, and its adequacy and inadequacies, is well understood and much described (34,90,91). It works best for radionuclides (e.g., ^{137}Cs) with high-energy γ-rays and for calculating doses in the angular sectors subtended by the points on the perpendicular bisectors of the long axis of the sources; it works less well in regions near the ends of the sources. Meli (91) notes that this model was used in seven of eight computer systems reviewed; Meigonni and Wallace's (92) review notes that it remains a popular representation for the dosimetry of linear sources. Generally, it is being replaced by TG-43 formalisms for low-energy γ-ray sources.

Generally, the integral is solved for a specific source design, and a table of reduced coordinates—the coordinates divided by the length of the source, with inverse

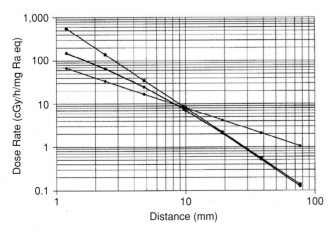

Figure 17.5. Dose rate (cGy/h/mg Ra eq) versus distance (mm) for a point source (—■—), a cesium 137 source of 12 mm active length (—●—), and a source with a theoretical inverse dependency on distance (—◆—). (Author's note: Nominally, 1 mg Ra eq = 7.227 μGy m^2 h^{-1}.)

TABLE 17.4	Dose Rate (cGy/h) for 7.227 cGy/h/U (1 mg Ra eq) ^{137}Cs Source with 20 mm total Length, 14 mm Active Length, Filtration; 1 mm Stainless Steel^a				
Data source	Distance along source (cm)	Distance away from source (cm)			
		0.5	1.5	3.0	4.5
Krishnaswamy	0	21.05	3.24	0.84	0.37
Modulex^b		21.38 (1.6%)	3.25 (0.3%)	0.84 (0.0%)	0.37 (0.0%)
Casal et^c		21.03		0.85	
Krishnaswamy	0.5	17.44	3.00	0.82	0.36
Modulex^b		17.45 (0.2%)	3.00 (0.0%)	0.82 (0.0%)	0.36 (0.0%)
Casal et^c		17.63		0.83	
Krishnaswamy	1.5	3.66	1.78	0.68	0.33
Modulex^b		3.63 (−0.6%)	1.78 (0.0%)	0.68 (0.0%)	0.33 (0.0%)
Casal et^c		3.71		0.69	
Krishnaswamy	3.0	0.79	0.69	0.42	0.25
Modulex^b		0.80 (1.3%)	0.69 (0.0%)	0.42 (0.0%)	0.25 (0.0%)
Casal et^c		0.80		0.43	

^{a}Divide all data by 7.227 to obtain cGy/h/U.
^{b}All Modulex percent errors normalized to Krishnaswamy data.
^{c}Published three significant digits rounded to two significant digits for this comparison.
Krishnaswamy V. Dose distributions about Cs-137 sources in tissue. *Radiology* 1972;105:181–184.
Casal E, Ballester F, Lluch JL, et al. Monte Carlo calculations of dose distribution around Amersham CDCS-M-Type Cs-137 source. *Med Phys* 2000;27:132–140.

square dependency removed—is generated for use. In reduced coordinates, all distances are expressed as multiples of the active length of the source; this eliminates direct dependency on the active length and sets the reduced active length to unity. Table 17.4 presents the results of such a calculation for a ^{137}Cs tube and compares the results with published literature (58,93). Analytic models of the integral, generally power law series expressions, are used in some computer algorithms.

Care must be exercised when selecting the air kerma rate constant or its analog for use in Equation 17.14. In many computer algorithms, the value needed is for an *unfiltered* source, not the filtered source, as the integral includes filtration corrections. Weaver notes that when the source is calibrated in terms of the exposure or air kerma rate measured on the transverse plane outside the filtered source, the integral must be multiplied by a positive exponential term to avoid correction for the filtration twice (53).

In the TG-43 and TG-43U1 formulations, $G(r,\theta)$, the geometry factor, accounts for the spatial distribution of the radioactive material within the source, neglecting self-absorption and attenuation in the source and attenuation and multiple scattering in the medium surrounding the

source. In TG-43U1, the notations "P" and "L" have been added to $G(r,\theta)$, such that the point-source approximation is $G_P(r,\theta) = r^{-2}$. The line source approximation is $G_L(r, \theta) = \beta[L \cdot r \cdot \sin \theta]^{-1}$, where β is the angle, in radian, subtended; this formula applies when $\theta = 0$ degree. At the ends of the source, where $\theta = 0$ degree, $G_L(r,\theta) = [r^2 - L^2/4]^{-1}$. The line source model can be applied to very short linear sources, such as seeds; however, this assumes that the orientation of the short sources can be determined in radiographs, so that the anisotropy factor $F(r,\theta)$ can be used. TG-43 (Table 17.5) gives example values of $G(r,\theta) \cdot r^2$ for a generic seed ~3 mm long. This table remains valid except where $\theta = 0$ degree; using TG-43U1, $G_L(r, \theta) = [r^2 - L^2/4]^{-1}$, which, presumably, would give different values than those in TG-43 Table 17.5. As previously noted, the TG-43 formalism is available on most isodose computation systems.

TISSUE EFFECTS

The medium around or near a radioactive source can generally be characterized as tissue (usually assumed to be water), air, or bone. As noted by Rivard et al. (32), assuming

TABLE 17.5	Some Mathematical Models of $T(r)$ Accounting for Attenuation and Multiple Scattering in a Medium Surrounding Radioactive Source	
Reference	**Model**	
Hale (95)	$D_W/D_A = (e^{-\mu r})(e^{[(+0.77/E0.029)\mu r]})$ (Model valid for $d < 1$; 0.25 MeV < E < 2 MeV)	
Kornelson and Young (96)	$D_W/D_A = (e^{-\mu r})[1 + k_a(\mu r)_b^k]$	
Meisberger et al. (98)	$X_W/X_A = A + Br + Cr^2 + Dr^3$ (valid to 10 cm)	
Van Kleffens and Star (99)	$f_2(r, \theta) = (1 + ar^2)/(1 + br^2)$	

D_W, dose to water; D_A, dose to air; X_W exposure in water; X_A exposure in air; r, distance in centimeters from source to point of calculation; θ, angular dependency term; μ, mass attenuation coefficient for water; E, average γ-ray energy in MeV; A, B, C, D, zero-, first-, second-, and third-order polynomial fitting coefficients; a, b, k_a, k_b fitting coefficients.

a tissue mass density of 1.06 g/cm³, for radionuclides with energies >0.1 MeV, the ratio of D_{water}/D_{tissue} is about 1.01; the absorbed dose to tissue is about 0.99 the absorbed dose to water. (Author's note: This is essentially the same 0.99 correction made when converting external beam absorbed dose in water to absorbed dose to muscle for RTOG protocols). For lower energy (about 0.015–0.05 MeV) radionuclides, the ratio of D_{water}/D_{tissue} is about 0.98 to 0.96. Historical practice is to report absorbed dose to water, neglecting the small variations in dose between the two mediums. However, this likely will change as Monte Carlo absorbed dose calculations become more common.

Historically, corrections for the absorbed dose to bone in or near an implant have not been made in brachytherapy. The brachytherapy sources with higher average energies—0.38 to 0.66 MeV (e.g., ^{192}Ir, [198]Au, ^{137}Cs)—produce ~4% less absorbed dose to bone than absorbed dose to water (94). The absorbed dose to tissue behind bone, however, is reduced several percent, depending on the relative geometry of the bone to the source; the greater density of bone has a modest shielding effect, depending on the bone density. For the lower-energy brachytherapy sources (e.g., [103]Pd, ^{125}I, [131]Cs, [169]Yb) that release energy by the photoelectric effect, the absorbed dose to bone can be twice the dose to water, and the bone shields the tissue behind it.

Numerous mathematical models have been used to describe the dose distributions in water around brachytherapy sources. For the higher-average-energy radionuclides, the simplest model, which neglects the presence of the tissue and assumes the region is occupied by air, is surprisingly accurate at regions near the source. In one-dimension, the radial dimension of a point source or along the perpendicular bisector of a short line source, the perturbing effects of tissue have commonly been expressed by the ratio of either the exposure or the absorbed dose in water to the exposure or absorbed dose in air as a function of radial distance from the source. Two competing phenomena, attenuation, or $A(r)$, and multiple scattering, more commonly called *buildup*, or $B(r)$, occur. Hence

$T(r) = A(r)B(r)$. The attenuation is commonly modeled as a simple negative exponential where a linear attenuation coefficient, μ_{en}, either is an average for the energy spectrum or is applied for each γ-ray energy in the spectrum. Hence, $A(r) = \exp(-\mu_{en}r)$. The buildup is a positive exponential in which the buildup coefficient is a complex energy-dependent term, as shown in Table 17.5 (95). Alternatively, the buildup can be expressed as a series expansion, $B(r) = 1 + k_a(\mu r)^{k_b}$, with the series coefficients specific to each radionuclide, also shown in Tables 17.5 and 17.6 (96). Often, it is necessary to estimate the absorbed dose to critical organs at distances >10 cm. Venselaar et al. provide fitting coefficients for k_a, k_b, and μ for 10 to 60 cm for ^{137}Cs and [192]Ir (97).

An alternative approach is to express $T(r)$—the product of $A(r)B(r)$—as one expression that models the combination of the two effects. A highly tested and widely used formulation is that of Meisberger et al. (98), also in Tables 17.5 and 17.6, in which the ratio of the exposure in water and tissue is expressed as a third-order polynomial that is a function of radial distance. Van Kleffens and Star (99) model the effect as a ratio of two terms. Generally, all of these models are spatially limited; some are normalized to unity at 1 cm and apply only in one-dimension perpendicular to the line source within several centimeters (usually up to 10 cm) from the source. In the original formulation of TG-43 (50), $T(r)$ is replaced by $g(r)$, a radial dose function that describes attenuation and multiple scattering in the medium along the transverse axis of the source. The radial doses are expressed as a fourth-order polynomial for certain models of ^{192}Ir seeds and as a fifth-order polynomial for specific models of ^{125}I seeds.

$$g(r) = a_0 + a_1r + a_2r^2 + a_3r^3 + a_4r^4 + a_5r^5$$

EQUATION (17.14)

The polynomial coefficients of TG-43 are listed in Table 17.7 (50). Mathematical fits to $g(r)$ are only valid

TABLE 17.6	Model Parameters for Tissue Attenuation and Multiple Scattering, $T(r)$				
Model	**Coefficient**	^{198}**Au**	^{192}**Ir**	^{137}**Cs**	^{60}**Co**
Meisberger et al. (98)	$A \times 10^0$	1.0306	1.0128	1.0091	0.99423
	$B \times 10^{-3}$	−8.1340	5.0190	−9.0150	−5.31800
	$C \times 10^{-3}$	1.1110	−1.1780	−0.3459	−2.61000
	$D \times 10^{-5}$	−15.9700	−2.0080	−2.8170	13.27000
Van Kleffens and Star (99)	A	—	—	0.0083	0.01000
	B	—	—	0.0108	0.01450
Kornelson and Young (96)	μ (cm^2/g)	0.1050	0.1130	0.0858	0.06320
	k_a	1.4800	1.5900	1.1400	0.89600
	k_b	1.3200	1.3600	1.2000	1.06300

over the range, r, of the fit, in this instance to ~10 cm. Outside that range, these polynomial yield nonphysical results, for example, a sharp *increase* of dose at $r > 10$ cm. Other mathematical equations (a double exponential and a sigmoid function) offer a more correct physical representation of $g(r)$ at $r > 10$ cm, but these equations have not been adopted in commercial isodose computation algorithms (100,101).

TG-43U1 adopts consensus $g(r)$ data for six ^{125}I seed models and two palladium seed models. An *erratum* to TG-43U1 corrects certain dose rate that is $g(r)$ dependent for Best Model 2301 (8). For line sources that exhibit measur-

able anisotropy created by end effects, these source-induced effects and the tissue effects must be expressed angularly in the plane of the long axis of the sources as well as radially. For interstitial sources in TG-43, these effects are commonly expressed in anisotropy tables, $F(r,\theta)$ normalized to unity at 1 cm from the perpendicular bisector ($\theta = 90$ degrees) of the source, for example, $F(1,90$ degrees$) = 1$. Table 17.8 presents the data for a stainless steel ^{192}Ir seed (50). TG-43 also presents $F(r,\theta)$ data—not given here because of space limitations—for the other three seed sources, model 6702 ^{125}I source, model 6711 ^{125}I source, and model 200 ^{103}Pd seeds (50).

TABLE 17.7	Recommended Coefficients for a Polynomial and Curve Fit to the Radial Dose Function $g(r) = a_0 + a_1 r + a_2 r^2 + a_3 r^3 + a_4 r^4 + a_5 r^5$			
Coefficient[a]	^{125}**I**[b] **Model 6711**	^{103}**Pd**[b] **Model 200**	^{192}**Ir**[c]	^{137}**Cs**[d]
Range of fit (cm)	0.5–10.0	0.5–10.0	0.5–9.0	0.15–20.0
a_0	1.0985	1.6160	9.8954×10^{-1}	1.0064
a_1	-4.88×10^{-2}	-7.597×10^{-1}	8.8139×10^{-3}	-5.4201×10^{-3}
a_2	-7.26×10^{-2}	1.398×10^{-1}	3.51778×10^{-3}	-9.6843×10^{-4}
a_3	1.69×10^{-2}	-1.16×10^{-2}	-1.46637×10^{-3}	1.9293×10^{-5}
a_4	-1.5×10^{-3}	4×10^{-4}	9.24370×10^{-5}	-8.0096×10^{-8}
a_5	5×10^{-5}			

[a]Warning: These coefficients are not applicable outside the stated ranges.
[b]Author's fit to data from 0.5 to 10 cm from TG-43. Rivard MJ, Coursey BM, DeWerd LA, et al. Update of AAPM Task Group 43 Report: a revised AAPM protocol for brachytherapy dose calculations. *Med Phys* 2004; 31:633–674.
[c]From Nath R, Anderson LL, Luxton G, et al. Meigooni AS. Dosimetry of interstitial brachytherapy sources: Task Group No. 43. *Med Phys* 1995;22:215.
[d]From Casal E, Ballester F, Lluch JL, et al. Monte Carlo calculations of dose-rate distributions around Amersham CDCS-M-type Cs-137 source. *Med Phys* 2000;27:139.

TABLE 17.8 Anisotropy Function, $F(r, \theta)$ and $\phi_{an}(r)$ for ^{192}Ir Source with Stainless Steel Encapsulation

r (cm)	0	10	20	30	40	50	60	70	80	$\phi_{an}(r)$
1.0	0.806	0.843	0.947	0.966	1.000	1.020	1.030	1.030	1.020	0.991
2.0	0.788	0.906	0.947	0.941	0.945	0.949	0.953	0.989	0.991	0.947
3.0	0.769	0.813	0.893	0.936	1.030	0.984	0.977	1.030	1.030	0.970
4.0	0.868	0.949	1.010	0.996	1.020	1.030	1.040	1.010	1.010	0.989
5.0	0.831	0.931	0.994	1.030	1.070	1.050	1.030	1.010	1.020	0.998
6.0	0.819	0.899	0.920	0.928	0.973	0.959	0.954	0.996	0.997	0.949
7.0	0.844	0.944	0.985	0.969	0.962	0.967	1.010	1.020	0.979	0.965

Reprinted from American Association of Physicists in Medicine. Report 43. Dosimetry of interstitial brachytherapy sources. *Med Phys* 1995;22:217. For $\theta = 90$ degrees, $F(r, \theta) = 1$ for $r = 1$–7; $\bar{\phi}_{an}(r) = 0.98$.

Table 17.9 reports $F(r,\theta)$ and $\phi_{an}(r)$, for ^{125}I Model 6711, Table 17.10 reports $F(r, \theta)$ and $\phi_{an}(r)$ for ^{103}Pd Model 200, and Table 17.11 reports $F(r, \theta)$ for a CDCS-M type ^{137}Cs source (7,58). TG-43U1 retains $F(r,\theta)$ and reports consensus $F(r,\theta)$ data for the six ^{125}I seed models and two palladium seed models (7). The *erratum* corrects erroneous $F(r,\theta)$ data for the Best Model 2301 (8). Recall that TG-43U1S1 (6) contains similar $F(r,\theta)$ for seven additional ^{125}I sources: Amersham model 6733, Draximage model LS-1, Implant Science model 3500, IBt model 1251 L, IsoAid model IAI-125 A, Mentor model SL-125/SH-125, and SourceTech Medical STM125I, and one ^{103}Pd source, the Best Medical Model 2335.

Recall that the dose-rate constant, Λ, in cGy/h/U, is the dose rate per unit air kerma strength at 1 cm along the transverse axis of the seed, and *is seed design specific*. Events too numerous to fully describe here have resulted in revisions to some of the reported Λ values in TG-43. The ^{192}Ir Λ, 1.12 cGy/h/U, for the Best Industries seed is unchanged, but new values, 0.965 and 0.686 cGy/h/U, are

recommended for ^{125}I Model 6711 and ^{103}Pd Model 200, respectively (7,8). Table 17.3 lists the dose-rate constant, Λ, in μGy/h/U at 1 m, including the still valid data for ^{192}Ir from TG-43, recommendations from TG-43U1, new data from TG-43U1S1, data for ^{131}Cs seeds, and example data for one model (X1267) ^{169}Yb. A complete review of TG-43, TG-43U1, TG-43U1S1, and reports for ^{131}Cs seeds is recommended before adopting any dosimetry data for computer use!

APPLICATOR EFFECTS

While some seeds (^{103}Pd, ^{125}I, ^{131}Cs, ^{169}Yb, ^{198}Au,) are implanted directly into tissue, other brachytherapy sources (^{125}I seeds and ^{131}Cs seeds in vicryl suture, ^{192}Ir seeds in nylon ribbons inserted into thin-walled plastic catheters, ^{137}Cs tubes in tandems) are in carriers or applicator. For ^{192}Ir seeds, the perturbing effects of the carrier are negligible. For ^{137}Cs tubes in gynecology applicators with bladder

TABLE 17.9 Anisotropy Function, $F(r, \theta)$ and $\phi_{an}(r)$ for Amersham Model 6711 ^{125}I Seed

r (cm)	0	10	20	30	40	50	60	70	80	$\phi_{an}(r)$
0.5	0.333	0.519	0.716	0.846	0.926	0.972	0.991	0.996	1.000	0.973
1.0	0.370	0.537	0.705	0.834	0.925	0.972	0.991	0.996	1.000	0.944
2.0	0.442	0.580	0.727	0.842	0.926	0.970	0.987	0.996	1.000	0.941
3.0	0.488	0.609	0.743	0.846	0.926	0.969	0.987	0.995	0.999	0.942
4.0	0.520	0.630	0.752	0.848	0.928	0.969	0.987	0.995	0.999	0.943
5.0	0.550	0.645	0.760	0.852	0.928	0.969	0.987	0.995	0.999	0.944

Reprinted from American Association of Physicists in Medicine. Update of AAPM Task Group Report 43 Report: a revised AAPM protocol for brachytherapy dose calculations. *Med Phys* 2004;31:645.

TABLE 17.10 Anisotropy Function, $F(r, \theta)$ and $\phi_{an}(r)$ for Amersham Model 200 ^{103}Pd Seed										
r (cm)	0	10	20	30	40	50	60	70	80	$\phi_{an}(r)$
0.25	0.619	0.284	0.496	0.775	0.917	0.945	0.976	0.981	0.992	1.130
0.5	0.694	0.496	0.442	0.586	0.734	0.837	0.906	0.929	0.955	0.880
1.0	0.541	0.487	0.501	0.593	0.727	0.834	0.912	0.964	0.972	0.855
2.0	0.526	0.504	0.501	0.593	0.727	0.834	0.912	0.964	0.972	0.870
3.0	0.504	0.519	0.547	0.633	0.750	0.853	0.931	0.989	1.017	0.884
4.0	0.497	0.530	0.585	0.667	0.778	0.881	0.960	1.008	1.046	0.895
5.0	0.513	0.544	0.605	0.683	0.784	0.886	0.964	1.004	1.037	0.897
7.0	0.547	0.590	0.642	0.719	0.820	0.912	0.974	1.011	1.043	0.918

Reprinted with permission from American Association of Physicists in Medicine. Update of AAPM Task Group Report 43 Report: a revised AAPM protocol for brachytherapy dose calculations. *Med Phys* 2004;31:647. See reference for additional data for $\theta = 1 - 5, 7, 12, 15, 25, 25, 75,$ and 85 degrees.

and rectal shields, the shields alter the radiation dose distribution dramatically (Fig. 17.6), reducing the dose by 25% to 50% around a single colpostat with an overall dose reduction of 10% to 20% when the dose contributions of the other colpostat and the intrauterine tandem are included (91,102,103). Modeling applicator effects falls into three broad categories: (a) ignoring the effect, (b) calculating the shielding effect with a simple approximate model, and (c) using a more exact model that approximates dose-altering effects of the applicator. If prior clinical observations and prescriptions neglected the applicator effects or represented them by simple models, one may safely continue to do so, even while knowing that a more current accurate dosimetry is being neglected. Physicians should not alter the classic brachytherapy prescriptions just because new computer algorithms can display the dosimetry of applicator shields. Often consistent dosimetry

applications over long time periods are more important than absolute dosimetry.

Isodose curves for gynecology applicators that neglect the effects of bladder and rectal shields continue to be used. In a 1995 review of the computational features of eight popular dose computation systems, only two had provisions for modeling the shields in applicators (91). While one may ignore the effect of shields, it is best to understand the magnitude of the effect being ignored. For example, thin-walled stainless steel tubing containing ^{192}Ir wire attenuates by <1%. However, this correction was never made by the originators of the Paris (Interstitial) System. Similarly, attenuation from ^{137}Cs sources in intrauterine tubes (tandems) measures as much as 5% depending on the angle but is a commonly neglected effect. Most accurate models of shielding effects around the applicators are derived from Monte Carlo computer calculations

TABLE 17.11 Anisotropy Function, $F(r, \theta)$ for Amersham CDCS-M Type ^{137}Cs Source										
r (cm)	0	10	20	30	40	50	60	70	80	90
0.25	—	—	—	1.022	0.969	1.003	1.008	1.005	1.001	1.000
0.5	—	—	1.023	1.02	0.969	1.003	1.008	1.005	1.001	1.000
1.0	—	0.898	0.980	0.980	0.986	0.991	0.994	0.997	0.999	1.000
2.0	0.888	0.878	0.951	0.974	0.985	0.989	9.992	0.995	0.998	1.000
3.0	0.875	0.881	0.950	0.975	0.987	0.991	0.994	0.996	0.998	1.000
4.0	0.845	0.894	0.954	0.977	0.987	0.992	0.995	0.997	0.999	1.000
5.0	0.855	0.904	0.956	0.978	0.987	0.992	0.995	0.997	0.999	1.000
7.0	0.900	0.908	0.956	0.978	0.988	0.992	0.995	0.997	0.999	1.000

Reprinted with permission from *Med Phys* 2000;27:138. See reference for additional data for $\theta = 1 - 9$ and 110–180 degrees and for $r = 0.15, 0.75, 1.25, 1.5,$ 6, 8, 10, and 15 cm. Authors note: $F(r, \theta)$ is *not* symmetrical for this source. Data for $\phi_{an}(r)$ is not provided.

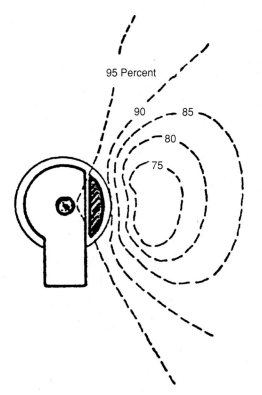

95 Percent

Figure 17.6. Transmission ratios (the fraction of the radiation transmitted through the tungsten shield) for a plane 1.2 cm from the top surface of the colpostat with cap show a 10% to 25% reduction in the dose of radiation delivered to the tissues screened by the shield. (Reprinted with permission from *Elsevier* (Copyright 1980); Hass JS, Dean RD, Mansfield CM. Evaluation of a new Fletcher applicator using cesium-137. *Int J Radiat Oncol Biol Phys* 1980;6:1593.)

documented with 3D dosimetry measurements (104–107). These measurements are used to construct 3D dosimetry tables that can be stored in the computer and recalled as required to reflect the dosimetry around a shielded applicator. The shielded dosimetry of ^{137}Cs in vaginal cylinders and in the popular Fletcher-Suit-Delclos applicator has been reported (103,104,106,107). The early design of the Weeks/Montana applicator (108–110) has evolved into a Weeks CT Mini-Ovoid CT compatible applicator that accepts conventional ^{137}Cs tubes. (Radiation Products Design, Inc, Albertville, MN) (see Chapter 8). However, the declining use of conventional ^{137}Cs tubes in conventional gynecology applicators (Fletcher-Suit-Delclos tandem and ovoids, Henschke tandem and ovoids, etc.) likely means there will be few new developments of CT or MR compatible conventional gynecologic applicators. Price et al. (111) reported on a prototype HDR cervical intracavitary applicator compatible with CT and MR imaging, and the discussion is relevant for LDR cervical intracavitary applicator.

General models for applicator heterogeneity corrections are more commonly found on isodose planning systems for specific sources (^{137}Cs spherical sources in Selectron LDR, ^{192}Ir HDR) rather than for LDR ^{137}Cs brachytherapy (112,113).

TARGET AND SOURCE LOCALIZATION

An anatomic target—diseased tissue surrounded by an acceptable margin of presumably normal tissue— must be determined before performing an implant. Unfortunately, this is not done easily. The radiation oncologist uses available conventional medical tools, including physical examination, plane film radiography and fluoroscopy, CT images, MRI, positron emission tomography (PET), ultrasonography, and nuclear medicine scans, to make this determination. The 3D imaging modalities, CT, MRI, and PET, offer the promise that the implanted radioactive sources and their resulting dose distribution can be superimposed in 3D on the target and normal anatomy. One can confirm over a true anatomical volume that the desired radiation dose distribution conforms to the target volume, that the target is treated to the specified dose within the degree of uniformity specified, and that the doses to adjacent normal tissue are within acceptable tolerances. Increasingly, the same modern analytic tools commonly used in external beam radiotherapy, including cumulative dose-volume histograms (CDVHs), differential dose-volume histograms (DDVHs), tumor control probabilities (TCP), and normal tissue complication probabilities (NTCP), discussed later, are being used to evaluate the quality of the implant and to ascertain the probability of success. Much progress has been made since Martel's 1995 review of the status of 3D imaging techniques in brachytherapy (114). Lief and Rownd offer reviews (115,116). Developments involve using modern image display tools, including solid surface displays, wire frames or mesh, multiple color displays, on–off display features, and isodose cages, target volumes, so that critical organs and other internal anatomy can be viewed from several directions (e.g., room view, applicator view), allowing dramatic visual displays of the implant and the isodose distributions relative to the anatomy. Virtual reality techniques allow the patient's surface anatomy to be displayed as well as the implant applicators or sources. Preliminary dose distributions can be studied as sources are turned on and off or as source spacing or activity is altered.

Erickson offers a succinct review of the potential and current status of image-based brachytherapy (117). Each (CT, MRI, PET) 3D imaging modality presents opportunities and challenges depending on anatomic site imaged and the type of brachytherapy. The prostate is the site most amenable to CT imaging—more commonly at some defined postimplant period to study prostate edema (118,119) and seed migration (120).

Commonly used metal applicators and simulated (dummy) metal sources generally are considered unsuitable for CT imaging. However, some facilities do perform CT scans of conventional shielded applicators and apply software corrections sufficient to yield corrected images sufficient for source localization. Specially fabricated applicators and dummy sources designed for CT imaging work best. They have been investigated, particularly for HDR treatments, but the material research is applicable to LDR brachytherapy (112). Serial CT scans are not always continuous; they can be separated by a few millimeters and may fail to show dummy sources lying between adjacent serial or reconstructed scans. However, the increasing use of spiral CT/simulator scanners—producing continuous images—eliminates this problem. CT 3D images for gynecologic tumors delineate gross anatomy well but do not sufficiently distinguish diseased tissue requiring treatment from normal healthy tissue (121,122).

Lerma and Williamson reported accurate localization of intracavitary applicators (123). Using postimplant 3D CT images, they report registering an accurate 3D model of the rigid applicator with the corresponding volume in the CT image set, allowing description of the applicator in the CT frame-of-reference. Known dose distributions for the source–applicator combination can then be mapped to the CT image set (123).

MRI allows localization of nonferromagnetic ^{125}I seeds postimplant, but not without difficulty, as reported by Thomas et al. who reported on the uncertainties in seed localization when using MR imaging (25). Magnetic resonance spectroscopy imaging (MRSI) allows localization of localized spots of tumor in the prostate (117).

MRI offers superior contrast resolution for gynecologic tumors compared with CT imaging (124,125) but image distortion can occur. Special nonferromagnetic applicators—usually carbon fiber or plastic—are required (112). Both CT and MRI images increasingly are used for source localization studies, and are slowly becoming the imaging standard in brachytherapy. PET has had limited use for imaging gynecologic tumors (117). Meli's 1995 review of eight computer systems used in brachytherapy dose computations revealed that none offered source reconstruction algorithms based on serial 3D images (126). Today, some general-purpose brachytherapy dose calculation algorithms still do not offer CT or MRI based source reconstruction algorithms.

The radiation oncologist's methods of determining target volumes can be classified as static (more common) or dynamic (less common). Static methods commonly involve physical measurements at the anatomical site combined with plane film radiography or other images of the anatomy, with simulated applicators or sources in position. Examples include simple measurements of the extent of exophytic lesions for surface implants or molds, sounding of the depth of the uterus for an intracavitary implant, measurement of lesion extent with placement of surgical clips during surgery to excise the bulk of the lesion or preparatory to permanent seed implants, and more recently preimplant volume studies with ultrasonography and fluoroscopy to plan needle placements for transperineal prostate implants. These and similar procedures allow the radiation oncologist to determine the general shape and gross dimensions of the target volume and possibly to estimate the physical volume of tissue to be treated.

Dynamic ultrasound imaging (with subsequent dynamic isodose computations) during prostate seed implants is increasingly popular—less common is performing prostate seed implants under CT image guidance. MRI-guided

prostate implants have been investigated (24)—plastic needles were superior to MRI compatible titanium needles.

The next step is to plan the distribution of the radioactive sources to achieve the desired dose distribution. To calculate absorbed dose distributions manually or by use of a computer, the positions and orientations of the radioactive sources relative to each other must be known as well as their position relative to the target volume. While there are still reports of use of classical radiographic plane films for imaging (127), film and film processors are rapidly disappearing from hospitals. Many have adopted other imaging methods, such as non-isocentric C-arm imaging (128–130). C-arm images are not necessarily isocentric—can suffer from image distortion—and yield poor quality lateral images in large patients. However, there are solutions to each of these problems (128–130).

(Author's note: As isocentrically obtained object images are independent of the medium [film or electronic digital image], I retain the explanation of reconstruction algorithms.) Classical radiographic methods fall into three broad categories: isocentric films, shift films, and nonisocentric films. Computer algorithms allow conversion of these source coordinates to a patient-based coordinate system. Lief and Meli offer useful reviews (115,126).

The most common isocentric method requires two orthogonal radiographs—taken from different perspectives—obtained simultaneously or sequentially with no movement of the sources, with the sources and a reference point visible on both images. Taken with the beam perpendicular to the radiographs and its central axis passing through the reference point, they yield the geometric relationship shown in Figure 17.7.

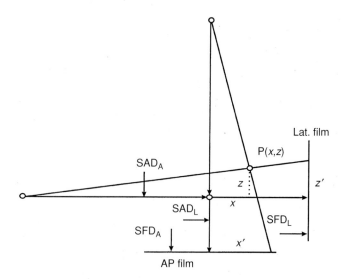

Figure 17.7. The geometry of orthogonal (anteroposterior and lateral) images. x' and z' are the displacements on the images of the point P(x,z), representing a seed or the tip or end of a source. The focus-to-axis distances are SAD; the focus-to-image distances are SFD. Lat., lateral; AP, anteroposterior. (Reprinted with permission from *Oxford University Press* (Copyright 1993); Modified from Arid EG, Williams JR. Brachytherapy. In: Williams JR, Thwaites DI, ed. *Radiotherapy physics.* Oxford: Oxford University Press, 1993:187–226, 192.)

If the distances from the focus to the origin are SAD_A and SAD_L with focus-to-image distances of SFD_A and SFD_L, and if x' and z' are the displacements of a point $P(x,z)$ from the origin, the coordinates of P are given thus:

$$x = x'[(SAD_A - z)/SFD_A]$$
$$= x'[(SAD - z)/SFD] \quad \text{EQUATION (17.15)}$$

$$z = z'[(SAD_L - x)/SFD_L]$$
$$= z'[(SAD - z)/SFD] \quad \text{EQUATION (17.16)}$$

where the second component of the equation applies if $SAD_A = SAD_L = SAD$ and $SFD_A = SFD_L = SFD$.

Equation solutions yield the following:

$$x = x'[(SAD_A SFD_L - z'SAD_L)/(SFD_A SFD_L - x'z')]$$
$$\text{EQUATION (17.17)}$$

$$z = z'[(SAD_L SFD_A - x'SAD_A)/(SFD_A SFD_L - x'z')]$$
$$\text{EQUATION (17.18)}$$

Again, if $SAD_A = SAD_L = SAD$ and $SFD_A = SFD_L = SFD$:

$$x = x'[(SAD \cdot SFDz'SAD)/(SAD^2 - x'z')]$$
$$\text{EQUATION (17.19)}$$

$$z = z'[(SAD \cdot SFD - x'SAD)/(SFD^2 - x'z')]$$
$$\text{EQUATION (17.20)}$$

If y' is the measured displacement from the origin on the anterior image, then the displacement, y, from the origin in the third dimension is given thus:

$$y = y'[(SAD_A SFD_L - z'SAD_L)/(SFD_A SFD_L - x'z')]$$
$$\text{EQUATION (17.21)}$$

Again, when $SAD_A = SADL$ and $SFD_A = SFD_L$:

$$y = y'[(SAD \cdot SFD - z'SAD)/(SFD^2 - x'z')]$$
$$\text{EQUATION (17.22)}$$

The radiographic magnification inherent in these exact equations is geometric reconstruction magnification, as it yields the coordinates (x, y, z) from the magnified coordinates (x', y', z') without approximations.

However, simpler equations arise if the implanted sources are closely grouped near isocenter and the displacements x' and z' measured on the images are much less than the distances from focus to origin and source to image. If the approximate magnification factors for the two images are $M_A = SFD_A/SAD_A$ and $M_L = SFD_L/SAD_L$, the approximate equations are as follows:

$$x = x'/M_A \quad z = z'/M_L \quad y = y'/M_A$$
$$\text{EQUATION (17.23)}$$

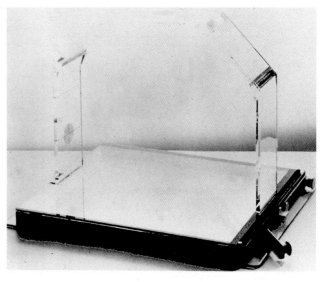

Figure 17.8. A reconstruction box or fiducial jig for reconstruction of nonorthogonal isocentric images. (Reprinted with permission from Nucletron Corporation, Columbia, MD.)

This average magnification method uses the magnification near the center of the sources near isocenter rather than the magnification of each source, and the magnification is often determined by placing a ring of known diameter (often 50 mm) as close as possible to the center of the sources and isocenter; one diameter of the ring is magnified without foreshortening, allowing a measurement of approximate magnification. Reconstruction boxes (Fig. 17.8) with fiducial markers can be used during the procedure to correct for small nonorthogonal errors that often occur if the radiographs are obtained nonorthogonally on portable x-ray units or C-arm devices.

Orthogonal radiographs afford accurate reconstruction equations but often in thick patients, lateral radiographs are poor in quality, and bony anatomy can obscure the views of the applicator or sources. *Semiorthogonal* (at angles < 90 degrees) radiographs, also called *semi-isocentric* radiographs, often allow better views, but the reconstruction algorithms are somewhat less accurate when average magnification is used. Some computer systems offer algorithms allowing for free reconstruction radiographs, obtained at any angle. A conventional simulator (rapidly disappearing from most radiation oncology facilities) or, more recently, the electronic portal imager on a linear accelerator, can be used to take two isocentric images at arbitrary but unknown angles that are selected to obtain optimal views of the sources. Sets of equations similar to those previously described allow reconstruction of the sources even if the angles are unknown. Generally, for both semiorthogonal and free reconstructions methods, a reconstruction device of some type is required.

Stereo radiographs, a double-exposure radiograph obtained either with the x-ray beam in two positions or on separate radiographs, use similar triangles for source localization, as shown in Figure 17.9 (99,131). Stereo

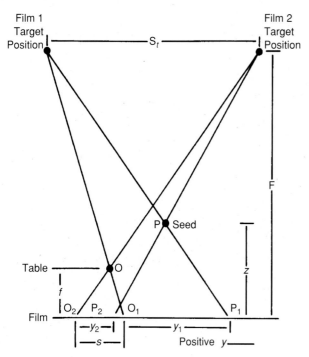

Figure 17.9. The geometry of stereo shift radiographs. y_1 is the distance on the first image between images of a seed at P and a tabletop reference point, which is seen as an origin at O. y_2 is the distance between images at the same points on the second image, taken from shifting the tube a distance S_t toward the patient's head (i.e., in the positive y direction). The image of the origin shifts a distance s in the opposite direction. From these distances and the target-to-image distances, F, and the tabletop distance, t, the vertical distance, z, of the seed from the image can be calculated. (Reprinted from Anderson LL. Dosimetry for interstitial radiation therapy. In: Hilaris BS, ed. *Handbook of interstitial brachytherapy*. Acton, MA: Publishing Sciences Group, 1975:87–115, with permission.)

radiographs are useful, as it is generally easier to match sources, particularly seeds, on the two radiographs. However, coordinate reconstruction errors, particularly in the vertical (z) dimension, can be large unless a large shift is used. The height, z, of a point P (a seed or source tip or end) follows from the application of similar triangle geometry in Figure 17.9. Namely:

$$[S_T/s] = [(F - f)/f] \qquad \text{EQUATION (17.24)}$$

$$[S_T/(y_1 + s - y_2)] = [(F - z)/z] \qquad \text{EQUATION (17.25)}$$

$$z = F[(F - f)(y_2 - y_1) - S_T f][(F - f)(y_2 - y_1) - S_T F]$$

$$\text{EQUATION (17.26)}$$

Large shifts of 60 cm minimize errors; 20-cm shifts (±10 cm from the center) with 100-cm source-to-film distances are common but not error-free. Generally, on a fixed x-ray unit the patient and the films (images) are shifted together—first in one direction from the center and then from the center to an equal distance in the opposite direction. Alternatively, if the x-ray unit moves along,

the patient and film (image) remained fixed and the x-ray tube is shifted in opposite directions to an equal distance from the center. Palvolyi reports the use of variable angle reconstruction method with a non-isocentric C-arm radiographic unit for reconstruction of the images a Fletcher-Suit-Delcols applicator (130).

Seed matching is difficult in permanent and template implants using several hundred seeds. Reconstruction algorithms requiring three radiographs allow reconstruction of seed implants without identifying the same seed in each radiograph. Random seed entry is used, and the algorithm is used to sort out and identify the same seeds in each radiograph. Methods include obtaining two orthogonal radiographs with one midway between them and the implant at isocenter (132), obtaining three radiographs at isocenter each separated 8 degrees (133), and obtaining three radiographs, one anteroposterior and two at angles < 45 degrees (134). Siddon and Chin (135) describe a two-film technique using films at arbitrary angles that are not necessarily coplanar and Todor et al. describe an operator-free method (136). The algorithms associated with each of these methods are complex and too lengthy to describe here. Generally, all of these methods yield the best matching results in small implants with few seeds. For larger implants with many seeds, more matching errors occur because seed images are more likely to be superimposed on the radiographs. Table 17.12 summarizes the features of source localization methods.

Image scanners now allow one to scan the images into computers for display and source identification rather than just digitizing the applicator or source coordinates from the images. Reconstruction of seed implant geometry from CT scans is increasingly common. Holupka et al. describe a seed finder for brachytherapy CT images based on the popular Hough transform (137). Such methods are increasingly common on most brachytherapy isodose computation computers.

STATIC-SOURCE INTRALUMINAL AND INTRACAVITARY DOSIMETRY SYSTEMS

Luminal LDR brachytherapy has largely been replaced by luminal HDR brachytherapy as it avoids patients' discomfort associated with long-duration LDR luminal treatments. The basic physics of LDR and HDR luminal treatments is similar. The dosimetry of nominally linear arrays of radioactive sources in lumens (the ducts or canals of tubular organs, e.g., the esophagus and bronchus) differs markedly from interstitial procedures. Depending on the anatomy and the diameter of the applicator, the sources may or may not be in contact with or near diseased tissue. In the smallest lumens, such as the bile duct, the diseased tissue may be within 5 mm of the lumen; in other anatomy, such as the vagina, the diseased tissue may be centimeters away. The source array can be as short as a single seed of a few millimeters or long as a vaginal applicator containing

TABLE 17.12 Image Methods of Target and Source Localization

Method of source identification	Number of images	Image orientation	Magnification method	Accuracy	Comment
Manual	2	Orthogonal (isocentric)	Geometric reconstruction (exact)	Excellent	Most accurate; limited only by patient movement between images and source digitization errors
			Average magnification (approximate)	Good	Works best for small sources closely grouped near isocenter
Manual	2	Arbitrary angle (isocentric)	Geometric reconstruction (exact)	Good	Can select angles to maximize source visibility; less accurate than true orthogonals
			Average magnification (approximate)	Modest	Less accurate, as it combines two less accurate methods
Manual	2	Stereo shift	Geometric reconstruction (exact)	Good	Even with an "exact" calculation, small (0.5 mm) localization errors yield measurable (2–3 mm) magnification errors in z
			Average magnification (approximate)	Modest	Less accurate, as it combines inherence shift errors with magnification errors
Auto	3	Implant near isocenter; orthogonal images with one 45 degrees between	Average magnification	Modest	Works best for closely spaced sources in small implants
Auto	3	One vertical image; two ±8 degrees from vertical images at isocenter	Geometric reconstruction	Good	Works best for closely spaced sources in small implants
Auto	3	One vertical 2, at 45 degrees or other arbitrary angles to vertical; need not have common isocenter	Geometric reconstruction	Good	Works best for closely spaced sources in small implants
Auto	2	Arbitrary angles not necessarily coplanar	Geometric reconstruction	Modest	Required location of tips and ends of each source

multiple tubes. Most lumens accommodate only one source array; because of the curved anatomy, the source array is not necessarily coplanar. The implants are temporary; the sources are in removable applicators of varying designs.

The inner diameter of the lumen and the thickness of diseased tissue around the lumen determine the radionuclide suitable for treatment. The lumen diameters are usually several millimeters and the target volumes around the lumens much thicker than a few millimeters. The lower

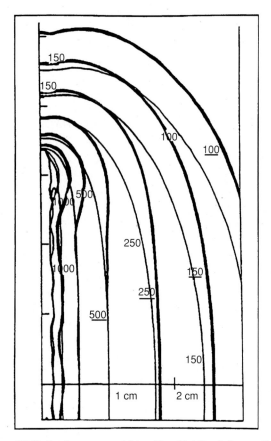

Figure 17.10. Isodose curves (*thin ellipsoidal lines*) from a linear array of equal activity point sources and isodose curves (*thick cylindrical lines*) representing an optimized treatment delivered at 1 cm by increasing the source activities near the end of applicator. Note the improved cylindrical shapes of the thicker lines and also the bulging of the thicker lines (higher doses) very close to the applicator. (Modified from Reis G. Lung and esophagus high dose rate treatment protocols. South China, ME: Health Service Consultants, 1993; 44.)

energy radioisotopes, ^{103}Pd, ^{125}I, ^{131}Cs, exhibit too much attenuation over even a few millimeters to be useful; the higher-energy radioisotopes, 137Cs, ^{169}Yb, ^{192}Ir, ^{198}Au, are more useful.

A simple linear array of equal-strength sources of any of these four radioisotopes produces a dose distribution somewhat ellipsoidal, depending on its length, as shown in Figure 17.10. The isodose curves budge out at the source center as the center section receives dose symmetrically from all segments of the array. Near the end of the array, most of the dose is contributed locally by the closer sources—source segments at the far end contribute little dose to the opposite end. Hence, the isodose curves taper off near the ends of the array. This isodose tapering can be offset by using seeds of higher activity near the ends of the array to yield a more uniform dose distribution along the entire length of the array.

The important and complex inverse relationship between distance and absorbed dose very near a linear source has been previously noted. Because of the sharp dose gradients close to the source, tissue a few millimeters thick is irradiated nonuniformly. A catheter should be as

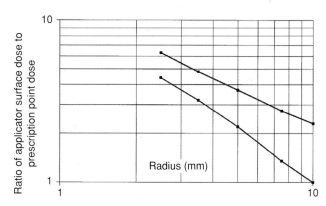

Figure 17.11. The ratio of applicator surface dose rate to prescription dose rate as a function of applicator radius. Upper curve denotes the ratio when the dose is prescribed as a distance from the applicator. The lower curve denotes the ratio when the dose is prescribed as a distance from the source in the center of the applicator. (Modified from Reis G. Lung and esophagus high dose rate treatment protocols. South China, ME: Health Service Consultants, 1993; 44.)

small as necessary to fit in a lumen, but as large in diameter as possible to improve the dose distribution around the lumen. Assuming the source is centered in the catheter, larger-diameter catheters, such as vaginal cylinders, improve the relative dose distribution around the catheter or applicator. Larger-diameter (2.0–3.0 cm) vaginal cylinders push the anatomy away from the source to distances for which the dose gradient is less sharp, improving the relative dose distribution and allowing more uniform irradiation of adjacent tissue.

The ratio of applicator surface dose to dose at some specified distance from the applicator decreases as the applicator diameter increases, as shown in Figure 17.11. For an 8-cm source with 7.227 μGy m²/h/cm (1 mg radium equivalent per centimeter), this graph shows the ratio of dose on the applicator surface to prescribed dose either 10 mm from the source axis (lower curve) or 10 mm from the applicator surface (upper curve). The dose gradient is less sharp for the upper curve. Understanding this relationship is particularly important, as use of too small an applicator can yield undesirably high surface doses. Moreover, clinically, one must be consistent with spatial dose prescriptions. Figure 17.11 shows how even the smallest variation in catheter size alters the surface dose at the catheter.

The largest cavity treated is the gynecological anatomy, the vagina, cervix, uterus, and adjacent tissue. Over the decades, numerous treatment philosophies have been used, widely described, and, in some instances, abandoned. Classical methods of treatment are well described by Potish et al. (138). The original Paris (Gynelogical) System (1920s) intracavitary treatments prescribed constant exposure, expressed in milligram hours, independent of tumor volume and source loadings. The Manchester system (1938) introduced reference points. Point A, originally defined to be 2 cm above the lateral vaginal fornix

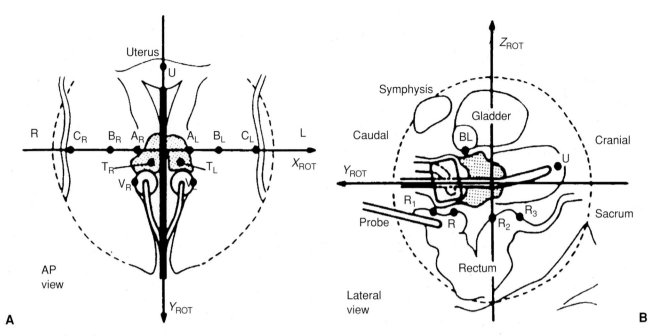

Figure 17.12. Anteroposterior (**A**) and lateral (**B**) views of an applicator and 19 specific dosimetry points. In the anteroposterior view, A and B are Manchester reference points; C, pelvic points; U, uterus point. In the lateral view R, R₁, R₂, and R₃ are rectum points; BL, a bladder point. The points A, B, C, and T lie in the rotated Z plane. (Reprinted with permission from Nucletron Corporation, Columbia, MD; Van der Laarse R. A dedicated treatment planning system [SPS]); Reprinted with permission from NucletronIn: Mould RF, ed. Brachytherapy 1984: Proceedings of the 3rd international selectron users meeting. Leersum, The Netherlands: Nucletron, 1985:180.)

and 2 cm lateral to the cervical canal, was considered to be a region of maximum radiation sensitivity. Point B, defined 3 cm lateral to point A, represented the doses to the pelvic wall. The clinical goal was—independent of implant size and loading—to achieve a reasonably constant dose rate at point A and subsequently constant duration treatment times for all patients. In 1953, point A was redefined to be 2 cm above the cervical os. Potish, Gerbi, and Engeler provide an excellent review of the numerous definitions of point A introduced over the years (138). The Fletcher system (1960s) combined elements of the Paris and Manchester systems. Depending on the anatomy to be treated, the implant was left in place until either a maximum milligram hours for small implants or a maximum duration in hours for larger implants was reached (138). Many radiation oncologists combined elements of the Manchester system (with numerous altered definitions of points A and B) and the Fletcher system and focused on limiting the doses to the bladder and the rectum.

The concept of point dose definitions—some relative to the patient's anatomy and some relative to the applicator—has been highly successful, with numerous additional points introduced, to better describe the dose distribution over this extended anatomy. Maruyuma et al. (139) introduced point T, 1 cm above the cervical marker (flange) and 1 cm lateral to the tandem to describe the tumor dose closer to the true origin of the tumor; point V describes the surface doses on the lateral surfaces of the ovoids, and point C describes the dose to the external iliac nodes at the lateral pelvis. A bladder (posterior bladder wall) dose, BL,

and rectal doses—R₁ (anterior rectal wall) and R₂ (sigmoid colon)—describe the doses to the critical organs. These points, with some modifications—the addition of point U, a dose to the uterus, and more rectal points (R₁, R, R₂, R₃), shown in Figure 17.12—are used in some dose computation systems as a method of dose specification.

The New York system of dosimetry (140) Figure 17.13 was designed for use with the Henschke applicator. In an anterior view, reference points REF_R, REF_L are 2 cm superior and 2 cm lateral from the cervical os, cervix points CVX_R, CVX_L are 1 cm superior and 1 cm lateral from the cervical os, uterine surface points UTE_R, UTE_L, are 1 cm inferior and 2 cm lateral from tandem tip, and vaginal surface points VG₁R, VG₁L are on the lateral surface of the ovoids. Other points of interest for which the dose is recorded are vaginal points VG₂R, VG₂L at 0.5 cm depth and obturator node points OBT_R, OBT_L, which are close to Manchester Point B. In the lateral view, tissue tolerance points consist of the five rectal points (R₁–R₅) determined with a rectal marker, bladder points in the center of the Foley catheter balloon BL₁, and BL₂, on the Foley balloon surface, and a sigmoid colon point, SC, midway between the applicator tip and the sacral promontorium. In the New York system, a dose optimization algorithm is used to determine the source distributions that produce the doses at the specified points.

To improve consistency in reporting absorbed doses, the American Brachytherapy Society has recommended specific dose-reporting points for cervix, Figure 17.14, and vaginal treatments, Figure 17.15 (141).

Figure 17.13. Dose points specified in the New York System. **A:** Anterior view. Reference points REF_R, REF_L; uterine surface points UTE_R, UTE_L; cervix points CVX_R, CVX_L; vaginal surface points VG_{1R}, VG_{1L}. Other points of interest for which the dose is recorded are vaginal points VG_{2R}, VG_{2L} at 0.5 cm depth and obturator node points OBT_R, OBT_L, which are close to Manchester Point B. **B:** In the lateral view tissue tolerance points consist of the five rectal points R_{1-5}, bladder points in the center of the Foley catheter balloon BL_1, and BL_2, on the Foley balloon surface, and a sigmoid colon point, SC, midway between the applicator tip and the sacral promontorium. (Reprinted with permission from Br J Radiol (Copyright 1977); Rosenstein LM. A simple computer program for optimization of source loading in cervical intracavitary applicators. *Br J Radiol* 1977;50:119–122.)

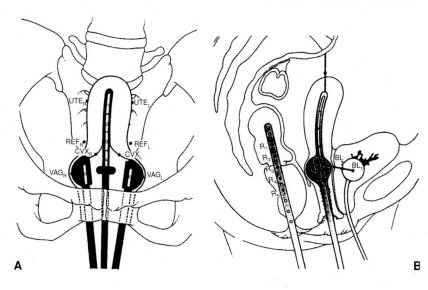

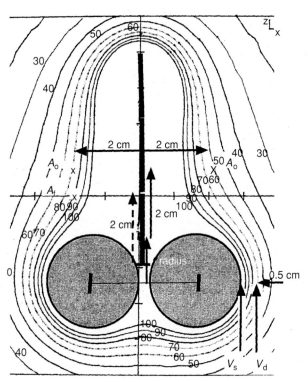

Figure 17.14. Left side: Variations of Point A based on definition. The point labeled A_o follows the original definition of 2 cm cephalad from the ovoid surface and 2 cm lateral. The point A_f begins at the flange instead of the ovoid surface. The latter point falls near the rapidly changing gradient in the cephalocaudal direction near the ovoids, whereas the former falls in a region where the dose changes little with changes in the direction along the tandem. Right side: Recommended reporting points for cervical cancer brachytherapy with a tandem and colpostat: point A, corresponding to the original Manchester definition (A_o); point V_s, on the lateral surface of the ovoid; and point V_d, 0.5 cm deep to point V_s, laterally. Reported doses should include the values on it *both* right and left sides of each point. (Reprinted with permission from Elsevier (Copyright 2002); Nag S, Chao C, Erickson B, et al. The American Brachytherapy Society Recommendations for low-dose-rate (LDR) brachytherapy for carcinoma of the cervix. *Int J Radiat Oncol Biol Phys* 2002;52:33–48.)

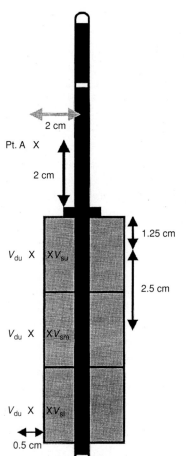

Figure 17.15. Dose-reporting points for cervical brachytherapy using a tandem with vaginal cylinders. Point A lies 2 cm cephalad along the tandem from the flange and 2 cm lateral (perpendicular) to the tandem. The upper vaginal dose points fall on the surface of the cylinder 1.25 cm below the bottom of the flange (V_s) and 0.5 cm lateral (perpendicular to the tandem) to that (V_d). The middle vaginal points fall 2.5 cm inferior parallel to the tandem of the upper points, and the lower vaginal points yet another 2.5 cm inferior. (Reprinted with permission from Elsevier (Copyright 2002); Nag S, Chao C, Erickson B, et al. The American Brachytherapy Society Recommendations for Low Dose-Rate Brachytherapy for Carcinoma of the Cervix. *Int J Radiat Oncol Biol Phys* 2002;52:33–48.)

Plane a

Plane b

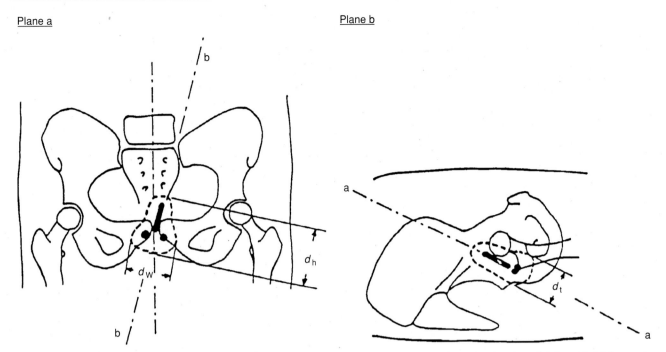

Figure 17.16. The reference isodose curve (and volume) dimensions of (Plane a) width, d_w, and height, d_h; and (Plane b) thickness, d_t. (Reprinted with permission from ICRU (Copyright 1985); Dose and volume specification for reporting intracavitary therapy in gynecology, ICRU Report No.38. Bethesda, MD: International Commission on Radiation Units and Measurements, 1985:10.)

Draw a line bisecting the colpostats. From the intersection of this line with the tandem, move superiorly along the tandem 2 cm *plus the radius of the colpostat.* Point A_{ABS} is defined 2 cm, laterally, perpendicular to the tandem. For a tandem used with vaginal cylinders, the distance along the tandem is measured from the flange on the tandem. For colpostats, lateral vaginal surface (mucosa) doses, $V_{s, ABS}$, and deep (0.5 cm) doses, $V_{d, ABS}$, are taken along the line bisecting the colpostats.

For tandems and cylinders, V_s and V_d are defined 1.25 cm inferior to the cervical os (flange location) and measured from the cylinder's surface. Depending on the vagina length (>4 cm), multiple V_s, V_d points (upper, middle, lower, e.g., V_{su}, V_{du}, V_{sm}, V_{dm}, V_{sl}, V_{dl}) can be defined at 2.5 cm intervals along the cylinder. Some dose computation systems use similar point definitions as a method of dose specification. The common feature in all of these systems is the identification of some points relative to the anatomy, some relative to the applicator, and some relative to devices (Foley catheter, rectal markers) used to delineate the critical organs and of course to determine the source array and its resulting dose distributions at these points. Hence, proper localization of these common points is required.

While point doses are widely used for specification and reporting of doses for gynecologic treatments in the United States, in Europe recommendations made by the International Commission on Radiation Units and Measurements (ICRU) Report 38 for dose reporting are used (46). The ICRU Report 38 methodology has been widely reviewed and is only briefly summarized here (35,37,142).

The method includes definitions of four tissue volumes (target, treatment, irradiated, and reference) and determination of the reference volume, shown in Figure 17.16, and its dose level. It reports the absorbed doses at reference points (bladder, rectum, lymphatic trapezoid, pelvic wall), the total reference air kerma (in micrograys)—the product of the air kerma rate (micrograys per hour) at 1 m times the duration (in hours) of treatment—and a description (sources and their strengths, applicator, and the time-dose pattern) of the technique. The reference volume is determined from the simple product of two major dimensions of the reference isodose curve of the oblique frontal or tilted coronal plane, which passes through the center of the ovoids and presumably contains the intrauterine tandem, and the thickness of the reference isodose curve of the oblique sagittal plane, which passes through the internal os and the center of the ovoids and presumably contains the intrauterine tandem. The weakness of this method is the difficulty in visualizing and determining a target volume. Hanson and Graves notes that it is important to take great care to ensure that these planes are properly determined, or the volume information obtained will be erroneous (143).

Three-dimensional (3D) imaging (CT images, MR images) offers new opportunities for prescribing and reporting brachytherapy dosimetry. The Gynaecological (GYN) GEC-ESTRO Working Group (I) focused on the assessment of gross target volume (GTV) and clinical target volume (CTV) *via* MR imaging (125) over the course of external beam and brachytherapy. They concluded it was necessary to distinguish between volumes at *diagnosis*

TABLE 17.13	GEC-ESTRO Working Group (II)

Recommendations for recording and reporting 3D gynecological brachytherapy

Complete description of clinical situation including anatomy and pathology and imaging examination
    Dimensions and volume of GTV at diagnosis and at time of brachytherapy
    Dimensions and volume of HR CTV and IR CTV, respectively

Complete description of 3D sectional imaging technique and contouring procedure

Complete description of brachytherapy technique
    Radionuclide; source type (wire, stepping source); source strength; applicator type; type of afterloading (manual or remote); description of additional interstitial needles, if any

Treatment prescription and treatment planning
    Applicator reconstruction technique, standard loading pattern, dose specification method,
    Optimization method, if applied

Prescribed Dose

Total Reference Air Kerma (TRAK)

Dose at point A (right, left, mean)

D100, D90 for GTV and HR CTV and IR CTV, respectively

Dose to bladder and rectum for ICRU reference points

$D_{0.1cc}$, D_{1cc}, D_{2cc} for organs at risk (e.g., rectum, sigmoid, bladder) (Vagina)[a]

D_{5cc}, D_{10cc} for organs at risk if contouring of organ walls is performed

Complete description of time-dose pattern; physical and biologically weighted doses

(α/β = 10 Gy for GTV and CTV; α/β = 3 Gy for OAR; $T_{1/2}$ = 1.5 hours for GTV, CTV, and OAR)

[a]For vagina dose-volume parameters still need to be defined.

(GTV_D, CTV_D) and *brachytherapy* (GTV_B, CTV_B) as well as distinguishing CTV by for recurrence as *high risk* (HR CTV) and *intermediate risk* (IR CTV). Work Group (II) (144) focused on dose-volume parameters for describing and reporting 3D dosimetry. The report combines the older reporting concepts, Total Reference Air Kerma (a modern expression of the milligram-hour concept), doses at Point A, and bladder and rectum ICRU reference points with new concepts. They specifically recommended CDVH for evaluating complex dose heterogeneity, reporting the minimum doses delivered to 90% (D90) and 100% (D100) of the GTV, HR CTV, and IR CTV. High dose-volume assessment is *via* reports of volumes enclosed by 150% (V150) and 200% (V200) of the prescribed dose. For organs-at-risk (OAR) (e.g., rectum, sigmoid, and bladder), they recommend reporting the minimum dose in the most irradiated tissue volumes of 0.1 cc ($D_{0.1\ cc}$), 1 cc ($D_{1\ cc}$), 2 cc ($D_{2\ cc}$), and 5 cc ($D_{5\ cc}$) and 10 cc ($D_{10\ cc}$) if organ walls are contoured, along with complete description of time-dose patterns. Table 17.13 summarizes the recommendations. Careful study of all of the many definitions in Work Group II is required to accurately report 3D dosimetry (144). Numerous papers have investigated the relationship between dosimetry reported by various point-based systems and the dosimetry that arises from image volume-based systems (145–149). Conclusions regarding the merits of the older point-dose systems versus the 3D dosimetry systems can depend on the type (CT, MR) of 3D imaging used for comparison, as, previously noted, MR is superior to CT for certain anatomic studies.

Interestingly, the American Brachytherapy Cervical Cancer Guidelines (48) adopts prescriptions (milligram-hours or cGy to Point A) from the earlier eras and reporting from the Work Group (II) recommendations. It appears that even as more anatomic information is visually displayed for analysis, historical precedents and concepts continue to guide prescriptions for gynecological treatments.

STATIC-SOURCE INTERSTITIAL DOSIMETRY AND DOSE SPECIFICATION SYSTEMS

The primary task of the radiation oncologist is to establish a therapeutic goal and identify methods of achieving that goal. A defined volume of tissue is to be irradiated using interstitially implanted radioactive sources. How should it be done? How should needles be spaced? Is absorbed dose uniformity desired or should the absorbed dose distribution be nonuniform to preferentially irradiation-diseased areas to different absorbed doses? Brachytherapy has a long history of answers to these basic questions, and new answers are always under development.

Interstitial brachytherapy can be broadly characterized by historical systems of dosimetry independent of computers and those that use modern computer calculations independent of system rules. This categorization is not clean; the dose distributions resulting from system rules obviously can be displayed by computers. Conversely, use of a computer, even with dose optimization, does not preclude use of the features of established systems in planning an implant. Anderson simply but elegantly describes the basic problem (150). Placing a single radioactive source in the center of a defined target surrounded by normal tissue produces a highly nonuniform dose in the target but is likely to spare the normal tissue. Conversely, placing multiple radioactive sources in the normal tissue around the target is likely to yield a reasonably uniform dose across the target but unacceptable dose to the normal tissue. The desired therapeutic goal lies somewhere between these two extremes, and numerous dosimetry systems have been developed to achieve various stated therapeutic goals. However, one message remains abundantly clear: *after the physical implant,* no computer optimization algorithm can correct for physical errors in the planned geometrical arrangement of the sources and/or applicators. Generally, *a poorly planned or executed implant cannot be salvaged by computer optimization methods.* Hence, there is great value in having radiation oncologists who perform implants understand the classical systems of implantation, their many rules, and apply, during the physical implant, the one they select for a particular case, to the best of their ability. In most anatomic sites, diseased tissue is highly irregular in shape. To quote Burns, "The best laid plans of mice and men oft go awry." And, the best preplanned implants can suffer a similar fate. To start an implant without a conceptual plan and desired therapeutic endpoints is a formula for disaster!

A system denotes "a set of rules taking into account source strengths, geometry, and method of application obtain suitable dose distributions over the volume(s) to be treated" (143). The classical interstitial systems (Manchester—also known as Paterson and Parker, Quimby, Paris [Interstitial], Memorial) are well described in numerous textbooks as are modern variations of their applications (33,35,151–154) Space limits the review to brief, general, relevant comments about their features and use, as, for example, focusing on their continued use and modern applications, serving as a method of independently hand-checking computer dose calculations for both conventional static-source arrays.

The Manchester (UK) system's stated objective is a uniform dose, within 10% of a stated minimum dose,

throughout the target region, achieved by the nonuniform distribution of ^{226}Ra sources of specific design (different linear activities) that allows system goals to be achieved. The system prescribes source distribution rules for surface molds, single-plane implants, and double-plane implants for anatomical thicknesses up to 2.5 cm (33,35). Volume implants of planned geometrical seed arrays—cube, cylinder, and sphere—distribute the sources, so that dose uniformity is still maintained to within 10%. Unfortunately, most large target volumes do not have such geometric regularity.

As ^{226}Ra sources with only one linear activity were originally available in the United States, Quimby devised a system for molds, interstitial planar implants, and for volume implants using a uniform distribution of these sources that produced a nonuniform radiation distribution in the target region (33,35). For planar implants, the dose—a maximum dose within the specified target plane—is specified on the central axis of the perpendicular bisector; however, for volume implants, the dose specification is a minimum dose within the specified volume. Anderson's excellent review (151) notes that for both Manchester and Quimby systems, source oblique filtration effects were neglected, as were tissue attenuation and multiple scattering, and that the systems, suitable for higher-energy radium equivalent radionuclides, are not suitable for radioactive sources (^{125}I, ^{103}Pd) producing photons of <200 keV.

Both systems depend on knowledge of the extent (area or volume) of the anatomical region and use tables of cumulated source strength (originally in milligram hours) to yield a specified dose (originally 1,000 R) as a function of area or volume. Modern tables reflect many changes in the dosimetry parameters (specific γ-ray constants, f factor, oblique filtration corrections, to list only a few) associated with the use of ^{226}Ra (33). Anderson conveniently restructures some tables to provide not only milligram hours, but also the integrated reference air kerma (IRAK) in units of centigrays square centimeter recommended by the American Endocurietherapy Society (AES) (150,155,156). Anderson also notes that both systems apply particularly well for use of ^{192}Ir sources, as these sources exhibit little oblique filtration, and that attenuation and multiple scattering in tissue are nearly compensatory within several centimeters of a source (151). Moreover, as many ^{192}Ir seed implants in the United States have been performed using uniform-intensity seeds with uniform spacing implanted in regularly spaced arrays—essentially the Quimby system—there is a substantial clinical experience in treating anatomical targets with prescribed minimal doses with measurable "hot" centers arising from that dose distribution.

The Paris interstitial system (157)—to distinguished from the original Paris system of treatment of intracavitary tumors—uses simple but elegant designs of parallel arrays of equidistant rigid straight ^{192}Ir wire sources of uniform and identical linear activity. Useful reviews of its many rules are available (33,152,153,158). The book, *A Practical Manual of Brachytherapy*, is an excellent resource text fully describing brachytherapy *with a French twist!* (159) This system spaces sources according to the length of the treated region—the greater the length to be treated, the greater the spacing between the sources. Also, the system derives its dose specification from the minimum dose prescribed, not the maximum.

Since ^{192}Ir wire sources have never been manufactured in the United States and the sources must be shipped from Europe, ^{192}Ir wire sources have had limited use in the United States. While numerous articles on its application to ^{192}Ir 3-mm long seeds spaced on 1-cm centers with between-the-seed gaps of 7 mm have appeared, it is generally accepted that the Paris system can be used accurately only if the seeds are spaced with only 1 mm to at most 2-mm gaps between the seeds—an uncommon practice in the United States. Moreover, for many reasons, in many sites where templates are difficult to use, curved seed arrays that conform to the anatomy are more commonly used in the United States. Neither does this system address the question of volume implants that involve more than two planes of sources.

The Memorial system of interstitial implants evolved from operative procedures in which—because the lesion was unresectable—it was decided to implant the lesion permanently, at the time of surgery, with a quantity of radioactive material in proportion to the average dimension of the lesion; this requires determining the lesion's three dimensions during the operative procedure (140). The evolution of this system from its earliest application for ^{222}Rn seeds, ^{125}I seeds, and, most recently, ^{103}Pd and ^{131}Cs seeds involves numerous dosimetry details best described by those who developed and used the system (140). However, the key concept involves matching the volume of the implanted region to the volume of a selected isodose curve encompassing the region, giving rise to the term matched peripheral dose. The original concepts and application nomogram are the basis of the dosimetry for the popular ^{125}I retropubic interstitial implants (140).

All systems described, from which doses are determined, assuming systems rules are followed from tables or nomograms, without computers, represent many years of development and work. Many patients have been systemically treated using these systems; there are published clinical experiences and outcome studies based on these systems. Hence, these systems can be used with confidence by those relatively inexperienced in brachytherapy; if they follow the rules, they will achieve outcomes similar to those previously reported. However, mixing the rules of the various systems, no matter how appealing, generally is not advised.

The advent of computers, discussed in the final section, markedly changed many radiation oncologists' attitudes regarding interstitial implants. The ability to visualize the dose distributions resulting from an implant, or to plan an implant using the computer and dose optimization algorithms, has been a contributing factor to the renewed interest in brachytherapy. However, as previously stressed, no computer optimization algorithm can correct for physical errors of a poorly planned or implanted geometrical arrangement of the sources or applicators. Again, *a poorly planned or executed implant cannot be salvaged by computer optimization methods.*

The simplest method of dose prescription postimplant—matching the three orthogonal dimensions of isodose curves to the three orthogonal dimensions of the target volume and observing the isodose coverage in cross-sectional cuts—is a direct result of computer calculations. For calculations of treatment duration, one selects the isodose-rate curve in which no breaks or gaps occur when isodose-rate curves are displayed over closely spaced (0.5 or 1 cm) cross-sectional cuts of the target, obtained by CT imaging or other methods. There are no requirements regarding dose uniformity, source placement, or other requirements similar to those stated in classical systems. This is more of a clinical practice than a well-defined dosimetry system; it is an alternative approach to matching respective tumor and isodose volumes. A common application of this practice is to perform the match on only the three central cross-sectional cuts that bisect the target volume. However, failure to inspect the isodose-rate curves in off-central-axis cuts can allow serious under doses and/or overdoses in these regions if the selected curve does not adequately cover the target volume or encompasses too much normal tissue. Moreover, it is imperative that the highest dose-rate isodose curves be displayed, so the maximum doses and volumes to tissue treated to these doses are known.

The basic difficulty associated with any of the systems described is confirmation that the resulting dose distribution conforms to the defined target volume as identified during the localization procedure—no system works unless the sources are positioned as planned and the desired degree of dose uniformity (or nonuniformity) has been achieved. The placement of surgical clips and markers that demarcate target boundaries and can be visualized along with simulated sources during localization procedures is highly recommended.

The use of so many different systems of interstitial and intracavitary dosimetry prompted the AES in 1991 to make recommendations for dose specifications in brachytherapy (155,156), including suggested dosimetry summary forms for recording all details of the treatment. The recommendations emphasize that the absorbed dose should be specified in relation to an identified target volume—delineated, if possible by surgical clips or other marking methods—defined as accurately as possible by the means available, that is, with localization films, CT or MRI images. Target volumes are estimated from the three orthogonal dimensions of the target by multiplying their product by a shape factor, $\pi/6$ for an ellipsoid, $\pi/4$ for a cylinder, and so forth (155,156) The planning system or method of planning must be described, as must the absorbed dose prescribed and the way the dose was defined—minimum dose throughout the volume, matched peripheral dose, or other prescription. The absorbed dose rate and treatment duration prescribed is reported, and sketches of the implant geometry are recommended. An evaluation of the treatment determines how well the plan was executed by evaluating how well the plan parameters—dose rate, volume, specified dose, and so on—were achieved. Absorbed doses to special interest points (critical organs) also are evaluated. The AES recommendations are significant, as they represent one of the few attempts to bring standard reporting methodology to brachytherapy (155,156).

Another attempt to unify the reporting of interstitial implant dosimetry is the ICRU report "Dose and volume specification and reporting on interstitial therapy" (160). Megooni offers a useful review (161). The report uses previously established ICRU nomenclature for gross (actual tumor mass) target volume, clinical (tumor mass plus occult disease) target volume, and treatment volume (tissue encompassed by a peripheral isodose surface). Users are not to change their practices of performing implants and stating prescribed dose (the dose the physician intends to deliver and states in the medical record) but are encouraged to adopt the ICRU terminology reporting recommendations. Four definitions of dose are presented:

1. Peripheral dose—the minimum dose encompassing the treatment volume
2. Mean central dose—the arithmetic mean of the doses at middle distances between each pair of adjacent sources (single-plane implant) or between each triad of adjacent source (multiple-plane implant)
3. Low-dose region, whose target volume receives 90% or less of peripheral dose
4. high-dose region, whose target volume receives 150% of the mean central dose

Measures of dose uniformity recommended include reporting the spread in the individual central doses used to obtain the mean central dose and calculating the ratio of the peripheral dose to the mean central dose. Recommendations for reporting the techniques, types of sources, dose rates, duration, total reference air kerma, and other dosimetry data are similar to the AES recommendations. Hanson and Graves reviewed the use of the reporting system for 47 breast implants and concluded the methodology was satisfactory (143).

First used in the early 1980s, ^{125}I seed permanent implants—now using ^{103}Pd or ^{131}I as well—to treat early stage prostate cancer are common. We focus on only the most recent developments in the nearly 30-year evolution of the use of prostate seed implants. AAPM Task Group 137 recommendations on dose prescription and reporting methods (4) provides uniform standards for dose prescription and reporting methods. The American Brachytherapy Society Prostate Low-Dose Rate Task Group (162) offers clinical guidelines for dose prescription by disease stage,

and includes 79 references to guide the uninitiated. Originally, ^{125}I seeds ($T_{1/2}$ = 59.4 d), Model 6702, were used exclusively. ^{103}Pd was used next with a perception that its shorter half-life ($T_{1/2}$ = 16.9 d) and higher initial absorbed dose rate might be advantageous for treating more rapidly growing tumors. In 2004, ^{131}Cs seeds ($T_{1/2}$ = 9.7 d) were introduced. The role of ^{131}Cs has been questioned (163–166) and knowledge of its dosimetry is evolving—consensus data is not available. Nevertheless, ^{131}Cs seed use continues, as there is a perception it may reduce prostate edema postimplant (119,167,168). Developments in prostate implants include the use of ultrasound and CT imaging for postimplant dosimetry (118), study of the effects of seed migration (120), the dosimetry of interseed attenuation and tissue composition (169), new algorithms to help solve the problem of seed matching (170,171), analysis of seed number with variability in prostate dosimetry (172), the use of angulated needles to avoid pubic arch interference (173) and the use of mixed radionuclide implants (20,71) to achieve numerous dosimetry endpoints.

THE CHANGING ROLE OF COMPUTERS IN BRACHYTHERAPY

Computers have been used for brachytherapy dose computations for 50+ years (since 1958). Numerous brachytherapy computational software programs with different dose calculations algorithms are in use. Computers are wonderful tools when properly used; *improperly used, they allow one to quickly make grievous computational errors yielding serious clinical consequences of long duration!*

Users must be exceedingly well versed in the details of the specific computer algorithms they use lest they make serious errors by entering incorrect source parameters or fail to understand whether particular corrections, such as tissue attenuation and multiple scattering, are made by their system's algorithms. It is not sufficient to know *how* to "run the program"; the *user must understand software and the physical effects the software algorithms purport to represent!*

As previously discussed, 3D imaging and treatment planning have changed methods of planning implants and of reporting and evaluating the treatments (125,144). Five features—3D displays, optimization algorithms, cumulative and DDVHs, uniformity indices, and tumor and normal tissue control probabilities—all now available, have a role in brachytherapy. Limited observations are offered about each topic.

Dose optimization algorithms, generally featured on remote-afterloading isodose computation systems, are less commonly employed for static brachytherapy sources. They can, of course, be useful in preplanning for the placement and distribution of static-sources, and they now have a role in fluoroscopy-based intra-operative prostate implant procedures. Interstitial brachytherapy optimization algorithms fall into two broad categories: those associated with distance (single- or double-catheter treatments or single plane) implants and those associated with volume (two or more planes) implants. For distance implants the source or sources—usually with fixed activities—are allowed specified fixed positions, while the boundary conditions (constraint points, dose points) on or near the applicator are specified by the user. The goal is to obtain a stated isodose curve or surface coincident with the dose points. The solutions follow from a linear system of equations solved by numerical techniques or using singular value decomposition that results in minimization of the sum of the squares of the differences between the specified doses and calculated doses at the dose points. In volume implants, dose points alone around the periphery are not sufficient to solve the nonlinear system of equations required to achieve a homogeneous dose among the catheters or applicators in the volume. However, it is possible to use source positions as additional constraint points (geometric optimization). Variations in optimizations technique that are too complex to describe here (geometric optimization on either distance or volume) allow solutions to certain geometries. Similar mathematical algorithms apply in gynecologic brachytherapy optimization algorithms.

Users of optimization algorithms are cautioned to remember that it is impossible to obtain certain isodose distributions. Moreover, optimization for one set of boundary conditions may produce unacceptable isodose curves at other boundaries. For example, boundary conditions that produce relatively uniform (cylindrical) isodose curves at a specified distance from a catheter—achieved by increased source activities near the end of the catheter relative to its center position—close to the catheter ends produce isodose curves much higher than those near the center of the catheter, as shown in Figure 17.10. Also, the different recipes for optimization produce different results. Fast optimization methods are for quick previews of isodose curves and generally are not as accurate as full optimization methods.

Dose-volume relationships are displayed by either cumulative (integral) dose-volume histograms (CDVHS)—percentage volume (*y*-axis) receiving a total dose (*x*-axis)—or by differential (per dose interval) dose-volume histograms (DDVH)–volume per dose interval (*y*-axis) versus dose intervals or dose (*x*-axis). As different volumes can be identified, these displays allow visual inspection of the volumes of targets (GTV, CTV, etc.) or critical organs (bladder, rectum, sigmoid colon, small bowel, etc.) receiving stated doses. (156,160). Examples of each are shown in Figures 17.17 and 17.18.

Uniformity indices are another evaluation tool readily applied with computers. Many such indices have been proposed for use in brachytherapy, but few have gained any widespread acceptance or use (156). Simpler uniformity measures include the ratio of average dose to treatment dose recommended by the AES and the two methods—spread in the individual minimum doses used to obtain mean central dose and ratio of peripheral dose to mean central dose—described by the ICRU (155,156,160). The natural dose-volume histogram developed by Anderson

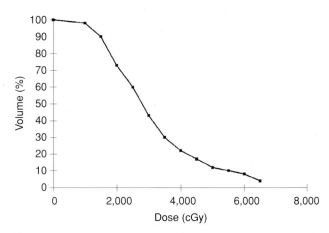

Figure 17.17. A cumulative dose-volume histogram (CDVH). The abscissa is generally expressed as dose (cGy) or dose rate (cGy/h); the ordinate generally is expressed either as absolute volume (cm³) or percentage volume.

defines a baseline variable, $u = (\text{dose})^{-3/2}$, and volume, V, enclosed by a specified isodose surface (151). The histogram is a plot of dV/du versus u, a uniformity index, not given here because of its complexity, is associated with the resulting plot. A single point source (poor uniformity) yields a straight line; a perfectly uniform dose distribution yields a step function (sharp peak) plot. This particular model is gaining acceptance as a computer evaluation tool for determining the uniformity of implants.

TCP and NTCPs, originally proposed for applications of external beam radiotherapy, have been applied to some interstitial implants (174,175). Use of TCP and NTCPs is likely to gain greater acceptance in future years as more accurate biological response data for tumor and normal tissue become available from patients treated with brachytherapy. As shown in Table 17.12, Work Group II recommends reporting biologically weighted dose (144).

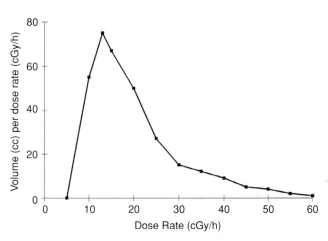

Figure 17.18. A differential dose-volume histogram (DDVH). The abscissa is generally expressed in small increments (e.g., 100 cGy) of dose or small increments (e.g., 10 cGy/h) of dose rate; the ordinate is generally expressed in volume (either cm³ or mm³) per dose or dose-rate increment displayed on the abscissa.

TABLE 17.14			Comparison of Dose Rate from a ^{192}Ir Seed as Calculated by a Computer Model and Compared with Task Group 43 Data (50)		
d (cm)	$g(r)$	$\phi_{an}(r)$	TG-43 Data (cGy/h)^a	μ (cm^{-1})	CMS Computer model (cGy/h)^b
0.5	0.994	0.98	31.182	+0.024900	31.260
1.0	1.000	0.98	7.842	0.000000	7.842
2.0	1.010	0.98	1.980	−0.000497	1.990
4.0	1.010	0.98	0.495	−0.000250	0.497
8.0	0.912	0.98	0.112	+0.001020	0.113

^{a}TG-43 data) converted to mg Ra eq.
^bD(cGy/h) $= A$(mg Ra eq.)$\cdot(\Gamma_\delta)_{Ra}\cdot g(r)\,\bar{\phi}_{an}(r)e^{-\mu x}/d^2$ (cm).
$(\Gamma_\delta)_X = 4.69$ R cm^2/h/mCi; $f_{water/air} = 0.970$ cGy/R.
$(\Gamma_\delta)_{Ra} = 8.25$ R cm^2/h/mCi.
D(cGy/hr) $= A$(mg Ra eq.)$\cdot(\Gamma_\delta)_X\cdot g(r)\,\bar{\phi}_{an}(r)/d^2$ (cm).
TG-43 = Task Group 43.

Advanced 3D planning, or inverse planning, using anatomy-based 3D images from various modalities, as described by Pouliot et al. (176), is analogous to external beam inverse planning. From 3D images, critical structures and target volumes are contoured and limiting doses and desired therapeutic doses assigned to these structures. Using inverse planning optimization methods, the computer algorithms, using an optimization engine (simulated annealing), search for the desired applicator or catheter placements, with assignment of source strengths within catheters or applicators. The method appears particularly promising for HDR brachytherapy treatments of all sites, including the cervix and vagina, but has been applied as well to permanent seed implants of the prostate (175). Future clinical applications are promising.

Other computational developments included application of micro-beam ray tracing to represent single-scatter events (177), application of "Greedy Heuristic" for dose optimization (22), and numerous applications of Monte Carlo calculations (20,178,179,180). BrachyDose is rapid-calculation EGSnrc Monte Carlo code that now has been "benchmarked tested" against the PTRAN Monte Carlo code (181).

I conclude by stressing the importance of testing computer algorithms for correctness. Baseline testing and subsequent quality assurance testing of the dosimetry of single and multiple source arrays, typical gynecological source loadings, and other commonly performed cases is critical to ensure that computations are both precise and accurate. There is a natural evolution of knowledge over time as we learn more and more about the dosimetry of radioactive sources. Moreover, data from different publications may be in conflict. Nevertheless, a data set must be adopted and used to test the computer. One must identify, for each radionuclide, usually of a specific model design, the best known and most widely accepted dosimetry data from published literature or other sources. For example, Table 17.4 compares the doses at points around a ^{137}Cs tube, model 6D6 C-CA (3M, St. Paul, MN), calculated by a CMS Modulex (Computerized Medical Systems, St. Louis, MO) computer with the doses at these same points from published Monte Carlo calculations (58,93). Neither of these data set may be absolutely correct, but this comparison validates the computer calculation. Table 17.14 is a similar comparison for the radial dose from a ^{192}Ir seed using the seed algorithm for that same computer against data from TG-43 (50). The excellent agreement was obtained by using the dummy values listed for the requested attenuation coefficients at each centimeter in the algorithm. While space does not allow presentation of other data for other radionuclides, one cannot emphasis enough the importance of such tests to confirm that the computer yields correct dosimetry results for a single source.

Neblett (182) and Wesick and Li (183) offer extensive suggestions for quality assurance of the brachytherapy isodose computation and planning processes. These simple examples stress just one point: *test, test, test, and test again that all aspects of a brachytherapy computational system are working properly for each type of brachytherapy performed.* Numerous misadministrations in manual brachytherapy reported by the United States Nuclear Regulatory Commission in recent years were associated with users failing to understand or properly use features of their brachytherapy programs.

CONCLUSION

The conclusion of a chapter always triggers Writer's Remorse! Why couldn't I better say more?

The mind races with omitted ideas, tables, and figures that neither space nor time allows inclusion! The knowledgeable reader recognizes the chapter's omissions, deficiency, and shortcomings. To these readers I can only say that I trust the ideas I selected to review are (I hope) without error! To those readers new to brachytherapy, know that it is literally more than 110 years old, with the continued promise of offering hope and benefit to patients treated with either its older methods or continuingly evolving newer methods. I trust this small offering has explained basic concepts, identified some important (but certainly not all!) references, and provided core data and parameters needed for isodose planning in LDR brachytherapy. *Plan Carefully and Well*!

REFERENCES

1. Williamson JF. Brachytherapy technology and physics practice since 1950: a half-century of progress. *Phys Med Biol* 2006;51:R303–R325.
2. Thomadsen BR, Williamson JF, Rivard MJ, et al. Anniversary paper: past and current issues, and trends in brachytherapy physics. *Med Phys* 2008;35:4708–4723.
3. Ibbott G, Ma CM, Rogers DWO, et al. Anniversary Paper: fifty years of AAPM involvement in radiation dosimetry. *Med Phys* 2008;35:1418–1427.
4. Nath R, Bice WS, Chen Z, et al. AAPM recommendations on dose prescription and reporting methods for permanent interstitial brachytherapy for prostate cancer: Report of Task Group 137. *Med Phys* 2009;36:5310–5322.
5. Li Z, Das RK, DeWerd LA, et al. Dosimetric prerequisites for routine clinical use of photon emitting brachytherapy sources with average energy higher than 50 keV. *Med Phys* 2007;34:37–40.
6. Rivard MJ, Butler WM, DeWerd LA, et al. Supplement to the 2004 update of the AAPM Task Group No. 43 Report. *Med Phys* 2007;34:2187–2205.
7. Rivard MJ, Coursey BM, DeWerd LA, et al. Update of AAPM Task Group No. 43 report: a revised AAPM protocol for brachytherapy dose calculations. *Med Phys* 2004; 31:633–674.
8. Rivard MJ, Butler WM, DeWerd LA, et al. Erratum: update of AAPM Task Group No. 43 Report: a revised AAPM protocol for brachytherapy dose calculations. *Med Phys* 2004;31:3532–3533.
9. Papagiannis P, Sakelliou L, Anagnostopoulos G, et al. On the dose rate constant of the selectSeed ^{125}I interstitial brachytherapy seed. *Med Phys* 2006;33:1522–1523.
10. Papagiannis P, Pantelis E, Georgiou E, et al. Polymer gel dosimetry for the TG-43 dosimetric characterization of a new ^{125}I interstitial brachytherapy seed. *Phys Med Biol* 2006;51:1201–2111.
11. Pirchio R, Galiano E, Savari M, et al. On the physical, spectral, and dosimetric characteristics of a new ^{125}I brachytherapy source. *Med Phys* 2007;34:2801–2806.
12. Rivard MJ. Monte Carlo radiation dose simulations and dosimetric comparison of the model 6711 and 9011 ^{125}I brachytherapy sources. *Med Phys* 2009;36:486–491.
13. Usher-Moga J, Beach SM, DeWerd LA. Spectroscopic output of ^{125}I and [103]Pd low dose rate brachytherapy sources. *Med Phys* 2009;36:270–278.

14. Chen ZJ, Nath R. Photon spectrometry for the determination of the dose-rate constant of low-energy photon-emitting brachytherapy sources. *Med Phys* 2007; 34:1412–1430.
15. Wittman RS, Fisher DR. Multiple-estimate Monte Carlo calculation of the dose rate constant for a cesium-131 interstitial brachytherapy seed. *Med Phys* 2007;34: 49–54.
16. Rivard MJ. Brachytherapy dosimetry parameters calculated for a [131]Cs source. *Med Phys* 2007;34:754–762.
17. Wang J, Zhang H. Dosimetric characterization of model CS-1 cesium-131 brachytherapy source in water phantoms and human tissues with MCNP5 Monte Carlo simulation. *Med Phys* 2008;35:1571–1579.
18. Tailor R, Tolani N, Ibbott GS. Thermoluminescence dosimtery measurements of brachytherapy sources in liquid water. *Med Phys* 2008;35:4063–1469.
19. Tailor R, Ibbott GS, Lampe S, et al. Dosimetric characterization of a [131]Cs brachytherapy source by thermoluminescence dosimetry in liquid water. *Med Phys* 2008; 35:5861–5868.
20. Bice WS, Prestidge BR, Kurtzman SM, et al. Recommendations for permanent prostate brachytherapy. with 131Cs: a consensus report from the Cesium Advisory Group. *Brachytherapy* 2008;7:290–296.
21. Nuttens VE, Lucas S. AAPM TG-43U1 formalism adaptation and Monte Carlo dosimetry simulations of multiple-radionuclide brachytherapy sources. *Med Phys* 2006; 33:1101–1107.
22. Chaswal V, Yoo S, Thomadsen BR, et al. Multi-species prostate implant treatment plans incorporating ^{192}Ir and ^{125}I using a Greedy Heuristic based 3D optimization algorithm. *Med Phys* 2007;34:436–444.
23. Nuttens VE, Lucas S. Determination of the prescription dose for biradionuclide permanent prostate brachytherapy. *Med Phys* 2008;35:5451–5462.
24. Lagerburg V, Moerland MA, Seppenwoolde JH, et al. Simulation of the artefact of an iodine seed placed at the needle tip in MRI-guided prostate brachytherapy. *Phys Med Biol* 2008;53:N59–N67.
25. Thomas SD, Wachowicz K, Fallone BG. MRI of prostate brachytherapy seeds at high field: a study in phantom. *Med Phys* 2009;36:5228–5234.
26. Meli J. The need for a dose calibration protocol for brachytherapy sources. *Med Phys* 2007;34:367–368.
27. Yue NJ, Haffty BG, Yue J. On the assay of brachytherapy sources. *Med Phys* 2007;34:1975–1982.
28. Butler WM, Bice WS Jr, DeWerd LA, et al. Third-party brachytherapy sources calibrations and physicist responsibilities: Report of the AAPM Low Energy Brachytherapy Source Calibration Working Group. *Med Phys* 2008; 35:3860–3865.
29. Thomadsen BR, Rivard MJ, Butler WM, eds. *Brachytherapy physics. Joint AAPM/American Brachytherapy Society Summer School.* Madison, WI: Medical Physics Publishing, 2005.
30. Wigg DR. *Applied radiobiology: continuous irradiation and brachytherapy.* Madison, WI: Medical Physics Publishing, 2008.
31. Baltas D, Sakelliou L, Zamboglou N. *The physics of modern brachytherapy for oncology.* New York, NY: Taylor & Francis, 2007.

32. Rivard MJ, Venselaar JLM, Beaulieu L. The evolution of brachytherapy treatment planning. *Med Phys* 2009;36: 2136–2153.

33. Glasgow GP, Perez C. Physics of brachytherapy. In: Perez C, Brady LW, eds. *Principles and practices of radiation oncology*, 2nd ed. Philadelphia, PA: JB Lippincott Co, 1992:265–299.

34. Williamson JF. Semi-empirical dose-calculation models in brachytherapy. In: Thomadsen BR, Rivard MJ, Butler WM, eds. *Brachytherapy physics*, 2nd ed. Joint AAPM/ American Brachytherapy Society Summer School. Madison, WI: Medical Physics Publishing, 2005.

35. Meigooni AS, Wallace RE. Treatment planning considerations of brachytherapy procedures. In: Thomadsen BR, Rivard MJ, Butler WM, eds. *Brachytherapy physics*, 2nd ed. Joint AAPM/American Brachytherapy Society Summer School. Madison, WI: Medical Physics Publishing, 2005.

36. Khan FM. *The physics of radiation therapy*, 3rd ed. Baltimore, MD: William & Wilkins, 2003:357–400.

37. Aird EG, Williams JR. Brachytherapy. In: Williams JR, Thwaites DI, eds. *Radiotherapy physics in practice*. Oxford: Oxford Medical Publications, 1993.

38. Bureau International des Poids et Measures. *Le Systeme International d'Unites (SI). French and English texts.* Servres, France: Bureau International des Poids et Measures, 1991.

39. Papagiannis P, Baltas D, Granero D, et al. Radiation transmission data for radionuclides and materials relevant to brachytherapy facility shielding. *Med Phys* 2008; 35:4898–4906.

40. Williamson JF, Coursey BM, DeWerd LA, et al. On the use of apparent activity (A$_{app}$) for treatment planning of ^{125}I and ^{103}Pd interstitial brachytherapy sources: recommendations of the AAPM Radiation Therapy Committee Subcommittee on low-energy brachytherapy source dosimetry. *Med Phys* 1999;26:2529–2530.

41. International Commission on Radiological Units and Measurements. *Radiation quantities and units, Report 10 a*. Washington, DC: International Commission on Radiological Units and Measurements, 1962.

42. International Commission on Radiological Units and Measurements. *Radiation quantities and units, Report 19*. Washington, DC: International Commission on Radiological Units and Measurements, 1971.

43. Glasgow GP. Specific γ-ray constant and exposure rate constant of ^{192}Ir. *Med Phys* 1979;6:49–52.

44. Glasgow GP. Exposure rate constants for filtered ^{192}Ir sources. *Med Phys* 1981;8:502–503.

45. International Commission on Radiological Units and Measurements. *Radiation quantities and units, Report 33*. Washington, DC: International Commission on Radiological Units and Measurements, 1980.

46. International Commission on Radiation Units and Measurements (ICRU). *Dose and volume specification for reporting intracavitary therapy in gynecology, Report No. 38*. Bethesda, MD: ICRU, 1985.

47. American Association of Physicists in Medicine. *Recommendations of AAPM Task Group 32: specification of brachytherapy source strength, Report No. 21*. New York: American Institute of Physics, 1987.

48. American Brachytherapy Society Cervical Cancer Brachytherapy Task Group. Available from americanbrachytherapy. org/guidelines/index.ctu/1/28/2010.

49. Interstitial Collaborative Working Group. *Interstitial brachytherapy*. New York: Raven Press, 1990.

50. Nath R, Anderson LL, Luxton G, et al. Dosimetry of interstitial brachytherapy sources: recommendations of the AAPM Radiation Therapy Committee Task Group No. 43. *Med Phys* 1995;22:209–233.

51. Taylor REP, Rogers DWO. More accurate fitting of ^{125}I and ^{103}Pd radial dose functions. *Med Phys* 2008;35:4242–4250.

52. Patterson MS. Medical physics top ten. *Med Phys* 2004; 31:682.

53. Weaver K. Dose calculation models in brachytherapy. In: Williamson JF, Thomadsen BR, Nath R, eds. *Brachytherapy physics, AAPM summer school*. Madison, WI: Medical Physics Publishing, 1995.

54. Williamson JF. Monte Carlo-based dose rate tables for the Amersham CDCS. J and 3M Model 6500 Cs-137 Tubes. *Int J Radiat Oncol Biol Phys* 1998;41:959–970.

55. Pérez-Calatayud J, Granero D, Ballester F, et al. Technical note: Monte Carlo derivation of TG-43 dosimetric parameters for radiation therapy resources and 3M Cs-137 sources. *Med Phys* 2005;32:2464–2470.

56. Pérez-Calatayud J, Ballester F, Serrano-Anders MA, et al. Dosimetry characteristics of the CDC-type miniature cylindrical Cs-137 brachytherapy source. *Med Phys* 2002;29:538–543.

57. Ballester F, Lluch JL, Limami Y, et al. A Monte Carlo investigation of the dosimetric characteristics of the CSM11 Cs-137 sources from CIS. *Med Phys* 2000;27:2182–2189.

58. Casal E, Ballester F, Lluch JL, et al. Monte Carlo calculations of dose rate distributions around the Amersham CDCS-M-type Cs-137 source. *Med Phys* 2000;27:132–140.

59. Liu L, Prasad SC, Bassano DA. Determination of Cs-137 dosimetry parameters according to the AAPM TG-43 formalism. *Med Phys* 2004;31:477–483.

60. Melhus CS, Rivard MJ. Approaches to calculating AAPM TG-43 brachytherapy dosimetry parameters for ^{137}Cs, ^{125}I, ^{192}Ir, ^{103}Pd, and ^{169}Yb sources. *Med Phys* 2006; 33:1729–1737

61. Vianello EA, deAlmeida CE. Experimental derivation of the fluence non-uniformity correction for air kerma near brachytherapy linear sources. *Med Phys* 2008;35:3389–3392.

62. Meigooni AS, Wright C, Koona RA, et al. TG-43 U! based dosimetric characterization of model 67–6520 Cs-137 brachytherapy source. *Med Phys* 2009;36:4711–4719.

63. Pérez-Calatayud J, Lliso F, Carmona V, et al. Monte Carlo calculation of dose rate distributions around 0.5 and 0.6 mm in diameter Ir-192 wires. *Med Phys* 1999; 26:395–401.

64. Karaiskos P, Papagiannis P, Angelopoulos L, et al. Dosimetry of ^{192}Ir wires for LDR interstitial brachytherapy following the AAPM TG-43 dosimetric formalism. *Med Phys* 2001;28:156–166.

65. Van Der Laarse R, Granero A, Pérez-Calatayud J, et al. Dosimetry characterization of ^{192}Ir LDR elongated sources. *Med Phys* 2008;35:1154–1161.

66. Ballester F, Granero D, Pérez-Calatayud J, et al. Monte Carlo dosimetric study of Best Industries and Alpha Omega Ir-192 brachytherapy seeds. *Med Phys* 2004;31:3298–3305.

67. Papagiannis P, Angelopoulos A, Pentelis E, et al. Dosimetry comparison of Ir-192 sources. *Med Phys* 2002;29: 2239–2246.

68. Anctil JC, Clark BG, Arsenault CJ. Experimental determination of the dosimetry functions of Ir-192 sources. *Med Phys* 1998;25:2279–2287.

69. Melchert C, Kohr P, Schmidt R. Calculation of dose decrease in a finite phantom of a ^{192}Ir point source. *Med Phys* 2007;34:3943–3950.

70. Tedgren AC, Carisson GA. Influence of phantom material and dimensions on experimental ^{192}Ir dosimetry. *Med Phys* 2009;36:2228–2235.

71. Glasgow GP, Dogan N, Mohideen N. Is an ^{192}Ir permanent seed implant feasible for prostate brachytherapy? *Brachytherapy* 2002;1:195–203.

72. Dauffy LS. Dosimetry characteristics and a standard for the Au-198 seed used in interstitial brachytherapy. *Med Phys* 2004;31:683 (Abst).

73. Dauffy LS, Braby LA, Berner BM. Dosimetry of the Au-198 source used in interstitial brachytherapy. *Med Phys* 2005;32:1579–1588.

74. Meigooni AS, Zhang H, Clark JR, et al. Dosimetry characteristics of the new RadioCoil™ Pd-103 wire line source for use in permanent brachytherapy implants. *Med Phys* 2004;31:3095–3105.

75. Rivard MJ, Melhus CS, Kirk BL. Brachytherapy dosimetry parameters calculated for a new Pd-103 source. *Med Phys* 2004;31:2466–2470.

76. Paxton AB, Culberson WS, deWerd LA, et al. Primary calibration of coiled ^{103}Pd brachytherapy sources. *Med Phys* 2008;35:32–38.

77. Sadeghi M, Raisali G, Hosseini SM, et al. Monte Carlo calculations and experimental measurements of dosimetric parameters of the IRA-^{103}Pd brachytherapy source. *Med Phys* 2008;35:1288–1294.

78. Abboud F, Scalliet P, Vynckier S. An experimental palladium-103 seed (OptiSeed^{exp}) in a biocompatible polymer without a gold marker: characterization of dissymmetric parameters including the interseed effect. *Med Phys* 2008; 35:5841–5850.

79. Murphy MK, Piper RK, Greenwood LR, et al. Evaluation of the new Cesium-131 seed for use in low-energy x-ray brachytherapy. *Med Phys* 2004;31:1529–1538.

80. Chen Z, Bongiorni P, Nath R. Dose rate constant of a Cesium-131 interstitial brachytherapy seed measured by thermoluminescent dosimetry and gamma ray spectrometry. *Med Phys* 2005;32:3279–3295.

81. Yue N, Heron DE, Komanduri K, et al. Prescription dose in permanent Cs-131 seed prostate implants. *Med Phys* 2005;32:2496–2502.

82. Granero D, Pérez-Calatayud J, Ballester F, et al. Broadbeam transmission data for new brachytherapy sources, Tm-170 and Yb-169. *Radiat Prot Dosim* 2005;118: 11–15.

83. Lymperopoulou G, Papagiannis P, Sakelliou L, et al. Comparison of radiation shielding requirements for HDR brachytherapy using ^{169}Yb and ^{192}Ir sources. *Med Phys* 2006;33:2541–2547.

84. Mainegra E, Capote R, López E. Dose rate constants for ^{125}I, ^{103}Pd, ^{192}Ir, and ^{169}Yb brachytherapy sources. *Phys Med Biol* 1998;43:1557–1566.

85. Karaiskos P, Sakelliou L, Sandilos P, et al. Limitations of the point and line source approximations for the determination of geometry factors around brachytherapy sources. *Med Phys* 2000;27:124–128.

86. Baltas D, Karaiskos P, Papagiannis P, et al. Beta versus gamma dosimetry close to Ir-192 brachytherapy sources. *Med Phys* 2001;28:1875–1882.

87. Iwata K, Yue NJ, Nath R. Near field dosimetry of I-125 sources for interstitial brachytherapy implants measured using thermoluminescent sheets. *Med Phys* 2004; 31:3406–3416.

88. Ballester F, Granero D, Pérez-Calatayud J, et al. Evaluation of high-energy brachytherapy source electronic equilibrium and dose from emitted electrons. *Med Phys* 2009; 36:4250–4256.

89. Nath R, Chen ZJ. Silver fluorescent x-ray yield and its influence on the dose rate constant for nine low-energy brachytherapy source models. *Med Phys* 2007;34: 3785–3793.

90. Karaiskos P, Angelopoulos A, Baras P, et al. dose rate calculations around Ir-192 brachytherapy. Sources using a sievert integration model. *Phys Med Biol* 2000;45:383–398.

91. Meli JA. Dosimetry of some interstitial and intracavitary sources and their applicators. In: Williamson JF, Thomadsen BR, Nath R, eds. *Brachytherapy physics, AAPM summer school.* Madison, WI: Medical Physics Publishing, 1995.

92. Meigooni AS, Wallace RE. Treatment planning considerations of brachytherapy procedure. In: Thomadsen BR, Rivard MJ, Butler WM, eds. *Brachytherapy physics,* 2nd ed. Joint AAPM/America Brachytherapy Society Summer School. Madison, WI: Medical Physics Publishing, 2005.

93. Krishnaswamy V. Dose distribution about cesium-137 sources in tissue. *Radiology* 1972;105:181–184.

94. Willamson JF, Pevera H, Li Z, et al. Comparison of calculated and measured heterogeneity correction factors for I-125, Cs-137, and Ir-192. *Med Phys* 1993;20:209–222.

95. Hale J. The use of interstitial dose rate tables for other radioactive isotopes. *Am J Roentgenol* 1958;79:49–53.

96. Kornelson RO, Young MES. Brachytherapy buildup factors. *Br J Radiol* 1981;54:136.

97. Venselaar JLM, Van Der Giessen PH, Dries WJF. Measurement and calculation of the dose at large distances from brachytherapy sources: Cs-137, Ir-192, and Co-60. *Med Phys* 1996;23:537–543.

98. Meisberger LL, Keller RJ, Shalek RJ. The effective attenuation in water of the y-rays of gold-198, iridium-192, radium-226, and cobalt-60. *Radiology* 1968;90:953–957.

99. Van Kleffens HJ, Star WM. Application of stereo x-ray photogrammetry in the determination of absorbed dose values during intracavitary radiation therapy. *Int J Radiat Oncol Biol Phys* 1979;5:557–563.

100. Furhang EE, Anderson LL. Functional fitting of interstitial brachytherapy dosimetry data recommended by the AAPM Radiation Therapy Committee Task Group 43. *Med Phys* 1999;26:153–160.

101. Moss DC. Technical note: improved analytic fit to the TG-43 radial dose function, g(r). *Med Phys* 2000;27: 659–661.

102. Hass JS, Dean RD, Mansfield CM. Evaluation of a new Fletcher applicator using cesium-137. *Int J Radiat Oncol Biol Phys* 1980;6:1593–1600.

103. Williamson JF. Dose calculations about shielded gynecological copostats. *Int J Radiat Oncol Biol Phys* 1990; 19:167–178.

104. Sloboda RS, Wang R. Combined experimental and Monte Carlo verification of Cs-137 brachytherapy plans for vaginal applicators. *Phys Med Biol* 1998;43:3495–3507.

105. Daskalov GM, Kirov AS, Williamson JF. Analytical approach to heterogeneity correction factor calculation for brachytherapy. *Med Phys* 1998;25:722–735.

106. Williamson JF, Meigooni AS. Quantitative dosimetry methods in brachytherapy. In: Williamson JF, Thomadsen BR, Nath R, eds. *Brachytherapy physics, AAPM summer school.* Madison, WI: Medical Physics Publishing, 1995.

107. Parsai EI, Zhang Z, Feldmeier JJ. A quantitative three-dimensional dose attenuation analysis around Fletcher-Suit-Delclos due to stainless steel tube for high-dose-rate brachytherapy by Monte Carlo calculations. *Brachytherapy* 2009;8:318–323.

108. Weeks KJ, Dennett JC. Dose calculations and measurements for a CT-compatible version of the Fletcher applicator. *Int J Radiat Oncol Biol Phys* 1990;18:1191–1198.

109. Weeks KJ, Montana GS. Three-dimensional applicator system for carcinoma of the uterine cervix. *Int J Radiat Oncol Biol Phys* 1997;37:455–463.

110. Weeks KJ. Monte Carlo dose calculations for a new ovoid shield system for carcinoma of the uterine cervix. *Med Phys* 1998;25:2288–2294.

111. Price MJ, Jackson EF, Gifford KA, et al. Development of prototype shielded cervical intracavitary brachytherapy applicators compatible with CT and MR imaging. *Med Phys* 2009;36:5515–5524.

112. Gifford KA, Horton JL Jr, Jackson EF, et al. Comparison of Monte Carlo calculations around a Fletcher Suit Delclos ovoid with radiochromic film and normoxic polymer gel dosimetry. *Med Phys* 2005;32:2288–2294.

113. Tedgren-Carlsson AK, Ahnesjo A. Accounting for high Z shields in brachytherapy using collapsible factor calculation for brachytherapy. *Med Phys* 2003;30:2206–2217.

114. Martel MK. Three-dimensional imaging techniques. In: Williamson JF, Thomadsen BR, Nath R, eds. *Brachytherapy physics, AAPM summer school.* Madison, WI: Medical Physics Publishing, 1995.

115. Lief EP. Localization, Part I: radiographic methods and accuracy. In: Thomadsen BR, Rivard MJ, Butler WM, eds. *Brachytherapy physics,* 2nd ed. Joint AAPM/America Brachytherapy Society Summer School, Madison, WI: Medical Physics Publishing, 2005.

116. Rownd J. Localization, Part II. Volume imaging techniques and accuracy for brachytherapy dosimetry. In: Thomadsen BR, Rivard MJ, Butler WM, eds. *Brachytherapy physics,* 2nd ed. Joint AAPM/America Brachytheraphy Society Summer School, Madison, WI: Medical Physics Publishing, 2005.

117. Erickson B. Imaged-based brachytherapy: a forum for collaboration between radiation oncologists and diagnostic radiologists. *J Am Coll Cardiol* 2005;2:735–758.

118. Ali I, Algan O, Thompson S, et al. A comparative study of seed localization and dose calculation on pre- and post-implantation ultrasound and CT images for low-dose-rate prostate brachytherapy. *Phys Med Biol* 2009;54:5595–5611.

119. Villeneuve M, Leclerc G, Lessard E, et al. Relationship between isotope half-life and prostate edema for optimal prostate dose coverage in permanent seed implants. *Med Phys* 2008;35:1970–1977.

120. Gao M, Wang JZ, Nag S, et al. Effects of seed migration on post-implant dosimetry of prostate brachytherapy. *Med Phys* 2007;34:471–480.

121. Fellner C, Potter R, Knocke TH, et al. Comparison of radiography- and computed tomography-based treatment planning in cervix cancer in brachytherapy with specific attention to some quality assurance aspects. *Radiother Oncol* 2001;5:53–62.

122. Viswanathan AN, Dimopoulos J, Kiristis C, et al. Computed tomography versus magnetic resonance imaging-based contouring in cervical cancer brachytherapy: Results of a prospective trial and preliminary guidelines for standardized contours. *Int J Radiat Oncol Biol Phys* 2007;68:491–498.

123. Lerma FA, Williamson JF. Accurate localization of intracavitary brachytherapy applicators from CT imaging studies. *Med Phys* 2002;29:325–333.

124. Wachter-Gerstner N, Wachter S, Reinstadler E, et al. Bladder and rectum dose defined from MRI based treatment planning for cervix cancer brachytherapy: comparison of dose-volume histograms for organ contours and organ wall, comparison with ICRU rectum and bladder reference points. *Radiother Oncol* 2003;68:269–276.

125. Haie-Meder C, Pötter R, Van Limbergen E, et al. Recommendations from Gynaecological (GYN) GEC-ESTRO Working Group (I); concepts and terms in 3D image based 3D treatment planning in cervix cancer brachytherapy with emphasis on MRI assessment of GTV and CTV. *Radiother Oncol* 2005;74:235–245.

126. Meli JA. Source localization. In: Williamson JF, Thomadsen BR, Nath R, eds. *Brachytherapy physics, AAPM summer school.* Madison, WI: Medical Physics Publishing, 1995.

127. Harris T, Hunter RJ, Skoczny J, et al. The variance of bladder and rectal doses calculated from orthogonal and simple stereo films in cervix high-dose-rate brachytherapy. *Brachytherapy* 2007;6:304–310.

128. Fung AYC. C-arm imaging for brachytherapy source reconstruction: geometrical accuracy. *Med Phys* 2002;29:724–726.

129. Liu L, Bassano DA, Prasad SC, et al. The use of C-arm fluoroscopy for treatment planning in high dose rate brachytherapy. *Med Phys* 2003;30:2297–2302.

130. Palvolgi J. Multiparametric fit method in reconstruction of Fletcher-Suit-Delclos applicator. *Med Phys* 2006;33:69–75.

131. Anderson LL. Dosimetry for interstitial radiation therapy. In: Hilaris BS, ed. *Handbook of interstitial brachytherapy.* Acton, MA: Publishing Sciences Group, 1975:87–116.

132. Rosenthal MS, Nath R. An automatic seed identification technique for interstitial implants using three isocentric radiographs. *Med Phys* 1983;10:475–479.

133. Amols HI, Rosen II. A three-film technique for reconstruction of radioactive seed implants. *Med Phys* 1981;8:210–214.

134. Biggs PJ, Kelly DM. Geometric reconstruction of seed implants using a three-film technique. *Med Phys* 1983;10:701–704.

135. Siddon RL, Chin LM. Two-film brachytherapy reconstruction algorithm. *Med Phys* 1985;12:77–83.

136. Todor DA, Cohen GN, Amlos HI, et al. Operator-free, film based 3D seed reconstruction in brachytherapy. *Phys Med Biol* 2002;47:2031–2048.

137. Holupka EJ, Meskell PM, Burdette EC, et al. An automatic seed finder for brachytherapy CT postplans based on the Hough transform. *Med Phys* 2004;31: 2672–2679.

138. Potish RA, Gerbi BJ, Engeler GP. Dose prescriptions, dose specifications, and applicator geometry in intracavitary therapy. In: Williamson JF, Thomadsen BR, Nath R, eds. *Brachytherapy physics, AAPM summer school.* Madison, WI: Medical Physics Publishing, 1995.

139. Maruyuma Y, Van Nagell JR, Wrede DF, et al. Approaches to optimization of dose in radiation therapy of cervix carcinoma. *Radiology* 1976;10:389–398.

140. Hilaris BS, Nori D, Anderson LL. *Atlas of brachytherapy.* New York: McMIllian, 1998.

141. Nag S, Chao C, Erickson B, et al. The American Brachytherapy Society recommendations for low-dose rate brachytherapy for carcinoma of the cervix. *Int J Radiat Oncol Biol Phys* 2002;52:33–48.

142. Thomadsen BR. ICRU reporting for cervical brachytherapy. In: Thomadsen BR, Rivard MJ, Butler WM, eds. *Brachytherapy physics,* 2nd ed. Joint AAPM/America Brachytheraphy Society Summer School. Madison, WI: Medical Physics Publishing, 2005.

143. Hanson WF, Graves M. ICRU recommendations on dose specification in brachytherapy. In: Williamson JF, Thomadsen BR, Nath R, eds. *Brachytherapy physics, AAPM summer school.* Madison, WI: Medical Physics Publishing, 1995.

144. Pötter R, Haie-Meder C, Van Limbergen E, et al. Recommendations from Gynaecological (GYN) GEC-ESTRO Working Group (II): concepts and terms in 3D image-based treatment planning in cervix cancer – 3D dose volume parameters and aspects of 3D imaged-based anatomy, radiation physics, radiobiology. *Radiother Oncol* 2006;78:67–77.

145. Kim RY, Pareek P. Radiography-based treatment planning compared with computed tomography (CT)-based treatment planning for intracavitary brachytherapy in cancer of the cervix: analysis of dose-volume histograms. *Brachytherapy* 2003;2:200–206.

146. Pelloski CE, Palmer M, Chronowski GM, et al. Comparison between CT-based volumetric calculations and ICRU reference-point estimates of radiation doses delivered to bladder and rectum during intracavitary radiotherapy for cervical cancer. *Int J Radiat Oncol Biol Phys* 2004;62:131–137.

147. Shin KH, Kim TH, Cho, JK, et al. CT-guided intracavitary radiotherapy for cervical cancer: Comparison of conventional point A plan with clinical target volume-based three-dimensional plan using dose-volume parameters. *Int J Radiat Oncol Biol Phys* 2005;62:197–204.

148. Kirisits C, Pötter R, Lang S, et al. Dose and volume parameters for MRI treatment planning in intracavitary brachytherapy for cervical cancer. *Int J Radiat Oncol Biol Phys* 2005;62:901–911.

149. Kim RY, Shen S, Duan J. Image-based three-dimensional treatment planning of intracavitary brachytherapy for cancer of the cervix: dose-volume histograms of the bladder, rectum, sigmoid colon, and small bowel. *Brachytherapy* 2007;6:187–194.

150. Anderson LL. Dose specification and quantification of implant quality. In: Williamson JF, Thomadsen BR, Nath R, eds. *Brachytherapy physics, AAPM summer school.* Madison, WI: Medical Physics Publishing, 1995.

151. Anderson LL, Presser JE. Classical systems I for temporary interstitial implants. In: Williamson JF, Thomadsen BR, Nath R, eds. *Brachytherapy physics, AAPM summer school.* Madison, WI: Medical Physics Publishing, 1995.

152. Gillin MJ, Albano KS, Erickson B. Classical systems II for planar and volume temporary interstitial implants. In: Williamson JF, Thomadsen BR, Nath R, eds. *Brachytherapy physics, AAPM summer school.* Madison, WI: Medical Physics Publishing, 1995.

153. Gillin MJ, Mourtada F. Systems 1B: Manchester planar and volume implants and the Paris system. In: Thomadsen BR, Rivard MJ, Butler WM, eds. *Brachytherapy physics,* 2nd ed. Joint AAPM/America Brachytheraphy Society Summer School. Madison, WI: Medical Physics Publishing, 2005.

154. Zwicker RD. Quimby-based brachytherapy systems. In: Thomadsen BR, Rivard MJ, Butler WM, eds. *Brachytherapy physics,* 2nd ed. Joint AAPM/America Brachytheraphy Society Summer School. Madison, WI: Medical Physics Publishing, 2005.

155. Anderson LL, Nath R, Olch AJ, et al. American Endocurietherapy Society recommendations for dose specification in brachytherapy. *Endocurieth Hyperth Oncol* 1991;7:1–12.

156. Anderson LL. Brachytherapy planning and evaluation. *Endocurieth Hyperth Oncol* 1991;7:139–146.

157. Piequin B, Wilson JF, Chassagne D. *Modern brachytherapy.* New York: Masson, 1987.

158. Gooden TS. *Physical aspects of brachytherapy. Medical physics handbook 19.* Bristol: Adam-Hilger, 1988.

159. Pierquin B, Marinello G. *A practical manual of brachytherapy.* Madison, WI: Medical Physics Publishing, 1997.

160. International Commission on Radiation Units and Measurements. *Dose and volume specification for reporting interstitial brachytherapy. Report No. 58.* Bethesda, MD: International Commission on Radiation Units and Measurements, 1997.

161. Meigooni AS. ICRU recommended dose and volume specifications for brachytherapy. In: Thomadsen BR, Rivard MJ, Butler WM, eds. *Brachytherapy physics,* 2nd ed. Joint AAPM/America Brachytherapy Society Summer School. Madison, WI: Medical Physics Publishing, 2005.

162. American Brachytherapy Society Prostate Low-Dose Rate Task Group. Available from americanbrachytherapy. org/guidelines/index.ctu/1/28/2010.

163. Bice WS. Point: cesium-131: ready for prime time? *Brachytherapy* 2009;8:1–3.

164. Butler WM. Counterpoint: cesium-131: not ready for prime time? *Brachytherapy* 2009;8:6.

165. Bice WS. Rebuttal to Dr. Butler. *Brachytherapy* 2009;8:7.

166. Butler WM. Rebuttal to Dr. Bice. *Brachytherapy* 2009; 8:8.

167. Chen Z, Deng J, Roberts K, et al. Potential impact of prostate edema on the dosimetry of permanent seed implants using the new ^{131}Cs (model CS-1) seeds. *Med Phys* 2006;33:968–975.

168. Wang JZ, Mayr NA, Nag S, et al. Effect of edema, relative biological effectiveness, and dose heterogeneity on prostate brachytherapy. *Med Phys* 2006;33: 1025–1032.

169. Carrier JF, Beauileau L, Therriault-Prouix F, et al. Impact of interseed attenuation and tissue composition for permanent implants. *Med Phys* 2006;33:595–604.

170. Siebert FA, Srivastav A, Kliemann L, et al. Three-dimensional reconstruction of seed implants by randomized rounding and visual evaluation. *Med Phys* 2007;34:967–975.

171. Su Y, Davis BJ, Furutani KM, et al. Prostate brachytherapy seed reconstruction using an adaptive grouping technique. *Med Phys* 2007;34:2975–2984.

172. Su Y, Davis BJ, Furutani KM, et al. Dosimetry accuracy as a function of seed localization uncertainty in permanent prostate brachytherapy: increased seed number correlates with less variability in prostate dosimetry. *Phys Med Biol* 2007;52:3105–3119.

173. Fu L, Liu H, Ng WS, et al. Hybrid dosimetry: feasibility of mixing angulated and parallel needles in planning prostate brachytherapy. *Med Phys* 2006;33:1192–1198.

174. Ling CC, Roy JN. Radiophysical aspects of brachytherapy. In: Williamson JF, Thomadsen BR, Nath R, eds. *Brachytherapy physics, AAPM summer school.* Madison, WI: Medical Physics Publishing, 1995.

175. Strigari L, Orlandini LC, Andriani I, et al. A mathematical approach for evaluating the influence of dose heterogeneity on TCP for prostate cancer brachytherapy treatments. *Phys Med Biol* 2008;53:5045–5049.

176. Pouliot J, Lessarde E, Hsu I. Advanced 3D Planning. In: Thomadsen BR, Rivard MJ, Butler WM, eds. *Brachytherapy physics,* 2nd ed. Joint AAPM/America Brachytheraphy Society Summer School. Madison, WI: Medical Physics Publishing, 2005.

177. Wang R, Sloboda RS. Brachytherapy scatter dose calculation in heterogeneous media: I. A microbeam ray-tracing method for the single-scatter contribution. *Phys Med Biol* 2007;52:5619–5636.

178. Rivard MJ, Melhus CS, Granero D, et al. An approach to using conventional brachytherapy software for clinical treatment planning of complex, Monte Carlo-based brachytherapy dose distributions. *Med Phys* 2009;36:1968–1975.

179. Pérez-Calatayud J, CabaNero DG, Pallares FB. Monte Carlo applications in brachytherapy. In: Lemoigne Y, Caner A, eds. *Radiotherapy and brachytherapy. NATO science for peace and security series B: physics and biophysics.* Dordrecht, The Netherlands: Springer Netherlands, 2009.

180. Chibani O, Williamson JF. MCPI: a sub-minute Monte Carlo dose calculation engine for prostate implants. *Med Phys* 2005;32:3688–3698.

181. Taylor REP, Yegin G, Rogers DWO. Benchmarking brachydose: voxel based EGSnrc Monte Carlo calculations of TG-43 dosimetry parameters. *Med Phys* 2007;34:445–457.

182. Neblett DL, Wesick JS. Quality assurance of computer-assisted planning. In: Williamson JF, Thomadsen BR, Nath R, eds. *Brachytherapy physics, AAPM summer school.* Madison, WI: Medical Physics Publishing, 1995.

183. Li Z. Quality review of brachytherapy treatment systems. In: Thomadsen BR, Rivard MJ, Butler WM, eds. *Brachytherapy physics,* 2nd ed. Joint AAPM/America Brachytherapy Society Summer School. Madison, WI: Medical Physics Publishing, 2005.

CHAPTER 18

High Dose-Rate Brachytherapy Treatment Planning

Bruce R. Thomadsen

GENERAL CONSIDERATIONS OF HIGH DOSE-RATE BRACHYTHERAPY TREATMENTS

High dose-rate (HDR) brachytherapy forms a special method of delivering brachytherapy where the treatment session lasts a short time. What constitutes "a short time" is considered below, but in the overview, the treatment session takes from 20 minutes to a couple of hours, as opposed to a day to several days for conventional, low dose-rate (LDR) brachytherapy. Most of treatment planning for HDR brachytherapy remains identical to that for general brachytherapy, which is covered in Chapter 8. This chapter will only consider those aspects of treatment planning that are either unique for, or of much greater importance to, HDR planning. The discussion that follows does not go in order of steps to perform for an HDR application. For example, planning a brachytherapy procedure, which constitutes the first step, comes late in the chapter. One reason for not following the procedural order is that the order varies depending on the nature of the procedure. However, the main reason is that the principles covered early in this chapter must be understood before applying them in planning.

Several methods have been used in the past to deliver the treatment in the short time, but all units currently use the same principal—a very intense radioactive source on a computer-controlled cable steps through the target volume, pausing for specified periods at particular locations along the way. The pausing locations are referred to as *dwell positions,* and the duration for which the source pauses are *dwell times.* Often, the dwell times are normalized to a particular dwell time location or the maximum, in which case the normalized values are called *dwell weights.* A unit that operates in such a manner is called a *stepping source device.* The radioactive source for most units is ^{192}Ir, although some use ^{169}Yb, or two sources, one each of iridium and ytterbium. Some very old units use ^{60}Co. The operation of HDR units is discussed in detail in many texts (1,2). Since this chapter deals with the treatment-planning aspect of HDR brachytherapy, further description of the units proper is left to the reader's initiative.

HDR brachytherapy offers several advantages over LDR brachytherapy.

1. **Improved dose optimization capability.** In an HDR brachytherapy application, the dwell positions perform the same role as the source positions do for LDR brachytherapy. For example, the same locations where individual iridium sources would fall in an LDR gynecological implant, the single HDR source would pause for a dwell position. Such an LDR implant could, and should, be "optimized." "Optimization," in this context, means adjusting the strength or positions of the sources to obtain a dose distribution with specified, desired characteristics (3). One optimization goal often is simply that a specified isodose surface covers a target volume. Other optimization criteria might include a specified required homogeneity for the dose through the target volume, or the maximum dose allowed to other anatomical structures. Optimization of a medium size LDR implants often requires 8 to 10 different source strengths, which sometimes becomes difficult to obtain from a supplier. For a similar HDR unit, the dwell times at each dwell position, on the other hand, commonly may vary in increments of 0.1 second from 0 to 999 seconds. Thus, satisfying the optimization requirements becomes easier with the great flexibility in relative strength at each dwell position. Optimization plays such an important part in HDR treatment planning that a section of this chapter is devoted to this topic.

2. **More stable positioning.** For intracavitary insertions, HDR applicators usually lock into their treatment positions through fixation to the treatment couch. With the patient essentially immobilized (e.g., in stirrups and strapped to the table), the applicator moves little between imaging for dosimetry calculations and the completion of the treatment session. One series studying the movement of HDR tandem and ovoid applications reported an average movement based on skeletal anatomy of 2 mm (4). This compares with an average of 2 cm movement for LDR tandem and ovoids (5).

3. **Adding distance to normal tissue.** For some HDR treatments—notably gynecological intracavitary insertions or head and neck interstitial implants—normal tissue structures can be pushed away from the path of the source during the treatment, reducing their dose. While not every treatment site can use this technique, in those for which it applies the dose reduction to normal structures can be marked. In general, the discomfort that similar tissue displacement would cause over the multiple-day treatments for LDR brachytherapy would be intolerable.

4. **Outpatient treatment.** The driving force that led to the wide use of HDR brachytherapy was the economic shift in reimbursement it produced from the inpatient hospital to the clinical facility that delivers the HDR treatments. This occurs because most HDR treatments are delivered on an outpatient basis. In addition to changing the revenue patterns, outpatient treatments usually are much more convenient and comfortable for the patients than confinement in a hospital room in radiation isolation.

5. **Smaller applicators.** For gynecological intracavitary applications, the tandem used for HDR treatment of uterine cancer has only a 3-mm diameter compared with the 7-mm diameter tandem used for LDR brachytherapy. The dilation required to insert the LDR tandem forms the most painful part of the treatment procedure. By comparison, the sound used to measure the length of the uterine cavity before dilation takes place is also 3-mm in diameter and often requires no anesthesia.

6. **Intraoperative and perioperative treatments.** For interstitial cases, HRD brachytherapy treatment can commence immediately following insertion of the applicator or catheters, localization imaging, and dose calculations. LDR brachytherapy cases usually require ordering the sources, or if sources were ordered ahead, performing the implant as planned without the possibility of modifications based on new information noted during the operative procedure. This ability to treat immediately after placement, along with the short duration of treatment, opens the possibility of using HDR brachytherapy during operative cases (intraoperative) for irradiation of tumor beds during resection or for wider use of image-guided implants (6).

7. **Reduction of radiation exposure to health care providers.** The final advantage of HDR brachytherapy is that all personnel leave the treatment room for the actual delivery of the radiation, and with adequately shielded walls and doors, the radiation exposure to staff should remain minimal.

HDR Brachytherapy also has disadvantages compared with LDR brachytherapy.

1. **Treatment unit complexity.** Compared with the usual LDR brachytherapy situation of sources manually inserted into an applicator, the HDR situation seems much more complicated. With the treatment unit, transfer tubes to guide the source between the unit and the applicator, transferring treatment programs between the treatment planning computer and the treatment unit computer, HDR brachytherapy entails a host of considerations not applicable to LDR brachytherapy.[1]

2. **Compressed time frame.** Adding to the complexity of HDR brachytherapy, much of the action takes place in time frames short compared with LDR brachytherapy. For example, after insertion of a tandem and ovoids for cervical cancer therapy, making images and calculating the treatment program, the actual delivery of the treatment frequently takes 10 to 30 minutes. If there were an error in the treatment program, it would be easy for the error to be executed before detection. The situation with LDR treatments provides some latitude for detecting errors. The long duration of the treatment gives more opportunity to spot and correct errors well before the end of treatment, when corrective actions could prevent serious injury.

3. **Radiobiological disadvantage.** The most serious disadvantage for HDR brachytherapy results from radiobiology. Radiobiology is also such an important aspect of HDR brachytherapy that it has its own section below. In the current discussion, it suffices to say that compared with LDR brachytherapy, radiation delivered at a HDR produces a greater increase in damage to normal tissue compared to cancerous tissue.

4. **The potential for very high radiation doses resulting from mechanical failure.** The HDR source cable can become stuck or snagged, or the source can break free from the cable. In either case, the patient could receive an injurious amount of radiation in about 1 minute. While the operator is unlikely to receive an injurious amount of radiation removing the stuck source from the patient, there is a real potential for receiving exposures in excess of allowed limits.

RADIOBIOLOGICAL CONSIDERATIONS

Therapeutic Ratio

Accomplishing the goal of radiotherapy requires inflicting more damage to diseased cells than to normal tissue cells. The therapeutic ratio is an important measure involved in the planning for the goal of uncomplicated cure of disease. The therapeutic ratio could be defined as the ratio of the damage to tumor cells to that to normal cells for the same delivered dose, or

$$\text{Therapeutic ratio} = \frac{\text{Damage to tumor cells}}{\text{Damage to normal cells}}\bigg|_{\text{Same dose}}$$

EQUATION (18.1)

Since it becomes difficult to grade damage, and the damage to cells is not linear with dose, a more common equivalent expression often forms the basis for the calculation of this ratio, determining the ratio of the doses required for the same biological endpoint, for example, five logs of cell kill. The equation becomes

$$\text{Therapeutic ratio} = \frac{\text{Dose to normal cells}}{\text{Dose to tumor cells}}\bigg|_{\substack{\text{Same biological} \\ \text{endpoint}}}$$

EQUATION (18.2)

---

[1] *The exception to this generalization is the use of a LDR remote afterloader—a device that moves LDR sources into applicators while the patient lies in a hospital bed. Since marketing of these units recently terminated, remote afterloading LDR brachytherapy will not be considered in this chapter.*

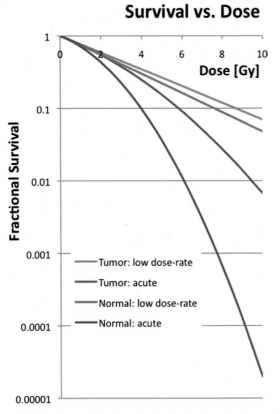

Figure 18.1. A cell survival curve, plotting the fraction of cells surviving a single exposure to radiation as a function of the dose delivered. The curves are based on $\alpha = 0.25$ Gy^{-1}, $\beta_{tumor} = 0.025$ Gy^{-2}, $\beta_{normal\ tissue} = 0.083$ Gy^{-2}, $\mu_{repair} = 1.5$ h^{-1}. Cell proliferation has been ignored.

The more effective the radiation is at killing a certain type of cell, the lower the dose required to reduce a population of cells to a given level.

Figure 18.1 shows a typical curve relating the survival of cells to dose of radiation. In general, the relationship between cell survival, S, and cell killing can be modeled as

$$S = e^{-\alpha D - \beta D^2},\qquad \text{EQUATION (18.3)}$$

where D indicates the dose delivered. Equation 18.3 is just a model, and should not be taken as the true description of the physical and biological process. In the figure, the lines labeled "Normal Acute" and "Tumor Acute" indicate the response of typical normal tissue and typical tumor cells to a single dose of radiation. For any dose level, the tumor cells show an increased survival—not a desirable feature for radiotherapy. The other curves indicate responses for a conventional LDR treatment regimen, delivering the dose at approximately 0.5 Gy/h. For both tissue types, the survival increases due to repair of sublethal damage during the radiation delivery. However, the difference in survival between the two curves at any dose decreases compared with the acute curves. Looking at it the other way, compared to LDR delivery, the difference in response between normal tissue and tumor tissues becomes worse for HDR delivery.

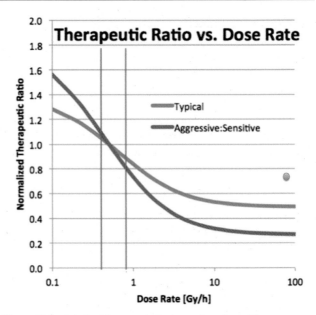

Figure 18.2. Relative Therapeutic Ratio as a function of dose rate, normalized to a dose rate of 0.5Gy/h. Each line assumes a particular ratio for the α and β in Equation 18.3 for tumor cells and normal cells. The blue line represents a typical situation, with $\alpha/\beta = 10$ Gy for the tumor and 3 Gy for normal tissue. The red line applies to and aggressive tumor, with an α/β of 20 Gy and normal tissue with α/β or 2 Gy. The vertical green lines indicate the LDR region. The blue dot indicates the normalized therapeutic ratio for fractionated HDR treatments.

Figure 18.2 illustrates the loss in therapeutic ratio with an increase in dose rate, and the loss in therapeutic ratio can be significant. Figure 18.2 also shows another interesting feature. The therapeutic ratio changes slowly with dose rate over the LDR portion of the curve (0.4–0.8 Gy/h, shown as green vertical lines in the figure), which accounts for historic LDR treatments giving similar results regardless of the exact dose rate. In that region, the therapeutic ratio does not change with absolute dose, only dose rate. At high dose rates, above 20 Gy/h, the therapeutic ratio again varies little with the actual dose rate. Most high dose-rate units deliver a dose at 1 cm at a rate of 100–500 Gy/h, but because much of an implant lies farther away than 1 cm at least some of the treatment time, the dose rate can fall well below that, but seldom below 12 Gy/h. Over any realistic HDR application, the dose rates anywhere in a volume of interest remain in the flat region of the curve. However, the biological dose distribution for an HDR application depends on the absolute dose level, and so differs from the physical dose distribution.

A very different situation obtains in the middle, transition region. In this case, the biological effectiveness of the radiation varies greatly with the actual dose rate, and the biological effectiveness of a given amount of dose varies with position in the treated volume. Often, treatments using nominally LDR remote afterloaders actually deliver doses at this middle dose-rate range. High precision is required with these devices to avoid exceeding tolerance of normal tissues.

The flat response in the HDR region of the curve traces back to the definition of "high dose-rate." In Equation 18.3

the term α in the exponent does not depend on the rate of dose delivery. This term is often associated with single-track killing, that is, one charged particle passing near the DNA strand produces sufficient ionization in the right location to break both sides of the DNA "ladder." Such a double-sided break can produce a biological effect, including cell death.[2] The term β can be thought of representing the situation where the break on each side results from different charged particles. The cell can repair a single-sided break because the remaining side provides the template for the missing side. T_r, the half-time for repair of sublethal damage, characterizes this repair giving the time required to repair half of single-sided breaks. Measured values of T_r vary widely, but a typical value is 1 to 2 hours for both normal and tumor cells. Some normal tissues exhibit repair with two components, one with a half-time of approximately the value above but also a shorter component of about 20 minutes (7), although other models of repair kinetics fit the data better (8). Tumor cells seem not to have this faster component of repair, which gives another therapeutic advantage to the use of low dose rates. For the simple, single-component model for repair, the repair coefficient, μ, can be calculated as

$$\mu = 0.693/T_r. \qquad \text{EQUATION (18.4)}$$

Because the breaks repair over time, the probability for a second-sided break at the same location as the first depends how compact in time the radiation is delivered. When all the radiation passes through the DNA in a short period, the likelihood that the second side will break before the first side repairs increases compared with a long delivery. In this case, a "short" time relates to the half-time for repair of sublethal damage. Regardless of the actual dose rate, HDR treatment refers to a treatment where essentially all the breaks occur before any significant repair takes place. In general, HDR treatments should be completed within a half hour of commencement.

Fractionation

While reducing the dose rate is one method to improve the therapeutic ratio, another is fractionation. Figure 18.3 shows survival curves for the same parameters as Figure 18.1, but includes the survival curves for delivering the doses in 2-Gy fractions. The fractionation reduces the effectiveness of the radiation at killing cells, but it also reduces the differences between the responses of the tumor and the normal tissues.

HDR brachytherapy generally fractionates the treatment course to mitigate the problem of loss of therapeutic ratio with the increase in dose rate. Figure 18.4 shows the improvement in the therapeutic ratio by using one more

---

[2]For more information, the reader may consult any basic radiobiology textbook, such as Hall EJ, Giaccia AJ. Radiobiology for radiologists, 6th ed. Philadelphia, PA: Lippincott Williams & Wilkins, 2005.

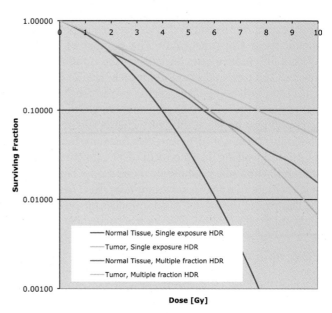

Figure 18.3. Survival curves using the same parameters as in Figure 18.1 for acute (single fraction) exposures and for 2-Gy acute fractions.

fraction. For example, if a plan is called for the use of three fractions, the therapeutic ratio would improve by 4.7% by using four fractions instead. If five fractions were used instead of four, the therapeutic ratio would improve another 4% above the 4.7% improvement from increasing from three to four. As can be seen, each additional fraction improves the therapeutic ratio, but by less than the addition of the fraction before. In external-beam treatment, which is definitely HDR therapy, the number of fractions maybe 35, which would provide a great benefit in the therapeutic ratio, and the addition or deletion of one or two fractions would not make much a difference. Brachytherapy is both taxing on the patient and a drain on the personnel and resources

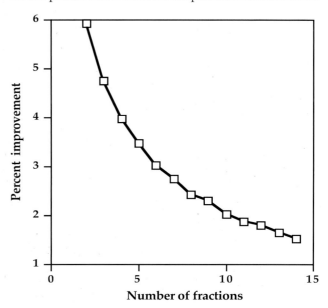

Figure 18.4. The percentage improvement in therapeutic ratio by the addition of one more fraction.

of the facility, and the use of a high number of fractions such as common in external-beam therapy, is not an option. Thus, a compromise must be made between improved therapeutic ratio and practicality. The number of fractions selected for curative cases depends on the amount of work involved and patient discomfort for each fraction. For interstitial cases with needle-like catheters in place, such as a prostate implant, three fractions are common. On the opposite extreme, breast implants with soft catheters and little patient discomfort often use 10, twice-a-day fractions. Intracavitary insertions involving the placement of a treatment appliance at each fraction often use five or six fractions. Tandem and ring applications using an indwelling Smit sleeve (a sheath for the tandem) in the uterine canal simplifies the procedure to the point to which 12 fractions have been used (9).

Prescription Doses

Because the biological effectiveness of radiation changes going from LDR treatments to fractionated HDR treatments, the absolute dose prescribed also has to change to obtain the same therapeutic endpoint. As Equation 18.3 shows, cell survival has a more or less exponential relationship to dose, so dose proper is not the best variable to use when evaluating or predicting biological effects. Of several approaches, one of the most practical begins by taking the log of both sides of the dose response curves from Equation 18.3,

$$Ln(S) = -\alpha D - \beta D^2, \qquad \text{Equation (18.5)}$$

and then divided by $-\alpha$ to have at least the first term in dose alone, to give

$$BED = \frac{Ln(S)}{-\alpha} = D + \frac{\beta}{\alpha} D^2 = D\left(1 + \frac{D}{\alpha/\beta}\right)$$

Equation (18.6)

BED stands for biological equivalent dose. An equivalent term seen in the literature is the RDE, radiological dose equivalent. Equation 18.6 holds for acute, single exposures. For multiple HDR exposures of n fractions of d Gy/fraction, the BED becomes

$$BED_{HDR} = n \cdot d\left(1 + \frac{d}{\alpha/\beta}\right) - \frac{0.693T}{\alpha T_{pot}}. \quad \text{Equation (18.7)}$$

Equation 18.7 holds when each fraction is short compared with the half-time for repair for cellular sublethal damage, and the time between fractions is long compared with this same half-time. As above, the duration of the treatment should be less than half hour, and the time between should be about 4 half-times, or about 6 hours. The newly included last term in Equation 18.7 gives the effect of cellular proliferation on the BED, where T is the total duration of the n fractions and T_{pot} is the potential doubling time for the cells. The equation shows that proliferation decreases the

effectiveness of the radiation. This latter factor often is not known well; however, a compilation of values gleaned from the literature has recently been published (10). Conventionally, due to the uncertainty in this parameter, the proliferation is often ignored. For interstitial cases, the total therapy duration often remains the same; and therefore also the proliferation effect, whether the treatment chosen is HDR or LDR brachytherapy, as discussed below.

Protracted LDR therapy with some repair of sublethal damage taking place during treatment follows Equation 18.8 (11),

$$BED_{LDR} = D\left[1 + \left(\frac{2\dot{D}}{\frac{\alpha}{\beta}\mu}\right) \cdot \left(\frac{1 - e^{-\mu T}}{\mu T}\right)\right] - \frac{0.693T}{\alpha T_{pot}},$$

Equation (18.8)

where $\dot{D}$ is the dose rate.

Assuming that the dose has been established for LDR treatments, the equation to produce the same biological effect with HDR brachytherapy can be calculated. The first step entails selecting the number of HDR fractions to use. As discussed above, this selection is an arbitrary compromise between improving the therapeutic ratio and practical utilization of resources. The next step sets the BED for each modality equal:

$$BED_{HDR} = BED_{LDR}, \qquad \text{Equation (18.9)}$$

or

$$n \cdot d\left(1 + \frac{d}{\alpha/\beta}\right) - \frac{0.693T}{\alpha T_{pot}}$$

$$= D_{LDR}\left[1 + \left(\frac{2\dot{D}}{\frac{\alpha}{\beta}\mu}\right) \cdot \left(\frac{1 - e^{-\mu T}}{\mu T}\right)\right] - \frac{0.693T}{\alpha T_{pot}}.$$

Equation (18.10)

If the total times are similar, then the last terms on each side cancel. Even if they are not similar, since the values needed for their calculation are not well known, they often are simply ignored, giving

$$n \cdot d\left(1 + \frac{d}{\alpha/\beta}\right) = D_{LDR}\left[1 + \left(\frac{2\dot{D}}{\frac{\alpha}{\beta}\mu}\right) \cdot \left(\frac{1 - e^{-\mu T}}{\mu T}\right)\right].$$

Equation (18.11)

The remaining unknown term in Equation 18.11 is the dose per fraction, d. Solving for d gives

$$d = \frac{-\left(\frac{\alpha}{\beta}\right) + \sqrt{\left(\frac{\alpha}{\beta}\right)^2 + \left(\frac{4D_{LDR}\left(\frac{\alpha}{\beta}\right)}{n}\right)\left[1 + \frac{2\dot{D}}{\frac{\alpha}{\beta}}\left(\frac{1 - e^{-\mu T}}{\mu^2 T}\right)\right]}}{2}$$

Equation (18.12)

TABLE 18.1	Equivalent Treatments for LDR and HDR Brachytherapy			
LDR regimen (0.5 Gy/h)		**HDR regimen (2 fractions/day)**		
Dose (Gy)	Duration (day)	Number of fractions	Dose/fraction (Gy)	Total dose (Gy)
20	1.7	4	3.99	16.0
30	2.5	6	3.88	23.3
40	3.3	7	4.25	29.7
50	4.2	8	4.51	36.1
60	5.0	10	4.35	43.5

BED depends on the tissue characteristics, as embodied in the values for α and β. Thus, the equivalence between LDR and HDR brachytherapy only applies to a single type of tissue—tumor or normal tissue. The dose cannot be equivalent for both simultaneously. An equivalent regimen must be selected to produce the same cure rate (equivalent for tumor) or the same normal-tissue reaction (equivalent for normal tissues). If the choice becomes too difficult, a compromise can be made—but at the cost of not being equivalent to the LDR regimen in any way. In general, making the HDR regimen equivalent to the LDR regimen for tumor tends to be the more common choice, since sacrificing cure rate would argue strongly against performing HDR brachytherapy, and physical techniques often can mitigate the increased effects on the normal structures. Early in HDR brachytherapy experience, Orton suggested that doses do not exceed 7 Gy/fraction to avoid normal tissue complications (12). The suggestion came from the review of a survey asking practitioners about their HDR experience. While the responses did indicate that complications increase with fraction sizes exceeding 7 Gy, the total doses for the cases in the survey were not controlled based on the linear-quadratic equations given here and commonly accepted in the present.

Complicating further the attempt to make an HDR brachytherapy treatment similar to one performed with LDR brachytherapy, notice that in Equation 18.12 the dose per HDR fraction, d, depends on the LDR dose to which it should be equivalent. This means that an HDR brachytherapy dose *distribution* can never be equivalent to an LDR brachytherapy dose *distribution*. Thus, to achieve a similar biological dose distribution, an HDR treatment should *not* duplicate the LDR physical dose distribution.

With interstitial implants, higher doses require more fractions to maintain normal tissues within tolerance doses. If the treatment catheters remain in place for the whole therapy, treatments frequently are given twice a day (BID). Table 18.1 relates LDR doses delivered at the rate of 0.5 Gy/h with the equivalent regimen with two HDR fractions per day. In general, the overall treatment duration—time with the catheters in place—remains about the same.

The patient, however, need not be in radiation isolation with the HDR treatments.

For Intracavitary insertions, the prescribed dose often falls at an unambiguous (although often arbitrary) location, for example, Point A for cervical cancer, the surface of a cylinder for vaginal cancer, or 1 cm from the center of the applicator for esophageal applications. Interstitial implants are sometimes less well determined. Take, for example, a post-tylectomy breast implant with a seroma visible on computer tomography (CT). The clinical target volume (CTV) might be the seroma plus a 1.5-cm margin, limited to remain 5 mm deep to the skin and not enter the pectoralis major. During the dosimetry process, the prescription-dose (100%) isodose surface ideally is set at the CTV. All these seem very straightforward. However, depending on where the source tracks fall with respect to the CTV, the 100% isodose may lie on the edge of the more or less uniform dose plateau of the implant or in the rapidly decreasing gradient. (It should be assumed that the 100% isodose surface would never fall beyond the rapidly decreasing gradient to where the dose decreases more slowly; that would be a poor plan indeed.) Thus, in actual cases, some of the CTV may not receive the full dose and some of the prescription isodose surface may fall outside the CTV. Some guidelines for specifying the prescription dose are given in the section on "Evaluation."

OPTIMIZATION

In brachytherapy, "optimization" generally connotes determination of some aspects of an application in order to achieve particular goals. For example, optimization may have as a goal delivering a minimum dose to a target volume with a specified homogeneity. With permanent implants of the prostate, optimization usually generates a pattern for locations of the sources to deliver 90% of the prescription dose to the entire CTV,[3] limit the volume raised to 300% of the prescription dose, and avoid doses to the rectum and

---

[3] *Definitions for the CTV and related terms can be found in Chapter 1.*

urethra that exceed their respective tolerances. In HDR brachytherapy, the most common optimization process determines the dwell times that produce the desired dose distribution—rarely does the process determine catheter location which usually is given. The assumption is that the planning of the implant, that is, where catheters or appliances should lie, occurs at a previous stage. This forms the basic difference between the HDR brachytherapy and the permanent implant cases—for permanent implants, optimization is a part of planning, while for HDR brachytherapy optimization is simply a part of dose computation.

The optimization problem in HDR brachytherapy tends to be simpler than for permanent implants with a single source strength, and can usually come closer to achieving the goals of the optimization. While the permanent implant problem can only decide whether or not to place a source in a given location, the HDR brachytherapy problem can begin assuming activation of all possible dwell locations, and then simply determine each dwell time. Sometimes, the easiest approach determines the dwell times relative to either the maximum time or some specific time (dwell weights) for each dwell position in order to achieve some uniformity, and then set the times in proportion to the dwell weights required for the dose. If solution for the problem does not require a particular dwell position, the optimization routine (optimizer) needs only set the weight to zero. There are several, very different approaches to optimization. Ezzell (13), and Ezzell and Luthmann (14) present excellent discussion on optimization theory and characteristics.

The optimization problem usually specifies a goal. A simple goal might be to deliver a particular dose to a particular location. More specific goals might include delivering the same dose to a set of points or a surface. Even more complex goals not only specify the dose to a surface, but the homogeneity of the dose through the bounded volume and maximum doses allowed to neighboring sensitive normal structures. With the more involved goals, one of the features of the optimization approach includes how to specify the problem and determine the importance of all the varied, and often conflicting, requirements. Many of the optimization approaches use an *objective function* to wrap all the goals into a single measure. And example of an objective function, OF, for a prostate implant could be

$$OF = w_t \sum_{\substack{all \\ target}} \left[(D_{prescribed} - D_t)^2 \text{ if } (D_t < D_{prescribed}) \right]$$

$$+ w_h \sum_{\substack{all \\ target}} \left[(2D_{prescribed} - D_t)^2 \text{ if } (D_t > 2D_{prescribed}) \right]$$

$$+ w_r \sum_{\substack{all \\ rectum}} \left[(D_{rectal\ limit} - D_r)^2 \text{ if } (D_r > D_{rectal\ limit}) \right]$$

$$+ w_u \sum_{\substack{all \\ urethra}} \left[(D_{urethra\ limit} - D_u)^2 \text{ if } (D_u > D_{urethra\ limit}) \right]$$

EQUATION (18.13)

where D stands for doses and w for weighting for the term. The first term considers the target voxels, denoted by subscript t. The first goal would be to deliver the prescribed dose to the target. Any voxels falling below the prescribed dose would add to the objective function. Homogeneity, indicated by the subscript h, also applies to the target voxels, and in the second term, voxels exceeding twice the prescribed dose add to the OF. The last two terms address dose to the rectum and urethra, and increase the OF for voxels that exceed a specified limit for the respective organ. The goal of an optimization could be to minimize this objective function. Objective functions (sometimes called cost functions) can be simpler or more complicated, and can be set such that the goal may be to minimize or maximize the function.

Considering the function above, there maybe many combinations of dwell times that satisfy all the requirements, so there would not be a unique solution. In the subset of all solutions, some may be better than others. If the differences in solutions make a difference in the perceived quality of the treatment plan, then the objective function should be modified to reflect the additional requirements or tighten the specifications. If the differences in the solution remain unimportant, then the first solution found could be used.

While there are many approaches to optimization, they tend to fall in general categories. The actual distinctions between the categories seldom are as clear as it seems they should be, and into which category a given approach falls often remains debatable. Nevertheless, the discussion below considers the characteristics of some of the major categories.

Deterministic Approaches

Deterministic approaches to optimization always find the same solution to the same problem, and generally solve equations to find the dwell times.

Heuristic Approaches

Heuristic approaches use pragmatic search techniques to construct solutions to the optimization problem. The search techniques may use surrogates for the optimized quantities if they are useful. Optimization purists might maintain that heuristics are not true optimization approaches because they tend not to produce a true optimum but merely a satisfactory result. For clinical problems, satisfactory results often serve the patient needs well. In any case, the results of the optimization must be evaluated for appropriateness.

For HDR brachytherapy, one of the most widely used heuristic approach is *geometric optimization*, developed by Edmundson (15). Geometric optimization assumes the goal is a uniform dose distribution, and further assumes a distribution of dwell positions through the volume to receive the uniform dose. The first step in the optimization process recognizes that the dose to the region of the target around a dwell position results not only from the radiation emanating from that dwell, but from all the other dwell positions as well. Looking first at what dose is received at a given dwell position from all the other dwell positions, the weighting of the dwell under consideration should be inversely proportional to the dose from the other positions. Thus, dwell positions that receive large doses from the other dwell positions should have shorter dwell times and those with little contribution from other dwells should have long times. Mathematically,

$$w_i = \left(\sum_{\substack{\text{all} \\ j \neq i}} D_{j \to i} \right)^{-1} , \qquad \text{EQUATION (18.14)}$$

where $D_{j \to i}$ is the dose from dwell position j delivered to dwell position i. The commercial versions of the programs approximate $D_{j \to i}$ with the inverse square relationship, using Equation 18.15,

$$w_i = \left[\sum_{\substack{\text{all} \\ j \neq i}} \left(1/r_{j \to i} \right)^2 \right]^{-1} . \qquad \text{EQUATION (18.15)}$$

Such an approximation is expedient but not necessary.

One problem with geometric optimization in the form of Equation 18.14 is that the optimization assumes equal dwell times during the calculation of the dwell weights, but then uses the calculated weights for the treatment. Thus, the treatment does not match the conditions for the optimization. This problem could be rectified through an iterative procedure, where the dwell weights for current iteration used those calculated in the last, such as

$$\underset{k+1}{\text{iteration}} w_i = \left[\sum_{\substack{\text{all} \\ j \neq i}} \left(\underset{k}{\text{iteration}} \, w_j / r_{j \to i} \right)^2 \right]^{-1} . \; \text{EQUATION (18.16)}$$

The iteration would continue until the dwell weights changed less than some specified percentage. Geometric optimization tends to underweight the periphery of implanted volumes. The iterative procedure could rectify this shortcoming.

A refinement of the approach ignores the contribution of those dwell positions within a specified radius of the one being calculated, assuming that the influence of very close dwells may unduly influence the resultant weights. Applying this technique of ignoring the nearby dwell positions goes by the name *volume optimization*. In practical implementation, often the calculation of the dose to a dwell position ignores the contributions from dwells along the same catheter track. When optimizing few source tracks, such as single catheters for esophageal treatments or a tandem and ovoid, all dwell positions would be included in Equation 18.14—a process then known as *distance optimization*.

Convergent Searches

Also called "downhill searches," convergent searches minimize the objective function iteratively (16,17). At each iteration, the program decides which direction to make changes and how much change to make, based on the differential of the objective function with respect to the parameter being optimized in that pass. These methods tend to get stuck in local minima if they occur between the starting condition and the true minimum. At the time of writing, no commercial brachytherapy planning system uses this technique, although given the popularity of downhill searches in optimization for intensity-modulated radiotherapy the method may move into HDR brachytherapy.

Point-Dose Optimization

Geometric optimization works without reference to an actual dose distribution. Point-dose optimization forms the most direct optimization approach actually to address doses. For this approach, the operator specifies doses to deliver to particular points (*optimization points*). The process then straightforwardly establishes a set of equations for the doses to the optimization points, of the form

$$D_a = \sum_{\substack{\text{all dwells} \\ i}} f_{i \to a} t_i , \qquad \text{EQUATION (18.17)}$$

where $f_{i \to a}$ denotes the function that describes the dose at optimization point a resulting from the source at dwell position i per unit dwell time. The dwell time, t_i, becomes the unknown in the equation. Each optimization point forms one equation, and each dwell time an unknown. Together they form a set of simultaneous equations. Unfortunately, solution of the set of equations presents two problems. The first problem is nonphysical solutions. Consider the situation with the same number of unknown dwell times and optimization points—a determined system. For a very simple case as shown in Figure 18.5 with 12 dwell positions, separated by 1 cm, and 12 optimization points, where each point falls 3 cm above the dwell position.

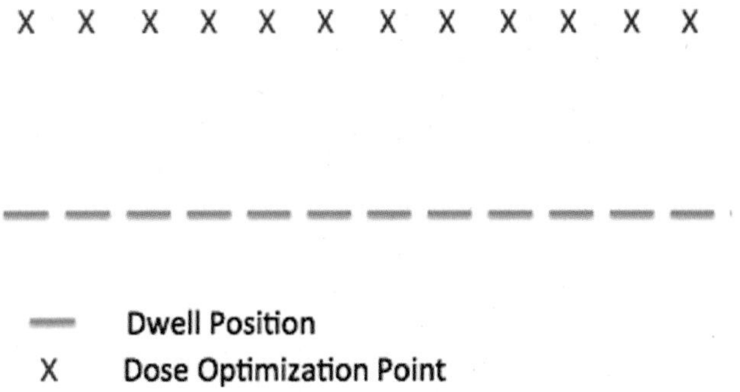

X X X X X X X X X X X X

━ ━ ━ ━ ━ ━ ━ ━ ━ ━ ━ ━

━ **Dwell Position**

X   **Dose Optimization Point**

Figure 18.5. An example for optimization: a single catheter with 12 dwell positions at 1 cm intervals, and 12 optimization points, each 3 cm below every dwell position.

Further, to simplify the problem, approximate the source as a point so the dose rate only depends on the source strength, S_K, the dose-rate constant, Λ, and the inverse of the distance, r. (For ^{192}Ir the other factors are minor and could be ignored for the example.) Assume that all the optimization points should receive the same dose. The system of equations becomes

$$D_i = S_K \Lambda \sum_{j=1}^{12} \frac{t_j}{(j-i)^2 + (3 \text{ cm})^2}, \quad \text{EQUATION (18.18)}$$

where every D_i = the dose at point i = the prescribed dose, and j indicates the source dwell position. Solving this system gives relative dwell weights of:

1.00, 0.08, −0.18, 0.26, 0.50, −0.02, −0.02, 0.50, 0.26, −0.18, 0.08, 1.00.

The negative dwell weights are necessary to satisfy the dose requirements. Simply deleting those dwell times, or increasing all the times by the amount of the most negative fails to produce the uniform dose.

A method to deal with the potential negative values for the dwell times developed by van der Laarse adds a constraint to reduce the variation between adjacent dwell times (18). With control of the variation of dwell times, the equation for optimization becomes

$$X^2 = \sum_{\substack{\text{all dose} \\ \text{points } a}} \left[\sum_{\substack{\text{all dwells} \\ i}} \left| D_a - f_{i \to a} t_i \right|^2 \right]$$

$$+ w_t \sum_{\substack{\text{dwell times} \\ i<n \text{ along a catheter}}} (t_i - t_{i+1})^2, \quad \text{EQUATION (18.19)}$$

where w_t is the dwell-time gradient weighting factor, a measure of the importance of minimizing the differences between adjacent dwell times, and n is the number of dwell positions along a catheter. The first term aims to minimize the differences between the desired doses at the optimization points and the calculated doses. The optimization process then becomes minimizing the chi-square, χ^2. Delivery of any dose requires the net dwell time summation to be positive, so there is no concern that the process might yield all negative times. Minimizing the differences between adjacent dwell times only makes sense locally, that is, along a catheter. Each catheter starts a new comparison of times. The best correlation between desired and calculated doses comes with the smallest value of w_t that eliminates negative dwell times. The values for w_t have no limiting range, although increasing the value above approximately 0.8 has little effect on the dose distribution.

Adding a dwell-time gradient control factor to the problem in Figure 18.5 and Equation 18.19 produces the dwell weight pattern of:

1.00, 0.31, 0.04, 0.10, 0.37, 0.22, 0.22, 0.37, 0.10, 0.04, 0.31, 1.00.

All the dwell weights have become positive. The value for the dwell weight gradient control factor in this example was just 0.01. A small amount of control makes a marked difference. The uniformity suffered slightly in this case. With the negative dwell weights, the dose at the end optimization points fell −4% below the average dose to the points, but the remaining points were within ±1%. With the control of the dwell times, the end points improved to −3%, but the rest of the points varied between −1% and +3%. The results of any optimization always require evaluation to assure that the clinical needs are met.

Approaching the problem as a minimization of chi-square also addresses another problem. While the single catheter example above had the same number of dwell positions and optimization points, real cases often have more dwell position than optimization points (making an underdetermined system of equations) or fewer (overdetermined)—either posing a situation that cannot be solved exactly just by manipulating the equations. The chi-square approach gives the best approximation to a solution. Underdetermined cases have many possible solutions. A useful criterion for selecting the best of the solutions controls the overall treatment time. While simply selecting the solution that minimizes the sum of the dwell times provides a straightforward method to achieve this, minimizing the sum of the squares of the dwell times tends to provide a more uniform distribution of dwell times, and likely of dose (19).

The results from optimization algorithms always need evaluation. The algorithms, of course, do what they are instructed, but the instructions may not be exactly the operator's intention. Consider the simple example of three dwell positions around a point, as shown in Figure 18.6, based on an example of van der Laarse. Point optimization simply specifying the dose to the point could result in the use of only one of the dwell positions, when the intention probably was to use all three and cover a larger volume. Either using a high value for the dwell-time gradient weighting factor or adding optimization points at locations where the dose is actually desired would solve the problem.

A further reason to review the results of the optimization carefully is that the optimization requirements may not have a solution. The line problem of Figure 18.5 had no solution that produced the prescribed dose at each of the optimization points. Depending on the problem, the solutions may be close to the specifications or not. Particularly for underdetermined problems, where the

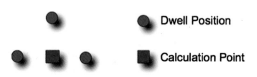

Figure 18.6. Three dwell positions around a point, based on an example case from van der Laarse.

number of optimization points exceeds the number of dwell positions, the probability of obtaining the desired dose at all points becomes low. Evaluation procedures are covered in the section on "Evaluation."

Modern brachytherapy, as with external-beam radiotherapy, tends to specify doses to the surface of a target volume rather than a few points. Programs often approximate surfaces with a collection of closely spaced points. Controlling the dose within a volume often requires more points. This proliferation of optimization points (equations) takes a greatly increased amount of computer resources. Direct algebraic approaches become less appealing.

Polynomial Optimization

A typical (not large) interstitial implant may have 25 catheters, each with 15 dwell positions, resulting in a total of 375 dwell positions. As noted at the end of the last paragraph, the number of optimization points in this case may also become exceedingly large—likely approximating the number of dwell positions. Thus, the system could have 375 equations—each with as many unknowns. This could take some time to solve. Van der Laarse proposed that with the dwell-time gradient weighting factor, the dwell times in a catheter could be constrained to the point that a polynomial could describe their pattern (19). The advantage of fitting the dwell times along a catheter is the reduction in parameters from the number of dwell times to the fitting parameters. Van der Laarse suggests that for n dwell positions in a catheter, a polynomial of order p could model the dwell times, where

$$p = 2\sqrt{n} - 1.$$ EQUATION (18.20)

Using the polynomials, the dwell time at position i along a catheter, at the distance x_i from the beginning of the catheter, becomes

$$t_i(x_i) = \sum_{j=1}^{p} a_j x_i^j.$$ EQUATION (18.21)

The optimization then substitutes Equation 18.21 in Equation 18.19, and sets $\frac{\delta X^2}{\delta a_j} = 0$ to find the optimum fit for the polynomials.

Polynomial optimization as implemented in the Nucletron[4] planning systems uses geometric optimization to give a first-pass value for the dwell times for volume implants, sums the resulting dwell times along each catheter, and divvies that time to each dwell position in proportion to the values resulting from Equation 18.21 divided by the total of the $t_i(x_i)$ for the given catheter.

[4]Nucletron BV, Veenendaal, The Netherlands.

Stochastic Approaches

Stochastic approaches to optimization search for solutions by starting with a possible solution to the problem (in this case, the dwell times for all dwell positions), but not necessarily (or likely) the optimum solution. The objective function is calculated for this solution. Then changes are made to the solution, and the objective function calculated for the new solution. Another new solution would then be formed—guided by whether the value for the objective function improved or degenerated. The nature of the search pattern differs for the various optimization programs, but all the stochastic approaches have some element of randomness in the search pattern. Because of this randomness, the programs may find different solutions with each run.

The only stochastic approach currently used in commercial HDR brachytherapy treatment planning are simulated annealing (20–22) and the genetic algorithm (23,24). Again, Ezzell (13) and Pouliot (25) present more detail on optimization techniques. For simulated annealing, the search makes somewhat random changes in the dwell times. The changes are not truly random, however. At first the changes may be large. With each iteration, the sizes of the changes decrease. If after the change the objective function improves, the next change pushes toward that same direction. On the other hand, if the objective function becomes worse, a more random change is made. This process hones in on a "best" solution, but can get stuck in a local optimum, rather than the global optimum. To prevent a local trapping, occasionally, the program makes a very large change. If the new region of solutions does not seem promising after some tries, the program goes back to the place it left off before the big jump. Even though the process is computationally intensive because of the iterative nature of the search, as implemented commercially at the time of writing, optimization for a HDR prostate implant only takes a few seconds.

Manual Reoptimization

Optimization programs often satisfy the specified criteria but fail to produce the dose distribution that the operator had in mind. Manual reoptimization remedies such a situation. Each commercial planning system for HDR includes a tool for adjusting the path of the isodose surfaces. With these tools, an isodose curve on a particular image slice can be grabbed by the cursor and moved to the desired position. The program then changes the dwell times to produce the change. The operator can choose to have the changes adjust just a single dwell position (local), all of the dwell positions (global), or any amount between. Global changes actually just renormalize the dose distribution to make a new dose as the prescription dose. Figure 18.7 shows manual optimization in action. Figure 18.7A shows the isodose distribution before adjustment, where the 100% isodose exceeds the target region of interest. Figure 18.7B shows

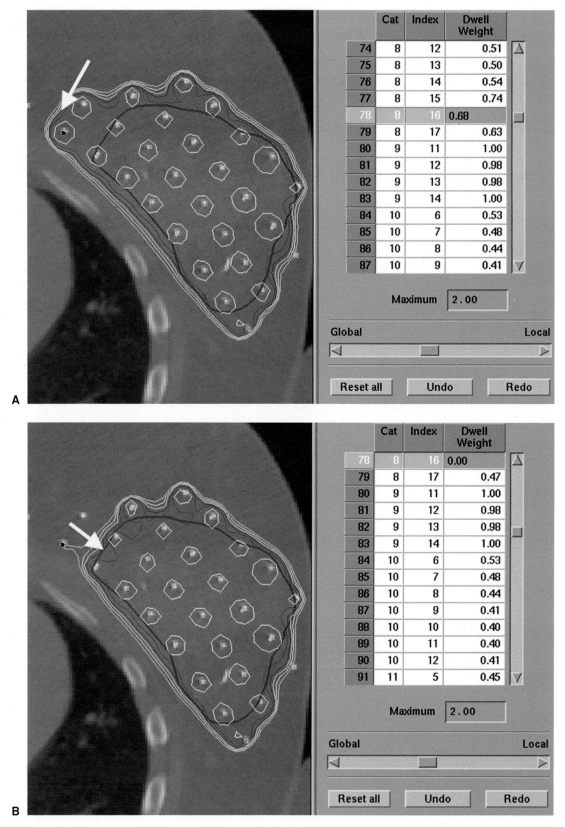

Figure 18.7. An example of manual optimization. **A:** The isodose distribution before adjustment. **B:** The result of the movement. The arrows follow the 100% isodose line (outer of the two darker, thin lines) as it moves to the edge of the target.

the result of moving the 100% isodose curve to the target. For this example the change level was set to "local." Even though the change is local, it still affects the dose distributions in other image cuts. Manual reoptimization must always be practiced iteratively, changing the dose distribution through a series of images and going back and adjusting them again, correcting the first cuts changes for the effects of the later. At some point, the changes become small enough that further reoptimization becomes unnecessary.

Reoptimization requires caution. Increasing the size of the 100% isodose also increases the size of all the other isodose surfaces. In particular, the high-dose region can become large as a result. Manual reoptimization should only be performed with the high-dose isodose lines visible on the images—following changes in one image, other images must be checked for unintended consequences.

Cervical Cancer Intracavitary Applications

While interstitial implants may vary in approach between facilities, for the most part the optimization follows extremely similar criteria. Approaches to optimization for gynecological applications very much more widely. Early work in HDR cervical applications attempted to duplicate the loading of LDR applications (26). As noted in the discussion above on radiobiology, duplicating the *physical dose distribution* does not duplicate the *biologically effective dose distribution*.

Figure 18.8 shows two more current approaches. The one on the left (from Jason Rownd, Medical College of Wisconsin) using the tandem and ring starts with the first optimization point 12 mm lateral to the first dwell position. The remaining optimization points each fall successively 0.5 cm more inferior: the second, the third, and the fourth lateral to the tandem 14 mm, 16 mm, and 18 mm, respectively. From the fifth point on through Point A, the points lie 20 mm lateral to the tandem. The ring optimization points fall 6 mm from the source track at the surface of the cap, specified as 140% of the dose to Point A. This optimization point pattern produces a slowly tapering pear shape with a narrow base.

The optimization pattern on the right (modified from the Madison System (4) as practiced at the time of writing) usually leaves the first centimeter of possible dwell positions inactive to provide space to reduce the dose to the superior bowel, depending on the patient's presentation. The first optimization point falls 1 cm below and 18 mm lateral to the first activated dwell position. From there, the optimization points fall successively 1 cm more inferior, and all at 20 cm lateral to the tandem. Regardless of the distance from the previous optimization point, points are added at the position of Point A and 0.25 cm inferior to Point A. Optimization points are added lateral to the ovoids at the surface. This optimization pattern produces a more squared-top dose distribution that is used at the Medical College of Wisconsin that also reaches further laterally at the position of the ovoids.

The two distributions represent different treatment philosophies. HDR intracavitary treatments require deciding on the shape of the desired dose distribution before determining the dwell times. The treatment planning system needs to know the doses to the optimization points for the dwell time calculation. To perform that optimization, sufficient number of optimization points need to be entered for the optimization routine to know how to shape the distribution.

Inhomogeneity Correction

Until recently, the effect of inhomogeneities in brachytherapy had been ignored, mostly because the effectiveness of heterogeneity corrections in brachytherapy treatment planning has always lagged behind that of external beam radiotherapy. However, for several forms of intracavitary treatments, the effects of inhomogeneities have shown to be important. Sometimes the inhomogeneities result in erroneous dose calculations, such as from bone or resulting from the shields in vaginal ovoids (27–29). In other cases, the inhomogeneity may perturb the geometry of the application, such as air pockets trapped on the surface of a vaginal applicator or on or within intracavitary breast applicator (30–32). While for many years the hope had been for incorporation of full Monte Carlo simulations into brachytherapy treatment planning systems, for various reasons this has not happened. However, recently a discrete-ordinate, grid-based solver for the Boltzmann's transport problem became available in a commercial treatment planning system.[5] The evaluations of this program indicate that it compares well with Monte Carlo simulations and differs importantly from calculations that ignore heterogeneities (33–35). Figure 18.9 compares treatment plans with and without correction for heterogeneities. Such programs likely will become common in brachytherapy as they are in external-beam radiotherapy treatment planning. The use of correction software requires imaging with CT or magnetic resonance, which also has become more common.

A Final Word on Optimization

Optimization assists a planner achieve the goals of a treatment. The first step to achieving the goals is to place the treatment appliance in the ideal position. While optimization can sometimes compensate for a less-than-ideal placement, optimization cannot make a good treatment from a bad placement. Poor placement of an appliance results in poor homogeneity of the dose distribution, even with the best optimization.

---

[5]*The program Acuros in BrachyVision, Varian Associates, Palo Alto, CA, based on Attila, Transpire Inc., Gig Harbor, WA.*

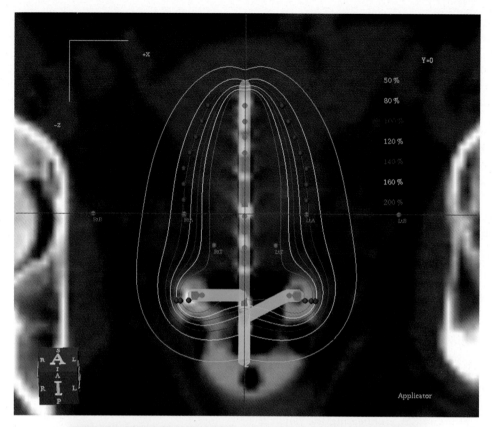

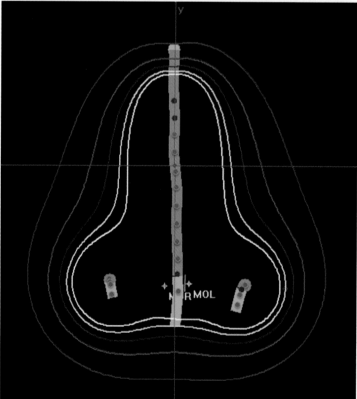

Figure 18.8. Two examples of optimization for cervical cancer intracavitary applications. Top: narrow-top pear shaped (Courtesy of Jason Rownd, Medical College of Wisconsin). Bottom: squared-off pear (University of Wisconsin).

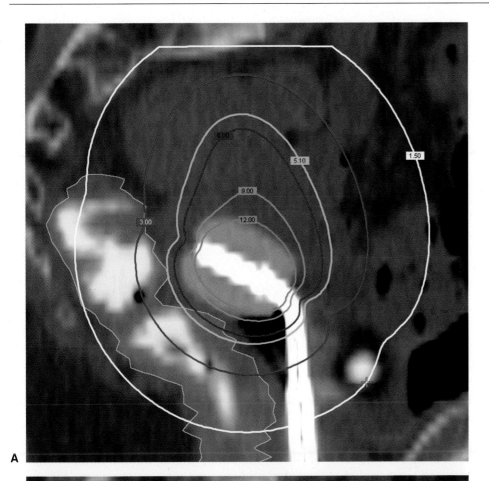

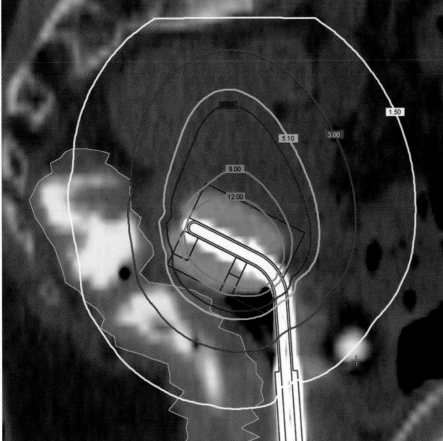

Figure 18.9. An illustration of inhomogeneity correction using a discrete-ordinates algorithm. **A:** A plan performed assuming all space is water. **B:** The same plan but corrected for the shielding in the ovoids using the Acuros program. The plans differ in the dose to the rectum due to the rectal shields. Images courtesy of Firas Mourtada.

EVALUATION

The generation of a treatment plan involves many steps—some fairly complicated—presenting many pathways and opportunities for errors to creep into the planning and be propagated into a treatment error. The next section on "Quality Assurance" addresses error prevention. The complexity of the treatment plan also presents situations where choices have to be made or data entered, and on occasion, an entry, while not obviously wrong, may possibly be less than ideal. As noted in the section on "Optimization," the results of the optimization program may not be quite that expected. For all these reasons, careful evaluation of an HDR treatment plan becomes very important. A fine line separates quality management and treatment plan evaluation, and the evaluation serves as the first step in quality assurance (QA).

Dose Prescription

The items to check do not have an unambiguous order. This discussion addresses the items from the more obvious to the more subtle.

The Absolute Dose to a Reference Location

Often, the dose distribution for brachytherapy shows isodose surfaces of particular dose. During evaluation, however, considering the absolute dose to a point or a set of points, and then the isodose distribution as doses relative to the absolute point clarifies the two-step process involved with most dose prescription. Assessing the absolute doses to specified points forms one of the first checks to perform. For the most part, if the operator entered particular points for dose specification, the programs will set the absolute dose to those points accurately. Problems that can arise include the following:

a. Selecting the wrong point from among those entered for dose specification, for example, accidentally selecting the rectal point instead of Point A for a cervical treatment.
b. Having entered the specification point incorrectly, either through poor digitization or through misinterpretation of the anatomy.
c. Specifying the dose to a set of points with a wide variation in dose between.

While the first two problems represent errors, the last may be either a poor judgment or a bad presentation in the patient. A very simple example would be a treatment with a tandem and ovoids in a patient with a severely tipped uterus. The dose at Point A on the right and left side will be very different, and simply specifying the dose to the average of the two points could result in excessive dose on one side and too little dose on the other. A more involved situation would be specifying the dose to a set of points on the surface of a tumor with catheters running through. Depending on the geometry, the points may have too wide a variation in doses to provide a good basis for the absolute dose specification.

In most situations, the reference location should relate to the dose target, rather than regions of concern for normal tissues. Consideration of normal structures comes later.

Part of checking the prescribed dose includes review of the fractionation schema. The dose for the fraction should correspond to the total dose divided by the number of fractions. As part of this verification, the dose should also be checked against any relevant protocol that may change the dose based on concomitant external-beam therapy (in an era of satellite facilities and specialty referrals, such concomitant treatments may not be obvious to the treatment planner) or chemotherapy.

Relative Doses to Specified Volumes

The optimization process required some specification of locations that should receive some faction of the prescription dose. In intracavitary cases, this may be a few points, for example, along an esophageal applicator or along a tandem and lateral to a vaginal ring. For a volume implant, it may be the target volume surface. In any case, these points define the goal for the treatment and satisfaction of the prescription requires conformance of the dose distribution to these specifications. For the simpler cases, review of each optimization point may be performed, but volume implants probably require a dose-volume histogram (DVH), as discussed below.

The dose to all the optimization points likely will not equal the specify dose, as noted above, but should be within some defined tolerance of that specified. Failure to adequately shape the dose distribution raises three possibilities: accepting the results if compatible with the treatment objectives; change the optimization parameters and try optimizing the plan again; or manually intervening, as discussed in the section on "Optimization."

Limitations

The doses to limiting normal structures should be checked to assure that they remain below tolerance. Assessment of the doses to normal structures falls under the next section.

Visual Evaluation of Dose Distributions

Adequate coverage of the target usually involves visual inspection of the isodose lines on multiple cuts or projections. While a DVH (see subsequent text) shows failure to include all target within the prescription isodose surface, the DVH does not show where the failures occur or whether the volumes that fall below the prescription dose are contiguous (a potentially serious problem) or widely dispersed (often not significant). The same can be said for high dose volumes (HDVs). When possible, the inspection of the isodose lines should be superimposed on images, such as from CT.

Much of the evaluation of the dose homogeneity comes in the next section using DVH. However, two tools that assess the uniformity of the doses only apply when visually evaluating the isodose distribution for implants. The *maximum significant dose* (MSD) refers to the highest-level isodose surface that encompasses more than one needle track. The dose very near the source track can be very high, but the body seems to tolerate these local HDVs. The MSD provides a convenient criterion for when small HDVs become "significant" and likely to produce biological consequences. For an implant taken to normal tissue tolerance, the MSD corresponds to the tolerance dose. For what fraction of the prescription isodose surface the MSD becomes limiting depends on several factors. The first is the volume of the implant—the tolerated level for the MSD decreases with volume. The second factor is where in the gradient around the implanted volume the prescription dose falls. Much of the modern experience with implants comes through the use of the Paris System (discussed below). With that system, the prescription dose (Reference Dose in the System's parlance) equaled 85% of the Basal Dose, that is, the mean of the local minima between needle tracks in the central plane. The Paris System further defined a HDV as that volume raised to 200% of the prescription dose (170% of the Basal Dose), and suggested that this dose tightly conform to the needle tracks. Thus, for Paris System implants, the MSD would be somewhat less than 200% of the prescription dose. Translating this MSD to HDR treatments requires a few steps. First, assume an LDR treatment of 60 Gy delivered at 0.5 Gy/h. From Equation 18.8 the BED using an $\alpha/\beta = 10$ Gy^{-1}, appropriate for tumor cells, would be 72.8 Gy$_{10}$.[6] The limitation on high doses in the target volume likely applies to normal tissue tolerances, since it is normal tissue breakdown that results in complications. Thus, the BED for the 200% dose, using $\alpha/\beta = 3$ Gy^{-1}, equals 290 Gy$_3$. Many HDR regimens could be used for this treatment, but this example assumes six fractions of 5.25 Gy each, which gives the same biological effect for the tumor. The physical dose that gives the same biological effectiveness for normal tissue as the MSD above is 8.45 Gy, or 160% of the prescription dose. This result highlights a general rule of HDR brachytherapy: *the variation in dose through the treated volume must remain markedly less than with LDR brachytherapy.* That rule just restates the relative increase in the sensitivity of normal tissue with the change to HDR treatments. The value of MSD of 160% matches well experience with breast implants that use the 150% isodose surface for the MSD, and that exceeding this level increases the probability of complications. This also agrees well with experience with large gynecological implants that the MSD should stay below 125% of the Basal Dose (3, 36). For small implants, the percentage of the prescription dose selected for the MSD can increase, but there is not as much data for small volume implant complications as for the large.

Another tool, developed by Neblett, considers the other boundary of the isodose distribution, finding the *maximum contiguous dose* (MCD), or the highest value for an isodose surface that completely surrounds the implanted needle tracks (37). Isodose levels higher than the MCD break into small islands of high dose with lower doses separating volumes enclosed. The prescription dose should not exceed the MCD, but should not fall much outside the MCD isodose surface.

Evaluation of dose distributions for intracavitary insertions, for the most part, remains as visual inspection of isodose plots. The concepts that measure uniformity or HDVs find little relevance in intracavitary applications because the dose always becomes high near the sources and falls continuously with distance. The question in evaluating the dose distribution becomes simply whether or not an adequate dose covers the target or targets and avoids excessive doses to limiting structures. One exception to this is intracavitary breast treatments with multi-lumen applicators. In these cases, tailoring the distribution to the patient often reduces the uniformity of the dose through the defined target volume, and measures of the homogeneity of the dose, as discussed below, provide insights into the quality of the treatment.

For intracavitary and interstitial cases, target evaluation should be considered a three-dimensional process. However, three-dimensional views often become difficult to interpret. Figure 18.10 shows the target for a breast implant and the 100% isodose surface as a veil draped over the target. This presentation clearly shows where the 100% isodose surface fails to cover the target (indicated by the white arrows). In many cases, however, the three-dimensional images may seem confusing to those with little experience looking at them, and sometimes to those

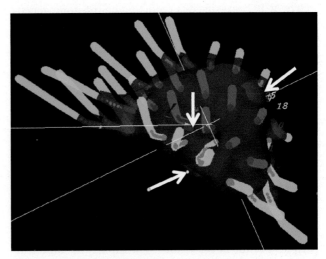

Figure 18.10. A three-dimensional view of the target and the 100% isodose surface for a breast implant.

[6]*Convention dictates that the units for BED indicate the α/β as a following subscript.*

with experience. Limiting the number of structures shown to a region of interest and one isodose surface helps during the interpretation.

Quantitative Assessment of Implants

The discussion below relates mostly to interstitial implants. For a much more detailed discussion of evaluation parameters, see Thomadsen (38). Assessment requires precise terminology. The following terms may be useful:

Recommendations for Interstitial Implant Reporting by the International Commission on Radiation Units and Measurements

For interstitial implants, the International Commission on Radiation Units and Measurements (ICRU) defines the following (39):

The *Mean Central Dose* is defined as the arithmetic mean of the local minimum doses between all adjacent sources in the implant. This concept is well known in the Paris system (approximating the basal dose), but is less well known in the USA.

Peripheral Dose is the minimum dose at the periphery of the CTV, and should be the minimum dose decided upon by the clinician as adequate to treat the target. This dose is similar to the typical "prescribed dose" used by many American clinicians.

A *Low-Dose Region* is a region within the CTV where the dose is less than 90% of the peripheral dose. The maximum dimensions of this volume are reported. This obviously relates to an underdosed volume of the target, so should correlate with treatment failure.

A *High-Dose Region* should correlate with complications. The high-dose region is defined as the volume encompassed by the isodose line equal to 150% of the mean central dose. The maximum dimensions of this volume in all planes calculated should be reported.

The ICRU also suggests reporting on the homogeneity of the dose by specifying the following:

1. *Spread*—the difference between the maximum and the minimum local minimum doses divided by the mean central dose
2. *Peripheral-mean ratio (PMR)*—the ratio of the peripheral dose to the mean central dose

Hanson points out that "the first gives a measure of nonuniformity within the implant and may be a measure of how well the implant was accomplished (40). The second is related to proper spacing of the source lines relative to the peripheral 'reach' of the implant."

Another useful quantifier is the *mean peripheral dose* (MPD), which equals, as it says, the mean dose on the periphery of the target volume. The capital "M" differentiates this from the minimum peripheral dose, simply called the peripheral dose by the ICRU, which is often denoted by

mPD. Neither of these quantities should be confused with the *matched peripheral dose*, which was a concept used before imaged-based dosimetry was available that specified the dose for a distribution of radioactive sources compared with the dose it would deliver to the periphery of an ellipse with the same average diameter as the volume implanted (41).

Dose-Volume Histograms

The first step in quantitative evaluation calculates the DVH. Several very different presentations of very different information fall under the category of DVH. The histograms in all cases display some function related to volume on the ordinate with dose (or a function of dose) on the abscissa. Many of the presentations apply to dosimetry of implants performed without correlation to volume imaging information (i.e., CT, MR, or ultrasound), and thus, have no information regarding the treatment relative to any target or normal structures. Such DVH consider the implant as a whole, and are called "unlimited" because they make no reference to a limiting region of interest. Because the current standard of care would discourage brachytherapy implants in the absence of imaging information, unlimited DVH will not be considered further. While they still prove interesting for evaluating the technical execution of an implant, they find little application in treatment planning. For more information of such DVH, the reader should consult Thomadsen (38).

Figure 18.11 shows a relative, cumulative DVH for an HDR prostate implant for a boost following external-beam therapy. The ordinate records the fraction of a structure that receives at least that dose shown on the abscissa. The normalization of the volume to the total volume of the region of interest makes the histogram "relative." Ideally, the curve labeled "prostate" would run along the top of the graph at 1.0 for all the doses until the prescription dose, indicating that the entire target receives at least the target dose, and then the curve rapidly falls. Of course the fall cannot be very sharp because there will always be HDVs around the source path. The entire prostate may not receive the prescription dose either. Depending on the limitations on dose to the rectum, and potentially on the placement of the catheters due to the pelvic arch, some regions of the prostate may fall shy of the prescription dose.

Figure 18.11 also shows a curve for the rectum. Unlike the target, only part of the rectal contour usually is entered into the computer. Thus, the histogram actually shows the fraction of the *contoured* volume that receives the given dose. Some organs may be completely contoured during planning, and the fraction of the whole organ receiving particular doses may relate to complications or other treatment limitations. For long tube-like organs, complete contouring not only may be unlikely, but unnecessary. Some evidence indicates that rather than the fraction of the rectum being the critical variable, that the absolute volume may be important. Various volumes have been proposed from 0.1 to 5 cm^3 (42–47). The value of interest for these volumes would be the minimum dose, since the

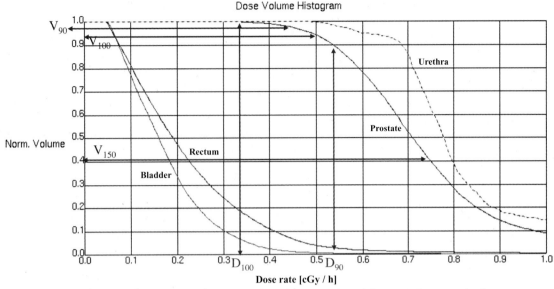

Figure 18.11. A cumulative, relative, dose-volume histogram (DVH) for an HDR prostate implant.

maximum dose would be just a point, and not change for any of the volumes. For volumes less than 5 cm³, it makes little difference if the contour simply encircles the whole rectal cross section or specifically just outlines the wall, as in Figure 18.12 (45).

Figure 18.13A shows an example of a relative differential DVH. In this case, the ordinate gives the change in the percent of the volume per dose, which is closely related to the fractional volume of the region of interest that actually receives the dose on the abscissa. The differential DVH sometimes proves useful in selecting the prescription dose, assessing whether the prescribed dose adequately covers the target and the uniformity of the dose through the target.

DVH assist in evaluation of implants by calling attention to the fraction of the tumor that may receive less than the treatment dose or whether a neighboring structure exceeds tolerance. They can also help distinguish between plans that would better concentrate the dose in the target. However, as noted above, while presenting this information for rapid detection, DVH lose special information, such as *where* the target dose may be low.

Figures of Merit

The DVH distills the information from the isodose distributions to simplify some evaluations. The DVH still

presents much of the data in a two-dimensional format, sometimes complicating some assessments. *Figures of Merit* provide numerical values for particular aspects of implants, and can assist in evaluations and facilitate communication about the treatments. More detailed discussions can be found in Saw and Suntharalingam (48) and Thomadsen (38). Below are some of the quantities most useful for HDR treatment planning.

Target Coverage

The first assessment should be whether the plan adequately covers the target. Several measures for that exist, each telling a slightly different story.

D_x, $V_x – D_{x\%}$ refers to the dose that covers $x\%$ of the target volume. Ideally, the prescription dose covers 100% of the target, although as mentioned before, that often cannot be the case. Recognizing this, many protocols call for the prescription dose to cover some particular fraction of the target volume, such as 95%. In such cases, $D_{95\%}$ becomes a value of great interest since it often defines the prescription. The companion quantity, V_x gives the volume receiving a dose equal or to x. This quantity assumes different forms depending on the conventions used for a treatment protocol. Most often the volume refers to the fraction of the CTV receiving the dose x, but at other times it is the absolute volume. The dose, x, may refer to the absolute dose, or it may be a fraction of the prescribed dose. The convention in use requires clarification. Again, ideally $V_{100\%}$ should equal 1 in an ideal implant if V equals the fraction of the target volume with x normalized to the prescribed dose. For the remainder of this discussion, the convention will specify doses explicitly as either a percent of the prescription dose labeled with "%" or an absolute labeled with "Gy." Reference volumes will be percent, again labeled as "%" or absolute with units of cm³. Finally, the volume to which the quantity refers will be a leading subscript, to give quantities such as $_{CTV}D_{90\%}$ or $_{rectum}V_{60}$ Gy.

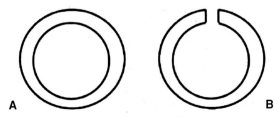

Figure 18.12. Examples of contouring the rectal wall: (**A**) for planning systems that can designate the region between the outer wall and the inner wall and (**B**) for systems that cannot.

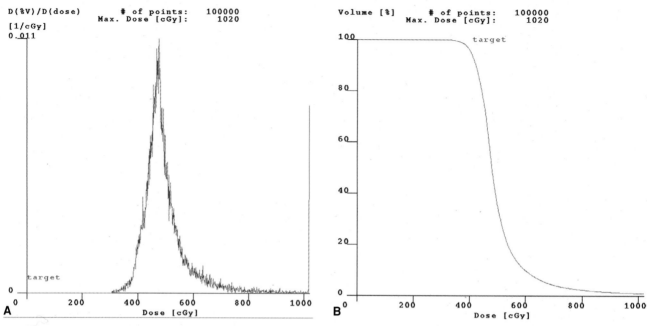

Figure 18.13. A: A relative, differential dose-volume histogram (DVH) for a breast implant. This presentation shows the volume that receives a particular dose. **B:** The cumulative DVH for the same implant.

The *Coverage index* (CI) specifies the fraction of the target volume receiving a dose equal to, or greater than, the target dose (49). The CI corresponds to the value on the relative, cumulative DVH for the CTV at the prescription dose. Thus, $CI = {}_{CTV}V_{100\%}$.

Dose Uniformity

After assessing the adequacy of target coverage, the next question focuses on the uniformity of the dose through the target volume. As discussed above, the MSD must be controlled, but other measures also can help in this evaluation.

The section on "Recommendations for Interstitial Implant Reporting by the International Commission on Radiation Units and Measurements" introduced the ICRU term high-dose region as the volume encompassed by the 150% isodose surface. This concept came from the HDV of the Paris System, which used a cut-off of 200% of the prescription dose. Zwicker makes the factor a variable, p, used during optimization (50). In the discussion above, converting from the LDR treatments to an HDR regimen, the Paris System's factor of 200% becomes 160%. Using an LDR factor of 150% leads to an HDR factor of 123%. Limiting the MSD to 123% is seldom possible in a real implant. The rest of this discussion uses a value of 150% to define the HDV for HDR implants. Figure 18.14 shows a schematic of a section through the CTV, a prescription isodose surface as the $V_{100\%}$ and the surface corresponding to 1.5 times the prescription dose, $V_{150\%}$. In this figure much of the $V_{100\%}$ and the CTV coincide, but some of the CTV remains below the prescribed dose while some of the prescribed dose falls outside the target. Some of the target and

normal tissues receive in excess of 150%, which is very undesirable for the normal tissue and uselessly high for the tumor. Thus, the most desirable region has the CTV receiving doses between the 100% and the 150%. This figure may be helpful during the following discussion.

The *relative dose homogeneity index* (HI) measures the uniformity of the dose through the target volume as the fraction of the target volume receiving a dose between the target dose and the high dose level, or (51)

$$HI = {}_{CTV}V_{100\%} - {}_{CTV}V_{150\%} \qquad \text{EQUATION (18.22)}$$

In Equation 18.22, both volumes are the fraction of the CTV raised to at least the percent of the prescription dose given. Originally, the HI referred only to the prescription isodose volumes without regard to the target, dating from when target information usually was not available. Most often nowadays, equation 18.22 is used.

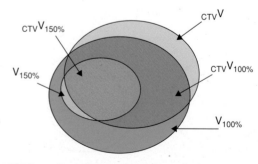

Figure 18.14. A schematic showing a section of a clinical target volume (CTV) (gray) and two isodose surfaces corresponding to 100% (single hatched) and 150% (cross hatched) of the prescribed dose.

A very similar index, the *dose nonuniformity ratio* (DNR) equals ratio of the HDV to that volume taken to at least the target dose (52),

$$\text{DNR} = \frac{_{CTV}V_{150\%}}{_{CTV}V_{100\%}}.$$ EQUATION (18.23)

This quantity indicates the price paid (in HDV) to set the prescription dose to cover the target. Obviously, the DNR and HI are related as HI = 1 − *DNR*, so specification of both quantities becomes duplicative.

Yu defines a somewhat more comprehensive quantity, the *uniformity number* (UN) (53). The derivation begins with defining the *harmonic treatment dose (HTD)* as

$$\text{HTD} = \frac{\int\limits_{CTV} D(v)\,dv}{_{CTV}V},$$ EQUATION (18.24)

where $D(v)$ is the dose to a voxel element dv, giving a quantity related to the mean dose through the target, and the *harmonic peripheral dose* (HPD) as

$$\text{HPD} = \frac{\int\limits_{\substack{CTV \\ Surface}} D(s)\,ds}{_{CTV}S},$$ EQUATION (18.25)

with $D(s)$ being the dose in a small element on the surface of the CTV, ds. From these, Yu determines the UN as

$$\text{UN} = \frac{\text{HPD}}{\text{HTD}},$$ EQUATION (18.26)

The UN tends toward greater stability and robustness in the face of small variations in the geometry of an implant.

Dose Outside the Target

As a measure of the dose outside the target, the *external volume index* (EI) equals the volume of nontarget tissue receiving doses equal to or greater than the target dose, as a fraction of the target volume (49,54). Thus,

$$EI = \frac{_{100\%}V - _{CTV}V_{100\%} \cdot _{CTV}V}{_{CTV}V}$$ EQUATION (18.27)

Here, $V_{100\%}$ indicates the entire volume enclosed by the prescription isodose surface and $_{CTV}V$ is the absolute volume of the CTV.

Since $_{CTV}V_{100\%}$ is the fraction of the CTV volume raised to at least 100% of the prescription dose, the product, $_{CTV}V_{100\%} \cdot _{CTV}V$, gives the absolute volume of the CTV raised to at least 100% of the prescription dose.

Conformity

The *conformation number* (CN) measures of the conformance of the prescription dose to the target (55,56),

$$\text{CN} = \left(\frac{_{CTV}V \cdot _{CTV}V_{100\%}}{V_{100\%}}\right) \cdot \left(\frac{_{CTV}V \cdot _{CTV}V_{100\%}}{_{CTV}V}\right)$$
$$= \left(\frac{_{CTV}V \cdot _{CTV}V_{100\%}}{V_{100\%}}\right) \cdot _{CTV}V_{100\%}$$

EQUATION (18.28)

The numerator of each factor gives the total volume of the CTV within the 100% isodose surface, as the volume of the CTV times the fraction of the CTV raised to the 100% dose. The first factor gives the dose within the CTV as a fraction of the whole 100% dose volume, a measure of the efficiency of the dose deposition. The second factor is related the coverage of the target. Together they indicate how closely the prescription dose matches the target.

The *peripheral uniformity number* (PUN) also addresses the conformity at the target but at the periphery, specifying (53)

$$\text{PUN} = \frac{\text{ICRU peripheral dose}}{\text{HPD}}.$$ EQUATION (18.29)

Figure of Merit Summary

Each of these figures of merit provides useful information about the implant. Several of them are redundant and which should be used becomes the user's preference. None of these quantities tells the entire story for a given implant. No single index or quantity perfectly characterizes any implant—evaluation requires consideration of many different aspects, not all of which optimize for the same conditions. Final decisions and the quality of an implant require consideration of the large overview of the implant.

QUALITY ASSURANCE

Quality assurance, QA, for the treatment plan assesses first the adequacy of the generated treatment plan—the measures which were addressed in the section on "Plan Evaluation." The evaluation process includes verification that the plan delivers the right dose to the right location. The other purpose for QA is to detect and correct errors in the treatment plan before treatment delivery. QA, by definition, provides indication that the plan contains no errors and is of the quality intended.

Before performing QA, quality control (QC) works to keep errors from happening in the first place. For HDR brachytherapy treatment planning, the most useful and effective QC tool is a form for recording and transmitting the important and requested information. Such a form may serve as the prescription, since it should contain the information of the dose—fractionation and normal structure limitation—as well as a description of the application and any other relevant information. A treatment planning protocol serves as the other very important QC tool. The protocol is a standard operating procedure that dictates routine planning decisions for most cases. Examples of information contained in a protocol include the definition used to find Point A for cervical intracavitary insertions and the step size for breast implants.[7]

"Independent verification" forms an invaluable part of QA. Having someone other than the person who generated a treatment plan check it increases greatly the probability of detecting errors. In addition, just as a form for recording and transmission of information helps prevent errors, forms to guide the plan evaluation also prevent omissions during the verification. Guidance for developing forms can be found in Thomadsen (38). If a having an independent person check the plan is not an option at a facility, the use of forms and a fixed verification protocol becomes even more important.

Indicators of Reasonableness

One major challenge in QA is to judge whether the planner made a significant error. One approach to assess the plan for errors compares some value related to the plan with standards or expectations. The standards derive from previous experience or from the literature. The sections below consider some examples. For a more detailed discussion, again see Thomadsen (38).

Intraluminal Tests

Intraluminal cases generally use a single catheter, such as for endobronchial, endoesophageal, or biliary treatments. Some of the tests discussed below also apply for vaginal cylinder applications. Thomadsen reported an index (57)

$$\text{Index} = \frac{\begin{array}{c}\text{Sum of all dwell times (s)} \cdot \\ \text{Source strength (Gy m}^2\text{ h}^{-1}\text{)}\end{array}}{\begin{array}{c}\text{Prescription dose (Gy)} \cdot \\ \text{Length of prescription dose (cm)} \cdot \\ \text{Distance to prescription dose (cm)}\end{array}}$$

EQUATION (18.30)

where the index should fall between 0.133 and 0.167 ([Gy m² s]/[Gy cm² h]) Obviously, the index actually has no

true units since with multiplying by appropriate constants, the units cancel. However, for convenience, the equation keeps the units most likely used for each variable. This index increases above these limits for short treatment lengths compared to the prescription distance.

Kubo (58) and Kubo and Chin (59) calculate the approximate total treatment time (±2%) based on a linear fit as,

$$\text{Time(s)} = \frac{0.1\left[\text{s} \times \text{Ci/cGy}\right] \cdot \text{Dose(Gy)} \cdot}{\begin{array}{c}(2.67 \text{ Length (mm)} + 78.6 \text{ mm})\\ \hline \text{Source strength (Ci)} \cdot \\ \text{Prescription distance (mm)}\end{array}}$$

EQUATION (18.31)

where "length" equals the active length along the catheter. They also derived a quadratic fit for the treatment duration for lengths (L) between 50 and 200 mm and prescription distance, d (60):

$$\begin{aligned}\text{Time (s)} = &\left(\frac{\text{Dose (Gy)} \cdot 2 \text{ (Ci/Gy)}}{\text{Source strength (Ci)}}\right) \\ &\times \Bigg[(-5.24 + 8.80d + 0.263d^2) \\ &+ \left(\frac{L - 50 \text{ mm}}{L - 200 \text{ mm}}\right) \\ &\times (-9.66 + 22.4d - 0.027d^2)\Bigg]\end{aligned}$$

EQUATION (18.32)

Ezzell calculates the dose to points 10 cm distant from the approximate center of the sources, along a line approximately perpendicular to the catheter, in opposite directions (61). He calculated a *dose index*, defined as

$$\text{Dose index} = \frac{100(\text{Dose}_{+10\text{cm}} + \text{Dose}_{-10\text{cm}})/2}{\text{Source strength} \cdot \text{Total time}},$$

EQUATION (18.33)

which should fall between:

- 0.95 to 1.10 for long treatment lengths (such as esophagus)
- 1.10 to 1.20 for short treatment lengths (such as vaginal cylinders)
- 1.05 to 1.20 for endobronchial treatments (lower if highly elongated, higher if curved)

For any of these checks, the source strength should come from a separate table rather than from the treatment plan.

Tandem and Ovoids

Indices similar to those discussed above have been used in gynecological applications, but because the constraints for optimization vary greatly between facilities, the actual

---

[7] *The step size becomes very important in many implant cases. Large step sizes give less ability to optimize the dose distribution. Small step sizes with very short dwell times cause some unit to void a treatment plan following a source change if the automatically recalculated dwell times become shorter than the shortest time programmable.*

values used with any such index must be developed locally. Two indices developed for use with the Madison System (4) assess whether a given tandem and ovoid application falls within the normal range (57):

$$\text{Index 1} = \frac{\text{Source strength (Gy m}^2\text{ h}^{-1})\cdot}{\text{Dwell time 1 cm from tip-most dwell (s)}}{\text{Prescribed dose (Gy)}},$$

EQUATION (18.34)

and

$$\text{Index 2} = \frac{\text{Source strength (Gy m}^2\text{ h}^{-1})\cdot}{\text{Total dwell time (s)}}{\text{Prescribed dose (Gy)}\cdot}{\text{Number of dwell positions}}.$$

EQUATION (18.35)

The location for the first index dwell falls far from the ovoids to consider mostly the loading of the tandem. The dwell times for the tip-most position varies greatly between patients and thus, do not serve well for measures of application consistency. The dwell 1 cm inferior to the first dwell position used becomes quite stable. Index 1 tells whether this one position falls within a normal range. Index 2 considers the application as a whole. The numerator simply gives the integrated reference air kerma (IRAK, which numerically equals the total reference air kerma, TRAK, of the ICRU (62)). The use of IRAK parallels the conventional mgRaeq.h customary for evaluating the normalcy of LDR applications. Following the Madison System optimization pattern, the limits for the indices in units of ([Gy m² s]/[Gy h]) become:

∎ Index 1—0.139 to 0.180
∎ Index 2
    ∎ For small ovoids—0.098 to 0.123
    ∎ For medium ovoids—0.123 to 0.147
    ∎ For large ovoids—0.135 to 0.180

The indices also apply to applications using tandem with cylinders in the vagina, where Index 2 values become:

∎ For 2.0 cm diameter—0.098 to 0.139
∎ For 2.5 cm diameter—0.114 to 0.147
∎ For 3.0 cm diameter—0.109 to 0.160
∎ For 3.5 cm diameter—0.143 to 0.168

Interstitial Implants

Common optimized HDR implants conceptually tend to follow a cross between Manchester and Paris implants. The implants behave much like Manchester implants in that the differential source-strength distribution pattern varies much like in the Manchester rules. However, unlike the Manchester system, where the dose tends to corre-spond to the Paris System's Basal Dose, most practitioners specify the prescription to a Reference Dose outside the limits of the implant, much like the Paris System. With this in mind, the Manchester implant tables can be modified to apply to ^{192}Ir HDR implants by multiplication of the source strengths by 1.11 to set the Reference Dose to 90% of the Basal Dose, and converting from mgRaeq · h to ^{192}Ir IRAK. For a given treatment plan, the total duration of the treatment calculated by the planning computer can be compared with the time given by

$$\text{Time} = \frac{\text{Dose (Gy)}\cdot R_V\text{ (Gy} \times \text{m}^2 \times \text{h}^{-1} \times \text{s/Gy)}}{\text{Source strength (Gy} \times \text{m}^2 \times \text{h}^{-1})}$$

EQUATION (18.36)

where in this equation $R_V = 0.00321$ $_{\text{Manchester}}R_V$, that is the R_V in the original Manchester tables, so

$$R_V = 0.1091 V^{2/3}e0.007^{(E-1)},$$ EQUATION (18.37)

where E is the longest dimension/shortest orthogonal dimension. Experience with breast implants show that this formula generally agrees with the time calculated by the treatment-planning computer within 5%.

A similar approach holds for modifying the R_A values from the Manchester table to verify the calculations for planar implants. Alternatively, Ezzell developed a formula that gives the expected time for a dose at a specified distance from an implant plane (63) as:

$$\text{Time (s)} = \frac{\text{Dose}(r)\text{ (cGy)}\cdot\text{Area (cm}^2)}{\text{Source strength (Ci)}\cdot(a+bE+cE^2)},$$

EQUATION (18.38)

where r is the distance from the plane where the prescribed dose falls, E is the equivalent square of the planar area = 4·area/perimeter, and a, b, and c are fitting parameters that depend on the distance, r, given in Table 18.2.

Unified Index

Das et al. considered predicting the treatment duration based on the volume of the prescription isodose surface, V_{100} (64). Beginning with a point source approximation, he derived the equation

$$Time[\text{s}] = \frac{\text{Prescribed dose [cGy]}\cdot K[\text{U}\cdot\text{s}\cdot\text{cGy}^{-1}\cdot\text{cm}^{-2}]\cdot V_{100\%}^{2/3}[\text{cm}^2]\cdot EC}{\text{Source strength [U]}}$$

EQUATION (18.39)

where EC is the elongation correction, approximated as $1 + 0.06(E - 1)^{1.26}$, and K is a constant depending on the number of catheters:

∎ 1 catheter, $K = 1{,}267$ U s/(cGy cm²)
∎ 2 or 3 catheters, $K = 1{,}182$ U s/(cGy cm²)
∎ More than three catheters, $K = 928$ U s/(cGy cm²)

TABLE 18.2	Fitting Parameters for Equation 18.38		
r (cm)	a (cGy·cm^2/[Ci·s])	b (cGy·cm/[Ci·s])	c (cGy/[Ci·s])
1.5	0.402	0.923	−0.0171
2.0	−0.258	0.836	−0.0148
2.5	−0.619	0.751	−0.0126
3.0	−0.822	0.673	−0.0106

a, b, and c are fitting parameters that depend on the distance, r.

Treatment Unit Programming and Pretreatment Checks

Once the treatment plan passes the evaluation and QA tests, the treatment plan must be passed to the treatment unit in the form of a treatment program specifying all the treatment information: channel lengths (distance to the first dwell position), step size or sizes, and the dwell time pattern for each channel. Verification of the program checks the items most likely to be in error.

The most likely error is selecting the wrong program for a given patient if there are more than one program under the patient's identity. This situation frequently arises in regimens where new plans are generated at each fraction, such as gynecological intracavitary applications. Such plans may differ subtlety, so checking the plan entails verifying each dwell position. Fortunately, intracavitary plans generally contain few dwell positions. Large volume implants with more catheters than treatment unit channels form another common treatment with multiple files under a patient's identity. In this case, enough details of the file must be checked to assure selection of the correct file for the treatment underway. To prevent using the wrong patient's file for a treatment, the name on the program must be matched with the patient's identity.

Regardless of the number of files a patient has, the first fraction for any file must include a verification of the length for each catheter, particularly if the length differs from the default value. The most common error with HDR brachytherapy is unintended treatment with the default length when a customized length was intended. The step size also forms a simple, but very important parameter to check. Once these have been verified, and a sampling of the dwell time pattern checked, the program can be approved. On subsequent treatment fractions, the checks to verify programming with the correct file suffice.

PLANNING AN IMPLANT

Planning is actually what goes before the action, or at least, what *should* go before. In the context of brachytherapy, before performing an implant or an insertion, planning entails determining the desired location of the treatment appliance. Optimization can often (but not always) make the prescription isodose surface cover the target in many cases following a less-than-optimum implant; however, the price paid becomes larger HDVs, increasing the probability of complication.

The initial steps for planning a brachytherapy procedure follow the same pattern as for any type of radiotherapy treatment: determining the target volumes. Earlier chapters discusses target delineation, so it will not be addressed here, other than to say that in brachytherapy the expansion from the CTV to form a planning target volume (PTV) usually remains small. Such an expansion needs to consider the ability to place the applicator in the desired location, and, for implants, the constraints placed on the location of needles by the implant pattern to conform to the CTV. As an example of the latter constraint, consider a template guided implant where the edge of the CTV falls between needle rows. Covering the CTV may require an additional needle in the row outside of the CTV, thus effectively expanding the CTV to a PTV.

Appliance Selection and Placement

Planning where to place the treatment appliance depends heavily on the form of the brachytherapy.

Intracavitary Insertions

Intraluminal insertions allow little selection in the treatment appliance or location. For example, the only variable in endobronchial applications would be how far past the target to insert the tip of the treatment catheter. Possibly the diameter of the catheter may be selectable from two sizes, and in some cases the stiffness of the catheter. More applicators are available for endoesophageal applications because of the size of the lumen. These applicators have various thicknesses of the walls and number of channels, running from one in the center (giving a more penetrating dose distribution) to many around the periphery (allowing some tailoring of the dose distribution to the CTV).

Gynecological applications present a greater opportunity to select the appliance most appropriate to the patient from a wide variety. For cervical cancer, the standard

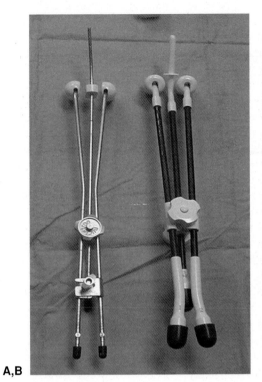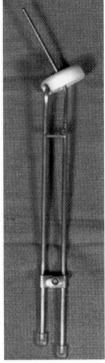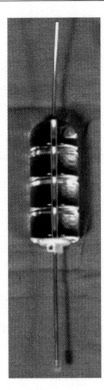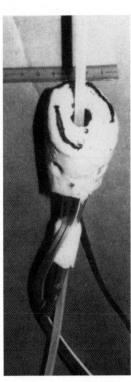

A,B **C,D**

Figure 18.15. Applicators for cervical cancer intracavitary insertions: **A:** Tandem and ovoid, on the left the conventional and on the right for CT or MR localization. **B:** A tandem and ring. **C:** A tandem and cylinder. **D:** A tandem and custom vaginal mold.

approach places a long tube (a tandem) in the uterus and channels for the source in the vagina, just as with the LDR treatments. While the tandem for all applicators remains mostly the same, the vaginal source channels differ greatly between applicators. The vaginal part of the appliance for four applicators will be compared for examples—ovoids, a ring, cylinders and custom molds. Figure 18.15 shows examples of these applicators. The source travels through ovoids in a tube running axially through either ellipsoidal (from which the term ovoid derives) or cylindrical piece of plastic. Some ovoids contain shielding in the direction of the rectum and bladder, as do LDR ovoids, and some do not. Ovoids come in three sizes, generally 1 cm, 1.25 cm, and 1.5 cm radius, sometimes with a "mini" size that maintains the 1-cm radius laterally but only a few millimeters medially to fit a smaller vagina. Some of these applicators have no fixed relationship between the tandems and ovoids, however some do. The nonfixed applicators allow better conformance with the patient's anatomy, while the fixed systems maintain a standard geometry. The best dose distribution comes from using the largest size ovoids that fit in the vagina. This gives the greatest distance between the source track and the vaginal mucosa and thus, the greatest depth dose, just as increasing the source to surface distance in external-beam radiotherapy increases the fractional depth dose. Spreading the ovoids should be avoided because that leads to reduced doses to the cervix proper.

In the ring applicator, the vaginal source path follows a circle centered on the tandem. The ring comes in several

diameters (26–34 cm). Typical cases only use the dwell positions in the lateral parts of the ring—somewhat simulating the dwell positions used in the ovoids. A plastic cap about 5 mm thick slips over the ring to provide spacing between the source track and the vaginal mucosa, reducing the local dose. Because the cap provides only half the spacing as the smallest ovoid, the ring projects the dose less deeply laterally. The smaller size of the ring applicator and the fixation to the tandem make insertion easier than ovoids.

Patients with very narrow vagina—not uncommon after high doses of radiation therapy—may not accommodate a tandem and ovoids. One approach places plastic cylinders around the tandem where it passes through the vagina. While this approach allows for treatment, the dose distribution fails to provide the coverage of tandems and ovoids. The difference results from constraining the source track to the tandem instead of spreading the tracks laterally, with a concomitant reduction in the coverage to the lateral aspects of the uterus.

Custom vaginal moulds have been used to provide applications tailored to individual patients. These applicators use an impression of the patient's vagina with tracks drilled to accommodate catheters for the source tubes (65–69). Figure 18.15D shows such a mould. In concept, these mould applicators should provide improved fit and stability for the applicators compared with standard ovoids or a ring. The advantage at the price of increased time commitments for construction of the mould.

Postoperative endometrial cancer treatments form one of the most common brachytherapy procedures in the United States. The treatment delivers radiation to the anastigmatic site at the superior end of the vagina following removal of the uterus, with the goal of preventing tumor recurrences in the surgical site. HDR treatments generally use either ovoids (without the tandem, since the uterus is gone) or cylinders. The ovoids tend to produce a dose distribution that conforms closely to the target at risk, while maintaining relatively low doses to the bladder and rectum. Cylinders give more dose to the rectum and the bladder than ovoids partially because of the orientation of the source places these organs near the perpendicular bisector of the sources and the maximum of the anisotropy of the source. Using cylinders, the axis of the source, where the anisotropy function is relatively low, points toward the target at the end of the cylinder. For ovoids, the situation is reversed, with the low values of the anisotropy toward the bladder and the rectum and the maximum toward the target. However, Pearcey and Petereit report that relatively low doses (50 Gy$_{10}$ or an LDR equivalent of 44 Gy) to the target produce control rates of greater than 98%, with complications not appearing until normal tissue doses of 100 Gy$_3$ (LDR equivalent of 60 Gy) (70). Uncomplicated control is the norm with this form of treatment. Thus, the differences between the applicators mean little with regard to the treatment outcome. There are, however, cylinders with source pathways forming a circle at the top, and rings without the tandem, that can combine the beneficial orientation of the source with the simplicity of the cylinder.

Interstitial Implants

Determining the needle pattern for an implant can be the most important decision for an implant. Many of the older systems developed rules for needle placement that still provide good guidance (71–76). Most of the rules that apply for LDR implants also apply for HDR procedures.

Many of the conventional, LDR brachytherapy approaches give rules for implants with uniform source distribution, that is, source material not differentially distributed. The Manchester System forms the exception. It becomes more difficult to achieve relative dose uniformity when all sources have the same strength per centimeter along a needle track, and rules for needle track placement were developed to produce a dose as uniform in a plane of volume as possible given that constraint (75,76). Beginning the planning for needle placement by following these rules generally requires less modulation of optimized dwell times to achieve the uniformity goals for the plan. Minimizing the required modulation of the dwell times reduces the likelihood of large high-dose regions. For most HDR multi-planar and volume implants, a needle separation of 1.5 cm results in a lower HDV than 1 cm, but larger separations increase the HDV again.

Most commonly, an approach similar to the Paris System (76,77) is followed assuming that the prescription

dose, as the Reference Dose, falls outside of the actual implanted volume. The change to optimized HDR treatments carries also the need to adjust the Paris system's specifications a bit. Optimization reduced the higher doses that occur in the interior of the implant although increases the high doses near the ends of needle tracks. While the Paris system used a Reference Dose (RD—surrounding the implanted volume) equal to 85% of the Basal Dose (BD—mean of the local dose minima in the central plane), reducing the higher doses in the interior reduces the mean of the dose minima, and that means that the percentage relating the BD and the RD must increase to maintain the same location and value of the Reference Dose. Further, the change to HDRs accentuates differences in dose, so the percentage must increase further. For a typical optimized HDR implant to give a similar biological Reference Dose as an LDR implant, the RD = 93% BD (36). The higher ratio of BD to RD implies that the needles should be placed slightly closer to the edge of the target volume for HDR implants.

For planar implants or volumes made from planes, following a strict grid pattern with uniform loading often results in a region of low dose between the outlying needles and the rest of the implanted volume, essentially wasting the space implanted near the outliers, as demonstrated in Figure 18.16A, from Neblett (78). Optimization can fill in this region but at the cost of increasing the HDV. Neblett recommends moving the corner needles closer to the main body of the implant than the regular spacing pattern would dictate, as demonstrated in Figure 18.17—a practice called tight-end loading (78). Figure 18.16B shows the resultant dose distribution, with the prescription isodose surface encompassing the whole implant. Tight-end loading increases the MCD, reducing the HDV.

Unfortunately, some implants, particularly those with irregular shapes, require needles outside the target volume to assure adequate coverage. Figure 18.18 shows one CT image of a breast implant. This implant uses needles outside the target volume to boost the dose near the edge of the implant in several locations. Optimization would not need these needles to cover the target except for the restriction to hold the MSD to 150%. Without that restriction, the dwell times near the boundary would simply increase to extend the dose to the target edge. This case trades the extension of dose to tissue outside the implant for reducing the HDV inside the implant.

Dwell Position

Optimization often allows keeping the dwell positions all inside the target volume. The Paris system and all the derivative systems for LDR treatments using uniform strength sources require that the sources extend beyond the target volume to assure adequate coverage. Optimization increases the relative dwell times on the ends of source tracks so the end dwell positions project the dose to the edge of the target. Increasing the dwell times at the ends of

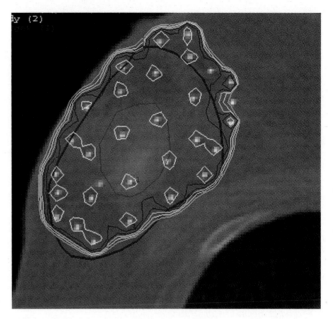

Figure 18.18. A breast implant, showing the necessity for needles outside the target volume in this image.

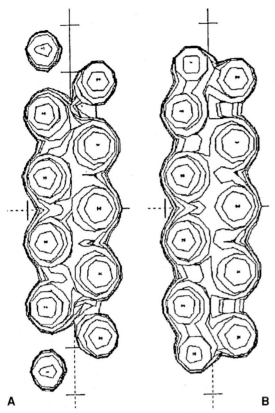

Figure 18.16. A: A planar implant with evenly spaced, uniformly loaded needles showing the failure of the prescription isodose surface to include the volume between the main body of the implant and the corner needles. B: The same implant as in A except with the corner needles moved inward slightly, eliminating the low-dose region. (From Neblett D. Clinical techniques and applicators available for interstitial implantation. In: Williamson JF, Thomadsen BR, Nath R, eds. *Brachytherapy physics.* Madison, WI: Medical Physics Publishing, 1995, with permission from Medical Physics Publishing.)

the tracks does require vigilance to prevent large HDV. This process simulates the crossing needles of the Manchester System.

For those with experience with linear sources, such as ^{192}Ir wire or ^{137}Cs needles, placing seed-type sources, such as an HDR brachytherapy source to give dose distribu-

tions similar to those from linear sources, requires some care. Figure 18.19 demonstrates that for equivalency—the dwell positions should not start and stop at the same location as the ends of the line source. Going to the stepping source, the activity of the line would be cut into the small pieces that become the dwell positions. Because the total length of source is smaller with the dwell pattern because of the gaps between positions, the linear activity density for the dwells has to be greater than for the wire. Thus, the strength of the wire is condensed into the dwells. Each dwell could be thought of as having a sphere of influence that commands the space around it until halfway to the next dwell. For the end dwells, this sphere also projects outward, and it is the edge of this sphere that should fall at the location equivalent to the end of the wire. While this concept is well oversimplified and does not account for the fact that all of the wire's length contributes to the dose everywhere as do all of the dwell positions, the rapid gradient in the dose from an element of source does make this learning presentation useful.

Although an HDR plan can be made equivalent to an LDR plan with continuous wire or ^{137}Cs needles, usually that would not be desirable. In wire-based implants or those with uniform linear strength such as used in the Paris System, the sources must extend beyond the target due to the low doses near the ends. With optimization, the

Triangular cells

Tight Side Spacing

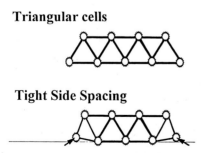

Figure 18.17. A demonstration of the process for tight end loading. (From Neblett D. Clinical techniques and applicators available for interstitial implantation. In: Williamson JF, Thomadsen BR, Nath R, eds. *Brachytherapy physics.* Madison, WI: Medical Physics Publishing, 1995, with permission from Medical Physics Publishing.)

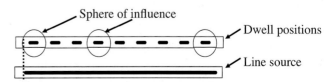

Figure 18.19. Placement of seeds or dwell positions to simulate a line source.

source material can remain within the target while delivering the dose to the periphery. As a general guidance for a starting point in planning dwell positions for an optimized implant, the distance from the surface of the target to the first dwell position in the target should be half the space between dwell positions (57).

REFERENCES

1. Das RK, Thomadsen BR. High dose rate brachytherapy sources and delivery systems. In: Thomadsen BR, Rivard MJ, Butler WM, eds. *Brachytherapy physics, 2nd*. Madison, WI: Medical Physics Publishing, 2005.
2. Das RK, Thomadsen BR. High dose rate brachytherapy. In: Webster J, ed. *Encyclopedia of medical devices and instrumentation*. Hoboken, NJ: John Wiley & Sons, 2006.
3. Thomadsen BR, Shahabi S, Buchler DA. Differential loadings of brachytherapy templates. *Endocurietherapy/Hypertherm Oncol* 1990;6:197–202.
4. Thomadsen BR, Shahabi S, Stitt JA, et al. High dose rate intracavitary brachytherapy for carcinoma of the cervix: the Madison system: II. Procedural and physical considerations. *Int J Radiat Oncol Biol Phys* 1992;24(2):349–357.
5. King CC, Stockstill TF, Bloomer WD, et al. Point dose variations with time in brachytherapy for cervical carcinoma. *Med Phys* 1992;19:777.
6. Gao S, Delclos ME, Tomas LC, et al. High-dose-rate remote afterloaders for intraoperative radiation therapy. *AORN J* 2007;86(5):827–836; quiz 837–840.
7. van den Aardweg GJ, Hopewell JW. The kinetics of repair for sublethal radiation-induced damage in the pig epidermis: an interpretation based on a fast and a slow component of repair. *Radiother Oncol* 1992;23(2):94–104.
8. Fowler JF. Repair between dose fractions: a simpler method of analyzing and reporting apparently biexponential repair. *Radiat Res* 2002;158(2):141–151.
9. Han I, Malviya V, Chuba P, et al. Multifractionated high-dose-rate brachytherapy with concomitant daily teletherapy for cervical cancer. *Gynecol Oncol* 1996;63(1):71–77.
10. QUANTEC Committee. Quantitative analyses of normal tissue effects in the clinic. *Int J Radiat Oncol Biol Phys* 2010;76(3S):S1–S160.
11. Dale RG. The application of the linear-quadratic dose-effect equation to fractionated and protracted radiotherapy. *Br J Radiol* 1985;58(690):515–528.
12. Orton CG, Seyedsadr M, Somnay A. Comparison of high and low dose rate remote afterloading for cervix cancer and the importance of fractionation. *Int J Radiat Oncol Biol Phys* 1991;21(6):1425–1434.
13. Ezzell G. Optimization in brachytherapy. In: Thomadsen BR, Rivard MJ, Butler W, eds. *Brachytherapy physics, 2nd*. Madison, WI: Medical Physics Publishing, 2005.
14. Ezzell G, Luthmann RW. Clinical implementation of dwell time optimization techniques. In: Williamson JF, Thomadsen BR, Nath R, eds. *Brachytherapy physics, 2nd*. Madison, WI: Medical Physics Publishing, 1995.
15. Edmundson GK. Geometry based optimization for stepping source implants. In: Martinez AA, Orton CG, Mould RF, eds. *Brachytherapy HDR and LDR*. Columbia, MD: Nucletron Corporation, 1990:184–192.
16. Shewchuk JR. *An introduction to the conjugate gradient method without the agonizing pain*. Pittsburgh, PA: Carnegie Mellon University, 1994.
17. Holmes T, Mackie TR, Simpkin D, et al. A unified approach to the optimization of brachytherapy and external beam dosimetry. *Int J Radiat Oncol Biol Phys* 1991; 20(4):859–873.
18. Thomadsen B, Houdek P, van der Laarse R. Treatment planning and optimization. In: Nag S, ed. *Textbook and high dose rate brachytherapy*. Armonk, NY: Futura Publishing Co, 1994.
19. van der Laarse R, Edmundson GK, Luthmann RW, et al. Optimization of HDR brachytherapy dose distributions. Activity 1991;5:94–101.
20. Lessard E, Pouliot J. Inverse planning anatomy-based dose optimization for HDR-brachytherapy of the prostate using fast simulated annealing algorithm and dedicated objective function. *Med Phys* 2001;28(5):773–779.
21. Lessard E. Development and clinical introduction of an inverse planning dose optimization by simulated annealing (IPSA) for high dose rate brachytherapy (Thesis abstract). *Med Phys* 2004;31:2935.
22. Hsu IC, Lessard E, Weinberg V, et al. Comparison of inverse planning simulated annealing and geometrical optimization for prostate high-dose-rate brachytherapy. *Brachytherapy* 2004;3(3):147–152.
23. Yu Y, Schell MC. A genetic algorithm for the optimization of prostate implants. *Med Phys* 1996;23(12):2085–2091.
24. Yang G, Reinstein LE, Pai S, et al. A new genetic algorithm technique in optimization of permanent 125I prostate implants. *Med Phys* 1998;25(12):2308–2315.
25. Pouliot J, Lessard E, Hsu I-C. Advanced 3D planning. In: Thomadsen BR, Rivard MJ, Butler W, eds. *Brachytherapy physics 2nd*. Madison, WI: Medical Physics Publishing, 2005.
26. Houdek PV, Schwade JG, Abitbol AA, et al. Optimization of high dose-rate cervix brachytherapy; Part I: dose distribution. *Int J Radiat Oncol Biol Phys* 1991;21(6): 1621–1625.
27. Mohan R, Ding IY, Martel MK, et al. Measurements of radiation dose distributions for shielded cervical applicators. *Int J Radiat Oncol Biol Phys* 1985;11(4):861–868.
28. Mohan R, Ding IY, Toraskar J, et al. Computation of radiation dose distributions for shielded cervical applicators. *Int J Radiat Oncol Biol Phys* 1985;11(4):823–830.
29. Watanabe Y, Roy JN, Harrington PJ, et al. Three-dimensional lookup tables for Henschke applicator cervix treatment by HDR 192IR remote afterloading. *Int J Radiat Oncol Biol Phys* 1998;41(5):1201–1207.
30. Richardson S, Palaniswaamy G, Grigsby PW. Dosimetric effects of air pockets around high-dose rate brachytherapy vaginal cylinders. *Int J Radiat Oncol Biol Phys* 2010; 78(1):276–279.
31. Huang YJ, Blough M. Dosimetric effects of air pocket sizes in MammoSite treatment as accelerated partial breast irradiation for early breast cancer. *J Appl Clin Med Phys* 2009;11(1):2932.
32. Richardson S, Pino R. Dosimetric effects of an air cavity for the SAVI™ partial breast irradiation applicator. *Med Phys* 2010;37(8):3919–3926.
33. Gifford KA, Price MJ, Horton JL Jr, et al. Optimization of deterministic transport parameters for the calculation

of the dose distribution around a high dose-rate 192Ir brachytherapy source. *Med Phys* 2008;35(6):2279–2285.

34. Zourari K, Pantelis E, Moutsatsos A, et al. Dosimetric accuracy of a deterministic radiation transport based ^{192}Ir brachytherapy treatment planning system. Part I: single sources and bounded homogeneous geometries. *Med Phys* 2010;37(2):649–661.

35. Mikell J, Mourtada F. Dosimetric impact of an ^{192}Ir brachytherapy source cable length modeled using a grid-based Boltzmann transport equation. *Med Phys* 2010; 37: 4733–4743.

36. Thomadsen BR. Clinical implementation of remote-afterloading, interstitial brachytherapy. In: Williamson JF, Thomadsen BR, Nath R, eds. *Brachytherapy physics.* Madison, WI: Medical Physics Publishing, 1995.

37. Neblett D, Syed AMN, Puthawala AA, et al. An interstitial implant technique evaluated by contiguous volume analysis. *Endocurietherapy/Hyperthem* 1985;1:213–221.

38. Thomadsen BR. *Achieving quality in brachytherapy.* London: Taylor & Francis, 1999.

39. I.C.O.R.U.A.M. ICRU *Report 58: dose and volume specification for reporting interstitial therapy.* Report No. 58. Bethesda, MD: International Commission on Radiation Units and Measures, 1997.

40. Hanson WF, Graves M. ICRU Recommendations on dose specification. In: Williamson JF, Thomadsen BR, Nath R, eds. *Brachytherapy physics.* Madison: Medical Physics Publishing, 1995.

41. Hilaris BS, Nori D, Anderson LL. *Atlas of brachytherapy.* New York, NY: Macmillan Publishing Company, 1988.

42. Schoeppel SL, LaVigne ML, Martel MK, et al. Three-dimensional treatment planning of intracavitary gynecologic implants: analysis of ten cases and implications for dose specification. *Int J Radiat Oncol Biol Phys* 1994; 28(1):277–283.

43. Saarnak AE, Boersma M, van Bunningen BN, et al. Inter-observer variation in delineation of bladder and rectum contours for brachytherapy of cervical cancer. *Radiother Oncol* 2000;56(1):37–42.

44. Fellner C, Potter R, Knocke TH, et al. Comparison of radiography- and computed tomography-based treatment planning in cervix cancer in brachytherapy with specific attention to some quality assurance aspects. *Radiother Oncol* 2001;58(1):53–62.

45. Wachter-Gerstner N, Wachter S, Reinstadler E, et al. Bladder and rectum dose defined from MRI based treatment planning for cervix cancer brachytherapy: comparison of dose-volume histograms for organ contours and organ wall, comparison with ICRU rectum and bladder reference point. *Radiother Oncol* 2003;68(3):269–276.

46. Kirisits C, Potter R, Lang S, et al. Dose and volume parameters for MRI-based treatment planning in intracavitary brachytherapy for cervical cancer. *Int J Radiat Oncol Biol Phys* 2005;62(3):901–911.

47. Van den Berg F, Meertens H, Moonen L, et al. The use of a transverse CT image for the estimation of the dose given to the rectum in intracavitary brachytherapy for carcinoma of the cervix. *Radiother Oncol* 1998;47:85–90.

48. Saw CB, Suntharalingam N. Quantitative assessment of interstitial implants. *Int J Radiat Oncol Biol Phys* 1991; 20(1):135–139.

49. Saw CB, Waterman FM, Ayyangar K, et al. Quantitative evaluation of planar ^{192}Ir implants [Abstract]. *Med Phys* 1986;13:580.

50. Zwicker RD, Schmidt-Ullrich R. Dose uniformity in a planar interstitial implant system. *Int J Radiat Oncol Biol Phys* 1995;31(1):149–155.

51. Wu A, Ulin K, Sternick ES. A dose homogeneity index for evaluating 192Ir interstitial breast implants. *Med Phys* 1988;15(1):104–107.

52. Saw CB, Suntharalingam N, Wu A. Concept of dose nonuniformity in interstitial brachytherapy. *Int J Radiat Oncol Biol Phys* 1993;26(3):519–527.

53. Yu Y. A nondivergent specification of the mean treatment dose in interstitial brachytherapy. *Med Phys* 1996;23(6): 905–909.

54. Saw CB, Suntharalingam N. Reference dose rates for single- and double-plane ^{192}Ir implants. *Med Phys* 1988; 15(3):391–396.

55. van't Riet A, Mak AC, Moerland MA, et al. A conformation number to quantify the degree of conformality in brachytherapy and external beam irradiation: application to the prostate. *Int J Radiat Oncol Biol Phys* 1997;37(3): 731–736.

56. Baltas D, Kolotas C, Geramani K, et al. A conformal index (COIN) to evaluate implant quality and dose specification in brachytherapy. *Int J Radiat Oncol Biol Phys* 1998; 40(2):515–524.

57. Thomadsen BR. Clinical implementation of HDR intracavitary and transluminal brachytherapy. In: Williamson JF, Thomadsen BR, Nath R, eds. *Brachytherapy physics.* Madison, WI: Medical Physics Publishing, 1995.

58. Kubo HD. Verification of treatment plans by mathematical formulas for single catheter HDR brachytherapy. *Med Dosim* 1992;17(3):151–155.

59. Kubo HD, Chin RB. Simple mathematical formulas for quick-checking of single-catheter high dose rate brachytherapy treatment plans. *Endocurietherapy/Hypertherm Oncol* 1992;8:165–169.

60. Rogus RD, Smith MJ, Kubo HD. An equation to QA check the total treatment time for single-catheter HDR brachytherapy. *Int J Radiat Oncol Biol Phys* 1998;40(1): 245–248.

61. Ezzell GA. Acceptance testing and quality assurance for high dose-rate remote afterloading systems. In: Martinez AA, Orton CG, Mould RF, eds. *Brachytherapy HDR and LDR.* Columbia, MD: Nucletron Corporation, 1990: 138–159.

62. International Commission on Radiation Units and Measurements. ICRU *Report 38: dose and volume specification for reporting intracavitary therapy in gynecology.* Bethesda, MD: International Commission on Radiation Units and Measures, 1985.

63. Ezzell GA. Quality assurance of treatment plans for optimized high dose rate brachytherapy–planar implants. *Med Phys* 1994;21(5):659–661.

64. Das RK, Bradley KA, Nelson IA, et al. Quality assurance of treatment plans for interstitial and intracavitary high-dose-rate brachytherapy. *Brachytherapy* 2006;5(1): 56–60.

65. Twombly GH, Rosh R. A new method for applying radium in the vagina in cases of carcinoma of the uterine cervix. *Cancer* 1955;8:1016–1020.

66. Chassagne D. La plesiocurietherapie des cancers du cavum avec support-moule et Yridium 192. *Annales de Radiologie* 1963;6:719–726.

67. Lewis GC. Acrylic molds for vaginal radium application. *Radiology* 1963;80:282–284.

68. Peracchia G, Salti C. A simple method of preparing custom molds for intracavitary treatment of gynecological cancer. *Int J Radiat Oncol Biol Phys* 1982;8(1):141–143.

69. Bertoni F, Bertoni G, Bignardi M. Vaginal molds for intracavitary: a new method of preparation. *Int J Radiat Oncol Biol Phys* 1983;9(10):1579–1582.

70. Pearcey RG, Petereit DG. Post-operative high dose rate brachytherapy in patients with low to intermediate risk endometrial cancer. *Radiother Oncol* 2000;56(1):17–22.

71. Paterson R. A dosage system for gamma ray therapy: Part I [Clinical]. *Br J Radiol* 1934;7:592–612.

72. Parker H. A dosage system for gamma ray therapy. Part II: physical aspects. *Br J Radiol* 1934;7:612–632.

73. Meredith WJ. *Radium dosage.* Edinburgh, London: E. & S. Livingstone, 1967.

74. Kwan DK, Kagan AR, Olch AJ, et al. Single- and double-plane iridium-192 interstitial implants: implantation guidelines and dosimetry. *Med Phys* 1983;10(4):456–461.

75. Zwicker RD, Schmidt-Ullrich R, Schiller B. Planning of Ir-192 seed implants for boost irradiation to the breast. *Int J Radiat Oncol Biol Phys* 1985;11(12):2163–2170.

76. Pierquin B, Marinello G. *A practical manual of brachytherapy.* Madison, WI: Medical Physics Publishing, 1997.

77. Pierquin B, Dutreix A. For a new methodology in curietherapy: the system of Paris (endo- and plesioradiotherapy with non-radioactive preparation). A preliminary note. *Ann Radiol (Paris)* 1966;9(9):757–760.

78. Neblett D. Clinical techniques and applicators available for interstitial implantation. In: Williamson JF, Thomadsen BR, Nath R, eds. *Brachytherapy physics.* Madison, WI: Medical Physics Publishing, 1995.

CHAPTER 19

Radiation Therapy Using High-Energy Electron Beams

Bruce J. Gerbi

INTRODUCTION

High-energy electrons have been commonly available in radiation therapy for the treatment of cancer since the early 1950s and their availability in modern radiation therapy departments is simply expected. The most useful electron energies in clinical settings range from 6 to 20 MeV with the intermediate beam energies being the most clinically useful. Electrons are used for specific purposes within a radiation therapy department mainly due to their precise depth of penetration and ability to deliver a high dose to the superficial regions of the body. They are most useful for treatments of the skin, scars, chest wall treatments post-mastectomy, and for superficial nodal treatments. They are also particularly well suited for treatments of targets that lie above sensitive structures such as the spinal cord, lung, or heart.

The energy of a clinical beam is described by the most probable energy at the surface at the standard treatment distance (usually 100 cm source–skin distance [SSD]) and represents the energy possessed by the majority of the incident electrons at that location. Thus, when a particular electron energy is selected for use on a linear accelerator, this is the closest integer value to the actual energy of the electron beam hitting the patient's surface.

HIGH-ENERGY ELECTRON CHARACTERISTICS

Electrons are directly ionizing particles that possess a negative charge and are low in mass compared to protons and neutrons. As charged particles, they interact directly with the absorbing material, being attracted to positive charges and repelled by negative charges. These forces of attraction or repulsion are called Coulomb interactions and result directly in ionizations and excitations within the absorbing medium. Because the mass of an electron is ~1/2,000 of the mass of protons and neutrons, its direction of travel can be easily changed by interactions with these more massive particles. Thus, electrons are easily scattered by the absorbing medium. As electrons pass through a material, their average energy decreases due to either collisions or radiative processes until they are eventually captured by the atoms of the absorbing material. It is the location at which these electrons scatter, where

bonds are broken, and where ionization and excitation take place that dictates where radiation dose is deposited within a medium, or more importantly, within patients.

Change in Central Axis Percentage Depth-Dose with Change in Beam Energy

The central axis (CA) percentage depth-dose curve is a display of the dose at depth along the CA of the beam compared to the dose at the depth of maximum dose. The CA percentage depth-dose characteristics of electron beams are fundamentally dependent upon the types of interactions that incident high-energy electrons undergo, as described above. From a clinical standpoint, the shape of the CA percentage depth-dose curve for an electron beam depends most notably on beam energy, field size, the angle of beam incidence, collimation, and SSD. Figure 19.1 shows typical CA percentage depth-dose curves in water for 10×10 cm^2 electron beams from a Varian 2300CD linear accelerator. The plot shows beam energies for 6, 9, 12, 15, 18, and 22 MeV electrons. As can be seen in the figure, the dose at the surface for electron beams is much higher than what is exhibited by photon beams. The surface dose (which is the dose in the first 0.05 cm) is ~75% for 6 MeV electrons increasing with energy to over 90% at the surface for the 22 MeV electron beam. This increase in surface dose with increasing beam energy occurs because lower energy electrons are scattered more easily and through larger angles than are electron beams of higher energy. This causes the dose to increase more rapidly and over shorter distances for low-energy electron beams at the surface. As electrons penetrate more deeply into the medium, the depth of maximum dose is reached. Contrary to megavoltage photon beams, the depth at which the maximum dose occurs for electron beams does not follow a specific trend of increasing with increasing beam energy. The depth of maximum dose is also dependent on linear accelerator design and the accessories used for the treatment. Beyond the depth of d_{max}, higher energy electrons penetrate more deeply and falloff less rapidly per centimeter than lower energy electrons. At depths greater than the practical range, R_p, the CA electron percentage depth-dose curve decreases slowly with depth since the dose in this region is contributed mainly by straggling electrons and bremsstrahlung radiation. The practical

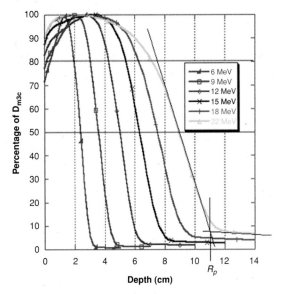

Figure 19.1. Electron central axis percentage depth-dose curves for a Varian 2300CD, 10×10 cm^2 cone, 100 cm SSD.

range of the beam is defined as the depth at which the straight line decreasing portion of the electron CA percentage depth-dose curve intersects a line describing the photon contamination of the beam. A good estimate of the practical range of the beam in centimeters can be obtained by taking the energy of the beam, in MeV, and

dividing it by 2. An R_{p} of 11 cm is shown in Figure 19.1 for the 22 MeV electron beam. The photon contamination is ~1% for 6 MeV rising to approximately 6% to 7% for the 22 MeV beam. This photon contamination is the result of electron interactions with the exit window of the linac, the scattering foils, the beam ion-chamber, the collimator jaws, or treatment apparatus. Additional x-rays can also be produced within the patient, although the magnitude of this contribution is not very large.

Change in Central Axis Percentage Depth Dose with Change in Field Size

Standard electron cone sizes for linear accelerators typically range from 6×6 to 25×25 cm^2. There is significant change in CA percentage depth dose with field size when the field size decreases to less than the practical range for that electron beam energy. This is because of the loss of side scatter with decreasing field size, and is shown by the data in Figure 19.2. There is a shift in both the depth of dose maximum and the D_{90} dose toward the surface with decreasing field size but the R_{p} is unchanged. Clinical data for an Elekta Synergy linear accelerator is shown in Table 19.1. For the 6 MeV beam data, the CA percentage depth dose is the same for all field sizes within the measurement accuracy of the data. For the more energetic 18 MeV beam, the CA percentage depth dose is slightly less for the 6×6 cm^2

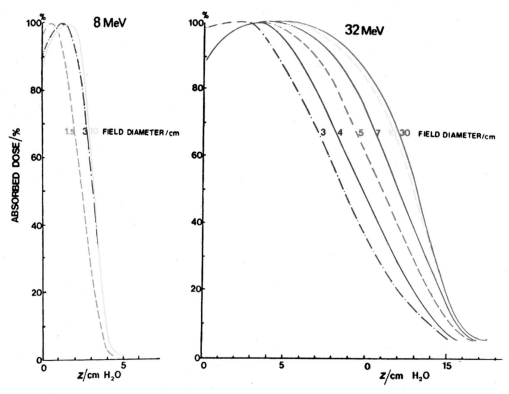

Figure 19.2. The change in percentage depth dose for high-energy electrons with change in field size. *Source:* From ICRU. International commission on radiation units and measurements, radiation dolsimetry: electron beams with energies between 1 and 50 MeV, ICRU Report 35. Bethesda, MD: International Commission on Radiation Units and Measurement, 1984.

| TABLE 19.1 | **Central Axis Percentage Depth Doses for 6 and 18 MeV Electrons from an Elekta Synergy Linear Accelerator** | | |

6 MeV Electrons

| Depth (cm) | Buildup dose (%)[a] | | |
	6 × 6 cone	14 × 14 cone	25 × 25 cone
Surface	68.0	70.7	72.0
0.5 cm	78.9	82.0	81.2
1.0 cm	90.8	92.7	92.6

| Dose (%) | Depth (cm)[b] | | |
	6 × 6 cone	14 × 14 cone	25 × 25 cone
100	1.5	1.5	1.5
95	1.9	1.9	1.9
90	2.0	2.0	2.0
80	2.2	2.2	2.2
70	2.4	2.3	2.4
60	2.5	2.5	2.5
50	2.6	2.6	2.6
40	2.8	2.7	2.8
30	2.9	2.9	2.9
20	3.0	3.0	3.0
10	3.3	3.2	3.3
Photon contamination	1	1	1

18 MeV Electrons

| Depth (cm) | Buildup dose (%)[a] | | |
	6 × 6 cone	14 × 14 cone	25 × 25 cone
Surface	88.3	86.3	87.4
0.5 cm	95.0	92.1	91.8
1.0 cm	98.1	95.0	95.0

| Dose (%) | Depth (cm)[b] | | |
	6 × 6 cone	14 × 14 cone	25 × 25 cone
100	3.9	3.9	3.9
95	4.9	5.4	5.4
90	5.5	5.8	5.8
80	6.0	6.2	6.3
70	6.4	6.6	6.6
60	6.8	6.9	6.9
50	7.1	7.2	7.2
40	7.4	7.5	7.5
30	7.7	7.8	7.8
20	8.1	8.3	8.3
10	8.7	8.8	8.8
Photon contamination	3.4%	3.7%	3.7%

[a]Measured using the Attix plane-parallel ionization chamber in a solid water phantom.
[b]Measured using a Therados electron diode, Scandatronix water phantom.

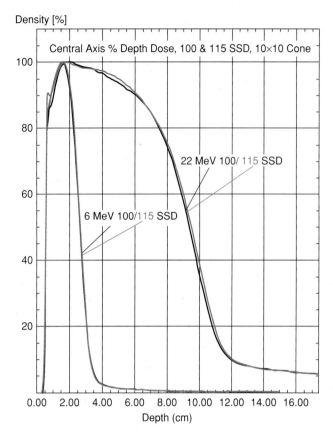

Figure 19.3. Central axis percentage depth-dose curve for 100 and 115 cm SSD. The slight difference in central axis percentage depth dose observed for the 22 MeV beam is due to field size differences rather than SSD effects.

cone size as compared to the two larger cone sizes since the practical range of the 18 MeV beam is ~9 cm. The data in the build-up region were taken using an Attix plane–parallel ionization chamber in a solid water phantom while the data deeper than the d_{max} point was taken using a Therados electron diode.

Change in Central Axis Percentage Depth Dose with Change in SSD

There is only a slight change in the CA percentage depth-dose values at extended treatment distances. In the buildup region of the curve, the difference between the 100 and 115 cm SSD data is clinically insignificant (Fig. 19.3). At depths deeper than the location of d_{max}, no difference is observed in the 100 cm SSD curve versus the 115 cm SSD data. For the 20 MeV data, the 80% to 95% isodose lines beyond the depth of the d_{max} show very slight but clinically insignificant differences between the 100 and the 115 cm SSD curves. This is because the 10×10 cm^2 field at 100 cm diverges to an 11.5×11.5 cm^2 field at 115 cm SSD.

Change in Central Axis Percentage Depth Dose due to Inhomogeneities

The CA percentage depth-dose curve can be significantly changed from those measured in water by the presence of non-unit density inhomogeneities such as lung, bone, air cavities, or other non-unit density materials. For small inhomogeneous regions, it is difficult to calculate accurately the dose distribution because of the complicated nature of the scatter in and around these areas. For larger regions of inhomogeneous material, the amount of change in the CA percentage depth-dose curve depends on the electron density of the material compared to the electron density of water. For lung tissue and air cavities whose electron density is lower than that of water, the electrons penetrate to a deeper depth than they would in a water medium. This change in the depth of penetration is shown in Figure 19.4 using cork to represent lung tissue. For compact bone whose electron density is greater than water, a proportionate decrease in the depth of penetration of the electrons is seen.

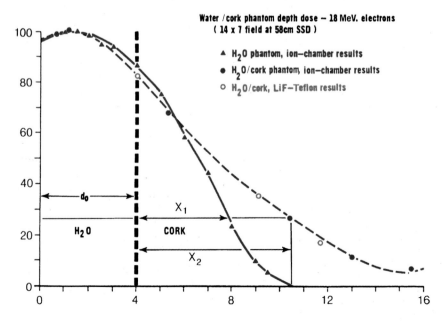

Figure 19.4. Depth-dose distribution in water and water-cork phantoms. *Source:* Modified from Almond P, Wright A, Boone M. High-energy electron dose perturbations in regions of tissue heterogeneity. *Radiology* 1967;88: 1146.

TWO- AND THREE-DIMENSIONAL DOSE DISTRIBUTIONS FOR ELECTRON BEAMS

Off-Axis Beam Characteristics: Flatness and Symmetry

A uniform intensity across the electron-beam field is a requirement for clinical use of high-energy electrons in radiation therapy. As with photon beams, the off-axis ratio (OAR) relates the dose at any point in a plane perpendicular to the CA of the beam to the dose at the CA of the beam. A plot of the OAR versus distance from the CA is called a dose profile (Fig. 19.5). According to the AAPM Task Group 25 report, both symmetry and flatness should be verified on each of the principle and diagonal axis of the beam for the largest field for each applicator. Flatness specifications should be checked at several collimator and gantry angles. The reference plane is defined in TG-25 report "as a plane, parallel to the surface of the phantom and perpendicular to the CA of the beam at the depth of the 95% isodose beyond the depth of dose maximum." "The flatness of the bean normalized to the CA should not exceed ±5% (optimally within ±3%) over an area within lines 2 cm inside the geometric edge of fields that are equal to or larger than 10×10 cm^2." The symmetry of the beam in the reference plane should not differ by >2% at any pair of points symmetrically located at an equal distance from the CA of the beam. These measurements of flatness and symmetry should be done at the time of linac installation and should be verified monthly and following any major service of the linear accelerator (1–3).

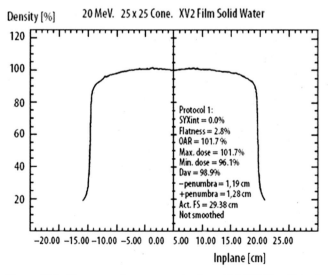

Figure 19.5. Flatness and symmetry plot for a 20 MeV, 25×25 cm^2 electron cone. The data is derived from an irradiated piece of Kodak XV2 film placed at the depth of maximum for the beam and scanned using a Wellhofer film scanner using WP700 software. *Source:* From Gerbi BJ. Clinical applications of high-energy electrons. In: Levitt SH, Purdy JA, Perez CA, et al., eds. *Technical basis of radiation therapy: practical clinical applications*, 4th ed. Berlin: Springer, 2006; Figure 7–6.

Isodose Curves for Normal Beam Incidence

Isodose curves are a collection of lines that join points of equal dose that show the variation in dose as a function of depth and distance away from the CA. The depth-dose data for fixed SSD beams are normalized to the point of maximum dose on the CA of the beam and are drawn at 10% intervals. Figure 19.6 shows typical isodose curves for electron beams (6 and 22 MeV) for a 10×10 cm^2 field from a Varian 2300CD accelerator. Isodose curves for electron beams are dependent on the beam energy, field size, collimation, and SSD. The 50% isodose curve almost follows beam divergence from the surface while the 90% and 80% isodose curves are pinched in toward the CA of the beam. Isodose curves lower than 50%, bow out, away from the CA, producing the distinctive isodose curve shape for high-energy electron beams. In clinical situations, the field size should be larger than the borders of the target by at least 1 cm to ensure that it is adequately covered by the 90% isodose line.

Isodose Distributions at Extended Treatment Distances

Figure 19.7 shows 9 and 20 MeV electron isodose curves at 100 and 115 cm SSD illustrating the influence of increasing the treatment distance on the shape of the isodose curves incident on a flat phantom. Because of the increased distance from the end of the electron cone, electrons scatter out of the beam resulting in a loss of sharpness in the edge of the beam both outside the 50% isodose line and inside the 50% line. The loss of field sharpness has critical clinical importance in both matching electron fields at extended distances and when choosing field sizes to cover the target region.

The final shape of the isodose curves can be influenced by factors such as patient curvature, inhomogeneities such as lung, bone, high-Z materials, and field-shaping devices such as cerrobend inserts, lead cutouts that are placed on the patient's skin surface, and internal shields designed to protect sensitive or normal tissues.

Isodose Distributions for Curved and Irregular Surfaces

Radiation fields are seldom incidents on flat surfaces. The more common situation is that the beam is incident on a curved surface, surfaces with multiple changes in contour, or on oblique surfaces. This is clearly evident in treatments of the post-mastectomy chest wall, extremities, the scalp, areas in and around the eyes, nose, or ears, or where complex skin folds are involved. Surgical areas can also create abrupt changes and irregularities in the patient's surface. Treatments of any of these areas of the body dramatically change the isodose characteristics of electron beams from what is measured for normally incident electron beams on flat surfaces. Figure 19.8 shows isodose

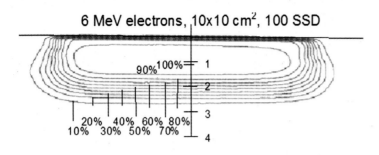

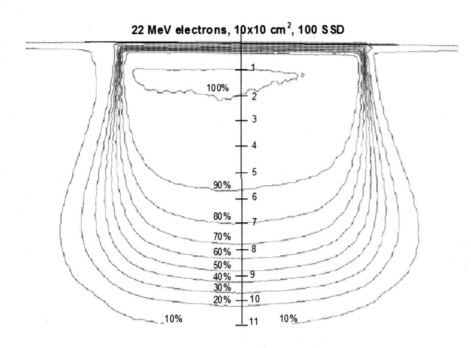

Figure 19.6. Typical 6 and 22 MeV electron curves, 10×10 cm^2 electron cone, 100 SSD, Varian 2300CD. The data was taken using Kodak XV2 film placed parallel to the incident beam in a solid water phantom and scanned using a Wellhofer film scanner using WP700 software.

curves for an electron beam incidents on a curved surface such as a post-mastectomy chest wall. The isodose curves follow roughly the curvature of the external contour but there are other changes due to attenuation of the beam, obliquity effects, loss of scatter, and decrease in the beam intensity due to inverse square decrease with increased distance from the end of the electron applicator. As the angle of beam incidence becomes more oblique, the maximum dose moves more toward the surface, and the shape of the CA percentage depth-dose curve changes dramatically, but the depth of maximum penetration of the beam stays essentially the same. Table 19.2 from Khan (4), shows numerically the change in the CA percentage depth dose as a function of the angle of electron beam incidence for various electron energies for angles of incidence of 30, 45, and 60 degrees.

Isodose Distributions Involving Inhomogeneities

High-energy electrons are greatly affected by the presence of inhomogeneities in the body. The effects of the presence of bone, lung, air, teeth, and implanted materials greatly influence the scattering and interactions of electrons and

consequently the final distribution of dose within the body. Electron depth-dose distributions are dependent on the electron density of the materials through which the beam passes and ultimately on the physical density of these materials. Because lung is one-fourth to one-third the density of normal tissue (5), high-energy electrons travel three to four times farther in this material than in unit density material. When using electrons for treatment of the post-mastectomy chest wall, the desire is to put the 80% isodose line at the lung chest-wall interface. This adequately treats the tissues of the chest wall but can lead to a high dose to the underlying lung. Figure 19.9 illustrates the challenges associated with the use of electrons in this region and shows the enhanced penetration in lung as compared to normal tissue. Bolus is often used to ensure not only that the 80% isodose line lies at the chest wall–lung interface, but also that a high dose is given to the skin surface.

Bones are often present in the treatment region when using electrons. Bone density can vary in density from approximately 1.0 to 1.1 g/cm^3 for spongy bone to 1.5 to 1.8 g/cm^3 for compact bone found in the skull, mandible, or the long bones that provide strength and support in the body. The ribs are also quite important to consider when

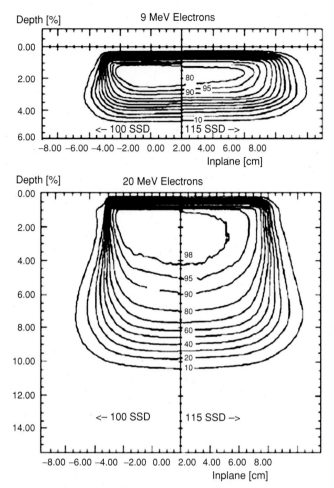

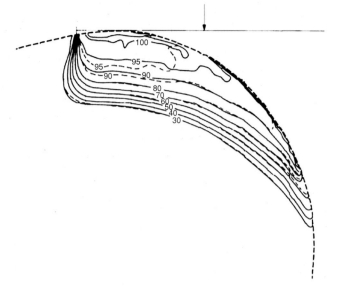

Figure 19.8. Electrons incident on a curved surface.

Figure 19.7. Electron isodose curves for 9 and 22 MeV electrons at 100 and 115 cm SSD produced with a 10 × 10 cm² cone.

treating the chest wall. Figure 19.10 shows the difference in the shape of the isodose distribution of 17 MeV electrons when a slab of bone is present in the beam as compared to the isodose distribution produced in a unit density phan-

tom. With the bone present, the electron isodose curves are shifted toward the surface because of the extra attenuation in bone. In addition, the dose is increased at the edges of the bone due to the enhanced scattering of electrons into this region. Underneath the bone edge, there is an area of decreased dose due to the loss of side scatter equilibrium.

The presence of air cavities ($\rho = 0.0013$ g/cm³) in the path of electron beams has a large effect on the final distribution of electrons within the body. Because of complicated scattering at the tissue–air interfaces, a significant reduction in dose to the tissues adjacent to the air cavity can lead to underdosing of 10% or more (6). This could result in an inadequate dose being delivered to the target region. Figure 19.11 (6) shows the electron distribution for treatments in the nasal region when both bone and air cavities are taken into account. In comparison to an electron dose distribution, which assumes the region to be

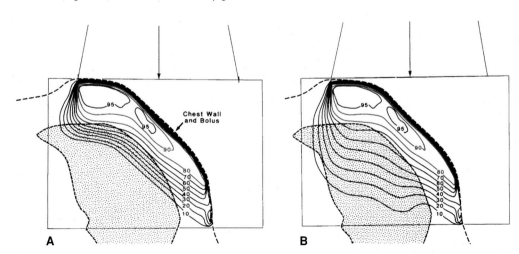

Figure 19.9. An example of chest wall irradiation using 13 × 15 cm², 10 MeV electrons (effective SSD = 68 cm) showing enhanced penetration into lung. **A:** Calculated isodose curves uncorrected for lung density. **B:** Calculated isodose curves corrected for lung density ($\rho = 0.25$ g/cm³). Bolus was added to the surface to even out chest wall thickness and maximize the surface dose.

TABLE 19.2	**Obliquity Factors for Electron Beams. These Factors Show the Relative Change in the Beam Intensity at Angle θ Compared with that at Normal Beam Incidence ($\theta = 0$ degree)**					

	E_0 (MeV)					
Z^a/R_p	22	18	15	12	9	6
(a) $\theta = 30$ degrees						
0.0	1.00	0.98	0.98	1.00	0.94	1.01
0.1	1.00	1.00	1.00	1.00	1.00	1.08
0.2	1.00	1.00	1.01	1.02	1.05	1.11
0.3	1.01	1.00	1.02	1.03	1.05	1.06
0.4	1.01	1.01	1.02	1.00	1.00	0.96
0.5	1.00	1.00	0.98	0.96	0.92	0.86
0.6	0.95	0.94	0.92	0.90	0.86	0.79
0.7	0.92	0.90	0.87	0.86	0.86	0.83
0.8	0.93	0.85	0.82	0.90	1.00	0.96
0.9	1.09	1.00	1.20	1.11	1.44	1.00
1.0	1.42	1.54	1.50	1.50	1.30	1.00
(b) $\theta = 45$ degrees						
0.0	1.03	1.02	1.03	1.05	0.98	1.14
0.1	1.03	1.04	1.04	1.06	1.10	1.14
0.2	1.05	1.06	1.07	1.11	1.12	1.12
0.3	1.06	1.07	1.09	1.09	1.05	1.07
0.4	1.04	1.04	1.04	1.01	0.93	0.92
0.5	1.00	0.99	0.92	0.92	0.80	0.77
0.6	0.93	0.90	0.86	0.82	0.70	0.69
0.7	0.84	0.84	0.82	0.77	0.70	0.76
0.8	0.87	0.83	0.85	0.86	0.83	1.10
0.9	1.30	1.00	1.43	1.20	1.40	1.46
1.0	2.17	2.31	2.19	2.50	2.00	2.14
(c) $\theta = 60$ degrees						
0.0	1.06	1.06	1.10	1.14	1.14	1.30
0.1	1.10	1.12	1.17	1.20	1.23	1.21
0.2	1.12	1.14	1.15	1.16	1.17	1.08
0.3	1.07	1.07	1.07	1.0	0.98	0.90
0.4	1.00	0.96	0.93	0.86	0.79	0.70
0.5	0.87	0.84	0.79	0.74	0.67	0.56
0.6	0.75	0.74	0.69	0.63	0.58	0.51
0.7	0.70	0.68	0.67	0.62	0.57	0.56
0.8	0.75	0.71	0.67	0.74	0.77	0.87
0.9	1.21	1.00	1.29	1.14	1.60	1.40
1.0	2.31	2.46	2.75	3.0	3.2	2.45

$^a Z$ indicates perpendicular depth below the surface of the phantom (cm), and R_p indicates the practical range of the electron beam (cm). Data taken using a Varian Clinac 2500 linear accelerator.
Source: From Khan FM, Deibel FC, Soleimani-Meigooni A. Obliquity correction for electron beams. *Med Phys* 1985; 12:749–753.

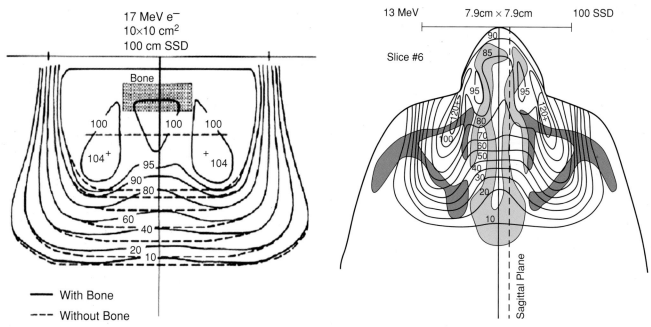

17 MeV e⁻
10×10 cm²
100 cm SSD

Bone

100   100   100

104⁺   ⁺104
      95
      90
      80
      60
      40
      20 10

—— With Bone
--- Without Bone

Figure 19.10. The effect of compact bone on 17 MeV electron isodose curves. *Source:* From Hogstron K. Dosimetry of electron heterogeneities. In: Wright A, Boyer A, eds. Advances in radiation therapy treatment planning. New York, NY: American Institute of Physics, Inc., 1983:223–243.

13 MeV   7.9cm × 7.9cm   100 SSD

Slice #6

Sagittal Plane

Figure 19.11. The effect of the abrupt change in surface contour by the nose and the effect on the final isodose distribution. The plan is done assuming unit density material and not taking into account the air cavities in this region of the body. *Source:* From Chobe R, McNeese M, Weber R, et al. Radiation therapy for carcinoma of the nasal vestibule. *Otolaryngol Head Neck Surg* 1988;98:67–71.

unit density, a much higher dose to the brain stem, brain, and underlying anatomy is actually delivered than what would be expected if only unit density materials were used in the calculation.

High-Z materials can also be present in electron beams in the form of implanted prosthetic devices (7), fillings for dental cavities, or deliberately as internal shields designed and used to limit the dose to underlying tissue. Implanted devices and materials most commonly consist of advanced polymers, ceramic materials, stainless steel, and titanium. Internal shields are fabricated from several materials and can consist of aluminum, lead, tungsten, and gold or a combination of these materials. The classic graph of electron backscatter versus atomic number, Z (Fig. 19.12) (8)

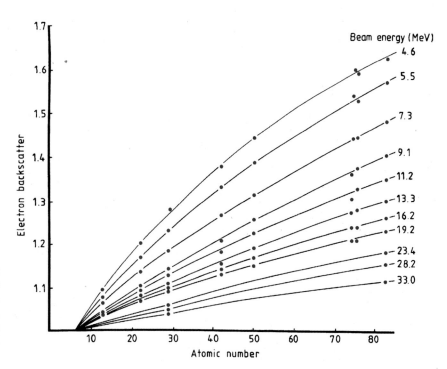

Beam energy (MeV)
4.6
5.5
7.3
9.1
11.2
13.3
16.2
19.2
23.4
28.2
33.0

Figure 19.12. The relative amount of electron backscatter for various electron beam energies above different atomic number materials. *Source:* From Klevenhagen SC, Lambert GD, Arbabi A. Backscattering in electron beam therapy for energies between 3 and 35 MeV. *Phys Med Biol* 1982;27:363–373.

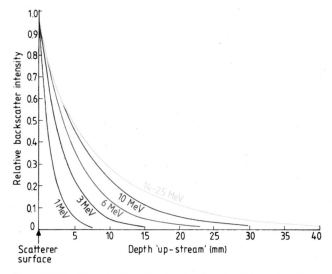

Figure 19.13. The intensity of backscatter from lead through polystyrene for different electron beam energies. *Source:* From Lambert G, Klevenhagen S. Penetration of backscattered electrons in polystyrene for energies between 1–25 MeV. *Phys Med Biol* 1982;27:721.

shows the relative amount of backscatter observed from different atomic number materials as a function of electron beam energy at the interface. This shows that there is increased backscatter with increasing Z and decreasing energy of the electrons at the interface. Figure 19.13 shows the intensity of the backscattered electrons from lead transmitted through polystyrene in the upstream direction of the incident electron beam (9). Whether designing internal shields for the protection of underlying material or when dealing with implanted materials used from the treatment of other medical conditions, the effects of these high-Z materials on the final dose distribution must be carefully evaluated.

CLINICAL USE OF ELECTRON BEAMS

Dose Prescription—ICRU 71

Report 71 of the International Commission on Radiation Units and Measurements (ICRU) was published in 2004. This report described new recommendations for "prescribing, recording, and reporting electron beam therapy" (10). They recommended that the same dose prescription approach be used for electron treatments as for photons as specified in ICRU Reports 50 and 62 for photon beams (11,12). The concepts of gross tumor volume (GTV), clinical target volume (CTV), planning target volume (PTV), treated volume, organs at risk, and planning organ at risk volume (PRV) were defined as for photon beam treatment planning purposes. The treatment was to be specified completely, including time-dose characteristics making no adjustments in the relative biological effectiveness differences between photons and electrons. For reporting electron doses, they recommended the selection of a reference

point referred to as the "ICRU reference point." This point should always be chosen at the center (or central part) of the PTV and should be clearly described. In general, the beam energy is selected so that the maximum of the depth-dose curve on the beam axis is located at the center of the PTV. If the peak dose does not fall in the center of the PTV, then the ICRU reference point for reporting should be selected at the center of the PTV and the maximum dose should also be reported. For reference electron irradiation conditions, they also recommend that the following dose values be reported (10):

■ The maximum absorbed dose to water.
■ The location of and dose value at the ICRU reference point if not located at the level of the peak absorbed dose.
■ The maximum and minimum doses in the PTV, and dose(s) to OARs derived from dose distributions and/or dose–volume histograms. For small and irregularly shaped beams, the peak absorbed dose to water for reference conditions should be reported. It is also recommended that when corrections for oblique incidence and inhomogeneous material are applied, the application of these corrections should be reported.

Dose reporting guidelines for the special techniques of intraoperative radiation therapy (13) and total skin irradiation (TSI) are also provided in ICRU Report 71. The treatment goal for TSI is to deliver a uniform dose to the total skin surface. For patients with superficial disease, TSI can be delivered with one electron energy. However, the thickness of the skin disease may vary with stage, pathology, and location on the body surface. For such cases, several CTVs need to be identified and different electron beam energies may be required to treat the various regions. For each anatomical site, an ICRU reference point at or near the center of the PTVs/CTVs has to be selected for reporting. The reference point may be at the level of the peak dose if it is located in the central part of the PTV. In addition, an ICRU reference point that is clinically relevant and located within the PTV can be used for the entire PTV.

ICRU Report 71 recommended the reporting of the following dose values:

■ The peak absorbed dose in water for each individual electron beam
■ The location of and dose value at the ICRU reference point for each anatomical area
■ The best estimate of maximum and minimum dose to each anatomical area
■ The location and absorbed dose at the ICRU point for the whole PTV, and best estimate of the maximum and minimum doses for the whole PTV
■ Any other dose value considered as clinically significant

IORT is used after surgical intervention to deliver a large single-fraction dose of high-energy electrons to a well-defined anatomical location. ICRU Report 71 recommends that all devices that are used for IORT need to be reported. This includes the IORT applicator system specifying type, shape, bevel angle, and size of the applicator. The ICRU reference point for reporting is always selected in the center or central part of the PTV, and at the level of the maximum dose on the beam axis, when possible.

The ICRU recommended that the following dose values be reported for IORT (10):

■ The peak absorbed dose to water, under reference conditions, for each individual beam (if the beam axis is perpendicular to the tissue surface).
■ The maximum absorbed dose in water on the "clinical axis" for oblique beam.
■ The location of and dose value at the ICRU reference point (if different from above).
■ The best estimate of the maximum and minimum doses to the PTV. Usually, the irradiation conditions (electron energy, field size, etc.) are selected so that at least 90% of the dose at the ICRU reference point will be delivered to the entire PTV.

Output Determination

For clinical treatments, the determination of dose per monitor unit for each electron treatment is critical. The first step in this determination is the proper calibration of each electron beam energy according to an accepted calibration protocol. The AAPM Task Group 51 report (14) describes in detail the steps that need to be taken to determine the dose rate in terms of gray (Gy) per monitor unit (U) at a reference point in an electron beam for a specified field size and treatment distance. The IAEA TRS Report 398 was developed in parallel with AAPM TG-51 and is very similar in its calibration approach (15). Both calibration protocols use a dose to water calibration factor. For these calibration protocols, the dose rate in water is determined at the depth of d_{ref} at 100 cm SSD along the central axis of the electron beam. The calibration field size is 10×10 cm^2 unless the R_{50}, the depth of the 50% isodose line, is >8.5 cm. A 20×20 cm^2 field or larger is to be used for these higher beam energies. The calibration is to be performed at the depth of d_{ref}, which is defined as $0.6\ R_{50} - 0.1$ cm. The depth of d_{ref} is close to the depth of d_{max} for electron energies below about 12 MeV but is deeper than d_{max} for electron beams of higher energy. This is important to note since the electron CA percentage depth-dose curves are all normalized to the depth of d_{max}.

The output for each electron beam energy of a linac for a 10×10 cm^2 cone is set to deliver 1.0 cGy per monitor unit at the depth of d_{max}. The output for every other electron cone is expressed as a ratio of the output of the 10×10 cm^2 cone. Thus, if the measured output at d_{max} for a 15 $\times$ 15 cm^2 cone when operated at 6 MeV is 1.008 cGy per monitor unit, then the 15×15 cm^2 electron cone factor would be 1.008 cGy/U divided by 1.000 cGy/U equaling a cone factor of 1.008. A general expression for the output

factor from AAPM Report 99 from Task Group 70 is, "... the output factor S_e for a particular electron field size r_a at any treatment SSDr_a is defined as the ratio of the dose per monitor unit, D/U (Gy/MU), on the central axis at the depth of maximum dose for that field, $d_{max}(r_a)$, to the dose per monitor unit for the reference applicator, or field size r_0, and standard SSDr_0 at the depth of maximum dose for the reference field used in calibration, $d_{max}(r_0)$. In equation form:

$$S_e(d_{max}(r_a), r_a, SSD_{r_a}) = \frac{D/U(d_{max}(r_a), r_a, SSD_{r_a})}{D/U(d_{max}(r_0), r_0, SSD_{r_0})}.\text{" (16)}$$

Output Determination: Blocked/Restricted Fields

When electron treatment fields are small, irregular in shape, or both, or when the field is smaller than or close to the minimum radius required for lateral scatter equilibrium, the depth of maximum dose moves toward the surface, the central axis percentage depth dose decreases, and the output decreases as compared to the unrestricted field. This minimum radius, R_{eq}, has been shown (17) to be well represented by the equation

$$R_{eq} \cong 0.88\sqrt{E_{p,0}}$$

where R_{eq} is in centimeters and $E_{p,0}$ is expressed in MeV. $E_{p,0}$ is the most probable energy at the phantom surface (18) and is given by the equation

$$E_{p,0} = 0.22 + 1.98R_p + 0.0025R_p^2$$

for water with the practical range, R_p, given in centimeters. Either custom measurements should be performed or analytical approaches described in the historical literature should be done for electron fields whose size is below this minimum radius. Alternatively, a collection of measured outputs for various irregularly shaped fields can be assembled against which a new irregularly shaped field can be compared. Actual measurements of dose rate, depth dose, and isodose distributions can be performed with ionization chambers, diodes, or various films but film can be the most efficient detector to quickly capture this information. A single film in a water equivalent solid phantom can be irradiated parallel to the electron beam with the patient cutout in place and used to determine the depth of d_{max} for the restricted field. This film can then be used to indicate the shape of the isodose curves for the field in that measurement plane to help assess if the electron field adequately covers the target to be treated. Once the d_{max} for the restricted field is determined from this first film, a second piece of film can be irradiated perpendicular to the incident electron beam at this depth in a water equivalent solid phantom with the cutout in place. The optical density on this film can be compared to a third film placed perpendicular to the beam at the depth of d_{max} for the unrestricted field and irradiated with the 10×10 cm^2 cone in place. By comparing the optical density of the 10×10 cm^2 film with that of the optical density of the film for the restricted field, the output in terms of dose per monitor unit for the restricted field can be determined. In addition, the isodose curves for the restricted field can be well described by the data represented on the two films taken with the restricted field cutout in place using automated film scanning software.

Small and irregular electron fields can be assessed using verified computational techniques (17,19–24) in place of direct measurements. Several analytical approaches are available in the historic literature that describe how to determine output, the shift in d_{max}, and the central axis percentage depth dose values for restricted fields. The CA depth-dose values for a rectangular electron field whose sides measure X and Y can be determined by taking the square root of the product of the depth doses for the square fields whose sides are X and Y (25) as shown by the equation:

$$\%dd(d, r_{X,Y}) = \sqrt{\%dd(d, r_{X,X}) \cdot \%dd(d, r_{Y,Y})}$$

The output factor, $S_e(d_m, r_{X,Y})$, at d_{max} for a rectangular field of dimensions X and Y, follows a similar relationship where the output factor for the rectangular field at d_{max} is equal to the square root of the product of the output factors at d_{max} for the square fields of dimension X and Y (26):

$$S_e(d_m, r_{X,Y}) = \sqrt{S_e(d_m, r_{X,X}) \cdot S_e(d_m, r_{Y,Y})}$$

For irregularly shaped fields that are not rectangular in nature, algorithms that use a sector integration technique (17,19,21–23,27,28) or discrete pencil-beam models (29–31) have been shown to be accurate in calculating output factors. The approach using lateral buildup ratios (LBRs) (17,23,28) is based on the electron pencil-beam model and is able to predict the shift in the depth of d_{max}, the change in the output factor at d_{max}, and the change in the CA depth dose for the irregularly shaped field. Alternatively, treatment planning systems based on the current models or on Monte Carlo codes may be accurate in the determination of output factors, depth dose, and isodose characteristics of small and irregularly shaped electron fields (32).

The Use of Bolus in Electron Beam Treatments

There are many uses for bolus during electron beam treatments. It can be used to increase the dose to the skin surface, as a replacement for missing tissue to compensate for surface irregularities, and as a compensating material to conform the radiation dose as closely as possible to the target volume. For modern linear accelerators, the dose at

the surface for the lower electron beam energies can be as low as 70% to 80% of the value at d_{max}. Bolus material would be required in almost all cases to ensure that a superficial target is covered by the 90% isodose line.

Many materials are currently used as bolus for electron treatments. These include paraffin wax, polystyrene, acrylic (polymethylmethacrylate), Super Stuff™, Superflab™, and Superflex™. Solid sheets of thermoplastic materials can also be used quite effectively as bolus since they conform very well to the skin surface. They are also transparent when hot, which is a distinct advantage since skin marks as well as anatomical features can be accurately transferred to the surface of the plastic at this time. The material is also very easy to cut while hot and this is the perfect time to make modifications to the final shape and conformation of the bolus. It has a density greater than water but this can be taken into account accurately by modern treatment planning systems using CT scan data with the material in place during the scan. Since it conforms so well to the patient's surface, the problem of small air gaps between the bolus and underlying skin surface can be greatly reduced or eliminated altogether.

For more demanding clinical situations, custom compensating bolus can be designed either by hand or by computerized techniques (33,34). The manual method of compensating bolus fabrication is the primary means available to most clinics. Hand techniques for creating custom compensating bolus have been described that use individual CT scans (35) or ultrasound imaging (36). For these techniques, an electron energy is selected so that the depth of penetration of the beam covers the deepest portion of the target to be treated to at least the 90% isodose line. Bolus is added to the entrance surface of each CT slice to create an equal depth of penetration along fan lines on all scans to cover the target (Fig. 19.14) (34). The proposed bolus is added to each individual CT scan and a computerized treatment plan is completed to confirm the acceptability of the bolus design. The technique is repeated until a final, acceptable bolus design based on the treatment plan is achieved. A grid describing the bolus location on the patient and the thickness of the bolus at those locations is produced and the compensator is made to these specifications (Fig. 19.15) (34). The custom bolus is then made from several thicknesses of bolus material according to the grid pattern. The grid also serves as an alignment tool so that the compensating bolus can be placed accurately on the patient from one treatment to the next. The constructed final bolus is put in place on the patient and a verification CT scan series is performed to ensure that the position of the bolus is correct and to perform a final, verification treatment plan for the patient with the custom bolus in place. This manual technique is very time-consuming.

Computerized techniques to perform this operation have been devised that take multiple Coulomb scattering into account and the three-dimensional (3D) nature of the problem (33,34). Using this technique, bolus that is

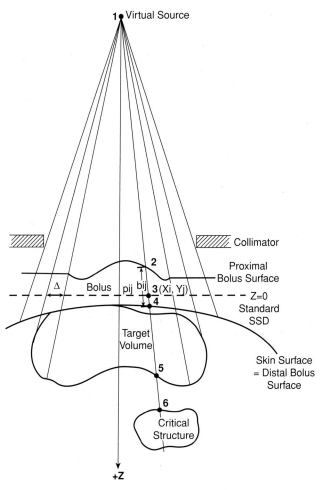

Figure 19.14. Diagram showing the patient contour, target volume, and the compensating bolus designed to optimize the irradiation of the target while minimizing the dose to the underlying critical structure. *Source:* From Low DA, Starkschall G, Bujnowski SW, et al. Electron bolus design for radiotherapy treatment planning: bolus design algorithms. *Med Phys* 1992;19:115–124.

much more effective in conforming the dose to the target and sparing underlying normal tissue can be produced. Treatment planning software with this capability has not been incorporated into the most common commercial systems but this capability does exist commercially through an alternate vendor (.decimal, Inc., 121 Central Park Place, Sanford, FL 28771). An example of this custom compensating bolus and the isodose coverage possible with its use for the head and neck region is shown in Figure 19.16.

Electron Field Matching and Abutment

Electron fields are abutted on the skin surface either to span a larger region or to treat a curved surface while trying to provide a homogeneous dose. Whether matching electron fields on a flat or a curved surface, care must be taken to ensure that the entire region is given an adequate and uniform dose, and that hot spots >20% are not created where the fields are abutted. Figure 19.17A shows

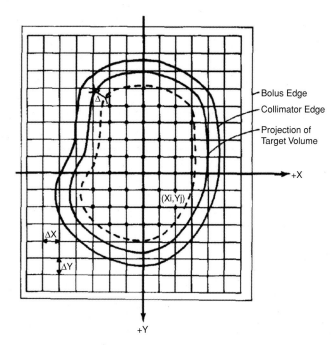

Figure 19.15. A compensating bolus diagram used for construction and placement of the bolus for patient treatment. *Source:* From Low DA, Starkschall G, Bujnowski SW, et al. Electron bolus design for radiotherapy treatment planning: bolus design algorithms. *Med Phys* 1992;19:115–124.

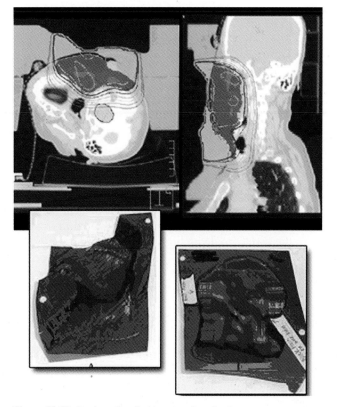

Figure 19.16. Isodose distributions produced using custom compensating bolus optimized using computerized software (.decimal, Inc., 121 Central Park Place, Sanford, FL 3277) is shown for a transverse (*upper left*) and sagittal contour (*upper right*) for the head and neck region. The *top* and *bottom* surfaces of the custom bolus is shown in the lower two illustrations.

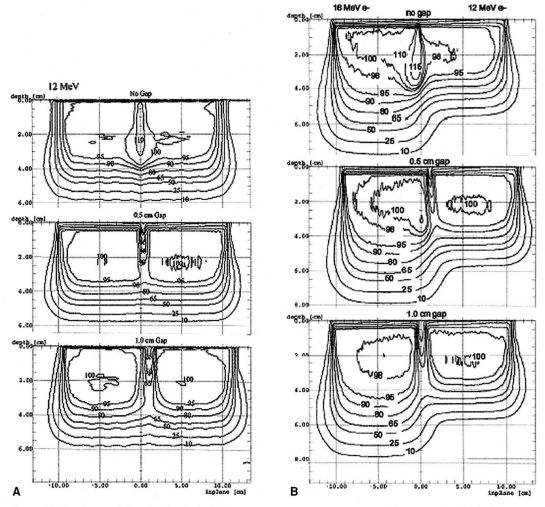

Figure 19.17. Electron field matching for a Varian 2100 c, 10 × 10 cone, 100 SSD; (**A**) two 12 MeV fields, (**B**) 16 MeV (*left*), 12 MeV (*right*) fields with no gap on the skin surface (*top*), 0.5 cm gap on the surface (*middle*), and 1.0 cm gap on the surface (*bottom*). Isodose values are 10, 25, 50, 65, 80, 90, 95, 100, and 110%. Data taken using Kodak XV-2 film in a solid water cassette and scanned using a Wellhofer isodensitomer and WP700 software.

two, 12 MeV 10 × 10 cm² electron fields from a Varian 2100 C abutted on a flat surface. The top figure shows the combined isodose curves when no gap is present between fields. The entire 20 cm long region is treated uniformly from the surface to depth but a high-dose region of 110% is created because of the bowing-out of the lower isodose curves from one field into the other. If a 0.5 or 1.0 cm gap on the skin is introduced, the 110% high-dose region is eliminated, but a region of low dose near the surface is introduced instead. If electron beams of different energy are abutted, such as the 16 and 12 MeV beams in Figure 19.17B, the magnitude of the high-dose region increases to 115%. Increasing the field separation to 0.5 or 1.0 cm reduces this high-dose region but again introduces a region of underdosage near the surface.

If electron fields are to be abutted, moving the junction location between the beams provides a safe means to reduce the overall magnitude of the high-dose region. The number of junction changes depends on the total dose, the size of the high-dose region, and the magnitude of the dose in the over-

lap region. A shift in the location of the junction by 1 cm is adequate in most instances but the absolute amount depends on the size of the overlap region and the number of junction shifts to be made. The junction should be moved a sufficient number of times and by a sufficient distance to ensure that the high-dose region does not exceed the prescription dose by more than 15% to 20%. Usually, a 1 cm junction shift every 1,000 cGy will meet this expectation.

Multiple electron fields are often used to treat curved surfaces. Matching electron fields in these situations can produce overlap regions that are not only larger in size, but also have a higher dose in the overlap region. The magnitude of the dose in the overlap region tends to increase with decreasing radius of curvature of the external body contour but depends on beam energy and the individual beam characteristics. Situations such as those illustrated in Figure 19.18 should be closely monitored in the clinic and the location of the junction should be repositioned with sufficient frequency to limit the risk of a complication. Using 12 MeV electrons and the beam

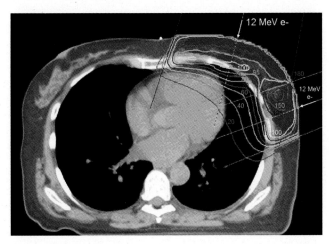

Figure 19.18. An illustration of the high-dose region (180% of the prescription dose) that can result when two electron fields abut at the skin surface. The diagram shows two, 12 MeV electron fields modeled on a pinnacle treatment planning system.

arrangement shown in the figure, the dose in the overlap region is 184% of the prescribed dose to d_{max}.

Electron Arc Technique

Electron arc techniques are an extension of the multiple matching electron field techniques described above and provide a solution to the high-dose regions generated using multiple, abutting electron fields. Electron arc techniques can be very effective in producing uniform dose distributions in areas of the body that have a consistent curvature throughout the entire region of treatment (Fig. 19.19). There are two basic approaches for electron arc therapy: the electron pseudoarc approach (37) and the electron arc technique (38,39) where the gantry is continuously rotating during the treatment. The pseudoarc technique employs a series of overlapping stationary electron fields and is usually easier to commission and use for patient planning. The amount of time required to commission and implement the continuously rotating electron arc technique for an individual patient is significantly greater. An excellent and detailed description of all aspects of electron arc therapy is given in the 1990 AAPM Summer School Proceedings (39).

Electron Pseudoarc Technique

The electron pseudoarc technique can be used to treat large areas of the chest wall or other curved surfaces of the body (37). Instead of using continuously rotating electron arc fields, several stationary electron fields are used to simulate an electron arc treatment. Several treatment examples where this technique could be useful are described below.

Chest Wall Irradiation

The pseudoarc technique as described by Boyer et al. can be effectively used to treat the post-mastectomy chest wall

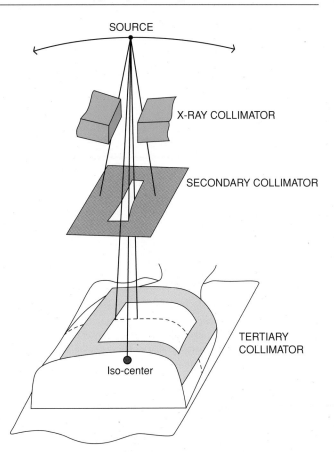

Figure 19.19. The field definition components required to perform electron arc irradiation. The secondary collimator is placed at a distance from the x-ray collimator and can vary in width to optimize the dose distribution at the patient surface. Tertiary collimation is required to restrict the electron scatter to the region being treated and to sharpen the electron dose distribution at the field edges. *Source:* From Khan FM, Fullerton GD, Lee JM, et al. Physical aspects of electron-beam arc therapy. *Radiology* 1977;124:497–500.

or any other body surface with a fairly consistent radius of curvature (37). Their technique is performed using the photon jaws to define the electron field size instead of using the electron cones. The region of treatment is outlined by lead or cerrobend shielding as with continuously rotating electron arcs. This is done to sharpen the field edges and to protect the tissues lying outside the treatment area. A field size of 10×35 cm^2 using the photon jaws was shown experimentally to provide the best combination of dose uniformity for phantom diameters of 16 to 40 cm and low amounts of photon contamination at the isocenter. The isocenter is positioned to provide a nearly constant distance from the isocenter to the skin surface and the fields are distributed along the patient's skin surface as indicated in Figure 19.20. The first electron field is situated with the CA of the beam on the shield with the field edge at the shield edge. The CA of the next field is placed at the edge of the former field and this sequence continues along the skin surface of the patient until the entire area is covered. The sequence is finished by adding a final field over the shielding at the end of the arc. The fields at the

Pseudo-Electron Arc

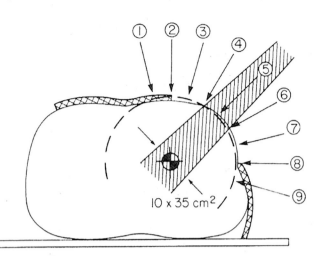

Figure 19.20. Schematic diagram of the shielding and placement of electron beams for a pseudo-electron arc treatment. The isocenter is placed below the surface of the patient at a location that is approximately equidistant to the patient's surface being treated. *Source:* From Boyer AL, Fullerton GD, Mira JG. An electron beam pseudoarc technique for irradiation of large areas of chest wall and other curved surfaces. *Int J Radiat Oncol Biol Phys* 1982;8:1969–1974.

beginning and ending of the string of fixed fields improve the uniformity of dose at the field edges. The resulting dose distribution obtained using this technique is very similar to what is produced from a continuously rotating electron arc (Fig. 19.21).

Total Limb Irradiation

Total limb irradiation is a subcategory of the pseudoarc technique used to treat the superficial regions of body extremities (40). This technique consists of the use of four to eight beams of 5 to 9 MeV electrons spaced at equal intervals around the periphery of the region to be treated. The field sizes used for the treatment should all be large enough to cover the entire region with falloff and extend both distally and proximally to cover the treatment area in

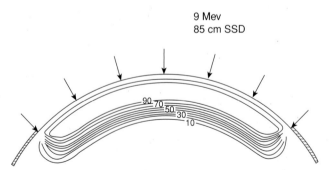

Figure 19.21. Dose distribution obtained using a 9 MeV electron pseudoarc technique with shielding on the skin surface to sharpen the distribution and define the treatment area. *Source:* From Boyer AL, Fullerton GD, Mira JG. An electron beam pseudoarc technique for irradiation of large areas of chest wall and other curved surfaces. *Int J Radiat Oncol Biol Phys* 1982;8:1969–1974.

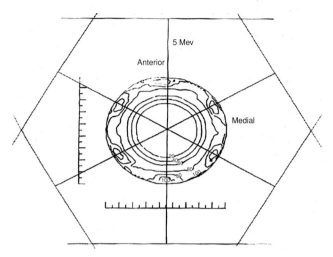

Figure 19.22. A 5 MeV, six-field electron beam arrangement to perform total limb irradiation. *Source:* From Wooden KK, Hogstrom KR, Blum P, et al. Whole-limb irradiation of the lower calf using a six-field electron technique. *Med Dosim* 1996;21:211–218.

those dimensions. Fields are all treated at one fixed SSD. Special shielding may be needed to confine the radiation only to the area of interest and this is most conveniently accomplished by the use of lead sheets placed on the patient's skin surface. Bolus may be required to ensure that the proper depth within the patient is treated. The use of bolus ensures that the skin dose is maximal but is not specifically needed for this purpose. The tangential incidence of the beams along with the use of multiple beams for this treatment deliver >90% of the maximum dose to the surface even without bolus. The penetration of the 90% isodose line for the multiple fields occurs at a shallower depth, however, than what would be measured for a single electron beam of the same energy. An idealized computer-generated dose distribution is shown in Figure 19.22 for six, equally spaced 17 cm wide, 5 MeV electron beams on a 9 cm diameter cylinder (40). The entire periphery of the cylindrical volume can be adequately treated to a known depth while still sparing a central core of tissue. Different beam energies, field sizes, and field arrangements can be chosen to optimize the dose distribution for a particular clinical situation.

To move this technique into clinical practice, the treatment positions and treatment region should be defined as completely as possible in the simulator. Since the technique involves fields that completely surround the extremity, a supine and prone treatment position may be required for treatments of a lower extremity since electron fields with cone attached cannot be delivered for the posterior and posterior oblique fields. Similar considerations need to be made for treating regions in the arms. Repositioning and immobilization aids are definitely required to ensure that the two treatment positions can be accurately reproduced for treatment. All superficial areas of clinical interest should be defined and marked so as to be visible on the treatment planning CT scan. A CT scan throughout the region should be performed and if the radio-opaque markers defining scars, field edges, involved areas, and the like cause artifacts on the scan or show as unusually high-Z areas, another scan should be taken with the markers removed so that an accurate electron calculation can be performed on the treatment planning computer. The CT scan without markers should be used for planning but fused with the CT scan set with markers. The PTV should be marked on the treatment planning CT scans, and computerized treatment planning should be done to ensure that the dose distribution throughout the entire region is adequate. This is important since the diameter of the extremity being treated often differs within the treatment region. For cases where a CT scan cannot be acquired in the treatment position, manually obtained contours representing the different diameter regions of the extremity should be taken and entered into the treatment planning computer. Measurements should be performed using a cylindrical phantom whose diameter is as close to the diameter of the extremities of the treatment situation to confirm the accuracy of the treatment plan and to define the output per monitor unit for the treatment. Once the patient starts treatment, TLDs should be used to ensure that the delivered dose is the same as the planned dose.

Total Skin Electron Therapy

Total skin electron therapy (TSET) was developed for the treatment of the entire skin surface to a uniform dose. It was primarily develop for the treatment of cutaneous T-cell lymphoma, which is a chronic progressive lymphoma often called mycosis fungoides. Management of this disease is reviewed by Hoppe (41,42). TSET is also useful in the treatment of Kaposi's sarcoma which is a radiosensitive cutaneous malignancy. Treatment typically uses electron beam energies of 4 to 10 MeV at the accelerator window, which translates into 3 to 7 MeV at the surface of the patient. Typical total doses range from 3,000 to 4,000 cGy delivered at 400 cGy per week delivered in four fractions

per week. Treatment, overall, is quite complex; it is time-consuming to develop and to deliver, involves numerous shielding requirements, boost fields, and a rigorous monitoring and quality assurance commitment. Performance of this technique requires special equipment, the ability to produce a large electron treatment field covering the entire body of the patient, a uniform dose over the entire skin surface with adequate penetration to cover the disease at depth, and a field arrangement that results in a small amount of photon contamination.

Special equipment includes a linear accelerator that is capable of operating in a high dose rate electron treatment mode (~900 cGy/min). A beam spoiler consisting of a 1 cm thick piece of acrylic large enough to intercept the beam (approximately 150×180 cm^2) should be available. Specialized cylindrical phantoms of 30 and 20 cm diameter are needed to determine output for the technique, the skin dose, the dose around the periphery of the patient, and the depth-dose distribution for the technique. A treatment stand along with specialized patient positioning devices is also required. Finally, various shields will be needed for the eyes, fingertips or the entire fingers, and for the toes or top of the feet.

Many techniques have been developed for the treatment of the total skin using electrons (41–49). The steps to take in commissioning this technique are listed in many reports and textbooks (43,50). Common to all these techniques is the need to produce a uniform (±10% flatness) electron field that is large enough to cover the entire patient. The most commonly used technique is the modified Stanford technique (47,48), which uses two fields angled above and below the horizontal (±θ) (Fig. 19.23) as the means to produce a treatment field large enough to encompass the entire patient. The amount of beam angulation is determined experimentally for the particular linac, treatment distance, and beam spoiler. For the treatment, each field is

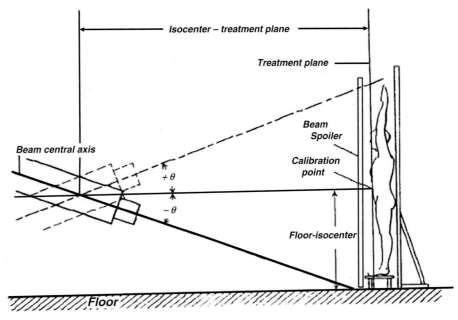

Figure 19.23. The modified Stanford Technique. Diagram illustrating total skin electron treatment position. Beam angulation provides a larger superior to inferior treatment field, along with extended treatment distance. The scatter plate (3/8 in. thick acrylic) is placed ~20 cm from the patient's surface while the treatment stand is designed to place umbilicus of the average-height patient at about the center of the overall treatment field.

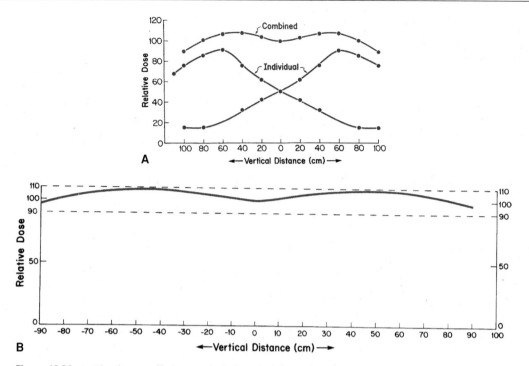

Figure 19.24. **A:** The dose profile in a vertical plane ($\pm y$) for each individual field and the final distribution obtained by both fields. **B:** The dose profile in the center of the two field electron in the right–left ($\pm x$) direction. *Source:* From Khan F. Total skin electron therapy: technique and dosimetry. In: Purdy JA, ed. Advances in radiation oncology physics AAPM Monograph No. 19. New York, NY: American Institute of Physics; 1990:466–479.

equally weighted. Figure 19.24A shows the Gaussian distributions for each angled beam plus the composite dose profile for both beams measured at the patient treatment plane in the floor to ceiling direction. Figure 19.24B shows the dose profile at the isocenter height of the two fields, total skin beam combination for the modified Stanford technique in the right–left ($\pm x$) direction.

Six different patient positions are used with the modified Stanford technique to ensure that the entire surface of the body is uniformly treated (Fig. 19.25A–D). Each patient position is rotated 60 degrees from the previous. Three of the six fields are treated per treatment session to reduce the treatment time per fraction. The anterior field along with the two posterior oblique fields is treated on day 1, while the posterior and two anterior oblique fields are treated on the second day (Fig. 19.25E). The technique developed at McGill University (51) rotates the patient using a motorized platform to uniformly treat the patient's skin surface. This eliminates the multiple patient position changes and reduces the time required to treat the patient.

The depth dose characteristics of the six combined electron fields are dramatically different than that of a single electron beam. This is due to oblique incidence of the beam plus the high angular distribution of the electrons scattered from the beam spoiler. The dose is essentially 100% on the skin surface, decreasing almost linearly to a depth of 3 cm which is indicative of the energy of the 6 MeV beam created by passing through the beam spoiler. The photon contamination associated with the treatment is approximately 1% to 2%. By placing strips of radio-

graphic film in ready pack around the outer periphery of the phantom along with packets of TLD chips at locations around the periphery, the output for the technique can also be determined.

Because of the large variations in skin contours for various areas of the body, TLD measurements need to be performed at multiple locations on the body to evaluate the dose received in those areas. Studies have shown (52,53) that there are often dose deficits at multiple locations such as the top of the head, the axillae, the perineum, and under the breasts (for women). These areas will need to be boosted with additional static electron fields to make up for the missing dose.

Continuously Rotating Electron Arc Technique

With continuously rotating electron arc treatments, establishing a treatment position that will allow a rotating electron arc is extremely important. A simulation is performed to determine the treatment position that is optimal to cover the entire area of interest in one rotation. The region is outlined in radio-opaque markers that are sufficiently small such that they do not negatively affect the accuracy of the computerized treatment planning. A treatment planning CT scan is taken for the determination of the rotational isocenter, to define clearly the PTV and to take into account the different radii of curvature present throughout the treatment region.

Treatment planning is performed to determine the energy of the treatment and to help define the amount of bolus that might be needed to provide adequate skin dose.

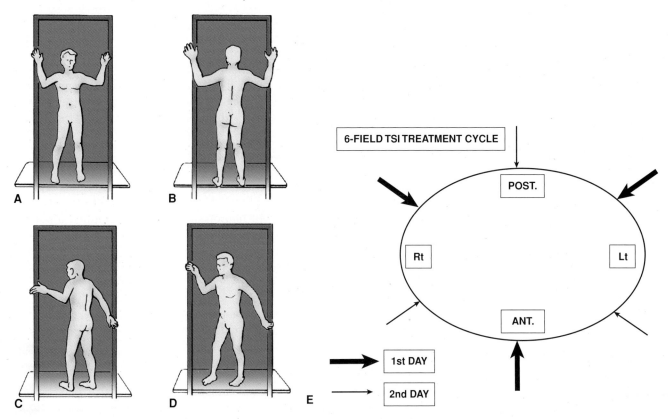

Figure 19.25. **A–D:** Four of the six patient treatment positions used for the modified Stanford total skin irradiation (TSI) technique. The remaining two fields not illustrated are the opposite to the oblique fields illustrated in C and D below. **E:** The six-field treatment cycle associated with the Stanford TSI technique. The anterior and two posterior fields are treated on the first day, while the posterior and two anterior oblique fields are treated on the second day of the 2-day cycle. *Source:* From Khan F. Total skin electron therapy: technique and dosimetry. In: Purdy JA, ed. Advances in radiation oncology physics AAPM Monograph No. 19. New York, NY: American Institute of Physics; 1990:466–479.

Currently, treatment planning of arc fields is done using several overlapping fixed fields usually placed at 10 degrees intervals since electron arc calculations are not possible on currently available treatment planning systems. In actual fact, photon arc treatment plans are also computed using a collection of fixed photon beams spaced at specific angular intervals. All areas of clinical importance are included in the plan (e.g., surgical incision sites) to ensure that the arc fields cover the entire area.

Three levels of field definition are used for electron arc treatments (Fig. 19.19). The first field definition is the x-ray jaw collimator opening. This is done automatically on the linear accelerator when the electron arc mode is selected with the field size opening being determined at the time the linac is installed. Any field width is theoretically acceptable but field widths of 4 to 8 cm are recommended. Smaller field widths have the disadvantage of lower dose per monitor unit, which results in a greater amount of photon contamination for an equivalent amount of delivered dose (38,54).

Secondary collimation is located between the x-ray jaws and the surface of the patient, is determined by the user, and fabricated to ensure that the correct dose based on planning or measurements is delivered to the patient. Its purpose is to produce a uniform dose throughout the

PTV. Since the chest wall radius tends to decrease toward the supraclavicular region, the dose in this region would be greater due to the focusing of the electrons because of the "velocity effect" (38). Reducing the width of the secondary collimator opening for the region that corresponds to this smaller radius of curvature leads to a more uniform dose throughout the entire treatment region. Differences in the radius of curvature throughout the treated region should be taken into account no matter what region of the body is being treated using electron arcs.

Tertiary collimation or shielding is placed on the patient's skin surface and is meant to confine the high-energy electrons to the treatment region. Figure 19.26 shows an example of an electron arc distribution both with and without a lead tertiary shield in place (38). This is needed because the electrons used for treatment need to extend beyond the end of the treatment region to ensure that a uniform dose is delivered throughout the region. Thus, the tertiary shielding serves to confine the electrons to the area of interest, sharpen the dose at the edge of the field, and to spare uninvolved regions that would be treated unnecessarily by the extended arc rotation. The tertiary shield can be made of either lead sheets or cerrobend but must be thick enough to protect against the electrons being used. These shields can be very heavy and

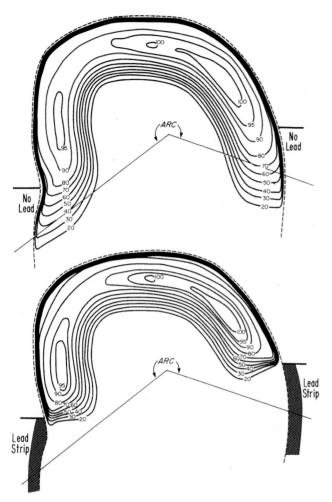

Figure 19.26. Isodose distributions taken in a Rando phantom using a 10 MeV, 236° electron arc, 10 cm average radius of curvature with both no lead at the ends of the arc rotation and with lead sheets in place. The lead sheets dramatically sharpen the electron distribution and provide shielding for the normal tissue at the ends of the arc. *Source:* From Khan FM, Fullerton GD, Lee JM, et al. Physical aspects of electron-beam arc therapy. *Radiology* 1977;124:497–500.

Alternatively, radiographic film such as Kodak XV2 can be sandwiched between the two halves of a cylindrical phantom and irradiated. The optical density of the exposed film can be compared to the film calibration curve for this electron beam energy. For the patient treatment, it is highly recommended that TLDs be used on the patient surface to verify the actual dose received by the patient once the treatment has been started.

Electron—Photon Field Matching

Internal Mammary Electrons—Intact Breast

Electron and photon fields are often abutted for treatments of the breast, for treatment in the head and neck region, and for treatments of the scalp. Figure 19.27 illustrates the match between tangential photon fields and internal mammary electron fields. Electrons are used to treat the internal mammary node chain of lymph nodes along with an internal mammary photon field so that the nodes are adequately treated, the heart is spared from excessive dose, and the dose to the skin surface is not excessive. If electrons were used alone, the heart would be maximally spared but the dose to the skin of the internal mammary field would be too high leading to unwanted consequences of treatment and a poor cosmetic result. At the University of Minnesota, 1,000 cGy is usually delivered to a depth of 3 cm for the internal mammary nodes followed by 4,000 cGy to d_{max} of electron irradiation.

Chest Wall Irradiation—Photons Plus Electrons

It is extremely challenging to treat extensive regions of the chest wall using electron fields alone. The use of combined photon and electron fields with moving junctions allows the treatment of a large amount of chest wall with acceptable high-dose regions. Figure 19.28A and B illustrates possible combinations of photon and electron fields to

must be supported so as not to be too uncomfortable for the patient or too heavy for the therapists to lift, handle, and position. Finally, scattering from the high-Z edges of the shield must be reduced by the use of a low-Z material. Strips of wax, aquaplast, or other low-Z material wrapped around the edge of the shield can address this problem and have the additional advantage of making the edges of the shield more comfortable for the patient (38,50).

Calibration of the dose rate for an electron arc treatment can be done in several ways. The most accurate measurement is conducted using an ionization chamber fitted into machined holes in a unit-density (e.g., polystyrene and solid water) cylindrical phantom. The holes should be positioned at the depth of d_{max} for the particular electron rotational field and the radius of curvature of the phantom should be within 2 to 3 cm of that of the treatment situation (38). TLDs can be placed on the surface of the phantom to quantify the surface dose for the treatment.

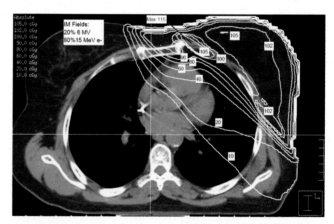

Figure 19.27. Dose distribution showing tangential 6 MV breast fields abutted to an internal mammary 6 MV photon field (20%) and 12 MeV electron field (80%). With proper beam angulation, the underlying heart can be spared with minimal high-dose region (115%) at the interface between the tangential breast and internal mammary fields.

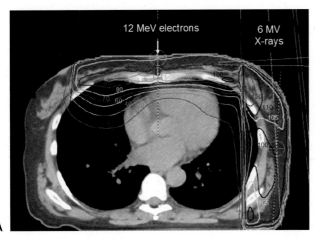
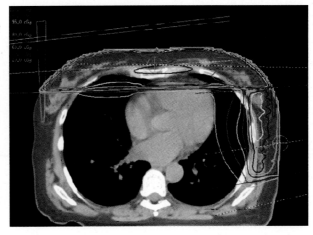

Figure 19.28. **A:** Treatment field arrangement for a large region of the chest wall. An anterior 12 MeV electron field is matched to an anterior/posterior 6 MV field combination. The prescription is to the 100% isodose line while the maximum dose is 140% for this field arrangement. The maximum dose for the overall treatment can be reduced by shifting the junction between the fields by 1 cm if desired. **B:** An alternate photon–electron field arrangement to cover the same region. A lateral, oblique 12 MeV electron field is matched to a right/left lateral 6 MV wedges field arrangement. The prescription is to the 100% isodose line resulting in a high-dose region of 120% at the junction between the photon and electron fields. Again the junction location can be shifted to reduce the high-dose region for the total treatment.

treat large regions of the chest wall. In Figure 19.28A, an anterior electron field is used to treat part of the left and right chest wall. Since disease involved the entire left lateral side of the chest wall, anterior–posterior photon fields were used to treat this region. The dose is prescribed to the 100% isodose line in this case and the high-dose region is 123%. This maximum can be reduced by shifting the junction between the photon and electron fields by 1 cm midway through treatment. Figure 19.28B shows the use of right–left lateral tangential photon fields matched with a left posterior oblique 12 MeV electron field to treat the left chest wall. The dose is delivered to the 100% isodose line resulting in a high-dose region of 112%. Both of these field arrangements make it possible to treat a large amount of the chest wall with a uniform dose and minimal high-dose regions. To reduce the size and magnitude of the high-dose regions, junction changes should be incorporated into the overall treatment plan. Using either photon beams or electron beams alone to treat this region would have resulted in unacceptable high-dose regions as in Figure 19.18. The illustrations represent the dose in only one plane, but these field arrangements have proven to be very useful in the clinic even taking the 3D characteristics of the PTV into account. These approaches, in theory, could be extended to treat the entire periphery of the chest wall, if necessary.

Electron–Photon Field Matching—Head and Neck Region

Treatments of the head and neck region commonly use abutted photon and electron fields. Right/left lateral 6 MV fields are used to treat the anterior neck, and electrons are used to boost the posterior neck nodes after the maximum dose is delivered to the cord via the lateral fields. A high-dose region is created at the junction location in the pho-

ton field and a corresponding low-dose region is created in 100 cm electron treatment distance. If the posterior neck electron fields are treated at an extended distance, for example, 115 to 120 cm SSD, the size of the high-dose region increases while the dose becomes less uniform within the treated electron field (55). In modern clinical practice, the above technique has been almost completely replaced by intensity-modulated radiation therapy (IMRT) (56) or TomoTherapy™ (57,58) treatment approaches.

Electron–Photon Field Matching—Total Scalp Irradiation

Total scalp treatments present a particularly challenging situation where the entire periphery of the scalp needs to be treated while sparing underlying brain tissue. Electron beams alone have been used to treat this area but involve very extensive field matching, special lead shielding, and junctioning techniques (59). In this technique, the junctions were shifted by 2 cm half way through the treatment to reduce the high-dose regions at the junction locations. This resulted in the use of 12 total treatment fields. A simpler technique using right/left lateral 6 MV photon fields matched with lateral electron fields was developed at the University of California, San Francisco (60) and later improved by Tung et al. (61). Figure 19.29 shows the field arrangement described by Tung et al. for the delivery of this technique. A common central axis for both the photon and the electron fields is chosen so that there is only one fixed patient treatment position for all the fields. They recommended that the first phase field junction be placed just inside the inner table of the skull and that an ~3 mm overlap between the matching photon and electron fields be used. This overlap improved the dose uniformity compared to the original technique, which recommended

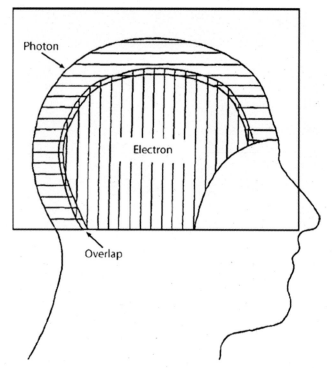

Figure 19.29. Combination of right–left lateral photon fields with abutting electron fields to treat the entire scalp region. The overlap between the photon and electron fields is ~3 mm. Both the photon and electron fields have a common central axis placed approximately in the center of the brain.

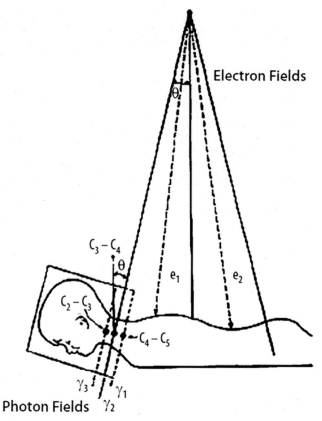

Figure 19.30. Craniospinal field arrangement showing the prone patient treatment position and the arrangement of the right/left lateral photon fields and the posterior electron fields. Two posterior spine electron fields are shown in the diagram but some patients are small enough that one posterior electron field is adequate to cover the entire spine. The lateral photon brain fields are rotated through an angle θ to match the divergence of the posterior electron field. The superior field edge of electron field "e1" is not moved during the treatment but the inferior border of the photon fields is shifted 9 mm to feather the junction location (positions y1, y2, and y3). The central axis of the photon beams is placed as close to the junction region as possible to eliminate divergence in the superior–inferior direction. *Source:* From Maor MH, Fields RS, Hogstrom KR, et al. Improving the therapeutic ratio of craniospinal irradiation in medulloblastoma. *Int J Radiat Oncol Biol Phys* 1985;11:687–697.

abutment of the photon and electron fields. A 1 cm shift in the junction location toward the CA is performed at least once during treatment to further reduce the dose in the abutment region between fields. At least a 6 mm thick bolus is used to increase the skin dose in the buildup region and the energy of the electron fields is chosen such that the 90% isodose line covers the scalp taking the bolus into account. Current competing techniques that can produce excellent dose distributions involve the use of IMRT or TomoTherapy (62–65).

Electron–Photon Field Matching— Craniospinal Irradiation

Irradiation of the craniospinal axis is used to treat medulloblastoma, malignant ependymoma, germinoma, infratentorial glioblastoma and other brain tumors that seed along the entire length of the cerebral spinal fluid (66). The patient is usually treated in a prone position using right/left lateral photon beams to the brain plus posterior photons to treat the spinal cord (67,68). Figure 19.30 shows the basic field arrangement for the technique developed at the University of Texas M. D. Anderson Cancer Center (66), which replaced the posterior photon beam with the use of high-energy electron beams. Using high-energy electrons to treat the posterior spine instead of photons can reduce greatly the dose to the upper thorax region, especially the heart, and the lower digestive tract. This can reduce both acute and late complications of

treatment and is especially important for pediatric patients. Making sure that the entire target is treated with a uniform dose minus excessive hot or cold spots is especially difficult when matching electron and photon beams throughout this region. The key concerns that must be taken into account when using a posterior electrons is that the depth of the spinal cord is not uniform from the neck to the inferior border. In addition, ensuring that the dose at the junction of the brain fields and the posterior spine field is done properly is a major concern. Just producing an electron field of adequate length to treat the posterior spine can be a challenge since the maximum electron cone size on modern linacs is 25×25 cm^2.

One technique using posterior spine electrons (66) has the lateral photon fields rotated through an angle θ to match the divergence of the posterior electron field. The central axis of the lateral brain fields are placed as close to the junction region as possible to eliminate beam divergence in the superior–inferior direction. The superior field edge of electron field, e1, is not moved during the treatment but the inferior border of the photon fields is shifted 9 mm to feather the dose at the junction location (positions $\gamma 1$, $\gamma 2$, and $\gamma 3$). To achieve the most uniform dose per fraction in the region of the junction, one-third of the photon treatments are delivered with the inferior border of the two photon fields coincident with the electron field edge. The next one-third of the photon treatments are delivered with the edge of one photon field moved 9 mm superior to the electron field edge and the edge of the second photon field moved 9 mm inferiorly to the electron field edge. The final one-third of the photon treatments are delivered with the edges of the photon fields reversed from their previous position.

The overall length of the cord to be treated often exceeds the field size that can be generated using a 25×25 cm² cone at either 110 or 115 cm SSD. A small increase in overall field size can be accomplished by rotating the collimator 45 degrees to produce a field size of approximately 30 to 35 cm in length at 115 cm SSD. If the entire length of the cord cannot be covered in one electron field, then a second posterior field is abutted to the inferior border of the first electron field. The addition of this second field requires that the couch be rotated 90 degrees and that the angle of the two electron fields be rotated by $\pm$ angle θ (Fig. 19.31) to account for the divergence of each of these electron fields and to produce a common field edge (66). A simulation of the patient is done to establish the treatment position and to properly place the photon and electron fields and to provide documentation for subsequent patient treatment.

The depth of the cord along its entire length must be described as well as the change in the SSD along the length

of the cord. The electron energy is selected such that the 90% isodose exceeds the maximum depth of the cord by 7 mm: 4 mm to account for the increased absorption of bone and 3 mm for a margin of error to ensure coverage of the target. If the depth of the spinal cord or the SSD to the patient skin surface varies significantly, bolus can be added to the spinal cord field to conform the 90% isodose surface to the anterior border of the cord. With modern 3D-treatment planning computers, the overall plan can be calculated before treatment is begun but the adequacy of the user's planning system to handle complex spinal geometry can be an issue (69). However, a recent study comparing TLD measurements in a pediatric anatomic phantom with calculations of a pencil-beam-based commercial system showed moderately good agreement (70). For the method described by Maor et al. (66) the dose in the junction region reaches a maximum of 36 to 37 Gy and a minimum of 27 Gy when 30 Gy is given to the posterior electron field, 30 Gy to the whole brain, plus 20 Gy to a posterior fossa boost.

The technique of Roback et al. (71) was developed to produce a posterior electron field long enough to treat the entire spinal cord in one field. Because electron fields become less sharp at the extended distances of 120 to 140 cm SSD (Fig. 19.7), a system of secondary field shaping was devised by these investigators. This system sufficiently sharpened the edges of the electron field in both the superior–inferior and the right–left lateral dimension to ensure that the field adequately covered the treatment region. Additional dosimetry must be performed when using this technique to describe the electron isodose shape, the depth of penetration of the beam, and the output per monitor unit at the extended, blocked field. An additional benefit of this technique is that tertiary collimation reduces the hot spot at the junction from 115% to 105% with zero skin gaps.

Clinical Treatment Techniques

Parotid Gland Treatments

Treatment of the parotid region was most commonly conducted using either a wedged pair combination of photon fields or by a combination of straight lateral photon and electron fields. With the increasing use of IMRT and TomoTherapy, these previous techniques are becoming less and less popular. This is due to the ability of these new approaches to both cover the PTV with a homogeneous dose and sparing the many sensitive structures that are present in this region (spinal cord, brain stem, eyes, pituitary gland, and oral cavity). A study performed by Yaparpalvi et al. (72) compared nine different non-IMRT/TomoTherapy techniques for treatment of the parotid region. They based their comparison between techniques on the homogeneous dose distribution throughout the region, the minimization of the dose to sensitive structures, and nonproduction of unacceptably high dose to the skin surface. They concluded that only three techniques

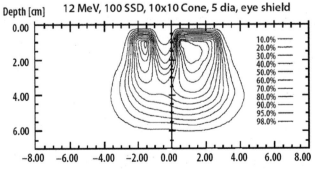

Figure 19.31. Isodose distribution produced using a Varian 2100 C, 12 MeV, 5 cm diameter circular electron field incident on a 2 cm thick, 1.2 cm diameter cylindrical cerrobend pencil eye shield in contact with a solid water phantom. The data is taken using Kodak XV2 film and scanned using a Wellhofer scanning densitometer system running WP700 software. *Source:* From Gerbi BJ. Clinical applications of high-energy electrons. In: Levitt SH, Purdy JA, Perez CA, et al., eds. *Technical basis of radiation therapy: practical clinical applications*, 4th ed. Berlin: Springer, 2006; Figure 7–19.

met acceptably all three criteria: (1) the ipsilateral wedge pair technique; (2) the three-field 6 MV photon technique consisting of anterior and posterior wedged fields plus a lateral photon field, and (3) the mixed straight lateral 6 MV photon plus 16 MeV electron field technique with beam weightings of 1:4 photon to electrons, respectively. The use of custom compensating bolus (73) can lead to dose distributions using this electron–photon combination that are more conformal than those achieved using wedged photon techniques and with consistently higher skin doses.

Facial Areas

Electrons have been used extensively in the treatment of the head and neck region. Common sites are in the nasal region, the eye, the eyelid, the buccal mucosa, and the oral cavity. These are all challenging sites to treat using electrons and require great attention to detail to produce the desired outcome.

Nose

For treatments in the nasal region, electron beams have often been combined with photon beams to produce adequate coverage of the target. High-energy photon beams were added to electron beams to reduce the skin dose to a tolerable level while covering the target and not delivering an excessive dose to the brain. Computerized treatment planning using corrections for inhomogeneous materials is essential in this region due to the severe surface irregularities around the nose and eyes, and the presence of air cavities, bone, and teeth that usually fall in this treatment region. Surface irregularities can be tamed by the use of box bolus (6) or custom compensating bolus designed using more sophisticated techniques (34,73). Bolus should be inserted into the nasal passages to ensure that the electrons are not preferentially scattered into the air cavities and that full dose is delivered to this region. Whenever custom bolus is to be used, a verification CT scan should be performed with the bolus in place on the patient to ensure that the bolus has been fabricated correctly, that it is properly positioned on the patient, and that there are no or limited air gaps between the bolus and the skin surface of the patient. An additional computerized treatment plan using this CT scan can be performed to confirm that the final calculated dose distribution covers the target volume as intended.

Eye

Eyelid. Treatment of the eye and eyelid can be done effectively with orthovoltage x-rays or low-energy electrons (74). The use of electrons for treatments in this region can be very complicated depending on the specifics of the disease and its location. For treatments of the eyelid, the lowest available electron energy (4–6 MeV) is most appropriate. The surface dose for these beam energies is ~75% depending on the specific linac so that bolus will be required to increase the surface dose to >90%. Shielding of the lens and underlying eye must also be taken into account. The entire decision process for producing effective eyelid treatment is to determine the region to be treated, the thickness of the eyelid, and the depth to which treatment is required. An electron energy adequate to cover this depth and the surface dose for that energy are selected. Enough bolus is added to the surface of the eyelid to ensure that the surface dose is >90%. An eye shield of sufficient thickness to protect the underlying lens and eye is selected based on the electron energy at the depth of the shield surface. For example, the energy of a 6 MeV beam after passing through 1 cm of unit density material is ~4 MeV. Thus, the shield thickness must be sufficiently thick to attenuate 4 MeV electrons. A shield made of lead would have to be 2 to 3 mm in thickness to provide adequate shielding. In addition, a lower Z material, such as aluminum of 1 mm thickness (8) should be added to the shield on the side facing the beam, to reduce the amount of backscatter from the lead surface. An acrylic coating should be applied to further reduce backscatter from the shield and to provide a protective coating between the lead and the patient's surface. Composite eye shields using lead as the primary attenuator have been replaced by commercially available eye shields containing tungsten. With a density of ~17 g/cm^3 versus a density of lead of 11.3 g/cm^3, these eye shields can be two-thirds of the overall thickness of lead eye shields while providing the same degree of protection. This results in an effective shield that is much more comfortable for the patient and easier for the physician or therapist to place for daily treatments. For all eye shields placed beneath the eyelid, the patient's eye needs to be anesthetized. Also, a noncorrecting contact lens should be placed below the shield to protect the cornea from being scratched by the insertion of the shield.

Eye and Orbit Treatments. Many beam arrangements using photons, photons plus electrons, and electrons alone have been described for treatment of the eye and orbit. Electrons of 12 to 18 MeV are required to adequately treat the entire orbit of adult patients. A single, en-face beam is used with a pencil eye shield in place to protect the lens of the eye. Rustgi et al. (75) showed that a 1 cm thick cerrobend shield, 1.3 cm in diameter placed 1 cm or closer to the surface of the eye was adequate to protect the lens for treatments using 6 to 9 MeV. Rykers et al. (76) showed that a 1.2 × 1.0 cm tapered oval shield suspended from the electron cutout and placed 1 cm from the eye surface was adequate to protect the lens while using 12 MeV electrons. The dose distribution shown in Figure 19.31 for 12 MeV electrons illustrates the protective effect of a 2 cm thick, 1.2 cm diameter cerrobend shield in contact with a solid water phantom. The dose to the lens is reduced to ~10% for this shielding arrangement. If areas posterior to the lens are to be treated, however, a 50% or greater dose deficit behind the lens will be affected by the placement of the shield.

Intraoperative Irradiation Using Electrons

Intraoperative radiotherapy (IORT) is the delivery of a single, high dose of radiation during the surgical procedure to a well-defined mass of tissue using high-energy electrons. The procedure is done by surgically exposing the region to be treated in the operating room or in a specially prepared linac treatment room, isolating the region to be treated, placing the treatment field to properly cover the target, delivering the radiation, and then finishing the surgical technique. The popularity of the stationary linac-based technique has waned over the years due to the complexity of coordinating several departments on the day of the procedure. With the advent of mobile irradiation devices, the technique has seen resurgence in popularity. IORT remains an effective treatment for post-surgical treatment of several cancer types most notably gastrointestinal and gynecological cancers (77–91). Using this technique, a high dose can be delivered directly to the tumor bed while minimizing the dose to adjacent and underlying normal tissues.

Whether performed in the Radiation Therapy Department using conventional fixed linacs or with modern mobile units, IORT remains a challenging and time-intensive technique. TG-48 of the AAPM (13) describes in great detail the program and personnel requirements for an IORT program using the fixed linacs typically available in a Radiation Therapy Department. The newer AAPM TG-72 report concentrates on the issues and concerns associated with mobile intra-op treatment units. Both AAPM reports describe specific quality assurance that should be performed and the prescription requirements for the technique. ICRU 71 describes the dose prescription and reporting guidelines from the international community (see above) while AAPM TG-72 recommends specifying the dose at the 90% isodose and reporting the 90% dose and the d_{max} dose.

Since the patient is under anesthesia for the entire operation and IORT treatment, data must be taken during commissioning that facilitates the efficient and accurate treatment of the patient. This data includes applicator or cone output factors, air-gap factors, central axis beam penetration characteristics, dose profile information at several depths, and the absolute calibration of the unit following AAPM TG-51 guidelines. Mobile IORT treatment unit commissioning may be more extensive than that required for stationary linac installations. Routine quality assurance should follow the recommendations made in AAPM Reports 48 and 72 and should represent a subset of the data taken at the time of commissioning. Additional testing may be required for mobile units to ensure that they are operating correctly before the operation begins. Quality assurance practices should also be instituted to ensure that the usual treatment planning and monitor

unit checks performed for routine treatment are also completed before IORT treatment commences. This is especially important since these are single-fraction treatments delivering a high dose where there is pressure to perform the treatment in as little time as possible.

REFERENCES

1. Kutcher GJ, Coia L, Gillin M, et al. Comprehensive QA for radiation oncology: report of AAPM Radiation Therapy Committee Task Group 40. *Med Phys* 1994;21:581–618.
2. Klein EE, Hanley J, Bayouth J, et al. Task Group 142 report: quality assurance of medical accelerators. *Med Phys* 2009;36:4197–4212.
3. Khan FM, Doppke KP, Hogstrom KR, et al. Clinical electron-beam dosimetry: report of AAPM Radiation Therapy Committee Task Group No. 25. *Med Phys* 1991;18:73–109.
4. Khan FM, Deibel FC, Soleimani-Meigooni A. Obliquity correction for electron beams. *Med Phys* 1985;12:749–753.
5. Van Dyk J, Hill R. Post-irradiation lung density changes measured by computerized tomography. *Int J Radiat Oncol Biol Phys* 1983;9:847–852.
6. Chobe R, McNeese M, Weber R, et al. Radiation therapy for carcinoma of the nasal vestibule. *Otolaryngol Head Neck Surg* 1988;98:67–71.
7. Menard CM, Bews J, Skoracki RI, et al. High-energy electron and photon therapy to the parotid bed: radiation dose perturbations with a titanium mandibular implant. *Australas Radiol* 1999;43:495–499.
8. Klevenhagen SC, Lambert GD, Arbabi A. Backscattering in electron beam therapy for energies between 3 and 35 MeV. *Phys Med Biol* 1982;27:363–373.
9. Lambert G, Klevenhagen S. Penetration of backscattered electrons in polystyrene for energies between 1–25 MeV. *Phys Med Biol* 1982;27:721.
10. Gahbauer R, Landberg T, Chavaudra J, et al. Prescribing, recording, and reporting electron beam therapy. *J ICRU* 2004:4(1):5–9.
11. ICRU. ICRU Report 50: prescribing, recording, and reporting photon beam therapy. Washington, DC: International Commission on Radiation Units and Measurements, 1993.
12. ICRU. ICRU Report 62: prescribing, recording and reporting photon beam therapy (supplement to ICRU Report 50). Washington, DC: International Commission on Radiation Units and Measurements, 1999.
13. Palta JR, Biggs PJ, Hazle JD, et al. Intraoperative electron beam radiation therapy: technique, dosimetry, and dose specification: report of task force 48 of the Radiation Therapy Committee, American Association of Physicists in Medicine. *Int J Radiat Oncol Biol Phys* 1995;33:725–746.
14. Almond PR, Biggs PJ, Coursey BM, et al. AAPM's TG-51 protocol for clinical reference dosimetry of high-energy photon and electron beams. *Med Phys* 1999;26:1847–1870.
15. IAEA. Absorbed dose determination in external beam radiotherapy. Technical Report Series No. 398. Vienna: International Atomic Energy Agency, 2000.

16. Gerbi BJ, Antolak JA, Deibel FC, et al. Recommendations for clinical electron beam dosimetry: supplement to the recommendations of Task Group 25. *Med Phys* 2009;36: 3239–3279.

17. Khan FM, Higgins PD, Gerbi BJ, et al. Calculation of depth dose and dose per monitor unit for irregularly shaped electron fields. *Phys Med Biol* 1998;43:2741–2754.

18. NACP. Procedures in external radiation therapy dosimetry with electron and photon beams with maximum energies between 1 and 50 MeV. *Acta Radiol* 1980;19:55.

19. Higgins PD, Gerbi BJ, Khan FM. Application of measured pencil beam parameters for electron beam model evaluation. *Med Phys* 2003;30:514–520.

20. Hogstrom KR, Mills MD, Meyer JA, et al. Dosimetric evaluation of a pencil-beam algorithm for electrons employing a two-dimensional heterogeneity correction. *Int J Radiat Oncol Biol Phys* 1984;10:561–569.

21. Jones D, Andre P, Washington JT, et al. A method for the assessment of the output of irregularly shaped electron fields. *Br J Radiol* 1990;63:59–64.

22. Jursinic PA, Mueller R. A sector-integration method for calculating the output factors of irregularly shaped electron fields. *Med Phys* 1997;24:1765–1769.

23. Khan FM, Higgins PD. Field equivalence for clinical electron beams. *Phys Med Biol* 2001;46:N9–14.

24. Mills MD, Hogstrom KR, Fields RS. Determination of electron beam output factors for a 20-MeV linear accelerator. *Med Phys* 1985;12:473–476.

25. Hogstrom KR, Mills MD, Almond PR. Electron beam dose calculations. *Phys Med Biol* 1981;26:445–459.

26. Mills MD, Hogstrom KR, Almond PR. Prediction of electron beam output factors. *Med Phys* 1982;9:60–68.

27. Dutreix A, Broit E. The development of a pencil beam algorithm for clinical use at the Institut Gustave Roussy In: Nahum A, ed. The computation of dose distributions in electron beams. Umea, Sweden: University of Umea, 1985:242–270.

28. Khan FM, Higgins PD. Calculation of depth dose and dose per monitor unit for irregularly shaped electron fields: an addendum. *Phys Med Biol* 1999;44:N77–N80.

29. Bruinvis IA, Mathol WA. Calculation of electron beam depth-dose curves and output factors for arbitrary field shapes. *Radiother Oncol* 1988;11:395–404.

30. Bruinvis IA, Van Amstel A, Elevelt AJ, et al. Calculation of electron beam dose distributions for arbitrarily shaped fields. *Phys Med Biol* 1983;28:667–683.

31. McParland BJ. A parameterization of the electron beam output factors of a 25-MeV linear accelerator. *Med Phys* 1987;14:665–669.

32. Cygler JE, Daskalov GM, Chan GH, et al. Evaluation of the first commercial Monte Carlo dose calculation engine for electron beam treatment planning. *Med Phys* 2004;31:142–153.

33. Antolak JA, Scrimger JW, Mah E. Optimization of a cord shielding technique for electrons. *Australas Phys Eng Sci Med* 1992;15:91–94.

34. Low DA, Starkschall G, Bujnowski SW, et al. Electron bolus design for radiotherapy treatment planning: bolus design algorithms. *Med Phys* 1992;19:115–124.

35. Archambeau JO, Forell B, Doria R, et al. Use of variable thickness bolus to control electron beam penetration

in chest wall irradiation. *Int J Radiat Oncol Biol Phys* 1981;7:835–842.

36. Beach JL, Coffey CW, Wade JS. Individualized chest wall compensating bolus for electron irradiation following mastectomy: an ultrasound approach. *Int J Radiat Oncol Biol Phys* 1981;7:1607–1611.

37. Boyer AL, Fullerton GD, Mira JG. An electron beam pseudoarc technique for irradiation of large areas of chest wall and other curved surfaces. *Int J Radiat Oncol Biol Phys* 1982;8:1969–1974.

38. Khan FM, Fullerton GD, Lee JM, et al. Physical aspects of electron-beam arc therapy. *Radiology* 1977;124:497–500.

39. Leavitt DD, Peacock LM, Gibbs FA Jr, et al. Electron arc therapy: physical measurement and treatment planning techniques. *Int J Radiat Oncol Biol Phys* 1985;11:987–999.

40. Wooden KK, Hogstrom KR, Blum P, et al. Whole-limb irradiation of the lower calf using a six-field electron technique. *Med Dosim* 1996;21:211–218.

41. Hoppe RT, Cox RS, Fuks Z, et al. Electron-beam therapy for mycosis fungoides: the Stanford University experience. *Cancer Treat Rep* 1979;63:691–700.

42. Hoppe RT, Fuks Z, Bagshaw MA. Radiation therapy in the management of cutaneous T-cell lymphomas. *Cancer Treat Rep* 1979;63:625–632.

43. AAPM. Report No. 23, Total skin electron therapy: technique and dosimetry. New York, NY: American Institute of Physics, 1987.

44. Bjarngard BE, Chen GT, Piontek RW, et al. Analysis of dose distributions in whole body superficial electron therapy. *Int J Radiat Oncol Biol Phys* 1977;2:319–324.

45. Edelstein GR, Clark T, Holt JG. Dosimetry for total-body electron-beam therapy in the treatment of mycosis fungoides. *Radiology* 1973;108:691–694.

46. Fraass BA, Roberson PL, Glatstein E. Whole-skin electron treatment: patient skin dose distribution. *Radiology* 1983;146:811–814.

47. Karzmark CJ. Large-field superficial electron therapy with linear accelerators. *Br J Radiol* 1964;37:302–305.

48. Karzmark CJ, Loevinger R, Steele RE, et al. A technique for large-field, superficial electron therapy. *Radiology* 1960;74:633–644.

49. Page V, Gardner A, Karzmark CJ. Patient dosimetry in the electron treatment of large superficial lesions. *Radiology* 1970;94:635–641.

50. Khan F. *The physics of radiation therapy*, 4th ed. Philadelphia: Wolters Kluwer/Lippincott Williams & Wilkins, 2010.

51. Podgorsak EB, Pla C, Pla M, et al. Physical aspects of a rotational total skin electron irradiation. *Med Phys* 1983;10:159–168.

52. Antolak JA, Cundiff JH, Ha CS. Utilization of thermoluminescent dosimetry in total skin electron beam radiotherapy of mycosis fungoides. *Int J Radiat Oncol Biol Phys* 1998;40:101–108.

53. Weaver RD, Gerbi BJ, Dusenbery KE. Evaluation of dose variation during total skin electron irradiation using thermoluminescent dosimeters. *Int J Radiat Oncol Biol Phys* 1995;33:475–478.

54. Kase KR, Bjarngard BE. Bremsstrahlung dose to patients in rotational electron therapy. *Radiology* 1979;133:531–532.

55. Johnson JM, Khan FM. Dosimetric effects of abutting extended source to surface distance electron fields with

photon fields in the treatment of head and neck cancers. *Int J Radiat Oncol Biol Phys* 1994;28:741–747.

56. Chou WW, Puri DR, Lee NY. Intensity-modulated radiation therapy for head and neck cancer. *Expert Rev Anticancer Ther* 2005;5:515–521.

57. Fiorino C, Dell'Oca I, Pierelli A, et al. Significant improvement in normal tissue sparing and target coverage for head and neck cancer by means of helical tomotherapy. *Radiother Oncol* 2006;78:276–282.

58. Sheng K, Molloy JA, Read PW. Intensity-modulated radiation therapy (IMRT) dosimetry of the head and neck: a comparison of treatment plans using linear accelerator-based IMRT and helical tomotherapy. *Int J Radiat Oncol Biol Phys* 2006;65:917–923.

59. Able CM, Mills MD, McNeese MD, et al. Evaluation of a total scalp electron irradiation technique. *Int J Radiat Oncol Biol Phys* 1991;21:1063–1072.

60. Akazawa C. Treatment of the scalp using photon and electron beams. *Med Dosim* 1989;14:129–131.

61. Tung SS, Shiu AS, Starkschall G, et al. Dosimetric evaluation of total scalp irradiation using a lateral electron-photon technique. *Int J Radiat Oncol Biol Phys* 1993;27:153–160.

62. Locke J, Low DA, Grigireit T, et al. Potential of tomotherapy for total scalp treatment. *Int J Radiat Oncol Biol Phys* 2002;52:553–559.

63. Bedford JL, Childs PJ, Hansen VN, et al. Treatment of extensive scalp lesions with segmental intensity-modulated photon therapy. *Int J Radiat Oncol Biol Phys* 2005;62:1549–1558.

64. Chan MF, Song Y, Burman C, et al. The treatment of extensive scalp lesions combining electrons with intensity-modulated photons. *Conf Proc IEEE Eng Med Biol Soc* 2006;1:152–155.

65. Orton N, Jaradat H, Welsh J, et al. Total scalp irradiation using helical tomotherapy. *Med Dosim* 2005;30:162–168.

66. Maor MH, Fields RS, Hogstrom KR, et al. Improving the therapeutic ratio of craniospinal irradiation in medulloblastoma. *Int J Radiat Oncol Biol Phys* 1985;11:687–697.

67. Dewit L, Van Dam J, Rijnders A, et al. A modified radiotherapy technique in the treatment of medulloblastoma. *Int J Radiat Oncol Biol Phys* 1984;10:231–241.

68. Miralbell R, Bleher A, Huguenin P, et al. Pediatric medulloblastoma: radiation treatment technique and patterns of failure. *Int J Radiat Oncol Biol Phys* 1997;37:523–529.

69. Ding GX, Cygler JE, Zhang GG, et al. Evaluation of a commercial three-dimensional electron beam treatment planning system. *Med Phys* 1999;26:2571–2580.

70. Hood C, Kron T, Hamilton C, et al. Correlation of 3D-planned and measured dosimetry of photon and electron craniospinal radiation in a pediatric anthropomorphic phantom. *Radiother Oncol* 2005;77:111–116.

71. Roback DM, Johnson JM, Khan FM, et al. The use of tertiary collimation for spinal irradiation with extended SSD electron fields. *Int J Radiat Oncol Biol Phys* 1997;37:1187–1192.

72. Yaparpalvi R, Fontenla DP, Tyerech SK, et al. Parotid gland tumors: a comparison of postoperative radiotherapy techniques using three dimensional (3D) dose distributions and dose-volume histograms (DVHS). *Int J Radiat Oncol Biol Phys* 1998;40:43–49.

73. Kudchadker RJ, Antolak JA, Morrison WH, et al. Utilization of custom electron bolus in head and neck radiotherapy. *J Appl Clin Med Phys* 2003;4:321–333.

74. Sinesi C, McNeese MD, Peters LJ, et al. Electron beam therapy for eyelid carcinomas. *Head Neck Surg* 1987;10:31–37.

75. Rustgi SN. Dose distribution under external eye shields for high energy electrons. *Int J Radiat Oncol Biol Phys* 1986;12:141–144.

76. Rykers K, Uden G, Thompson V. Orbital lymphoma: a simple treatment using electrons. *Med Dosim* 2003;28:95–98.

77. FA C, Aristu J, Azinovic I, et al. Intraoperative radiotherapy with accelerated electrons for urinary bladder carcinoma: principles and results. *Arch Esp Urol* 1999;52:649–654.

78. Calvo FA, Aristu JJ, Abuchaibe O, et al. Intraoperative and external preoperative radiotherapy in invasive bladder cancer: effect of neoadjuvant chemotherapy in tumor downstaging. *Am J Clin Oncol* 1993;16:61–66.

79. Crane CH, Beddar AS, Evans DB. The role of intraoperative radiotherapy in pancreatic cancer. *Surg Oncol Clin N Am* 2003;12:965–977.

80. del Carmen MG, Eisner B, Willet CG, et al. Intraoperative radiation therapy in the management of gynecologic and genitourinary malignancies. *Surg Oncol Clin N Am* 2003;12:1031–1042.

81. Gerard JP, Collin G, Ayzac L, et al. The role of IORT as salvage therapy for recurrent cervical and endometrial carcinoma. *Front Radiat Ther Oncol* 1997;31:260–262.

82. Gunderson LL, Nagorney DM, McIlrath DC, et al. External beam and intraoperative electron irradiation for locally advanced soft tissue sarcomas. *Int J Radiat Oncol Biol Phys* 1993;25:647–656.

83. Hashiguchi Y, Sekine T, Sakamoto H, et al. Intraoperative irradiation after surgery for locally recurrent rectal cancer. *Dis Colon Rectum* 1999;42:886–893; discussion 893–885.

84. Mahe MA, Gerard JP, Dubois JB, et al. Intraoperative radiation therapy in recurrent carcinoma of the uterine cervix: report of the French intraoperative group on 70 patients. *Int J Radiat Oncol Biol Phys* 1996;34:21–26.

85. Martinez-Monge R, Jurado M, Aristu JJ, et al. Intraoperative electron beam radiotherapy during radical surgery for locally advanced and recurrent cervical cancer. *Gynecol Oncol* 2001;82:538–543.

86. Nag S, Mills J, Martin E, et al. IORT using high-dose-rate brachytherapy or electron beam for colorectal carcinoma. *Front Radiat Ther Oncol* 1997;31:238–242.

87. Pisters PW, Ballo MT, Fenstermacher MJ, et al. Phase I trial of preoperative concurrent doxorubicin and radiation therapy, surgical resection, and intraoperative electron-beam radiation therapy for patients with localized retroperitoneal sarcoma. *J Clin Oncol* 2003;21:3092–3097.

88. Sanfilippo NJ, Crane CH, Skibber J, et al. T4 rectal cancer treated with preoperative chemoradiation to the posterior pelvis followed by multivisceral resection: patterns of failure and limitations of treatment. *Int J Radiat Oncol Biol Phys* 2001;51:176–183.

89. Shaw EG, Gunderson LL, Martin JK, et al. Peripheral nerve and ureteral tolerance to intraoperative radiation therapy: clinical and dose-response analysis. *Radiother Oncol* 1990;18:247–255.

90. Sindelar WF, Kinsella TJ. Studies of intraoperative radiotherapy in carcinoma of the pancreas. *Ann Oncol* 1999;10(Suppl 4):226–230.

91. Willett CG, Suit HD, Tepper JE, et al. Intraoperative electron beam radiation therapy for retroperitoneal soft tissue sarcoma. *Cancer* 1991;68:278–283.

92. ICRU. International commission on radiation units and measurements, radiation dolsimetry: electron beams with energies between 1 and 50 MeV, ICRU Report 35. Bethesda, MD: International Commission on Radiation Units and Measurement, 1984.

93. Almond P, Wright A, Boone M. High-energy electron dose perturbations in regions of tissue heterogeneity. *Radiology* 1967;88:1146.

94. Gerbi BJ. Clinical applications of high-energy electrons. In: Levitt SH, Purdy JA, Perez CA, et al., eds. *Technical basis of radiation therapy: practical clinical applications*, 4th ed. Berlin: Springer, 2006.

95. Hogstron K. Dosimetry of electron heterogeneities. In: Wright A, Boyer A, eds. *Advances in radiation therapy treatment planning*. New York, NY: American Institute of Physics, Inc., 1983:223–243.

96. Khan F. Total skin electron therapy: technique and dosimetry. In: Purdy JA, ed. *Advances in radiation oncology physics AAPM Monograph No. 19*. New York, NY: American Institute of Physics; 1990:466–479.

CHAPTER 20

Proton Beam Therapy

Hanne M. Kooy ∎ Judy A. Adams

INTRODUCTION

Proton beam radiotherapy further advances a central aim of radiation therapy: significant reduction in healthy tissue dose and, as a corollary, significant safe increase in malignant tissue dose. Proton beam radiotherapy is not new and was used as a definitive modality as early as 50 years ago. Its recent emergence as a viable, and even necessary, technology is a consequence of its historical success in treating otherwise incurable disease, the present desire for increased conformal radiation therapy, and the commercial availability of proton beam equipment.

The evolution of proton and photon radiotherapy is diametrically opposite. Proton radiotherapy was, *ab initio*, a conformal modality but only sparsely available; radiotherapy was a therapeutic analog to planar x-ray imaging and broadly available. Of course, brachytherapy also was, and is, a local conformal modality but has its own application and is in equal competition to proton and photon radiotherapy.

Proton radiotherapy from its inception required careful attention to detail as a consequence of the intrinsic precision afforded by the proton beam itself even while the supporting technologies were minimal. As a result, the early adopters of proton beam radiotherapy were neurosurgeons: Dr. Lars Leksell in Stockholm, Sweden and Dr. Raymond Kjellberg in Boston, USA. Neurosurgeons, by training, have an exquisite understanding of the cranial anatomy as visualized on x-rays, as CT was not yet available. The early use was in abnormalities visible on those x-rays such as pituitary and arterio-venous abnormalities. The x-ray information allowed effective use of the advantageous properties of the proton beam. Easy access to a proton beam, at the Harvard Cyclotron Laboratory at Harvard University, allowed Dr. Kjellberg to establish a proton radiosurgery program that continues to date. Dr. Leksell did not have this convenience and out of necessity looked for alternative conformal methods, which culminated in the gammaknife.

Treatment of ocular melanomas was another early adopter of proton beam therapy. Again, the orbital anatomy and the use of x-ray opaque markers at the target margin provided sufficient information to apply proton beams.

These early adopters used existing, post-nuclear research, cyclotrons. Many of these, at Clatterbridge, UK, for example, were of low energy and could only be used for ocular targets. A few cyclotrons, those at Harvard University (USA) and later in Orsay (France), for example, had sufficiently high energy to treat internal targets. The treatment of those targets, however, did not commence until the late 1970s when volumetric imaging with CT was available and the treatment planning tools for using those images had been developed (1). It is the treatment of those targets that introduced proton radiotherapy to the general practice of radiotherapy. Proton radiotherapy, as an intrinsically conformal modality, introduced many of the elements of "modern" conformal radiotherapy: attention to the details of imaging, setup, treatment planning and delivery.

CLINICALLY EFFECTIVE PROPERTIES OF THE PROTON BEAM

The clinical potential of a proton beam was recognized by Robert R. Wilson, then at the Harvard Cyclotron Laboratory, in his article of 1947 (2), in which the geometric and dosimetric localization properties of a mono-energetic proton beam were proposed for treating targets inside the body. The practicalities were in doubt, as available proton beams had insufficient penetrating energy: the first Harvard Cyclotron, built in 1937, had an energy of 12 MeV equal to 17 mm range! This cycolotron was moved, by Dr. Wilson, to Los Alamos for the Manhattan project in 1943, which allowed the construction of the second Harvard Cyclotron in 1947 with an initial energy of 90 MeV (6.4 cm range in water) and later upgraded to 160 MeV (17.7-cm range in water) in 1955. It was another 12 year before Dr. Wilson's vision became a reality (3).

A proton beam, as any charged particle, loses energy along its track as a function of the local stopping power. The stopping power, the energy loss per unit length, increases rapidly as the proton in water slows down and equals 5.2 MeV/cm at 160 MeV, 12.4 MeV/cm at 50 MeV, and 26.1 MeV/cm at 20 MeV. This rapid increase in energy loss per unit length results in a very large dose enhancement at the end of the particle track and results in the characteristic Bragg peak beyond which no dose is deposited (see Fig. 10.2). The large mass of the proton (938.3 MeV/c^2) results in tracks that deviate little from the initial proton direction and

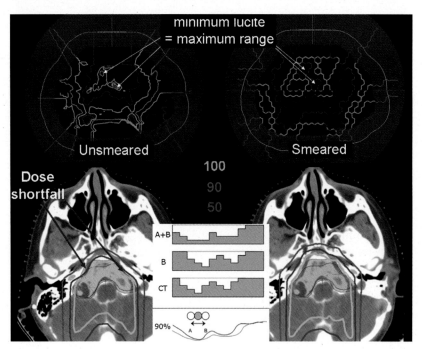

Figure 20.1. The use of range-compensators requires two steps, smearing and tapering, to achieve satisfactory target coverage. Smearing considers each point on the range-compensator and replaces the thickness of that point with the minimum thickness found at other points within a smearing radius of the point under consideration. This has the effect to "throw" the dose deeper into the patient (see *bottom-right* compared to *bottom-left*). The *middle insert* illustrates the example where the CT represents the unsmeared compensator, while **B** (and similarlly **A**) is the compensator if a shift were to occur. The composite compensator considers positions **A** and **B**. Smearing, originally, was introduced to compensate for geometric uncertainties by considering the "worst"-case penetration range within a region. Tapering considers range-compensator gradients along the aperture edge and applies a smoothing to those gradients to remove scattering artifacts. In general, support for smearing and tapering is poor within existing treatment planning systems and requires considerable knowledge on the treatment planner to achieve a satisfactory result.

thus all protons along the same direction yield Bragg peaks at the same depth and the overall dose distribution is, in essence, a simple addition of the dose distribution along a single track. This is in contrast to a beam of electrons where the small mass of the electron (0.511 MeV/c^2) results in tracks that lose any correlation with the initial direction and as a consequence the electron Bragg peak is "smeared" throughout the effective treatment volume and only a distinct distal fall-off remains (See Fig. 20.1). The intact or pristine Bragg peak characteristic of heavy charged particles and its large peak to entrance dose ratio offers the opportunity for localizing dose at a point in a target volume. Thus, a proton beam has intrinsic three-dimensional (3D) shaping features, in depth and laterally, compared to the two-dimensional (2D), lateral, controls in a photon beam.

The depth of the Bragg peak is a function of the initial proton beam energy and there is a direct correspondence between energy E (in MeV) and penetration depth or range R (in g/cm^2). The terms "energy" and "range" are interchangeable although the range is more effective in clinical communication. A consequence of the energy–range relationship is that the energy loss can be equated to material thickness. Thus, inserting a material of certain thickness in a proton beam results in a proportional energy reduction and a known shift downward of the range. The proton beam intensity, however, does not change: all entering protons exit. This is in contrast to a clinical photon beam where the mean energy is minimally affected while the intensity reduces exponentially as a function of thickness.

The near-straight tracks of the protons produce a beam whose penumbral edge is intrinsically sharp. The individual protons undergo (primarily) many multiple Coulomb scattering events, which result in a Gaussian-shaped broad-ening of an initially parallel proton beam. The Gaussian spread increases with depth and results in a depth-dependent penumbra (80/20%) (see Fig. 20.2 where the penumbra profile increases per depth).

The proton beam penumbra is intrinsically sharper compared to a single photon beam penumbra at depths below ~18 cm (in water). This single beam penumbra is relevant when one wishes to achieve the sharpest lateral fall-off of dose between the target and a critical structure. Thus, proton beam treatments in the head and neck achieve a sharper lateral fall-off, for example, in a target around the brainstem compared to a photon (intensity-modulated radiotherapy [IMRT]) beam treatment. On the other hand, a prostate or other deep-seated target does not show a penumbral advantage for a proton beam. Of course, other benefits may still favor the proton beam dosimetry.

In practice, however, it is the composite penumbra of multiple fields that is of relevance as it determines not only the sharpest achievable penumbra but also the integral dose "bath" throughout the patient. Photon beams have no localization ability along depth and "pass" through the target. Proton beams, in contrast, deposit no dose beyond the distal edge of the Bragg peak. This simple difference means that a composite of multiple proton beams will have approximately half the integral dose of a similarly arranged set of photon beams (see Fig. 20.3).

A single proton field, as the composite of multiple individual dose-weighted Bragg peaks, can deliver an arbitrary dose distribution to a target volume. Scattered proton fields, in clinical practice, are shaped to deliver homogeneous dose to all or part of the target volume. In the case of partial target coverage, a second field is used to fill-in or "patch" (see below) the remainder. Thus, a single proton

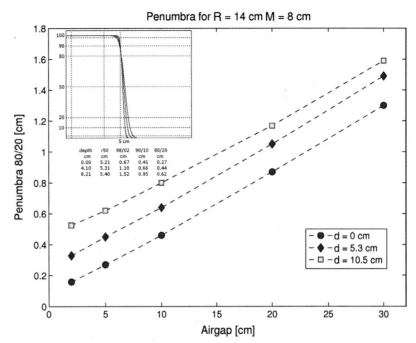

Figure 20.2. The effect of increasing the airgap in a scattered field results in an increase in penumbra because the projection of the effective source size, on the order of 7 cm in scattered proton fields, in the patient increases. The penumbra also increases, but much less so, as a consequence of the scatter in patient as a function of depth (depths of 0, 5.3 and 10.5 cm are shown for a field of 14-cm range and 8-cm modulation). The initial penumbra at a depth of 0 equals the projected source size only as the proton beam has not yet scattered in the patient. The *insert* (*top left*) shows the penumbra for this field as a function of depth for an airgap of 5 cm.

field can achieve the desired dose description. Such a single proton field can achieve superior dose shaping by virtue of the lateral penumbra and the distal fall-off that spares distal tissues. A single scattered proton field cannot control the entrance dose given the fixed modulation width of a spread-out Bragg peak (SOBP). An example of such a field is shown in Figure 20.3 in comparison to an IMRT treatment.

The distal fall-off of the Bragg peak has the sharpest dose gradient (about half of the lateral penumbra) and

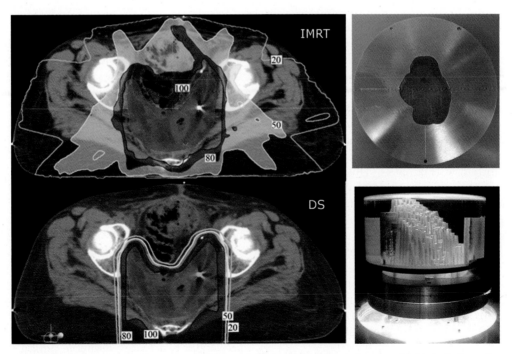

Figure 20.3. Treatment plans, intensity-modulated radiotherapy (IMRT) and scattered fields (DS), for endometrial nodal disease are compared. The IMRT plan uses seven fields and has an unavoidable dose bath (yellow between 50% and 80% isodose lines). The DS plan, in contrast, achieves superior coverage with a single posterior aperture and range-compensator field (examples of these devices, not those used for this treatment, are shown on the *right*). The aperture, as for a photon beam, achieves lateral beam's-eye-view conformance. The range-compensator shifts the proton penetration range in proportion to the local thickness to conform the dose to the distal surface of the target volume. Note that for a scattered field, the entrance dose cannot be controlled and results for this case in near, full skin dose.

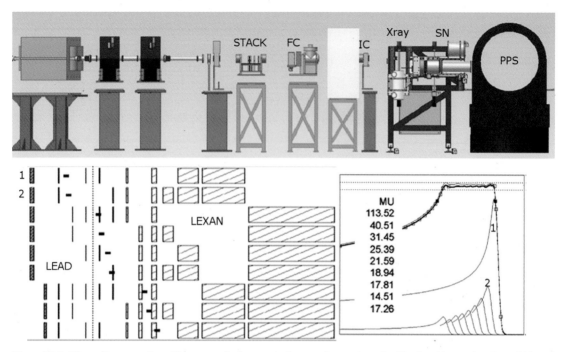

Figure 20.4. The radiosurgery beamline uses a single-scattered proton beam. A stack of lead and lexan absorbers shift and scatter the proton beam (of $R = 20.7$ cm) to the desired energy and fixed scattering angle. The reference ionization chamber (IC) counts the appropriate number of MU to create spread-out Bragg peaks (SOBPs) of the desired modulation. The patient is positioned on the patient positioner (PPS) at 450 cm from isocenter (the *dot* in the lamination pattern on left bottom). The position is verified with x-ray and the snout (SN) allows imaging of the full cranial anatomy and with the aperture. The beam energy is verified by a multi-layered Faraday cup (FC). A thick neutron absorber (*white*) between the FC and IC reduces the neutron dose well below the required levels at the patient.

should offer the best opportunity to achieve a dose differential between target and healthy tissues. In practice, however, the range in patient has an uncertainty estimated on the order of 3.5%. This uncertainty arises from the uncertainty in (relative) stopping power in the patient as derived in practice from CT. CT data measures, per voxel, the electron density in Hounsfield units. For proton radiotherapy treatment planning, the Hounsfield unit in each voxel is converted to stopping power using a tissue-dependent conversion curve (Fig. 20.4). This conversion is empirical and global, and ignorant of patient-specific variations. Proton radiotherapy planning assumes the worst-case scenarios concerning the possible position of the distal edge of the Bragg peak. In practice the distal edge is extended beyond the target volume by 3.5% of the distal range. The modulation, that is, the difference between distal and proximal (90–98%, in our practice), is extended by 7%. Most significantly, it means that the distal edge cannot be used to achieve a dose gradient between the target and a critical structure—doing so could imply a direct overshoot into the critical structure!

Proton dose distributions are biologically equivalent to photon dose distributions except for a constant relative–biological effect (RBE) factor of 1.1. That is, a photon dose of 54 Gy (Co60 equivalent) equals a physical—as measured in an ionization chamber (IC), proton dose of 54/1.1, or 49.1 Gy. Proton dose distributions are, therefore, stated as 54 Gy (RBE) (4) to indicate that the physical dose

has been corrected by the RBE factor and can be compared directly to an equivalent photon dose distribution of 54 Gy. Dose effect knowledge from photon radiotherapy can thus be transferred to proton radiotherapy. This is a major advantage in the clinical application of proton radiotherapy. In contrast, the RBE of heavier charged particles, that is, for Lithium and beyond, introduces significant complexities and unknowns in dose reporting.

GENERATION OF CLINICAL PROTON FIELDS

The proton pristine Bragg peak is too narrow, on the order of 6 mm, to be clinically useful. Thus, many Bragg peaks must be added and distributed through the target volume to achieve a clinical dose distribution.

Accelerators

The generation of a clinical proton beam requires an accelerator to achieve a desirable clinical energy range of up to about 250 MeV. The latter corresponds to about 38 cm in water and is considered good maximum choice given the deepest seated targets. The lowest minimum range is about 3 to 4 cm (60 MeV) and is needed for orbital and other shallow targets.

Current accelerating technologies are cyclotrons and synchrotrons. A cyclotron accelerates a proton beam when it crosses repeatedly over a gap over which a strong cyclical (of a period equal to the proton traversal time between gap crossings) electrical field is applied. The proton beam is in a constant magnetic field $B = B_T$ and the accelerating proton beam assumes an ever-increasing radial orbit R, that is, $R = R(E)$. At the highest design energy, that is, at the maximum radius $T = R(E_{MAX})$ of the cyclotron cavity, the proton beam is extracted from the cyclotron. Thus, a cyclotron produces a single energy beam E_{MAX} and the proton beam must pass through a carbon or beryllium (i.e., a low scatter material) variable thickness degrader to achieve the desired clinical energy. A synchrotron accelerates the proton beam by passing it through an accelerating cavity and keeps the beam in a constant-radius orbit T by synchronizing (and increasing) the magnetic field with the proton energy, that is, $B = B(E)$ such that the proton bending radius equals T. A synchrotron can produce any energy E, proportional to the number of passes through the cavity and limited by the maximum magnetic field B, without the need for post-extraction degradation.

The primary difference between a synchrotron and cyclotron is the need for energy degradation of the latter. The degrading material, however, scatters the beam, which results in a large emittance, that is the position and momentum phase space, for a cyclotron. This, in turn, affects the beam transport design and the ability to achieve a narrow beam at the patient. The choice of cyclotron was preferred due to their simpler operation and higher beam current. The latter is to compensate for proton loss in scattered fields where a large portion of protons (between 50% to 90%) is lost to scatter and field collimation within the scattered field radius. The emerging preference for scanned beam technology, however, places different requirements on the beam parameters compared to scattered beams and the choice between synchrotron and cyclotron may shift in favor of the synchrotron.

The generated beam is transported to the treatment delivery device using a magnetic beamline. A distributed beamline allows a single accelerating device to supply multiple treatment rooms which reduces the overall facility cost.

Scattered Proton Fields

An initially narrow proton beam of a given energy is shifted to lower energies and spread in depth by different thickness absorbers, broadened and flattened laterally by carefully designed scatterers, and "stacked" with appropriate weights by synchronizing absorber insertion with monitor units (MU) or another integrated beam-current measure (see Fig. 10.2). Such composite and scattered proton fields are labeled SOBP fields and, in general, produce homogeneous dose per field over a desired modulation width up to a maximum range.

Single Scattering

A proton beam scattered by a series of flat absorbers is labeled a single-scattered beam. The scattered beam

profile is Gaussian and, with a large SAD and sufficiently large scattering angle, a near-uniform collimated field can be created over a radius at the top of this profile. An example of such a system is the radiosurgery beamline at the F H Burr Proton Therapy Center (see Fig. 20.4). An incoming proton beam of 185 MeV (22 cm range in water) is centered on a binary stack of lexan and lead absorbers. Lexan is a low-Z material and is an efficient energy absorber with low relative scatter (1 g/cm^2 has a mean angle of 0.0072 radian at 130 MeV) while lead is a high-Z material with high scatter (1 g/cm^2 has a mean angle 0.021 rad) and low relative absorption. The stack has 10 lexan absorbers with thicknesses from 0.022 to 11.5 g/cm^2, where each subsequent thickness is twice the previous, and five lead absorbers from 0.088 to 1.403 g/cm^2, again with doubling of thickness. Combinations of lexan and lead produce pristine Bragg peaks between 4 and 22 cm, where each emerging beam is scattered into a Gaussian profile within which a 10-cm diameter field has a minimum intensity of 95% relative to the center. By switching combinations of lexan and lead absorbers for appropriate beam-on times, as measured in an IC, for example, SOBP fields of arbitrary modulation widths can be created.

Double Scattering

A common mechanical method for creating SOBP fields uses a rotating wheel where the thickness of a particular angular interval encodes the pull-back of the pristine peak in an SOBP and the width of the angular interval encodes the weight of the pristine peak (see Fig. 20.5). Such a wheel can be constructed of a lexan and lead combination to create a constant-scatter angle as a function of rotation and combined with a second scatterer to increase the efficiency of the proton beam and to broaden and flatten the field. The second scatterer, again, is constructed of two, low-Z/high-Z, materials and is contoured along its radius to uniformly absorb the proton energy. The scatterer is shaped differentially to scatter the protons to create a uniform field. A photon scatterer, in contrast, is shaped differentially to absorb photons.

Dual-scattering systems have been the primary technology, up to now, for proton-radiotherapy field delivery. Here we summarize, briefly, the operation of the IBA[1] dual-scattering nozzle at the F H Burr Proton Therapy Center as an example (see Fig. 20.5 top). In such a system, one wishes to minimize the number of scatterers and modulators to reduce complexity. The system is fully automated, efficient to operate, but not necessarily optimal in terms of proton efficiency or field parameters due to pragmatic operational considerations. The IBA nozzle offers SOBP ranges between 3 and 30 cm in water with a field diameter of up to 24 cm for ranges <25 cm and up to 12 cm for ranges >25 cm.

---

[1] *IBA LTD, Louvain la Neuve, Belgium.*

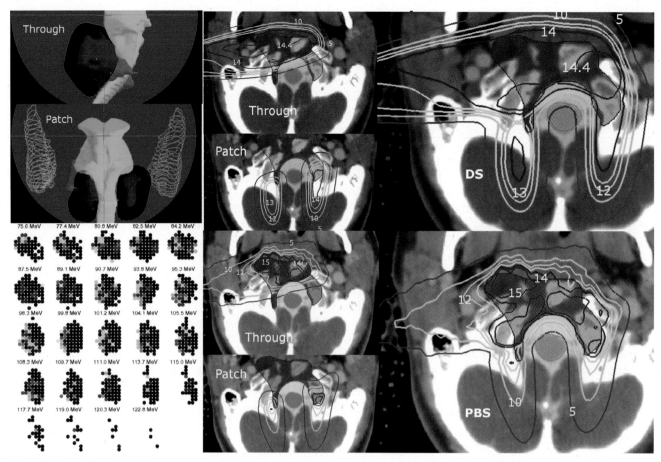

Figure 20.5. Patching of fields is a necessary technique in scattered fields to wrap the dose distributions around a target. In the above example, the through-field (*left-top* where the circle is a 12-cm aperture) covers the anterior part of the GTV and the patch field covers the posterior "horns." The *top-right* three figures show the dose distributions for the scattered (DS) fields. The bottom-right three figures show the result using the DS-field apporaches and using the pencil-beam scanning (PBS) optimization to achieve a total dose distribution without the benefit of either apertures or range-compensators. In the PBS optimization, all fields are optimized as an ensemble. The desired prescription dose is 14.4 Gy (RBE). The construction of patching fields in DS is tedious as the field parameters—range, modulation and aperture size—must be carefully tweaked to achieve a dose distribution that covers the partial volumes to yield coverage of the total volume. For example, the through-field for the DS plan shows a distinct softening at its distal edge which makes it harder for the patch field to cover that volume. The PBS patching, by virtue of its simultaneous optimization of all fields and its ability to vary local intensity, achieves a much more satisfactory result. In addition, the posterior lateral gradient of the PBS through-field is not as sharp compared to the DS through-field. The PBS gradient is defined by the varying pencil-beam intensities while the DS gradient is defined by the field edge. Thus, the PBS patch is probably less sensitive to errors. The PBS fields used a total of 1,600 pencil-beams with an initial spread of $\sigma = 5$ mm and with ranges between 4.5 and 14.5 cm (in water). The *bottom-right* figure shows the 1,103 spots for each of 24 energy layers for the Through PBS beam. The color indicates the number of gigaprotons (Gp) in each spot.

The nozzle has three rotating modulator wheels, each of which has three tracks. The nozzle defines eight combinations of modulator wheel track and scatterer where each combination, called an option, covers a particular clinical-range interval of about 3 to 4 cm. A total of eight options thus cover the desired clinical minimum and maximum ranges. In theory, a pair of modulator wheel track and scatterer only produces a flat field, laterally and in depth, for the design energy. Below that energy, the field is "over"-scattered, and above it "under"-scattered. The nozzle has a set of thin-foiled lead insertable scatterers upstream from the modulator track that increases the mean scatter angle and flattens the field as the energy increases in the option interval.

The SOBP depth dose plateau flatness (better than ±1% in our practice) can be controlled by modulating the cyclotron beam current during the rotation (at 10 Hz) of the modulator track. This is a convenient property of a cyclotron which acts as a continuous and variable current source. The SOBP flatness is determined by the set of weights for each of the pristine Bragg peaks in the SOBP. These weights of each peak's contribution to the SOBP are hard-coded in the modulator track but are not "exact" for a particular SOBP range. The modulation of the beam-current adjusts the weight by varying the number of protons that pass through an angular segment. The use of current modulation reduces the complexity of modulator track design, which now can be "corrected", and allows a

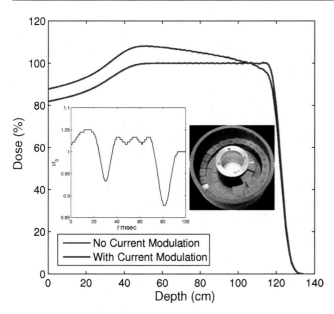

Figure 20.6. The ability to control the current (relative to the current I_0 set for a specific dose rate) as a function of the rotation time (100 ms) of the modulator wheel allows a track to be "tuned" to produce a perfectly flat spread-out Bragg peak (SOBP) (*blue*) compared to that produced with a constant current (*red*).

particular track to be applied well outside its initial design interval (see Fig. 20.6).

The beam-current control also controls the width of the SOBP field. The modulator track, over its full rotation, achieves a maximum constant pullback SOBP width. The current can be turned off at an angle within the full rotation to allow for arbitrary modulation up to the maximum pullback to deliver the desired modulation width for a particular patient field.

Field-Shaping Devices

Scattered fields are shaped laterally by apertures, as photon fields, and in depth by range-compensators (Fig. 20.3). Apertures are collimated to the beam's-eye-view projection of the target volume and require a distance of 7 to 10 mm between the target and aperture edges to account for the depth-dependent penumbra. The apertures must have sufficient thickness to absorb the incident range as a proton field does *not* change in intensity as it passes through an absorber. Thus, insufficient thickness will result in full dose to the patient! The range-compensator is unique to proton and heavy charged particles. The range-compensator adjusts the range across the lateral field profile such that the resultant distal dose surface closely matches the distal target volume surface. A range-compensator thus spares tissues distal to the target.

The thickness of the target volume, measured as the difference between the deepest and shallowest radiological path-lengths in the target volume, determines the desired maximum range of the SOBP field and the modulation width. The combination of an aperture and range-compensator can thus achieve, for a single SOBP field,

lateral and distal conformation and homogeneous dose in the target volume (see Fig. 20.3).

The aperture is placed as close as possible to the patient to reduce the effect of the large effective proton source, whose size is on the order of 5 to 10 cm, due to scattering material in the beam, compared to 1 to 2 mm for a photon beam! The penumbra of this source can only be mitigated by, first, placing it as far as possible from the patient, typically at an SAD ~ 300 cm, and demagnify it by the aperture–patient distance over the aperture–source distance. Thus, in clinical practice, the effective source size is demagnified 40-fold and its contribution to the penumbra for double-scattered fields is on the order of 5% (see Fig. 20.2).

The design of the range-compensator considers individual radiological path-lengths from the source to the distal surface and sets the range-compensator thickness such that the distal fall-off of the SOBP is just beyond the target distal surface. Consider an "open" field of range R_d that reaches, as measured from the source to that point, just beyond the deepest point P_d on the target distal surface. We wish to insert material for every other point P_i on the target distal surface equal to $T_i = R_d - R_i$ where R_i is radiological path-length to point P_i. The range-compensator is constructed with the thicknesses T_i. The result is that the range R_d as it passes through the range-compensator is shifted along each ray from the source such that the distal edge of the proton composite dose distribution lies just beyond the target distal surface (see Fig. 20.3).

Known uncertainties in the patient or target position, caused by setup errors or otherwise, create variations in path-lengths that could lead to an underdose of the target or an overshoot into the healthy tissues. The range-compensator profile is, therefore, "smeared" where each point is assigned the largest range (or least thickness) from among the points in its neighborhood within a radius corresponding to the total expected variation (see Fig. 20.1). This ensures worst-case coverage of the distal target surface in the presence of these variations. It does, however, push the distal fall-off dose further into the healthy tissues. This, and the inherent uncertainty in range stated above, means that the distal fall-off of the SOBP cannot be used to shape a gradient between the target volume and a critical structure.

Absolute Dosimetry

The relationship between dose in patient and number of protons produced by the cyclotron is not trivial for scattered fields. The number of protons, as usual, is monitored by a reference IC placed upstream of the collimated field which produces a signal proportional to the proton flux. In general, we can refer to proton beam flux in terms of absolute number of protons, that is, gigaprotons or Gp, or in terms of the IC response in MU as the two are related by the stopping power S_{air}, that is, $MU \propto S_{air} \times G$ for G protons passing through the collection volume of the IC. For scanning beams, discussed below, the use of Gp is recommended. For scattered fields in a continuous system such as a dual-scattered system with a rotating modulator wheel, the target volume receives the fractional prescription dose at every wheel rotation interval (i.e., 0.1 s). Thus, MU is proportional to the fraction of prescription dose in patient. A delivery interruption (within 0.1 s) results in the whole volume receiving partial prescription dose. For the single scattered system described above, however, an IC count interval corresponds to the delivery of an individual pristine peak in the set of peaks of the SOBP. In such a system, a delivery interruption results in some parts of the target volume receiving full dose, while other parts receive incomplete dose. Resumption of such fields much be accurately handled in the delivery system.

The relationship between physical dose (in Gy) in the SOBP plateau and MU is complicated. In principle, one could calibrate each pristine Bragg peak in units of Gy per number of protons (or MU). This relationship for scattered fields is impractical except for the simplest beamlines. In general, the complex secondary interactions in a dual-scattering system and the variability of mechanical device settings preclude such a calibration or derivation.

One can establish a semitheoretical relationship for the output factor Ψ (in Gy/MU) between MU and physical dose in water. The SOBP output factor is the ratio between dose D_p in the plateau and dose (i.e., MU) measured in the IC. The latter, in turn, is proportional to the entrance dose D_0 of the SOBP. Thus Ψ is proportional to the ratio of D_p/D_0, which can be derived from a mathematical description of the Bragg peak and equals

$$\Psi(R,M) = \Psi_R \times \frac{D_0^R}{D_0(R,M)} = \Psi_R \times \frac{D_0^R}{100/(1+a \cdot r^b)}$$

EQUATION (20.1)

where D_0^R is the SOBP entrance dose of the reference SOBP which has an output factor Ψ_R, and the entrance dose of the SOBP of interest, with range R and modulation M, is $D_0(R,M)$ and described by the two-parameter function characterized by a form factor $r = (R - M)/M$. The function parameters, a and b, have the theoretical values of 0.44 and 0.6, respectively. In practice, these differ due to the secondary effects in the nozzle.

In clinical practice, the applicability of Equation 20.1 depends very much on the construction details of the delivery system. In our practice, the formula is successfully applied to both the single-scattering beamline and our dual-scattering gantry nozzle. The parameters a and b are obtained from calibration and are constant for each option. In general, Equation 20.1 will apply to a constant configuration of a nozzle where the SOBP shaping devices do not change, which is the case in the IBA nozzle for each option.

Scanned Proton Fields

The clinical practice of proton radiotherapy, about 50,000 patients to date, has been based almost exclusively on scat-

tered field technology. The use of scattered fields to achieve complex dose distributions requires considerable manual planning and time. Scanned proton beam technology is clinically viable, as by the PSI team, and should become the future of proton radiotherapy. Only scanned proton fields can match the level of automation and complexity integration that now is expected in photon radiotherapy considering technologies enabled by IMRT and treatment planning optimization.

Scanned proton fields use a narrow beam of protons of variable energy, to control depth penetration, and which is moved in the lateral dimensions by magnetic fields (Fig. 10.8 bottom). Thus, an almost arbitrary 3D dose distribution can be created inside the patient without the aid of mechanical beam modifiers or field-shaping devices such as apertures and range-compensators. The latter, however, may continue to have clinical use or benefit and their use should not be considered voided.

There are two clinical modes of using pencil-beam scanning (PBS) technology. The first mode, labeled single-field uniform dose (SFUD) (5), is analogous to the clinical use of SOBP fields. In this mode, each PBS field is designed to deliver a homogeneous dose, like an SOBP field, to the target volume. Unlike an SOBP field of constant modulation width, the dose to the volume proximal to the target volume now conforms as well. This offers further healthy tissue sparing compared to scattered SOBP fields. The second mode uses two or more fields and optimizes the dose as a composite for all fields. This mode is analogous to IMRT field optimization, where each individual field delivers inhomogeneous dose, and is labeled intensity-modulated proton therapy (IMPT).

The clinical application of PBS to date (at PSI) has been primarily with SFUD fields and not IMPT fields. The reason is twofold. First, IMPT fields have uncertainties in the precise knowledge of the end-of-range of the pencil-beam and also require precise knowledge of the sources of geometric errors. These uncertainties could cause the individual fields not to "mesh" correctly to yield the desired composite dose. Second, the optimization problem for IMPT is significantly more complex compared to IMRT optimization. In IMPT optimization, the number of variables is one or two orders of magnitude larger compared to IMRT and requires a substantial increase in numerical computing power which only has become available recently with the advent of 64-bit computing architectures.

The optimization unit for IMPT, that is, the pencil-beam itself, also complicates the convergence of conventional optimization algorithms as it presents to the optimizer a sharp distal fall-off and a coarser (by a factor of 2) lateral fall-off. This causes conventional optimization algorithms, that is, those based on squared dose differences, to prefer the distal edge fall-off which exacerbates the problem of distal edge uncertainty. SFUD field optimization only considers a single field at a time and avoids these problems.

Thus, the successful clinical introduction of IMPT requires new optimization technologies that consider the robustness of the final treatment plan. The robustness of a treatment plan measures its invariance against the known and specified sets of uncertainties that have been included in the optimization methodology. For IMPT plans, this set includes range and positional uncertainties, including those of target motion (6). The positional uncertainties, especially, are significant for SOBP fields in general and for IMPT in particular. For both, the local motion of a target volume, such as may be present, in the lung, causes significant changes in radiological path-lengths and cannot be considered by a simple expansion of the clinical target volume (CTV) into a planning target volume (PTV). Such an expansion can be used for the lateral extent, that is, in the BEV plane. Along the depth dimension, however, the final beam profile, managed with a range-compensator for SOBP fields and by differential pencil-beam intensities for IMPT, must ensure coverage of the target for all phases of motion. The correct consideration of these effects requires a computation over all phases instead of a geometric assumption such as the ITV concept.

Multi-criteria Optimization

In current clinical practice, optimization algorithms use a quadratic cost-function F of the form

$$F = \sum_k \sum_{j \in k} a_k (D_k - d_j)^2 \qquad \text{EQUATION (20.2)}$$

which specifies, for each organ of interest, the prescription dose D_k and weight factor a_k as an indicator of the significance of meeting the prescription dose. The function F is minimized for all dose point d_j that contribute dose to the organ k. This methodology, in practice, yields treatment plans that approximate the desired solution, that is, the "optimal" treatment plan, but often require arbitrary recalculations that "tweak" the parameters a_k and D_k to achieve the physician's intent. This intent is typically not specifiable as it depends on a trade-off analysis by the physician which can only be done, given the actual possibilities.

Recent developments in optimization introduce the use of multi-criteria optimization (MCO) which consider multiple trade-offs simultaneously (7). The MCO approach, at least in our practice, computes all "possible" treatment plans, each of which is optimal within the choice of trade-offs. In MCO, the physician specifies a set of absolute constraints, such as minimum and maximum doses allowed to the target and or structures, and a set of objectives, such as "minimize the mean to the lung" or "minimize the maximum to the GTV." The MCO optimizer generates a set of plans, each of which meets the constraints, of sufficient number to sample all the possibilities of the stated objectives. These optimal treatment plans lie on the Pareto trade-off surface which is a multi-dimensional surface (of dimension proportional to the number of objectives) formed by those points whose values are the optimal trade-offs. That is, chang-

ing one trade-off (such as increasing the target dose) will decrease another trade-off (such as higher critical structure dose). The user traverses this surface to select the desired set of trade-offs. Consider the example in Figure 20.7 that shows the Pareto surface (a curve in this case of two objectives) of a chest-wall target volume with a desired optimal dose of 70 Gy (RBE) but where a minimum of 40 Gy (RBE) was set to allow sufficient "room" to assess lung dose. The two objectives are "minimize the mean lung dose" and "maximize the minimum dose to the GTV." An optimal plan that lies on the curve means that improving lung dose will degrade target dose and *visa versa*.

Absolute Dosimetry

PBS dosimetry is, in essence, simple as one only considers the interaction of a pure proton beam in medium. The proton pencil-beam control parameters are its lateral deflection as defined in the reference plane and measured in a positional IC, its energy as defined by the accelerator, and its instantaneous or integrated current. All these parameters must be specified by the treatment planning system as the final dose calculation must consider, at a minimum, the exact relative dose contribution from each pencil-beam. Figure 20.8 shows a set of pristine Bragg peaks as a function of range which have been carefully calibrated for treatment planning to match those delivered on the equipment. The peaks are specified in units of Gy (RBE) mm^2/Gp. These units allow the treatment planning system to relate the dose in patient directly in terms of a delivery system control parameter, that is, the number of protons (in Gp). This relation between dose in patient and the beam charge (assuming a pure Gaussian model, see Chapter 10, Proton Dose Calculations) is

$$D(x,y,z) = \sum_i \frac{G_i}{2\pi\sigma_i^2(z)} \exp\left(\frac{r_i^2(x,y,z)}{2\sigma_i^2(z)}\right) D_i^\infty(z)$$

$$\text{EQUATION (20.3)}$$

where $\sigma_i(z)$ is the spread of pencil-beam i at depth at z (in the pencil-beam coordinate system with z equal to pencil-beam axis), $r_i(x,y,z)$ is the lateral displacement of the calculation point with respect to the pencil-beam axis, G_i is the number of protons in the pencil-beam, and $D_i^\infty(z)$ is the pristine Bragg-peak depth dose. The index i includes summation over pencil-beams of different energies and positions. The pencil-beam spread $\sigma_i(z)$ includes both the in-patient scatter due to (primarily) multiple Coulomb interactions and the initial spread of the pencil-beam prior to entering the patient as produced in the delivery equipment. The final dose thus has the correct units of Gy. It is the responsibility of the treatment planning optimization system to compute the set G_i to be delivered by the delivery equipment. The pencil-beam energies and deflections are typically pre-computed given the target shape and location.

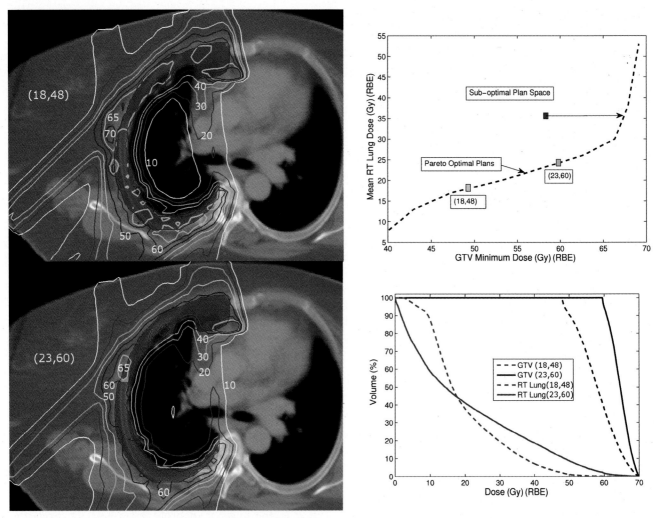

Figure 20.7. The challenge of selecting the "optimal" plan is illustrated by the above hypothetical, proton pencil-beam scanning (PBS) irradiation of a chestwall. The PBS treatment uses three beams: a posterior (gantry 170), anterior (gantry 350), and right posterior oblique (gantry 225). The GTV (*in red*) is constrained to a dose range of 40 to 70 Gy (RBE) and the competing objectives are to "maximize the minimum GTV dose" and to "minimize the mean to the right lung" (note that there is *no* contralateral lung dose concern as the proton beams have no exit dose). The *top right* figure shows the Pareto surface of optimal plans (a curve in this case given two objectives). The Pareto optimizer computes a mathematical representation of all plans that lie on the curve. This representation allows a rapid computation of any plan that corresponds to a point on the curve. The "red" plan is a suboptimal plan because, given its mean RT lung dose, it should allow a GTV dose of 68 Gy (RBE; *arrow*); a Pareto optimizer would not yield such a plan by definition. The "cyan" and "green" plans (labeled 18,48 and 23,60 for the curve coordinates) are Pareto-optimal plans. Note how the GTV dose can be significantly increased in the central curve region with only a modest increase in lung dose. The analysis afforded by the multi-criteria optimization (MCO) is essential for PBS given the higher level of variability in a treatment plan because of the large number of PBS pencil-beams (on the order of 10^3–10^4). The corresponding dose distributions and DVHs are shown on the *left* and *bottom-right*, respectively.

CLINICAL CASE ANALYSIS

Our example is a pediatric cervical chordoma. This site has as critical structures: brainstem, cord, cochlea, and chiasm. The prescription dose is 50.4 Gy (RBE) to the CTV and 79.2 Gy(RBE) to the GTV, while keeping the chiasm below 62 Gy (RBE), brainstem and cord center (surface) below 55 (67) Gy (RBE), and the cochlea below 60 Gy (RBE). The treatment approach reflects a long experience in sequencing the fields.

The first set of five fields to the CTV have gantry angles of 70, 100, 230 and 260 at a couch angle of 0 and a gantry angle of 155 at a couch angle of 90. The main objective of this field arrangement is to reduce the dose to the parotid glands but little to the spinal cord. Each field, in the scattered-field (DS) delivery, covers the CTV to homogeneous dose. The DS fields are not all delivered at each treatment session. Instead, triplets of rotating combinations are used. Figure 20.8 shows the normalized dose distribution for a single field and the composite dose distributions for all five fields.

The GTV fields, as a consequence of the full CTV dose inclusion, must avoid the brainstem and spinal cord. For DS fields, this can only be achieved by patch combinations. A patch combination is the proton equivalent of field edge matching. Given the finite range of the proton,

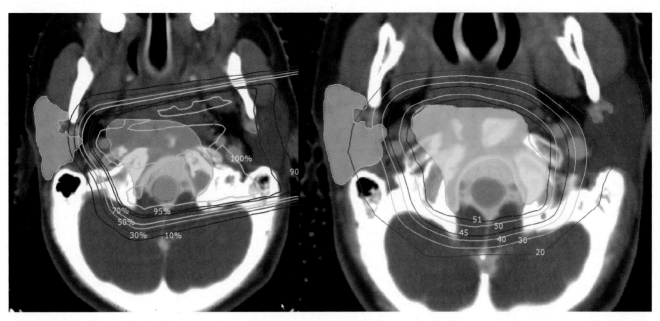

Figure 20.8. An example of a double-scattered field delivery to the clinical target volume (CTV) (*green*). Each of the five fields achieve full target coverage (>98% isodose line—not shown). Note how each field arrangement (one of which is shown on the *left*) spares the contra-lateral parotid. The full complement of five fields reduces the parotid dose to about 20% of 50 Gy (RBE) as only one field passes through each parotid. Note that the fixed modulation of the DS SOBP cannot control the entrance dose (as visible in left figure where the 95% isodose line crosses the parotid). The composite dose distribution (in Gy (RBE)) is on the right. The maximum dose to the CTV is 51 Gy (RBE) and indicates the high degree of homogeneity achievable with SOBP fields.

one can now also patch the distal edge of one field to the penumbral edge of another field. Each field delivers full dose within its subtarget volume and the combination of patch fields achieves full dose to the target volume. As noted before, however, the uncertainty in the distal range can lead to a cold or a hot spot. As a consequence, patch combinations are always "switched" around to feather this hot or cold spot. The construction of patch-field combinations for scattered SOBP fields is cumbersome in spite of some available support in treatment planning systems. For illustrations purposes (Fig. 20.5), we use one of the three DS patch-field combination (in fact a "double" patch) and use the PBS optimization engine to "auto-patch" the field without the use of an aperture and range-compensator. The result is (probably) more robust to cold or hot spots as the individual field dose distributions present a more gradual distal fall-off compared to the "true" pristine peak dose fall-off. Thus, any over- or undershoot effect is minimized by the lower gradient. We expect, in the clinical practice of PBS and subject to further validation, to continue to use the DS-field approaches as these have inherent robust properties such as target avoidance with the penumbral edge and distal edges away from critical structures. Even with available robust optimization techniques, these DS-field approaches retain their use.

Figures 20.9 and 20.10 show the total, CTV + GTV, dose distributions for both the IMPT and DS plans. The IMPT plan does significantly improve on the parotid glands which are primarily located in the integral dose region, which—as stated before—can be reduced on average by 50% with protons and even more with IMPT compared to photons. In general, however, the DS plan is competitive with the IMPT plan and, in general, we do not expect as dramatic a change between IMPT and DS compared to

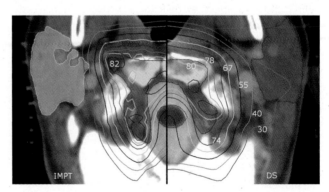

Figure 20.9. The figure shows a near symmetric chordoma wrapping around the spinal cord in this transverse image. The GTV is shown in *red*, the spinal cord in *purple*, and the parotid glands in *cyan* and *purple*. Isodose values are shown in Gy (RBE). The desired prescription dose for the GTV is 78 Gy (RBE). The left half of the picture shows an IMPT treatment plan, and the right half shows a scattered field (DS) treatment plan. Both plans used the identical beam angles, as created for the DS plan. The choice of the DS beams inherently selects "robust" approaches (see text). Distinctive features in favor of the intensity-modulated proton therapy (IMPT) plan are (1) tighter and more complete coverage of the GTV especially into the posterior tails (see 78 Gy (RBE) isodose), (2) better sparing of the parotid (see 30 Gy (RBE) isodose), (3) significant less spinal cord dose (see 55 Gy (RBE) isodose), and (4) lower integral dose as apparent from the 30 and 40 Gy (RBE) isodose lines. Overall, however, the scattered field approach achieves a very comparable treatment plan.

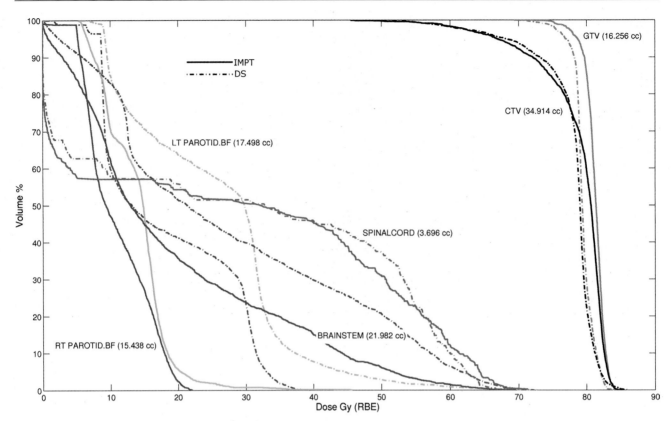

Figure 20.10. The dose-volume histograms for the parotid glands and brainstem show significant reduction in dose. This is primarily a consequence of the fact that pencil-beam scanning (PBS) fields reduce the proximal dose that cannot be controlled in a scattered field. The spinal cord does not show an overall reduction for the PBS approach as the field approaches deliberately, per convention and per need to avoid the parotids, pass through it.

IMRT and 3D conformal. Instead, we expect PBS to significantly reduce the treatment planning overhead required to create the numerous fields (12 for this case) required to achieve superior DS dose distributions in patient.

REFERENCES

1. Goitein M, Abrams M, Rowell D, et al. Multi-dimensional treatment planning: II. Beam's eye-view, back projection, and projection through CT sections. *Int J Radiat Oncol Biol Phys* 1983;9:789–797.
2. Wilson RR. Radiological use of fast protons. *Radiology* 1946;47:487–491.
3. Richard W. *A brief history of the Harvard University cyclotrons.* Cambridge: Harvard University Press, 2004. Available from http://physics.harvard.edu/~wilson/cyclotron/history.html.
4. ICRU Report 78. Prescribing, recording, and reporting proton-beam therapy. *J ICRU* 2007;7(2).
5. Lomax A. Intensity modulation methods for proton radiotherapy. *Phys Med Biol* 1999;44:185.
6. Lomax AJ. Intensity modulated proton therapy and its sensitivity to treatment uncertainties 2: the potential effects of inter-fraction and inter-field motions. *Phys Med Biol* 2008;53:1043.
7. Monz M, Küfer KH, Bortfeld TR, et al. Pareto navigation—algorithmic foundation of interactive multi-criteria IMRT planning. *Phys Med Biol* 2008;53:985.

CHAPTER 21

Fractionation: Radiobiological Principles and Clinical Practice

Colin G. Orton

INTRODUCTION

From the very beginning of radiotherapy, treatments were fractionated. For example, on January 29, 1896, just 1 month after Roentgen announced his momentous discovery of x-rays to the world, Emil Grubbé in Chicago was reported to have begun administration of a course of 18 daily 1-hour fractions of radiotherapy to a patient with cancer of the breast (1). More fractions would have been delivered, but treatment had to be terminated when the patient developed a virulent dermatitis. Within a few years, hundreds of patients had been treated with fractionated radiotherapy worldwide.

In these early years just about all radiotherapy was fractionated, but fractionation was used not because it was known that this was the appropriate way to deliver high doses without exceeding normal tissue tolerance—as we know today—but because of the very low output from the early x-ray machines available at that time. To deliver a single dose sufficient to destroy a tumor would have required several hours—sometimes even days—so treatments had to be given in several sessions. Single-fraction radiotherapy did not become feasible until 1914 with the advent of the Coolidge hot cathode tube, with its high output, adjustable tube current and reproducible exposures. The ensuing two decades witnessed a period of uncertainty as to the proper way to fractionate. Reportedly, there were two schools of thought: Erlangen and Paris (2). Wintz, from Erlangen, led a group of radiotherapists who believed that single doses were necessary to cure cancer, and they referred to fractionated treatment as "decisively inferior and . . . to be considered weak irradiation or the primitive method." Their rationale for single-fraction radiotherapy was based on their interpretation of the Bergonié–Tribondeau Law of radiation sensitivity, published in 1906, which concluded: "From this law, it is easy to understand that roentgen radiation destroys tumors without destroying healthy tissues." Therefore, it appeared that there was an inherent advantage of roentgen irradiation that might be lost if cancer cells were allowed time to recover. Wintz and his colleagues argued that "recovery from radiation injury depends on cellular metabolism and a rapidly growing tumor cell is better able to affect recovery from injury than a connective tissue cell. Therefore, the difference in recovery will favor the tumor if the cancerocidal dose is not applied in the first treatment" (1).

The Paris School, on the other hand, used the radiobiological experiments of Regaud on the effect of fractionation on the sterilization of rams to justify the need to fractionate. Regaud found that it was possible to sterilize rams by irradiation of their testes without excessive damage to the skin of the scrotum only if the treatments were fractionated. When single doses were given, such sterilization was possible only with induction of unacceptable skin damage. Regaud postulated that the testes could be considered a good model to simulate a rapidly dividing cancer and, therefore, fractionation ought to allow a cancerocidal dose to be delivered without exceeding normal tissue tolerance. This led to a careful study of fractionated radiotherapy by Henri Coutard at the Curie Institute in Paris (2).

The debate over fractionation was not settled until 1932, when Coutard published the excellent results he had obtained using fractionated radiotherapy (3). Fractionation was thereafter established as the standard of practice of radiotherapy. However, it is only relatively recently that the radiobiological rationales for fractionated radiotherapy have been fully understood.

RADIOBIOLOGICAL PRINCIPLES OF FRACTIONATION

The basic principle of radiotherapy is the destruction of all cancer cells without killing so many normal cells as to exceed tolerance. Thus, cell survival and the shape of cell survival curves is of utmost importance in radiotherapy.

Cell Survival Curves

A plot of the fraction of surviving cells as a function of dose for acutely irradiated cells is shown in Figure 21.1. Note that surviving fraction is plotted on a log scale. This is partly because, as we will see later, the shape of the log-linear survival curve for specific cell types tells us something about the important radiobiological properties of these cells, and partly because much of the important information about cell survival is contained within the low and high dose extremes of the survival curve (regions A and B in Fig. 21.1). Plotting cell survival on a log scale helps us visualize and

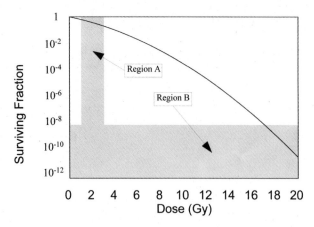

Figure 21.1. Graph showing the surviving fraction of cells (log scale) as a function of dose. The two shaded areas represent the regions of most interest in fractionated radiotherapy for which doses per fraction normally range from 1 to 3 Gy (region A) and the cell-surviving fraction required to control a typical tumor containing 10^8 to 10^{10} cells must be on the order of 10^{-8} to 10^{-12} (region B). This hypothetical graph has been constructed according to the linear quadratic (LQ) model with parameters $\alpha = 0.4$ Gy^{-1}, $\alpha/\beta = 10$ Gy.

study the shape of the survival curve in these regions. It is low doses per fraction (in region A) that are used for fractionated radiotherapy (1–3 Gy/fraction) and, to cure a tumor with typically 10^8 to 10^{10} cells, cell-surviving fractions as low as 10^{-8} to 10^{-12} are required (region B).

Since the shapes of cell survival curves are so important, it is necessary to have a mathematical model that can predict these shapes. Currently, the model of choice is the linear quadratic (LQ) theory of cell survival.

Linear Quadratic Theory

The basis of the LQ theory is that a cell is inactivated only when both strands of a deoxyribonucleic acid (DNA) molecule are damaged. Actually, this is a gross oversimplification of the highly complex chemical and biological responses triggered by irradiation of cells, but this was the basic assumption made when the LQ model was first devised (4) so, for simplicity, we will adopt this approach here. Readers interested in a more thorough (and accurate) discussion of the complex events that occur when cells are irradiated are referred to an excellent review by Wouters and Begg (5).

On this simple model, double-strand breaks can be produced either during the passage across the cell of a single ionizing particle or by independent interactions by two separate ionizing particles. Such events are random and, because there are large numbers of cells, the probability that any specific cell will be inactivated will be extremely low. Under such conditions, the statistics of rare events (Poisson statistics) prevails. According to Poisson statistics, the probability of there being no such lethal events, that is, the surviving fraction, S, of cells, is given by the expression (6):

$$S = e^{-p} \qquad \text{EQUATION (21.1)}$$

where p is the mean number of hits per cell. For single-particle events, p is a linear function of dose, D, so the mean number of hits/cell can be expressed as αD. Then, Equation 21.1 can be written as:

$$S = e^{-\alpha D} \qquad \text{EQUATION (21.2)}$$

where α is the average probability per unit dose that such a single-particle event will occur. In order for a single particle to damage both arms of the DNA in a single passage across the molecule, it has to be fairly densely ionizing, that is, high linear energy transfer (LET). With photon and electron irradiation, it is only the slow electrons that are responsible for most of these interactions. Conversely, when cells are irradiated with high-LET radiations, such as α-particles and heavy ions, almost all the events will be by single particles, so cell survival will be governed by Equation 21.2 and cell survival curves will be practically linear.

For the two separate ionizing particle events of the LQ theory, the mean probability of one particle causing damage in one arm of a DNA molecule in any specific cell is linearly proportional to dose, as also is the mean probability that a second particle will have such an interaction in the adjacent arm of this same DNA molecule. Therefore, the mean probability of both events occurring is βD^2, so the probability that no such two-particle events will occur is given by:

$$S = e^{-\beta D^2} \qquad \text{EQUATION (21.3)}$$

where β is the mean probability per unit square of the dose that such complementary events will occur.

The overall LQ equation for cell survival is therefore:

$$S = e^{-\alpha D - \beta D^2} \qquad \text{EQUATION (21.4)}$$

This is illustrated in Figure 21.2, which shows how the two components of cell killing, α-damage and β-damage, combine to form the cell survival curve. It will be shown later that α-damage and β-damage relate to irreparable and repairable damage, respectively. For two-particle

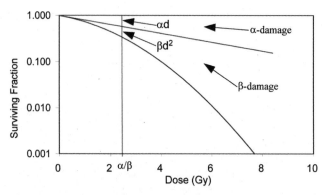

Figure 21.2. Linear-quadratic cell survival curve, with $\alpha = 0.22$ Gy^{-1} and $\alpha/\beta = 2.5$ Gy. Note that the log cell kill for α-type damage equals that for β-damage at a dose equal to α/β.

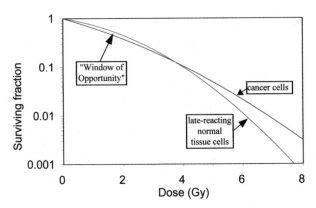

Figure 21.3. Typical survival curves for cancer and late-reacting normal tissue cells, superimposed for comparison. Compared with the cancer curve, the normal tissue cell survival curve has a shallower initial slope (lower α) and is "curvier" (lower α/β). Note that there is a "Window of Opportunity" below ~4 Gy (with the parameters used here) where normal tissue cells exhibit a higher survival than cancer cells. Parameters used to draw these hypothetical curves are as follows: tumor, $\alpha = 0.4$ Gy^{-1}, $\alpha/\beta = 10$ Gy; late-reacting normal tissues, $\alpha = 0.22$ Gy^{-1}, $\alpha/\beta = 2.5$ Gy.

events (β-type), if the damage from the second particle occurs before the lesion from the first particle has been repaired, the cell will be inactivated ("killed"). Since cellular repair half-times are of the order of 1 hour, this gives rise to the dose-rate effect: the higher the dose rate, the greater the effect.

Of special interest is the dose at which the log-surviving fraction for α-damage ($-\alpha D$) equals that for β-damage ($-\beta D^2$), that is, $\alpha D = \beta D^2$, or $D = \alpha/\beta$. This is also illustrated in Figure 21.2. This parameter, α/β, represents the curviness of the cell survival curve. Specifically, the higher the α/β, the straighter the curve. Similarly, a high α/β is characteristic of a type of cell that exhibits considerable irreparable damage and/or little repair (high α and/or low β). In contrast, a low α/β (low α and/or high β) indicates little irreparable damage and/or a high capability of repair. Here lies the major difference between the cells of tumors and those of late-responding normal tissues: α/β values tend to be high for cancers and low for late-reacting normal tissues. For example, typical α/β values determined for cancer cells range from 5 to 20 Gy (mean ~10 Gy), but for late-responding normal tissues the range is 1 to 4 Gy (mean ~2.5 Gy). There appear to be some exceptions, however. For example, the α/β values for prostate and breast cancer cells have been reported to be about 1.5 and 4 Gy, respectively (7,8).

Figure 21.3 shows typical survival curves for tumor and late-reacting normal cells, superimposed for comparison. The difference in the shapes of cell survival curves of cancer and normal cells provides the major rationale for fractionated radiotherapy.

Rationale for Fractionation

Radiotherapy, in general, is governed by the four Rs: repair, reoxygenation, repopulation, and redistribution, and so

also is fractionation. Following is a discussion of how each of the four Rs affects the practice of fractionation.

Repair

Of all the four Rs, repair is the most important in terms of the rationale for fractionation. As discussed in the preceding section, late-reacting normal tissue cells tend to exhibit a greater propensity for repair than do tumor cells. This is exhibited by their low α/β values and their curvier survival curves, as shown in Figure 21.3. In this illustration, the normal tissue and tumor cell curves cross at doses of the order of 4 Gy. At doses below the crossover point, cell survival for late-reacting tissues is greater than that for tumors, and the reverse is true above the crossover. This means that delivery of doses greater than ~4 Gy will be more destructive to normal tissues than to cancer cells. There is essentially a "Window of Opportunity" centered at ~2 Gy within which normal cells have a greater survival than cancer cells. However, doses far in excess of 4 Gy are needed to control tumors. There are two ways to safely deliver such high doses. One is to deliver much higher doses to the tumor than to the normal tissues, such as with stereotactic radiosurgery (SRS), intensity-modulated radiation therapy (IMRT), and various other forms of conformal therapy. This will be discussed in detail later. The second option is to fractionate with doses/fraction within the "Window of Opportunity."

If a course of fractionated radiotherapy is delivered with time between fractions sufficient for complete repair (which clinical evidence has shown to be about 6 hours or more), all the cells that have been sublethally (but not lethally) damaged during the first exposure will have repaired before the second, and so on. This relates to the β-type damage in the LQ model. Then, at least to a first approximation, cell-surviving fractions for each successive treatment will be identical, that is, the shape of the survival curve will simply repeat for each fraction and the cell-surviving fraction equation becomes:

$$S = e^{-N\left(\alpha d - \beta d^2\right)}$$ EQUATION (21.5)

where N is the number of fractions and d is the dose/fraction. Then, if the dose per fraction is below the crossover point shown in Figure 21.3, the resultant cell survival curves gradually separate, with tumor cells suffering more damage than normal cells, as illustrated in Figure 21.4, which has been derived using Equation 21.5.

At least as far as repair is concerned, the optimal dose per fraction is that, which will produce the maximum separation of the two fractionated radiotherapy curves in Figure 21.4. However, the LQ model predicts that this maximum separation occurs with an infinite number of infinitely small dose fractions, each separated by sufficient time for complete repair. Clearly, this is not a realistic fractionation scheme, and in any event it ignores the influence of the other three Rs of radiotherapy, especially repopulation (see later discussion). With this in mind a better

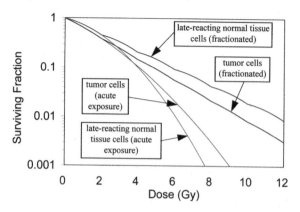

Figure 21.4. How fractionation with dose per fraction below the crossover point of the late-responding normal tissue and tumor cell survival curves in Figure 21.3 results in higher cell survival for the normal tissue cells as the total dose increases.

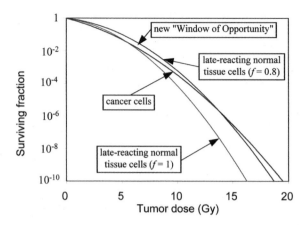

Figure 21.5. How the crossover point for single (acute) irradiations shown in Figure 21.3 moves to considerably higher tumor doses if there is even a modest amount of "geometrical sparing" of the normal tissues (the normal tissue curve moves 20% to the right). In this example, a 20% sparing ($f = 0.8$) causes the crossover point to move from ~4 Gy out to 14 Gy. The same linear quadratic (LQ) model parameters as for Figure 21.3 are used here.

definition of the optimal dose per fraction is where the rate of increase in separation of the two fractionated radiotherapy curves in Figure 21.4 per unit number of fractions is a maximum. It can be shown that this occurs at the point of maximum separation between the acute exposure tumor and normal tissue curves shown in Figure 21.3, which turns out to be at exactly 50% of the dose at the crossover point. For the parameters used to plot the survival curves in Figure 21.3, this dose is ~2 Gy. Hence, the optimal dose per fraction is about 2 Gy. If the α and β values for normal tissues and tumor were known for each patient, it would be possible to design patient-specific fractionation regimens but, unfortunately, the technology to do this is not refined enough at present. The alternative is to determine the optimal dose per fraction for specific types of disease for the average patient, and this has been the objective of numerous clinical trials of altered fractionation (2,7–17).

The situation is somewhat different for SRS and other forms of highly conformal radiotherapy, because the effective dose to normal tissues is usually kept well below that to the tumor, where the "effective dose" may be defined as the dose that, if delivered uniformly to the tissue in question, would result in the same probability of local control or complication as the actual inhomogeneous dose distribution in that tissue. Several methods to determine such effective doses from dose–volume data have been published (18–24) and these are reviewed in Chapter 23. For example, if f (the geometrical sparing factor) is the ratio of the effective dose in normal tissues to effective dose in tumor, even a modest sparing represented by $f = 0.8$ moves the crossover point to considerably higher doses and significantly widens the "Window of Opportunity," as shown in Figure 21.5. In this example, the crossover point moves from 4 Gy all the way out to about 14 Gy, so the optimal tumor dose per fraction becomes ~7 Gy. Interestingly, this is the typical tumor dose per fraction used for high dose-rate brachytherapy for cervix cancer, with which significant geometrical sparing inherent with the brachytherapy modality can be expected.

For SRS, single doses of the order of 20 Gy are used. It is readily shown that with the parameters used to plot Figures 21.3 to 21.6, this will be optimal if f equals ~0.6, not too unlikely, especially for small tumors. For large tumors, f may exceed 0.6, so fractionated radiotherapy might be required.

One concern with SRS and other types of radiotherapy such as IMRT, CyberKnife, and so on, for which the time it takes to deliver a treatment session can be of the same order of magnitude as the half-time for cellular repair, is that repair during irradiation might reduce the effectiveness of the treatment. Studies have shown that this effect might cause reductions in effective dose as much as about 12% if the time to deliver the treatment is as high as about 0.5 hours, with concomitant reductions in tumor control as much as 30% (25). Fortunately, it is possible that protraction of irradiation time during a treatment might reduce the effect on normal tissues more than on cancers (26). Hence, it might be possible to increase the total dose sufficiently to offset the effect of this intrafraction repair without increasing the damage to normal tissues.

All the foregoing discussions, and especially the dose per fraction estimates, are of course highly dependent on the α and β parameters assumed. They also totally ignore the effect of the other three Rs of radiotherapy.

Reoxygenation

Oxygen is the most powerful of all radiation sensitizers, so cells deprived of oxygen are relatively resistant to radiation and require approximately three times as much dose as well-oxygenated cells to destroy them. Such doses in a course of radiotherapy will likely exceed normal tissue tolerance unless highly conformal therapy is used. Furthermore, there is evidence that a significant proportion of human cancers contain hypoxic cells (27–32). It would be

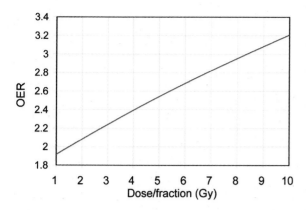

Figure 21.6. Illustration of the increase in oxygen enhancement ratio (OER) with increase in dose/fraction. Parameters used (see text) are those derived to fit clinical data for the treatment of prostate cancers by Nahum, et al. (30).

expected, therefore, that immediately after the exposure of a tumor to radiation, the fraction of the surviving cells that are hypoxic should increase because the sensitive, well-oxygenated cells will be killed preferentially. Indeed, this is exactly what has been observed in many animal *in vivo* experiments. However, in some of these experiments, the hypoxic-cell fraction rapidly returned to the much lower pre-irradiation levels, and this has been interpreted as reoxygenation (33). In that case, if enough time is allowed for reoxygenation between exposures in a course of fractionated radiotherapy (typically 24 hours is sufficient), the number of hypoxic cells in a tumor reduces to a level that can be handled by doses that do not exceed normal tissue tolerance. Hence, fractionation takes on added importance when treating tumors with a significant hypoxic-cell fraction. However, there is some evidence that fractionation does not always ensure sufficient reoxygenation to overcome hypoxic-cell radioresistance. For example, several clinical trials have demonstrated that pre-irradiation hypoxia significantly reduces local control even after an extended course of fractionated radiotherapy long enough to ensure reoxygenation (27–32). If complete reoxygenation were taking place between fractions, such reductions in local control would not be expected.

Another aspect of the effect of oxygen on fractionated radiotherapy relates to the effect of LET. When cells are exposed to high-LET radiation, the protective effect of hypoxia is greatly reduced (33). Hence, in the part of the cell survival curve where α (i.e., high-LET) damage predominates, that is, at low dose or low dose/fraction (see Fig. 21.2), the effect of hypoxia should be less than where β-damage predominates, that is, at high dose or high dose/fraction. This effect of dose or dose/fraction has been demonstrated by cell survival experiments (34,35) and has been shown to be consistent with clinical data (30).

The effect of O_2 is represented by the oxygen enhancement ratio (OER), where:

$$OER = \frac{dose\,under\,anoxic\,conditions}{dose\,under\,aerobic\,conditions} \quad \text{Equation (21.6)}$$

to produce the same biological effect, for example, cell survival. Low OER means that the protective effect of hypoxia on cell survival is little, and high OER means that the effect is great. The potential magnitude of the effect of dose/fraction on the OER can be illustrated using the LQ model using Equation 21.5: $S = e^{-N(\alpha d - \beta d^2)}$ and taking the natural logs of both sides giving:

$$-\ln S = Nd(\alpha + \beta d) \quad \text{Equation (21.7)}$$

Then, if subscripts a and h represent aerobic and hypoxic irradiation conditions, respectively, and equating values of $-\ln S$ for N fractions of dose d/fraction for equal biological effect:

$$N_a d(\alpha_a + \beta_a d) = N_h d(\alpha_h + \beta_h d) \quad \text{Equation (21.8)}$$

$$\therefore OER = \frac{N_h d}{N_a d} = \frac{\alpha_a + \beta_a d}{\alpha_h + \beta_h d} \quad \text{Equation (21.9)}$$

Figure 21.6 shows how OER varies with dose/fraction for prostate cancer using values of α and β that have been shown to fit clinical data (30): $\alpha_a = 0.26$ Gy^{-1}, $\beta_a = 0.0312$ Gy^{-2}, $\alpha_h = 0.149$ Gy^{-1}, and $\beta_h = 0.00293$ Gy^{-2}. This figure shows the trend of increasing OER as dose/fraction increases but it should be realized that the actual numbers depicted here represent just a single study for a single type of cancer. Data from other analyses of clinical results for prostate and other cancers will yield different OER versus dose/fraction curves, but the trend should be as shown in Figure 21.6. Similar observations of increasing OER with dose/fraction above 1 Gy/fraction have been made using modified versions of the LQ model and different parameters (36,37). This would indicate that, for the treatment of cancers that might contain significant numbers of hypoxic cells, low dose/fraction techniques, with of the order of 1 Gy/fraction, might have an advantage over conventional (about 2 Gy/fraction) and high dose/fraction (>2 Gy/fraction) regimes.

In summary, fractionation is essential for reoxygenation but, even with fractionated radiotherapy, not all cancers appear to reoxygenate. Furthermore, fractionation has the added benefit of keeping the OER low so as to not overly protect hypoxic cells.

Repopulation

By their very nature, all cancers contain dividing cells, with viable cancer cells usually dividing much faster than those of late-reacting normal tissues. Hence, during a course of radiotherapy, there is considerably more repopulation of cancer cells than cells of the late-responding normal tissues, so the longer a course of radiotherapy, the more difficult it becomes to control the tumor without exceeding normal tissue tolerance. Furthermore, some studies show that repopulation of cancer cells might accelerate during a course of fractionated radiotherapy (accelerated repopulation), with the faster rate of division kicking in after the first 2 to 4 weeks of treatment (38). On these grounds, therefore, repopulation appears to dictate that courses of radiotherapy should not be overly protracted and that accelerated repopulation, if it exists—there is some controversy about this (39)—even indicates that optimal schedules of treatment might be as short as 2 to 4 weeks. However, repopulation is not entirely detrimental. Acutely responding normal tissues need to repopulate during a course of radiotherapy to avoid exceeding acute tolerance. Hence, the length of a course of radiotherapy, and therefore the fractionation, must be controlled so as to not allow too much time for excessive repopulation of tumor cells, at the same time not treating so rapidly that acute tolerance is exceeded.

Redistribution

According to the cell cycle effect, cells irradiated during the mitotic (*M*) phase of the cell cycle are most sensitive, and during late synthesis (late *S*) they are most resistant, with a second peak of resistance in *G1* in some cells (40). For cells irradiated in the *M* phase, the survival curve is practically linear, indicating minimal repair. In contrast, for cells irradiated in late *S*, survival curves exhibit the greatest curvature, representing considerable repair. Consequently, cells surviving a single dose of irradiation tend to be partially synchronized, with an overabundance of surviving cells in late *S* moving into early *G2* immediately after exposure. If a second exposure is delivered some time after the first, the number of cells inactivated depends on how far this surviving bolus of cells has traveled around the cell cycle. For example, if they have reached the *M*

phase at the time of the second exposure, they will be most sensitive. It is this radiation-induced partial synchronization of cells that is known as redistribution (or reassortment).

Redistribution can be a benefit in a course of fractionated radiotherapy if the cancer cells can be caught in mitosis after each fraction, or detrimental if they have reached a resistant phase of the cell cycle. In theory, it ought to be possible to adjust the interval between fractions so as to gain maximum benefit from redistribution, but to date there has been no evidence that such an advantage can be obtained in practice. Consequently, potential effects of redistribution are generally ignored when designing fractionation strategies.

Fractionation Strategies

The radiobiological principles discussed in the foregoing sections have been used extensively to guide in the design of numerous clinical trials of altered-fractionation regimens. In this section, the rationale for various fractionation schemes will be presented. Table 21.1 lists a variety of fractionation schemes, their typical parameters, and some brief comments. Following is a detailed description of each of these fractionation schemes.

Conventional Fractionation

The most common fractionation for curative radiotherapy is about 1.8 to 2.2 Gy/fraction delivered at five fractions a week. This has evolved as the conventional fractionation regimen because it is convenient (no weekend treatments), efficient (treatment every weekday), and effective (high doses can be delivered without exceeding

TABLE 21.1	**Fractionation Schemes with Typical Parameters**			
Fractionation scheme	Dose/ fraction (Gy)	Fractions/ week	Total dose (Gy)	Comments
Conventional	1.8–2.2	5	~60	Used for most patients
Hyperfractionation	1.2–1.3	10	~70	Allows higher dose to tumors without increased late complications
Accelerated fractionation	2–2.2	7	~60	Used for rapidly proliferating cancers
	1.4–1.6	10	~54	Increased risk of late complications
	~2.5	5	~50	May need rest period because of acute reactions
Hyperfractionated accelerated radiotherapy	~1.5	15 (CHARTWEL)	~54	Used for rapidly proliferating cancers
		21 (CHART)		High risk of severe acute complications
Hypofractionation	3–10	1–5	10–30 (palliation)	For palliation
			40–60 (cure)	Used for cure with highly conformal radiotherapy

either acute or chronic normal tissue tolerance). The principal rationale for the prescription of conventional fractionation for a particular patient or disease is that most experience is with this type of fractionation, for which both tumoricidal and tolerance doses are well documented. Unless there is a good reason to change, radiation oncologists are reluctant to deviate from this tried-and-true method of treatment.

Hyperfractionation

A hyperfractionated course of radiotherapy is one in which more than one fraction is delivered each day but the overall treatment time remains similar to that for conventional fractionation. Typically, this means 1.2 to 1.3 Gy/fraction, two fractions a day, with an increase in total dose of the order of 20% to account for increased repair at the lower dose per fraction.

The major rationale for hyperfractionation is to take full advantage of the difference in repair capacity of late-reacting normal tissues compared with tumors. This was illustrated by the curvier cell survival curves for these normal tissues (Fig. 21.3) and the concomitantly lower α/β values. If conventional radiotherapy is not producing particularly good clinical results and no obvious reasons for this are evident, maybe the reason is that the dose per fraction that adequately separates the two fractionated radiotherapy curves in Figure 21.4 is below that used in conventional fractionation. With such a low dose per fraction, more than one fraction per day is necessary to keep the course of therapy short enough to avoid the risk of excessive tumor cell repopulation. Such hyperfractionation regimes will have to be delivered at about 1.2 to 1.3 Gy/fraction, two fractions a day. To treat with higher than 1.3 Gy/fraction at more than one fraction per day may exceed acute tolerance, and to use <1.2 Gy/fraction will require three fractions per day in order to not overly increase overall treatment time, with at least 6 hours between fractions required for complete repair, a treatment schedule that would be highly inconvenient.

Another potential advantage of hyperfractionation might be the reduced OER at low dose/fraction compared with that with conventional fractionation (see Fig. 21.6). This could be important for cancers that might be expected to contain significant numbers of hypoxic cells.

Accelerated Fractionation

For rapidly growing tumors with short potential doubling times of the viable cycling cancer cells (T_{pot}), accelerated treatment is desirable. This is especially important for types of tumors that exhibit accelerated repopulation (38).

There are several ways to achieve reduced overall treatment time. The simplest is to treat 6 or 7 days a week instead of the normal 5, keeping the dose per fraction the same as with conventional fractionation. This produces a modest acceleration that may be enough to influence clinical outcome. A more drastic acceleration can be achieved

by treating twice a day at 1.4 to 1.6 Gy/fraction, but only at the risk of exceeding acute normal tissue tolerance. Such accelerated fractionation regimens have been tried but have usually been unsuccessful because many patients had to be given a rest of 1 to 2 weeks during the course of therapy to allow acute reactions to subside, negating the intent to accelerate the treatments.

Another possibility is to increase the dose per fraction to ~2.5 Gy (often called rapid fractionation), but this risks losing the repair advantage of late-responding normal tissues. Increased late reactions usually occur unless the dose to the normal tissues can be reduced, such as with conformal therapy. Alternatively, for rapidly growing cancers it is possible to exploit the difference in repair between late-reacting normal tissues and tumors by hyperfractionating while accelerating the course of therapy by treating with three fractions per day. Such treatment is known as accelerated hyperfractionation.

Accelerated Hyperfractionation

A major problem with such accelerated fractionation is that cancerocidal doses delivered in such short overall times are likely to exceed acute tolerance unless a gap is included part way through treatment to allow early reactions to subside. One way around this is to complete the treatments in such a short time that the acute reactions reach their peak only after the radiotherapy has been completed. This was the rationale for the development of the continuous hyperfractionated accelerated radiotherapy (CHART) regimen at Mount Vernon Hospital in London (11). With CHART, treatments 6 hours apart are delivered three times a day, 7 days a week. With a dose fraction of 1.5 Gy, a total dose of 54 Gy can be delivered in 36 fractions over 12 successive treatment days including weekends. With this schedule, patients can complete treatment without a break because peak acute reactions occur approximately 2 weeks after the start of therapy. Although clinical results for the treatment of lung and head and neck cancers have been promising with CHART, they have been achieved with considerable trauma to the patients: many of these patients developed grade 3 or worse acute complications (41). CHART is also difficult for the staff, since delivery of three fractions per day 6 hours apart for 12 successive days, including weekends, is very inconvenient. Some of this inconvenience is reduced with an alternative form of CHART called CHARTWEL (CHART weekend less), wherein the 54 Gy at 1.5 Gy/fraction at three fractions per day is delivered over a total of 16 days without the weekend treatments (14). Clinical trials have shown that CHARTWEL is a viable alternative to CHART (42).

Hypofractionation

All the fractionation regimes presented above require the delivery of many fractions over many days. They are costly in terms of resources and are inconvenient for patients. These fractionation schemes were necessitated by the desire to "cure" cancers without exceeding normal tissue tolerance. However, not all radiotherapy is aimed at "cure." For many patients, the aim is to palliate the disease, so there is no need to employ the very high doses required for "cure" and hence no need to approach tolerance of normal tissues. For these patients it is, therefore, possible to design much more convenient and cost-effective treatments, which use far fewer fractions, that is, to employ hypofractionation. Typical hypofractionation schemes range from as many as 10 fractions of 3 Gy to as few as a single fraction of ~10 Gy, with anything from one to five fractions per week.

With conformal radiotherapy, because there is considerable geometrical sparing of normal tissues, the "Window of Opportunity" (Fig. 21.5) is widened such that the high doses/fraction needed for hypofractionated treatments can be used for curative radiotherapy. This has led to the development of many clinical trials of hypofractionation, especially for prostate and breast cancers for which the α/β ratio is lower than the 10 Gy, typically assumed for most cancers (8,15,17,43).

One potential disadvantage of hypofractionation relates to the increased OER that might be expected with high dose/fraction schedules (Fig. 21.6). Hence, unless otherwise demonstrated by clinical results, it seems prudent to not apply hypofractionation for the treatment of cancers thought to contain significant fractions of hypoxic cells.

One possible advantage of hypofractionation for cancers with a high α/β that might be exploited is the increase in intrafraction repair that takes place with long treatment times, which should benefit late-reacting normal tissues because of their lower α/β (prostate cancer might be an exception). This would require increasing the total dose to account for this increased repair just enough so as to not increase the risk of late complications. This could be determined by, for example, a carefully controlled dose-escalation clinical trial or, maybe, calculation of the appropriate dose using a bioeffect dose model. This exemplifies a major challenge with most modified fractionation regimens for which there is no previous experience: the determination of the appropriate total dose to use. Rather than just guessing, it has been a common practice to use mathematical bioeffect dose models to calculate these doses. The most popular of these is the biologically effective dose (BED) model.

The Biologically Effective Dose Model

The BED model for fractionated radiotherapy can be derived directly from the LQ equation for cell survival for fractionated irradiations presented earlier (Equation 21.7): $-\ln S = Nd(\alpha + \beta d)$.

This equation could be used to calculate treatment regimes that are equally effective biologically (constant $-\ln S$) but, to do so, we would need to know the values of the two parameters α and β for each tissue involved.

Unfortunately, it is hard enough to determine a single biological parameter from clinical data, let alone two. However, it is possible to reduce the number of unknown parameters to one by dividing both sides of the Equation 21.7 by α to derive a quantity known as the BED, originally called the extrapolated response dose (ERD) (44,45):

$$\frac{-\ln S}{\alpha} = \text{BED} = Nd\left(1 + \frac{d}{\alpha/\beta}\right) \quad \text{EQUATION (21.10)}$$

Fractionation schemes for which BEDs are equal will be equally effective biologically. Here, we have just one biological parameter, α/β, to determine from clinical data for each type of tissue involved where, as we saw earlier, α/β is the dose at which α-type and β-type damages are equal (Fig. 21.2).

Equation 21.10 was derived assuming acute radiation conditions (i.e., no time for repair during each fraction) and complete repair between fractions. This does not always prevail, however, since there may be occasions when the time between fractions is not sufficient for full repair, or the time to deliver each fraction is long enough for some repair to occur during irradiation. The former has been observed clinically with some of the early three fractions per day patients, for example, when less than 6 hours between fractions was sometimes used (46), and the latter probably occurs for some of the highly conformal therapy techniques such as with SRS, IMRT, and CyberKnife treatments (25,26,47). For these situations, a more complex form of the BED equation is needed that takes into account both the rate at which cells repair, the rate at which each part of the tissue is irradiated, and the time between fractions. The full BED equation for such fractionated therapy has been published (25,48,49) but it is extremely complicated and outside the scope of this chapter.

Equation 21.10 accounts for repair only, but cells, especially cancer cells, are known to repopulate during a course of therapy. If tumor cell repopulation is assumed to be an exponential function of time, with doubling time for repopulation of the cycling cells T_{pot}, then $\ln S$ will be increased by $(0.693/T_{pot})T$, so (50):

$$\ln S = -N(\alpha d + \beta d^2) + (0.693/T_{pot})T \quad \text{EQUATION (21.11)}$$

and hence the BED equation becomes:

$$\frac{-\ln S}{\alpha} = \text{BED} = Nd\left(1 + \frac{d}{\alpha/\beta}\right) - \frac{0.693T}{\alpha T_{pot}}$$
$$\text{EQUATION (21.12)}$$

However, since the two additional biological parameters T_{pot} and α are very difficult to determine from analysis of clinical data, it is useful to replace $0.693/\alpha T_{pot}$ by a single repopulation rate parameter, k, estimated from loss of local control when radiotherapy is prolonged (51). For example, if retrospective analysis of data shows that a patient has a rapidly repopulating tumor, a value of $k = 0.6$ BED units/day might be used. At the other extreme, for a slowly proliferating disease like prostate cancer, $k = 0.1$ BED units/day might be more appropriate. Note that it is usual to assume that $k = 0$ for late-responding normal tissues, since little or no repopulation of these cells would be expected to occur during a course of therapy. For acutely responding normal tissues, the value of k is probably in the range of 0.2 to 0.4 BED units/day (51).

One further refinement of the BED equation is required if cells are believed to exhibit accelerated repopulation after a kick-in time T_k. If it is assumed that repopulation is negligible before T_k and after that proceeds at a rate represented by k BED units/day (51):

$$\text{BED} = Nd\left(1 + \frac{d}{\alpha/\beta}\right) - k(T - T_k) \quad \text{EQUATION (21.13)}$$

where $k = 0$ for $T < T_k$.

A further useful application of the LQ model for comparison of different fractionation regimes is to calculate the equivalent dose at 2 Gy/fraction, because much of the clinical data used to represent tumor control and normal tissue complication probabilities has been published for 2 Gy/fraction treatment schedules (52–54). This is achieved by equating BEDs. For example, if we ignore repopulation effects, the 2 Gy/fraction total dose, D_2, equivalent to a regime of D_d Gy delivered at d Gy/fraction, is given by:

$$\text{BED} = D_2\left(1 + \frac{2}{\alpha/\beta}\right) = D_d\left(1 + \frac{d}{\alpha/\beta}\right) \quad \text{EQUATION (21.14)}$$

$$\therefore D_2 = D_d\left[\left(1 + \frac{d}{\alpha/\beta}\right)\bigg/\left(1 + \frac{2}{\alpha/\beta}\right)\right] \quad \text{EQUATION (21.15)}$$

Another useful application of the LQ model is to correct for errors in dose/fraction. For example, if the wrong dose/fraction is delivered for the first several fractions, Joiner showed that it is possible (with some obvious exceptions) to use the LQ model to calculate a treatment schedule to complete the course of treatment and achieve the same biologic effects that are originally planned for both tumor and normal tissues, provided repopulation effects can be ignored (55). He showed that, if the planned total dose was D_p Gy at d_p Gy/fraction but, due to an error, the first D_e Gy was delivered at dose/fraction d_e Gy, the course could be completed with dose D_c delivered at d_c Gy/fraction, where $D_c = D_p - D_e$ and

$$d_c = \frac{D_p d_p - D_e d_e}{D_p - D_e} \quad \text{EQUATION (21.16)}$$

Note that the total dose is unchanged ($D_p = D_e + D_c$) and that the solution is independent of the α/β of the tissues involved, which is why the effects on both tumor and normal tissues are the same as originally planned. Also, although not stated in Joiner's paper (55), it can be shown that the solution is independent of any geometrical sparing of normal tissues, that is, it is independent of geometrical sparing factor, f.

The following examples illustrate how these models can be applied to the solution of practical radiotherapy problems.

Examples

Problem 1: Gap in treatment: A patient with a rapidly growing cancer is planned to receive a course of 70 Gy in 35 fractions in 7 weeks. After 25 fractions the patient develops a severe acute reaction that necessitates a 2-week rest period. To complete the treatment in 10 more fractions in 2 weeks, what dose per fraction should be delivered?

Solution

Application of the LQ model to problems such as this is complicated since different solutions are possible for different tissues considered and several tissue-specific parameters have to be assumed. For this problem, assume the following parameters for this patient:

For tumor:

$$\alpha/\beta = 10 \text{ Gy}, \ T_k = 28 \text{ days}, \ k = 0.6 \text{ BED units/day}$$

For late-responding normal tissues:

$$\alpha/\beta = 2.5 \text{ Gy}, \ k = 0$$

Tumor solution. Before the break the BED is (using Equation 21.13):

$$\text{BED} = 50(1 + 0.2) - 0.6(35 - 28) = 55.8$$

After the break this reduces to:

$$55.8 - 0.6(14) = 47.4$$

The planned BED was:

$$70(1 + 0.2) - 0.6(49 - 28) = 71.4$$

Therefore, the residual BED that needs to be delivered is:

$$71.4 - 47.4 = 24.0$$

If d is the dose per fraction required to complete the treatment in 10 fractions over 2 weeks:

$$24.0 = 10d(1 + 0.1d) - 0.6(14)$$

Treatment Planning in Radiation Oncology

Therefore:

$$d^2 + 10d - 32.4 = 0$$

Solving this for d gives:

$$d = 2.58 \text{ Gy/fraction}$$

Late-responding normal tissue solution. Since no repopulation is assumed for late-responding normal tissues ($k = 0$), the break should have no effect, so the dose to complete the course of therapy should be unchanged. Therefore:

$$d = 2.00 \text{ Gy/fraction}$$

If it is assumed that the original course represented the maximum dose that could be delivered safely to this patient then, in order not to increase the risk of late normal tissue injuries, the treatment should be completed in 10 fractions of 2.0 Gy. However, since the dose per fraction required for the tumor (2.58 Gy) is much higher than this, it might be necessary to compromise the treatment of the normal tissues in order to not reduce tumor control too much. It might be decided to treat with more than 10 fractions of 2 Gy, but less than the number that would be required for the full tumor effect. This illustrates the undesirability of allowing rest periods during the treatment of rapidly proliferating cancers.

Problem 2: Hyperfractionation: A hyperfractionation regimen consisting of 2 fractions per day, 6 hours apart, for a total of 60 fractions in 6 weeks is designed to be equivalent to 60 Gy in 30 fractions in 6 weeks. What dose per fraction is required?

Solution
Assume all the same parameters as in the first problem. However, since the overall time is unchanged, no account need be taken of repopulation.

Tumor solution. Equating the conventional to the hyperfractionated regimens, the dose/fraction d is determined using Equation 21.10:

$$60(1 + 0.2) = 60d(1 + 0.1d)$$

or

$$6d^2 + 60d - 72 = 0$$

Solving for d gives:

$$d = 1.08 \text{ Gy/fraction}$$

Late-responding normal tissue solution. Equating the two regimens gives (using Equation 21.10):

$$60\left(1 + \frac{2}{2.5}\right) = 60d\left(1 + \frac{d}{2.5}\right)$$

or

$$24d^2 + 60d - 108 = 0$$

The solution to this is:

$$d = 1.21 \text{ Gy/fraction}$$

Note that the late-reacting tissues can tolerate doses much higher than that required for the tumor. This is a consequence of the low dose per fraction and is the major rationale for hyperfractionation. However, even though a course of 60 fractions at 1.21 Gy/fraction in 6 weeks is tolerable as far as late reactions are concerned, the risk of acute reactions might be higher than that for the conventional course of treatment because a total of 2.42 Gy will be delivered each day. But this might not be a problem if the risk of acute injuries is negligible for the conventional course. If these calculations are to be used as the basis for the design of a hyperfractionation regime for real patients, it might be prudent for the radiation oncologist to develop some experience by treating the first few patients with slightly fewer fractions and, if the acute reactions appear tolerable, to escalate the number of fractions to the required 60. Several national clinical trials of hyperfractionation have been designed using dose escalation in this way.

Problem 3: Accelerated fractionation: An accelerated fractionation scheme consisting of 40 treatments, twice a day for 4 weeks is to be equivalent to 60 Gy in 30 fractions in 6 weeks. What dose per fraction is required? Assume the same parameters as in Problem 1.

Tumor solution. The accelerated regimen is completed before the kick-in time for repopulation (28 days), and equating BEDs using Equation 21.13 to determine the dose/fraction d:

$$60(1 + 0.2) - 0.6(42 - 28) = 40d(1 + 0.1d)$$

or

$$4d^2 + 40d - 63.6 = 0$$

Solving this for d gives:

$$d = 1.40 \text{ Gy/fraction}$$

Late-responding normal tissue solution. No repopulation correction is needed, so (using Equation 21.10):

$$60\left(1 + \frac{2}{2.5}\right) = 40d\left(1 + \frac{d}{2.5}\right)$$

or

$$16d^2 + 40d - 108 = 0$$

The solution is:

$$d = 1.63 \text{ Gy/fraction}$$

According to these calculations, it would be safe to deliver the treatment at 1.63 Gy/fraction, which means that the effect on the tumor should be greater than that for the conventional fractionation scheme. This is the rationale for accelerated fractionation for such rapidly proliferating cancers. Note that the daily dose for the accelerated regime is 3.26 Gy, which might not be well tolerated acutely. As in the previous problem, it might prudent to start out using less than the desired 40 fractions of 1.63 Gy/fraction and to dose-escalate with this accelerated radiotherapy schedule, carefully watching out for excessive acute reactions.

Problem 4: Hypofractionation: What is the appropriate dose/fraction required for hypofractionated total breast radiotherapy in 13 fractions over 5 weeks in order for this to be equivalent in terms of tumor control to standard radiotherapy with 25 fractions of 2 Gy delivered over 5 weeks assuming α/β for breast cancer is 4 Gy?

Solution
Since the overall time is unchanged, there is no need to take repopulation into account, so Equation 21.10 can be used.

For the standard treatment the BED is $50(1 + 2/4) = 75$. Then, if d Gy is the dose/fraction needed for the hypofractionated treatments:

$$75 = 13d(1 + d/4)$$

Therefore:

$$3.25d^2 + 13d - 75 = 0$$

Solving this for d gives:

$$d = 3.20 \text{ Gy/fraction}$$

Hypofractionation regimes consisting of 13 fractions of about 3.2 Gy delivered over 5 weeks have been studied in clinical trials and found to be acceptable in terms of both tumor control and complications (8).

Problem 5: Correction of treatment error: A patient is planned to receive 30 daily fractions of 1.8 Gy but, due to an error, the first five fractions are delivered at 2 Gy/fraction. How can the treatment continue so as to result in the same effects on tumor and normal tissues as originally planned?

Solution
According to Equation 21.16, the remainder of the treatments should be delivered at a dose/fraction d_c given by:

$$d_c = \frac{D_p d_p - D_e d_e}{D_p - D_e} = \frac{54 \times 1.8 - 10 \times 2}{54 - 10}$$

$$= 1.75 \text{ Gy.}$$

The total dose remains as planned at 54 Gy, so the remaining 44 Gy has to be delivered in $44/1.75 = 25.1$ fractions. Since we cannot deliver 0.1 of a fraction, 25 fractions of $44/25 = 1.76$ Gy should be used.

Problem 6: Accelerated hyperfractionation: A CHART scheme consisting of 36 treatments, 3 times a day for 12 successive days with at least 6 hours between fractions is to be equivalent to 70 Gy in 35 fractions in 49 days as far as tumor control is concerned. What dose per fraction is required? With this treatment regime, will the effect on late-responding normal tissues exceed that expected from a conventional course of 30 fractions of 2 Gy in 42 days?

Solution
Assume the same parameters as before, except for the repopulation kick-in time for the tumor, which is assumed to be 0 (assume CHART is being tried for these patients because their cancers are rapidly proliferating right from the start of treatment).

For tumor: equating BEDs, the CHART dose/fraction d is given by (using Equation 21.13):

$$70(1 + 0.2) - 0.6(49) = 36d(1 + 0.1d) - 0.6(12)$$

or

$$3.6d^2 + 36d - 61.8 = 0$$

Solving this for d gives:

$$d = 1.49 \text{ Gy/fraction.}$$

For late-reacting normal tissues: the BED for the conventional regime is (using Equation 21.10):

$$\text{BED} = 60(1 + 2/2.5) = 108$$

and for the CHART treatments it is:

$$\text{BED} = 36 \times 1.49(1 + 1/2.5) = 85.6$$

Hence, the CHART treatments should be far more tolerable as far as late reactions are concerned. One would expect that, compared to conventional therapy with 60 Gy at 2 Gy/fraction, CHART should provide equivalent tumor control without the added risk of severe late reactions. However, because the daily dose is about 4.5 Gy, one would expect acute reactions to be very severe, as clinical results have demonstrated (14).

The Importance of Fractionation

The LQ model solutions to the second and third problems illustrate the important radiobiological principle that treatments regimens consisting of more fractions, at lower dose/fraction, typically allow higher BEDs to be delivered to the tumor without increasing the risk of late normal tissue injury. For example, in Problem 2, increasing the number of fractions from 30 to 60 makes the dose per fraction required for tumor control (1.08 Gy) much lower than that which the late-reacting normal tissues can tolerate (1.21 Gy). Similarly, in Problem 3, changing from 30 to 40 fractions caused the dose per fraction for tumor control (1.4 Gy) to be less than that corresponding to tolerance for late reactions (1.63 Gy). This, of course, was demonstrated by an analysis of cell survival curves earlier. An alternative way to study the importance of fractionation is to investigate how dose–response curves for local tumor control and normal tissue complications vary with dose per fraction. This can be done using the LQ model.

Figure 21.7 shows hypothetical dose–response curves for tumor control (upper curve) and late normal tissue injury (lower curve). These dose–response curves are not meant to represent any specific types of tumor or normal tissue, but are for illustrative purposes only. They have been derived using the logistic model, in which the probability of effect P is given by (24,56):

$$P = \frac{1}{1+(D_{50}/D)^{\kappa}}$$
EQUATION (21.17)

where D is the total dose, D_{50} is the total dose for 50% probability ($P=0.5$), and κ is a tissue-specific parameter that regulates the slope of the dose–response curve at dose $D = D_{50}$. Both D and D_{50} are for the same dose per fraction d (in Fig. 21.7 this is 2 Gy). Then, using Equation 21.10, these correspond to the following BEDs

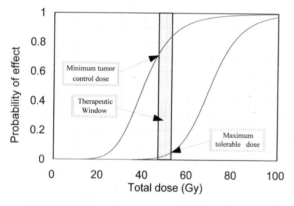

Figure 21.7. Probability of tumor control (left-hand curve) or severe late complications (right-hand curve) as a function of total dose delivered at 2 Gy/fraction. At a total dose of 50 Gy the local tumor control rate is assumed to be 80% and the risk of severe late complications 3%. The Therapeutic Window (shaded) shows the range of values of total dose within which acceptable treatment regimens could be designed (a maximum of 10% reduction in local control or 5% probability of serious late normal tissue injury). Assumptions: logistic dose–response model with $D_{80} = 50$ Gy and slope parameter $\kappa = 6.2$ for tumor; $D_{03} = 50$ Gy and $\kappa = 10.3$ for late reactions; α/β (tumor) = 10 Gy and α/β (late reactions) = 2.5 Gy.

(ignoring the effect of repopulation for simplicity for this demonstration):

$$BED = D\left(1+\frac{d}{\alpha/\beta}\right)$$
EQUATION (21.18)

and

$$BED_{50} = D_{50}\left(1+\frac{d}{\alpha/\beta}\right)$$
EQUATION (21.19)

Hence:

$$D_{50}/D = BED_{50}/BED$$
EQUATION (21.20)

So the logistic Equation 21.17 becomes:

$$P = \frac{1}{1+(BED_{50}/BED)^{\kappa}}$$
EQUATION (21.21)

To determine appropriate tumor values for BED_{50} and κ for this demonstration, the tumor-response curve has been normalized such that 80% local control is achieved at a total dose of 50 Gy at 2 Gy/fraction, which falls to 50% if the dose is reduced to 40 Gy. This gives values of BED_{50} and κ for tumor of 48 and 6.2, respectively, using $\alpha/\beta = 10$ Gy. Similarly, the late-responding normal tissue curves have been normalized such that the risk of severe injury is 3% at 50 Gy, rising to 50% at 70 Gy. The resulting values of BED_{50} and κ for these late-reacting tissues are 126 and 10.3, respectively, using $\alpha/\beta = 2.5$ Gy.

It is with these parameters that the dose–response curves for treatments delivered at 2 Gy/fraction in Figure 21.7 have been constructed. Since some radiation oncologists are willing to accept a slightly lower probability of tumor control to reduce the risk of injury, they tend to prescribe a lower total dose. If it is assumed that the "acceptable" limit is a 10% reduction in local control (from 0.8 to 0.72), the left-hand vertical line in Figure 21.7 represents the minimum acceptable tumor dose. On the other hand, more aggressive radiation oncologists may be willing to risk higher complication rates to improve local control. Assuming for this demonstration that the highest "acceptable" risk of severe normal tissue injury is 5%, the right-hand vertical line in Figure 21.7 represents the maximum acceptable normal tissue dose. Then it is possible to specify a "Therapeutic Window" of total dose within which "acceptable" treatment regimens can be designed. The width of this Therapeutic Window defines how much leeway the radiation oncologist has in the definition of the prescribed dose. The narrower this window, the more difficult it becomes to prescribe a safe and effective total dose, realizing that all patients are different: Some will have sensitive cancers, others resistant, and in some the normal tissues will be extra sensitive, in others not. Indeed, if the width of the window becomes negative, no total dose meets the constraints of the problem, and the treatment

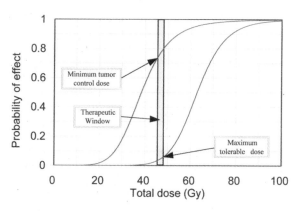

Figure 21.8. Same as Figure 21.7 but with dose per fraction 2.5 Gy. Note the decrease in the width of the therapeutic window (shaded).

regimen must either exceed tolerance or result in too low a local control rate.

Figures 21.8 and 21.9 show what happens as the dose per fraction rises to 2.5 and 3 Gy, respectively. The Therapeutic Window narrows as the dose per fraction increases and in fact becomes negative above about 3 Gy/fraction. This is illustrated by the lower of the two curves in Figure 21.10, which shows how the width of the Therapeutic Window varies with dose per fraction: for >3 Gy/fraction (shaded region with $f=1$) there is an unacceptable risk of excessive normal tissue injury and/or low tumor control.

In the calculations for the figures above, we have ignored the effect of geometrical sparing of normal tissues inherent with conformal radiotherapy such as IMRT. As we saw previously using cell survival curves and the "Window of Opportunity," the effect of geometrical sparing can be very significant. For example, if we assume just a modest geometrical sparing of 20% (i.e., a geometrical sparing factor f of 0.8), the Therapeutic Window increases significantly, as illustrated by the upper curve in Figure 21.10. With the parameters used here, tumor doses/fraction as high as 4.5 Gy can give "acceptable" results.

It should be noted that this analysis of the effect of fractionation uses generic values of the various parameters

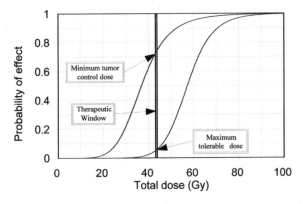

Figure 21.9. Same as Figure 21.7 but with dose per fraction 3 Gy. The therapeutic window has reached almost zero width at this dose per fraction.

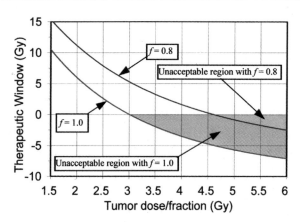

Figure 21.10. The width of the Therapeutic Window as a function of tumor dose per fraction. The lower of the two curves shows that, if there is no geometrical sparing of normal tissues ($f=1$), above ~3 Gy/fraction (*shaded region*) it is not possible to design a treatment schedule that will be sufficiently damaging to tumor cells without exceeding normal tissue tolerance. The upper curve shows that this cut-off dose/fraction moves out to ~4.5 Gy for a modest geometrical sparing of normal tissues ($f=0.8$). The parameters used are the same as those for Figure 21.7.

and therefore does not represent any specific type of tumor or normal tissue. The same applies to the six examples of the application of the LQ model presented earlier. The parameters used for these calculations have been selected to represent reasonable fits to typical clinical data. These LQ model parameters are not known accurately for any specific tumors or normal tissues and, in fact, they probably vary considerably from patient to patient. With such generic parameters as applied here, however, it is possible to use the LQ model to demonstrate some of the important radiobiological principles that govern fractionated radiotherapy for typical patients.

SUMMARY

Treatments have been fractionated from the very inception of radiotherapy a century ago, although it was not until the early 1930s that it was generally accepted that curative therapy required fractionation. Recent studies of the radiobiological principles of cell survival demonstrate that the major reason fractionation is so important is the difference in the capacity of tumor and late-responding normal tissue cells to repair damage at low doses per fraction. Specifically, normal tissue cells are more capable of repair than are tumor cells. This causes their cell survival curves to be curvier than those for tumors which, according to the LQ model, correspond to a lower value of the α/β ratio.

A second difference between tumor and late-reacting normal cells is repopulation. These normal cells repopulate little, if at all, during a course of fractionated radiotherapy, whereas tumor cells, especially those with a short potential doubling time, exhibit significant repopulation.

These repair and repopulation differences between normal and tumor cells provide the major rationale for clinical trials of several types of modified fractionation schemes, such as hyperfractionation, accelerated fractionation, and accelerated hyperfractionation.

One problem encountered whenever fractionation regimens are modified is how to decide on an appropriate total dose when little prior clinical experience is available. The most common way this has been done is by the use of the BED model. However, it must be realized that this model provides only approximate solutions to clinical problems. It represents a grossly oversimplified view of the extremely complex biological changes that occur during a course of fractionated radiotherapy. It is useful for demonstration of the effects of fractionation but, if applied to actual patient treatment calculations, it should be used with caution, preferably only when previous clinical experience is not available.

REFERENCES

1. Orton CG. Uses of therapeutic x-rays in medicine. *Health Phys* 1995;69:662–676.
2. Thames HD. On the origin of dose fractionation regimens in radiotherapy. *Semin Radiat Oncol* 1992;2:3–9.
3. Coutard H. Roentgen therapy of epitheliomas of tonsillar regions, hypopharynx, and larynx from 1920 to 1926. *Am J Roentgenol* 1932;28:313–331.
4. Chadwick KH, Leenhouts HP. A molecular theory of cell survival. *Phys Med Biol* 1973;18:78–87.
5. Wouters BG, Begg AC. Irradiation-induced damage and DNA damage response. In: Joiner M, van der Kogel A, eds. *Basic clinical radiobiology*, 4th ed. London: Hodder Arnold, 2009:11–26.
6. Tubiana M, Dutreix J, Wambersie A. *Introduction to radiobiology*. Bristol, PA: Taylor & Francis, 1990:97–104.
7. Fowler JF. The radiobiology of prostate cancer. *Acta Oncol* 2005;44:265–276.
8. Owen JR, Ashton A, Bliss JM, et al. Effect of radiotherapy fraction size on tumour control in patients with early-stage breast cancer after local tumour excision: long-term results of a randomised trial. *Lancet Oncol* 2006;7:467–471.
9. Cox JD. Clinical perspectives of recent developments in fractionation. *Semin Radiat Oncol* 1992;2:10–15.
10. Fowler JF. Intercomparisons of new and old schedules in fractionated radiotherapy. *Semin Radiat Oncol* 1992;2:67–72.
11. Saunders MI, Dische S. Continuous, hyperfractionated, accelerated radiotherapy (CHART). *Semin Radiat Oncol* 1992;2:41–44.
12. Stuschke M, Thames H. Hyperfractionation: where do we stand? *Radiother Oncol* 1998;46:131–133.
13. Kaanders J, Van Der Kogel A, Ang KK. Altered fractionation: limited by mucosal reactions? *Radiother Oncol* 1998;50:247–260.
14. Wilson EM, Williams JF, Lyn BE, et al. Comparison of two dimensional and three dimensional radiotherapy treatment planning in locally advanced non-small cell lung cancer treated with continuous hyperfractionated accelerated radiotherapy weekend less. *Radiother Oncol* 2005;74:307–314.
15. Khoo VS, Dearnaley DP. Question of dose, fractionation and technique: ingredients for testing hypofractionation in prostate cancer—the CHHip trial. *Clin Oncol* 2008;20:12–14.
16. Stuschke M, Thames HD. Hyperfractionated radiotherapy of human tumors: overview of the randomized clinical trials. *Int J Radiat Oncol Phys Biol* 1997;37:259–267.
17. Miles EF, Lee WR. Hypofractionation for prostate cancer: a critical review. *Semin Radiat Oncol* 2008;18:41–47.
18. Lyman JT. Complication probabilities as assessed from dose-volume histograms. *Radiat Res* 1985;104:S13–S19.
19. Kutcher GJ, Burman C, Brewster L, et al. Histogram reduction method for calculating complication probabilities for three-dimensional treatment planning evaluations. *Int J Radiat Oncol Phys Biol* 1991;21:137–146.
20. Mohan R, Mageras GS, Baldwin B, et al. Clinically relevant optimization of 3-D conformal treatments. *Med Phys* 1992;19:933–944.
21. Niemierko A, Goitein M. Calculation of normal tissue complication probability and dose–volume histogram reduction schemes for tissue with a critical element architecture. *Radiother Oncol* 1991;20:161–176.
22. Niemierko A. Reporting and analyzing dose distributions: a concept of equivalent uniform dose. *Med Phys* 1997;24:103–110.
23. Kwa S, Theuws J, Wagenaar A, et al. Evaluation of two dose-volume histogram reduction models for the prediction of radiation pneumonitis. *Radiother Oncol* 1998;48:61–69.
24. Moiseenko V, Battista J, Van Dyk J. Normal tissue complication probabilities: dependence on choice of biological model and dose-volume histogram reduction scheme. *Int J Radiat Oncol Biol Phys* 2000;46:983–993.
25. Wang JZ, Li XA, D'Souza WD, et al. Impact of prolonged fraction delivery times on tumor control: a note of caution for intensity-modulated radiation therapy (IMRT). *Int J Radiat Oncol Phys Biol* 2003;57:543–552.
26. Liao Y, Joiner M, Huang Y, et al. Hypofractionation: what does it mean for prostate cancer treatment? *Int J Radiat Oncol Phys Biol* 2010;76:260–268.
27. Fyles AW, Milosevic M, Wong R, et al. Oxygen predicts radiation response and survival in patients with cervix cancer. *Radiother Oncol* 1998;48:149–156.
28. Stadler P, Becker A, Feldmann HJ, et al. Influence of the hypoxic subvolume on the survival of patients with head and neck cancer. *Int J Radiat Oncol Biol Phys* 1999;44:749–754.
29. Brizel DM, Dodge RK, Clough RW, et al. Oxygenation of head and neck cancer: changes during radiotherapy and impact on treatment outcome. *Radiother Oncol* 1999;53:113–117.
30. Nahum AE, Movsas B, Horwitz EM, et al. Incorporating clinical measurements of hypoxia into tumor local control modeling of prostate cancer: implications for the α/β ratio. *Int J Radiat Oncol Biol Phys* 2003;57:391–401.
31. Nordsmark M, Bentzen SM, Rudat V, et al. Prognostic value of tumor oxygenation in 397 head and neck tumors after primary radiation therapy. An international multi-center study. *Radiother Oncol* 2005;77:18–24.

32. Movsas B, Chapman JD, Hanlon AL, et al. A hypoxic ratio of prostate pO_2/muscle pO_2 predicts for biochemical failure in prostate cancer patients. *Urology* 2002;60:634–639.
33. Hall EJ. *Radiobiology for the radiologist*, 5th ed. Philadelphia, PA: Lippincott Williams & Wilkins, 2000:112–123.
34. Chapman JD, Gillespie CJ, Reuvers AP, et al. The inactivation of Chinese hamster cells by x-rays: the effects of chemical modifiers on single- and double-events. *Rad Res* 1975;64:365–375.
35. Palcic B, Skarsgard LD. Reduced oxygen enhancement ratio at low doses of radiation. *Rad Res* 1984;100:328–329.
36. Daşu A, Denekamp J. New insights into factors influencing the clinically relevant oxygen enhancement ratio. *Radiother Oncol* 1998;46:269–277.
37. Daşu A, Denekamp J. Superfractionation as a potential hypoxic cell radiosensitizer: prediction of an optimal dose per fraction. *Int J Radiat Oncol Biol Phys* 1999;43:1083–1094.
38. Withers HR, Taylor JMG, Maciejewski B. The hazard of accelerated tumor clonogen repopulation during radiation therapy. *Acta Oncol* 1988;27:131–146.
39. Bentzen S, Thames HD. Clinical evidence for tumor clonogen regeneration: interpretations of the data. *Radiother Oncol* 1991;22:161–166.
40. Hall EJ. *Radiobiology for the radiologist*, 5th ed. Philadelphia, PA: Lippincott Williams & Wilkins, 2000:51–66.
41. Bentzen SM, Saunders MI, Dische S, et al. Radiotherapy-related early morbidity in head and neck cancer: quantitative clinical radiobiology as deduced from the CHART trial. *Radiother Oncol* 2001;60:123–135.
42. Saunders MI, Rojas A, Lyn BE, et al. Experience with dose escalation using CHARTWEL (continuous hyperfractionated accelerated radiotherapy weekend less) in non-small cell lung cancer. *Br J Cancer* 1998;78:1323–1328.
43. Fowler JF, Ritter MA, Chappell RJ, et al. What hypofractionated protocols should be tested for prostate cancer? *Int J Radiat Oncol Biol Phys* 2003;56:1093–1104.
44. Barendsen GW. Dose fractionation, dose-rate and isoeffect relationships for normal tissue responses. *Int J Radiat Oncol Biol Phys* 1982;8:1981–1997.
45. Dale RG. The application of the linear-quadratic dose-effect equation to fractionated and protracted radiotherapy. *Br J Radiol* 1985;58:515–528.
46. Bentzen SM, Ruifrok ACC, Thames HD. Repair capacity and kinetics for human mucosa and epithelial tumors in the head and neck: clinical data on the effect of changing the time interval between multiple fractions per day in radiotherapy. *Radiother Oncol* 1996;38:89–101.
47. Murphy MJ, Peck-Sun L. Intra-fraction dose delivery timing during stereotactic radiotherapy can influence the radiobiological effect. *Med Phys* 2007;34:481–484.
48. Narayana V, Orton C. Pulsed brachytherapy: a formalism to account for the variation in dose rate of the stepping source. *Med Phys* 1999;26:161–165.
49. Manning MA, Zwicker RD, Arthur DW, et al. Biologic treatment planning for high-dose-rate brachytherapy. *Int J Radiat Oncol Biol Phys* 2001;49:839–845.
50. Fowler JF. Brief summary of radiobiological principles in fractionated radiotherapy. *Semin Radiat Oncol* 1992;2:16–21.
51. Orton CG. Recent developments in time–dose modeling. *Austral Phys Eng Sci Med* 1991;14:57–64.
52. Emami B, Lyman J, Brown A, et al. Tolerance of normal tissue to therapeutic irradiation. *Int J Radiat Oncol Biol Phys* 1991;21:109–122.
53. Marks LB, Yorke ED, Jackson A, et al. Use of normal tissue complication models in the clinic. *Int J Radiat Oncol Biol Phys* 2010;76:S10–S19.
54. Kirkpatrick JP, Van Der Kogel AJ, Schultheiss TE. Radiation dose–volume effects in the spinal cord. *Int J Radiat Oncol Biol Phys* 2010;76:S42–S49.
55. Joiner MC. A simple α/β-independent method to derive fully isoeffective schedules following changes in dose per fraction. *Int J Radiat Oncol Biol Phys* 2004;58:871–875.
56. Schultheiss TE, Orton CG. Models in radiotherapy: definition of decision criteria. *Med Phys* 1985;12:183–187.

CHAPTER 22

Tolerance of Normal Tissue to Therapeutic Radiation

Bahman Emami and Eric Kielhorn

INTRODUCTION

Radiation therapy is an integral part of the treatment of patients inflicted with cancer. It is estimated that over 60% of patients with cancer will have radiotherapy as part of their total course of treatment (1). Radiation therapy affects both tumor cells and uninvolved normal cells; the former to the benefit and the later to the detriment of patients. With the goal of achieving uncomplicated local regional control of cancer, balancing between the two is both an art and a science of radiation oncology. Unfortunately, after over 100 years of practicing radiation oncology and in spite of much recent progress, knowledge on either of the two is far from perfect.

From a historical point of view, the first formal attempt to address at least one of the goals, namely normal tissue tolerance to radiation, was carried out by Rubin and Cassarett (2). Even though this publication was a collection of anecdotal reports, it has served radiation oncologists as a raw reference to build on their own experience. The decade of the 1980s was a quantum leap of progress in the field of radiation oncology. With the monumental work of researchers on four National Cancer Institute multi-institutional contracts, the science and practice of radiation oncology changed from a two-dimensional (2D) to a three-dimensional (3D)/volumetric process (3). During the work on these contracts, it became apparent to the clinicians that information on the tumoricidal doses of radiation as well as normal tissue complication doses, especially on partial volumes, is mostly empirical and totally inadequate. A committee was formed to address a part of this dilemma by comprehensively reviewing the available published data. In the process of this review by the committee, it became clear that much of the data is nonexistent and they would have to rely on the collective experience of eight clinicians from major institutions in the United States. Moreover, in order to shed some light on the volumetric aspect of these issues, it was decided that organs be divided into one-third, two-thirds, and whole organ volumes. In spite of the clear indication in the manuscript on the paucity of solid experimental/prospectively driven data, this publication, so-called Emami's paper, has gained much popularity. The main goal of this publication was to address a clinical need based on available information up to that time and points to the fact that there is a need for extensive and comprehensive research in this area. Obvious limitations of the publication were as follows: (1) It was a literature review up to 1991. (2) It completely pre-dated the 3D-CRT-IMRT-IGRT era. Even at that time dose-volume histograms were not in routine clinical use. (3) It was a tabulation of the estimates for three of the aforementioned arbitrary volumes. (4) It was only for external beam radiation with conventional fractionation. (5) Only one severe complication was chosen as an endpoint.

Over the last two decades, since the publication of "Emami's paper" the practice of radiation oncology has been completely revolutionized:

1. Multidisciplinary management of cancer has become the standard of care.
2. Choice of an endpoint for complication analysis and modeling has significantly altered.
3. There has been a major revolutionary change in technology:
   a. CT simulation has become routine along with the fusion of other modalities such as MRI, PET, and 4DCT.
   b. 3D-CRT/IMRT/IGRT has become standard with the array of evaluation tools.

As a result, dose distributions have become very complex and as of recent, the fourth dimension, namely time, has also been added to this complexity. Multiplicity and complexities of factors affecting radiation including normal tissue complications have made it impossible to have actual data for every clinical situation facing practicing radiation oncologists. Therefore, there is a need to have reasonable predictive models for plan evaluation, to improve tumor control, and to predict and hopefully prevent normal tissue injury. Optimally, databases on biophysical models should be used in summarizing complicated dose-volume data to help describe clinical outcomes and ultimately aid in the prediction of clinical toxicity.

During the last two decades, a vast amount of published information has become available to address the relationship between dosimetric parameters and the clinical outcomes of normal tissues. Because of different analytic methodologies, calculation methods, endpoints, grading schemes, etc., the data is noisy and sifting through these data for practicing radiation oncologists is a nearly impossible task. Realizing this difficulty and the obvious need for a simplistic format, a group of physicians and researchers were formed with the name "The Quantitative Analysis of Normal Tissue Effects in the Clinic (QUANTEC)." The first goal was to review the available literature of the last 18 years on volumetric/dosimetric information of normal tissue complication and provide a simple set of data to be used by the busy community practitioners of radiation oncology, physicists, and dosimetrists. The second goal of the QUANTEC group was to provide reliable predictive models on relationships between dose-volume parameters and the normal tissue complications to be utilized during the planning of radiation oncology. The result of several years of work by this group has recently been

published (4–27). Although these publications contain a comprehensive review of published information and can be a guide for future research on this issue, they still have many shortcomings mainly due to the basic complexity of the subject. This shortcoming has been clearly indicated in the QUANTEC publication and the need for much more data in the future has been emphasized. However, the presented data in the publication is still cumbersome and lacks the "user-friendliness," which is required to be used in the day-to-day practice of a busy community clinician. As shown in Table 22.1 there are numerous factors that affect the radiation-induced complications of normal tissues on any given clinical situation. Thus, the experience

TABLE 22.1	**Variables That Can Impact Normal Tissue Tolerance**	
I.	Host	Age Comorbid conditions Host response to radiation Smoking KPS

II	Organ	Pre-radiation organ condition (Poor PFTs; LFTs; COPD)
		Regional variation of radiosensitivity with the organ
		Impact of other organs
		Hierarchal organization of the organ:
		    Serial: dose effect: spinal cord
		    Parallel: volume effect: lung, liver
		    Both: kidney

III	Natural history of tumor	
IV	Treatment	A—Radiation Dose (max, min, mean) Fractionation (fractional dose): BED Dose rate Overall treatment time Treatment energy Volume (V dose: absolute or relative)
IV	Treatment	B—Nonradiation Chemotherapy (drug type, dose, schedule) Radiation modifiers (type, dose, schedule) Surgery (interval)
V	End points ACUTE	Type: Clinical LATE Radiographical: anatomical, functional Biochemical (blood test, functional test) Degree of severity Degree of frequency Impact on quality of life (QOL)
VI	Issues on reporting of toxicity	
VII	Genotype vs. molecular vs. phenotype	
VIII	Statistical methodology	

and judgment of the clinician still plays the most important role in treating patients. As for predictive models, the problem lies in finding a reasonable model, acquiring sufficient data, and applying the statistical methods properly. So far, in spite of major efforts, there is no model that has been demonstrated to predict radiation responses with sufficient accuracy for widespread clinical use. Most of the modeling at this point is still phenomenological and "descriptive" rather than predictive. The development of reliable and user-friendly predictive models is quite unlikely in the near future.

After reviewing the publication by the QUANTEC group, we attempt to provide the clinicians and the practitioners of radiation oncology a comprehensive but simpler, user-friendly set of data (Tables 22.2 and 22.3). It should be noted that the data is not intended to be extrapolated to pediatric patients. The data should be used only as a guide and does not substitute for a physician's clinical judgment. We believe, as indicated in the original paper of "Emami et al." and in the QUANTEC publication, that there is an urgent need for systematic research on this issue, which we hope will be forthcoming.

Word of Caution About BED

Recently, it has become popular (as in many sections of QUANTEC publication) to convert the dose-fractionation to a biological equivalent dose (BED) in order to compare various dosimetric parameters. A practical version of isoeffect formula based on the linear quadratic (LQ) model is:

$$D/D_{ref} = (\alpha/\beta + d_{ref})/(\alpha/\beta + d)$$

The index of α/β is calculated based on information from cell survival curves that has been extrapolated and extended to human tumor and normal tissues by some computerized scientists. Unverified assignment of an α/β ratio and using it to calculate a normal tissue tolerance dose can be misleading or at least should be experimentally validated before being recommended for routine clinical use (7,9,10). The following are some basic facts based on current knowledge:

Fact 1	Dose/fractionation has significant impact on normal tissue complications, e.g., central nervous system (CNS)
Fact 2	1.8–2.0 Gy per fraction, five fractions per week, is considered standard in the United States
Fact 3	In a majority of publications during last two decades an α/β ratio of 2 is used for CNS tissues (28,29)

Fact 4	In the QUANTEC publication an α/β of 3 is used to calculate BED for CNS tissues (7,9)
Fact 5	Using the power of IMRT technology, one can have any dose/fraction as a constraint for tissues such as CNS

The following example depicts the basic fallacies of using BED, calculated from the above formula in clinics.
Example:

Gy dose/ fractions	Dose/ fraction (Gy)	α/β for brain tissue	BED
60 Gy/30 Fr[a]	2	1	180
60 Gy/30 Fr[a]	2	2	120
60 Gy/30 Fr[a]	2	3	100

If we arbitrarily choose 1 Gy/fraction/day of brain tissue, then the conversion of BED to dose/fractionation of 1 Gy/day:

BED	Dose/ fraction (Gy)	α/β	Calculated total dose from formula (Gy)
180	1	1	90
120	1	2	80
100	1	3	75
180	3	1	45
120	3	2	48
100	3	3	51

In the authors' limited informal survey, no radiation oncologists would use 90 Gy at 1 Gy/day or 51 Gy at 3 Gy/day (despite being the same BED as 60 Gy in 30 fractions using an α/β of 1), thus limiting the applicability of BED for routine clinical use.

The following descriptive paragraphs of Tables 22.2 and 22.3 are presented as general guidelines.

STANDARD FRACTIONATION

Central Nervous System

Brain

Radiation necrosis of the brain typically occurs 3 months to several years after radiotherapy (median 1–2 years) (3,7). The original Emami publication estimated a 5% risk of radionecrosis at 5 years with a dose of 60 Gy to one-third of the brain with standard fractionation (3). More recently,

| TABLE 22.2 | Normal Tissue Tolerance for Standard Fractionation | | | | |

Organ	Endpoint	Rate (%)	Dose-volume parameter	D_{max} (Gy)	D_{mean} (Gy)
Brain	Symptomatic necrosis	<3		<60	
		<5		<65	
Brainstem	Necrosis or cranial neuropathy	<5	D100 <54 Gy		
		<5	D1–10 cc ≤59 Gy	<64 Point	
Spinal cord	Grade ≥2 myelopathy	<1		50	
Optic nerve & chiasm	Optic neuropathy	<3		<55	<50
		3–7		55–60	
Retina	Blindness	<1		<50	
Cochlea	Hearing loss	<15			≤45
Parotid 1	Grade 4 xerostomia	<20			<20
Parotid 2		<20			<25
Mandible	ORN	<5		<70 Point	
Pharyngeal constrictors	PEG tube dependent	<5			<50
	Aspiration	<5			<60
Larynx	Grade ≥2 edema	<20	V50 <27%		<44
Brachial plexus	Clinically apparent nerve damage	<5		<60	
Lung	Symptomatic pneumonitis	5	V5 <42%, V20 <22%		7
		10	V20 <31%		13
		20	V20 <40%		20
		30			24
		40			27
Esophagus	Grade ≥2 esophagitis	<30	V35 <50% V50 <40% V70 <20%	<74 Point	
	Grade ≥3 esophagitis	≤10	V60 <30%		<34
Heart	Pericarditis	<15	V30 <46%		<26
	Long-term cardiac mortality	<1	V25 <10%		
Liver	RILD, normal liver	<5			≤30
	RILD, liver disease	<5			≤28
Kidney 1	Renal dysfunction	<5	Equivalent of 1 kidney <18 Gy		
Kidney 2	Renal dysfunction	<5			<18
Stomach	Ulceration		D100 <50 Gy		
Small Bowel	Acute grade ≥3 toxicity	<10	V15 <120 cc		
	Late obstruction/perforation	<5	V50 <5%		
Rectum	Grade ≥2/≥3 late toxicity	<10/<15	V50 <50%		
	Grade ≥2/≥3 late toxicity	<10/<15	V60 <35%		
	Grade ≥2/≥3 late toxicity	<10/<15	V65 <25%		
	Grade ≥2/≥3 late toxicity	<10/<15	V70 <20%		
	Grade ≥2/≥3 late toxicity	<10/<15	V75 <15%		

(continued)

TABLE 22.2 Normal Tissue Tolerance for Standard Fractionation (*Continued*)

Organ	Endpoint	Rate (%)	Dose-volume parameter	D_{max} (Gy)	D_{mean} (Gy)
Bladder	Grade ≥3 late toxicity	<6 ?	D100 <65 Gy V65 ≤50% V70 ≤35% V75 ≤25% V80 ≤15%		
Penile bulb	Severe erectile dysfunction	<35			<50
Femoral head	Necrosis	<5	D100 <52 Gy		

Parotid 1, sparing single parotid gland; Parotid 2, combined parotid glands; Kidney 1, bilateral partial kidney RT; Kidney 2, bilateral whole kidneys; Vx, volume of the organ receiving ≥x Gy; Dx, minimum dose received by x% of the organ; D_{max}, maximum radiation dose; D_{mean}, mean radiation dose.

TABLE 22.3 Mostly Unvalidated Normal Tissue Dose Constraints for SBRT

Serial tissue	Volume (mL)	Volume max (Gy)	Max point dose (Gy)	Endpoint (≥grade 3)
Single-fraction treatment				
Brain	5–10	12[a]		Necrosis {<20%}
Optic pathway	<0.2	8	10 12	Neuritis Neuritis {<10%}
Cochlea			12 ≤14[a]	Hearing loss Hearing loss {<25%}
Brainstem	<1	10	15 <12.5[a]	Cranial neuropathy Cranial neuropathy {<5%}
Spinal cord	<0.25 <1.2	10 7	14 13[a]	Myelitis Myelitis {<1%}
Cauda equina	<5	14	16	Neuritis
Sacral Plexus	<3	14.4	16	Neuropathy
Esophagus	<5	14.5	19	Stenosis/fistula
Ipsilateral brachial plexus	<3	14.4	16	Neuropathy
Heart/pericardium	<15	16	22	Pericarditis
Great vessels	<10	31	37	Aneurysm
Trachea and ipsilateral bronchus	<4	8.8	22	Stenosis/fistula
Skin	<10	14.4	16	Ulceration
Stomach	<10	13	16	Ulceration/fistula
Duodenum	<5	8.8	16	Ulceration
Jejunum/ileum	<5	9.8	19	Enteritis/obstruction
Colon	<20	11	22	Colitis/fistula
Rectum	<20	11	22	Proctitis/fistula
Bladder wall	<15	8.7	22	Cystitis/fistula

(*continued*)

| TABLE | 22.3 | **Mostly Unvalidated Normal Tissue Dose Constraints for SBRT (*Continued*)** |

Serial tissue	Volume (mL)	Volume max (Gy)	Max point dose (Gy)	Endpoint (≥grade 3)
Penile bulb	<3	14	34	Impotence
Femoral heads (right and left)	<10	14		Necrosis
Renal hilum/vascular trunk	<2/3 volume	10.6		Malignant hypertension

Parallel tissue	Critical volume (mL)	Critical volume dose max (Gy)		Endpoint (≥grade 3)
Lung (right and left)	1,500	7		Basic lung function
Lung (right and left)	1,000	7.4		Pneumonitis
Liver	700	9.1		Basic liver function
Renal cortex (right and left)	200	8.4		Basic renal function

Three-fraction treatment

	Critical volume (mL)	Volume max (Gy)	Max point dose (Gy)	Endpoint (≥grade 3)
Optic pathway	<0.2	15 (5 Gy/fx)	19.5 (6.5 Gy/fx)	Neuritis
Cochlea			20 (6.67 Gy/fx)	Hearing loss
Brainstem	<1	18 (6 Gy/fx)	23 (7.67 Gy/fx)	Cranial neuropathy
Spinal cord	<0.25 <1.2	18 (6 Gy/fx) 11.1 (3.7 Gy/fx)	23 (7.67 Gy/fx)	Myelitis
Cauda equine	<5	21.9 (7.3 Gy/fx)	24 (8 Gy/fx)	Neuritis
Sacral Plexus	<3	22.5 (7.5 Gy/fx)	24 (8 Gy/fx)	Neuropathy
Esophagus	<5	21 (7 Gy/fx)	27 (9 Gy/fx)	Stenosis/fistula
Ipsilateral brachial plexus	<3	22.5 (7.5 Gy/fx)	24 (8 Gy/fx)	Neuropathy
Heart/pericardium	<15	24 (8 Gy/fx)	30 (10 Gy/fx)	Pericarditis
Great vessels	<10	39 (13 Gy/fx)	45 (15 Gy/fx)	Aneurysm
Trachea and ipsilateral bronchus	<4	15 (5 Gy/fx)	30 (10 Gy/fx)	Stenosis/fistula
Skin	<10	22.5 (7.5 Gy/fx)	24 (8 Gy/fx)	Ulceration
Stomach	<10	21 (7 Gy/fx)	24 (8 Gy/fx)	Ulceration/fistula
Duodenum	<5	15 (5 Gy/fx)	24 (8 Gy/fx)	Ulceration
Jejunum/ileum	<5	16.2 (5.4 Gy/fx)	27 (9 Gy/fx)	Enteritis/obstruction
Colon	<20	20.4 (6.8 Gy/fx)	30 (10 Gy/fx)	Colitis/fistula
Rectum	<20	20.4 (6.8 Gy/fx)	30 (10 Gy/fx)	Proctitis/fistula
Bladder wall	<15	15 (5 Gy/fx)	30 (10 Gy/fx)	Cystitis/fistula
Penile bulb	<3	21.9 (7.3 Gy/fx)	42 (14 Gy/fx)	Impotence
Femoral heads (right and left)	<10	21.9 (7.3 Gy/fx)		Necrosis
Renal hilum/vascular trunk	<2/3 volume	18.6 (6.2 Gy/fx)		Malignant hypertension

Parallel tissue	Critical volume (mL)	Critical volume dose max (Gy)		Endpoint (≥grade 3)
Lung (right and left)	1,500	10.5 (3.5 Gy/fx)		Basic lung function
Lung (right and left)	1,000	11.4 (3.8 Gy/fx)		Pneumonitis
Liver	700	17.1 (5.7 Gy/fx)		Basic liver function
Renal cortex (right and left)	200	14.4 (4.8 Gy/fx)		Basic renal function

(*continued*)

| TABLE 22.3 | **Mostly Unvalidated Normal Tissue Dose Constraints for SBRT (*Continued*)** |

Serial tissue	Volume (mL)	Volume max (Gy)	Max point dose (Gy)	Endpoint (≥grade 3)
Five-fraction treatment				
Optic pathway	<0.2	20 (4 Gy/fx)	25 (5 Gy/fx)	Neuritis
Cochlea			27.5 (5.5 Gy/fx)	Hearing loss
Brainstem	<1	26 (5.2 Gy/fx)	31 (6.2 Gy/fx)	Cranial neuropathy
Spinal cord	<0.25 <1.2	22.5 (4.5 Gy/fx) 13.5 (2.7 Gy/fx)	30 (6 Gy/fx)	Myelitis
Cauda equine	<5	30 (6 Gy/fx)	32 (6.4 Gy/fx)	Neuritis
Sacral Plexus	<3	30 (6 Gy/fx)	32 (6.4 Gy/fx)	Neuropathy
Esophagus	<5	27.5 (5.5 Gy/fx)	35 (7 Gy/fx)	Stenosis/fistula
Ipsilateral brachial plexus	<3	30 (6 Gy/fx)	32 (6.4 Gy/fx)	Neuropathy
Heart/pericardium	<15	32 (6.4 Gy/fx)	38 (7.6 Gy/fx)	Pericarditis
Great vessels	<10	47 (9.4 Gy/fx)		Aneurysm
Trachea and ipsilateral bronchus	<4	18 (3.6 Gy/fx)	38 (7.6 Gy/fx)	Stenosis/fistula
Skin	<10	30 (6 Gy/fx)	32 (6.4 Gy/fx)	Ulceration
Stomach	<10	28 (5.6 Gy/fx)	32 (6.4 Gy/fx)	Ulceration/fistula
Duodenum	<5	18 (3.6 Gy/fx)	32 (6.4 Gy/fx)	Ulceration
Jejunum/ileum	<5	19.5 (3.9 Gy/fx)	35 (7 Gy/fx)	Enteritis/obstruction
Colon	<20	25 (5 Gy/fx)	38 (7.6 Gy/fx)	Colitis/fistula
Rectum	<20	25 (5 Gy/fx)	38 (7.6 Gy/fx)	Proctitis/fistula
Bladder wall	<15	18.3 (3.65 Gy/fx)	38 (7.6 Gy/fx)	Cystitis/fistula
Penile bulb	<3	30 (6 Gy/fx)	50 (10 Gy/fx)	Impotence
Femoral heads (right and left)	<10	30 (6 Gy/fx)		Necrosis
Renal hilum/vascular trunk	<2/3 volume	23 (4.6 Gy/fx)		Malignant hypertension

Parallel tissue	Critical volume (mL)	Critical volume dose max (Gy)		Endpoint (≥grade 3)
Lung (right and left)	1,500	12.5 (2.5 Gy/fx)		Basic lung function
Lung (right and left)	1,000	13.5 (2.7 Gy/fx)		Pneumonitis
Liver	700	21 (4.2 Gy/fx)		Basic liver function
Renal cortex (right and left)	200	17.5 (3.5 Gy/fx)		Basic renal function

Reproduced from Timmerman (61) with permission.
[a]Data from QUANTEC (4)
{} rate of endpoint.

QUANTEC conducted an extensive review of the modern literature and published new dose constraints for the brain (6,7). The review was based on a heterogeneous group of studies with varied dose and fractionation schemes. Studies were compared using the BED with an α/β ratio of 3. A dose–response relationship was found to exist. For standard fractionation, the incidence of radionecrosis appears to be <3% for a dose of <60 Gy. The incidence increases to 5% with a dose of 72 Gy and 10% with a dose of 90 Gy. However, these doses were based on studies with widely varying parameters (target volumes, sample size, brain region, etc.). It should be noted that an α/β ratio of 3 is greater than the values frequently used in the literature and caution should be used when converting to BED (see above discussion). In our practice, we strive to achieve very homogeneous dose distributions with a Dmax (point dose) ≤ 65 Gy with only rare occurrences of symptomatic radiation necrosis.

Brainstem

RT-induced brainstem toxicity can be incapacitating and potentially lethal. The initial estimates by Emami et al. (3) were of a TD 5/5 of 50 Gy to the entire brainstem and 60 Gy to one-third of the brainstem. These estimates were based on the scant amount of data in the literature at that time and on clinical experience. The QUANTEC review identified additional modern series focusing on brainstem dose and dose-volume measures (6,9). The review included series that treated patients with photons, protons, or both. The QUANTEC review concluded that the original Emami constraint of 50 Gy was overly conservative. The entire brainstem can tolerate up to 54 Gy with a <5% risk of brainstem necrosis or neurologic toxicity. Small volumes (1–10 cc) can tolerate up to 59 Gy while a point (<<1 cc) may receive up to 64 Gy.

Spinal Cord

Spinal cord injury due to irradiation, though rare, can be extremely debilitating resulting is paralysis, sensory, deficits, pain, and bowel/bladder incontinence (10,30). Schultheiss (30) published an extensive review of the literature regarding de novo irradiation of the spinal cord. Among the reviewed studies, a wide range of fractionation regimens were used (2–9 Gy/fraction). An α/β ratio of 0.87 was estimated for the spinal cord and corresponding 2-Gy equivalent doses were calculated. The review estimated the risk of myelopathy to be 0.2% at 50 Gy and 5% at 59.3 Gy. Similar conclusions regarding α/β ratio and dose-volume limits were published by QUANTEC (6,10). It should be noted that an α/β ratio of 0.87 is less than the values frequently used in the literature and caution should be used when converting to BED (see above discussion).

Chiasm and Optic Nerves

Radiation-induced optic neuropathy (RION) is infrequent but usually results in rapid painless visual loss (8). The initial Emami review listed a TD 5/5 of 50 Gy to the whole organ without partial volume tolerance data (3).

Again, this was based primarily on clinical experience and sparse published data. Many more studies are now published and were reviewed by QUANTEC (6,8). Based on the QUANTEC review, a whole organ dose of 50 Gy is associated with <1% risk of blindness. In fact, blindness was quite rare until a dose of ≥55 Gy. Between 55 and 60 Gy, the risk of blindness is approximately 3% to 7%. At doses >60 Gy, the risk of RION greatly increases.

Head and Neck

Retina

Radiation retinopathy, resulting in loss of vision or visual acuity, presents similarly to diabetic retinopathy often within 5 years of radiotherapy. Parsons (31,32) reported only one instance of retinopathy with a dose <50 Gy to at least half the posterior pole of the eye with a steep dose–response curve at doses >50 Gy. Subsequently, Parsons (33) demonstrated no cases of retinopathy at doses below 45 Gy but a steep dose curve at doses >45 Gy. More recently, Monroe et al. reported a 4% rate of retinopathy after <50 Gy was received by at least 25% of the globe with conventional fractionation and modern conformal techniques (34). Using hyperfractionation, the rate of retinopathy decreased from 37% to 13% with doses ≥50 Gy. Takeda et al. reported no cases of retinal complications when the D_{max} was <50 Gy (35). Clearly, the dose tolerance of the retina is dependent upon multiple factors including predisposing comorbidities, the fractionation schema employed, and the volume that is irradiated. Multiple publications have demonstrated a steep dose–response curve for doses >50 Gy (33–35). Using modern treatment planning techniques and standard fractionation, we recommend limiting the retina to a D_{max} <50 Gy.

Cochlea

Damage to the cochlea may result in sensorineural hearing loss (SNHL). As summarized by QUANTEC, high frequency hearing loss is much more common than low-frequency hearing loss (11). Cisplatin-based chemotherapy can have an additional adverse effect on SNHL. The definition of clinically significant SNHL varies throughout the literature but is generally considered to be an increase in bone conduction threshold of 10 to 30 dB. The QUANTEC review examined several series and suggested a mean dose constraint of ≤45 Gy (6,11). Chan et al. conducted a longitudinal study of 87 consecutive patients treated for nasopharyngeal carcinoma, mostly treated with cisplatin-based chemoradiotherapy (36). A mean dose of ≤47 Gy to the cochlea resulted in <15% rate of SNHL. Therefore, based on a review of the literature with modern treatment planning techniques and concurrent cisplatin chemoradiotherapy we believe that a cochlear mean dose constraint of ≤45 Gy will result in a <15% rate of SNHL.

Parotid

Late salivary dysfunction is a common toxicity from radiotherapy for head and neck cancer that can take up to

2 years to recover (37,38). Xerostomia has been widely defined in the literature from patient-reported outcomes to objective salivary flow. Quantifiably, xerostomia is defined by the LENT-SOMA scale. Grade 4 xerostomia consists of an objective reduction of ≥75% of baseline salivary function. The QUANTEC review (6,12) summarized the literature including the Washington University experience (37). Blanco demonstrated that sparing (mean dose <20 Gy) of at least one parotid gland minimized the incidence grade 4 xerostomia. Likewise, limiting both parotids to a mean dose of <25 Gy resulted in minimal grade 4 xerostomia. Dose to the parotids should be reduced as much as clinically allowable as lower mean doses generally result in better salivary function (12).

Mandible

The rates of osteoradionecrosis (ORN) of the mandible have decreased over the past few decades (39). The risk of ORN is dependent on several factors including radiation dose, use of chemotherapy, dental hygiene, tumor location, mandibular surgery, and radiation technique (39–44). Ben-David et al. (40) demonstrated a steep dose falloff across the mandible when IMRT is employed. In their study, ≥50% of the patients in their study received ≥70 Gy to ≥1% of the mandibular volume with no cases of grade ≥2 ORN. Additional studies, including IMRT for oral cavity cancers, demonstrate a rate of ORN near 5% (41–43). Therefore, we recommend limiting the mandible to a D_{max} (point dose) ≤70 Gy when using IMRT.

Pharyngeal Constrictors

Treatment intensification for head and neck cancer has resulted in an increased rate of late sequela including dysphagia and aspiration. Modern treatment planning has allowed the study of various components of the swallowing apparatus. The results in the literature in this burgeoning area of research are variable as summarized in the QUANTEC review (6,13). Several groups have found the dose to the superior and/or middle pharyngeal constrictor muscles to be of paramount importance. Others have demonstrated the dose to the inferior pharyngeal constrictors or larynx to be of importance. Feng et al. (45) found no patients to have aspiration when the pharyngeal constrictors were limited to a mean dose of <60 Gy. We base our practice primarily on the findings from the University of Michigan and limit the superior pharyngeal constrictors to a mean dose of <60 Gy whenever clinically possible.

Larynx

Toxicity from radiotherapy to the larynx can include vocal dysfunction and laryngeal edema. The original Emami publication (3) addressed the risk of cartilage necrosis; however, this is rarely seen in modern radiotherapy and is not as relevant of an endpoint as vocal function and laryngeal edema. The QUANTEC publication reviewed several studies involving vocal dysfunction, concluding doses to multiple structures

(e.g., larynx, pharynx, and oral cavity) play an important role in voice function (6,13). Radiotherapy is commonly used for treatment of early-stage glottic cancer, employing doses >60 Gy, with a good voice outcome. A single publication (46) on laryngeal edema was reviewed, which found <20% incidence of ≥grade 2 edema when the mean laryngeal dose was <43.5 Gy and the V50 <27%.

Thorax

Brachial Plexus

Brachial plexopathy can manifest as pain, paresthesias, or motor deficits of the upper extremity (47). Muscular atrophy and edema may develop. Emami et al. (3) suggested that the TD 5/5 to the entire brachial plexus was 60 Gy. More recently, several studies with over 20 years of follow-up have suggested that the incidence of brachial plexopathy continues to rise after 5 years and may not be apparent for up to 20 years after radiotherapy (47,48). The brachial plexus appears to be especially sensitive to fractionation schedules, with the risk of injury much higher for larger fractions despite equivalent BED (49). With standard fractionation the risk of clinically apparent nerve damage seems to be <5%, after 5 years of completing radiotherapy, when the brachial plexus is limited to 60 Gy.

Lung

Symptomatic radiation pneumonitis (RP) is one of the most common toxicities in patients treated with radiation for cancers of the lung, breast, and mediastinal lymphatics. The risk of RP often limits the dose delivered for treatment of these malignancies. Since the initial Emami publication (3) there has been an extensive amount of research attempting to relate many different dose-volume parameters to RP. The QUANTEC publication reviewed >70 published articles looking at both mean lung doses and Vx parameters (6,14). This comprehensive review demonstrated no clear threshold dose for symptomatic RP. The compiled data showed a mean dose–response curve with a 20% risk of RP for a mean lung dose of 20 Gy. In addition, multiple Vx values have been investigated for predicting RP but the data are not as consistent as the data for mean lung doses. Using 3D techniques, Graham found the V20 to be the most useful parameter for predicting the risk of RP (50). When Vx values are used, the V20 is the most commonly incorporated parameter.

Esophagus

Acute esophagitis commonly occurs during radiotherapy for thoracic malignancies and can lead to hospitalizations, procedures, and treatment breaks (16). Most series in the literature report rates of RTOG grade ≥2 esophagitis. The QUANTEC review summarized 11 studies that used 3D treatment planning (6,16). A single best parameter was not identified due to the diverse range of dose-volume metrics that correlated with acute esophagitis (51–53). As demonstrated in the QUANTEC publication, there appears to be a trend demonstrating increased rates of acute esophagitis for volumes receiving >40 to 50 Gy. Currently, the ongoing RTOG 0617 is collecting V60 data on all patients and recommends keeping the mean dose <34 Gy (54).

Heart

Clinical pericarditis and long-term cardiac mortality are the two most relevant cardiac toxicities. Since the original Emami publication (3), there remains a paucity of data reporting rates of pericarditis with dose-volume parameters. Indeed, several current RTOG protocols continue to use constraints similar to the original Emami TD 5/5 dose-volume estimates for the heart (54–56). As reviewed by QUANTEC (6,15), two esophageal cancer studies (57,58) assessed 3D-derived data with both studies demonstrating a rate of pericarditis <15% when the mean pericardial dose was <26 Gy. In addition, Wei found the pericardial V30 <46% to be significant on multivariate analysis. Long-term cardiac mortality has been demonstrated in multiple studies, most commonly in the treatment of breast cancer and Hodgkin's lymphoma (15). A joint analysis of the Hodgkin's and breast cancer data (59,60), summarized by QUANTEC, produced a dose–response curve for cardiac mortality. QUANTEC proposed a conservative approach, predicting that a V25 <10% of the heart will be associated with a <1% probability of cardiac mortality at 15 years after radiotherapy.

Abdomen

Liver

Radiation-induced liver disease (RILD) typically occurs between 2 weeks and 3 months after radiotherapy. Preexisting liver disease may render patients more susceptible to RILD (17). The findings by QUANTEC (6,17) are very similar to the original estimates by Emami et al. (3), suggesting a <5% rate of RILD when the mean liver dose is ≤30 Gy in patients without preexisting liver disease or primary liver cancer. The mean liver dose should be ≤28 Gy in those patients with preexisting liver disease.

Kidney

Radiation-induced renal dysfunction can be expressed in various ways including symptomatic expression, biochemical changes, or radiologic findings. As summarized by QUANTEC, a wide array of endpoints has been used in the literature from a decrease in creatinine clearance to renal failure (6,19). For bilateral whole kidney irradiation, a pooled analysis by Cassady (61) concluded a mean dose of 18 Gy corresponded to a 5% risk of injury at 5 years. For bilateral partial kidney irradiation, the data is less clear with a multitude of dose-volume metrics studied by several investigators (19). Small volumes of the kidney can tolerate relatively high doses of radiation. QUANTEC estimated a <5% risk of injury when the mean kidney dose is limited to <18 Gy. In addition, the current common practice of limiting the equivalent of one kidney to

<20 Gy seems to be reasonable and is frequently used in our practice.

Stomach

Late radiation-induced toxicity to the stomach can include dyspepsia and ulceration. Since the original Emami publication (3), few studies have reported severe RT-related gastric toxicity. The QUANTEC publication reviewed these studies, primarily pancreatic cancer trials, and concluded that a whole organ dose of 50 Gy has been associated with a 2% to 6% risk of severe late toxicity (6,18) (similar to Emami et al.).

Small Bowel

Small-bowel toxicity can be greatly affected by the use of concurrent chemotherapy and prior abdominal surgery. In particular, concurrent chemotherapy can impact the rates of acute small-bowel toxicity. Modern series employing 3D-conformal RT or IMRT have demonstrated that the volume of small bowel receiving relatively low doses of radiation plays a significant role in the rate of acute toxicity (18). When contouring individual bowel loops, the most robust dose-volume metric is the V15. The rate of grade ≥3 acute toxicity is <10% when the V15 <120 cc (62,63). When the entire potential space within the peritoneal cavity is contoured, a V45 <195 cc results in <10% acute toxicity (64). Late small-bowel toxicity, consisting of obstruction or perforation, can be influenced by prior abdominal surgery. Modern series reviewed by QUANTEC generally confirm the Emami et al. (3) TD5/5 estimate for partial organ irradiation (6,18). In practice, we limit the volume of the small bowel receiving 50 Gy to much less than one-third. We generally limit the V50 <5% based on the clinical scenario.

Pelvis

Rectum

The treatment of prostate cancer has evolved such that the great majority of patients will be alive for many years after radiotherapy. Late rectal toxicities from radiotherapy can significantly impact quality of life (QOL). Since Emami et al. (3), numerous studies have employed dose escalation using 3D-CRT or IMRT for the treatment of prostate cancer. These trials have resulted in the publication of many dose-volume analyses as summarized by the QUANTEC review (6,21). The dose-volume results are surprisingly consistent suggesting that high doses are most important in determining risk of toxicity.

Bladder

The bladder frequently receives radiation during the treatment of commonly encountered pelvic malignancies such as prostate, cervical, and bladder cancer. Due to the distensibility of the bladder it is difficult to conduct robust dose-volume analyses. The QUANTEC publication was unable to find any reliable data for partial bladder volume constraints in the treatment of prostate cancer and recommended using RTOG 0415 dose limits (6,20,65). In the treatment of bladder cancer, where the entire organ is targeted, rates of severe late bladder toxicity are varied (20). Shipley et al. (66) reported the pooled results of multiple RTOG trials demonstrating a grade ≥3 toxicity rate of ≤6% when treating the bladder to a dose of 64 to 65 Gy.

Penile Bulb

Erectile dysfunction can have a significant detrimental effect on QOL after treatment for prostate cancer. QUANTEC summarized the published studies correlating the dose and volume of the penile bulb that is irradiated with rates of erectile dysfunction (22). The results for various dose-volume parameters are conflicting. There is some data to support limiting the D70 <70 Gy and D90 <50 Gy. However, the strongest data supports the recommendation of limiting the penile bulb to a mean dose of <52 Gy without compromising target coverage (67).

Femoral Head

Toxicity of radiation treatment to the pelvis includes femoral head necrosis, femoral neck fracture, or long-term sequela resulting in hip replacement surgery. Besides radiation dose and volume, additional risk factors may include preexisting osteoporosis/osteopenia and androgen deprivation therapy (68–70). Emami et al. (3) suggested a TD 5/5 of 52 Gy to the whole femoral head. Grigsby et al. published the Washington University experience and documented a 4.8% incidence of femoral neck fracture following groin irradiation (68). Of note, there was only one case of femoral neck fracture when the whole femoral neck received ≤50 Gy. There is0 little data describing femoral toxicity when higher doses are delivered to small volumes of the femoral head or neck (71–74). We generally limit the entire femoral head to <50 Gy in an attempt to limit femoral head/neck toxicity to <<5%.

Hypofractionation

Some of the earliest radiotherapy treatments were delivered in a hypofractionated fashion. As technology and radiobiology advanced, protracted fractionation schemes became the norm. Eventually, hypofractionation was again pursued and used to treat intracranial lesions. Stereotactic radiosurgery (SRS) has been used for decades and its success led to the use of hypofractionated treatment outside the brain. Over the past 15 years, the use of stereotactic body radiotherapy (SBRT) has become widespread and utilized to treat a number of cancers. The QUANTEC group reviewed the literature pertaining to SRS and published tolerance doses for some CNS organs at risk (6–11). The most comprehensive review to date was published by Timmerman (75). Both intracranial and extracranial organ tolerances were reviewed and adjusted for either single-fraction, three-fraction, or five-fraction treatments. Because the data in this burgeoning modality is relatively

limited, the dose constraints are not validated. Rather, they are based on a combination of published data, clinical observations, modeling, and educated guessing. Despite these caveats, the dose constraints published by Timmerman provide an excellent starting point for clinical use.

CONCLUSION

From the pioneering work of Rubin and Cassarett, to the monumental work by Emami et al. and now the exhaustive review by QUANTEC, great progress has been made in the field of normal tissue tolerance to therapeutic radiation. Despite these efforts, many questions still remain. Normal tissue tolerance is an extremely complex issue and multifactorial in nature. There continues to be an urgent need for comprehensive and collaborative research. The dose-volume parameters within this chapter should be used only as a guide. For instance, there are clinical scenarios where a 5% rate of a particular toxicity is unacceptable. In contrast, there may be cases where one is willing to accept the risk a 20% rate of a particular side effect in order to obtain a desired clinical outcome. Therefore, it is imperative that the clinical judgment of the treating physician prevails in the treatment decision-making process.

REFERENCES

1. Halperin EC, Perez CA, Brady, LW. Preface to the first edition. In: Halperin EC, Perez CA, Brady LW, eds. *Perez and Brady's principles and practice of radiation oncology*, 5th ed. Philadelphia, PA: Lippincott Williams & Wilkins, 2008:xxi.
2. Rubin P, Cassarett G. A direction for clinical radiation pathology. In: Vaeth JM, et al., eds. *Frontiers of radiation therapy and oncology VI*. Baltimore, MD: University Park Press, 1972:1–16.
3. Emami B, Lyman J, Brown A, et al. Tolerance of normal tissue to therapeutic irradiation. *Int J Radiat Oncol Biol Phys* 1991;21(1):109–122.
4. Marks LB, Ten Haken RK, Martel MK. Guest editor's introduction to QUANTEC: a users guide. *Int J Radiat Oncol Biol Phys* 2010;76(3 Suppl):S1–S2.
5. Bentzen SM, Constine LS, Deasy JO, et al. Quantitative Analyses of Normal Tissue Effects in the Clinic (QUANTEC): an introduction to the scientific issues. *Int J Radiat Oncol Biol Phys* 2010;76(3 Suppl):S3–S9.
6. Marks LB, Yorke ED, Jackson A, et al. Use of normal tissue complication probability models in the clinic. *Int J Radiat Oncol Biol Phys* 2010;76(3 Suppl):S10–S19.
7. Lawrence YR, Li XA, el Naqa I, et al. Radiation dose-volume effects in the brain. *Int J Radiat Oncol Biol Phys* 2010;76(3 Suppl):S20–S27.
8. Mayo C, Martel MK, Marks LB, et al. Radiation dose-volume effects of optic nerves and chiasm. *Int J Radiat Oncol Biol Phys* 2010;76(3 Suppl):S28–S35.
9. Mayo C, Yorke E, Merchant TE. Radiation associated brainstem injury. *Int J Radiat Oncol Biol Phys* 2010;76 (3 Suppl):S36–S41.

10. Kirkpatrick JP, Van Der Kogel AJ, Schultheiss TE. Radiation dose-volume effects in the spinal cord. *Int J Radiat Oncol Biol Phys* 2010;76(3 Suppl):S42–S49.

11. Bhandare N, Jackson A, Eisbruch A, et al. Radiation therapy and hearing loss. *Int J Radiat Oncol Biol Phys* 2010; 76(3 Suppl):S50–S57.

12. Deasy JO, Moiseenko V, Marks L, et al. Radiotherapy dose-volume effects on salivary gland function. *Int J Radiat Oncol Biol Phys* 2010;76(3 Suppl):S58–S63.

13. Rancati T, Schwarz M, Allen AM, et al. Radiation dose-volume effects in the larynx and pharynx. *Int J Radiat Oncol Biol Phys* 2010;76(3 Suppl):S64–S69.

14. Marks LB, Bentzen SM, Deasy JO, et al. Radiation dose-volume effects in the lung. *Int J Radiat Oncol Biol Phys* 2010;76(3 Suppl):S70–S76.

15. Gagliardi G, Constine LS, Moiseenko V, et al. Radiation dose-volume effects in the heart. *Int J Radiat Oncol Biol Phys* 2010;76(3 Suppl):S77–S85.

16. Werner-Wasik M, Yorke E, Deasy J, et al. Radiation dose-volume effects in the esophagus. *Int J Radiat Oncol Biol Phys* 2010;76(3 Suppl):S86–S93.

17. Pan CC, Kavanagh BD, Dawson LA, et al. Radiation-associated liver injury. *Int J Radiat Oncol Biol Phys* 2010;76(3 Suppl):S94–S100.

18. Kavanagh BD, Pan CC, Dawson LA, et al. Radiation dose-volume effects in the stomach and small bowel. *Int J Radiat Oncol Biol Phys* 2010;76(3 Suppl):S101–S107.

19. Dawson LA, Kavanagh BD, Paulino AC, et al. Radiation-associated kidney injury. *Int J Radiat Oncol Biol Phys* 2010;76(3 Suppl):S108–S115.

20. Viswanathan AN, Yorke ED, Marks LB, et al. Radiation dose-volume effects of the urinary bladder. *Int J Radiat Oncol Biol Phys* 2010;76(3 Suppl):S116–S122.

21. Michalski JM, Gay H, Jackson A, et al. Radiation dose-volume effects in radiation-induced rectal injury. *Int J Radiat Oncol Biol Phys* 2010;76(3 Suppl):S123–S129.

22. Roach M 3rd, Nam J, Gagliardi G, et al. Radiation dose-volume effects and the penile bulb. *Int J Radiat Oncol Biol Phys* 2010;76(3 Suppl):S130–S134.

23. Jaffray DA, Lindsay PE, Brock KK, et al. Accurate accumulation of dose for improved understanding of radiation effects in normal tissue. *Int J Radiat Oncol Biol Phys* 2010;76(3 Suppl):S135–S139.

24. Jeraj R, Cao Y, Ten Haken RK, et al. Imaging for assessment of radiation-induced normal tissue effects. *Int J Radiat Oncol Biol Phys* 2010;76(3 Suppl):S140–S144.

25. Bentzen SM, Parliament M, Deasy JO, et al. Biomarkers and surrogate endpoints for normal-tissue effects of radiation therapy: the importance of dose-volume effects. *Int J Radiat Oncol Biol Phys* 2010;76(3 Suppl):S145–S150.

26. Deasy JO, Bentzen SM, Jackson A, et al. Improving normal tissue complication probability models: the need to adopt a "data-pooling" culture. *Int J Radiat Oncol Biol Phys* 2010;76(3 Suppl):S151–S154.

27. Jackson A, Marks LB, Bentzen SM, et al. The lessons of QUANTEC: recommendations for reporting and gathering data on dose-volume dependencies of treatment outcome. *Int J Radiat Oncol Biol Phys* 2010;76(3 Suppl): S155–S160.

28. Veninga T, Langendijk HA, Slotman BJ, et al. Reirradiation of primary brain tumours: survival, clinical response and prognostic factors. *Radiother Oncol* 2001;59:127–137.

29. Mayer R, Sminia P. Reirradiation tolerance of the human brain. *Int J Radiat Oncol Biol Phys* 2008;70(5): 1350–1360.

30. Schultheiss TE, Kun LE, Ang KK, et al. Radiation response of the central nervous system. *Int J Radiat Oncol Biol Phys* 1995;31:1093–1112.

31. Parsons F. The effect of radiation on normal tissues in management of head and neck cancer. In: Million R, Cassisi N, eds. *Management of head and neck cancer: a multidisciplinary approach, chapter 14.* Philadelphia, PA: Lippincott Williams & Wilkins, 1984:183–184.

32. Parsons JT, Fitzgerald CR, Hood CI, et al. The effects of irradiation on the eye and optic nerve. *Int J Radiat Oncol Biol Phys* 1983;9609–9622.

33. Parsons JT, Bova FJ, Fitzgerald CR, et al. Radiation retinopathy after external-beam irradiation: analysis of time-dose factors. *Int J Radiat Oncol Biol Phys* 1994;30(4):765–773.

34. Monroe AT, Bhandare N, Morris CG, et al. Preventing radiation retinopathy with hyperfractionation. *Int J Radiat Oncol Biol Phys* 2005;61(3):856–864.

35. Takeda A, Shigematsu N, Suzuki S, et al. Late retinal complications of radiation therapy for nasal and paranasal malignancies: relationship between irradiated-dose area and severity. *Int J Radiat Oncol Biol Phys* 1999;44(3): 599–605.

36. Chan SH, Ng WT, Kam KL, et al. Sensorineural hearing loss after treatment of nasopharyngeal carcinoma: a longitudinal analysis. *Int J Radiat Oncol Biol Phys* 2009;73(5): 1335–1342.

37. Blanco AI, Chao KSC, El Naqa I, et al. Dose-volume modeling of salivary function in patients with head-and-neck cancer receiving radiotherapy. *Int J Radiat Oncol Biol Phys* 2005;62:1055–1069.

38. Eisbruch A, Kim KM, Terrell JE, et al. Xerostomia and its predictors following parotid-sparing irradiation of head-and-neck cancer. *Int J Radiat Oncol Biol Phys* 2001; 50:695–704.

39. Jereczek-Fossa BA, Orecchia R. Radiotherapy-induced mandibular bone complications. *Cancer Treat Rev* 2002; 28(1):65–74.

40. Ben-David MA, Diamante M, Radawski JD, et al. Lack of osteoradionecrosis of the mandible after intensity-modulated radiotherapy for head and neck cancer: likely contributions of both dental care and improved dose distributions. *Int J Radiat Oncol Biol Phys* 2007;68(2):396–402.

41. Gomez DR, Zelefsky MJ, Wolden SL, et al. Osteoradionecrosis (ORN) of the mandible in head/neck cancer treated with intensity modulated radiation therapy (IMRT). *Int J Radiat Oncol Biol Phys* 2008;72(1 Suppl):S410.

42. Gomez DR, Zhung JE, Gomez J, et al. Intensity-modulated radiotherapy in postoperative treatment of oral cavity cancers. *Int J Radiat Oncol Biol Phys* 2009;73(4): 1096–1103.

43. Eisbruch A, Harris J, Garden AS, et al. Multi-institutional trial of accelerated hypofractionated intensity-modulated radiation therapy for early-stage oropharyngeal cancer (RTOG 00–22). *Int J Radiat Oncol Biol Phys* 2010;76(5):1333–1338.

44. Lee IJ, Koom WS, Lee CG, et al. Risk factors and dose-effect relationship for mandibular osteoradionecrosis in oral and oropharyngeal cancer patients. *Int J Radiat Oncol Biol Phys* 2009;75(4):1084–1091.

45. Feng FY, Kim HM, Lyden TH, et al. Intensity-modulated radiotherapy of head and neck cancer aiming to reduce dysphagia: Early dose–effect relationships for the swallowing structures. *Int J Radiat Oncol Biol Phys* 2007;68:1289–1298.

46. Sanguineti G, Adapala P, Endres EJ, et al. Dosimetric predictors of laryngeal edema. *Int J Radiat Oncol Biol Phys* 2007;68:741–749.

47. Bajrovic A, Rades D, Fehlauer F, et al. Is there a life-long risk of brachial plexopathy after radiotherapy of supraclavicular lymph nodes in breast cancer patients? *Radiother Oncol* 2004;71(3):297–301.

48. Johansson S, Svensson H, Denekamp J. Dose response and latency for radiation-induced fibrosis, edema, and neuropathy in breast cancer patients. *Int J Radiat Oncol Biol Phys* 2002;52(5):1207–1219.

49. Powell S, Cooke J, Parsons C. Radiation-induced brachial plexus injury: follow-up of two different fractionation schedules. *Radiother Oncol* 1990;18(3):213–220.

50. Graham MV, Purdy JA, Emami B, et al. Clinical dose-volume histogram analysis for pneumonitis after 3D treatment for non-small cell lung cancer (NSCLC). *Int J Radiat Oncol Biol Phys* 1999;45:323–329.

51. Bradley J, Deasy JO, Bentzen S, et al. Dosimetric correlates for acute esophagitis in patients treated with radiotherapy for lung carcinoma. *Int J Radiat Oncol Biol Phys* 2004;58:1108–1113.

52. Singh AK, Lockett MA, Bradley JD. Predictors of radiation-induced esophageal toxicity in patients with non-small cell lung cancer treated with three-dimensional conformal radiotherapy. *Int J Radiat Oncol Biol Phys* 2003;55:337–341.

53. Kim TH, Cho KH, Pyo HR, et al. Dose–volumetric parameters of acute esophageal toxicity in patients with lung cancer treated with three-dimensional conformal radiotherapy. *Int J Radiat Oncol Biol Phys* 2005;62:995–1002.

54. RTOG Protocol. Available from: http://rtog.org/members/protocols/0617/0617.pdf. Last accessed September 20, 2010.

55. RTOG Protocol. Available from: http://rtog.org/members/protocols/0436/0436.pdf. Last accessed September 20, 2010.

56. RTOG Protocol. Available from: http://rtog.org/members/protocols/0623/0623.pdf. Last accessed September 20, 2010.

57. Martel MK, Sahijdak WM, Ten Haken RK, et al. Fraction size and dose parameters related to the incidence of pericardial effusions. *Int J Radiat Oncol Biol Phys* 1998;40:155–161.

58. Wei X, Liu HH, Tucker SL, et al. Risk factors for pericardial effusion in inoperable esophageal cancer patients treated with definitive chemoradiation therapy. *Int J Radiat Oncol Biol Phys* 2008;70:707–714.

59. Gagliardi G, Lax I, Ottolenghi A, et al. Long-term cardiac mortality after radiotherapy of breast cancer—application of the relative seriality model. *Br J Radiol* 1996;69:839–846.

60. Eriksson F, Gagliardi G, Liedberg A, et al. Long-term cardiac mortality following radiation therapy for Hodgkin's disease: analysis with the relative seriality model. *Radiother Oncol* 2000;55:153–162.

61. Cassady JR. Clinical radiation nephropathy. *Int J Radiat Oncol Biol Phys* 1995;31:1249–1256.

62. Baglan KL, Frazier RC, Yan D, et al. The dose-volume relationship of acute small bowel toxicity from concurrent 5-FU-based chemotherapy and radiation therapy for rectal cancer. *Int J Radiat Oncol Biol Phys* 2002;52:176–183.

63. Robertson JM, Lockman D, Yan D, et al. The dose-volume relationship of small bowel irradiation and acute grade 3 diarrhea during chemoradiotherapy for rectal cancer. *Int J Radiat Oncol Biol Phys* 2008;70:413–418.

64. Roeske JC, Bonta D, Mell LK, et al. A dosimetric analysis of acute gastrointestinal toxicity in women receiving intensity modulated whole-pelvic radiation therapy. *Radiother Oncol* 2003;69:201–207.

65. RTOG Protocol. Available from: http://rtog.org/members/protocols/0415/0415.pdf. Last accessed September 20, 2010.

66. Shipley WU, Bae K, Efstathiou JA, et al. Late pelvic toxicity following bladder-sparing therapy in patients with invasive bladder cancer: analysis of RTOG 89–03, 95–06, 97–06, 99–06. *Int J Radiat Oncol Biol Phys* 2007;69 (3 Suppl):S8.

67. Roach M, Winter K, Michalski JM, et al. Penile bulb dose and impotence after three-dimensional conformal radiotherapy for prostate cancer on RTOG 9406: Findings from a prospective, multi-institutional, phase I/II dose-escalation study. *Int J Radiat Oncol Biol Phys* 2004;60:1351–1356.

68. Grigsby PW, Roberts HL, Perez CA. Femoral neck fracture following groin irradiation. *Int J Radiat Oncol Biol Phys* 1995;32(1):63–67.

69. Katz A, Eifel PJ, Jhingran A, et al. The role of radiation therapy in preventing regional recurrences of invasive squamous cell carcinoma of the vulva. *Int J Radiat Oncol Biol Phys* 2003;57(2):409–418.

70. Shahinian VB, Kuo YF, Freeman JL, et al. Risk of fracture after androgen deprivation for prostate cancer. *N Engl J Med* 2005;352:154–164.

71. Fiorino C, Valdagni R, Rancati T, et al. Dose-volume effects for normal tissues in external radiotherapy: pelvis. *Radiother Oncol* 2009;93(2):153–167.

72. Bedford JL, Khoo VS, Webb S, et al. Optimization of coplanar six-field techniques for conformal radiotherapy of the prostate. *Int J Radiat Oncol Biol Phys* 2000;46(1):231–238.

73. Marion CM, Zelefsky MJ, Paoli J, et al. Predictors of late femoral head toxicity after high-dose 3D-conformal radiotherapy and intensity modulated radiotherapy. *Int J Radiat Oncol Biol Phys* 2002;54(2 Suppl):S111.

74. Jereczek-Fossa BA, Vavassori A, Fodor C, et al. Dose escalation for prostate cancer using the three-dimensional conformal dynamic arc technique: analysis of 542 consecutive patients. *Int J Radiat Oncol Biol Phys* 2008;71(3):784–794.

75. Timmerman RD. An overview of hypofractionation and introduction to this issue of seminars in radiation oncology. *Semin Radiat Oncol* 2008;18(4):215–222.

Andrew Jackson ■ Gerald J. Kutcher

INTRODUCTION

Interest in understanding and developing methods of plan evaluation has burgeoned over the past two decades. This has been driven in part by the development of three-dimensional (3D) treatment planning systems, and consequent introductions of 3D conformal radiation therapy (3DCRT) and intensity-modulated radiation therapy (IMRT). On the one hand, the substantial amounts of data generated by 3D planning systems have necessitated new methods of presenting and condensing the voluminous information in an understandable format. On the other hand, even with a condensed dose representation like dose-volume histograms (DVHs), the balance between tumor control and normal organ toxicity, so important, for example, in dose escalation, also needs to be addressed. Conventional evaluation of treatment plans, which judges a "best treatment plan" using tradition and practical knowledge alone, is no longer adequate to answer the issues that continually arise in modern practice. For example, should we escalate the dose to the prostate to the highest nonuniform dose or to a lower, more uniform, target dose? Can the rectum and bladder tolerate a high localized dose to a small volume? And if so, how small a volume and how high a dose? And finally, how should we balance tumor control and the risk of normal tissue complications?

In this chapter, we describe two general sets of tools for plan evaluation, one based upon physical endpoints, namely DVHs, and the other based on biologic indices, tumor control probabilities (TCPs), and normal tissue complication probabilities (NTCPs). First, we describe briefly and in schematic form the basic structure of these tools, and then describe some applications. In the penultimate section, we review the clinical data for three sites: lung, liver, and rectum.

DOSE-VOLUME HISTOGRAMS

DVHs were introduced over two decades ago (11) and are now a routine planning tool. DVHs may be represented in either differential or integral form. The former represents the volume of the organ receiving a dose within a specified dose interval, whereas the latter is defined as the volume receiving at least dose D as a function of D. The volume is either represented as the percent (or fraction) of the total volume of the organ or as the volume in cubic centimeters. The differential form lends itself well to rapid visual inspection of the range and uniformity of dose. This works well in finding cold spots in the target volume or hot spots in normal organs. The integral form facilitates the assessment of the total volume of tissue in such hot or cold spots and is the preferred format.

Suppose an integral DVH for plan A lies to the left of one for plan B. If the organ is a nontarget tissue, then plan A is better; if the organ is the target, then plan B is better. A more complex comparison is given in Figure 23.1 where integral DVHs for a normal organ planned with a parallel-opposed (traditional) and multifield 3D plan are shown. Although the volume irradiated to any dose level can be used to quantitatively compare the treatment plans, the location of high-dose (or other) regions cannot be determined from the DVHs. Moreover, in the example shown, the DVHs cross one another so that it is not obvious which DVH is better. This suggests augmenting DVHs to account for biologic effects.

BIOLOGIC INDICES

Biologic indices represent an alternative method for evaluating treatment plans. In this section, we will describe NTCP and TCP.

Normal Tissue Complication Probability

The use of a complication probability (CP) factor to rank rival treatment plans was first discussed by Dritschilo (22). Since then, a number of techniques have been developed for estimating NTCPs. These NTCP models aim to predict the probability of a complication as a function of the dose (or biologically equivalent dose) and volume.

Existing models can be distinguished by their descriptions of the volume effect. The phenomenological model of Lyman (33–55) augmented by Kutcher and Burman (LKB)[1] seeks to describe the tolerance doses and volume effects in

---

[1] *Although the Lyman model was designed for uniform irradiation of partial volumes, it can be extended for inhomogeneous dose distribution using the dose-volume reduction scheme of Kutcher and Burman (6,7).*

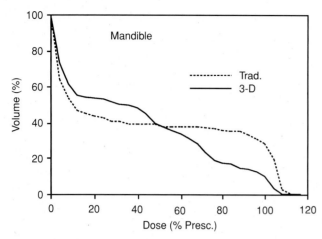

Figure 23.1. Dose-volume histograms (DVHs) for the mandible. *Source:* Reprinted from Kutcher GJ. Quantitative plan evaluation. In: Purdy JA, Simpson LR, eds. Advances in radiation oncology physics: dosimetry, treatment planning, brachytherapy. New York, NY: American Institute of Physics, 1992:998–1021, with permission.

terms of four parameters. In this model, partial volume tolerance doses are related to each other through a power law in volume. This implies that there is always a partial volume dose for which there is a given probability that complication will occur, no matter how small the partial volume.

Other models are based on the tissue architecture of organs (88,99), with different volume effects specific to the functional organization. Serial (critical element) models assume that certain organs are organized like chains; when one link (a functional subunit) is damaged the entire chain is broken (10,11). A candidate for a serial organ is the spinal chord. Organs with this architecture have a small volume effect. For the parallel model (also called *critical volume*) a complication does not occur until a significant fraction of independent functional subunits (functional reserve) have been incapacitated (9,12–14). The volume effect in these tissues is large, because a complication does not occur if less than the functional reserve is irradiated (12,13). This behavior is not reflected in the LKB models unless augmented by an additional parameter such as a critical volume below which there is no complication. We now describe these models in more detail.

Empirical Models: Uniform Irradiation

Lyman (33) represents the NTCP for uniform partial volume irradiation of an organ with an error function of dose and volume.

$$\text{NTCP} = (1/\sqrt{2\pi}) \int_{-\infty}^{t} \exp(-t^2/2)\,dt \quad \text{EQUATION (23.1)}$$

$$v = V/V_{\text{ref}} \quad \text{EQUATION (23.2)}$$

$$t = [D - \text{TD}_{50}(v)] / [m \cdot \text{TD}_{50}(v)] \quad \text{EQUATION (23.3)}$$

$$\text{TD}_{50}(1) = \text{TD}_{50}(v) \cdot v^n \quad \text{EQUATION (23.4)}$$

The model contains four parameters: TD_{50} (11), the tolerance dose for whole organ irradiation; m, the steepness of the dose–response curve; V_{ref}, the reference volume, which in some cases may be the whole volume of the organ; n, which relates the tolerance doses for uniform whole and uniform partial organ irradiation. This latter parameter represents the volume effect. When n is near unity, the volume effect is large[2] and when it is near zero, the volume effect is small. A value of $n \sim 1$ implies that NTCP correlates with the mean dose, whereas a small volume effect implies a correlation with the peak organ dose. The NTCP for partial organ irradiation in the Lyman model was originally based on clinical estimates of partial organ tolerance doses. An early compilation by Emami et al. (15) was fitted to the model by Burman et al. (16). Although many of the parameter values he obtained are still in use, values resulting from maximum likelihood fit of DVH and complication data from 3D conformal dose escalation protocols are available for a growing list of organs. This will be described in more detail in the section on "Supporting Data for Biologic Models."

For statistical models, described in the subsequent text, the analog of an organ with large n would be a parallel architecture organ and the analog of one with small n would be a serial organ.

Nonuniform Irradiation—Histogram Reduction and Equivalent Uniform Dose

The approach in the preceding text has been extended to inhomogeneous irradiation by converting the organ's DVH into an "equivalent" uniform one using the effective volume method (77). The DVH is transformed into one in which the partial volume, v_{eff}, which is equal to or less than the whole organ volume, receives a dose equal to the peak organ dose. This effective volume transformation is self-consistent with the power law model for uniform irradiation in that it can be derived from just two hypotheses: The organ is homogeneous in response and each element of the organ obeys the same power law relationship as the whole organ. Moreover, there is a family of equivalent uniform DVHs with effective volume and dose related through the defining power law relationship. This method was extended to calculate the effective whole volume dose (d_{eff}) by Mohan et al. (17). More recently, use of the equivalent uniform dose (EUD) (18–20) has become popular. This quantity is calculated in an identical fashion to d_{eff} (in the EUD formalism, the LKB model parameter n is replaced by the parameter a, they are related by $n = 1/a$).

These models rely on clinical data, which for some organs is still quite sparse and unreliable. This is due to a number of historical factors including the inevitably poor statistics of complication data from individual treatment protocols, uncertain dose specification in the literature, lack of 3D dose

---

[2]*Nothing prevents n being greater than 1, in which case greater emphasis is placed on large volumes exposed to lower doses.*

distributions, poorly specified endpoints, and poor statistical analysis. With the advent of 3DCRT, as outlined in the section on "Supporting Data for Biologic Models," considerable improvements have been made. These include the prospective collection of dose distribution and complication data, and better statistical methods of analysis.

Statistical Models

Statistical models use binomial statistics in combination with an idea proposed by Withers (88) that normal tissues are composed of independent functioning subunits (FSUs) defined either architecturally (e.g., nephrons of the kidney) or operationally (e.g., FSUs of the skin). Moreover, it is possible to consider that tumors consist of some type (or more likely, types) of elementary units (EUs) or tumorlets as well. NTCP and TCP can then be derived in these models by considering the radiobiology of the EUs and their architectural arrangement—that is, the probability of eradicating an EU and how many need to be disabled, respectively. The former represents local dose–response and the later organ complication.

To derive NTCP/TCP we require a 3D dose distribution and a local dose–response function (12). We then derive a risk histogram, the fractional volume of the organ as a function of the probability of eradicating the EUs in that volume. Finally, we calculate the damage distribution, $P(M)$, the probability of eradicating M and only M EUs. A generalized CP (NTCP for normal organs and 1-TCP, the recurrence probability, for tumors) is obtained by summing up the damage distribution from a lower limit L (the minimum number of eradicated EUs required to realize a complication) to N (the total number of EUs in the organ).

$$\text{CP} = \sum_{M=L}^{N} P(M) = 1 - \sum_{M=0}^{L-1} P(M) \quad \text{EQUATION (23.5)}$$

If $L = 1$, then we obtain a serial complication model where at least one EU must be eradicated. If all the EUs must be killed, $L = N$, then Equation 23.5 yields the recurrence probability, 1-TCP. If L is between these limits, we have a parallel complication model in which at least L EUs must be eradicated for a complication. Because the number of EUs is usually quite large, typically 10^4 to 10^9 (21), the derived dose–response curves will be much steeper than observed. However, if we average in some fashion over a heterogeneous population, then more realistic dose–response curves are obtained. For example, TCP calculations can be averaged over the population distribution of radiosensitivities (e.g., the distribution of the dose that controls 50% of tumors [TCD50]), whereas NTCP may be averaged over a distribution of normal organ functional reserves. Such an approach leads to models with at least four parameters, two for local response and two for the population distribution, although more may be required for the parallel model (99) and less are possible for a serial model (22). For further discussion see subsequent text and Jackson et al. (12).

Serial Organs

The description in the preceding text is somewhat formal and general. We can obtain some insight by deriving NTCP in the serial chain model. For uniform irradiation of N FSUs, the probability of eradicating at least one is given by one minus the probability of not eradicating any:

$$\text{NTCP} = 1 - (1 - p)^N \quad \text{EQUATION (23.6)}$$

where p is the probability of eradicating a single FSU. This relationship yields a sigmoid curve of NTCP versus dose, which shifts to the left as the number of irradiated FSUs, which is proportional to the volume, increases. This serial model can be extended to nonhomogeneous irradiation (22). Moreover, while the predictions of the serial model differ from LKB models, they agree at low CP; that is the clinically significant domain.

Parallel Organs

In parallel element tissues, which have also been modeled using binomial statistics (12–14), a complication occurs if the fraction of eradicated FSUs exceeds a threshold fraction, the functional reserve of the organ. The kidney, liver, and lung are conjectured to behave as parallel organs. Because the number of FSUs is always large in these organs (21), the functional reserve can be defined by the fraction rather than the number of eradicated FSUs. Furthermore, as remarked before, the large number of FSUs leads to unrealistically large gradients of NTCP with dose in the region of NTCP = 50%. To remedy this population averaging is invoked, which requires additional parameters. For example, if the functional reserve and the FSU radiosensitivity (defined by the dose required for 50% FSU death) vary among a population of patients, then two additional parameters are required to represent the widths of these distributions. In addition, intraorgan variation in radiosensitivity may also be considered. Fortunately, it can be demonstrated that intraorgan variability has a negligible effect on the slope of the local dose–response curve (12).

A further simplification is possible if the width of the distribution of radiosensitivities is narrower than that of the functional reserve. In this limit the NTCP is given by the integral of the functional reserve up to the mean fraction of eradicated FSUs, that is, up to the fraction damaged (12). This form is quite useful for fitting clinical complication data as will be shown in the section on "Applications."

NTCP models for parallel organs demonstrate a threshold effect such that a complication occurs only if at least a critical volume of the organ is irradiated to sufficient dose to eradicate the FSUs. Moreover, parallel models have a large volume effect such that NTCP correlates more closely with the mean dose rather than the peak organ dose as in the serial model. Power law models with n near unity also have a large volume effect although the functional relationship between NTCP and volume differs in detail from

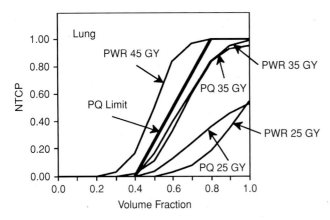

Figure 23.2. Normal tissue complication probabilities (NTCP) versus lung volume. PQ denotes the parallel model and PWR denotes the Lyman power law model. *Source:* Redrawn from Yorke ED, Kutcher GJ, Jackson A, et al. Probability of radiation-induced complications in normal tissues with parallel architecture under conditions of uniform whole or partial organ irradiation. *Radiother Oncol* 1993;26:226–237.

the parallel model (13). This is demonstrated in Figure 23.2, which compares calculated NTCPs for the lung for the power law and parallel models as a function of the fraction of lung uniformly irradiated to various doses. At lower doses the parallel model yields higher complications for the same fraction of irradiated lung. However, as dose is increased a limiting curve is reached, which reflects the fact that if only a fraction of the organ is irradiated, then the entire functional reserve cannot be destroyed so that the CP is less than unity. For details on this example, see Yorke et al. (13).

Tumor Control Probability

The central assumption of all TCP models is that a tumor is destroyed if all viable clonogenic cells within it are killed (23). From this Brahme (24) and Goitein (25) derive TCP from the product of probabilities that individual clonogens (or tumorlets) are killed. The simplest form of these models assumes that clonogens in a tumor have identical radiosensitivities and are uniformly distributed. If the dose D to each tumorlet is homogeneous and each responds independently, then $\mathrm{TCP}(v, D)$, the TCP for each tumorlet with partial volume v, can be inferred from the TCP for uniform irradiation of the whole tumor, $\mathrm{TCP}(1, D)$.

$$\mathrm{TCP}(v, D) = \mathrm{TCP}(1, D)^v \qquad \text{(TCP 1)}$$

It then follows that the TCP of an inhomogeneously irradiated tumor is given by the product of tumorlet TCPs.

$$\mathrm{TCP} = \prod_{i=1}^{N} \mathrm{TCP}(v_i, D_i) = \prod_{i=1}^{N} [\mathrm{TCP}(1, D_i)]^{v_i} \quad \text{(TCP 2)}$$

where $\mathrm{TCP}(v_i, D_i)$ is the TCP for the ith tumorlet receiving dose D_i and N is the number of tumorlets.

Several features of the model emerge immediately. The probability of controlling a tumor is dominated by any clonogens with low probability of being killed, thus TCP is very sensitive to cold spots in the dose distribution. Given the large numbers of clonogens in a tumor, when the dose is uniform the probability of destroying any individual clonogen must be very close to one for TCP to be appreciable. Given reasonable values for radiosensitivities of tumor cells, the model implies a very sharp dose response not seen in clinical studies. This discrepancy is not explainable by variations in tumor size (26,27).

Goitein and others (26,28–32) propose that the radiosensitivity of tumors differs from patient to patient and that the averaging over this difference results in the relatively broad dose response seen in clinical studies of TCP. Site-, stage-, and grade-specific parameters that describe the radiosensitivity of individual tumors and their variation in the patient population have been collected from clinical studies and summarized by Okunieff et al. (33). As a consequence of a distribution in radiosensitivities among patients, Zagars, Schultheiss, and Peters (32) and Thames et al. (34) point out that an escalation in dose is most effective for patients with intermediate sensitivity. Those whose tumors are most sensitive do not require such a high prescribed dose, and those who are least sensitive rarely require a dose in excess of normal tissue constraints. This implies that assays predicting radiosensitivity would be useful in identifying patients who would benefit from dose escalation.

There are other possible explanations for the discrepancy between predicted and clinical dose responses. Bentzen (29), and Bentzen and Thames (27) point out that the number of clonogens in a tumor may not scale according to the volume. Alternatively, if the number of clonogens in tumors is small, then dose–response curves will be shallow. In this case, stochastic effects arising from repopulation may need to be considered (35).

Heterogeneity in the probability of killing clonogens within a patient arises for both dosimetric and biologic reasons. Planned dose distributions in external beam radiotherapy are traditionally designed to give uniform dose distributions within the target. However, because of setup errors and organ motion, delivered dose distributions may contain unquantified cold spots that adversely affect clinical outcome. These dosimetric uncertainties cannot be accounted for at present, although efforts to measure them are underway at several institutions (36–38). More difficult to account for is the biologic heterogeneity of tumors. Significant variations of radiosensitivity are thought to exist within individual patients. These may arise from regions of hypoxia (39), or from genetic variation within the clonogen population. The existence of radioresistant clonogens and their location with respect to hot or cold spots in the delivered dose distribution may determine clinical outcome. Kallman et al. (40) propose a modification of the basic TCP model that attempts to account for radioresistant clonogens uniformly distributed throughout the tumor. Not surprisingly, they find that TCP is dominated by the probability of killing the most radioresistant fraction of the clonogens. If the number of highly radioresistant clonogens is small enough, this can flatten the dose response. In addition, attempts have been made to describe the effects of variations in the density of clonogens within the tumor (41).

The uncertainty in defining tumor boundaries, uncertainty in clonogenic tumor cell densities, heterogeneous colonogen radiosensitivity, and the interaction between these uncertainties and the unknown inhomogeneities in delivered dose distributions make it difficult to test TCP models of the effects of cold spots against clinical data. Two studies attempting this indicate that the results of such efforts may be site dependent. Terahara et al. (42) studied the effects of dose inhomogeneity on local control using DVH and outcome data from 115 patients treated for skull base chordomas with combined photons and protons. In these patients, with relatively small positional uncertainties and relatively large dose inhomogeneities in the target, a Cox multivariate analysis showed that the models (including gender) and the minimum target dose were significantly associated with outcome. In contrast, Levegrun et al. (43,44) studied the effects of dose distributions and prognostic factors on biopsy outcome in a series of 132 patients treated with 3DCRT for prostate cancer. In this patient population, the clinical target volume (CTV) was defined as the prostate gland and seminal vesicles, although it is likely that the tumor clonogens were confined to subvolumes of the CTV. In addition, positional uncertainty on the order of 1 cm can be expected in the CTV location during treatment due to setup error and organ motion. The relationship between locations of cold spots in the planning target volume (PTV) and the positions of tumor clonogens was unknown. Finally in contrast with the chordoma patients, the PTV was treated relatively homogeneously. In these circumstances, the mean (but not the minimum) PTV dose was found to be significantly correlated with biopsy outcome (43), and the TCP model fits showed that there was considerable degeneracy in model parameters that were able to describe the data (44) (similar degeneracies have been found when attempting to fit such models to clinical data when DVHs were not used, see for example, Buffa et al.) (45). In an additional paper (46) studying 103 of these patients treated without hormones, the dose response was shown to be dependent on the risk group, providing evidence that the shallow dose responses seen clinically arise, at least in part, from patient heterogeneity.

APPLICATIONS

We consider three applications of the models as follows:

1. Fitting the parallel model to clinical complication data
2. The application of NTCP models, in this example, v_{eff}, to the design of dose escalation studies
3. The evaluation of target dose distributions using the TCP model

Fitting the Parallel Model to Clinical Complication Data

Biophysical models can be used to try to fit clinical data. Such an approach is a starting point to suggest further developments in the collection and analysis of clinical data. We describe here one example in which a parallel model (described in preceding text) and the method of maximum likelihood is used to fit DVHs and complication data for radiation hepatitis of 93 patients treated for tumors of the liver (47–49).

The method of maximum likelihood can be applied as follows. The DVH[3] for each patient is used to calculate NTCP by first assigning a best guess for the model parameters. The predicted probability of a complication for each patient is then compared against the observed grade of complication in that patient. The overall likelihood L of the observations is then modeled according to:

$$L(\gamma_1, \gamma_2, \ldots) = \prod_{\substack{m \\ \text{complication}}} O_m(t_m, \gamma_1, \gamma_2, \ldots)$$

$$\prod_{\substack{n \\ \text{no complication}}} [1 - O_n(t_n, \gamma_1, \gamma_2, \ldots)]$$

EQUATION (23.7)

where

$$O_m(t_m, \gamma_1, \gamma_2, \ldots) = O(t_m)\, \text{NTCP}_m(\gamma_1, \gamma_2, \ldots)$$

EQUATION (23.8)

where L is the likelihood, $O(t_m)$ is the probability that a complication will manifest itself after the follow-up time t_m for the mth patient—calculated from complication and follow-up time data with the Kaplan-Meier method (50)—and $\gamma_1, \gamma_2, \ldots$ indicates the model parameters. The likelihood function is then maximized with respect to the model parameters. Note that the likelihood is essentially the probability in the model of the observed complication pattern.

Furthermore, it is convenient to assume, as described earlier, that the organ has a functional reserve described with two parameters (whose values are to be obtained from the maximum likelihood fit) and that NTCP is given by the integral of the functional reserve up to the mean fraction of eradicated FSUs, that is, up to the fraction damaged (12). For each patient, the fraction damaged is calculated by summing up the product of the fractional

---

[3]*Doses were reexpressed as biologically equivalent doses delivered in 2 Gy fractions using the linear quadratic model with an α/β ratio of 4 Gy, suitable for late reacting tissues (21).*

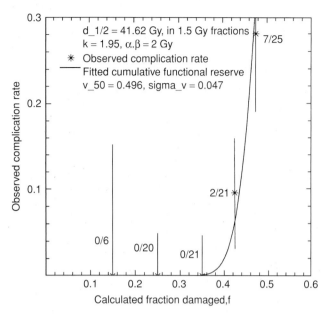

Figure 23.3. Observed complication rate for radiation hepatitis versus calculated fraction damaged. *Source:* Reprinted from Jackson A, Ten Haken RK, Robertson JM, et al. Analysis of clinical complication data for radiation hepatitis using a parallel architecture model. *Int J Radiat Oncol Biol Phys* 1995;31:883–891, with permission.

volume of each voxel of the organ and the probability of damage. The latter can be calculated using each patient's DVH and an assumed local response function with two parameters (whose values are to be obtained from the maximum likelihood fit).

The results of applying such an analysis to the hepatitis data is shown in Figure 23.3 for observed complication rate as a function of the calculated fraction of the liver that is damaged. The observed complications for this data set show a threshold effect with a steep response, which is described well with the parallel model. In this application, the best-fit functional reserve distribution and their confidence intervals predict that irradiation of less than one-third of the liver volume leads to negligible complications (47). That is, the threshold volume is about one-third. A more detailed analysis of the fit revealed that the uncertainties in the width of the functional reserve distribution and radiosensitivity of functional subunits were correlated. This arose because complications were seen only in the cohort of patients who received a whole liver irradiation as part of the treatment course. The lack of complications among patients given only partial volume irradiation suggested that an attempt to increase local control through dose escalation was feasible. After follow-up of subsequently treated patients, some of whom had received 90 Gy, Dawson et al. analyzed data from 138 patients, including 19 with radiation-induced liver disease (RILD). Observation of complications in patients with only partial volume irradiation helped to resolve the correlated uncertainties in the model parameters and the threshold limit was revised down from one-third to one-fourth (51,52).

Design of Dose Escalation Protocols

NTCP models can also be used to design dose escalation protocols. This is a reasonable manner in which to use such models, that is, to suggest strategies, which are then tested in a tried and true clinical manner based on clinical judgment and clinical outcome data.

The value of an escalation, which uses a model including volume effects reveals itself quite readily. For example, most dose escalation protocols stratify patients only in terms of the prescription dose, and these studies are terminated when the incidence of complication of the entire group exceeds a specific limit. A major disadvantage of this approach is the possibility that the tolerance of a high-risk subpopulation will, in effect, limit the dose escalation. Recognizing this, a dose escalation scheme for the lung was developed, which prospectively incorporated dose volume dependencies of critical structures into the protocol (48,49,53,54). In this approach, patients with smaller volumes of irradiated critical tissue are escalated to higher doses, even when patients with larger irradiated volumes have reached their tolerances. As a result, the boundary of safe treatment is more thoroughly explored in both prescribed dose and the volume of irradiated normal tissue. In one dose escalation scheme for the treatment of lung tumors (53,54), the LKB model (33,44,66) was used to calculate the effective lung volume irradiated for each patient:

$$v_{\text{eff}} = \sum_i \left[v_i \left(\frac{d_i}{d_p} \right)^{1/n} \right] \qquad \text{Equation (23.9)}$$

On the basis of calculated v_{eff}, the plan is assigned to one of five v_{eff} bins and given a corresponding prescription dose (judged clinically acceptable). When a sufficient number of patients have been accrued to the v_{eff}-dose bins, the decision to escalate the prescription dose is made independently for each bin. To ensure that dose escalation proceeds in a timely fashion, the dose is increased after three patients have been successfully treated without serious complications. If a complication occurs at the next level, the dose is returned to the previous level and eight more patients are added, and if no complications are seen, escalation is reattempted (54).

Evaluation of Target Dose Using Tumor Control Probability Models

An important consequence of tumor modeling has been derived by Brahme (24), who expanded the TCP in a Taylor series about the mean tumor dose

$$\text{TCP} = \text{TCP}(\bar{D}) - \frac{\gamma^2}{2\text{TCP}(\bar{D})} \left(\frac{\sigma_D}{\bar{D}} \right)^2 \quad \text{Equation (23.10)}$$

$$\sigma_D^2 = \frac{\int [D(r) - \bar{D}]^2 \, dm}{\int dm} \qquad \text{Equation (23.11)}$$

where $\bar{D}$ is the mean tumor dose, $D(r)$ is the 3D dose distribution, γ is the measure of the steepness of the tumor control curve (more precisely, $\gamma = (1/D) \, \Delta TCP/\Delta D$), and the integrals are carried out over each element, dm, of the tumor mass. We note that when the tumor dose distribution is near uniform, that is, the variance of tumor dose, σ_D^2, is near zero, then TCP is determined by the mean tumor dose.

The implications of the statistical TCP model and the analysis in the preceding text is that tumor control is better correlated with the mean rather than the minimum target dose, as long as the tumor dose distribution does not differ significantly from a homogeneous distribution (24). This conclusion differs starkly from convention where the minimum dose is the *sine qua non* of plan evaluation. The replacement of minimum by mean dose is a crucial, although unproven supposition because it provides a rationale for dose escalation with inhomogeneous dose distributions. For example, if a critical organ abuts the tumor and the dose has reached organ tolerance, then according to conventional ideas no further escalation is possible. However, according to the analysis in the preceding text, TCP may be further improved by increasing dose to most of the tumor while respecting organ tolerance with a lower dose near the tumor–normal organ interface.

SUPPORTING DATA FOR BIOLOGIC MODELS

Over the past 10 years, statistical fits of NTCP models to clinical outcome data (47) from 3DCRT and IMRT treatment protocols have accumulated for a number of organs, notably for radiation pneumonitis in lung (55–62); RILD (47,52,63,64), and rectal bleeding (65–75). We will review these in subsequent paragraphs. In addition, studies of xerostomia (76–80), hearing loss (81–83), spinal cord tolerance (84,85), and brain necrosis (86–88) have been published. These studies have supplanted many of the estimates of partial volume tolerance doses of Emami et al. (15) (and the corresponding parameter estimates for the Lyman model of Burman et al. (16)), which were based on clinical experience from patient series with unquantified volumes of irradiated normal tissues. Summaries of the analyses of the major data sets through 2001 are contained in an issue of Seminars in Radiation Oncology devoted to partial organ irradiation (51,89–91).

Radiation Pneumonitis

Travis (92) and Marks (93) reviewed clinical evidence for lung tolerance doses before conformal radiation therapy. Whole volume tolerance doses have been deduced from patients treated with single-dose hemi-body irradiation (94); after corrections to account for fractionation, these doses are generally consistent with those deduced from patients treated with various fractionation schedules to volumes in excess of 75% (92,95). Few quantitative data for partial volume tolerances were available before the advent of conformal treatment techniques, although data did exist to indicate that the probability of pneumonitis is significantly correlated with the volume of lung irradiated (96–100). On the basis of this and similar data, Emami et al. concluded that the volume effect in the lung was very large (15). The Burman et al. fit to these estimates gave a value of n of 0.87 (16).

Martel et al. (58) and Graham et al. (101) used DVHs to analyze pneumonitis in patients treated with conformal radiation therapy techniques. Martel et al. analyzed nine and five cases of pneumonitis ($\geq$Grade I) from 42 patients with lung cancer and 21 patients with Hodgkin's disease, respectively. Graham et al. analyzed results from 70 patients with lung cancer, containing nine cases of $\geq$Grade III and eight cases of Grade II pneumonitis. Both groups compared this data with the predictions of the LKB model (using total lung volume and the Burman parameters). Correlations were found between calculated and observed CP, confirming the large volume effect in the lung predicted by the model, although in neither case was a formal statistical analysis given. Graham et al. fit the LKB model "by eye" and found that large values for the volume effect parameter of $n \geq 0.9$ were favored by their data. They also noted that in six of the nine patients with $\geq$Grade III pneumonitis, >37% of total lung volume received >20 Gy.

Prospective dose escalation studies in non-small-cell lung cancer (NSCLC), which based the prescription dose on model-dependent measures of the volume of involved lung, either v_{eff} (53) or f_{dam} (59,60,102) reached prescription doses >100 Gy to isocenter (103), or 94 Gy to isodoses surrounding the tumor (102) for small tumors. This is a strong indication that the volume effect for radiation pneumonitis must be large, because the whole volume tolerance dose is a factor of 4 to 5 times lower than these doses (Emami et al. (15) give 17.5 Gy as the whole lung 5% tolerance dose).

Studies from different institutions have analyzed their data using different models of pneumonitis, including V_{20} (the volume of lung receiving at least 20 Gy) (61); LKB d_{eff} (with $n = 0.87$ (16)); f_{dam} (59,60); and mean dose (56). In several studies, mean dose has been found to be associated with pneumonitis (56,59,60,104). Use of mean dose in the lung receives additional support from the observation that the dose response of local function (found after comparing pre- and posttreatment perfusion or ventilation scans) is approximately linear over the clinical range of doses (105,106). Kwa (107) analyzed pooled mean dose data from five institutions, consisting of 540 patients including 73 cases of $\geq$Grade III pneumonitis, and calculated the mean dose response (although at low mean doses, subtraction of an ~10% complication rate was necessary to account for residual complications occurring in the data from three of the institutions). Examining data from patients with breast and lung lymphoma, Kwa pointed out that strong correlations exist between the clinical values of different model predictors of pneumonitis (108). Similar correlations have been found between dose-volume parameters (such as V_{20} and V_{30}, the volumes getting at least 20 and 30 Gy, respectively) (60). These correlations, together with small numbers of complications occurring in single institution studies, make it difficult to distinguish between models.

The only study claiming that one model of pneumonitis is significantly better than another is that by Seppenwoolde (56), who fitted a generalized parallel model to the data of 380 patients including 44 cases of ≥Grade II pneumonitis from Netherlands Cancer Institute (NKI) and University of Michigan. The best-fit model was equivalent to a mean dose model, which was found to be a significantly better model that the best dose volume parameter V_{13} (the volume receiving at least 13 Gy) although the authors noted that mean dose and V_{13} were still highly correlated.

In contrast, distinguishing between sensitivity of different regions in the lung has been relatively straightforward. Liao et al. (109) showed that the base of mouse lung is more radiosensitive than the apex. If such a large difference was seen in clinical data, then for equal numbers of tumors in the base and apex, when the overall complication rate is 20%, we would estimate that the complication rate for tumors in the base of the lung would be on the order of 30% higher than for tumors in the apex. Following this, several studies found indications of the same effect in patients undergoing radiotherapy for NSCLC. Graham et al. (101,110) found that incidence of ≥Grade III pneumonitis was 6% in 49 patients with upper lobe tumors and 29% in 21 patients with middle or lower lobe tumors. Martel et al. (58) reported that of 42 patients with lung cancer who were studied, all nine with pneumonitis (≥Grade I) had tumors in the middle or lower lobes. Yorke et al. (59,60) found significant correlation between model-dependent predictors evaluated in the lower and ipsilateral lungs, but no correlation when the same predictors were evaluated in the upper and contralateral lung. Although lack of correlation of dose to the contralateral lung is likely the result of treatment plans that spare the contralateral lung, this is not the case for the upper lung, because most of the patients in the study had tumors in the upper lung. Seppenwoolde et al. (55) found that pneumonitis was significantly correlated with mean dose to the posterior, lower, ipsilateral, central, and peripheral lung. No correlation was found for the mean dose to the anterior, cranial, and contralateral lung. Correlation was improved if the relevant lung subvolumes were weighted with local perfusion values.

Radiation-Induced Liver Disease

Most quantitative data on RILD comes from a pioneering series of dose escalation studies conducted at the University of Michigan (53,111–113), which culminated in a phase II trial treating patients to the maximum dose consistent with an NTCP between 10% and 15% (114). This resulted in prescription doses up to 90 Gy for the smallest tumors, a factor of 3 greater than the 5% whole volume tolerance dose of 30 Gy estimated by Emami et al. (15). Again, this indicates a very large volume effect in the liver.

Analysis of RILD incidence in the early trials by Lawrence et al. (49) found that a "by hand" estimate yielded a value of 0.69 for the Lyman model parameter n, as compared with the value of 0.32 estimated by Burman (16) from the partial volume tolerances of Emami et al. (15). As described earlier, in the section on "Applications," Jackson et al. (47) fit a parallel model to this data and found that the best-fit model predicted complication rates <5% as long as <40% of the liver was irradiated. Subsequent model fits to larger data sets by Dawson et al. (51,52) reduced this portion to 25%. First Lawrence et al. (49) and subsequently Dawson et al. (63) found that mean dose also provided a good fit to the data, noting that no cases of RILD had occurred in patients receiving mean liver doses <30 Gy; indeed a maximum likelihood fit of the LKB model to the DVH and complication data from 138 patients, including 19 with RILD, yielded a value of 0.94 for the volume effect parameter n (a value of 1.0 would be exactly equivalent to a mean dose model).

Rectal Bleeding

The tubular, deformable nature of the rectal wall, interacting with differences in clinical practice from institution to institution (in endpoint definition, contouring, set up, margin size, and beam geometry), make it difficult to form a coherent picture of the dose-volume dependence of rectal bleeding. Individual clinical studies have concentrated on establishing dose-volume limits for safe treatment, and strictly speaking, these limits are applicable only to the particular clinical techniques from which they derive. Although this *caveat* is generally true for all organs, it is essential to bear this in mind when considering complications occurring in the rectal wall. Nevertheless, some general observations can be made concerning the dose-volume limits that have been published in the last 15 years or so.

Quantitative evidence for a volume effect in the rectum has been nonexistent before conformal therapy. Emami et al. estimated a whole volume 5% tolerance dose of 60 Gy with no volume effect (15). Initial high-dose 3DCRT protocols quickly established the technique dependence of rectal bleeding rates (115–120), and that the incidence of rectal bleeding rose rapidly for prescription doses above 70 Gy (117,118,120). DVH-based studies showed that restriction of the volume of rectal wall receiving doses >70 Gy was essential in controlling this. Benk et al. (121) and Hartford (122) published clinical studies of 41 patients, including 13 with rectal bleeding, treated for prostate cancer with photons and protons. The exposed volume of the rectum was well determined for these patients because the whole rectum received 50.4 Gy given by photons, and in addition, the anterior portion of the rectum (immobilized with a rectal probe) received a proton boost. A statistically significant increase in the probability of Grade II rectal bleeding was demonstrated when >40% of the anterior portion of the rectal wall receives at least 75 Cobalt Gray Equivalent (CGE). These observations were confirmed by later studies (75,123–125).

Skwarchuk et al. (125) and Jackson et al. (75) showed that volumes receiving lower doses (approximately 40–50 Gy) are also associated with rectal bleeding, perhaps indicating that a "dose bath" effect is involved. A proliferation of other studies (67,69,72–74,126,127) have confirmed that lower doses (in some cases, much lower (70)) are also implicated in rectal bleeding. Following introduction of IMRT at prescription doses >80 Gy, Zelefsky et al. noted a drastic decrease in rectal toxicity (128).

An explanation for the differences in the dose-volume limits obtained by various studies is implied in the work of Le Crevoisier et al. (129), who noted the lower local control rates and lower rectal bleeding rates in patients whose rectums were full (as opposed to empty) at the time of the planning scan. This work implies that the motion of the rectal wall interacts with various clinical techniques to determine which planned dose-volume limits will correlate with rectal bleeding. Initial attempts to deal with this difficult problem have been made by Fenwick et al. (130,131).

Despite an increase in the quantity and quality of such data in recent years, individual clinical series almost always contain small numbers of complications, and studies based on them are seriously limited by statistics. Meta-analysis of published data is hindered by lack of common endpoint (107) and dose definitions, and heterogeneity in the predictive parameters examined (132). Recently, Jackson et al. (133) have proposed dose-volume (and model-dependent) atlases of complication incidence as tools with which to facilitate interinstitutional meta-analysis and comparison of treatment techniques.

CONCLUSIONS

We have described dosimetric and biologic endpoints and some applications. We have also described some recent findings in human and animal data to be used in the biologic models. Both dosimetric and biologic endpoints have their place in treatment plan evaluation, although biologic models are more provocative.

For example, the volume effect in both normal organs and tumors can have important implications for the design of treatment strategies. If we consider a tissue with a small volume effect it may be advantageous to decrease the dose by distributing it over a larger volume, whereas for some parallel organs it might be preferable to use a small number of fields to keep the total local damage below the organ's functional reserve. The volume effect for normal organs, therefore, has a direct influence on treatment strategy. Target distributions can be produced by using a large number of uniform photon fields, or alterna-

tively with a smaller number of intensity-modulated photons, or with high-energy protons or electrons. Therefore, the technique of choice should consider, in addition to target dose, the architecture of the surrounding normal organs (134,135).

Another example is that for tumors, as we have discussed, TCP increases with the mean dose and decreases in proportion to its variance. This implies that, for a uniform tumor cell density, the ideal dose distribution is uniform. However, when critical organs are located nearby, the minimum target dose is constrained by the normal organ tolerance. The TCP models suggest that dose escalation with a nonuniform target dose may be preferable in that better tumor control may be obtained while maintaining normal organ constraints.

Although NTCP and TCP models and dose-volume constraints described here are undoubtedly biologically crude, they have proved their usefulness in radiotherapy by enabling and guiding dose escalation protocols safely to high prescription doses—doses between 90 and 100 Gy in some cases. In the past 10 years, utilizing DVH and complication data from these dose escalation protocols together with statistical methods of analysis, considerable progress has been made in understanding the dose-volume effects in organs such as lung, liver, parotid, spinal cord, and rectum.

REFERENCES

1. Shipley WU, Tepper JE, Prout GR, et al. Proton radiation as boost therapy for localized prostatic carcinoma. *JAMA* 1979;241:1912–1915.
2. Dritschilo A, Chaffer JT, Bloumon WD, et al. The complication probability factor: a method of selection of treatment plans. *Br J Radiol* 1978;51:370–374.
3. Lyman JT. Complication probabilities as assessed from dose-volume histograms. *Radiat Res* 1985;104:S13–S19.
4. Lyman JT, Wolbarst AB. Optimization of radiation therapy. III. A method for assessing complication probabilities from dose-volume histograms. *Int J Radiat Oncol Biol Phys* 1987;13:103–109.
5. Lyman JT, Wolbarst AB. Optimization of radiation therapy. IV. A dose volume reduction algorithm. *Int J Radiat Oncol Biol Phys* 1987;13:103–109.
6. Kutcher GJ, Burman C, Brewster L, et al. Histogram reduction method for calculating complication probabilities for three dimensional treatment planning evaluations. *Int J Radiat Oncol Biol Phys* 1991;21:137–146.
7. Kutcher GJ, Burman C. Calculation of complication probability factors for non uniform normal tissue irradiation: the effective volume method. *Int J Radiat Oncol Biol Phys* 1989;16:1623–1630.
8. Withers HR, Taylor JMG, Maciejewski B. Treatment volume and tissue tolerance. *Int J Radiat Oncol Biol Phys* 1988;14:751–759.
9. Wolbarst AB, Chin LM, Svensson GK. Optimization of radiation therapy: integral-response of a model biological system. *Int J Radiat Oncol Biol Phys* 1982;8:1761–1769.

10. Schultheiss TE, Orton CG, Peck RA. Models in radiation therapy: volume effects. *Med Phys* 1983;10:410–415.

11. Wolbarst AB. Optimization of radiation therapy. II. The critical voxel model. *Int J Radiat Oncol Biol Phys* 1984;10:741–745.

12. Jackson A, Kutcher GJ, Yorke ED. Probability of radiation induced complications for normal tissues with parallel architecture subject to non-uniform irradiation. *Med Phys* 1993;20:613–625.

13. Yorke ED, Kutcher GJ, Jackson A, et al. Probability of radiation induced complications in normal tissues with parallel architecture under conditions of uniform whole or partial organ irradiation. *Radiother Oncol* 1993;26:226–237.

14. Niemierko A, Goitein M. Modeling of normal tissue response to radiation: the critical volume model. *Int J Radiat Oncol Biol Phys* 1993;25:135–145.

15. Emami B, Lyman JT, Brown A, et al. Tolerances of normal tissues to theraputic radiation. *Int J Radiat Oncol Biol Phys* 1991;21:109–122.

16. Burman C, Kutcher GJ, Emami B, et al. Fitting normal tissue tolerance data to an analytic function. *Int J Radiat Oncol Biol Phys* 1991;21:123–135.

17. Mohan R, Mageras GS, Baldwin B. Clinically relevant optimization of 3D conformal treatments. *Med Phys* 1992;19:933–944.

18. Niemierko A. Reporting and analyzing dose distributions: a concept of equivalent uniform dose. *Med Phys* 1997;24:103–110.

19. Niemierko A. A generalized concept of equivalent uniform dose (EUD). *Med Phys* 1999;26:1100 (abstr).

20. Wu Q, Mohan R, Niemierko A. Optimization of intensity-modulated radiotherapy plans based on the equivalent uniform dose. *Int J Radiat Oncol Biol Phys* 2002;52:224–235.

21. Thames HD, Hendry JH. *Fractionation in radiotherapy.* London: Taylor & Francis, 1987.

22. Niemierko A, Goitein M. Modeling of normal tissue response to radiation: the critical volume model. *Int J Radiat Oncol Biol Phys* 1992;20:135–145.

23. Munro TR, Gilbert CW. The relation between tumour lethal doses and the radiosensitivity of tumour cells. *Br J Radiol* 1961;34:246–251.

24. Brahme A. Dosimetric precision requirements in radiation therapy. *Acta Radiol Oncol* 1984;23:379–391.

25. Goitein M. Causes and consequences of inhomogeneous dose distributions in radiation therapy. *Int J Radiat Oncol Biol Phys* 1986;12:701–704.

26. Goitein M. The probability of controlling an inhomogeneously irradiated tumor. In: Zink S, ed. Evaluation of treatment planning for particle beam radiotherapy, NCI Contract Report. Bethesda, MD: National Cancer Institute, 1987.

27. Bentzen SM, Thames HD. Tumor volume and local control probability: clinical data and radiobiological interpretations. *Int J Radiat Oncol Biol Phys* 1996;36:247–251.

28. Niemierko A, Goitein M. Implementation of a model for estimating tumor control probability for an inhomogeneously irradiated tumor. *Radiother Oncol* 1993;29:140–147.

29. Bentzen SM. Steepness of the clinical dose-control curve and variation in the *in vitro* radiosensitivity of head and neck squamous cell carcinoma. *Int J Radiat Oncol Biol Phys* 1992;62:417–423.

30. Suit H, Skates S, Taghian A, et al. Clinical implications of heterogeneity of tumor response to radiation therapy. *Radiother Oncol* 1992;25:251–260.

31. Dutreix J, Tubiana M, Dutreix A. An approach to the interpretation of clinical data on the tumor control probability-dose relationship. *Radiother Oncol* 1988;11:239–248.

32. Zagars G, Schultheiss T, Peters L. Inter-tumor heterogeneity and radiation dose control curves. *Radiother Oncol* 1987;8:353–362.

33. Okunieff P, Morgan D, Niemierko A, et al. Radiation dose-response of human tumors. *Int J Radiat Oncol Biol Phys* 1995;32:1227–1237.

34. Thames H, Schultheiss T, Hendry J, et al. Can modest escalation of dose be detected as increased tumor control? *Int J Radiat Oncol Biol Phys* 1991;22:241–246.

35. Zaider M, Minerbo GN. Tumour control probability: a formulation applicable to any temporal protocol of dose delivery. *Phys Med Biol* 2000;45:279–293.

36. Cho BC, van Herk M, Mijnheer BJ, et al. The effect of set-up uncertainties, contour changes, and tissue inhomogeneities on target dose-volume histograms. *Med Phys* 2002;29:2305–2318.

37. Beaulieu L, Aubin S, Taschereau R, et al. Dosimetric impact of the variation of the prostate volume and shape between pretreatment planning and treatment procedure. *Int J Radiat Oncol Biol Phys* 2002;53:215–221.

38. Mageras GS, Pevsner A, Yorke ED, et al. Measurement of lung tumor motion using respiration-correlated CT. *Int J Radiat Oncol Biol Phys* 2004;60:933–941.

39. Kaanders JH, Wijffels KI, Marres HA, et al. Pimonidazole binding and tumor vascularity predict for treatment outcome in head and neck cancer. *Cancer Res* 2002;62:7066–7074.

40. Kallman P, Agren A, Brahme A. Tumor and normal tissue response to fractionated non-uniform dose delivery. *Int J Radiat Biol* 1992;62:249–262.

41. Web S, Nahum A. A model for calculating tumor control probability in radiotherapy including the effects of inhomogeneous distributions of dose and clonogenic cell density. *Phys Med Biol* 1993;38:653–666.

42. Terahara A, Niemierko A, Goitein M, et al. Analysis of the relationship between tumor dose inhomogeneity and local control in patients with skull base chordoma. *Int J Radiat Oncol Biol Phys* 1999;45:351–358.

43. Levegrun S, Jackson A, Zelefsky MJ, et al. Analysis of biopsy outcome after three-dimensional conformal radiation therapy of prostate cancer using dose-distribution variables and tumor control probability models. *Int J Radiat Oncol Biol Phys* 2000;47:1245–1260.

44. Levegrun S, Jackson A, Zelefsky MJ, et al. Fitting tumor control probability models to biopsy outcome after three-dimensional conformal radiation therapy of prostate cancer: pitfalls in deducing radiobiologic parameters for tumors from clinical data. *Int J Radiat Oncol Biol Phys* 2001;51:1064–1080.

45. Buffa FM, Fenwick JD, Nahum AE. An analysis of the relationship between radiosensitivity and volume

effects in tumor control probability modeling. *Med Phys* 2000;27:1258–1265.

46. Levegrun S, Jackson A, Zelefsky MJ, et al. Risk group dependence of dose-response for biopsy outcome after three-dimensional conformal radiation therapy of prostate cancer. *Radiother Oncol* 2002;63:11–26.

47. Jackson A, Ten Haken RK, Robertson JM, et al. Analysis of clinical complication data for radiation hepatitis using a parallel architecture model. *Int J Radiat Oncol Biol Phys* 1995;31:883–891.

48. Lawrence TS, Tesser RJ, Ten Haken RK. An application of dose volume histograms to the treatment of intrahepatic malignancies with radiation therapy. *Int J Radiat Oncol Biol Phys* 1990;19:1041–1047.

49. Lawrence TS, Ten Haken RK, Kessler ML, et al. The use of 3D dose volume analysis to predict radiation hepatitis. *Int J Radiat Oncol Biol Phys* 1992;23:781–788.

50. Kaplan EL, Meier P. Nonparametric estimation from incomplete observations. *J Am Stat Assoc* 1958;53:457–816.

51. Dawson LA, Ten Haken RK, Lawrence TS. Partial irradiation of the liver. *Semin Radiat Oncol* 2001;11:240–246.

52. Dawson LA, Ten Haken RK. Partial volume tolerance of the liver to radiation. *Semin Radiat Oncol* 2005;15:279–283.

53. Ten Haken RK, Martel MK, Kessler ML, et al. Use of v_{eff} and iso-NTCP in the implementation of dose escalation protocols. *Int J Radiat Oncol Biol Phys* 1993;27:689–695.

54. Hazuka MB, Turrisi AT, Martel MK, et al. A phase I dose escalation study of conformal three dimensional radiation therapy in patients with unresectable, locally advanced no-small cell lung cancer. UMMC 9204 1993.

55. Seppenwoolde Y, De Jaeger K, Boersma LJ. Regional differences in lung radiosensitivity after radiotherapy for non-small-cell lung cancer. *Int J Radiat Oncol Biol Phys* 2004;60:748–758.

56. Seppenwoolde Y, Lebesque JV, de Jaeger K. Comparing different NTCP models that predict the incidence of radiation pneumonitis. Normal tissue complication probability. *Int J Radiat Oncol Biol Phys* 2003;55(3):724–735.

57. Hernando ML, Marks LB, Bentel GC. Radiation-induced pulmonary toxicity: a dose-volume histogram analysis in 201 patients with lung cancer. *Int J Radiat Oncol Biol Phys* 2001;51:650–659.

58. Martel MK, Ten Haken RK, Hazuka MB. Dose-volume histogram and 3D treatment planning evaluation of patients with pneumonitis. *Int J Radiat Oncol Biol Phys* 1994;28:575–581.

59. Yorke ED, Jackson A, Rosenzweig KE. Dose-volume factors contributing to the incidence of radiation pneumonitis in non-small-cell lung cancer patients treated with three-dimensional conformal radiation therapy. *Int J Radiat Oncol Biol Phys* 2002;54:329–339.

60. Yorke ED, Jackson A, Rosenzweig KE, et al. Correlation of dosimetric factors and radiation pneumonitis for non-small-cell lung cancer patients in a recently completed dose escalation study. *Int J Radiat Oncol Biol Phys* 2005;63:672–682.

61. Graham MV, Purdy JA, Emami B. Clinical dose-volume histogram analysis for pneumonitis after 3D treatment for non-small cell lung cancer (NSCLC). *Int J Radiat Oncol Biol Phys* 1999;45:323–329.

62. Bradley J, Graham MV, Winter K. Toxicity and outcome results of RTOG 9311: a phase I-II dose-escalation study using three-dimensional conformal radiotherapy in patients with inoperable non-small-cell lung carcinoma. *Int J Radiat Oncol Biol Phys* 2005;61:318–328.

63. Dawson LA, Normolle D, Balter JM. Analysis of radiation-induced liver disease using the Lyman NTCP model. *Int J Radiat Oncol Biol Phys* 2002;53:810–821.

64. Dawson LA, Biersack M, Lockwood G. Use of principal component analysis to evaluate the partial organ tolerance of normal tissues to radiation. *Int J Radiat Oncol Biol Phys* 2005;62:829–837.

65. Peeters ST, Lebesque JV, Heemsbergen WD. Localized volume effects for late rectal and anal toxicity after radiotherapy for prostate cancer. *Int J Radiat Oncol Biol Phys* 2006;64:1151–1161.

66. Vargas C, Yan D, Kestin LL. Phase II dose escalation study of image-guided adaptive radiotherapy for prostate cancer: use of dose-volume constraints to achieve rectal isotoxicity. *Int J Radiat Oncol Biol Phys* 2005;63:141–149.

67. Akimoto T, Muramatsu H, Takahashi M. Rectal bleeding after hypofractionated radiotherapy for prostate cancer: correlation between clinical and dosimetric parameters and the incidence of grade 2 or worse rectal bleeding. *Int J Radiat Oncol Biol Phys* 2004;60:1033–1039.

68. Rancati T, Fiorino C, Gagliardi G. Fitting late rectal bleeding data using different NTCP models: results from an Italian multi-centric study (AIROPROS0101). *Radiother Oncol* 2004;73:21–32.

69. Zapatero A, Garcia-Vicente F, Modolell I. Impact of mean rectal dose on late rectal bleeding after conformal radiotherapy for prostate cancer: dose-volume effect. *Int J Radiat Oncol Biol Phys* 2004;59:1343–1351.

70. Tucker SL, Cheung R, Dong L. Dose-volume response analyses of late rectal bleeding after radiotherapy for prostate cancer. *Int J Radiat Oncol Biol Phys* 2004;59:353–365.

71. Koper PC, Heemsbergen WD, Hoogeman MS. Impact of volume and location of irradiated rectum wall on rectal blood loss after radiotherapy of prostate cancer. *Int J Radiat Oncol Biol Phys* 2004;58:1072–1082.

72. Greco C, Mazzetta C, Cattani F. Finding dose-volume constraints to reduce late rectal toxicity following 3D-conformal radiotherapy (3D-CRT) of prostate cancer. *Radiother Oncol* 2003;69:215–222.

73. Wachter S, Gerstner N, Goldner G. Rectal sequelae after conformal radiotherapy of prostate cancer: dose-volume histograms as predictive factors. *Radiother Oncol* 2001;59:65–70.

74. Fenwick JD, Khoo VS, Nahum AE. Correlations between dose-surface histograms and the incidence of long-term rectal bleeding following conformal or conventional radiotherapy treatment of prostate cancer. *Int J Radiat Oncol Biol Phys* 2001;49:473–480.

75. Jackson A, Skwarchuk MW, Zelefsky MJ. Late rectal bleeding after conformal radiotherapy of prostate

cancer. II. Volume effects and dose-volume histograms. *Int J Radiat Oncol Biol Phys* 2001;49:685–698.

76. Blanco AI, Chao KS, El Naqa I. Dose-volume modeling of salivary function in patients with head-and-neck cancer receiving radiotherapy. *Int J Radiat Oncol Biol Phys* 2005;62:1055–1069.

77. Chao KS, Deasy JO, Markman J. A prospective study of salivary function sparing in patients with head-and-neck cancers receiving intensity-modulated or three-dimensional radiation therapy: initial results. *Int J Radiat Oncol Biol Phys* 2001;49:907–916.

78. Johnson TD, Taylor JM, Ten Haken RK. A Bayesian mixture model relating dose to critical organs and functional complication in 3D conformal radiation therapy. *Biostatistics* 2005;6:615–632.

79. Eisbruch A, Dawson LA, Kim HM. Conformal and intensity modulated irradiation of head and neck cancer: the potential for improved target irradiation, salivary gland function, and quality of life. *Acta Otorhinolaryngol Belg* 1999;53:271–275.

80. Schilstra C, Meertens H. Calculation of the uncertainty in complication probability for various dose-response models, applied to the parotid gland. *Int J Radiat Oncol Biol Phys* 2001;50:147–158.

81. Honore HB, Bentzen SM, Moller K, et al. Sensorineural hearing loss after radiotherapy for nasopharyngeal carcinoma: individualized risk estimation. *Radiother Oncol* 2002;65:9–16.

82. Pan CC, Eisbruch A, Lee JS, et al. Prospective study of inner ear radiation dose and hearing loss in head-and-neck cancer patients. *Int J Radiat Oncol Biol Phys* 2005;61:1393–1402.

83. Chen WC, Jackson A, Budnick AS, et al. Sensorineural hearing loss in combined modality treatment of nasopharyngeal carcinoma. *Cancer* 2006;106:820–829.

84. Schultheiss TE, Kun LE, Ang KK. Radiation response of the central nervous system. *Int J Radiat Oncol Biol Phys* 1995;31:1093–1112.

85. Marucci L, Niemierko A, Liebsch NJ, et al. Spinal cord tolerance to high-dose fractionated 3D conformal proton-photon irradiation as evaluated by equivalent uniform dose and dose volume histogram analysis. *Int J Radiat Oncol Biol Phys* 2004;59:551–555.

86. Chin LS, Ma L, DiBiase S. Radiation necrosis following gamma knife surgery: a case-controlled comparison of treatment parameters and long-term clinical follow up. *J Neurosurg* 2001;94:899–904.

87. Flickinger JC, Lunsford LD, Wu A, et al. Predicted dose-volume isoeffect curves for stereotactic radiosurgery with the 60Co gamma unit. *Acta Oncol* 1991;30:363–367.

88. Levegrun S, Hof H, Essig M, et al. Radiation-induced changes of brain tissue after radiosurgery in patients with arteriovenous malformations: correlation with dose distribution parameters. *Int J Radiat Oncol Biol Phys* 2004;59:796–808.

89. Seppenwoolde Y, Lebesque JV. Partial irradiation of the lung. *Semin Radiat Oncol* 2001;11:247–258.

90. Jackson A. Partial irradiation of the rectum. *Semin Radiat Oncol* 2001;11:215–223.

91. Eisbruch A, Ship JA, Kim HM. Partial irradiation of the parotid gland. *Semin Radiat Oncol* 2001;11:234–239.

92. Travis EL. Lung morbidity of radiotherapy. In: Plowman PN, McElwin TJ, Meadows AT, eds. *Complications of cancer management.* Stonehan MA: Butterworth-Heinemann, 1991:232–249.

93. Marks LB. The pulmonary effects of thoracic irradiation. *Oncology* 1994;8:89–100.

94. Van Dyk J, Keane TJ, Khan S, et al. Radiation pneumonitis following large single dose irradiation: a re-evaluation based on absolute dose to lung. *Int J Radiat Oncol Biol Phys* 1981;7:461–467.

95. Wara WM, Phillips TL, Margolis LW, et al. Radiation pneumonitis: a new approach to the deterioration of time dose factors. *Cancer* 1973;32:547–552.

96. Perez CA, Stanley K, Rubin P, et al. A prospective randomized study of various irradiation doses and fractionation schedules in the treatment of inoperable non-oat-cell carcinoma of the lung. *Cancer* 1980;45:2744–2753.

97. Seydel HG, Diener-West M, Urtasun R, et al. Radiation Therapy Oncology Group (RTOG). Hyperfractionation in the radiation therapy of unresectable non-oat cell carcinoma of the lung: preliminary report of an RTOG pilot study. *Int J Radiat Oncol Biol Phys* 1985;11:1841–1847.

98. Rothwell RI, Kelly SA, Joslin CAF. Radiation pneumonitis in patients treated for breast cancer. *Radiother Oncol* 1985;4:9–14.

99. Brady LW, German PA, Cancer L. The effects of radiation therapy on pulmonary function in carcinoma of the lung. *Radiology* 1965;85:130–134.

100. Brady LW, Cancer L, Evans GC, et al. Carcinoma of the lung: results of supervoltage radiation. *Arch Surg* 1965;90:90–94.

101. Graham MV, Drzymala RE, Jain NL, et al. Confirmation of dose-volume histograms and normal tissue complication probability calculations to predict pulmonary complications after radiotherapy for lung cancer, reprint of talk given at 33rd Astro Meeting. *Int J Radiat Oncol Biol Phys* 1994;30(Suppl. 1):198.

102. Rosenzweig KE, Fox JL, Yorke E. Results of a phase I dose-escalation study using three-dimensional conformal radiotherapy in the treatment of inoperable nonsmall cell lung carcinoma. *Cancer* 2005;103:2118–2127.

103. Kong FM, Ten Haken RK, Schipper MJ, et al. High-dose radiation improved local tumor control and overall survival in patients with inoperable/unresectable non-small-cell lung cancer: long-term results of a radiation dose escalation study. *Int J Radiat Oncol Biol Phys* 2005;63:324–333.

104. Marks LB. Dosimetric predictors of radiation-induced lung injury. *Int J Radiat Oncol Biol Phys* 2002;54:313–316.

105. Marks LB, Munley MT, Spencer DP, et al. Quantification of radiation-induced regional lung injury with perfusion imaging. *Int J Radiat Oncol Biol Phys* 1997;38:399–409.

106. Theuws JC, Kwa SL, Wagenaar AC, et al. Dose-effect relations for early local pulmonary injury after irradiation for malignant lymphoma and breast cancer. *Radiother Oncol* 1998;48:33–43.

107. Kwa SL, Lebesque JV, Theuws JC. Radiation pneumonitis as a function of mean lung dose: an analysis of

pooled data of 540 patients. *Int J Radiat Oncol Biol Phys* 1998;42:1–9.

108. Kwa SL, Theuws JC, Wagenaar A. Evaluation of two dose-volume histogram reduction models for the prediction of radiation pneumonitis. *Radiother Oncol* 1998; 48:61–69.

109. Liao ZX, Travis EL, Tucker SL. Damage and morbidity from pneumonitis after irradiation of partial volumes of mouse lung. *Int J Radiat Oncol Biol Phys* 1995; 32:1359–1370.

110. Graham MV, Purdy JA, Emami B, et al. Preliminary results of a prospective trial using three dimensional radiotherapy for lung cancer. *Int J Radiat Oncol Biol Phys* 1995;33:993–1000.

111. Lawrence TS, Dworzanin LM, Walker-Andrews SC, et al. Treatment of cancers involving the liver and porta hepatis with external beam irradiation and intraarterial hepatic fluorodeoxyuridine. *Int J Radiat Oncol Biol Phys* 1991;20:555–561.

112. McGinn CJ, Ten Haken RK, Ensminger WD, et al. Treatment of intrahepatic cancers with radiation doses based on a normal tissue complication probability model. *J Clin Oncol* 1998;16:2246–2252.

113. Dawson LA, McGinn CJ, Normolle D, et al. Escalated focal liver radiation and concurrent hepatic artery fluorodeoxyuridine for unresectable intrahepatic malignancies. *J Clin Oncol* 2000;18:2210–2218.

114. Ben-Josef E, Normolle D, Ensminger WD, et al. Phase II trial of high-dose conformal radiation therapy with concurrent hepatic artery floxuridine for unresectable intrahepatic malignancies. *J Clin Oncol* 2005;23:8739–8747.

115. Sandler HM, Perez-Tamayo C, Ten Haken RK, et al. Dose escalation for stage C (T3) prostate cancer: minimal rectal toxicity observed using conformal therapy. *Radiother Oncol* 1992;23:53–54.

116. Sandler HM, McLaughlin PW, Ten Haken RK, et al. Three dimensional conformal radiotherapy for the treatment of prostate cancer: low risk of chronic rectal morbidity observed in a large series of patients. *Int J Radiat Oncol Biol Phys* 1995;33:797–801.

117. Schultheiss TE, Hanks GE, Hunt MA, et al. Incidence of and factors related to late complications in conformal and conventional radiation treatment of cancer of the prostate. *Int J Radiat Oncol Biol Phys* 1995;32:643–649.

118. Schultheiss TE, Lee WR, Hunt MA, et al. Late GI and GU complications in the treatment of prostate cancer. *Int J Radiat Oncol Biol Phys* 1997;37:3–11.

119. Zelefsky MJ, Leibel SA, Kutcher GJ, et al. The feasibility of dose escalation with three dimensional conformal radiotherapy in patients with prostatic carcinoma. *Cancer J* 1995;1:142–150.

120. Zelefsky MJ, Cowen D, Fuks Z, et al. Long term tolerance of high dose three-dimensional conformal radiotherapy in patients with localized prostate carcinoma. *Cancer* 1999;85:2460–2468.

121. Benk VA, Adams JA, Shipley WU, et al. Late rectal bleeding following combined x-rays and proton high dose irradiation for patients with stages T3-T4 prostate carcinoma. *Int J Radiat Oncol Biol Phys* 1993;26:551–557.

122. Hartford AC, Niemierko A, Adams JA. Conformal irradiation of the prostate: estimating long-term rectal bleeding risk using dose-volume histograms. *Int J Radiat Oncol Biol Phys* 1996;36:721–730.

123. Boersma LJ, Van Den Brink M, Bruce AM, et al. Estimation of the incidence of late bladder and rectum complications after high-dose (70–78 GY) conformal radiotherapy for prostate cancer, using dose-volume histograms. *Int J Radiat Oncol Biol Phys* 1998;41:83–92.

124. Storey MR, Pollack A, Zagars G, et al. Complications from radiotherapy dose escalation in prostate cancer: preliminary results of a randomized trial. *Int J Radiat Oncol Biol Phys* 2000;48:635–642.

125. Skwarchuk MW, Jackson A, Zelefsky MJ, et al. Late rectal toxicity after conformal radiotherapy of prostate cancer (I): multivariate analysis and dose-response. *Int J Radiat Oncol Biol Phys* 2000;47:103–113.

126. Fiorino C, Sanguineti G, Cozzarini C, et al. Rectal dose-volume constraints in high-dose radiotherapy of localized prostate cancer. *Int J Radiat Oncol Biol Phys* 2003;57(4):953–962.

127. Cozzarini C, Fiorino C, Ceresoli GL, et al. Significant correlation between rectal DVH and late bleeding in patients treated after radical prostatectomy with conformal or conventional radiotherapy (66.6–70.2 Gy). *Int J Radiat Oncol Biol Phys* 2003;55:688–694.

128. Zelefsky MJ, Fuks Z, Hunt M, et al. High-dose intensity modulated radiation therapy for prostate cancer: early toxicity and biochemical outcome in 772 patients. *Int J Radiat Oncol Biol Phys* 2002;53:1111–1116.

129. de Crevoisier R, Tucker SL, Dong L, et al. Increased risk of biochemical and local failure in patients with distended rectum on the planning CT for prostate cancer radiotherapy. *Int J Radiat Oncol Biol Phys* 2005;62:965–973.

130. Fenwick JD, Nahum AE. Impact of dose-distribution uncertainties on rectal NTCP modeling. I: Uncertainty estimates. *Med Phys* 2001;28:560–569.

131. Fenwick JD. Impact of dose-distribution uncertainties on rectal NTCP modeling. II: uncertainty implications. *Med Phys* 2001;28:570–581.

132. Rodrigues G, Lock M, D'Souza D. Prediction of radiation pneumonitis by dose-volume histogram parameters in lung cancer–a systematic review. *Radiother Oncol* 2004;71:127–138.

133. Jackson A, Yorke ED, Rosenzweig K. Atlas of Complication Incidence: a proposal for a new standard for reporting the results of radiotherapy protocols. *Semin Radiat Oncol* 2006;16(4):260–268.

134. Kutcher GJ, Niehaus A, Yorke ED. The effect of normal organ architecture on 3D conformal strategies. In: Hounsell AR, Wilkinson JM, Williams PC, eds. *Proceedings of the XIth international conference on the use of computers in radiotherapy.* Manchester: Northwestern Medical Physics Department, 1994:10–11.

135. Jackson A, Yorke ED. NTCP and TCP for treatment planning. In: Fuks Z, Leibel S, Ling C, eds. *A practical guide to intensity modulated radiation therapy.* Madison, WI: Medical Physics Publishing, 2003:287–316.

136. Kutcher GJ. Quantitative plan evaluation. In: Purdy JA, Simpson LR, eds. *Advances in radiation oncology physics: dosimetry, treatment planning, brachytherapy.* New York, NY: American Institute of Physics, 1992:998–1021.

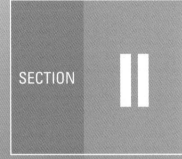

SECTION **II**

Treatment Planning for Specific Cancers

CHAPTER 24

Cancers of the Gastrointestinal Tract

Matthew D. Callister ■ Jonathan B. Ashman

INTRODUCTION

Radiotherapy in combination with chemotherapy has a significant role in the treatment of cancers of the anus, rectum, pancreas, stomach, and esophagus. The role of combined-modality therapy in the treatment of these diseases has been defined largely as a result of several prospective clinical trials conducted over the past 20 years. This chapter reviews the technical aspects of treatment of gastrointestinal cancer, with particular emphasis on anatomic target definitions and modern treatment planning techniques.

ANAL CANCER

In 2009, there were an estimated 5,290 new cases on anal cancer diagnosed in the United States (1). Given the favorable results of radiotherapy, either alone or in combination with chemotherapy, a sphincter-preserving approach is the standard of care for this disease.

Diagnostic Evaluation

The patient history and a thorough physical examination are essential for a successful treatment planning for patients with anal cancer. Risk factors for HIV infection should be reviewed with a low threshold for ordering laboratory testing if indicated. Careful review of gastrointestinal and genitourinary symptoms may indicate extension of tumor beyond what is clinically or radiographically detected.

The physical examination should give particular attention to the inguinal-femoral lymph nodes and anorectal canal. Inguinal nodes which contain gross metastatic disease on exam or imaging will be treated to a higher radiotherapeutic dose than areas requiring only elective treatment. Therefore, consideration should be given to fine needle aspiration of groin nodes of indeterminate size (≥1–1.5 cm) prior to treatment planning. Thorough examination of the perianal skin and anorectal canal is imperative for accurate treatment planning as it often reveals disease beyond what is visible on imaging studies alone. When patients have severe anal discomfort that inhibits adequate examination, such examination can be scheduled under anesthesia. Attention should be made to the proximal and distal extent of the tumor in relation to the anal margin as well as any perianal extension of disease. Among

female patients, the radiation oncologist should perform a complete pelvic examination given the proximity of the anal canal to the lower posterior vaginal wall. In addition, the anatomic extent of disease reported on anoscopy or proctoscopy should be carefully reviewed.

Imaging studies should complement the history and physical examination in defining the extent of local-regional disease as well as detection of distant metastases. The abdomen and pelvis must be evaluated with either magnetic resonance imaging (MRI) or computed tomography (CT). Positron emission tomography (PET) may be of value in detecting regional or distant spread of disease not discernable by CT (2) and may alter radiotherapy field design (3). Endoscopic ultrasound (EUS) gives more accurate determination of the depth of tumor invasion than physical exam and may be of prognostic value (4), but is not required for treatment planning or staging.

Treatment Options

Patients with carcinoma of the anal canal should generally be treated with definitive radiotherapy. Chemotherapy is administered concurrently for all patients except those who are medically unfit or have very small tumors. The addition of mitomycin-C and 5-fluorouracil (5-FU) to radiotherapy has been shown to improve local control, colostomy-free survival, and disease-free survival (5–7). Patients who are HIV positive may be considered for combined-modality therapy if they are sufficiently immunocompetent (as defined by CD4 count). Carcinoma *in situ* and tumors of the perianal skin (which do not extend past the anal verge), should initially be considered for local excision. When these lesions cannot be excised adequately without significantly compromising anal function, definitive RT alone is an efficacious option. Abdominoperineal resection is reserved as salvage treatment for patients with persistent or recurrent disease after radiotherapy.

Treatment Planning

Simulation

The patient is simulated in the supine or prone position depending on the treatment technique selected (see section on "Radiotherapy Fields and Techniques"), though prone positioning may be less reproducible. The bladder may be distended to decrease the amount of small bowel within the pelvis. To reduce skin toxicity, cutaneous folds within the medial groin may be minimized by moderately abducting the patient's legs and using an immobilization device to ensure setup reproducibility of the lower extremities. The clinical extent of any visible or palpable perianal tumor should be demarcated with radiopaque markers as it may not be apparent on simulation imaging. The anal verge should also be marked and the rectum may be visualized with rectal contrast. The amount of exposed anal tumor posteriorly can vary significantly depending on degree of perineal extension, body habitus, and leg positioning. This should be noted at the time of simulation to ensure proper beam selection and occasionally bolus may be indicated with posterior beams in a thin patient due to exposed tumor. Oral contrast assists in small-bowel visualization. The use of CT-based targeting and treatment planning is critical for accurate treatment of the inguinal lymph nodes and to complement the findings of physical examination in regards to the extent of the primary tumor.

Radiotherapy Target

The radiotherapy target includes the primary tumor, clinically involved lymph nodes, as well as perianal tissues and regional lymphatics at risk for subclinical spread of disease. All diagnostic information should be used together (imaging, physical exam, and endoscopy) to define the maximal extent of the gross tumor volume (GTV) for the primary lesion and any involved lymph nodes. Treatment planning that relies solely on the images from a planning CT risks underestimation of the full extent of tumor involvement.

The clinical target volume(s) includes inguinal-pelvic lymphatics and perianal tissues. Adjacent to the primary anal tumor, the CTV should include a 1 to 2 cm radial margin of surrounding soft tissue. Longitudinally, it should include any portions of the anal canal not involved by tumor, including at least 2 cm of normal mucosal or skin margin. The CTV also includes the inguinal and pelvic lymph nodes. Data from abdominoperineal resection series document a pelvic nodal involvement rate of 35% and a subsequent inguinal nodal failure rate of 13% (8) (without dissection). Similarly, an inguinal nodal failure rate of 15% is reported in a radiotherapy series without elective groin treatment (9).

Traditional radiotherapy fields have included inguinal lymph nodes generally based on bony landmarks and palpation. Accurate definition of this nodal station by CT imaging requires more than just identifying the femoral blood vessels. The inguinal lymph nodes are located within the fatty tissue throughout the femoral triangle. The medial border of this triangle is the pubic tubercle and the adductor longus muscle. The lateral border is the sartorius muscle, including the fatty tissues underneath this muscle. The inferior apex of the femoral triangle is where the sartorius and adductor longus muscle intersect in the sagittal plane (generally where the deep branches of the femoral artery and vein originate). The superior extent of the femoral triangle is the inguinal ligament. The ligament is difficult to delineate by CT, but can be reproduced as a line from the pubic tubercle to the anterior superior iliac spine. The floor of the femoral triangle is the flexor muscles of the hip, but the lymph nodes lay in the fatty tissue at and anterior to the level of the femoral vessels. Extension of radiotherapy fields to cover the far lateral inguinal region adjacent to the anterior superior iliac spine may be of little benefit based on lymphangiogram and surgical dissection data (10).

Pelvic lymph nodes included in the CTV are the external and internal iliac, perirectal, and presacral nodal regions. As the superior extent of traditional fields for pelvic nodal treatment is generally the L5–S1 interspace, the lower portion of the common iliac lymph nodes may be included as well. In defining these nodal areas, contouring should not be limited to pelvic vasculature alone. The adjacent soft tissues of the pelvic sidewall and presacral area must be included (see section on "Radiotherapy Target" under section "Rectal Cancer"). A Radiation Therapy Oncology Group (RTOG) panel prepared detailed excellent review of the CTV for lower gastrointestinal cancers which serves as an excellent reference in target definition during treatment planning (11).

The planning target volume (PTV) should be an expansion of the CTV sufficient to account for organ motion and patient setup error. A minimum PTV of 1 cm beyond the CTV is appropriate, though smaller margins may be used if image-guided radiotherapy (IGRT) is employed.

Normal Tissue Tolerances

The amount of small bowel treated to >45 Gy should be minimized. Although this is generally achievable due to the inferior location of the boost target volume, large volumes of bowel receiving even moderate doses of radiation (as low as 15–30 Gy) probably contribute to acute toxicity (12) and should be minimized when possible. The femoral heads and necks should receive <45 Gy (13), and preferably <40 Gy. The perianal skin develops significant moist desquamation as a result of combined-modality therapy. Dosimetric hot spots in this region should be avoided. Although treatment breaks are commonly employed in the treatment of anal cancer due to acute skin toxicity (as well as gastrointestinal and hematological side effects), prolongation of overall treatment time has been associated with a detriment in local control (14,15). In the absence of infection, treatment breaks for skin toxicity alone should not be systematically scheduled, but instead should be avoided when possible, with aggressive supportive measures.

Radiotherapy Dose

The appropriate dose for elective nodal sites has not been well defined. In RTOG 87-04, 30.6 Gy in 1.8 Gy fractions was delivered to initial pelvic fields with the superior border placed at the L4–L5 interspace (5). Subsequently, the superior field borders were reduced to the bottom of the sacroiliac joints, and the pelvis and inguinal nodes continued treatment to 36 Gy. Finally, 10 × 10 cm fields which included the primary tumor and lowermost pelvis were treated to cumulative doses of 45 to 50.4 Gy. In RTOG 98–11, the initial pelvic fields were treated to 30.6 Gy with the superior border placed at L5–S1 (16). Reducing the superior border to the bottom of the sacroiliac joints, the lower pelvis was treated to 45 Gy. The inguinal lymph nodes electively received 36 Gy. Although successive pelvic field reductions probably address the gradient of risk for micrometastatic disease within lymph nodes, retrospective series suggest that doses as low as 30 Gy with concurrent chemotherapy may be sufficient to achieve control of subclinical disease within nodes or at the primary site after excisional biopsy of small lesions (17–19). When concurrently treating multiple targets at different doses per fraction (i.e., IMRT), higher total doses may be indicated for regions receiving <1.8 Gy/day (20).

Only small primary tumors that have completely responded to radiation should be treated to 45 to 50.4 Gy. Larger tumors (T3/T4) and incompletely responding tumors should receive 54 to 59 Gy. Multiple retrospective series have reported superior local control rates in this dose range compared to lower doses (9,17,21). For patients treated with radiotherapy alone, the primary tumor should receive a cumulative dose of 60 to 63 Gy (22).

Radiotherapy Fields and Techniques

The treatment of patients with anal cancer can be technically challenging given the complex geometric distribution of targets, particularly the inguinal nodes, in relationship to normal pelvic structures. Most of the reported techniques have been devised to enable safe treatment of the inguinal lymph nodes overlying the femoral heads, while there has been less emphasis on techniques to minimize unnecessary dose to the genitalia, bladder, and small bowel. The risk of femoral neck fracture is rare at doses below 45 Gy, but significantly increases after 50 Gy (13). Treatment designed to treat inguinal lymph nodes but spare the femoral head and neck should be done cautiously. The deep inguinal lymph nodes (defined at the depth of the femoral vessels) are generally much deeper than has been historically appreciated. These nodes are routinely deeper than 3 cm and in the majority of patients may lie 5 to 6 cm from the surface (23–25), beyond the effective treatment depth of some electron techniques. Care must be taken to determine the depth of the inguinal vessels on the treatment planning CT and choose an appropriate treatment technique. Patient body habitus may influence not only depth of lymph nodes, but also the selection of the optimal technique for delivery of radiation (26).

Below is discussion of some of the common external beam techniques for treating anal cancer. Each approach has relative advantages and disadvantages, which are somewhat dependent on the radiation dose prescribed to elective nodes.

1. 3D/IMRT: There are only limited reports of treatment of anal cancer with more sophisticated treatment planning techniques, but improvements in conformality of dose to targets could lead to reductions in normal tissue complications. Vuong et al. (27) have reported encouraging acute toxicity outcome among 30 patients with anal cancer treated with a complex 3D conformal technique.

   Initial dosimetric analysis of the use of IMRT in treating anal cancer has also shown promise in regards to conformality and sparing of the genitalia, small bowel, bladder, bone marrow, and femoral necks (see Fig. 24.1)

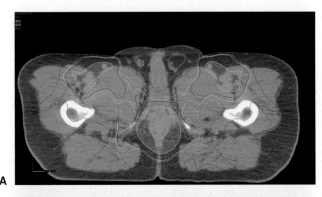
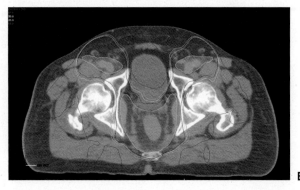
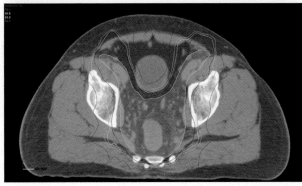

Figure 24.1. A 64-year-old male with a T_2N_0 SCC of the anal canal, treated with an eight-field IMRT technique. Representative axial dosimetry in the groin (**A**), lower pelvis (**B**), and mid-pelvis (**C**). (CTV is shown in *blue*; *red, yellow, green,* and *purple lines* represent 95%, 90%, 85%, and 65% isodose lines, respectively.)

(28–31). Actual treatment with IMRT has been reported in a limited number of series with favorable toxicity and clinical outcomes (32,33). Preliminary results of RTOG 0529, a phase II trial of IMRT with concurrent chemotherapy, showed an encouraging reduction in the expected rate of gastrointestinal, genitourinary, and dermatologic toxicity (20). While attempting to spare normal tissues with these techniques, precise contouring of treatment targets is critical in order to avoid inadvertently undertreating regions of risk previously included in clinical trials.

2. Wide AP/Narrow PA (see Fig. 24.2): A wide AP photon field, which includes the inguinal lymph nodes is simulated with a narrow PA field that excludes the femoral neck (may include a small sliver of the medial femoral head for margin on the obturator nodes). Due to divergence, it is occasionally possible to match the lateral exit of the narrow PA beam with the surface entrance of the wide AP photon beam and provide sufficient dosimetric

coverage of the groins (26). More commonly, however, supplemental anterior electrons are indicated. The lateral exit of the narrow PA field is marked anteriorly on the patient's groins (easily done at time of fluoroscopic simulation). This serves as the medial border for each electron supplement. The lateral border of each electron supplement is placed at or 1 cm lateral (due to beam constriction) to the surface entrance of the wide anterior photon beam. Particular attention must be made during treatment to any shifts made with the PA field to ensure similar movement in the anterior electron field junctions. Radiopaque wire place on these junctions may assist proper setup when porting the PA field. To reduce the complexities associated with electron groin setups, photons have also been used to supplement the lateral inguinal lymph nodes using the same AP photon field and setup. This can be achieved by the use of a central (pelvic) partial-transmission block (34) or with multi-leaf collimation (35,36).

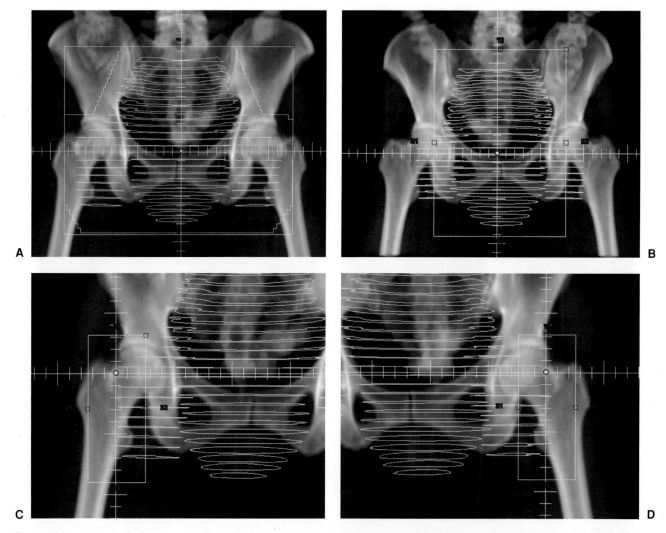

Figure 24.2. A 61-year-old female with T₃N₂ SCC of the anal canal treated with a "wide" AP (**A**) and "narrow" PA (**B**) photon fields which encompass the primary anal tumor (GTV not shown) and inguinal/pelvic lymph nodes (CTV). *Right* (**C**) and *left* (**D**) electron groin fields supplement the lateral inguinal regions excluded from the PA field. The lateral borders of the electron field extend slightly beyond the "wide" AP photon field to account for beam convergence.

3. Wide AP/Wide PA: Photon fields are devised to encompass the primary tumor and pelvis and laterally extend to encompass the inguinal lymph nodes ("wide") in both the AP and PA fields (13,17). This field arrangement is the most simple as it requires no field matching, reducing the chance of technical error or underdosing the inguinal lymph nodes. Without the use of electrons, patients can be treated in the prone position, possibly reducing the amount of small bowel in the pelvis. The obvious disadvantage is that there is no sparing of the femoral neck, genitalia, and bladder. However, if moderate doses are selected for elective nodal irradiation, doses to these structures may be kept well within organ tolerance. Series from the M.D. Anderson Cancer Center have reported the use of this technique (17,37). The initial 30.6 Gy of radiation (pelvis and groins) is delivered with wide photon AP–PA fields. Subsequently the patient's lower pelvis is resimulated with prone positioning on a belly-board using a three-field technique (narrow PA excluding lateral groins and lateral fields) for an additional 19.8 Gy. During this phase, inguinal lymph nodes are supplemented with anterior electrons (patient flipped supine), only if initially involved with tumor. Finally, the primary tumor is boosted to an appropriate final dose.

4. Four-field Technique: With this technique, three of the photon fields (AP and laterals) include the pelvis and inguinal region while the PA field is kept "narrow" to exclude the femurs. With appropriate beam weighting and energy selection, sufficient dose can usually be delivered to the inguinal nodes, as verified with computerized treatment planning. Patients may be treated in the prone position, reducing bowel within the pelvis. There are two variations of a four-field technique. First, an AP field is simulated "wide" and the PA field is kept "narrow" as above. The lateral fields, however, exclude the inguinal region (anterior border is placed at the pubic symphysis) and anterior electrons groin fields are then used to supplement the wide AP field (38). In the other variation, the patient may be treated prone on a belly-board with a wide PA field which exists through the groins and lateral fields which exclude the inguinal lymph nodes (three fields) (39). Supplementation of the groins with anterior electron fields is administered in the supine position. Although these techniques often reduce dose to the medial inguinal skin and genitalia, they both require complex setup and creation of a somewhat imprecise internal junction between the distal electron dose gradient and the lateral photon beams edges.

Boost Planning

With the exception of dose-painted intensity-modulated radiation therapy (IMRT), the GTV (both the primary tumor and the involved lymph nodes) should be boosted with reduced fields encompassing tumor with a 2 to 3 cm margin to the field edge. Using 3D definitions, a boost PTV of at least 1 to 1.5 cm around the GTV is appropriate with additional dosimetric margin to the field edge. When possible, a composite representation of dose between the initial and boost treatments should be created to ensure normal organ tolerance is not exceeded during the boost phase of treatment. A variety of beam arrangements may be used. Separate boost fields for involved inguinal lymph nodes are usually necessary but care should be taken not to concurrently overlap any tissues irradiated by the boost treatment to the anus. Boosting the primary lesion with a perineal field precludes CT planning in the treatment position and should be reserved for tumors that can be completely exposed to ensure coverage (e.g., tumors of the anal margin).

Chemotherapy

Careful coordination of the timing of concurrent chemotherapy with the delivery of radiation is important for successful treatment of anal cancer. The addition of mitomycin-C (10 mg/m^2 on days 1 and 29 of radiotherapy) to 5-FU (1 g/m^2/day for 96 hours on days 1–4 and 29–32 of radiotherapy) was established as the standard of care by the results of RTOG 87-04 (5), which compared both drugs to concurrent 5-FU alone. Treatment should begin on a Monday or Tuesday so that radiotherapy may be given on each day of chemotherapy delivery (4 days of 5-FU). As an alternative to mitomycin-C, multiple institutions have reported excellent results and with cisplatin and 5-FU concurrent with radiation (37,40). However, in RTOG 98-11, cisplatin and 5-FU, given as induction therapy and concurrent with RT, have not been found superior to RT concurrent with mitomycin-C and 5-FU (16).

Prognosis

The outcome of patients treated with combined-modality therapy is well described from the results of randomized trials (5–7,16). Favorable outcome is somewhat dependent clinical stage but long-term local control, colostomy-free survival, and overall survival are approximately 70%, 70%, and 60% to 70%, respectively among patients receiving combined-modality therapy. Among patients who fail treatment locally, 50% have been salvaged with surgical resection (5).

COLORECTAL CANCER

In 2009, there were an estimated 106,100 cancers of the colon and 40,870 cancers of the rectum diagnosed in the United States (1). Collectively, these cancers account for 9% of overall cancer incidence and death among both men and women. Radiotherapy plays an important neoadjuvant or adjuvant role in the management of rectal cancers, which penetrate bowel wall or spread to adjacent lymph nodes, but is uncommonly indicated in the treatment of colon cancer.

Diagnostic Evaluation

Careful diagnostic evaluation is essential not only for accurate staging and selection of patients for neoadjuvant strategies, but also to assist appropriate target definition during treatment planning. During the patient history, careful attention should be given not only to bowel-related symptoms, but also to indicators of local tumor extension into other pelvic structures (bladder/prostate or pelvic wall). The radiation oncologist's digital rectal examination should assess the distance of the tumor from the anal verge, size and location, degree of circumferential involvement, and palpable morphology. The mobility of palpable lesions is described as mobile, tethered, or fixed, the latter implying initial unresectability. Proximal rectal cancers that are not palpable are referenced to the anal verge by endoscopy. Measurements from flexible endoscopies should be relied upon with caution as they are notoriously imprecise and inconsistent between exams. Measurements from rigid proctoscopy tend to be more reliable.

Pretreatment imaging is not only important to rule out distant metastases, but also to determine patients who are candidates for neoadjuvant chemoradiotherapy. EUS or MRI has been reported superior to CT in both determination of tumor depth of penetration (T stage) and detection of perirectal adenopathy (41). High-resolution MRI may be of particular benefit in predicting involvement of circumferential resection margin (42,43). Pelvic CT or MRI is indicated for the evaluation of pelvic lymphatic stations beyond perirectal lymph nodes. Among patients with locally advanced disease, PET has detected liver metastases in up to 8% of patients, which were not identified by other modalities (44). PET does not have sufficient spatial resolution to determine depth of tumor penetration nor consistently distinguish perirectal adenopathy from adjacent tumor.

Treatment Options

The use of adjuvant or neoadjuvant radiotherapy is generally reserved for patients whose tumors penetrate the bowel wall ($\geq$T3) or are node positive. Among such patients, randomized trials clearly support the benefit adjuvant combined-modality therapy (pelvic radiotherapy and 5-FU-based chemotherapy) in regards to both local control and overall survival (45–47). The German Rectal Cancer Study Group reported improvement in local control with preoperative chemoradiotherapy versus similar postoperative treatment (5-year local relapse rate of 6% vs. 13%, $p = 0.006$) (48). In addition, randomized trials of hypofractionated pelvic radiotherapy versus surgery alone have shown improvement in overall survival (49) as well as local control, even among patients undergoing total mesorectal excision (TME) (50). The presence of node positivity or penetration of tumor through the bowel wall needs to be determined by EUS or MRI in order to justify a neoadjuvant approach.

Adjuvant radiotherapy for patients with colon cancer is not indicated. Although retrospective series have shown favorable local control outcomes with the use of adjuvant radiotherapy among patients with T4 tumors and selected T3 tumors, and positive lymph nodes (51,52), this has not be corroborated in clinical trials. Among such patients, Martenson et al. (53) reported the results of a randomized trial, which studied the use of adjuvant chemoradiotherapy but did not detect a benefit to patient survival. Preoperative treatment may be considered in patients whose tumors are considered unresectable at presentation.

Treatment Planning

Simulation

Proper patient positioning can significantly reduce the amount of small bowel within the pelvis and limit toxicity from treatment. In addition to decreasing the volume of bowel receiving maximal organ tolerance (45–50 Gy), reduction of bowel receiving doses as low as 5 Gy has been associated with improved patient tolerance to pelvic radiation (12,54,55). Maximal displacement of small bowel out of the pelvis is achieved with prone positioning and bladder distension. Without the use of a belly-board or lower abdominal wall compression, however, ~25% of patients will have *more* small bowel in the pelvis with prone positioning compared to supine (more commonly in obese patients) (56). Multiple studies have documented significant reduction in pelvic small-bowel volume with use of a belly-board device (57–59) or lower abdominal wall compression (56). Bladder distension may actually contribute more to bowel displacement than a belly-board, but the effect of each method appears additive (60) and concurrent use of both techniques should be considered. Although these efforts displace bowel from the pelvis, they may also be less reproducible and be associated with variation in patient setup, which is undesirable when employing highly conformal radiation techniques.

Although small-bowel series are useful during fluoroscopic simulation, CT-based planning provides more complete identification of bowel, especially any that does not opacify with contrast (61). Small bowel has been shown to be more mobile in patients treated preoperatively than after surgical intervention (61). To ensure there has been no significant change in bowel positioning during treatment, consideration may be given to repeat CT-imaging at the time of boost planning for patients whose total pelvic radiation doses approach or exceed bowel tolerance.

Simulation in the prone position enables access for digital rectal examination. This allows verification of lower and middle rectal lesion location in relationship to the anal verge, while maintaining the treatment position. The anal verge should be marked with a radiopaque marker and rectal contrast instilled into the rectum to assist radiographic identification of the primary lesion. Insufflation of a small amount of air into the rectum (50 cc) may further assist in identification of the rectal mass (62). Taping the buttocks laterally may reduce their self-bolusing effect on the perianal skin during treatment, but is of questionable reproducibility. Patients who have undergone abdominoperineal resection must have the perineal scar marked and included in the initial pelvic fields, with appropriate bolus utilized posteriorly if exposed. Perineal recurrence has been described in 8% to 30% of patients in the absence of adjuvant RT (63–65), but as low as 2% when the scar is adequately treated (66).

Radiotherapy Target

For patients treated preoperatively, the GTV includes the primary tumor and any radiographically enlarged lymph nodes. All clinical, endoscopic, and imaging information must be used to define the maximal extent of the rectal tumor. Relying solely on one modality risks underestimation of the tumor extent and inaccurate field design (especially within boost portals). Although not mandatory in treatment planning, the addition of PET to CT in GTV contouring has been shown to increase the target size by an average of 25% (67) and lead to change in treatment fields in 17% of patients (68). Soft-tissue extension or suspected infiltration of rectal tumors into adjacent mesorectal fat should be included within the GTV, particularly posteriorly.

The CTV encompasses all the perirectal tissue, presacral space, and lymphatics of the internal iliac chain (which are not commonly dissected at the time of surgery). A report of 269 cases of rectal cancer that recurred in the pelvis after surgery alone emphasized the predilection for rectal cancer recurrence in the posterior pelvis, specifically the presacral space. Among patients undergoing anterior resection, 93% recurred at or posterior to the colorectal anastomosis (69). Other studies of rectal cancer failure patterns have also shown infrequent recurrence above the S1–S2 interspace, lateral pelvic nodes, or in the anal sphincter (70,71).

Accurate contouring of the pelvic CTV involves more than simply identifying the internal iliac vessels. A study comparing locations of external and common pelvic lymphatics (by lymphangiography) to vessel location revealed that lymph nodes are not directly superimposable upon vasculature (72). Myerson et al. (62) and Roels et al. (73) provide an excellent review of CT-based treatment planning for rectal cancer. In the upper pelvis, the CTV should extend cephalad to include the sacral promontory, posteriorly to include the anterior wall of the sacrum, and laterally it should encompass vasculature and presacral soft tissue to the border of the iliopsoas muscles. In the mid-pelvis, the CTV includes similar tissues with care taken to include perirectal fat anterior to the rectum. In addition, 1 to 2 cm of posterior bladder or uterus may be included if at risk of subclinical extension of disease for patients who have adjacent, locally advanced lesions. In the lower pelvis, the CTV includes all the perirectal fat inferiorly and laterally extending to the levator ani muscles. It should extend to the posterior wall of the prostate or vagina as well. A larger margin of anterior pelvic organs is indicated for tumors with documented invasion (T4). The CTV should also include 2 cm of normal rectum cephalad and caudad to the primary tumor. With a subsequent PTV expansion of at least 1 cm

(without IGRT) around the CTV, this will provide a minimum 4 cm longitudinal margin from GTV to block edge (assuming an additional 1 cm beyond PTV to block edge for dosimetric buildup). Given the distensibility of the rectum, more PTV margin may be indicated anteriorly, especially for anterior wall tumors of the mid- and upper rectum. Bladder, small bowel, and femoral heads should also be contoured for evaluation of normal tissue tolerance.

The inclusion of the external iliac lymph nodes is generally reserved for patients with T4 tumors, which extend into anterior organs of the pelvis (prostate, bladder, vagina, and cervix/uterus) for whom these nodes are at risk. This modification is supported by failure patterns (69) from patients treated with surgery alone. However, in a series of patients with T4 rectal cancers where external iliac lymph nodes were not routinely included within RT portals, regional recurrence of disease still occurred almost exclusively within the radiotherapy field (74).

Tumors of the lower rectum, which extend to the dentate line of the anal canal, have a theoretical risk of failure in the inguinal lymph nodes. A report of 184 patients with such lesions revealed only six groin failures (5-year actuarial rate of 4%) without elective radiotherapy to the inguinal lymph nodes (75). Thus, for patients with low-lying rectal cancers, careful attention should be given to the groins during initial staging, but the added toxicity of treatment does not seem justified if the inguinal nodes are clinically negative.

In the postoperative setting, treatment volumes are similar except that with the removal of the primary lesion, the entire preoperative tumor bed must be reconstructed and included within the CTV (often identified separately as a boost volume—CTV2). Review of preoperative imaging, operative reports and surgical clip placement is imperative. As mentioned above, the perineal scar must be included in the initial fields for patients who have undergone abdominoperineal resection.

To account for internal target motion and patient setup variability, a PTV is delineated beyond the CTV. In the absence of IGRT, PTV margin of at least 1 cm is appropriate. However, retrospective study of interfraction variability has shown that in the patient setup without IGRT can easily approach these margins, especially among patients with large body mass index treated in the prone position (76). Intrafraction movement of the mesorectum has also been evaluated and found on average to move <4 mm in various dimensions, but significant individual variability is observed (77).

Normal Tissue Tolerances

The amount of small bowel receiving 45 Gy should be minimized without compromising target coverage. Any small bowel within the boost volume of treatment should be limited and not receive beyond 50 Gy. In addition to maximum dose, acute intestinal side effects from pelvic radiotherapy have been found to correlate with volume of bowel receiving all dose levels to as low as 5 Gy (54,55). Thus, bowel exposure at any dose should be minimized.

The femoral heads and necks should receive <45 Gy (13), and preferably <40 Gy. Blocking in the lateral fields excludes the anterior genitalia in addition to small bowel.

Radiotherapy Dose

There is very little data in literature regarding the optimal radiotherapy dose in the treatment of rectal cancer. One retrospective study supporting current dosing guidelines is from Brizel and Timmerman (78) who observed superior local control with adjuvant radiotherapy doses ≥45 Gy compared to patients who received less dose. Forty-five Gy, given in 1.8 Gy fractions, is the currently accepted dose and fractionation for initial pelvic fields based on its repeated use in clinic trial designs (47,79). After the initial 45 Gy, a boost of 5.4 Gy is generally given to the GTV in preoperative cases and a 5.4 to 9 Gy boost is delivered to the tumor bed (CTV2) in the postoperative setting with careful attention to minimize small bowel within the field. Treating beyond a cumulative dose of 50 Gy should only be considered when small bowel can be completely excluded from this high-dose region of treatment.

Radiotherapy Fields and Techniques

Patients are commonly treated with a three-field technique consisting of a PA and laterals (see Fig. 24.3). When inclusion of the anterior pelvis is indicated (e.g., treatment of the external iliac lymph nodes), an additional AP field may be advantageous dosimetrically. High energy photons and appropriate beam wedging and weighting are mandatory to ensure a homogenous dose distribution within the pelvis.

Traditional field design has been based on boney landmarks, the location of contrast-enhanced bowel/rectum and the anal verge. The superior border of the PA (and AP) fields generally covers the sacral promontory while the inferior border is placed at least 3 to 4 cm distal to the rectal cancer. For upper rectal cancers, the distal border need not include the entire anal canal, but should extend to the dentate line (about 2 cm from the anal verge) so that all the mesorectum is encompassed. The lateral borders of the PA field should include 1.5 to 2 cm margin beyond the pelvic brim, with appropriate blocking of almost all of the femoral head. Lateral fields should cover the anterior bony margin of sacrum with 1.5 to 2 cm margin posteriorly to allow for setup error and dosimetric coverage. Anteriorly, the field includes the internal iliac lymph nodes by placing its border on the posterior edge of pubic symphysis. Care is taken, however, when devising this border to ensure at least 3 cm coverage of the primary tumor anteriorly. In the superior-anterior portion of the field, it is usually possible to block a portion of small bowel. Similarly, the anterior genitalia in most patients should be blocked in the lateral fields. Custom boost fields are devised that include the GTV (or tumor bed) with a 2- to 3 cm margin. A three-field technique or laterals alone will often suffice.

Traditional field orientations (PA and laterals) are usually adequate for three-dimensional reconstructed targets. Although similar in shape to traditionally simulated fields, field shaping (blocking) can be more precisely individualized based on a CT-defined CTV. After CTV expansion of at least 1 cm to create a PTV (without IGRT), field borders are generally expanded another 5 to 10 mm in order to achieve sufficient dosimetric target coverage.

Possible benefits of treatment of rectal cancer with IMRT include dose escalation to the GTV and construction of a concave dose distribution that reduces small-bowel dose, in addition to bladder and bone marrow (see Fig. 24.4). Dosimetric studies comparing IMRT to traditional techniques in rectal cancer have shown clinically significant reductions in dose to bowel (80,81) as well as

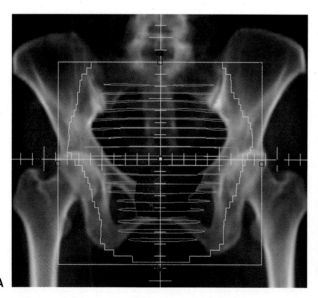
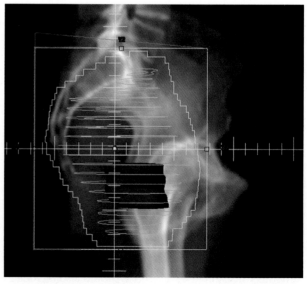

Figure 24.3. Preoperative fields for a 63-year-old female with a cT_3N_0 adenocarcinoma of the distal rectum, treated with a PA (**A**), *right* (**B**) and *left* (not shown) lateral fields. GTV and CTV shown in *red* and *green*, respectively (PTV not shown).

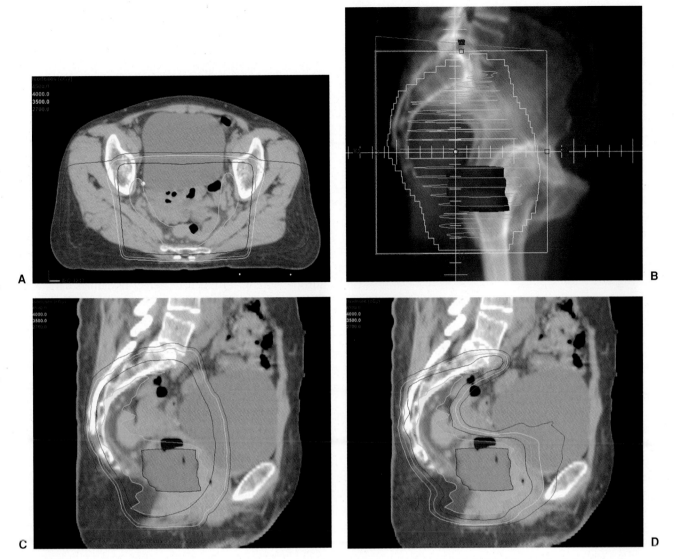

Figure 24.4. Axial and sagittal dosimetry in the mid-pelvis using a three-field (**A, C**) and nine-field IMRT (**B, D**) plans in the preoperative treatment of a cT$_3$N$_0$ distal rectal cancer with daily image guidance. GTV (*red*) and CTV (*blue*) shown with 45 (*red*), 40 (*green*), 35 (*yellow*), and 27 Gy (*purple*) isodose lines (PTV not shown).

bladder and femoral heads (82). The successful implementation of IMRT in the management of rectal cancer has been reported from multiple institutions generally with dose escalation to the GTV by and large with favorable outcomes (83–85). A retrospective review of 92 patients treated at the Mayo Clinic in Arizona demonstrated a 32% incidence of ≥ grade 2 gastrointestinal toxicity among patients treated with IMRT compared to 62% (*p* = 0.006) among patients treated with conventional fields during the same era (86). In view of the challenges of internal movement and distensibility pelvic organs (rectum, bowel, and bladder) as well as the dose inhomogeneity produced by some treatment planning systems, caution should be used before undertaking IMRT in rectal cancer.

Chemotherapy

Adjuvant or neoadjuvant radiotherapy is generally delivered with concurrent 5-FU. In the postoperative setting, protracted venous infusion (PVI) of 5-FU (225 mg/m^2/

day) throughout the course of pelvic radiotherapy has been shown to decreased tumor recurrence and improve overall survival compared to the administration of bolus 5-FU and is the current standard of care (79). In contrast, Intergroup 0144 subsequently showed no significant difference in outcome between PVI regimens and bolus 5-FU with leucovorin during radiotherapy (avoiding the need for central catheterization) (87). Multiple studies have reported encouraging results with the use of capecitabine, an orally administered premetabolite of 5-FU, in conjunction with pelvic radiation for rectal cancer (88–91). NSABP R-04 is currently investigating its use in comparison to PVI of 5-FU during preoperative radiotherapy.

Treatment Planning for Colon Cancer

Patients treated with radiotherapy for colon cancer are treated with the same chemotherapeutic and radiation principles as rectal cancer. The initial CTV generally includes the tumor bed and adjacent pelvic/retroperitoneal lymphatics, with a subsequent boost to the tumor bed (or tumor preoperatively). Review of preoperative imaging, operative reports, and identification of surgical clips demarcating the tumor bed are essential in order to define targets and design fields that may impact local control and the prognosis of this disease.

Prognosis

The prognosis of patients with rectal cancer who receive adjuvant treatment has been well defined by Gunderson et al. (92), based on T and N stage. The 5-year survival for patients with intermediate risk cancers (pT1–2N1, T3N0) is 74% to 83%, 44% to 80% for moderately high-risk (T1–2N2, T3N1, T4N0) patients, and 29% to 57% for high-risk patients (T3N2, T4N1–2).

PANCREATIC CANCER

In the year 2009, the American Cancer Society estimated 42,470 new pancreatic cancers in the United States (1). They also predicted 35,240 deaths from this disease, highlighting the unfavorable prognosis of this cancer at any stage and the need for more effective therapies.

Diagnostic Evaluation

The pretreatment diagnostic evaluation is crucial for selection of patients who are candidates for surgical resection, those with unresectable disease who may be treated with chemoradiotherapy, and patients who are not candidates for aggressive local therapy due to distant metastases. Abdominal CT or MRI remains the most useful modalities for defining local extent of disease and to detect metastasis within the abdomen. Tumor involvement of the celiac, hepatic, or superior mesenteric arteries or encasement of the superior mesenteric vein/occlusion of the portal-venous confluence indicates surgical unresectability. Refinements in abdominal CT imaging, such as acquisition of thin sections, dual-phase contrast imaging, 3D reconstruction, and use of multidetector CT, have greatly improved the accuracy in defining local tumor extension. With these techniques, accurate prediction of resectability has been reported in up to 87% of patients (93). In addition to CT or MRI, EUS in experienced hands may add further information regarding tumor extent, vascular involvement, and regional adenopathy, but probably is most useful in obtaining cytological diagnosis when other methods are unsuccessful. Imaging from endoscopic retrograde cholangiopancreatography (ERCP) should also be reviewed as it may assist in defining tumor boundaries during treatment planning based on abnormalities of the biliary and/or pancreatic ducts.

Although PET imaging has been reported to have a high sensitivity in detecting pancreatic carcinomas (94), its poor anatomic resolution limits its usefulness for local staging (surgical resectability or nodal involvement) but may be more sensitive than other modalities in detecting distant metastases (95).

Treatment Options

Given the poor prognosis associated with any stage of this disease, whenever possible patients should be considered for enrollment on a clinical trial. When a patient is medically fit and their tumor is anatomically resectable, surgical resection is clearly indicated as it is the only strategy that contributes to long-term survival in this disease.

After surgical resection, patients not only have a high-risk distant metastasis, but local failure as well. A local component of disease failure after surgery has been reported in large majority of patients who recur (96,97). A small randomized trial conducted by the GITSG reported a doubling in median survival (10.9 vs. 21.0 months) among patients treated with adjuvant chemoradiotherapy compared to patients undergoing surgical resection alone (98). A subsequent four-arm randomized trial from Europe (ESPAC-1) failed to detect patient benefit with such treatment (99). Both studies should be interpreted with caution given the split course radiotherapy in both trials, the small numbers of the GITSG trial, and the lack of radiotherapy quality assurance or standardized specimen review in the ESPAC-1 trial. Recent retrospective analysis of large cohorts of patients from Mayo Clinic and Johns Hopkins Hospital strongly support the use of postoperative chemoradiotherapy in the management of resected pancreas cancer (100,101). Thus, postoperative chemoradiotherapy may be considered part of the overall adjuvant treatment plan in medically fit patients.

Multiple series have reported the feasibility and outcome of patients with resectable tumors treated with preoperative chemoradiotherapy (102–105). Some of the theoretic advantages of this strategy include local tumor downstaging to improve resectability, better oxygenation of the target tissues during radiation and chemotherapy, reduced risk of intraoperative seeding, better selection of patients for surgery, and improved treatment tolerance compared to adjuvant therapy in the postoperative setting (106). Preoperative chemoradiotherapy, however, has not been sufficiently studied or established as a treatment standard by prospective randomized trial.

Patients with unresectable cancers who have a favorable functional status should be considered for chemoradiotherapy. With the exception of one randomized trial (107), the use of combined-modality therapy has been associated with improved overall survival compared to radiotherapy alone (108), chemotherapy alone (109,110), or supportive care (111). Patients who present with metastatic disease are candidates for systemic chemotherapy. Short palliative courses of radiotherapy for symptoms such as pain may be beneficial in some instances.

Treatment Planning

Simulation

Patients should be simulated in the supine position with arms over the head using a wing-board or similar device to ensure reproducibility and to allow treatment of lateral fields. Oral contrast during fluoroscopic simulation allows identification of the duodenal C-loop as an important reference for field design. Using water rather than oral contrast during CT imaging often improves mucosal resolution of the stomach and duodenum compared to when oral contrast agents are used. Intravenous contrast during CT planning will aid in detection of vascular landmarks and target definition, but generally planning CT images are inferior to a diagnostic scans optimized for pancreas imaging (acquisition during arterial and portal-venous phases of contrast). Therefore, diagnostic films should be reviewed in conjunction with planning CT images whether or not IV contrast is used at simulation.

Radiotherapy Target

Accurate target definition is important not only to impact locoregional control with radiation, but also to reduce toxicity of treatment. For unresectable tumors or those treated neoadjuvantly, the GTV includes the primary tumor (including vessels encased by tumor) and any radiographically enlarged lymph nodes. The CTV includes any areas of potential subclinical extension of local disease as well as regional lymph nodes. A 1 to 2 cm margin of soft tissue around the primary tumor should be included in the CTV. This margin, however, is usually within the volume required to include the peripancreatic lymph nodes. Given the proximity of the pancreatic head to duodenum, the adjacent medial wall is included. The entire circumference should be included for tumor with gross duodenal invasion. Given the predominance of tumor recurrence within radiotherapy ports even when small local fields are used (112), some have questioned the value of treating the regional lymph nodes in patients with unresectable pancreatic cancer. Initial reports have described treating the primary tumor only with stereotactic body radiotherapy (SBRT) (113). Although local control was encouraging, toxicity was significant. SBRT has also been used as a boost after initial standard fractionation (114). Given that pathologic nodal involvement is reported in up to 76% of patients undergoing surgical resection (115,116), elective treatment of regional lymphatics seems justified, unless directed otherwise on an investigational trial, since previous randomized trials have employed this practice. SBRT techniques in the setting of pancreatic cancer are still best performed in the context of a clinical trial.

Brunner et al. (115) have provided an excellent analysis of nodal regions at risk based on pathologic specimens from 175 cancers of the pancreatic head. Peripancreatic nodal regions at >5% risk of nodal metastasis include (in order of decreasing frequency): posterior pancreaticoduodenal area, superior/inferior border of the pancreatic head, anterior pancreaticoduodenal area, hepatoduodenal ligament (porta hepatis), superior margin of pancreatic body, and superior mesenteric artery. Thus, a CTV that includes a small rim of peripancreatic soft tissue in all directions of the pancreatic head and neck will include all

but the nodes along the porta hepatis, SMA, aorta, and celiac artery, which should also be included within the CTV. Attention to a biliary stent may assist in locating the porta hepatis during target contouring. Although the location of the celiac artery and SMA has traditionally been described in relationship to T12 and L1, respectively, data from angiography (117) suggests that there is enough individual variability that identification should be based on CT-imaging rather than relying solely on boney landmarks.

Although the paraaortic lymph nodes are considered a distant site of disease for staging purposes, given the over 20% risk of subclinical metastases (115), they should be included in the CTV. With respect to the inferior vena cava and aorta, in >90% of cases, retroperitoneal metastases are anterior to these vessels, between them, or lateral to the aorta (<5% metastases are retrocaval/retroaortic or lateral to the cava) (118). In the craniocaudad dimension, the majority of paraaortic nodal involvement is between the celiac artery superiorly and the level of the renal veins inferiorly (except for tumors >3 cm, where CTV where volume should extend inferiorly to level of inferior mesenteric artery) (116).

The principles for defining the CTV for pancreatic tail lesions are similar, except that the suprapancreatic lymph nodes (along splenic vessels) and splenic hilum should be included. Elective treatment of inferior pancreaticoduodenal lymph nodes may be excluded in these patients, sparing radiation exposure to the right kidney.

Postoperatively the CTV for elective nodal coverage is similar, though preoperative imaging, the operative report, and surgical clips should be reviewed during its construction. Location of biliary-enteric and gastro-enteric anastomoses should also be noted. For boost planning, a CTV2 should be devised, that is, a reconstruction of the preoperative tumor volume.

Normal Tissue Tolerances

The amount of small bowel receiving 45 Gy should be minimized without compromising target coverage. Any small bowel within the boost volume of treatment should be limited and not receive beyond 50 Gy, though up to 55 Gy may be cautiously delivered to small portions of the duodenum wall if clinically indicated. At least 75% of one kidney or the composite of one whole kidney should be kept below 18 to 20 Gy. If the large majority of one kidney will receive doses beyond 20 Gy, consideration should be given to a quantitative renal scan prior to treatment to ensure sufficient function of the other kidney. Sixty percent of the liver should be kept below 30 Gy and the whole liver should not receive >25 Gy. The spinal cord should not receive >45 Gy.

Radiotherapy Dose

The only data from randomized trials regarding radiotherapy dose in pancreatic cancer is the GITSG trial for unresectable tumors. No difference in patient outcome was detected between 40 and 60 Gy (split course schedule with concurrent 5-FU) (108). The radiotherapy and imaging techniques of this trial would be considered outdated by current standards and so current radiotherapy dose guidelines are based on normal organ tolerance to upper abdominal radiation rather than the results of this trial. Elective nodal stations (CTV) are treated to 45 Gy at 1.8 Gy/fraction. A subsequent boost of 5.4 Gy is delivered to the GTV or CTV2 (postoperatively). Higher boost doses may be considered for unresectable patients or those with positive margins when dose can be delivered within the constraints of normal organs (especially small bowel).

Radiotherapy Fields and Techniques

The pancreas is commonly treated with a four-field technique with disproportionate weighting of the anterior and posterior fields to reduce dose to the liver from the lateral fields (see Fig. 24.5A and B). While maintaining a 2 to 3 cm margin on the primary tumor (or tumor bed), traditional fields typically encompass T11 superiorly through L3 inferiorly. The left field edge is at least 2 cm from the left vertebral body edge (or past the splenic hilum for pancreatic tail lesions). The right field border is extended to cover the duodenum and porta hepatis. With the lateral fields, the posterior border generally splits the vertebral bodies,

while the anterior border is placed at least 2 cm anterior to the tumor, maintaining a 3 to 4 cm margin anterior to the vertebral bodies to ensure coverage of paraaortic lymph nodes. These boundaries should be customized based on patient differences in target volumes as well as normal structure location. Boost fields encompass unresected tumor or original tumor bed with 1.5 to 2 cm margins.

With a 3D reconstruction of carefully defined CT-based target volumes, field borders can be refined, which reflect individual tumor and patient anatomy. A four-field technique is often still appropriate with optimization of field weighting with computer dosimetry. To account for setup error and target movement, a minimum PTV of 1 cm is advised. Given the movement of upper abdominal organs due to respiration, greater margin in the superior to inferior dimension may be prudent (119). Field edges are devised at an additional 5 to 10 mm beyond the PTV to provide dosimetric coverage.

The use of highly conformal radiotherapy techniques should be used cautiously due to substantial *inter-* and *intrafraction* variations in the pancreas position. Study of pancreas movement by cine MRI has shown that changes in pancreas position are larger and more variable than often

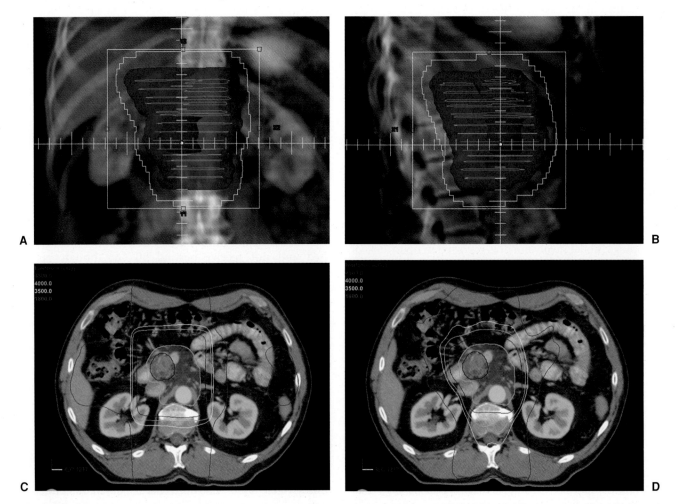

Figure 24.5. A 69-year-old male with an unresectable carcinoma of the head of pancreas, treated with a four-field technique. AP (**A**), right lateral (**B**) (PA and left lateral not shown). GTV (*red*), CTV (*green*), PTV (*blue*). Axial dosimetry from four-field plan (**C**) and eight-field non-coplanar IMRT plan (**D**). 45 (*red*), 40 (*green*), 35 (*yellow*), and 18 Gy (*purple*) isodose lines (PTV not shown).

appreciated, especially in the cranio-caudad dimension and do not necessarily correlate well with diaphragm location (120). Similarly, image-guidance based on boney landmarks has been found to correlate with accurate pancreas target setup in only 20% of treatments when compared to tumor fiducial markers even when using respiratory gating (121).

3D treatment planning with four to six non-coplanar beams has been objectively compared to traditional four-field techniques and may provide some dosimetric advantages (122), particularly in sparing the kidneys (123). Deviation from traditional field orientations may be considered when the target has been accurately defined and normal tissues are carefully evaluated by dose-volume histograms. Such techniques may be of particular value among patients with dosimetric challenges due to atypical target volumes or normal organs (e.g., one kidney).

The use of IMRT for pancreatic cancers has been clinically described and may also provide some dosimetric advantages by sparing kidneys, bowel, and liver (124–126) (see Fig. 24.5C and D) as well as enabling possible dose escalation to the GTV (127). A few institutions have reported patient outcome after treatment with IMRT with favorable tolerance and expected survival (124,128). Care must be taken when employing this modality to account for target motion, avoid dosimetric hot spots, and be certain the devised plan is clinically superior to that which could be achieved with less advanced techniques.

Chemotherapy

Among unresectable patients, a randomized trial conducted by the GITSG established the superiority of bolus 5-FU concurrent with radiotherapy over radiotherapy alone (108). Prolonged venous infusion of 5-FU is now more commonly given with radiation, with a maximum tolerated dose of 250 mg/m^2/day defined by a prospective phase I study (129). Although gemcitabine has been repeatedly studied concurrently with radiation both among unresectable patients and in the postoperative setting, it has not been established as the standard of care, despite one small randomized trial which reported a better outcome compared to 5-FU and radiation (130). Toxicity from this approach is dependent on the inverse relationship between gemcitabine schedule and dose related to radiation field size and dose (131). Without standardized parameters or large trials showing benefit over 5-FU and radiation, gemcitabine and radiation should be considered investigational.

Prognosis

The prognosis of this disease is poor, yet somewhat dependent on stage of disease. Among resectable patients, the median survival is 20 months (98), with a 5-year overall survival rate of 8% to 20% (99). Among unresectable patients who receive combined-modality therapy, median survival is 8 to 10 months (107,109). Although a few long-term survivors have been reported among patients with small unresectable tumors who have undergone chemoradiotherapy and intraoperative radiation (132), long-term survival is not anticipated in patients with inoperable tumors. The median

survival for patients presenting with metastatic cancer treated with chemotherapy is less than 6 months (133).

GASTROESOPHAGEAL CANCER

In 2009, there were an expected 37,500 cases of gastroesophageal cancer in the United States and ~25,150 deaths attributed to this disease (1). Gastric cancer and esophageal cancer have generally been considered as two distinct diseases anatomically, etiologically, and therapeutically. In 1991, Blot et al. (134) described an alarming increase in the incidence of adenocarcinomas of the esophagus and proximal stomach compared to previous histological and anatomic patterns of disease presentation. A subsequent update has confirmed this finding, reporting a marked increase in the number of patients developing these tumors, particularly white males (135). Due to this increased incidence of tumors at or near the gastroesophageal junction (GEJ), radiation oncologists frequently have to synthesize the principles of treatment planning for both esophageal and gastric cancer for a given patient with a tumor near or at this junction. For this reason, treatment planning is combined into one section for these previously distinct malignancies.

Diagnostic Evaluation

As with other gastrointestinal malignancies, a complete diagnostic workup is crucial in defining the maximal extent of locoregional disease prior to treatment. Due to the limitations of each of the diagnostic modalities in staging this disease, no single study should be relied on solely to define the extent of tumor during treatment planning.

Description of the mucosal extent of disease is best defined optically by upper endoscopy and not infrequently it will define tumor beyond what is appreciated by imaging modalities. Review of endoscopy reports and/or discussion with the gastroenterologist is imperative. Measurements of tumor extent in the esophagus are referenced by their endoscopic distance from the incisors. These measurements may be inconsistent and imprecise between exams, but they should be noted and compared to radiologic findings to ensure general consistency between modalities. The distance from the incisors to the thoracic inlet is generally 18 cm (beginning of upper thoracic esophagus), the carina is located at ~24 cm (demarcating the beginning of the mid-esophagus), and the lower esophagus begins at 32 cm and ends at ~40 cm (GEJ) (136). Imaging with barium swallow and/or upper gastrointestinal series may also assist in defining the extent of disease, but in no way obviates the need for endoscopy and axial imaging.

As with rectal cancer, EUS is an established modality in experienced hands for staging local and adjacent regional spread of disease. The accuracy of EUS in determining correct T-stage is generally reported above 80% for both gastric (137,138) and esophageal cancers (139–142), especially for tumors which penetrate the muscularis propria (T3). Regional staging by EUS, which characterizes both nodal size and architecture, is also of clinical benefit but less consistently accurate than determination of T-stage. Fine-needle aspiration may augment the accuracy of the procedure for determining lymph node involvement by tumor.

Axial imaging of the chest and abdomen with CT (or MRI) is also imperative for locoregional staging and to evaluate for distant metastases. Such imaging will not only detect distant disease, but also image regional nodal stations beyond the range of EUS. The results of PET imaging for gastric (143,144) and GEJ/esophagus (145–147) cancers have been studied by comparison to surgical findings. The primary benefit of PET imaging appears to be the detection of distant metastases not appreciated by other modalities. Compared to EUS, these studies have reported a lower sensitivity of PET in detecting perigastric and periesophageal adenopathy (<40%), likely due to the inferiority of PET in distinguishing primary tumor from adjacent lymph nodes because of the poor spatial resolution of the imaging. PET, however, likely has a higher specificity than other modalities for lymph-node metastases (146) and may be more sensitive than other studies in detecting lymphadenopathy distant from the primary lesion (145).

Among patients with concerning respiratory symptoms at presentation, bronchoscopy should be considered to evaluate for fistula with the tracheobronchial tree prior to treatment planning. Although presence of a fistula has traditionally been considered a contraindication to radiotherapy, there are multiple reports of irradiating these patients successfully (148–151). At times the fistula may even close with treatment (151) and the survival of irradiated patients appears superior to patients treated with chemotherapy or supportive care alone (150). Consideration should be given to endoscopically stenting these patients, decreasing the daily dose to 150 cGy (149) and/or incorporating treatment breaks.

Treatment Options

The optimal coordination of surgery, chemotherapy, and radiotherapy continues to be studied by large multi-institutional studies in patients with gastroesophageal cancers. Surgical resection remains the foundation of curative strategies for locoregionally confined gastric and GEJ cancers. All patients with transmural penetration of tumor (pT3) or whose tumors are node positive should be considered for postoperative chemoradiotherapy based on the overall survival benefit demonstrated in Intergroup 0116 (median survival 27 vs. 36 months) (152). In addition to gastric tumors, this study also included patients with adenocarcinoma of the GEJ. The gastroesophageal anastomoses for these tumors are often located high within the thorax or neck, requiring larger postoperative radiotherapy fields. For this reason, there is interest and rationale for treating these tumors preoperatively, extrapolating from the neoadjuvant chemoradiotherapy experience in esophageal cancer. Although theoretic advantages exist, there have been no clinical trials directly comparing neoadjuvant chemoradiotherapy for gastric and GEJ cancers with the postoperative therapy established by Intergroup

0116. It should also be noted that a minimum caloric intake of 1,500 kcal/day was required for enrollment on Intergroup 0116. Thus, given the rigors of treatment of the upper abdomen with chemoradiation, close attention to patient nutritional intake prior to treatment is mandatory.

The reported overall survival rates of surgical resection and definitive chemoradiotherapy for esophagus cancer appear similar (153–156). Because of the relatively high risk of locally recurrent/persistent disease with either strategy, preoperative radiotherapy and preoperative chemoradiotherapy have been studied. The use of preoperative radiotherapy has not consistently shown benefits over surgical resection alone (157–159). Neoadjuvant *chemo*radiotherapy, however, has been evaluated in at least seven randomized trials (160–166). Two of these trials detected a patient survival benefit with the addition of neoadjuvant chemoradiotherapy to surgical resection alone (164,165). Surgical resection may not benefit all patients after chemoradiotherapy. Randomized trials of the addition of surgical resection to initial chemoradiotherapy for locally advanced squamous cell carcinomas of the esophagus has not revealed improvement patient survival (167,168). Strategies in the multimodality management of locally advanced esophageal cancer continue to evolve with completion of clinical trials.

The benefit of postoperative radiotherapy for esophageal cancer has not been detected in randomized trials (169–171). A possible benefit to postoperative *chemo*radiotherapy for selected patients has been reported from at least one non-randomized prospective study (172), but has not been evaluated by randomized trial. Thus, adjuvant chemoradiotherapy should be reserved for patients on clinical trials. However, postoperative chemoradiotherapy is indicated for esophageal adenocarcinomas extending to the GEJ of appropriate stages based on Intergroup 0116 (152).

Patients with early mucosal disease (T1/T2N0) of the stomach or esophagus are preferentially treated with surgery alone. Definitive radiation with or without chemotherapy is reserved for those who are medically unfit for surgery. Although patients with metastatic disease are candidates for only palliative treatment, the presence of M1 disease (celiac nodes for lower esophageal cancers and cervical nodes for upper esophageal cancers) represents an exception. Although these distant nodal sites correlate with poorer patient prognosis, the results of treatment with definitive intent are not universally dismal with this stage of disease and thus patients may be considered for curative approaches (136). It should be noted that the celiac nodal station represents a regional nodal site for cancers of the GEJ rather than a site of distant disease.

Treatment Planning

Simulation

Patients are generally simulated in the supine position with arms extended over the head using a wing-board or similar device to ensure reproducibility and to allow treatment of oblique or lateral fields. Although prone positioning is less reproducible, it may be advantageous for some patients with middle or lower esophageal lesions. Prone positioning is reported to move the esophageal lumen anteriorly, an average of 1.7 cm from the spinal cord compared to supine positioning (173). It should be noted that despite such maneuvers, periesophageal tissue posterior to the esophagus still remains fixed to the vertebral column. If treatment fields will encompass any stomach, the patient should be both simulated and treated with an empty stomach (minimum 4 h) to reduce gastric distension and improve target reproducibility. Although CT-based planning is essential, fluoroscopic simulation is a useful step for identifying surgical staple lines, clips, as well as administration of oral contrast to aid in localizing the mucosal extent of gastroesophageal cancers. In addition, respiratory movement of the left hemidiaphram can be noted and incorporated into parameters of the PTV for GEJ and proximal stomach tumors. Studies of 4D CT-simulation (4DCT) of esophageal cancers has demonstrated significant primary tumor as well as nodal (celiac) movement with respiration in all directions (174,175). Given wide patient variation in such target motion, individual assessment of target motion is preferred to standardized internal target margins for all patients.

CT-based treatment planning is imperative not only for accurate identification of target, but also for proper evaluation of dose to upper abdominal and thoracic normal structures. Both local and regional diseases may extend significantly beyond what is appreciated with simulation techniques that rely on oral contrast alone to define fields. At least one institution has reported not only an increase in field size associated with CT-based planning compared to conventional techniques, but also a statistically significant improvement in long-term patient survival (176).

Radiotherapy Target

For patients treated neoadjuvantly or definitively with radiotherapy, the GTV includes the maximal extent of gross disease as defined by the combination of all staging modalities. Dependence on upper gastroesophageal radiography alone at the time of simulation will certainly underestimate both the radial tumor margin and regional nodal disease. CT is better at defining the radial and regional extent of gross disease, but longitudinal tumor boundaries may not be distinct. In addition, small tumors (T1 or T2) are often not discernable on CT. Upper endoscopy may provide the most accurate assessment of longitudinal tumor boundaries, but it is impossible to precisely correlate these measurements with a planning CT. EUS is probably the best modality for defining both longitudinal and radial extent of the primary tumor. By coordinating with the endoscopist, the superior and inferior boundaries of tumor can be referenced to an intrathoracic structure such as the top of the aortic arch rather than just the incisors (177). Measurements relative to the aortic arch can thereby be translated with some accuracy to the treatment-planning CT and reflected in GTV contouring.

PET imaging is also useful in defining the GTV. With clinical judgment, the GTV may be expanded to include FDG-avid tissue not appreciated as tumor with other imaging. At times, other imaging modalities may define greater extent of tumor volumes than defined by PET. For example, the longitudinal extent of tumor is often perceived greater on CT than PET (147). However, given the risks of a false-negative imaging, target contours should not be reduced to include only abnormal volumes defined by PET (178).

The CTV includes areas of microscopic risk of disease from either primary tumor extension or nodal metastases not detected by clinical staging. The lymphatic drainage of the esophagus is primarily longitudinal with channels extending some distance before perforating the muscularis propria to communicate with adventitial lymphatics (179). Autopsy studies in patients dying of esophageal cancer have found lymphangitic carcinomatosis of the esophageal wall in up to one-third of patients, with *in situ* or invasive skip lesions at a distance of 2 to 10 cm in 13% of patients (180). Thus, in the preoperative or definitive setting, radiotherapy ports for esophageal cancer have traditionally included a generous longitudinal margin of mucosa. Refinements in pretreatment staging of gross disease have not obviated the need for generous longitudinal margin for the CTV. Although initial ports in RTOG 85–01 treated the entire esophagus for 30 Gy (154), subsequent trials have limited this margin to 5 cm (181). With 3D target definition, this 5 cm margin is comparable to a 3 to 4 cm CTV of longitudinal margin of esophagus from the GTV (assuming 1 cm PTV and 0.5 to 1 cm to block edge for dosimetric buildup). For tumors of the lower esophagus and GEJ, a 3 to 4 cm inferior extension of the CTV often includes proximal stomach. Pathologic study of resected SCC and ACA has shown risk of microscopic extension to be limited to 3 and 5 cm, respectively (182). Similarly, primary gastric tumors treated preoperatively require adequate longitudinal margin which may extend into the lower esophagus for proximal lesions. In addition to longitudinal extensions, the CTV includes radial expansion from the GTV as well. Although this radial expansion of CTV around the GTV should include 1 to 2 cm of adjacent soft tissue, generally this is well within the CTV boundary required for regional nodal coverage.

The regional lymphatics included within the CTV depend on the anatomic location of the primary tumor. For primary tumors of the esophagus, the CTV should be extended radially to include periesophageal lymph nodes around GTV and normal esophagus included within the CTV for as longitudinal margin (see Fig. 24.6). The periesophageal lymph nodes lie in the posterior mediastinum in the soft tissue immediately surrounding the esophagus. Although conventional radiotherapy fields have accommodated these nodes by a 2 to 2.5 cm margin on the esophagus, such guidelines do not account for the often asymmetric and variable distribution of this tissue surrounding the esophagus. Thus, the CTV should be contoured based on individual patient anatomy. In the mid-esophagus, the subcarinal lymph-node region should be included in the CTV if esophagus or tumor is included to this axial level as a target volume. Similarly, if the upper

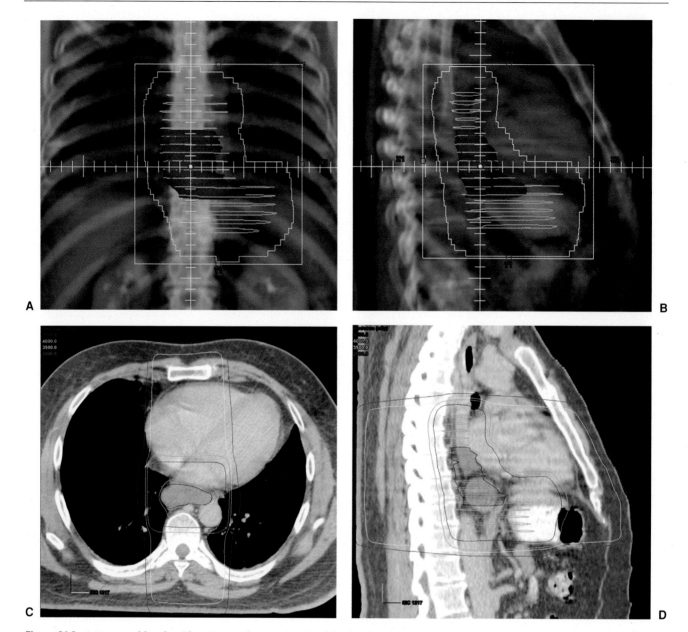

Figure 24.6. A 54-year-old male with a cT3N0 adenocarcinoma of the distal esophagus treated with neoadjuvant chemoradiotherapy treated with a four-field technique. AP (**A**), right lateral (**B**) (PA and left lateral not shown). GTV (*red*), CTV (*green*), PTV (not shown). Axial (**C**) and sagittal (**D**) dosimetry, with 45 (*red*), 40 (*green*), 35 (*yellow*), and 20 Gy (*purple*) isodose lines.

esophagus is within the CTV, adjacent paratracheal lymphatics should be included in addition to periesophageal tissue. Given a >40% rate of subclinical metastases to the supraclavicular lymph nodes for upper esophageal cancers as defined by surgical dissections (183), extension of the CTV to this region is also indicated for tumors in this location. Similarly, for lower esophageal lesions, the CTV may be extended to include the celiac nodes. Treatment of the thoracic hilar or anterior mediastinal lymph nodes is not indicated unless they are grossly involved on pretreatment imaging.

Esophageal tumors that extend to involve the GEJ pose a threat to upper abdominal lymph nodes. Pericardial lymph nodes (medial and lateral borders of gastric cardia)

and celiac lymph nodes are included in the CTV. Splenic hilar lymph nodes are at risk for T3 or T4 GEJ tumors (184). With extension of tumor inferiorly/laterally into the gastric cardia, lymph nodes of the entire celiac axis are at risk. Nodal tissue within the porta hepatis, gastrohepatic ligament, left gastric artery, along the splenic artery (suprapancreatic nodes) and splenic hilum should be included in the CTV. In addition, perigastric lymph nodes (along the inner and outer gastric curvatures) that are adjacent to normal gastric wall included for longitudinal margin will be within the CTV.

For primary gastric tumors, local and regional tissues at risk for recurrence have been well defined from multiple reports, including the University of Minnesota re-operation series (185). The CTV includes all the peri-gastric lymph nodes along the inner and outer curvatures of the stomach. Although adequate normal mucosal margin within the CTV should be generated, the inclusion of the perigastric lymph nodes in a preoperative scenario generally ensures such. For proximal gastric tumors, 3 to 4 cm extension of CTV cranially may include distal esophagus with associated periesophageal lymphatics. For very distal gastric cancers, similar caudal extension including a portion of the duodenum is appropriate. Tumors of the gastric cardia or fundus (especially if T3) should include the medial left hemidiaphram.

In addition to the perigastric lymph nodes, nodal stations to be included in the CTV for gastric tumors include the celiac, porta hepatis (including gastrohepatic and hepatoduodenal), suprapancreatic (along the splenic artery), splenic hilar, supra- and infrapyloric (above and below the pylorus), pancreaticoduodenal (tissue around and posterior to the pancreatic head), and local paraaortic/retroperitoneal lymph nodes (along the cranial-caudad extent of the stomach).

Similar principles for target identification exist in the postoperative setting for gastroesophageal cancers with some notable points. Using preoperative staging studies and operative findings, the original extent of the primary cancer (and gross nodal disease) must be reconstructed on the planning CT and included within the CTV. In addition, the gastroesophageal anastomosis must be identified and included. Although there may be temptation to exclude the anastomosis among patients where it lies high in the thorax or even lower neck, such an omission has been associated in one series with a 29% anastomotic recurrence rate (compared to 0% with treatment) (186). Among gastric tumors that involve only the upper one-third of the stomach and who have minimal lymphatic tumor involvement *pathologically*, cautious consideration can be given for exclusion of the infrapyloric and pancreaticoduodenal lymph nodes (187). Similarly, lesions of the lower one-third of the stomach may have a lower propensity for involvement of the splenic hilar lymph nodes (187).

Normal Tissue Tolerances

The amount of small bowel receiving 45 Gy should be minimized without compromising target coverage. Any small bowel within a possible boost volume of treatment should be of limited and not receive beyond 50 Gy. At least 75% of one kidney or the composite of one whole kidney should be kept below 18 to 20 Gy. If the large majority of one kidney will receive doses beyond 20 Gy, consideration should be given to a quantitative renal scan prior to treatment to ensure sufficient function of the other kidney. Sixty percent of the liver should be kept below 30 Gy and the whole liver should not receive >25 Gy. The percentage of total lung receiving >20 Gy should be kept to <30%, and preferably <25%. Among patients treated neoadjuvantly, postoperative pulmonary complications has been inversely associated with the absolute volume of lung spared 5 Gy (188,189). The whole heart should not receive beyond 30 Gy. One-half of the heart should be restricted to 40 Gy or less. Doses of 50 Gy or slightly beyond may be delivered to a maximum of 30% of heart volume, but attempt should be made to limit high doses to the left ventricle when possible. The spinal cord should not receive >45 Gy.

Radiotherapy Dose

RTOG 95–05 (181) evaluated the radiotherapy dose for definitive treatment of esophageal cancer in conjunction with concurrent chemotherapy. No difference in locoregional control or overall survival was detected between the 50.4 and 64.8 Gy arms of the trial. Thus, 50.4 Gy given at 1.8 Gy/fraction is the recommended dose for patients with esophageal cancer treated definitively with radiation. Without concurrent chemotherapy, a total dose of 60 Gy with standard fractionation seems appropriate. In the neoadjuvant setting, 45 Gy at 1.8 Gy/fraction is delivered to the CTV. Consideration of a 5.4 Gy boost to gross disease is reasonable, if it is possible to respect organ tolerance.

In the postoperative setting, 45 Gy at 1.8 Gy/fraction was delivered to patients with gastric and GEJ tumors in Intergroup 0116 (152). Boost treatment beyond 45 Gy for such indications as close or involved surgical margins may be considered cautiously, with regard given to normal tissue and patient tolerances.

Radiotherapy Fields and Techniques

Common field arrangements for the treatment of esophageal cancers usually involve some consideration for limitation of total dose to the spinal cord. AP–PA techniques radiate the least amount of normal lung but, care must be taken with lower esophageal/GEJ tumors where such a field arrangement can include a significant amount of heart. Supplementation with lateral or oblique fields which avoid the spinal cord is required to deliver doses beyond 45 Gy to the thorax, but will generally lead to increased doses to the lung. A four-field technique (AP, PA, and laterals) usually enables a satisfactory dose distribution when the weighting of lateral fields is limited according to lung tolerance (see Fig. 24.6A–C). Alternatively, patients may be treated with AP–PA until cord tolerance and then treated with either lateral or oblique fields, which avoid the spinal cord. Oblique ports include less lung than lateral fields, but depending on orientation may include more heart (173). Another option is to treat the patient with a three-field technique (AP and posterior obliques), with at least one field not contributing to spinal cord dose.

Traditional field borders for esophageal cancers have generally been defined with 2 cm lateral (radial) margins beyond the esophagus and a 5 cm longitudinal margin from tumor (superior–inferior) (181). 3D treatment planning allows for further optimization of field shaping and orientation compared to 2D techniques. However, the transition from 2D field definitions to 3D definition of target must be done with caution in order to avoid undertreatment of tissues at risk, which were previously included in multi-institutional trials (190). The PTV should be a minimum of 1 cm expansion of the CTV and GTV to account for setup error and target movement. Greater expansion of the PTV should be considered for targets involving the lower esophagus and proximal stomach given their movement with respiration. Without the aid of more sophisticated technologies, fluoroscopy with upper gastrointestinal contrast may assist in defining this expansion as such internal movement may not simply be limited to the superior and inferior dimensions. 4DCT is an ideal technology to assess target motion. Conforming field borders should then be devised that allow dosimetric coverage of the PTV (usually another 5–10 mm to the field edge). Dosimetric study of conventional versus 3D treatment planning for esophageal cancer has suggested some possible benefits such as dose escalation (191), but the application of such has not yet been supported by prospective trial.

Following the results of the Intergroup 0116, Smalley et al. (187) provided an excellent review of radiation treatment planning for gastric cancer based on surgical considerations and published pattern of failure data. It should be emphasized that since the total radiotherapy dose in this trial was 45 Gy, the majority of patients were successfully treated with an AP–PA field arrangement. The superior field border includes the left hemidiaphram, though it may be significantly higher for proximal gastric tumors whose anastomoses are in the thorax. In order to include the infrapyloric and pancreaticoduodenal nodes, the inferior field border is generally located at L3. The left lateral border extends sufficiently to include the lateral border of the perigastric lymph nodes of the greater curvature and the splenic hilum. The medial border is placed to include the porta hepatis and the medial extent of the preoperative tumor volume. Using this technique, the addition of lateral or oblique fields to AP–PA ports may have limited benefit. The gastric fundus and adjacent perigastric lymph nodes often extend posteriorly enough that straight lateral fields are unable to spare the entire spinal cord or a significant amount of kidney. In addition, more liver is irradiated with such fields and so if used they must be weighted to ensure their contribution is <20 Gy. The anterior borders of lateral and oblique fields must cover the preoperative extent of the ventral gastric wall.

Given the large postoperative treatment volumes required for gastric cancer, it seems 3D treatment planning could provide more conformal dose delivery and reduce irradiation of normal structures compared to simpler techniques. However, determination of preoperative tumor volumes is often imprecise and gastric nodal drainage is anatomically complex. Attempts at more sophisticated planning should take place only after assurance that all target tissues included in Intergroup 0116 are contoured within the CTV. Prospective study has confirmed significant variation in gastric field design among radiation oncologists with both 2D and 3D treatment planning (190).

Similar to esophageal cancer, a minimum of 1 cm expansion of the CTV to create a PTV is appropriate during 3D treatment planning. Greater expansion should be considered for target along the left hemidiaphram to accommodate respiratory movement. When considering the limitations discussed above, a four-field technique may be advantageous for some patients depending on the anatomic extent of target. Oblique fields optimized to avoid spinal cord or kidney while covering the PTV may often prove superior to straight lateral fields. 3D treatment planning with five or more fields has been studied in comparison to the AP–PA technique used in Intergroup 0116 with reported dosimetric gains in regards to normal structures (192) and favorable clinical assessment of toxicity (193). The dosimetric benefit achieved was from reduction in kidney and spinal cord doses, at the expense of small increases in dose to the liver.

Given the complex geometric targets associated with gastroesophageal cancers and the proximity of normal organs, the increased conformality of IMRT may provide dosimetric advantages compared to standard radiotherapy techniques. However, this technology must be employed with care, given the challenges of respiratory and cardiac motion, the intolerance of large volumes of the lung to even modest doses of radiation, and the undesirability of dose inhomogeneity within the CTV. Dosimetric studies of IMRT in the postoperative treatment of gastric cancer have reported a possible improvement target coverage and sparing of critical structures (194), most notably in reducing kidney exposure (195–198) compared to conventional techniques. However, clinically apparent renal dysfunction has not been described as a common problem after treatment with more conventional techniques, such as among patients treated in Intergroup 0116 (152). There is limited clinical experience with the use of IMRT in the treatment of esophageal cancer (see Fig. 24.6D). Its careful implementation has been associated with decreased exposure of the lungs and heart compared to traditional techniques (199–202). Observed clinical benefit of IMRT over 3D conformal treatment for gastroesophageal cancer is yet to be reported.

Chemotherapy

Intergroup 0116 employed an adjuvant/concurrent regimen of 5-FU for gastric and GEJ cancers (152). Patients initially received 5-FU (425 mg/m^2) with leucovorin (20 mg/m^2) for 5 days. Chemoradiotherapy began 28 days later with reduced doses of 5-FU (400 mg/m^2) and leucovorin on the first 4 days and last 3 days of radiotherapy. Two more monthly cycles of chemotherapy were given a month after completion of radiotherapy.

For patients treated with definitive chemoradiotherapy of the esophagus, both cisplatin and 5-FU are used concurrently with radiation. RTOG 85–01 established the clear superiority of chemoradiotherapy over radiotherapy alone for patients with squamous cell carcinoma of the esophagus (154). Cisplatin (75 mg/m^2) was administered on the first and fifth week of radiotherapy with 5-FU (1,000 mg/m^2) for 4 days. Two additional cycles of cisplatin and 5-FU we administered after completion of radiotherapy. All four randomized trials of neoadjuvant chemoradiotherapy for esophageal cancer have similarly included various schedules of concurrent cisplatin (161–164), generally with 5-FU as well.

Prognosis

The outcome of patients with gastroesophageal cancers treated with curative intent has been defined by randomized clinical trials. For locally advanced esophageal cancers, the 5-year overall survival after definitive chemoradiotherapy was 27% in RTOG 85–01 (153) and similar survival rates have been reported with surgery alone (155). Five-year survival among patients undergoing trimodality therapy has been reported to exceed 30% (164,165). Surgical treatment of T1 and T2, N0 esophageal cancer has been associated with an 86% and 34% 5-year survival, respectively (203). Among patients with T3 or node-positive gastric treated with adjuvant chemoradiotherapy, the 5-year survival is >40% (152).

REFERENCES

1. Jemal A, Siegel R, Ward E, et al. Cancer statistics, 2009. *CA Cancer J Clin* 2009;59(4):225–249.
2. Cotter SE, Grigsby PW, Siegel BA, et al. FDG-PET/CT in the evaluation of anal carcinoma. *Int J Radiat Oncol Biol Phys* 2006;65(3):720–725.
3. Winton E, Heriot AG, Ng M, et al. The impact of 18-fluorodeoxyglucose positron emission tomography on the staging, management and outcome of anal cancer. *Br J Cancer* 2009;100(5):693–700.
4. Giovannini M, Bardou VJ, Barclay R, et al. Anal carcinoma: prognostic value of endorectal ultrasound (ERUS). Results of a prospective multicenter study. *Endoscopy* 2001;33(3):231–236.
5. Flam M, John M, Pajak TF, et al. Role of mitomycin in combination with fluorouracil and radiotherapy, and of salvage chemoradiation in the definitive nonsurgical treatment of epidermoid carcinoma of the anal canal: results of a phase III randomized intergroup study. *J Clin Oncol* 1996;14(9):2527–2539.
6. Bartelink H, Roelofsen F, Eschwege F, et al. Concomitant radiotherapy and chemotherapy is superior to radiotherapy alone in the treatment of locally advanced anal cancer: results of a phase III randomized trial of the European Organization for Research and Treatment of Cancer Radiotherapy and Gastrointestinal Cooperative Groups. *J Clin Oncol* 1997;15(5):2040–2049.
7. Epidermoid anal cancer: results from the UKCCCR randomised trial of radiotherapy alone versus radiotherapy, 5-fluorouracil, and mitomycin. UKCCCR Anal Cancer Trial Working Party. UK Co-ordinating Committee on Cancer Research. *Lancet* 1996;348(9034):1049–1054.
8. Boman BM, Moertel CG, O'Connell MJ, et al. Carcinoma of the anal canal. A clinical and pathologic study of 188 cases. *Cancer* 1984;54(1):114–125.
9. Ferrigno R, Nakamura RA, Dos Santos Novaes PE, et al. Radiochemotherapy in the conservative treatment of anal canal carcinoma: retrospective analysis of results

and radiation dose effectiveness. *Int J Radiat Oncol Biol Phys* 2005;61(4):1136–1142.
10. Nicklin JL, Hacker NF, Heintze SW, et al. An anatomical study of inguinal lymph node topography and clinical implications for the surgical management of vulval cancer. *Int J Gynecol Cancer* 1995;5(2):128–133.
11. Myerson RJ, Garofalo MC, El Naqa I, et al. Elective clinical target volumes for conformal therapy in anorectal cancer: a radiation therapy oncology group consensus panel contouring atlas. *Int J Radiat Oncol Biol Phys* 2009;74(3):824–830.
12. Baglan KL, Frazier RC, Yan D, et al. The dose–volume relationship of acute small bowel toxicity from concurrent 5-FU-based chemotherapy and radiation therapy for rectal cancer. *Int J Radiat Oncol Biol Phys* 2002;52(1):176–183.
13. Grigsby PW, Roberts HL, Perez CA. Femoral neck fracture following groin irradiation. *Int J Radiat Oncol Biol Phys* 1995;32(1):63–67.
14. John M, Pajak T, Flam M, et al. Dose escalation in chemoradiation for anal cancer: preliminary results of RTOG 92–08. *Cancer J Sci Am* 1996;2(4):205.
15. Weber DC, Kurtz JM, Allal AS. The impact of gap duration on local control in anal canal carcinoma treated by split-course radiotherapy and concomitant chemotherapy. *Int J Radiat Oncol Biol Phys* 2001;50(3):675–680.
16. Ajani JA, Winter KA, Gunderson LL, et al. Fluorouracil, mitomycin, and radiotherapy vs fluorouracil, cisplatin, and radiotherapy for carcinoma of the anal canal: a randomized controlled trial. *Jama* 2008;299(16):1914–1921.
17. Rich TA, Ajani JA, Morrison WH, et al. Chemoradiation therapy for anal cancer: radiation plus continuous infusion of 5-fluorouracil with or without cisplatin. *Radiother Oncol* 1993;27(3):209–215.
18. Hu K, Minsky BD, Cohen AM, et al. 30 Gy may be an adequate dose in patients with anal cancer treated with excisional biopsy followed by combined-modality therapy. *J Surg Oncol* 1999;70(2):71–77.
19. Hatfield P, Cooper R, Sebag-Montefiore D. Involved-field, low-dose chemoradiotherapy for early-stage anal carcinoma. *Int J Radiat Oncol Biol Phys* 2008;70(2):419–424.
20. Kachnic L, Winter KA, Myerson RJ, et al. RTOG 0529: A phase II evaluation of dose-painted IMRT in combination with 5-fluorouracil and mitomycin-C for reduction of acute morbidity in carcinoma of the anal canal. *Int J Radiat Oncol Biol Phys* 2009;75(3):S5.
21. Constantinou EC, Daly W, Fung CY, et al. Time-dose considerations in the treatment of anal cancer. *Int J Radiat Oncol Biol Phys* 1997;39(3):651–657.
22. Martenson JA Jr, Gunderson LL. External radiation therapy without chemotherapy in the management of anal cancer. *Cancer* 1993;71(5):1736–1740.
23. McCall AR, Olson MC, Potkul RK. The variation of inguinal lymph node depth in adult women and its importance in planning elective irradiation for vulvar cancer. *Cancer* 1995;75(9):2286–2288.
24. Koh WJ, Chiu M, Stelzer KJ, et al. Femoral vessel depth and the implications for groin node radiation. *Int J Radiat Oncol Biol Phys* 1993;27(4):969–974.
25. Kalidas H. Influence of inguinal node anatomy on radiation therapy techniques. *Med Dosim* 1995;20(4):295–300.

26. Brown PD, Kline RW, Petersen IA, et al. Irradiation of the inguinal lymph nodes in patients of differing body habitus: a comparison of techniques and resulting normal tissue complication probabilities. *Med Dosim* 2004; 29(3):217–222.

27. Vuong T, Devic S, Belliveau P, et al. Contribution of conformal therapy in the treatment of anal canal carcinoma with combined chemotherapy and radiotherapy: results of a phase II study. *Int J Radiat Oncol Biol Phys* 2003; 56(3):823–831.

28. Chen YJ, Liu A, Tsai PT, et al. *Organ sparing by conformal avoidance instensity modulated radiation therapy for anal cancer, #4257.* Paper presented at the ASCO annual meeting, Orlando, FL, 2005.

29. Ahmad M, Song H, Moran M, et al. IMRT of whole pelvis and inguinal nodes: Evaluation of dose distributions produced by an inverse treatment planning system. *Int J Radiat Oncol Biol Phys* 2004;60(1):S484–S485.

30. Menkarios C, Azria D, Laliberte B, et al. Optimal organ-sparing intensity-modulated radiation therapy (IMRT) regimen for the treatment of locally advanced anal canal carcinoma: a comparison of conventional and IMRT plans. *Radiat Oncol* 2007;2:41.

31. Mell LK, Schomas DA, Salama JK, et al. Association between bone marrow dosimetric parameters and acute hematologic toxicity in anal cancer patients treated with concurrent chemotherapy and intensity-modulated radiotherapy. *Int J Radiat Oncol Biol Phys* 2008;70(5):1431–1437.

32. Milano MT, Jani AB, Farrey KJ, et al. Intensity-modulated radiation therapy (IMRT) in the treatment of anal cancer: toxicity and clinical outcome. *Int J Radiat Oncol Biol Phys* 2005;63(2):354–361.

33. Salama JK, Mell LK, Schomas DA, et al. Concurrent chemotherapy and intensity-modulated radiation therapy for anal canal cancer patients: a multicenter experience. *J Clin Oncol* 2007;25(29):4581–4586.

34. Rosenthal DI, Chang CH, Orr KY. Transmission blocks for lower neck and inguinal lymph node radiotherapy. *Med Dosim* 1998;23(1):1–4.

35. Dittmer PH, Randall ME. A technique for inguinal node boost using photon fields defined by asymmetric collimator jaws. *Radiother Oncol* 2001;59(1):61–64.

36. Watson BA, Tatro DS, Ten Haken RK, et al. Use of segmental boost fields in the irradiation of inguinal lymphatic nodes. *Med Dosim* 1999;24(1):27–32.

37. Hung A, Crane C, Delclos M, et al. Cisplatin-based combined modality therapy for anal carcinoma: a wider therapeutic index. *Cancer* 2003;97(5):1195–1202.

38. Lee WR, McCollough WM, Mendenhall WM, et al. Elective inguinal lymph node irradiation for pelvic carcinomas. The University of Florida experience. *Cancer* 1993;72(6):2058–2065.

39. Minsky BD. Anal canal cancer. In: Leibel SA, Phillips TL, eds. *Textbook of radiation oncology,* 1st ed. Philadelphia: W.B. Saunders Co., 1998:703–709.

40. Gerard JP, Ayzac L, Hun D, et al. Treatment of anal canal carcinoma with high dose radiation therapy and concomitant fluorouracil-cisplatinum. Long-term results in 95 patients. *Radiother Oncol* 1998;46(3):249–256.

41. Kim NK, Kim MJ, Yun SH, et al. Comparative study of transrectal ultrasonography, pelvic computerized tomography, and magnetic resonance imaging in preoperative staging of rectal cancer. *Dis Colon Rectum* 1999; 42(6):770–775.

42. MERCURY Study Group. Diagnostic accuracy of preoperative magnetic resonance imaging in predicting curative resection of rectal cancer: prospective observational study. *BMJ* 2006;333(7572):779.

43. MERCURY Study Group. Extramural depth of tumor invasion at thin-section MR in patients with rectal cancer: results of the MERCURY study. *Radiology* 2007; 243(1):132–139.

44. Calvo FA, Domper M, Matute R, et al. 18 F-FDG positron emission tomography staging and restaging in rectal cancer treated with preoperative chemoradiation. *Int J Radiat Oncol Biol Phys* 2004;58(2):528–535.

45. Prolongation of the disease-free interval in surgically treated rectal carcinoma. Gastrointestinal Tumor Study Group. *N Engl J Med* 1985;312(23):1465–1472.

46. Douglass HO Jr, Moertel CG, Mayer RJ, et al. Survival after postoperative combination treatment of rectal cancer. *N Engl J Med* 1986;315(20):1294–1295.

47. Krook JE, Moertel CG, Gunderson LL, et al. Effective surgical adjuvant therapy for high-risk rectal carcinoma. *N Engl J Med* 1991;324(11):709–715.

48. Sauer R, Becker H, Hohenberger W, et al. Preoperative versus postoperative chemoradiotherapy for rectal cancer. *N Engl J Med* 2004;351(17):1731–1740.

49. Improved survival with preoperative radiotherapy in resectable rectal cancer. Swedish Rectal Cancer Trial. *N Engl J Med* 1997;336(14):980–987.

50. Kapiteijn E, Marijnen CA, Nagtegaal ID, et al. Preoperative radiotherapy combined with total mesorectal excision for resectable rectal cancer. *N Engl J Med* 2001; 345(9):638–646.

51. Willett CG, Tepper JE, Skates SJ, et al. Adjuvant postoperative radiation therapy for colonic carcinoma. *Ann Surg* 1987;206(6):694–698.

52. Willett CG, Goldberg S, Shellito PC, et al. Does postoperative irradiation play a role in the adjuvant therapy of stage T4 colon cancer? *Cancer J Sci Am* 1999;5(4):242–247.

53. Martenson JA Jr, Willett CG, Sargent DJ, et al. Phase III study of adjuvant chemotherapy and radiation therapy compared with chemotherapy alone in the surgical adjuvant treatment of colon cancer: results of intergroup protocol 0130. *J Clin Oncol* 2004;22(16):3277–3283.

54. Robertson JM, Lockman D, Yan D, et al. The dose-volume relationship of small bowel irradiation and acute grade 3 diarrhea during chemoradiotherapy for rectal cancer. *Int J Radiat Oncol Biol Phys* 2008;70(2):413–418.

55. Tho LM, Glegg M, Paterson J, et al. Acute small bowel toxicity and preoperative chemoradiotherapy for rectal cancer: investigating dose-volume relationships and role for inverse planning. *Int J Radiat Oncol Biol Phys* 2006;66(2):505–513.

56. Gallagher MJ, Brereton HD, Rostock RA, et al. A prospective study of treatment techniques to minimize the volume of pelvic small bowel with reduction of acute and late effects associated with pelvic irradiation. *Int J Radiat Oncol Biol Phys* 1986;12(9):1565–1573.

57. Martin J, Fitzpatrick K, Horan G, et al. Treatment with a belly-board device significantly reduces the volume of small bowel irradiated and results in low acute toxicity

in adjuvant radiotherapy for gynecologic cancer: results of a prospective study. *Radiother Oncol* 2005;74(3):267–274.

58. Olofsen-van Acht M, Van Den Berg H, Quint S, et al. Reduction of irradiated small bowel volume and accurate patient positioning by use of a bellyboard device in pelvic radiotherapy of gynecological cancer patients. *Radiother Oncol* 2001;59(1):87–93.

59. Pinkawa M, Gagel B, Demirel C, et al. Dose-volume histogram evaluation of prone and supine patient position in external beam radiotherapy for cervical and endometrial cancer. *Radiother Oncol* 2003;69(1):99–105.

60. Kim TH, Chie EK, Kim DY, et al. Comparison of the belly board device method and the distended bladder method for reducing irradiated small bowel volumes in preoperative radiotherapy of rectal cancer patients. *Int J Radiat Oncol Biol Phys* 2005;62(3):769–775.

61. Nuyttens JJ, Robertson JM, Yan D, et al. The position and volume of the small bowel during adjuvant radiation therapy for rectal cancer. *Int J Radiat Oncol Biol Phys* 2001;51(5):1271–1280.

62. Myerson R, Drzymala R. Technical aspects of image-based treatment planning of rectal carcinoma. *Semin Radiat Oncol* 2003;13(4):433–440.

63. Moossa AR, Ree PC, Marks JE, et al. Factors influencing local recurrence after abdominoperineal resection for cancer of the rectum and rectosigmoid. *Br J Surg* 1975;62(9):727–730.

64. Roberson SH, Heron HC, Kerman HD, et al. Is anterior resection of the rectosigmoid safe after preoperative radiation? *Dis Colon Rectum* 1985;28(4):254–259.

65. Ciatto S, Pacini P. Radiation therapy of recurrences of carcinoma of the rectum and sigmoid after surgery. *Acta Radiol Oncol* 1982;21(2):105–109.

66. Schild SE, Martenson JA Jr, Gunderson LL, et al. Postoperative adjuvant therapy of rectal cancer: an analysis of disease control, survival, and prognostic factors. *Int J Radiat Oncol Biol Phys* 1989;17(1):55–62.

67. Bassi MC, Turri L, Sacchetti G, et al. FDG-PET/CT imaging for staging and target volume delineation in preoperative conformal radiotherapy of rectal cancer. *Int J Radiat Oncol Biol Phys* 2008;70(5):1423–1426.

68. Anderson C, Koshy M, Staley C, et al. PET-CT fusion in radiation management of patients with anorectal tumors. *Int J Radiat Oncol Biol Phys* 2007;69(1):155–162.

69. Hruby G, Barton M, Miles S, et al. Sites of local recurrence after surgery, with or without chemotherapy, for rectal cancer: implications for radiotherapy field design. *Int J Radiat Oncol Biol Phys* 2003;55(1):138–143.

70. Syk E, Torkzad MR, Blomqvist L, et al. Local recurrence in rectal cancer: anatomic localization and effect on radiation target. *Int J Radiat Oncol Biol Phys* 2008;72(3):658–664.

71. Yu TK, Bhosale PR, Crane CH, et al. Patterns of locoregional recurrence after surgery and radiotherapy or chemoradiation for rectal cancer. *Int J Radiat Oncol Biol Phys* 2008;71(4):1175–1180.

72. Chao KS, Lin M. Lymphangiogram-assisted lymph node target delineation for patients with gynecologic malignancies. *Int J Radiat Oncol Biol Phys* 2002;54(4):1147–1152.

73. Roels S, Duthoy W, Haustermans K, et al. Definition and delineation of the clinical target volume for rectal cancer. *Int J Radiat Oncol Biol Phys* 2006;65(4):1129–1142.

74. Sanfilippo NJ, Crane CH, Skibber J, et al. T4 rectal cancer treated with preoperative chemoradiation to the posterior pelvis followed by multivisceral resection: patterns of failure and limitations of treatment. *Int J Radiat Oncol Biol Phys* 2001;51(1):176–183.

75. Taylor N, Crane C, Skibber J, et al. Elective groin irradiation is not indicated for patients with adenocarcinoma of the rectum extending to the anal canal. *Int J Radiat Oncol Biol Phys* 2001;51(3):741–747.

76. Robertson JM, Campbell JP, Yan D. Generic planning target margin for rectal cancer treatment setup variation. *Int J Radiat Oncol Biol Phys* 2009;74(5):1470–1475.

77. Tournel K, De Ridder M, Engels B, et al. Assessment of intrafractional movement and internal motion in radiotherapy of rectal cancer using megavoltage computed tomography. *Int J Radiat Oncol Biol Phys* 2008;71(3):934–939.

78. Brizel HE, Tepperman BS. Postoperative adjuvant irradiation for adenocarcinoma of the rectum and sigmoid. *Am J Clin Oncol* 1984;7(6):679–685.

79. O'Connell MJ, Martenson JA, Wieand HS, et al. Improving adjuvant therapy for rectal cancer by combining protracted-infusion fluorouracil with radiation therapy after curative surgery. *N Engl J Med* 1994;331(8):502–507.

80. Engels B, De Ridder M, Tournel K, et al. Preoperative helical tomotherapy and megavoltage computed tomography for rectal cancer: impact on the irradiated volume of small bowel. *Int J Radiat Oncol Biol Phys* 2009;74(5):1476–1480.

81. Guerrero Urbano MT, Henrys AJ, Adams EJ, et al. Intensity-modulated radiotherapy in patients with locally advanced rectal cancer reduces volume of bowel treated to high dose levels. *Int J Radiat Oncol Biol Phys* 2006;65(3):907–916.

82. Callister M, Ezzell GA, Gunderson LL. IMRT reduces the dose to small bowel and other pelvic in the preoperative treatment of rectal cancer. *Int J Radiat Oncol Biol Phys* 2006;66(3):S290.

83. De Ridder M, Tournel K, Van Nieuwenhove Y, et al. Phase II study of preoperative helical tomotherapy for rectal cancer. *Int J Radiat Oncol Biol Phys* 2008;70(3):728–734.

84. Freedman GM, Meropol NJ, Sigurdson ER, et al. Phase I trial of preoperative hypofractionated intensity-modulated radiotherapy with incorporated boost and oral capecitabine in locally advanced rectal cancer. *Int J Radiat Oncol Biol Phys* 2007;67(5):1389–1393.

85. Aristu JJ, Arbea L, Rodriguez J, et al. Phase I-II trial of concurrent capecitabine and oxaliplatin with preoperative intensity-modulated radiotherapy in patients with locally advanced rectal cancer. *Int J Radiat Oncol Biol Phys* 2008;71(3):748–755.

86. Samuelian JM, Callister M, Ashman JB, et al. *Does intensity-modulated radiotherapy (IMRT) reduce acute bowel toxicity in patients treated for rectal cancer?* Paper presented at 2010 gastrointestinal cancers symposium, Orlando, FL, 2010.

87. Smalley SR, Benedetti JK, Williamson SK, et al. Phase III trial of fluorouracil-based chemotherapy regimens plus radiotherapy in postoperative adjuvant rectal cancer: GI INT 0144. *J Clin Oncol* 2006;24(22):3542–3547.

88. Corvo R, Pastrone I, Scolaro T, et al. Radiotherapy and oral capecitabine in the preoperative treatment of patients with rectal cancer: rationale, preliminary results and perspectives. *Tumori* 2003;89(4):361–367.

89. Dunst J, Reese T, Sutter T, et al. Phase I trial evaluating the concurrent combination of radiotherapy and capecitabine in rectal cancer. *J Clin Oncol* 2002;20(19): 3983–3991.

90. Kim JC, Kim TW, Kim JH, et al. Preoperative concurrent radiotherapy with capecitabine before total mesorectal excision in locally advanced rectal cancer. *Int J Radiat Oncol Biol Phys* 2005;63(2):346–353.

91. Kim JS, Kim JS, Cho MJ, et al. Preoperative chemoradiation using oral capecitabine in locally advanced rectal cancer. *Int J Radiat Oncol Biol Phys* 2002;54(2): 403–408.

92. Gunderson LL, Sargent DJ, Tepper JE, et al. Impact of T and N stage and treatment on survival and relapse in adjuvant rectal cancer: a pooled analysis. *J Clin Oncol* 2004;22(10):1785–1796.

93. Vargas R, Nino-Murcia M, Trueblood W, et al. MDCT in Pancreatic adenocarcinoma: prediction of vascular invasion and resectability using a multiphasic technique with curved planar reformations. *AJR Am J Roentgenol* 2004;182(2):419–425.

94. Zimny M. Diagnostic imaging of pancreatic cancer—the role of PET. *Front Radiat Ther Oncol* 2004;38:67–75.

95. Kauhanen SP, Komar G, Seppanen MP, et al. A prospective diagnostic accuracy study of 18 F-fluorodeoxyglucose positron emission tomography/computed tomography, multidetector row computed tomography, and magnetic resonance imaging in primary diagnosis and staging of pancreatic cancer. *Ann Surg* 2009;250(6): 957–963.

96. Griffin JF, Smalley SR, Jewell W, et al. Patterns of failure after curative resection of pancreatic carcinoma. *Cancer* 1990;66(1):56–61.

97. Tepper J, Nardi G, Sutt H. Carcinoma of the pancreas: review of MGH experience from 1963 to 1973. Analysis of surgical failure and implications for radiation therapy. *Cancer* 1976;37(3):1519–1524.

98. Further evidence of effective adjuvant combined radiation and chemotherapy following curative resection of pancreatic cancer. Gastrointestinal Tumor Study Group. *Cancer* 1987;59(12):2006–2010.

99. Neoptolemos JP, Stocken DD, Friess H, et al. A randomized trial of chemoradiotherapy and chemotherapy after resection of pancreatic cancer. *N Engl J Med* 2004; 350(12):1200–1210.

100. Hsu CC, Herman JM, Corsini MM, et al. Adjuvant chemoradiation for pancreatic adenocarcinoma: the Johns Hopkins hospital-Mayo clinic collaborative study. *Ann Surg Oncol* 2010;17(4):981–990. Published online Jan 20.

101. Corsini MM, Miller RC, Haddock MG, et al. Adjuvant radiotherapy and chemotherapy for pancreatic carcinoma: the Mayo Clinic experience (1975–2005). *J Clin Oncol* 2008;26(21):3511–3516.

102. Spitz FR, Abbruzzese JL, Lee JE, et al. Preoperative and postoperative chemoradiation strategies in patients treated with pancreaticoduodenectomy for adenocarcinoma of the pancreas. *J Clin Oncol* 1997;15(3):928–937.

103. Evans DB, Rich TA, Byrd DR, et al. Preoperative chemoradiation and pancreaticoduodenectomy for adenocarcinoma of the pancreas. *Arch Surg* 1992;127(11): 1335–1339.

104. Hoffman JP, Lipsitz S, Pisansky T, et al. Phase II trial of preoperative radiation therapy and chemotherapy for patients with localized, resectable adenocarcinoma of the pancreas: an Eastern Cooperative Oncology Group Study. *J Clin Oncol* 1998;16(1):317–323.

105. Lowy AM, Lee JE, Pisters PW, et al. Prospective, randomized trial of octreotide to prevent pancreatic fistula after pancreaticoduodenectomy for malignant disease. *Ann Surg* 1997;226(5):632–641.

106. Crane CH, Evans DB, Wolff RA, et al. The pancreas. In: Cox JD, Ang KK, eds. *Radiation oncology: rationale, technique, results.* St. Louis, MO: Mosby, Inc., 2003: 465–480.

107. Klaassen DJ, MacIntyre JM, Catton GE, et al. Treatment of locally unresectable cancer of the stomach and pancreas: a randomized comparison of 5-fluorouracil alone with radiation plus concurrent and maintenance 5-fluorouracil–an Eastern Cooperative Oncology Group study. *J Clin Oncol* 1985;3(3):373–378.

108. Moertel CG, Frytak S, Hahn RG, et al. Therapy of locally unresectable pancreatic carcinoma: a randomized comparison of high dose (6000 rads) radiation alone, moderate dose radiation (4000 rads + 5-fluorouracil), and high dose radiation + 5-fluorouracil: The Gastrointestinal Tumor Study Group. *Cancer* 1981;48(8):1705–1710.

109. Treatment of locally unresectable carcinoma of the pancreas: comparison of combined-modality therapy (chemotherapy plus radiotherapy) to chemotherapy alone. Gastrointestinal Tumor Study Group. *J Natl Cancer Inst* 1988;80(10):751–755.

110. Loehrer PJ, Powell ME, Cardenes HR, et al. A randomized phase III study of gemcitabine in combination with radiation therapy versus gemcitabine alone in patients with localized, unresectable pancreatic cancer: E4201. *J Clin Oncol* 2008;29(S):4506.

111. Shinchi H, Takao S, Noma H, et al. Length and quality of survival after external-beam radiotherapy with concurrent continuous 5-fluorouracil infusion for locally unresectable pancreatic cancer. *Int J Radiat Oncol Biol Phys* 2002;53(1):146–150.

112. Tokuuye K, Sumi M, Kagami Y, et al. Small-field radiotherapy in combination with concomitant chemotherapy for locally advanced pancreatic carcinoma. *Radiother Oncol* 2003;67(3):327–330.

113. Chang DT, Schellenberg D, Shen J, et al. Stereotactic radiotherapy for unresectable adenocarcinoma of the pancreas. *Cancer* 2009;115(3):665–672.

114. Seo Y, Kim MS, Yoo S, et al. Stereotactic body radiation therapy boost in locally advanced pancreatic cancer. *Int J Radiat Oncol Biol Phys* 2009;75(5):1456–1461.

115. Brunner TB, Merkel S, Grabenbauer GG, et al. Definition of elective lymphatic target volume in ductal carcinoma of the pancreatic head based on histopathologic analysis. *Int J Radiat Oncol Biol Phys* 2005;62(4):1021–1029.

116. Kayahara M, Nagakawa T, Ohta T, et al. Analysis of paraaortic lymph node involvement in pancreatic carcinoma: a significant indication for surgery? *Cancer* 1999;85(3):583–590.

117. Kao GD, Whittington R, Coia L. Anatomy of the celiac axis and superior mesenteric artery and its significance in radiation therapy. *Int J Radiat Oncol Biol Phys* 1993;25(1):131–134.

118. Nagakawa T, Kobayashi H, Ueno K, et al. Clinical study of lymphatic flow to the paraaortic lymph nodes in carcinoma of the head of the pancreas. *Cancer* 1994;73(4):1155–1162.

119. Bussels B, Goethals L, Feron M, et al. Respiration-induced movement of the upper abdominal organs: a pitfall for the three-dimensional conformal radiation treatment of pancreatic cancer. *Radiother Oncol* 2003;68(1):69–74.

120. Feng M, Balter JM, Normolle D, et al. Characterization of pancreatic tumor motion using cine MRI: surrogates for tumor position should be used with caution. *Int J Radiat Oncol Biol Phys* 2009;74(3):884–891.

121. Jayachandran P, Minn AY, Van Dam J, et al. Interfractional uncertainty in the treatment of pancreatic cancer with radiation. *Int J Radiat Oncol Biol Phys* 2010;76(2):603–728.

122. Higgins PD, Sohn JW, Fine RM, et al. Three-dimensional conformal pancreas treatment: comparison of four- to six-field techniques. *Int J Radiat Oncol Biol Phys* 1995;31(3):605–609.

123. Steadham AM, Liu HH, Crane CH, et al. Optimization of beam orientations and weights for coplanar conformal beams in treating pancreatic cancer. *Med Dosim* 1999;24(4):265–271.

124. Ben-Josef E, Shields AF, Vaishampayan U, et al. Intensity-modulated radiotherapy (IMRT) and concurrent capecitabine for pancreatic cancer. *Int J Radiat Oncol Biol Phys* 2004;59(2):454–459.

125. Milano MT, Chmura SJ, Garofalo MC, et al. Intensity-modulated radiotherapy in treatment of pancreatic and bile duct malignancies: toxicity and clinical outcome. *Int J Radiat Oncol Biol Phys* 2004;59(2):445–453.

126. Van Der Geld YG, van Triest B, Verbakel WF, et al. Evaluation of four-dimensional computed tomography-based intensity-modulated and respiratory-gated radiotherapy techniques for pancreatic carcinoma. *Int J Radiat Oncol Biol Phys* 2008;72(4):1215–1220.

127. Brown MW, Ning H, Arora B, et al. A dosimetric analysis of dose escalation using two intensity-modulated radiation therapy techniques in locally advanced pancreatic carcinoma. *Int J Radiat Oncol Biol Phys* 2006;65(1):274–283.

128. Fuss M, Wong A, Fuller CD, et al. Image-guided intensity-modulated radiotherapy for pancreatic carcinoma. *Gastrointest Cancer Res* 2007;1(1):2–11.

129. Whittington R, Neuberg D, Tester WJ, et al. Protracted intravenous fluorouracil infusion with radiation therapy in the management of localized pancreaticobiliary carcinoma: a phase I Eastern Cooperative Oncology Group Trial. *J Clin Oncol* 1995;13(1):227–232.

130. Li CP, Chao Y, Chi KH, et al. Concurrent chemoradiotherapy treatment of locally advanced pancreatic cancer: gemcitabine versus 5-fluorouracil, a randomized controlled study. *Int J Radiat Oncol Biol Phys* 2003;57(1):98–104.

131. Crane CH, Wolff RA, Abbruzzese JL, et al. Combining gemcitabine with radiation in pancreatic cancer: understanding important variables influencing the therapeutic index. *Semin Oncol* 2001;28(3 Suppl 10):25–33.

132. Willett CG, Del Castillo CF, Shih HA, et al. Long-term results of intraoperative electron beam irradiation (IOERT) for patients with unresectable pancreatic cancer. *Ann Surg* 2005;241(2):295–299.

133. Burris HA 3rd, Moore MJ, Andersen J, et al. Improvements in survival and clinical benefit with gemcitabine as first-line therapy for patients with advanced pancreas cancer: a randomized trial. *J Clin Oncol* 1997;15(6):2403–2413.

134. Blot WJ, Devesa SS, Kneller RW, et al. Rising incidence of adenocarcinoma of the esophagus and gastric cardia. *Jama* 1991;265(10):1287–1289.

135. Devesa SS, Blot WJ, Fraumeni JF Jr. Changing patterns in the incidence of esophageal and gastric carcinoma in the United States. *Cancer* 1998;83(10):2049–2053.

136. Esophagus. In: Green FL, et al., eds. *AJCC cancer staging handbook*, 6th ed. Philadelphia: Lippincott Raven Publishers, 2005:101–109.

137. Saito N, Takeshita K, Habu H, et al. The use of endoscopic ultrasound in determining the depth of cancer invasion in patients with gastric cancer. *Surg Endosc* 1991;5(1):14–19.

138. Caletti G, Ferrari A, Brocchi E, et al. Accuracy of endoscopic ultrasonography in the diagnosis and staging of gastric cancer and lymphoma. *Surgery* 1993;113(1):14–27.

139. Natsugoe S, Yoshinaka H, Morinaga T, et al. Ultrasonographic detection of lymph-node metastases in superficial carcinoma of the esophagus. *Endoscopy* 1996;28(8):674–679.

140. Hiele M, De Leyn P, Schurmans P, et al. Relation between endoscopic ultrasound findings and outcome of patients with tumors of the esophagus or esophagogastric junction. *Gastrointest Endosc* 1997;45(5):381–386.

141. Botet JF, Lightdale CJ, Zauber AG, et al. Preoperative staging of esophageal cancer: comparison of endoscopic US and dynamic CT. *Radiology* 1991;181(2):419–425.

142. Tio TL, Coene PP, den Hartog Jager FC, et al. Preoperative TNM classification of esophageal carcinoma by endosonography. *Hepatogastroenterology* 1990;37(4):376–381.

143. Yeung HW, Macapinlac H, Karpeh M, et al. Accuracy of FDG-PET in gastric cancer. Preliminary experience. *Clin Positron Imaging* 1998;1(4):213–221.

144. Chen J, Cheong JH, Yun MJ, et al. Improvement in preoperative staging of gastric adenocarcinoma with positron emission tomography. *Cancer* 2005;103(11):2383–2390.

145. Lerut T, Flamen P, Ectors N, et al. Histopathologic validation of lymph node staging with FDG-PET scan in cancer of the esophagus and gastroesophageal junction: A prospective study based on primary surgery with extensive lymphadenectomy. *Ann Surg* 2000;232(6):743–752.

146. Flamen P, Lerut A, Van Cutsem E, et al. Utility of positron emission tomography for the staging of patients with potentially operable esophageal carcinoma. *J Clin Oncol* 2000;18(18):3202–3210.

147. Konski A, Doss M, Milestone B, et al. The integration of 18-fluoro-deoxy-glucose positron emission tomography and endoscopic ultrasound in the treatment-planning process for esophageal carcinoma. *Int J Radiat Oncol Biol Phys* 2005;61(4):1123–1128.

148. Gschossmann JM, Bonner JA, Foote RL, et al. Malignant tracheoesophageal fistula in patients with esophageal cancer. *Cancer* 1993;72(5):1513–1521.

149. Yamada S, Takai Y, Ogawa Y, et al. Radiotherapy for malignant fistula to other tract. *Cancer* 1989;64(5):1026–1028.

150. Burt M, Diehl W, Martini N, et al. Malignant esophagorespiratory fistula: management options and survival. *Ann Thorac Surg* 1991;52(6):1222–1228; discussion 1228–1229.

151. Martini N, Goodner JT, D'Angio GJ, et al. Tracheoesophageal fistula due to cancer. *J Thorac Cardiovasc Surg* 1970;59(3):319–324.

152. Macdonald JS, Smalley SR, Benedetti J, et al. Chemoradiotherapy after surgery compared with surgery alone for adenocarcinoma of the stomach or gastroesophageal junction. *N Engl J Med* 2001;345(10):725–730.

153. al-Sarraf M, Martz K, Herskovic A, et al. Progress report of combined chemoradiotherapy versus radiotherapy alone in patients with esophageal cancer: an intergroup study. *J Clin Oncol* 1997;15(1):277–284.

154. Herskovic A, Martz K, al-Sarraf M, et al. Combined chemotherapy and radiotherapy compared with radiotherapy alone in patients with cancer of the esophagus. *N Engl J Med* 1992;326(24):1593–1598.

155. Kelsen DP, Ginsberg R, Pajak TF, et al. Chemotherapy followed by surgery compared with surgery alone for localized esophageal cancer. *N Engl J Med* 1998;339(27):1979–1984.

156. Chiu PW, Chan AC, Leung SF, et al. Multicenter prospective randomized trial comparing standard esophagectomy with chemoradiotherapy for treatment of squamous esophageal cancer: early results from the Chinese University Research Group for Esophageal Cancer (CURE). *J Gastrointest Surg* 2005;9(6):794–802.

157. Wang M, Gu XZ, Yin WB, et al. Randomized clinical trial on the combination of preoperative irradiation and surgery in the treatment of esophageal carcinoma: report on 206 patients. *Int J Radiat Oncol Biol Phys* 1989;16(2):325–327.

158. Gignoux M, Roussel A, Paillot B, et al. The value of preoperative radiotherapy in esophageal cancer: results of a study by the EORTC. *Recent Results Cancer Res* 1988;110:1–13.

159. Nygaard K, Hagen S, Hansen HS, et al. Pre-operative radiotherapy prolongs survival in operable esophageal carcinoma: a randomized, multicenter study of preoperative radiotherapy and chemotherapy. The second Scandinavian trial in esophageal cancer. *World J Surg* 1992;16(6):1104–1109; discussion 1110.

160. Apinop C, Puttisak P, Preecha N. A prospective study of combined therapy in esophageal cancer. *Hepatogastroenterology* 1994;41(4):391–393.

161. Burmeister B, Smithers B, Fitzgerald L, et al. A randomized phase III trial of preoperative chemoradiation followed by surgery (CR-S) versus surgery alone (S) for localized resectable cancer of the esophagus. *Lancet Oncology* 2005;6(9):659–668.

162. Bosset JF, Gignoux M, Triboulet JP, et al. Chemoradiotherapy followed by surgery compared with surgery alone in squamous-cell cancer of the esophagus. *N Engl J Med* 1997;337(3):161–167.

163. Urba SG, Orringer MB, Turrisi A, et al. Randomized trial of preoperative chemoradiation versus surgery alone in patients with locoregional esophageal carcinoma. *J Clin Oncol* 2001;19(2):305–313.

164. Walsh TN, Noonan N, Hollywood D, et al. A comparison of multimodal therapy and surgery for esophageal adenocarcinoma. *N Engl J Med* 1996;335(7):462–467.

165. Tepper J, Krasna MJ, Niedzwiecki D, et al. Phase III trial of trimodality therapy with cisplatin, fluorouracil, radiotherapy, and surgery compared with surgery alone for esophageal cancer: CALGB 9781. *J Clin Oncol* 2008;26(7):1086–1092.

166. Le Prise E, Etienne PL, Meunier B, et al. A randomized study of chemotherapy, radiation therapy, and surgery versus surgery for localized squamous cell carcinoma of the esophagus. *Cancer* 1994;73(7):1779–1784.

167. Stahl M, Stuschke M, Lehmann N, et al. Chemoradiation with and without surgery in patients with locally advanced squamous cell carcinoma of the esophagus. *J Clin Oncol* 2005;23(10):2310–2317.

168. Bedenne L, Michel P, Bouche O, et al. Chemoradiation followed by surgery compared with chemoradiation alone in squamous cancer of the esophagus: FFCD 9102. *J Clin Oncol* 2007;25(10):1160–1168.

169. Teniere P, Hay JM, Fingerhut A, et al. Postoperative radiation therapy does not increase survival after curative resection for squamous cell carcinoma of the middle and lower esophagus as shown by a multicenter controlled trial. French University Association for Surgical Research. *Surg Gynecol Obstet* 1991;173(2):123–130.

170. Fok M, Sham JS, Choy D, et al. Postoperative radiotherapy for carcinoma of the esophagus: a prospective, randomized controlled study. *Surgery* 1993;113(2):138–147.

171. Zieren HU, Muller JM, Jacobi CA, et al. Adjuvant postoperative radiation therapy after curative resection of squamous cell carcinoma of the thoracic esophagus: a prospective randomized study. *World J Surg* 1995;19(3):444–449.

172. Rice TW, Adelstein DJ, Chidel MA, et al. Benefit of postoperative adjuvant chemoradiotherapy in locoregionally advanced esophageal carcinoma. *J Thorac Cardiovasc Surg* 2003;126(5):1590–1596.

173. Corn BW, Coia LR, Chu JC, et al. Significance of prone positioning in planning treatment for esophageal cancer. *Int J Radiat Oncol Biol Phys* 1991;21(5):1303–1309.

174. Patel AA, Wolfgang JA, Niemierko A, et al. Implications of respiratory motion as measured by four-dimensional computed tomography for radiation treatment planning of esophageal cancer. *Int J Radiat Oncol Biol Phys* 2009;74(1):290–296.

175. Dieleman EM, Senan S, Vincent A, et al. Four-dimensional computed tomographic analysis of esophageal mobility during normal respiration. *Int J Radiat Oncol Biol Phys* 2007;67(3):775–780.

176. Sykes AJ, Burt PA, Slevin NJ, et al. Radical radiotherapy for carcinoma of the oesophagus: an effective alternative to surgery. *Radiother Oncol* 1998;48(1):15–21.

177. Thomas E, Crellin A, Harris K, et al. The role of endoscopic ultrasound (EUS) in planning radiotherapy target volumes for oesophageal cancer. *Radiother Oncol* 2004;73(2):149–151.

178. Vrieze O, Haustermans K, De Wever W, et al. Is there a role for FGD-PET in radiotherapy planning in esophageal carcinoma? *Radiother Oncol* 2004;73(3):269–275.

179. Sannohe Y, Hiratsuka R, Doki K. Lymph node metastases in cancer of the thoracic esophagus. *Am J Surg* 1981;141(2):216–218.

180. Mandard AM, Chasle J, Marnay J, et al. Autopsy findings in 111 cases of esophageal cancer. *Cancer* 1981;48(2):329–335.

181. Minsky BD, Pajak TF, Ginsberg RJ, et al. INT 0123 (Radiation Therapy Oncology Group 94–05) phase III trial of combined-modality therapy for esophageal cancer: high-dose versus standard-dose radiation therapy. *J Clin Oncol* 2002;20(5):1167–1174.

182. Gao XS, Qiao X, Wu F, et al. Pathological analysis of clinical target volume margin for radiotherapy in patients with esophageal and gastroesophageal junction carcinoma. *Int J Radiat Oncol Biol Phys* 2007;67(2):389–396.

183. Akiyama H, Tsurumaru M, Udagawa H, et al. Radical lymph node dissection for cancer of the thoracic esophagus. *Ann Surg* 1994;220(3):364–372; discussion 372–363.

184. Meier I, Merkel S, Papadopoulos T, et al. Adenocarcinoma of the esophagogastric junction: the pattern of metastatic lymph node dissemination as a rationale for elective lymphatic target volume definition. *Int J Radiat Oncol Biol Phys* 2008;70(5):1408–1417.

185. Gunderson LL, Sosin H. Adenocarcinoma of the stomach: areas of failure in a re-operation series (second or symptomatic look) clinicopathologic correlation and implications for adjuvant therapy. *Int J Radiat Oncol Biol Phys* 1982;8(1):1–11.

186. Yu E, Dar R, Rodrigues GB, et al. Is extended volume external beam radiation therapy covering the anastomotic site beneficial in post-esophagectomy high risk patients? *Radiother Oncol* 2004;73(2):141–148.

187. Smalley SR, Gunderson L, Tepper J, et al. Gastric surgical adjuvant radiotherapy consensus report: rationale and treatment implementation. *Int J Radiat Oncol Biol Phys* 2002;52(2):283–293.

188. Tucker SL, Liu HH, Wang S, et al. Dose-volume modeling of the risk of postoperative pulmonary complications among esophageal cancer patients treated with concurrent chemoradiotherapy followed by surgery. *Int J Radiat Oncol Biol Phys* 2006;66(3):754–761.

189. Wang SL, Liao Z, Vaporciyan AA, et al. Investigation of clinical and dosimetric factors associated with postoperative pulmonary complications in esophageal cancer patients treated with concurrent chemoradiotherapy followed by surgery. *Int J Radiat Oncol Biol Phys* 2006;64(3):692–699.

190. Chung HT, Shakespeare TP, Wynne CJ, et al. Evaluation of a radiotherapy protocol based on INT0116 for completely resected gastric adenocarcinoma. *Int J Radiat Oncol Biol Phys* 2004;59(5):1446–1453.

191. Bedford JL, Viviers L, Guzel Z, et al. A quantitative treatment planning study evaluating the potential of dose escalation in conformal radiotherapy of the oesophagus. *Radiother Oncol* 2000;57(2):183–193.

192. Leong T, Willis D, Joon DL, et al. 3D Conformal radiotherapy for gastric cancer-results of a comparative planning study. *Radiother Oncol* 2005;74(3):301–306.

193. Ringash J, Khaksart SJ, Oza A, et al. Post-operative radiochemotherapy for gastric cancer: adoption and adaptation. *Clin Oncol (R Coll Radiol)* 2005;17(2):91–95.

194. Ringash J, Perkins G, Brierley J, et al. IMRT for adjuvant radiation in gastric cancer: A preferred plan? *Int J Radiat Oncol Biol Phys* 2005;63(3):732–738.

195. Dahele M, Skinner M, Schultz B, et al. Adjuvant radiotherapy for gastric cancer: a dosimetric comparison of 3Dimensional conformal radiotherapy, tomotherapy and conventional intensity modulated radiotherapy treatment plans. *Int J Radiat Oncol Biol Phys* 2009;35(2):115–121.

196. Wieland P, Dobler B, Mai S, et al. IMRT for postoperative treatment of gastric cancer: covering large target volumes in the upper abdomen: a comparison of a step-and-shoot and an arc therapy approach. *Int J Radiat Oncol Biol Phys* 2004;59(4):1236–1244.

197. Verheij M, Oppedijk V, Boot H, et al. *Late renal toxicity following post-operative chemoradiotherapy in gastric cancer (#2).* Paper presented at the ASCO GI cancer symposium, Hollywood, FL, 2005.

198. Van Der Geld YG, Senan S, van Sornsen de Koste JR, et al. A four-dimensional CT-based evaluation of techniques for gastric irradiation. *Int J Radiat Oncol Biol Phys* 2007;69(3):903–909.

199. Mayo CS, Urie MM, Fitzgerald TJ, et al. Hybrid IMRT for treatment of cancers of the lung and esophagus. *Int J Radiat Oncol Biol Phys* 2008;71(5):1408–1418.

200. Chen YJ, Liu A, Han C, et al. Helical tomotherapy for radiotherapy in esophageal cancer: a preferred plan with better conformal target coverage and more homogeneous dose distribution. *Med Dosim* 2007;32(3):166–171.

201. Hsu FM, Lee YC, Lee JM, et al. Association of clinical and dosimetric factors with postoperative pulmonary complications in esophageal cancer patients receiving intensity-modulated radiation therapy and concurrent chemotherapy followed by thoracic esophagectomy. *Ann Surg Oncol* 2009;16(6):1669–1677.

202. Ashman JB, Callister MD, Ezzell GA, et al. Use of intensity-modulated radiotherapy (IMRT) for distal esophageal/esophagogastric junction cancer to reduce lund and heart doses in selected patients. #98. Paper presented at the gastrointestinal cancers symposium, Orlando, FL, 2010.

203. King RM, Pairolero PC, Trastek VF, et al. Ivor Lewis esophagogastrectomy for carcinoma of the esophagus: early and late functional results. *Ann Thorac Surg* 1987;44(2):119–122.

CHAPTER 25

Gynecologic Malignancies

Arno J. Mundt ■ Loren K. Mell ■ Catheryn Yashar

INTRODUCTION

Gynecologic cancers arise from organs throughout the female reproductive tract, including the ovaries, uterus, cervix, vagina and vulva. Gynecologic cancers represent the fourth most common malignant tumors diagnosed in women in the United States each year, with approximately 83,000 cases expected in 2010 (1). Worldwide, gynecologic cancers represent approximately 20% of all cancers, with nearly one million cases diagnosed per year (2).

Radiation therapy (RT) occupies an important role in the treatment of nearly all gynecologic malignances. Radiation is commonly used as definitive treatment in many early stage patients and in conjunction with surgery and/or chemotherapy in women with locally advanced disease. It is also frequently used to palliate patients when cure is no longer possible.

This chapter provides an overview of the role of RT in the treatment of gynecologic malignancies, with a focus on the planning of various radiotherapeutic approaches used in these patients, including external beam RT and brachytherapy. Novel technologies including intensity-modulated RT (IMRT) and image-guided RT (IGRT) as well as their emerging application in the treatment of these cancers are also discussed.

RADIOTHERAPEUTIC MANAGEMENT

Cervical Cancer

Radiation is commonly used in the treatment of nearly all stages of cervical cancer. Select early (microscopic) tumors (Stage IA) are treated primarily with surgery; however, when such patients are unable to undergo surgery due to advanced age and/or significant comorbidities, RT can be used and is associated with excellent results (3). Early stage patients with gross disease (stages IB–IIA) are managed well with either radical surgery or definitive RT, with cure rates exceeding 80% following either approach (4).

The choice of surgery versus radiation in early stage cervical cancer depends on a number of factors, including patient age, comorbidities and various tumor characteristics. Older women, particularly those with multiple comorbidities, are generally treated with RT, whereas younger women receive surgery. A common reason for favoring surgery in young women is the ability to preserve their ovarian function. However, it may be possible to preserve ovarian function in pre-menopausal patients by performing an ovarian transposition prior to RT (5). Another oft-stated reason for favoring surgery in young women is the commonly held belief that sexual function would be less adversely affected. However, prospective quality-of-life analyses have found equivalent sexual function following surgery compared to RT (6). Moreover, new approaches have been developed to address sexual dysfunction in irradiated women (7).

In general, RT is recommended over surgery in early stage cervical cancer patients as lesion size and vaginal involvement increase. As tumor diameter exceeds 4 cm, there is increased likelihood of tumor spread to surrounding organs and regional lymph nodes, necessitating the need for adjuvant RT following surgery. Randomized trials conducted by the Gynecologic Oncology Group (GOG) and other cooperative groups have found that postoperative RT is beneficial in many cervical cancer patients following surgery. GOG 92 noted an improved 2-year recurrence-free survival rate (88% vs. 79%, $p = 0.008$) comparing adjuvant RT versus no further therapy in node negative patients with high risk features (deep stromal invasion, bulky primary disease and/or lymphovascular invasion [LVI]) (8). GOG 109 compared adjuvant pelvic RT versus pelvic RT plus chemotherapy in women found to have involved pelvic nodes, parametrial invasion and/or positive margins and noted a superior 4-year overall survival (81% vs. 71%, $p = 0.007$) with the combined approach (9). Whether concomitant chemoradiotherapy is superior to RT alone in node negative patients with high-risk features is currently being evaluated by GOG 263, whereas the benefit of adjuvant chemotherapy following chemoradiotherapy in high-risk node positive patients is the subject of GOG 0724.

While a treatment option in early stage patients, radiation has long been the cornerstone of treatment in cervical cancer patients with locally advanced (stage IIB–IVA) disease. In these women, radiation is combined with concomitant chemotherapy in light of multiple prospective randomized trials demonstrating a survival advantage to the combined approach (10–12). Surgery is typically not utilized in patients with locally advanced disease, albeit some investigators have advocated pelvic exenteration in cases with bladder and/or rectal invasion (stage IVA) (13). Metastatic (Stage IVB) patients may also undergo RT, particularly those with a good response to chemotherapy or those requiring palliative treatment due to uncontrolled vaginal bleeding.

Definitive RT in cervical cancer is administered with a combination of pelvic RT and brachytherapy, except in earliest stage patients in whom brachytherapy alone is sufficient (3). Early stage patients (stage IB1) is standardly treated with radiation as there are currently no randomized trials demonstrating improved outcomes with the addition of chemotherapy. Early stage patients with bulky (>4 cm) tumors (stage IB2) are treated with a combination of pelvic RT and chemotherapy (14), with or without an adjuvant hysterectomy (15). Hysterectomy increases local control but does not alter survival. When delivered adjuvantly, most patients receive pelvic RT with or without chemotherapy. In women with locally advanced disease, pelvic fields are also used, except in those with documented paraortic lymph node involvement in whom extended field RT (EFRT) is administered. In the past, there was considerable interest in *prophylactic* para-aortic RT in locally advanced patients, following the superior survival rates reported on the Radiation Therapy Oncology Group (RTOG) trial using this approach (16). Today, however, EFRT is rarely used without evidence of paraortic involvement, except at some centers in woman with involvement of common iliac lymph nodes. Pelvic fields are extended to include the inguinal lymph nodes in patients with lower vaginal involvement and additional external beam RT is often delivered in patients with significant parametrial involvement and/or gross nodal disease.

Brachytherapy is commonly delivered in conjunction with pelvic RT in cervical cancer patients undergoing definitive treatment. In the adjuvant setting, brachytherapy is less commonly performed, except when patients are treated preoperatively. If brachytherapy is prescribed, most patients receive intracavitary brachytherapy (ICB). However, at some centers, interstitial brachytherapy is favored in women with unfavorable anatomy and/or significant parametrial involvement. See section on "Radiotherapeutic Techniques" for a full discussion of the various RT techniques used in cervical cancer patients.

Uterine Cancer

Although radiation has traditionally been delivered prior to surgery in many uterine cancer patients (17), the majority of patients today undergo upfront surgery, consisting of total abdominal hysterectomy and bilateral salpingo-oophorectomy (TAH-BSO), with RT delivered postoperatively to select patients based on pathologic features in the surgical specimen. In the United States, many uterine cancer patients undergo extended surgical staging (ESS) at the time of surgery as well, consisting of pelvic and para-aortic lymphadenectomies, despite the results of two randomized trials questioning its benefits in terms of survival (18,19).

The most common pathologic features used to determine the need for adjuvant RT in early stage (stage I–II) uterine cancer are tumor grade, histology, depth of myometrial invasion (MI), LVI, and cervical involvement. Some investigators also use tumor size and lower uterine segment (LUS) involvement, albeit the prognostic significance of such features, particularly in the absence of other more established adverse features, remains unclear (20). Multiple randomized trials have been performed by the GOG and other groups demonstrating that adjuvant RT in early stage uterine cancer patients with adverse pathologic features significantly reduces locoregional failure (21–24). Whether it improves survival, however, remains a matter of intense debate, despite the results of two large Surveillance Epidemiology and End Results (SEER) studies suggesting a survival benefit in most patients (25,26).

At many centers today, low-risk early stage uterine cancer patients (stage I, grade 1, no or minimal MI) are treated with surgery alone, while those with intermediate risk factors (grade 3 with superficial MI or grade 1 to 2 with deep MI, especially combined with advanced age and LVI) receive adjuvant RT. In the latter group, pelvic RT is currently reserved for patients who do not undergo ESS and vaginal brachytherapy is delivered in those who do (provided all nodes are negative)—a trend that appears to be increasing in the United States (27). It may be possible, however, to treat select intermediate risk patients with adjuvant vaginal brachytherapy alone even when ESS is not performed (28). In the adjuvant setting, either pelvic RT or vaginal brachytherapy are delivered. While commonly delivered together in the past, the routine use of both appears to only increase the risk of serious toxicity without improving local control and thus should be avoided whenever possible (29).

The optimal approach in high-risk early stage uterine cancer patients (deep MI and grade 3 disease, cervical stromal invasion, LVI) remains controversial. In Europe, the Postoperative Radiotherapy for Endometrial Carcinoma (PORTEC)-3 trial is comparing pelvic RT versus pelvic RT plus concomitant and adjuvant chemotherapy in these patients. In the United States, GOG 0249 is randomizing patients to pelvic RT versus vaginal brachytherapy plus chemotherapy.

In early stage uterine cancer patients unable to undergo surgery due to advanced age and/or multiple co-morbidities radiation can be used with curative intent and typically consists of a combination of brachytherapy with or without pelvic RT in grade 3 patients and brachytherapy alone in those with grade 1 to 2 disease (30). Pelvic magnetic resonance imaging (MRI) may be helpful in these women to evaluate MI and extra-uterine spread.

In stage III and IV uterine cancer, the standard approach has been for many years surgery followed by adjuvant RT, using a variety of techniques including pelvic RT, EFRT and whole abdominal RT (WART). Historically, select locally advanced patients with positive peritoneal cytology received intraperitoneal radioactive phosphorus (^{32}P) (31). Outcomes varied considerably in stage III–IV patients depending on the type and number of extrauterine sites involved, with the best results seen in patients with isolated adnexal involvement (32) and poorer outcomes in those with involvement of multiple extra-uterine sites, nodal involvement and/or residual disease (33).

Today, WART is rarely used in the United States following the publication of the GOG 122 trial randomizing stage III–IV patients to either WART or chemotherapy which noted a superior 5-year survival (55% vs. 42%) with adjuvant chemotherapy but inferior pelvic control (34). However, the question remains whether adjuvant RT has a role in conjunction with chemotherapy. Patterns of failure studies suggest that it does, given the high risk of loco-regional recurrence in women undergoing surgery and chemotherapy (35). At many centers today, stage III and select stage IV patients are treated with chemotherapy combined with limited volume RT (pelvic RT, EFRT and/or vaginal brachytherapy based on pathologic features), an approach known as "tumor volume-directed" RT, which was used in the GOG 184 trial (36). Of note, GOG 258 is currently randomizing locally advanced patients to chemotherapy versus chemoradiotherapy. The results of this important trial will help define the role of RT in these patients.

The role of RT in the treatment of patients with unfavorable histologies—notably papillary serous and clear cell tumors—is controversial. However, RT may help reduce the risk of locoregional recurrence in such patients who receive adjuvant chemotherapy following surgery (37). Patients with early stage uterine sarcomas, except those with low-grade endometrial stromal sarcoma, have traditionally been treated with adjuvant pelvic RT. Locally advanced sarcoma patients are treated at many centers with adjuvant chemotherapy without RT, due to the superior outcomes in patients undergoing chemotherapy compared to WART on the GOG 150 trial (38). Nonetheless, adjuvant RT still remains a common treatment of choice in these patients, particularly in elderly women and others who are unable to undergo adjuvant chemotherapy. See section on "Radiotherapeutic Techniques" for a full discussion of the various RT techniques used in patients with uterine cancer.

Ovarian Cancer

For many years, RT occupied an important role in the treatment of ovarian cancer. Following upfront surgery, consisting of an omentectomy, TAH-BSO, peritoneal sampling and cytoreduction of extra-ovarian disease throughout the abdomen and pelvis, and often pelvic and para-aortic lymph node dissection, adjuvant RT was routinely delivered in the form of intraperitoneal ^{32}P in high-risk early stage disease and WART in locally advanced disease patients.

Several randomized GOG studies have compared adjuvant ^{32}P versus chemotherapy (melphalan or cisplatin-cytoxan) in early-stage high risk disease (stages IA–B grade 3, stages IC–II) and found no differences in either relapse-free or overall survival rates (39,40). Moreover, in GOG 7602, chemotherapy was associated with higher toxicity rate compared to RT, including a higher rate of second malignancies (39). Despite these favorable results, few patients receive intraperitoneal ^{32}P today, apart from its use at some centers in select elderly high-risk early stage patients unable to receive chemotherapy, partly due to the development of peritoneal adhesions in some patients.

In locally advanced ovarian cancer patients who were optimally cytoreduced (previously defined as <2 cm residuum remaining following surgery), WART was long considered the standard adjuvant approach at many centers throughout the world. Published long-term outcomes have been highly favorable in such patients treated with WART, particularly in those with microscopic or no residual disease after cytoreductive surgery (41,42). Investigators at Stanford University reported a 15-year relapse-free survival rate of 50% in stage I–III optimally cytoreduced patients undergoing adjuvant WART (41). Despite these favorable results and even a prospective phase III MD Anderson Hospital randomized trial demonstrating identical survival rates following WART or chemotherapy (43), adjuvant WART has been largely abandoned at most centers today—at least in the United States. The standard adjuvant approach is currently combination chemotherapy. Unfortunately, a randomized trial comparing WART and chemotherapy regimens popular today will most likely never be performed.

Although no longer used alone following surgery, the question remains whether adjuvant adjuvant RT has a role in conjunction with chemotherapy and surgery in ovarian cancer. Several prospective trials have evaluated the role of "consolidative" RT in stage I-III patients following upfront surgery and adjuvant chemotherapy (44,45). No benefit was seen using intraperitoneal ^{32}P compared to observation in a GOG trial focused on stage I–III patients with microscopic residual disease following surgery and chemotherapy (44). In contrast, the Swedish-Norwegian Ovarian Cancer Study Group trial compared WART versus cisplatin-doxorubicin-epirubicin versus observation in stage III patients achieving a pathologic complete response and noted 5-year progression-free survivals of 56%, 36% and 35% in the WART, chemotherapy and observation groups, respectively (45). Although favorable results have been reported combining adjuvant RT with modern taxane-based adjuvant chemotherapy (46), whether adjuvant RT is truly beneficial in this setting remains unclear.

RT is occasionally used in the management of patients with non-epithelial ovarian cancers. Given its exquisite radiosensitivity, ovarian dysgerminoma may be treated with RT; however, in these patients as well, the standard practice today is adjuvant chemotherapy, particularly in those desiring fertility-sparing treatment. As in other gynecologic cancers, RT has an important role in the palliative treatment of ovarian cancer patients (47). See section on "Radiotherapeutic Techniques" for a discussion of the various RT techniques used in ovarian cancer.

Vulvar Cancer

The treatment of vulvar cancer at most centers today consists of upfront surgery, typically radical vulvectomy or radical wide local excision in select patients with small well-lateralized tumors (48), with RT delivered adjuvantly in patients with high-risk features including LVI, tumor invasion >5 mm, surgical margins < 8 mm, grade 3 disease, and microscopic positive margins (49,50). Most patients also undergo bilateral inguinofemoral dissections, particularly those found to have tumor invasion >3 mm, LVI and/or high-grade disease, due to their high risk of nodal involvement.

Although commonly used in many other gynecologic cancers, *prophylactic* nodal irradiation is rarely used to treat clinically negative regional lymph nodes in vulvar cancer. This practice is based on the GOG 88 trial which compared prophylactic inguinofemoral RT versus lymphadenectomy in clinically node negative patients and found a significantly higher rate of recurrence ($p = 0.03$) and death ($p = 0.04$) in the RT group (51). See section on "Radiotherapeutic Techniques" for a critique of this influential study.

In women with locally advanced but resectable disease, surgery is typically performed followed by adjuvant radiation or chemoradiation. Over 20 years ago, the GOG completed a landmark trial (GOG 37) comparing adjuvant RT versus pelvic node dissection in patients found to have involved inguinal nodes at the time of surgery (52). A significantly higher survival rate was noted in the RT group, with the greatest benefit seen in women with clinically suspicious and/or ≥2 pathologically involved nodes. Moreover, adjuvant RT significantly reduced the risk of recurrence in the inguinal nodes (5% vs. 24%, $p = 0.02$). This trial established adjuvant RT as the treatment of choice in these patients.

In unresectable vulvar cancer patients, RT has been used preoperatively with promising results (53,54). Considerable interest has been focused on further augmenting these results by combining RT with chemotherapy (50,55,56). GOG 101 evaluated preoperative chemoradiotherapy in locally advanced unresectable patients and found that nearly all patients (97%) became resectable, with only 16% ultimately failing locally (57).

Adjuvant RT in vulvar cancer is delivered using a variety of techniques, ranging from small electron fields directed solely at the primary site to generous fields encompassing the primary, pelvis plus one or both groins. The most common approach, however, is pelvic-inguinal irradiation, delivered with or without a midline block. Brachytherapy has a limited role in vulvar cancer, apart from patients with a positive vaginal margin or in medically inoperable patients in whom high doses are required

to control the primary tumor. However, at most centers, high dose central boosts are delivered in such patients using external beam techniques. A description of the various RT techniques used in vulvar cancer is provided below (see section on "Radiotherapeutic Techniques").

Vaginal Cancer

The treatment of choice in all stages of vaginal cancer is definitive RT. Select early stage patients, for example, those with small-volume disease limited to the upper vagina, however, can be treated with a variety of surgical approaches, including partial or radical vaginectomy (58).

Early stage vaginal cancer patients typically receive brachytherapy alone or is combined with external beam when tumors invade into the paravaginal tissues (59,60). Some investigators advocate the use of combined external beam and brachytherapy even in patients without paravaginal invasion (61). Overall, definitive RT is associated with excellent outcomes in most early stage vaginal cancer patients, particularly in those with stage I disease in whom locoregional control rates exceed 85% (60). Patients with locally advanced disease undergo pelvic RT and brachytherapy (59–61). At some institutions, chemotherapy is delivered concomitantly in these patients in an effort to improve tumor control and potential survival extrapolation from cervical cancer studies. Given the low number of vaginal cancer patients diagnosed each year, it is unlikely that randomized trials evaluating such approaches will ever be successfully conducted.

Brachytherapy in early stage vaginal cancer typically involves ICB, but in women with >0.5 cm tumor invasion or thickness, interstitial brachytherapy is recommended. Some investigators favor interstitial brachytherapy combined with ICB even in patients with superficial tumors to reduce the total vaginal dose and, in distal vaginal tumors, the rectal dose (61). If external beam is also delivered, vaginal cancer patients receive either pelvic irradiation, or in cases involving the lower one-third of the vagina, pelvic-inguinal RT. See section on "Radiotherapeutic Techniques" for a discussion of the various RT techniques used in patients with ovarian cancer.

RADIOTHERAPY TECHNIQUES

External-Beam Therapy

Whole Pelvic Radiotherapy

Pelvic RT is used in many gynecologic cancers to irradiate multiple target tissues within the pelvis, including the uterus/cervix (or the postoperative bed), the upper vagina, paracervical/parametrial tissues and the pelvic (internal, external and common iliac) lymph nodes. Pelvic RT fields have traditionally been designed using fluoroscopic simulation based on bony landmarks and are delivered with either two-field (opposed anterior-posterior:posterior-anterior

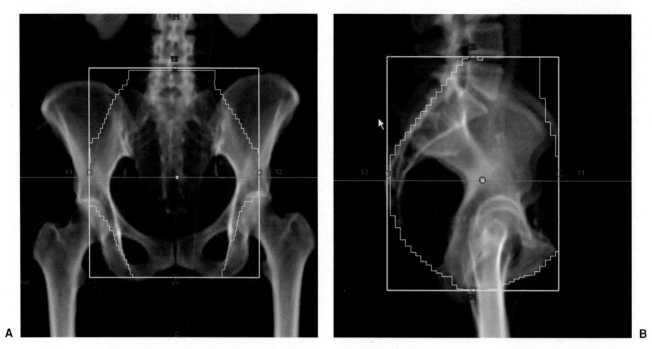

Figure 25.1. Anterior-posterior (AP) (**A**) and lateral fields (**B**) in a representative gynecologic cancer patient undergoing whole pelvic radiation therapy.

[APPA] fields) or four-field (APPA plus opposed lateral fields) techniques (Fig. 25.1). In recent years, however, most centers have moved away from APPA treatment (62), since four-field approaches allow considerably more normal tissue sparing, notably the anterior small bowel and posterior rectum. Some investigators still favor opposed APPA fields, however, in patients with locally advanced cervical cancer.

For many years, the superior border of the pelvic RT field was placed at the L5-S1 interspace; however, most investigators currently favor the L4–L5 interspace to include the common iliac lymph nodes. It is important to note, however, that the common iliacs in some patients may extend considerably higher, requiring an upper border as high as L2–L3 to ensure their full coverage. The lower pelvic RT border is typically placed at the inferior obturator foramen while the lateral borders are set 1–1.5 cm beyond the pelvic brim. The anterior border of the lateral field is at (or 1 cm anterior) the pubic symphysis to ensure coverage of the external iliac nodes; the posterior border is at the S2–S3 interspace. Previously, the posterior border was commonly set at the S1–S2 interspace; however, concerns were raised about adequate coverage of the attachment of the uterosacral ligament to the sacrum with this approach, particularly in locally advanced cervical cancer patients (63). Customized blocking is added to each field using either cerrobend or multileaf collimation to reduce dose to the surrounding normal tissues including the small bowel and rectum. Oral and rectal contrast may be administered at simulation to aid in the design of these blocks.

Various modifications can be done to the traditional pelvic RT fields, depending on the clinical scenario. In cer-

vical or uterine cancer patients with significant vaginal involvement, the lower border can be extended to the introitus ensuring irradiation of the entire vaginal canal. In such cases, it is helpful to place a radiopaque marker in the vagina at the time of simulation marking the inferior extent of disease. The superior border may be extended superiorly to fully encompass the common iliac lymph nodes, particularly in women with involvement of the external iliac lymph nodes, or may be lowered to the L5-S1 interspace, in patients undergoing ESS and found to have negative pelvic nodes. The posterior border of the lateral field can also be moved posterior to the sacrum in cervical cancer patients with bulky disease, whereas the anterior border may be moved anteriorly in women with an anteverted uterus and/or bulky external iliac nodes.

At many centers, patients undergoing pelvic RT are immobilized and simulated in the supine position. Prone positioning with a "belly board" is favored by some investigators to help reduce the volume of small bowel irradiated. Similarly, at some centers, patients are simulated and treated with a full bladder to displace small bowel. Whatever approach is used, it is important to strive for consistent bladder and rectal filling throughout treatment, given that the volume of these organs may impact on the position of the cervix/uterus (or vaginal cuff) (64,65).

Although pelvic RT fields have traditionally been designed based on bony landmarks, multiple investigators have demonstrated that such an approach may underdose the target tissues and/or inadequately shield surrounding normal tissues in many patients (66,67). Finlay and colleagues assessed the adequacy of nodal coverage of conventional pelvic RT fields in 43 cervical cancer patients (66). Pelvic vessels were contoured following computed tomography (CT)

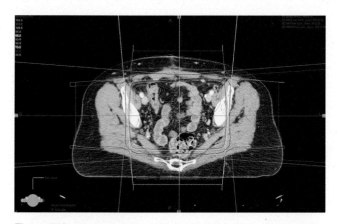

Figure 25.2. Treatment plan with isodose lines in a representative gynecologic cancer patient treated with whole pelvic radiation therapy.

simulation and used as surrogates for the pelvic lymph nodes. In 41 patients (95%), conventional fields inadequately covered various lymph node groups. Of note, in 24 (56%), conventional fields and blocks were found to be too generous. Others have similarly used three-dimensional (3D) imaging and found that conventional fields and blocking may result in inadequate target coverage in up to 50% of patients, particularly with the placement of the posterior field border of the lateral pelvic field at S2–S3(67). These results strongly support the design of pelvic RT field using CT simulation—a trend that is growing in the community.

Conventional pelvic RT fields are typically delivered using moderate-high energy (≥10 MV) photon beams. However, lower energies can be used in select thin patients. Wedges may be added to the lateral fields to reduce "hot spots" in the treatment plan. As example, pelvic RT plan is shown in Figure 25.2. Total doses prescribed typically range from 39.6–50.4 Gy delivered in 1.8–2 Gy/fractions, the higher doses used in patients undergoing external beam alone and lower doses in those treated with both external beam and brachytherapy.

In the past, there was considerable interest in the use of altered fractionation schedules in gynecologic cancer patients, including accelerated hyperfractionated RT as a means of escalating the pelvic radiation dose. However, the RTOG 88-05 trial using this approach in locally advanced cervical cancer patients failed to demonstrate a benefit in terms of tumor control or complications (68). Others have also reported high complication rates using a hyperfractionated approach (69). Moreover, twice daily treatment in an effort to boost the cervical tumor prior to brachytherapy has also been associated with an increased complications (70). In contrast, hypofractionated approaches, for example, 2.5–3 Gy daily fractions (total doses 30–35 Gy) have been used successfully in patients treated palliatively. Higher dose per fraction (up to 10 Gy) palliative regimens have also been explored (71,72).

Various blocks can be added to the conventional pelvic RT field. At some centers, a midline block is utilized allowing a higher proportion of the total dose to be delivered by brachytherapy in cervical cancer patients, typically placed after approximately 20 Gy (73). A midline block may also be placed following brachytherapy in cervical cancer patients with significant parametrial involvement and/or involved pelvic lymph nodes allowing an additional boost to be delivered, typically 10–12 Gy in five to six fractions.

At many centers, midline blocks are often standardized, but at others they may be customized based on the brachytherapy isodose distributions (Fig. 25.3). Wolfson and colleagues performed a survey of GOG institutions and reported that the percentages of centers using standard and customized midline blocks were 76% and 21%, respectively (74). Only 3% utilized step-wedge blocks as popularized by Perez and associates (73). The width of the midline block should fully encompass the colpostats on the anterior radiograph plus a margin since narrow mid-line blocks inadequately shield the ureters and are associated with increased complications (75). The inferior edge of the block should be coincident with the lower border of the pelvic field. However, various superior block edges can be used. In the GOG survey, the upper border of the midline block was set at the top of the pelvic field, the tip of the tandem plus a 1 to 2 cm margin or the level of the sacro-iliac joint by 29%, 38% and 33% of respondents, respectively (74).

IMRT is increasingly being used in the treatment of gynecologic cancers. Investigators at the University of Chicago were the first to compare conventional and IMRT planning in gynecologic cancer patients undergoing pelvic RT and found that IMRT reduced the volume of small bowel irradiated by a factor of two and the volume of both the bladder and rectum irradiated by 23% (76). Subsequently, others have confirmed these results, with reductions up to 70% seen with IMRT planning in terms of the volume of small bowel receiving the prescription dose (77–79). More recently, IMRT planning has been shown to be an effective means of reducing the volume of pelvic bone marrow irradiated in patients undergoing pelvic RT—an appealing approach particularly in patients receiving concomitant chemotherapy (80).

Patients undergoing pelvic IMRT are typically immobilized in the supine position and undergo CT simulation with thin (5 mm) slices, although at select centers prone positioning is favored (81). Contrast may be administered to aid in the delineation of the target and normal tissues; intravenous contrast is particularly useful since the pelvic vasculature is used as a surrogate for the lymph nodes in the planning process.

Following simulation, a gross tumor volume (GTV) and clinical target volume (CTV) are contoured on the planning CT scan, based on ICRU 50 guidelines (82). The GTV should include all demonstrable disease, including involved regional lymph nodes. A variety of imaging modalities can be used to aid in target design, with growing attention on positron emission tomography (PET) and MRI (83,84). Investigators at Washington University base their target volume definition on PET and contour a metabolically active tumor volume (MTV), specified at the 40% threshold level (85).

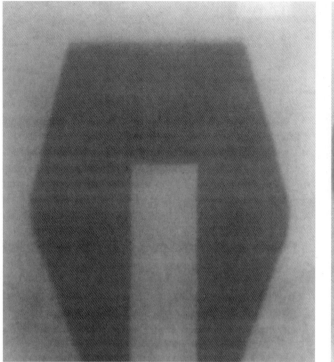 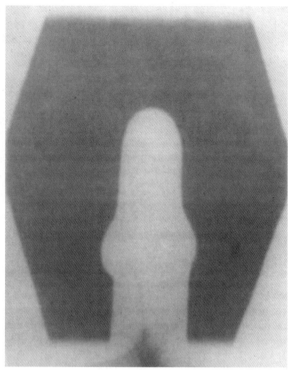

Figure 25.3. Example midline blocks used in patients with cervical cancer: (**A**) standard block and (**B**) customized block based on brachytherapy isodose distribution. *Source:* From Wolfson AH, Abdel-Wahab M, Markoe AM, et al. A quantitative assessment of standard versus customized midline shield construction for invasive cervical carcinoma. *Int J Radiat Oncol Biol Phys* 1997;37:237–242, with permission.

The CTV in most patients undergoing pelvic IMRT consists of the upper half of the vagina, uterus/cervix (if present), parametria, pre-sacral region and pelvic lymph nodes (internal, external and lower common iliac nodes). The most superior extent of the CTV is typically placed 1–1.5 cm inferior to the L4–L5 interspace to account for planning target volume (PTV) expansions. In uterine cancer patients without cervical involvement, the pre-sacral region need not be included. At some centers, a single CTV is drawn, whereas at others several CTVs are delineated. In a postoperative patient, for example, two CTVs may be delineated; the CTV$_{nodes}$ includes the common, external and internal iliac nodes and pre-sacral space, whereas the CTV$_{vagina}$ includes the vaginal cuff and paravaginal/parametrial tissues. At some centers, an integrated target volume (ITV) is generated by fusing empty and full bladder planning CT scans, encompassing contours of the cervix (or vaginal cuff in postoperative patients) on both scans, with patients treated with a full bladder or, at other centers, an empty bladder as maintaining a full bladder has not been shown to be reproducible. Normal tissues are contoured as well, including the small bowel, bladder, rectum and, at some centers, the sigmoid colon. The pelvic bones are used as a surrogate for the pelvic bone marrow in patients undergoing chemoradiotherapy. In the past, only the iliac crests were contoured; however, recent data suggest that the pelvic bones are a better surrogate for the bone marrow in the optimization process (86).

Consensus guidelines regarding CTV design in gynecologic cancer patients undergoing postoperative pelvic IMRT were developed for the RTOG 0418 phase II trial (Fig. 25.4) (87). These guidelines were based, in part, on

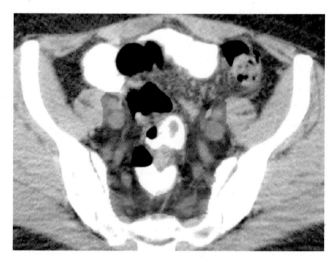

Figure 25.4. Mid-pelvic computed tomography (CT) image illustrating a clinical target volume (CTV) delineated in a patient with cervical cancer treated postoperatively based on guidelines developed for the Radiation Therapy Oncology Group (RTOG) 0418 trial. Upper external and internal iliac (red) and presacral region (blue). *Source:* From Small W Jr, Mell LK, Anderson P, et al. Consensus guidelines for delineation of clinical target volume for intensity-modulated pelvic radiotherapy in postoperative treatment of endometrial and cervical cancer. *Int J Radiat Oncol Biol Phys* 2008;71:428–434, with permission.

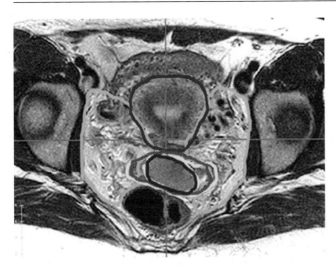

Figure 25.5. Axial view of a T2-weighted magnetic resonance (MR) images illustrating contours of the gross tumor volume (GTV) (red), cervix (pink), vagina (yellow), parametria (green) and uterus (blue) in a patient with intact cervical cancer undergoing intensity modulated radiation therapy (IMRT) based on the Radiation Therapy Oncology Group (RTOG) consensus conference. *Source:* From Lim K, Small W, Portelance L, et al. Consensus guidelines for delineation of clinical target volume for intensity-modulated pelvic radiotherapy for the definitive treatment of cervical cancer. *Int J Radiat Oncol Biol Phys* 2011;79:348–355, with permission.

work of Taylor et al. who mapped pelvic lymph node regions using iron oxide-enhanced MRI, a method to visualize benign lymph nodes (88). In an analysis of 20 patients using this technique, a modified margin of 7 mm around the major pelvic vessels was found to encompass 99% of the visualized lymph nodes. More recently, consensus guidelines have been developed for cervical cancer patients treated with an intact uterus based on MRI (Fig. 25.5) (89).

The next step in the IMRT planning process involves the expansion of the CTV to generate a PTV, accounting for patient setup uncertainty and organ motion. The optimal PTV expansion remains a matter of debate, particularly in patients with intact cervical cancer in which there may be considerable organ motion (64,65). A reasonable approach is to provide generous expansions around the cervical tumor (definitive patients) and the vaginal cuff (postoperative patients) on the order of 1.5–2 cm. Tighter expansions can be placed around the CTV in the upper pelvis (0.7–1 cm). Daily in-room image-guided RT (IGRT) techniques, notably cone-beam CT (CBCT) imaging, may help ensure adequate coverage of the target tissues on a daily basis (64).

No consensus exists regarding many IMRT planning parameters used in gynecologic cancer patients. At many centers seven to nine equally spaced 6-MV beams are used; however, others favor volumetric arc or tomotherapy approaches. As in conventional RT, the total dose prescribed is a function of the tumor site, stage and treatment volume. Most investigators deliver 45 Gy in 1.8 Gy daily fractions, particularly in women subsequently undergoing

brachytherapy. Higher doses (50.4 Gy) can be used in patients treated with pelvic IMRT alone (90). Some investigators are exploring the use of more sophisticated simultaneous integrated boost (SIB) approaches, particularly in women with grossly positive nodes (91).

Given the potential ability to safely deliver higher and potentially more efficacious doses, some investigators have explored using IMRT as a substitute for brachytherapy in cervical cancer (92,93). Investigators at the Princess Margaret Hospital recently presented a case study of a stage IIB cervical cancer patient unsuitable for brachytherapy treated with an IMRT boost (94). Using MRI guidance, a GTV was delineated consisting of the cervix and LUS. The GTV was expanded by a 10 mm margin (7 mm posteriorly) generating the CTV which was subsequently expanded by 5 mm (10 mm anteriorly) to generate the PTV. Six static 6 MV fields were used to deliver 25.2 Gy in 1.8 Gy daily fractions to the PTV. The resultant treatment plan was highly conformal; average doses delivered to 50% of the rectum, bladder and small bowel were 21, 13 and 5 Gy, respectively. Treatment was tolerated well without significant sequelae. Given the paucity of data using IMRT in lieu of brachytherapy, this approach should be considered experimental at the present time and only used in women unable to undergo brachytherapy.

The optimal dose–volume constraints for the PTV and normal tissues in gynecologic cancer patients undergoing pelvic IMRT remain unclear. Investigators at Washington University reported the use of the following constraints: PTV (100% to receive 95% of the prescription dose), small bowel (<40% to receive ≥30 Gy), rectum (<40% to receive ≥40 Gy), and femoral heads (<40% to receive ≥30 Gy) (95). In the original series from the University of Chicago, <40% of the small bowel, rectum and bladder were constrained to receive ≥36, ≥40 and ≥40 Gy, respectively. Moreover, >95% of the PTV needed to receive >95% of the prescribed dose (96).

In recent years, detailed normal tissue complication probability (NTCP) studies have been performed in gynecologic cancer patients undergoing pelvic IMRT which shed light on the optimal dose–volume constraints for various normal tissues (Fig. 25.6) (97–99). In update of the combined University of Chicago/University of California San Diego experience, the small bowel volume receiving ≥45 Gy was constrained to 250 cc and the volume of pelvic bone marrow (defined as entire pelvic bones) receiving ≥10 and ≥20 Gy were constrained to receive ≤90% and ≤75%, respectively (100). Current attention is focused on the use of more sophisticated image-guided approaches in an effort to further optimize IMRT planning (101).

Preliminary clinical outcome studies in gynecologic cancer patients undergoing pelvic IMRT have been extremely promising, with lower rates of acute and chronic toxicities reported compared to conventional techniques (96,98,100–103). Recent outcome studies have also reported excellent tumor control rates in both cervical

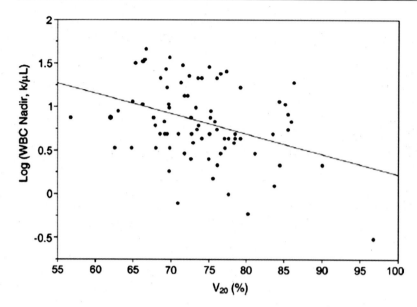

Figure 25.6. Plot of white blood cell count log (WBC nadir) versus bone marrow volume receiving 20 Gy or more (V_{20}) in a cohort of cervical cancer patients treated with combined chemoradiotherapy, supporting the use of bone marrow V_{20} as a constraint in the optimization process. Pelvic bones were used as a surrogate for pelvic bone marrow in this analysis. Regression coefficient (b) = −0.021 k/mL/%, p = 0.002. *Source:* From Rose BS, Aydogan B, Liang Y, et al. Normal tissue complication probability modeling of acute hematologic toxicity in cervical cancer patients treated with chemoradiotherapy. *Int J Radiat Oncol Biol Phys* 2010;78:912–919, with permission.

(95,100) and uterine (104) cancers. Favorable outcomes have also been reported using adjuvant pelvic IMRT on the RTOG 0418 prospective clinical trial (105,106). An international cooperative group trial evaluating pelvic IMRT in cervical cancer is currently under development (107).

Extended Field Radiotherapy

EFRT is used to treat the pelvic and para-aortic regions. A variety of techniques are currently utilized. At some centers, the entire volume is treated with large opposed APPA fields, extending from pelvis to the T12-L1 interspace. The para-aortic portion of these fields is typically 8–10 cm wide, depending on the patient's anatomy and disease extent. CT or PET/CT-based planning is helpful to ensure coverage of all enlarged lymph nodes. To reduce the small bowel dose, some favor using four-field approaches (APPA plus opposed laterals). However, when using such approaches, care needs to be taken to minimize the dose to the kidneys with variable weightings between the APPA and lateral fields ensuring a maximum kidney dose of 18 Gy or less. At some centers, the pelvis and para-aortic regions are treated separately with a place "gap" between fields. Select patients may need to be treated at an extended distance given the length of the fields treated.

Whichever field arrangement is used, moderate-high energy beams (≥10 MV) are indicated except in select thin women; all patients are simulated and treated in the supine position. Prescribed doses range from 39.6 to 45 Gy delivered in 1.8–2 Gy per fractions. In women with involved para-aortic nodes, a 5–10 Gy boost may be delivered via reduced fields. Select involved sites may be treated to 60 Gy or higher; however, care needs to be given to minimize the dose to the surrounding bowel and other normal tissues including kidneys and spinal cord.

Multiple centers have explored the use of IMRT planning in gynecologic cancer patients undergoing EFRT

(108–110). Compared to an APPA approach, investigators at Washington University noted that intensity-modulated EFRT (IM-EFRT) reduced the volume of small bowel, bladder and rectum receiving the prescription dose by 61%, 96% and 71%, respectively (108). Compared to a four-field approach, corresponding reductions were 60%, 93% and 56%, respectively. The following normal tissue constraints were used in the IM-EFRT planning: small bowel (<50% to receive ≥30 Gy), kidneys (<33% to receive ≥10 Gy) and spinal cord (<5% to receive ≥45 Gy). Lian and coworkers compared 3D conformal EFRT plans in 10 endometrial cancer patients to IMRT and helical tomotherapy (HT) plans (109). The following constraints were used in the IMRT and HT optimization process: bladder (<50% to receive ≥40 Gy), rectum (<40% to receive ≥40 Gy), bowel (<35% to receive ≥35 Gy), kidneys (<35% to receive 16 Gy) and spinal cord (maximum dose, 40 Gy). Overall, both IMRT and HT resulted in superior target coverage and significantly reduced normal tissue doses compared to 3D conformal planning; however, the HT achieved the best normal tissue sparing (Fig. 25.7).

A potentially important role for IMRT in gynecologic cancer patients undergoing EFRT is the ability to safely deliver higher than conventional doses to involved para-aortic lymph nodes. Using conventional techniques, doses above 60 Gy, except in patients with small volume disease, are difficult to deliver. However, the likelihood of controlling bulky para-aortic nodes with such doses is quite low. Multiple investigators have demonstrated that higher doses may be possible using SIB IMRT approaches in patients with involved para-aortic lymph nodes. Two different approaches have been proposed. Some investigators recommend that the entire para-aortic region be treated with conventional fraction sizes (1.8 Gy/day, 45 Gy total dose) and a SIB technique used to irradiate the involved nodes with *higher* than conventional fraction size (2.4 Gy/day, 60 Gy total dose) (111). Alternatively, conventional fractions can

3DCRT   IMRT   Tomotherapy

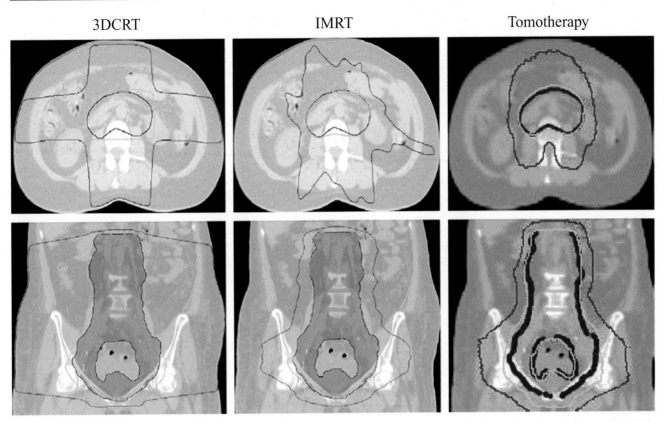

Figure 25.7. Comparison of planning target volume coverage by the 95% (green line) in 3-dimensional conformal radiotherapy (3DCRT), intensity-modulated radiotherapy (IMRT) and helical tomotherapy (HT) plans in a stage IIIC uterine cancer patient undergoing extended field irradiation. Blue indicates the 50% isodose line; red line or red area indicates planning target volume. *Source:* From Lian J, Mackenzie M, Joseph K, et al. Assessment of extended-field radiotherapy for stage IIIC endometrial cancer using three-dimensional conformal radiotherapy, intensity-modulated radiotherapy, and helical tomotherapy. *Int J Radiat Oncol Biol Phys* 2008;70:935–943, with permission.

be used for the SIB portion (1.8 Gy/day, 59.4 Gy total dose) and *lower* than conventional fractions used to treat the para-aortic region (1.53 Gy/day, 50.4 Gy total dose) (91).

Limited outcome data exist using IM-EFRT. Salama and coworkers treated 13 women to a total dose of 45 Gy in 1.8 Gy fractions (112). While 84% of patients experienced acute grade 2 bowel toxicity, no grade 3 or higher bowel or bladder sequelae were noted. Using the SIB approach with higher than conventional daily fractions (2.2 Gy/day, 55 Gy total dose) to PET-defined para-aortic nodes, investigators at the University of Pittsburgh noted acute grade 2 and 3 bowel sequelae in 10% and 0% of patients, respectively (113). Du and coworkers randomized 60 cervical cancer patients with involved para-aortic nodes to either IMRT or conventional RT to the para-aortic region (114). While the IMRT patients received a higher prescribed dose (58–68 Gy vs. 45–50 Gy) than the conventional RT patients, they experienced less acute and chronic toxicity. Moreover, IMRT patients had a superior 3-year survival (36.4% vs. 15.6%, $p = 0.016$) compared to the conventional RT patients.

Pelvic-Inguinal Radiotherapy

In women with vulvar cancer and other gynecologic cancer patients involving the lower vagina, pelvic-inguinal irradiation is used to irradiate the pelvis, vagina, vulva and bilateral inguinofemoral regions. Such patients are immobilized and simulated supine in the "frog leg" position to minimize skin folds and thus, the risk of acute perineal toxicity. Moderate-high energy beams (≥10 MV) are used.

The upper border of the conventional pelvic-inguinal field differs between institutions and is based on the disease extent. In vulvar cancer patients, some advocate the treatment of reduced pelvic fields ("true pelvis") with the upper border placed inferiorly to the sacro-iliac joints. Others place the upper border at the L5-S1 or L4-L5 interspace. In a survey of members of the Gynecologic Cancer Intergroup (GCIG), the most common upper border was L5-S1 followed by L4-L5 (50). In women with upper pelvic adenopathy, the upper border may need to be even higher. The lower border is typically placed approximately 5 cm inferior to the vulva/perineum to ensure coverage of the inguinofemoral lymph nodes.

A variety of treatment approaches have been used in patients undergoing pelvic-inguinal RT. One common approach is to use opposed APPA fields, with a "wide" AP field encompassing the pelvis and groin regions and a "narrow" PA field treating only the pelvis. Supplemental electron fields are used to treat the groins, reducing the dose received by the femoral heads. Alternatively, APPA fields can be equally wide with partial transmission blocks placed on the PA field minimizing dose to the femoral heads. A third approach is to prescribe high energy photons (10–24 MV) for the PA field and low energy photons (4–6 MV) for the AP field. A novel modified segmental boost technique has been developed using a wide AP field, narrow PA field and two-angled photon fields encompassing the bilateral groins (115). Whichever technique is used, attention needs to be given to avoid underdosing the vulvar region, particularly in patients treated preoperatively. Bolus is typically used with doses confirmed via thermoluminescence dosimetry (TLD). Total prescribed doses in patients undergoing pelvic-inguinal RT range from 45 to 50.4 Gy in 1.8–2 Gy daily fractions. Additional boosts may be delivered to the inguinal region in patients with involved lympyh nodes. In the GCIG survey, the mean pelvic and groin node doses were 48.1 Gy and 49.9 Gy, respectively (49).

When treating the inguinal lymph nodes with electrons, care needs to be taken to ensure the proper selection of beam energy. Routine use of low energy electron beams will likely underdose the groin nodes in a significant number of patients, particularly obese women. The depth of treatment should be tailored to the individual patient based on CT imaging, since the depth of the inguinofemoral nodes is highly variable with an average depth of 6.1 cm reported in one study (116). The high rate of nodal failures observed in the RT patients treated on GOG 88 comparing prophylactic RT versus lymphadenectomy in clinically node-negative vulvar cancer patients was likely due, at least in part, to the fact that the groins were treated via a single anterior field prescribed to a depth of 3 cm (50). Such an approach would significantly underdose the inguinal nodes in many patients. Prophylactic groin irradiation in clinically node-negative patients has been shown to be highly effective if properly planned and delivered (117). Care must also be taken to also ensure an adequate volume is irradiated given inguinal nodal metastases can occur throughout the groin region. Thus, small volume fields designed to irradiate the vessels with a limited margin are not recommended.

Considerable controversy exists regarding the use of a midline block in vulvar cancer patients undergoing pelvic-inguinal RT. In one highly quoted report, Dusenbery and coworkers noted a 48% central recurrence rate in 26 women treated with a midline block (118). However, all patients in this study had pathologically positive lymph nodes and many did not have wide negative margins. Of note, central recurrences were rare in the GOG 37 trial despite the use of a midline block (52). Thus, in the properly selected patient, a midline block may be reasonable, particularly in elderly, frail patients who are at high risk of requiring treatment breaks due to perineal toxicity if treated without a midline block.

Limited experience is available evaluating IMRT in gynecologic cancer patients undergoing pelvic-inguinal RT, with largest experience to date from the University of

Pittsburgh. Beriwal and colleagues compared IMRT and conventional planning in terms of normal tissue sparing in 15 vulvar cancer patients (119). Various IMRT techniques were used, with a median number of seven beams (range, 5–8). Normal tissue planning constraints included: small bowel (<35% to receive ≥35 Gy), rectum (<40% to receive ≥40 Gy) and bladder (<40% to receive ≥30 Gy). The plans were considered acceptable if <5% of the PTV received <100% of the prescribed dose and <10% received >110%. Mean preoperative and postoperative prescribed doses were 46.4 and 50.4 Gy, respectively. IMRT planning resulted in better sparing of the small bowel, rectum and bladder; however, unlike other reports (120), no significant difference was seen in volume of the femoral heads irradiated. Treatment was well tolerated, with only one patient experiencing acute grade 3 toxicity and none developing a grade ≥3 late toxicity. Two patients ultimately recurred locally, both were treated postoperatively.

Investigators at the University of Pittsburgh also reported their experience with preoperative chemotherapy and intensity-modulated pelvic-inguinal RT in 18 vulvar cancer patients (121). IMRT was delivered twice daily during the first and last treatment weeks. Overall, treatment was well tolerated with no grade ≥3 late toxicities. Moreover, no recurrences were seen in the nine patients achieving a pathologic complete response, whereas three of five partial responders failed locally.

Whole Abdominal Radiotherapy

WART involves the treatment of the entire peritoneal cavity. While in the past, due to the limitations of machine field size, treatment was delivered with a "moving strip" technique (122), WART is currently delivered at most centers using large opposed APPA techniques. Care needs to be taken at simulation to ensure that the upper border is placed sufficiently high (1–1.5 cm superior to the dome of the diaphragm) to cover the full excursion of the diaphragm during respiration. Laterally, the field borders are set 3 to 4 cm beyond the peritoneal reflection. Inferiorly, fields extend to the inferior obturator foramen. CT-based planning is particularly helpful to ensure complete coverage of the entire peritoneal cavity. Given the large volumes treated, select patients may need to be treated at an extended distance.

Patients undergoing WART are simulated in the supine position and immobilized with their arms overhead. Prescribed doses range from 25 to 30 Gy in 1.5 Gy daily fractions, generally followed by a boost to the pelvis (total pelvis dose, 45–50 Gy). Low-moderate beam energies are recommended (6 MV) to avoid underdosing the anterior peritoneal structures. At many centers, partial transmission blocks (two to five half value layers) are placed on the posterior field over the kidneys (with a 0.5 cm margin) to limit the kidney dose to ≤18 Gy. Some centers elect to limit the kidney dose to ≤15 Gy, particularly in women previously treated with chemotherapy. If the total prescribed dose exceeds 25 Gy, blocks are added at some centers to limit the liver dose to 25 Gy.

Various modifications to the conventional WART technique have been introduced over the years to boost select intra-abdominal and pelvic sites. Martinez and colleagues at Stanford developed a technique incorporating progressively shrinking fields delivering 30 Gy to the abdomen, 42 Gy to the para-aortics and medial diaphragm surface and 51 Gy to the pelvis (123). Others have focused on hyperfractionated techniques, delivering 0.8–1 Gy twice daily to 30–30.4 Gy (124).

Limited data are available evaluating IMRT in gynecologic cancer patients undergoing WART. Investigators at Memorial Sloan Kettering Cancer Center compared IMRT using five equally-spaced static fields and conventional large field APPA techniques in 10 endometrial cancer patients treated with WART (125). The target volume included a 1 cm rim of liver but completely excluded the bilateral kidneys, which were constrained to receive a maximum dose of 18 Gy. IMRT planning was associated with significantly better coverage of the peritoneal cavity and a 60% reduction in the volume of pelvic bones (a surrogate for pelvic bone marrow) irradiated (Fig. 25.8). Others have reported equally favorable early clinical results using volumetric arc IMRT techniques (126,127).

Stereotactic Body Radiotherapy

SBRT is a novel treatment approach used to deliver high, ablative doses of radiation in a limited number of fractions (typically three to five) to extracranial targets. Popularity is rapidly growing for this technique in the treatment of primary and metastatic tumors, particularly in the liver, lung and spine tumors (128). Initially delivered on conventional linear accelerators, SBRT today is currently delivered using specialized machines such as the Cyberknife (Accuray Inc., Sunnyvale, CA), Novalis (BrainLab AG, Feldkirchen, Germany), and the Trilogy or TrueBeam (Varian Medical Systems, Palo Alto, CA). Moreover, while originally developed using stereotactic localization methods, most SBRT approaches today instead rely on image-guidance, using either planar or volumetric-based imaging techniques (128).

In recent years, several investigators have begun exploring the potential of SBRT in gynecologic cancers. Choi and colleagues reported their experience using SBRT to treat recurrent para-aortic lymph nodes with the Cyberknife system (129). A total of 30 patients were treated with 33–45 Gy in three fractions, prescribed to the 73–87% isodose line (IDL). Prior to treatment, fiducial markers were placed in adjacent vertebral pedicles and used for on-line image-guidance. In all patients, the GTV consisted of the involved lymph node defined by either CT or PET/CT imaging and was expanded by 2 mm to generate the PTV. Treatment was well tolerated with few acute and chronic sequelae. Local control was excellent, particularly in small volume (≤ 17 cc) disease. A treatment plan in a representative patient from this series is shown in Figure 25.9.

The use of SBRT as a possible alternative to brachytherapy was reported by Molla and coworkers (130,131). In their studies, the CTV was defined as the vaginal vault, uterus/parametria, residual or recurrent tumor and was expanded by 6–10 mm to generate the PTV. Following external beam RT, patients were immobilized and simulated in the supine position with an endorectal probe in place to minimize internal organ motion (which was also used during treatment). Using 5–15 static IMRT fields, postoperative patients received 7 Gy × 2 while those with intact disease underwent 4 Gy × 5 using the Novalis System. At a median followup of 12.6 months, 15 of 16 patients remained locally controlled. Only one patient developed a late grade 3 or higher toxicity.

Brachytherapy

Intracavitary Brachytherapy

ICB in gynecologic cancer patients was initially performed by placing radioactive sources directly within the vagina and/or uterus. However, by the 1960s, *after-loading* techniques were introduced whereby an applicator was first

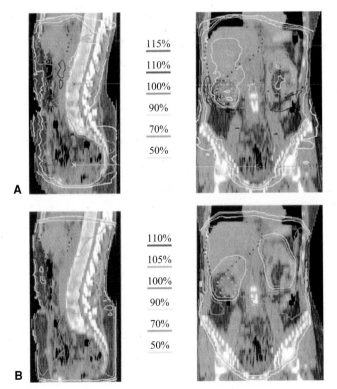

Figure 25.8. Isodose distributions from an intensity modulated whole abdominal radiotherapy (IM-WART) plan with five gantry angles in a patient with locally advanced uterine cancer. Isodose levels in%: (A) sagittal plane and (B) coronal plane. Also shown are isodose distributions from a conventional WART plan delivered with opposed anterior-posterior:posterior-anterior (APPA) fields in the patient: (C) sagittal plane and (D) coronal plane. *Source:* From Hong L, Alektiar K, Chui C, et al. IMRT of large fields: whole-abdomen irradiation. *Int J Radiat Oncol Biol Phys* 2002;54:278–289, with permission.

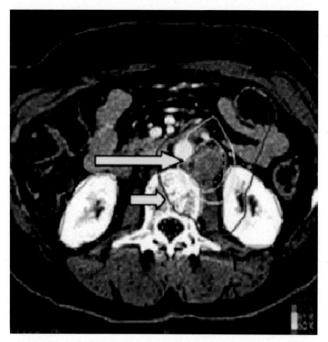

Figure 25.9. Treatment plan of a gynecologic cancer patient with an isolated para-aortic recurrence treated with stereotactic body radiation therapy (SBRT). The gross tumor volume (GTV) was defined as the visible tumor in the para-aortic lymph node region on computed tomography (CT) (innermost red line). The radiation dose was prescribed to the 81% isodose line of the maximum dose to cover the GTV + 2-mm margin (sky-blue line indicated by the *long arrow*). The outermost line is the 30% isodose line (blue line indicated by the *short arrow*). *Source:* From Choi CW, Cho CK, Yoo SY, et al. Image-guided stereotactic body radiation therapy in patients with isolated para-aortic lymph node metastases from uterine cervical and corpus cancer. *Int J Radiat Oncol Biol Phys* 2009;74:147–153, with permission.

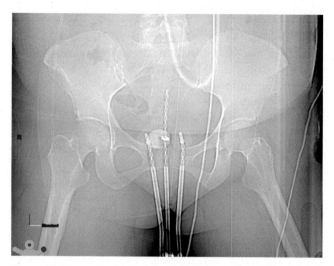

Figure 25.10. Tandem and ovoid applicator used for high-dose-rate (HDR) brachytherapy in patients with intact cervical cancer.

positioned within the patient while the sources were placed at a later time, typically after the patient had been transferred to an isolated (and often shielded) hospital room. Using this approach, radioactive sources were initially inserted manually but, more recently, remote-afterloading techniques have been developed, significantly reducing the exposure of the radiation oncologist and staff.

Various ICB applicators have been used in gynecologic cancer patients, depending on the specific clinical scenario. In cervical cancer patients treated with an intact uterus, the Fletcher-Suit-Delclos device based on the original Manchester system (132) is typically used, consisting of a curved tandem inserted into the uterus and two colpostats (ovoids) placed in the vaginal fornice. Various tandem lengths and colpostat diameters are available; most colpostats used today include shielding along the medial aspects of the anterior and posterior colpostat faces, reducing dose to the bladder and rectum (Fig. 25.10). A popular variation of the traditional tandem and ovoid system consists of a tandem and ring—a system particularly useful in patients with asymmetric fornices. Another ICB applicator used in the treatment of cervical cancer is the Henschke device (133). While medically inoperable uter-

ine cancer patients have historically been treated with intrauterine Heyman–Simon capsules (134), newer applicators have been developed, including the dual-tandem Rotte "Y" device (135). In patients treated postoperatively, a variety of applicators can be placed within the vagina, typically either a vaginal cylinder or colpostats. The MIRALVA vaginal applicator consists of two ovoid sources and a central tandem (136).

Gynecologic cancer patients undergoing ICB can be treated using either low dose rate (LDR) or high dose rate (HDR) techniques. According to the ICRU Report 38, LDR is defined as dose rates ranging from 0.4 to 2 Gy/hour while HDR utilizes dose rates of >12 Gy/hour, with modern HDR systems capable of delivering dose rates exceeding 400 Gy/hour (137). A variety of radioactive sources are used; however, the most popular are Cesium-137 (^{137}Cs) for LDR and high activity Iridium-192 (^{192}Ir) for HDR. Unlike LDR which is delivered in the hospital over several days, HDR is performed in the outpatient getting over several minutes obviating the need for anesthesia and prolonged bedrest, making it an ideal approach particularly in women with multiple medical comorbidities. Other advantages of HDR include increased ability to optimize treatment plans, reduced radiation exposure of personnel and better stability of the applicator during treatment. Disadvantages include increased number of treatment sessions and greater equipment cost. While some have argued that LDR is radiobiologically superior to HDR in terms of normal tissue effects, particularly in patients with an intact uterus (138), prospective randomized trials have demonstrated that the two techniques are similar in terms of both tumor control and toxicity (139,140). Some investigators favor the use of pulsed-dose-rate (PDR) brachytherapy whereby intermittent "pulses" of radiation (10–30 minutes/hour) are delivered using a machine similar to an after-loading HDR system. Proponents argue that PDR combines the logistic advantages of HDR with the potential radiobiological advantages of LDR. However, outcome data remain limited (141,142). Recently, others have explored the use of HDR electronic brachytherapy in gynecologic cancer patients (143).

Various doses and prescription points have been used for HDR and LDR ICB. In patients with intact cervical cancer, dose is typically prescribed to a reference point known as Point A. In the original Manchester formulation (132), Point A was defined as 2 cm lateral to the center of the intrauterine canal and 2 cm superior to the mucosal surface of the lateral fornix, presumably at the medial edge of the broad ligament where the uterine artery crosses the ureter. In the early 1950s, however, the definition of Point A was modified to be 2 cm superior to the external cervical OS and 2 cm lateral to the intrauterine canal. A second specified reference point in the Manchester system was Point B (3 cm lateral to Point A) which was felt to represent the location of the obturator lymph nodes, although CT-based studies reveal that this is rarely the case (144). Currently, the American Brachytherapy Society (ABS) recommends using a sidewall dose point rather than Point B and, in intact cervical cancer patients undergoing HDR ICB, Point H is the recommended prescription dose point (Fig. 25.11) (145). At select centers, alternative prescription points are used including Point M (146) and Point T (147). In postoperative cervical or uterine cancer patients or patients with vaginal cancer, ICB is prescribed to either the vaginal surface or at 0.5 cm depth. In uterine cancer patients treated with an intact uterus (either preoperatively or definitively), ICB was traditionally prescribed in terms of milligram-hours, but more recently most radiation oncologists prescribe to 2 cm from the midpoint of the intrauterine sources (148).

Additional points used in the planning of ICB of gynecologic cancer patients include bladder and rectal reference points. The bladder point is defined on planar orthogonal radiographs as the point on the surface of the Foley balloon (pulled snugly into the bladder trigone) receiving the highest dose, although volumetric studies have demonstrated that this point consistently fails to capture the true maximum bladder dose (149). A rectal reference point is defined 0.5 cm posterior to the posterior vaginal wall.

Intact cervical cancer patients undergoing LDR ICB are typically treated with two separate insertions, although comparable tumor control and complication rates have been reported with a single insertion, particularly in early stage patients (150). The first insertion should be performed as soon as pelvic geometry allows, typically during the second to fourth week of pelvic RT; the second 1 to 2 weeks later. Care should be taken to complete the entire course of treatment within 8 weeks, since more protracted courses have been associated with poorer outcomes (151).

Intact cervical cancer patients undergoing HDR typically receive four to six insertions. Given the increased number of fractions, HDR necessitates interdigitating pelvic RT and the initial HDR insertions to ensure that treatment is completed within 8 weeks, with the first treatment

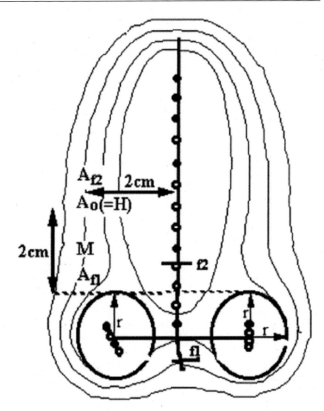

Figure 25.11. Relevant geometry for intracavitary brachytherapy dosimetry for a tandem and ovoid insertion. Finding Point H begins with drawing a line connecting the mid-dwell positions of the ovoids. From the intersection of this line with tandem, move superiorly along the tandem 2 cm plus the radius of the ovoids, and then 2 cm perpendicular to the tandem in the lateral direction. The figure also shows variations in the position of the conventional Point A based on its evolving definition. A_o located Point A in the original Manchester formulation. The position of A_{f1} and A_{f2} follow the revised definition and Point M is based on the Madison System. *Source:* From Nag S, Erickson B, Thomadsen B, et al. The American Brachytherapy Society recommendations for high-dose-rate brachytherapy for carcinoma of the cervix. *Int J Radiat Oncol Biol Phys* 2009;48:201–211, with permission.

delivered as soon as pelvic geometry allows. However, it is not recommended that both ICB and external beam RT or chemotherapy be delivered on the same day. For postoperative cervical and uterine cancer, vaginal cancer and medically inoperable uterine cancer, ICB is delivered with 1 to 2 LDR or 3–5 HDR insertions.

Treatment planning for patients undergoing ICB has traditionally been based on two-dimensional (2D) radiographs. More recently, CT-based planning with computerized dosimetry has come into wider use. In LDR patients, given the limited overall number of source activities and positions, treatment planning is typically performed manually by varying the various source activities and positions, focusing on the doses to Point A as well as normal tissues. Many radiation oncologists typical start with a "standard" loading, for example, 15-10-10 milligram radium equivalents (mg-Ra-eq) in the tandem and 10–15 mg-Ra-eq in both colpostats in a patient with intact cervical cancer. The goal is to deliver a total Point A

| TABLE 25.1 | American Brachytherapy Society Guidelines Definitive Radiation Therapy for Cervical Cancer LDR Intracavitary Brachytherapy |

	External beam irradiation (Gy)			LDR brachytherapy (Gy)	
Stage	**Pelvis**	**Pelvic wall**	**PMB**	**Point A dose**	**Total point A**
IA1	0	0	0	50–60	50–60
IA2	0	0	0	50–60	50–60
Select IB1[a]	0	0	0	60–70	60–70
IB1	19.8 or 45	50.4 or 45	0	55 or 30–35	75 or 75–80
IB2, IIA[b]	45	45	0	40	85
IIB	45	45	9–15	40	85
III	45–50	45–50	9–15	40	85–90
IIB,IIIB,IV[c]	50	50	9–15	40	90

[a]Superficial ulceration less than 1 cm in diameter or involving fewer than two quadrants.
[b]Alternative approach is to increase brachytherapy contribution to point A by delivering pelvic radiotherapy of 19.8– 30.6 Gy followed by pelvic radiotherapy with a step wedge midline shiled for an additional 19.8–30.6 Gy and intracavitary brachytherapy bringing point A to the recommended total dose levels.
[c]Poor pelvic anatomy, patient not readily treated with intracavitary insertions (barrel-shaped cervix not regressing, inability to locate external OS).
LDR, low-dose-rate.
Source: Adapted from Nag S, Chao C, Erickson B, et al. The American Brachytherapy Society recommendations for low-dose-rate brachytherapy for carcinoma of the cervix. *Int J Radiat Oncol Biol Phys* 2002;52:33–48.

dose (including the pelvic RT) of approximately 80–85 Gy for small tumors and 85–90 Gy for bulky tumors, while limiting the rectal and bladder doses to <80% of the Point A dose. Different investigators recommend different maximum acceptable rectal and bladder doses, typically <75–80 Gy for the bladder and <70–75 Gy for the rectum. Dose rates of 40–60 cGy/hour to Point A are used at most centers. Care must be taken not only to optimize the doses and dose rates at the various reference and normal tissue points, but to also review the isodose distributions themselves in an effort to obtain a classic "pear shape." Patients treated postoperatively to the vaginal cuff are typically treated with surface dose rates of 80–100 cGy/hour or 50–80 cGy/hour to 0.5 cm. Dose distributions in these patients should conform to the shape of the cylinder.

Given the increased number of potential dwell positions and times, HDR brachytherapy optimization lends itself to more sophisticated optimization approaches. In fact, several inverse planning approaches have been described in these patients (152). The ABS has provided detailed guidelines on the optimization of HDR brachytherapy treatments in patients with cervical cancer, using multiple optimization points along the tandem and vaginal surface (145).

A large variety of dose-fractionation schemes have been used for gynecologic cancer patients undergoing LDR and HDR ICB. Over the years, the ABS has published guidelines for LDR and HDR ICB for both cervical (145,153) and uterine (148) cancer (Tables 25.1–25.4). No guidelines

| TABLE 25.2 | American Brachytherapy Society Guidelines Definitive Radiation Therapy for Cervical Cancer HDR Intracavitary Brachytherapy |

EBRT (Gy)[a]	**No. of HDR fractions**	**HDR dose (Gy)/fraction**
Early stage		
20	6	7.5
20	7	6.5
20	8	6.0
45	5	6.0
45	6	5.3
Advanced stage		
45	5	6.5
45	6	5.8
50.4	4	7.0
50.4	5	6.0
50.4	6	5.3

[a]Delivered at 1.8 Gy/fraction.
HDR, high-dose-rate; EBRT, external beam radiotherapy.
Source: Adapted from Nag S, Erickson B, Thomadsen B, et al. The American Brachytherapy Society recommendations for high-dose-rate brachytherapy for carcinoma of the cervix. *Int J Radiat Oncol Biol Phys* 2009;48:201–211.

| TABLE 25.3 | American Brachytherapy Society Guidelines Postoperative Radiation Therapy for Uterine Cancer HDR Intracavitary Brachytherapy |

EBRT (Gy)[a]	No. HDR fractions	Dose (Gy)/ fraction	Dose-specific point
Brachytherapy alone			
N/A	3	7.0	0.5 cm depth
N/A	4	5.5	0.5 cm depth
N/A	5	4.7	0.5 cm depth
N/A	3	10.5	Vaginal surface
N/A	4	8.8	Vaginal surface
N/A	5	7.5	Vaginal surface
EBRT + brachytherapy			
45	2	5.5	0.5 cm depth
45	3	4.0	0.5 cm depth
45	2	8.0	Vaginal surface
45	3	6.0	Vaginal surface

[a]Delivered at 1.8 Gy/fraction.
HDR, high-dose-rate; EBRT, external beam radiation therapy.
Source: Adapted from Nag S, Erickson B, Parikh S, et al. The American Brachytherapy Society recommendations for high-dose-rate brachytherapy for carcinoma of the endometrium. *Int J Radiat Oncol Biol Phys* 2000;48:779–790.

| TABLE 25.4 | American Brachytherapy Society Guidelines Radiation Therapy for Inoperable Uterine Cancer HDR Intracavitary Brachytherapy |

EBRT (Gy)[a]	No. HDR fractions	Dose (Gy)/ fraction	Dose-specific point (cm)[b]
Brachytherapy alone			
N/A	4	8.5	2
N/A	5	7.3	2
N/A	6	6.4	2
N/A	7	5.7	2
EBRT + brachytherapy			
45	2	8.5	2
45	3	6.3	2
45	4	5.2	2

[a]Delivered at 1.8 Gy/fraction.
[b]From the midpoint of the intrauterine sources.
HDR, high-dose-rate; EBRT, external beam radiation therapy.
Source: Adapted from Nag S, Erickson B, Parikh S, et al. The American Brachytherapy Society recommendations for high-dose-rate brachytherapy for carcinoma of the endometrium. *Int J Radiat Oncol Biol Phys* 2000;48:779–790.

are available for ICB dose-fractionation schemes for vaginal cancer. Fortunately, a variety of LDR and HDR approaches have been published using these techniques (58–61,154,155).

Considerable interest has recently focused on the use of volumetric image-based treatment planning in intact cervical cancer patients. European investigators have pioneered MRI-based approaches in these patients. T2-weighted MRI using a pelvic coil provides excellent soft tissue resolution and differentiation between tumor and normal tissues, allowing more accurate assessment of parametrial and uterine tumor extension (156,157) and improved sparing of the bladder and rectum (158). Controversy exists, however, whether MRI is needed at every insertion or whether CT imaging during subsequent insertions is sufficient. Comparison studies have demonstrated that CT may overestimate tumor width (159,160). However, if MRI with each implant is infeasible, MRI may be used at the first insertion with CT-based planning at

subsequent implants for normal tissue delineation, relying on the initial MRI for tumor delineation (160).

Both the Group Europeen de Curietherapie-European Society for Therapeutic Radiology and Oncology (GEC-ESTRO) and North American IGRT Working Group have published recommendations for MRI-guided brachytherapy in cervical cancer (161,162). The nomenclature that has been adopted worldwide for treatment planning in these patients is based on work primarily performed by GEC-ESTRO (Fig. 25.12). GEC-ESTRO recommendations are to contour the GTV, high-risk CTV (HR-CTV), intermediate risk CTV (IR-CTV) and normal tissues including the bladder, rectum, sigmoid colon and small bowel. The HR-CTV includes the entire cervix as well as any macroscopic disease that persists in the parametria, uterus, rectum, bladder or vagina (but not to cross these anatomic boundaries without clear rationale). The prescription goal is 80–95 Gy to the HR-CTV. The IR-CTV includes the HR-CTV, with the intent to deliver 60 Gy to

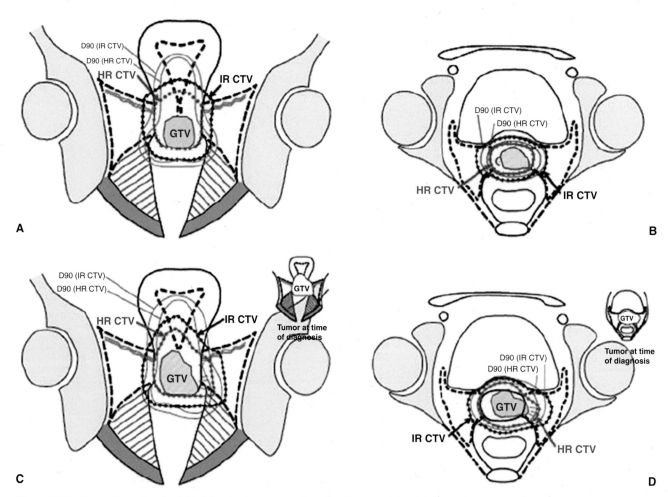

Figure 25.12. Group Européen de Curiethérapie–European Society for Therapeutic Radiology and Oncology (GEC-ESTRO) working group concepts and terms used for image-guided brachytherapy. Schematic diagram with coronal (**A,C**) and transverse (**B,D**) sections of an optimized treatment plan for limited (**A,B**) and advanced (**C,D**) disease with partial remission after external irradiation. GTV, gross tumor volume; HR CTV, high-risk clinical target volume; IR CTV, intermediate-risk clinical target volume. *Source:* From Haie-Meder C, Pötter R, Van Limbergen E, et al. Recommendations from Gynaecological (GYN) GEC-ESTRO Working Group (I): concepts and terms in 3D image based 3D treatment planning in cervix cancer brachytherapy with emphasis on MRI assessment of GTV and CTV. *Radiother Oncol* 2005;74:235–245, with permission.

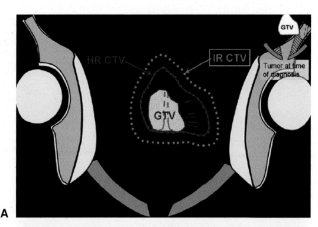

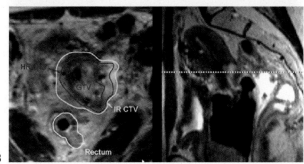

Figure 25.13. Target and organs at risk (OAR) delineation at the first magnetic resonance imaging (MRI)-guided brachytherapy insertion. (**A**) Volume delineated on a coronal view, using clinical drawings at the time of the first brachytherapy application. (**B**) Target and OAR delineation on the MRI according to the GEC ESTRO guidelines, axial cut, and the corresponding sagittal level identification (dotted line). *Source:* From Sturdza A, Dimopoulos J, Potter R. MR-guided target delineation in a patient with locally advanced cervical cancer undergoing brachytherapy (Case Study). In: Mundt AJ, Roeske JC, eds. *Image-Guided Radiation Therapy: A Clinical Perspective.* Shelton, CT: People's Medical Publishing House-USA, 2011:430–435, with permission.

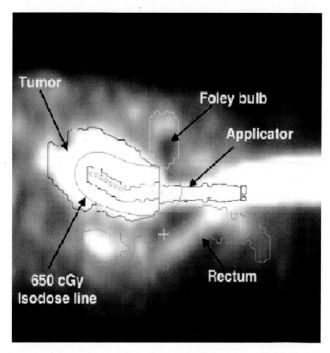

Figure 25.14. Positron-emission tomography (PET)-guided brachytherapy planning in a patient with cervical cancer. *Source:* From Malyapa RS, Mutic S, Low DA, et al. Physiologic FDG-PET three-dimensional brachytherapy treatment planning for cervical cancer. *Int J Radiat Oncol Biol Phys* 2002;54:1140–1146, with permission.

this volume. HR and IR-CTV contours in a representative cervial cancer patient are shown in Figure 25.13.

Recommendations for reporting and quality assurance in patients undergoing MRI-guided brachytherapy include calculation and reporting of the minimum dose to 90% and 100% of the contoured target volume (D_{90}, D_{100}). In addition, for evaluation within a single treatment scheme, the volume encompassed by the 100% IDL (V_{100}) should also be determined. For the normal tissues, reporting of the ICRU reference bladder and rectal points should continue for comparison with the dose–volume histogram (DVH) data. The minimum dose received by the maximally irradiated contiguous 0.1 cm^3, 1 cm^3 and 2 cm^3 of the bladder, rectum, sigmoid and small bowel, respectively, should also be calculated and reported. Dose should be expressed as bioequivalent doses given at 2 Gy per fraction, using the linear quadratic model, to standardize for different dose rates. Provisional dose–volume constraints for the normal tissues are to maintain the bladder below 85–90 Gy and the rectum and sigmoid below 75 Gy. There

have been validation for the recommendation for rectum, but there is a weaker basis for recommendations for bladder, sigmoid and vagina (163,164).

Several promising outcome reports have been published in cervical cancer patients undergoing MRI-guided HDR brachytherapy using the GEC-ESTRO guidelines (164–168). In a series of the first 145 patients (predominantly stages IIB-IIIB) treated at the University of Vienna, the 3-year actuarial local control was 85%. Local control was dependent on tumor size with best results (>90%) seen in 2–5 cm tumors. However, evaluating the most recent locally advanced patients with tumors >5 cm, the local control rate was 82%. Low rates of chronic treatment-related toxicities were also seen.

Investigators at Washington University have conducted several studies on PET-guided brachytherapy planning for cervical cancer, demonstrating the feasibility and dosimetric advantages of this approach over conventional techniques (Fig. 25.14) (84,169,170). The procedure involves scanning patients after both intravenous delivery of [18] F-fluorodeoxyglucose ([18] F-FDG) and insertion of tubes containing [18] F-FDG into the tandem and colpostats. To date, no outcome data are available using this novel approach.

Interstitial Brachytherapy

Interstitial brachytherapy involves implanting radioactive sources directly within the target tissues. Unlike ICB, interstitial implants may be temporary whereby sources are removed after the treatment or permanent with limited half-life sources left place. In gynecologic cancer patients undergoing interstitial brachytherapy, the great majority are treated with temporary implants. Similar to patients undergoing ICB, interstitial brachytherapy was previously performed using "live" sources but is now performed primarily using after-loading techniques. As noted in the ICB section above, after-loading approaches significantly reduce the radiation exposure of the medical and ancillary staff, particularly when performed using remote after-loading techniques.

While the great majority of gynecology patients undergoing brachytherapy receive ICB (171), interstitial brachytherapy is recommended in women in whom ICB would result in suboptimal dose distributions (145). Interstitial brachytherapy should also be considered in patients with extensive parametrial involvement, bulky primary tumors, narrow or distal vaginal involvement, post-hysterectomy central recurrence or a history of prior RT. Other indications are distal or extensive vaginal involvement (>0.5 cm thickness) or persistent disease following external beam RT and ICB.

Multiple after-loading commercial applicators are currently available for interstitial brachytherapy, the most popular of which are the Martinez Universal Perineal Interstitial Template (MUPIT) and the Syed–Neblett template. The MUPIT consists of two acrylic cylinders, an acrylic template with an array of equally spaced holes through which hollow needles are inserted and a cover plate (172). The Syed–Neblett template is comprised of a vaginal cylinder, two lucite plates with 38 holes through which hollow needles are introduced; six additional needles can be inserted into groves along the vaginal cylinder (173). The Vienna ring applicator allows placement of interstitial needles along with ICB brachytherapy (Fig. 25.15) (168).

Pre-planning using CT and/or MRI can be used in patients undergoing interstitial brachytherapy to help determine source number and placement, particularly in patients treated with LDR techniques which required ordering of radioactive seeds and/or wires. However, at the time of implant with the patient under anesthesia, physical examination should be performed to determine optimal applicator and needle placement, based on the patient's individual anatomy and tumor extent (Fig. 25.16) (174). Care needs to be taken to avoid perforation of adjacent organs including the small bowel, bladder and rectum. Intraoperative digital transrectal palpation is recommended not only to assess tumor extent but also to help avoid implanting needles into the rectum. Today, interstitial implants are performed at many centers under image and/or laparoscopic-guidance (175,176). Care also should be taken to avoid excessive doses to the vaginal mucosa. If needles are inserted along the periphery of the central cylinder of a Syed-Neblett template, vaginal dose can be reduced with the placement of a sleeve over the cylinder (177).

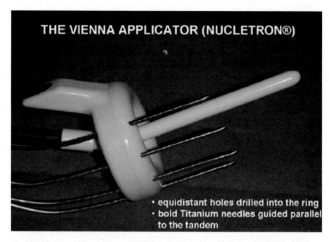

Figure 25.15. The Vienna Ring applicator that allows placement of interstitial needs in patients with residual parametrial involvement in conjunction with intracavitary brachytherapy. *Source:* From Sturdza A, Dimopoulos J, Potter R. MR-guided target delineation in a patient with locally advanced cervical cancer undergoing brachytherapy (Case Study). In: Mundt AJ, Roeske JC, eds. *Image-guided radiation therapy: a clinical perspective.* Shelton, CT: People's Medical Publishing House-USA, 2011:430–435, with permission.

As with ICB, interstitial brachytherapy can be delivered using LDR, HDR or PDR techniques (see earlier section on ICB for a discussion of the advantages and disadvantages of each approach). [192]Ir is the most common isotope currently used, with high activity sources used for HDR. Limited data are available using permanent [198]Au or [103]Pd interstitial implants in gynecologic cancer patients (178,179).

Various doses and prescription points have been used for interstitial brachytherapy in gynecologic cancer patients. The treatment volume is typically defined by the peripheral needles with or without an additional 5 mm margin, with the dose prescribed to an IDL encompassing this volume. Growing interest is focused on MRI-based treatment planning using the GEC-ESTRO guidelines in patients undergoing interstitial brachytherapy (180).

Computerized dosimetry is useful to ensure dose homogeneity throughout the implant. Maximum doses to the adjacent normal should be calculated and efforts made to spare the surrounding bladder and rectum as much as possible. No consensus exists regarding maximum allowable doses to these organs in patients undergoing interstitial brachytherapy. In a series of locally advanced cervical cancer patients treated with interstitial brachytherapy, Demanes and colleagues recommended bladder and rectal maximum doses <75% and <65% of the prescribed dose, respectively (181). Nag and coworkers treated 13 locally recurrent uterine cancer patients with salvage interstitial brachytherapy and optimized the treatment plans to ensure maximum rectal and bladder doses of 60% and 100% of the prescribed dose (174). Total rectal doses of >76 Gy were noted in one study to be highly correlated with the development of severe gastrointestinal toxicity including rectovaginal fistulae (182).

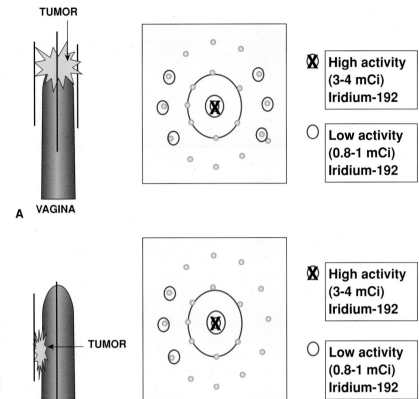

TUMOR

🞨	High activity (3-4 mCi) Iridium-192
○	Low activity (0.8-1 mCi) Iridium-192

A   VAGINA

Figure 25.16. Example customized implant plans for uterine cancer patients with (**A**) a vaginal vault recurrence and (**B**) recurrence in the right lateral vaginal wall. *Source:* From Nag S, Yacoub S, Copeland LJ, et al. Interstitial brachytherapy for salvage treatment of vaginal recurrences in previously unirradiated endometrial cancer patients. *Int J Radiat Oncol Biol Phys* 2002;54:1153–1539, with permission.

TUMOR

🞨	High activity (3-4 mCi) Iridium-192
○	Low activity (0.8-1 mCi) Iridium-192

B   VAGINA

Given the invasive nature of interstitial brachytherapy, an effort is made to minimize the number of implants performed. Most patients undergoing LDR interstitial brachytherapy are treated with a single insertion, which requires several days at bedrest in the hospital. Patients undergoing HDR interstitial brachytherapy undergo one to three implants, often with multiple fractions delivered during each implant. If multiple implants are performed in patients with intact cervical cancer, it is recommended to initiate brachytherapy during external beam RT, to avoid unnecessary treatment protractions (145). As with ICB, interstitial brachytherapy should not be performed on the same day as either external beam RT or chemotherapy.

No consensus currently exists regarding the optimal dose-fractionation schedule for gynecologic cancer patients receiving interstitial brachytherapy. In a series of 69 locally advanced/recurrent gynecologic cancer patients undergoing a single LDR interstitial implant, Gupta and colleagues at William Beaumont Hospital prescribed median doses of 32 Gy and 35 Gy in patients treated with and without external beam RT, respectively (183). Five-year actuarial local control rates were 54% and 44% in the entire group and the subset of primary cervical cancer patients, respectively. Severe complications (grade 4) were noted in 14% of patients. Demanes and colleagues at the California Endocurietherapy Center (CEC) presented the outcomes of 62 previously untreated locally advanced cervical cancer patients undergoing HDR interstitial brachy-

therapy (6 fractions of 5.5–6 Gy) combined with external beam RT (181). Overall, the local control of the entire group was 94%, with rates exceeding 90% even in stage IIB-IIIB patients. Severe (grade 3–4) late sequelae were seen in 6.5% of patients. The ABS has endorsed the dose-fractionation regimens employed at the CEC (Table 25.5) (145).

Other groups have published outcomes of patients treated with a variety of interstitial dose-fractionation regimens, including in cervical (180,184,185), vaginal (185–188), vulvar (189,190) and locally recurrent uterine (174,191) cancer, using predominantly HDR techniques. More limited data exist regarding PDR dose-fractionation regimens for interstitial brachytherapy (192).

Intraperitoneal ^{32}P

A pure β emitter with a relatively short half-life (14.3 days) and minimal tissue penetration (maximum 7 to 8 mm), ^{32}P has long been felt to be an attractive means of treating the peritoneal surfaces in patients with ovarian and uterine cancer without damaging the underlying parenchymal organs (liver, kidneys, etc.). Available as a chromic phosphate suspension and delivered in 10 mL vials containing 5–15 mCi, treatment is delivered via intraperitoneal or peritoneal dialysis catheters placed at the time of surgery or postoperatively.

Initially, 250 cc of normal saline is instilled into the peritoneal cavity. Peritoneal distribution is assessed by

TABLE 25.5	**California Endocureitherapy Cancer Center Guidelines Interstitial HDR Brachytherapy for Cervical Cancer**		
Stage	**EBRT (Gy)**	**Sidewall total (Gy)**	**HDR Dose × fractions**
IB/IIA (<4 cm)	25	50	6 Gy × 6
IB/IIA (>4 cm)	30	50	5.75 Gy × 6
IIB/IIIA/IIIB	36	50	5.5 Gy × 6

Note: the tumor doses presented can safely be administered only when brachytherapy doses to the rectum and bladder are limited to 65% and 75% of the tumor dose, respectively.
HDR, high-dose-rate; EBRT, external beam radiotherapy.
Source: Adapted from Nag S, Erickson B, Thomadsen B, et al. The American Brachytherapy Society recommendations for high-dose-rate brachytherapy for carcinoma of the cervix. *Int J Radiat Oncol Biol Phys* 2009;48:201–211.

performing a technetium-99 m (^{99m}Tc) scan or by the instillation of a small volume of dilute radiopaque contrast. Assessment of adequate peritoneal distribution is essential component of treatment for the presence of multiple loculations is a contraindication to ^{32}P therapy (193). Avoiding protracted delays between surgery and treatment is important due to the development of adhesions following surgery.

Once adequate distribution is determined, 15 mCi of ^{32}P in 500 cc normal saline is instilled followed by flushing the catheter with an additional 250 cc of normal saline. While most patients tolerate treatment well, some patients experience significant pain and reduced volumes of fluid may be necessary. The patient is then turned frequently, for example, every 10–15 minutes over 2 hours, to distribute the radiocolloid throughout the peritoneum. At some centers, four patient positions (supine, prone, right and left laterals) and three bed positions (flat, Trendelenburg, reverse Trendelenburg) are used. However, some postoperative patients may not tolerate the prone position for extended periods. In the published clinical trials, more limited positions are used (left lateral supine, Trendelenburg, reverse Trendelenburg and right lateral supine) (44,194).

FUTURE DIRECTIONS

Radiotherapeutic approaches and treatment planning in gynecologic cancer patients are rapidly evolving. Long-held techniques and concepts are rapidly giving way to ever newer ones. One area of current intense research is the development of adaptive RT in gynecologic patients. It is well known that in select patients, particularly woman with bulky cervical cancer, tumors rapidly regress throughout treatment and re-planning may be beneficial (195). However, sophisticated high-speed techniques are needed before adaptive RT can be introduced clinically (196,197). Novel image-guided approaches are also currently being explored which may further enhance IMRT treatment in these patients, including bone marrow-sparing techniques

which reduce dose to functionally active bone marrow sites (198). It is also possible in the future that novel approaches including SBRT (128,199) and even proton therapy (200), which are both growing in popularity throughout the world, will be increasingly applied to gynecologic cancer patients.

REFERENCES

1. http://www.cancer.org/Research/CancerFactsFigures/CancerFactsFigures/cancer-facts-and-figures-2010 (Accessed April 20, 2011).
2. Sankaranarayanan R, Ferlay J. Worldwide burden of gynaecological cancer: the size of the problem. *Best Pract Res Clin Obstet Gynecocol* 2006;20:207–225.
3. Grigsby PW, Perez CA. Radiotherapy alone for medically inoperable carcinoma of the cervix: stage IA and carcinoma in situ. *Int J Radiat Oncol Biol Phys* 1991;21:375–378.
4. Landoni F, Maneo A, Colombo A, et al. Randomised study of radical surgery versus radiotherapy for stage Ib-IIa cervical cancer. *Lancet* 1997;350:535--540.
5. Bloemers MC, Portelance L, Legler C, et al. Preservation of ovarian function by ovarian transposition prior to concurrent chemotherapy and pelvic radiation for cervical cancer. A case report and review of the literature. *Eur J Gyneacol Oncol* 2010;31:194–197.
6. Bergmark K, Avall-Lundqvist E, Dickman PW, et al. Vaginal changes and sexuality in women with a history of cervical cancer. *N Engl J Med* 1999;340:1383--1389.
7. Schroder M, Mell LK, Hurteau JA, et al. Clitoral therapy device for treatment of sexual dysfunction in irradiated cervical cancer patients. *Int J Radiat Oncol Biol Phys* 2005;61:1078–1086.
8. Sedlis A, Bundy BN, Rotman MZ, et al. A randomized trial of pelvic radiation therapy versus no further therapy in selected patients with stage IB carcinoma of the cervix after radical hysterectomy and pelvic lymphadenectomy: a Gynecologic Oncology Group Study. *Gynecol Oncol* 1999;73:177–183.
9. Peters WA III, Liu PY, Barrett RJ II, et al. Concurrent chemotherapy and pelvic radiation therapy compared

with pelvic radiation therapy alone as adjuvant therapy after radical surgery in high-risk early-stage cancer of the cervix. *J Clin Oncol* 2000;18:1606–1613.

10. Rose PG, Ali S, Watkins E, Thigpen JT, et al. Long-term follow-up of a randomized trial comparing concurrent single agent cisplatin, cisplatin-based combination chemotherapy, or hydroxyurea during pelvic irradiation for locally advanced cervical cancer: a Gynecologic Oncology Group Study. *J Clin Oncol* 2007;25:2804–2810.

11. Whitney CW, Sause W, Bundy BN, et al. Randomized comparison of fluorouracil plus cisplatin versus hydroxyurea as an adjunct to radiation therapy in stage IIB-IVA carcinoma of the cervix with negative para-aortic lymph nodes: a Gynecologic Oncology Group and Southwest Oncology Group study. *J Clin Oncol* 1999;17:1339–1348.

12. Morris M, Eifel PJ, Lu J, et al. Pelvic radiation with concurrent chemotherapy compared with pelvic and para-aortic radiation for high-risk cervical cancer. *N Engl J Med* 1999;340:1137–1143.

13. Ungar L, Palfalvi L, Novak Z. Primary pelvic exenteration in cervical cancer patients. *Gynecol Oncol* 2008; 111:S9–S12.

14. Keys HM, Bundy BN, Stehman FB, et al. Cisplatin, radiation, and adjuvant hysterectomy compared with radiation and adjuvant hysterectomy for bulky stage IB cervical carcinoma. *N Engl J Med* 1999;340:1154–1161.

15. Keys HM, Bundy BN, Stehman FB, et al. Radiation therapy with and without extrafascial hysterectomy for builky stage IB cervical carcinoma: a randomized trial of the Gynecologic Oncology Group. *Gynecol Oncol* 2003;89:343–353.

16. Rotman M, Pajak TF, Choi K, et al. Prophylactic extended-field irradiation of para-aortic lymph nodes in stages IIB and bulky IB and IIA cervical carcinomas. Ten-year treatment results of RTOG 79-20. *JAMA* 1995;274:387–393.

17. Kinsella TJ, Bloomer WD, Lavin PT, et al. Stage II endometrial carcinoma: 10-year follow-up of combined radiation and surgical treatment. *Gynecol Oncol* 1980;10:290--293.

18. Panici PB, Stefano S, Maneschi F, et al. Systematic pelvic lymphadenectomy vs no lymphadenectomy in early-stage endometrial carcinoma: randomized clinical trial. *J Natl Cancer Inst* 2008;100:1707–1711.

19. The writing committee on behalf of the ASTEC study group. Efficacy of systematic pelvic lymphadenectomy in endometrial cancer (MRC ASTEC trial): a randomized study. *Lancet* 2009;373:125–136.

20. Phelan C, Montag AG, Rotmensch J, et al. Outcome and management of pathological stage I endometrial carcinoma patients with involvement of the lower uterine segment. *Gynecol Oncol* 2001;83:513–517.

21. Aalders J, Abeler V, Kolstad P, et al. Postoperative external irradiation and prognostic parameters in stage I endometrial carcinoma. *Obstet Gynecol* 1980;56:419–421.

22. Creutzberg CL, van Putten WL, Koper PC, et al. Surgery and postoperative radiotherapy vs surgery alone for patients with stage-1 endometrial carcinoma: multicentre randomized trial. PORTEC Study Group, post operative radiation therapy in endometrial carcinoma. *Lancet* 2000;355:1404–1409.

23. ASTEC/EN.5 Study Group, Blake P, Swart AM, et al. Adjuvant external beam radiotherapy in the treatment of endometrial cancer (MRC ASTEC and NCIC CTG EN.5 randomized trials): pooled trial results, systematic review and meta-analysis. *Lancet* 2009;373:137–141.

24. Keys HM, Roberts JA, Brunetto VL et al. A phase III trial of surgery with or without adjunctive external pelvic radiation therapy in intermediate risk endometrial adenocarcinoma: a Gynecologic Oncology Group study. *Gynecol Oncol* 2004;92:744–751.

25. Lee CM, Szabo A, Shrieve DC, et al. Frequency and effect of adjuvant radiation therapy among women with stage I endometrial adenocarcinoma. *JAMA* 2006;295:389–392.

26. Wright JD, Fiorelli J, Kansler AL, et al. Optimizing the management of stage II endometrial cancer: the role of radical hysterectomy and radiation. *Am J Obstet Gynecol* 2009;200:419–423.

27. Naumann RW, Coleman RL. The use of adjuvant radiation therapy in early endometrial cancer by members of the Society of Gynecologic Oncologists in 2005. *Gynecol Oncol* 2007;105:7–11.

28. Nout RA, Smit VT, Putter H, et al. Vaginal brachytherapy versus pelvic external beam radiotherapy for patients with endometrial cancer of high-intermediate risk (PORTEC-2): an open-label, non-inferiority randomised trial. *Lancet* 2010;375:816–820.

29. Randall MR, Wilder J, Greven K, et al. Role of intracavitary cuff boost after adjuvant external irradiation in early endometrial carcinoma. *Int J Radiat Oncol Biol Phys* 1990;19:49–54.

30. Shenfield CB, Pearcey RG, Ghosh S, et al. The management of inoperable stage I endometrial cancer using intracavitary brachytherapy alone: a 20-year institutional review. *Brachytherapy* 2009;8:278–283.

31. Soper JT, Creasman WT, Clarke-Pearson DL, et al. Intraperitoneal chromic phosphate P 32 suspension therapy of malignant peritoneal cytology in endometrial carcinoma. *Am J Obstet Gynecol* 1985;153:191–196.

32. Connell PP, Rotmensch J, Waggoner S, et al. The significance of adnexal involvement in endometrial carcinoma. *Gynecol Oncol* 1999;74:74–79.

33. Greven KM, Lanciano RM, Corn B et al. Pathologic stage III endometrial carcinoma. Prognostic factors and patterns of recurrence. *Cancer* 1993;71:3697–3702.

34. Randall ME, Filiaci VL, Muss H, et al. Randomized phase III trial of whole-abdominal irradiation versus doxorubicin and cisplatin chemotherapy in advanced endometrial carcinoma: a Gynecologic Oncology Group Study. *J Clin Oncol* 2006;24:36–41.

35. Mundt AJ, McBride R, Rotmensch J, et al. Significant pelvic recurrence in high-risk pathologic stage I-IV endometrial carcinoma patients after adjuvant chemotherapy alone: implications for adjuvant radiation therapy. *Int J Radiat Oncol Biol Phys* 2001;50:1145.

36. Homesley HD, Filiaci V, Gibbons SK et al. A randomized phase III trial in advanced endometrial carcinoma of surgery and volume directed radiation followed by cisplatin and doxorubicin with or without paclitaxel: A Gynecologic Oncology Group study. *Gynecol Oncol* 2009;112:543.

37. Murphy KT, Rotmensch J, Yamada SD, et al. Outcome and patterns of failure in pathologic stages I-IV clear-cell carcinoma of the endometrium: implications for adjuvant radiation therapy. *Int J Radiat Oncol Biol Phys* 2003;55:1272–1276.

38. Wolfson AH, Brady MF, Rocereto T, et al. A gynecologic oncology group randomized phase III trial of whole abdominal irradiation (WAI) vs. cisplatin-ifosfamide and mesna (CIM) as post-surgical therapy in stage I-IV carcinosarcoma (CS) of the uterus. *Gynecol Oncol* 2007;107:177–185.

39. Young RC, Walton LA, Ellenberg SS, et al. Adjuvant therapy in stage I and stage II epithelial ovarian cancer. Results of two prospective randomized trials. *N Engl J Med* 1990;322:1021–1027.

40. Young RC, Brady MF, Nieberg RK, et al. Adjuvant treatment for early ovarian cancer: a randomized phase III trial of intraperitoneal 32P or intravenous cyclophosphamide and cisplatin–a gynecologic oncology group study. *J Clin Oncol.* 2003;21:4350–4355.

41. Martinez A, Schray MF, Howes AE, Bagshaw MA. Postoperative radiation therapy for epithelial ovarian cancer: the curative role based on a 24-year experience. *J Clin Oncol* 1985;3:901–911.

42. Fuller DB, Sause WT, Plenk HP, Menlove RL. Analysis of postoperative radiation therapy in stage I through III epithelial ovarian carcinoma. *J Clin Oncol* 1987;5:897–905.

43. Smith JP, Rutledge FN, Delclos L. Postoperative treatment of early cancer of the ovary: a random trial between postoperative irradiation and chemotherapy. *Natl Cancer Inst Monogr* 1975;42:149–153.

44. Varia MA, Stehman FB, Bundy BN, et al. Intraperitoneal radioactive phosphorus (32P) versus observation after negative second-look laparotomy for stage III ovarian carcinoma: a randomized trial of the Gynecologic Oncology Group. *J Clin Oncol* 2003;21:2849–2855.

45. Sorbe B. Consolidation treatment of advanced ovarian carcinoma with radiotherapy after induction chemotherapy. *Int J Gynecol Cancer* 2003;13 Suppl 2:192–195.

46. Dinniwell R, Lock M, Pintille M, et al. Consolidative abdominopelvic radiotherapy after surgery and carboplatin/paclitaxel chemotherapy for epithelial ovarian cancer. *Int J Radiat Oncol Biol Phys* 2005;62:104–110.

47. Corn BW, Lanciano RM, Boente M, et al. Recurrent ovarian cancer. Effective radiotherapeutic palliation after chemotherapy failure. *Cancer* 1994;74:2979–2983.

48. Burke TW, Stringer CA, Gershenson DM, et al. Radical wide excision and selective inguinal node dissection for squamous cell carcinoma of the vulva. *Gynecol Oncol* 1990;38:328–332.

49. Heaps JM, Fu YS, Montz FJ, et al. Surgical-pathologic variables predictive of local recurrence in squamous cell carcinoma of the vulva. *Gynecol Oncol* 1990;38:309–314.

50. Gaffney DK, Du Bois A, Narayan K, et al. Patterns of care for radiotherapy in vulvar cancer: a Gynecologic Cancer Intergroup study. *Int J Gynecol Cancer* 2009;19:163–167.

51. Stehman FB, Bundy BN, Thomas G, et al. Groin dissection versus groin radiation in carcinoma of the vulva: a Gynecologic Oncology Group study. *Int J Radiat Oncol Biol Phys* 1992;24:389–396.

52. Homesley HD, Bundy BN, Sedlis A, et al. Radiation therapy versus pelvic node resection for carcinoma of the vulva with positive groin nodes. *Obstet Gynecol* 1986;68:733–740.

53. Acosta AA, Given FT, Frazier AB, et al. Preoperative radiation therapy in the management of squamous cell carcinoma of the vulva: preliminary report. *Am J Obstet Gynecol* 1978;132:198–206.

54. Boronow RC. Combined therapy as an alternative to exenteration for locally advanced vulvo-vaginal cancer: rationale and results. *Cancer* 1982;49:1085–1091.

55. Landoni F, Maneo A, Zanetta G, et al. Concurrent preoperative chemotherapy with 5-fluorouracil and mitomycin C and radiotherapy (FUMIR) followed by limited surgery in locally advanced and recurrent vulvar carcinoma. *Gynecol Oncol* 1996;61:321–327.

56. Thomas G, Dembo A, DePetrillo A, et al. Concurrent radiation and chemotherapy in vulvar carcinoma. *Gynecol Oncol* 1989;34:263–267.

57. Moore DH, Thomas GM, Montana GS, et al. Preoperative chemoradiation for advanced vulvar cancer: a phase II study of the Gynecologic Oncology Group. *Int J Radiat Oncol Biol Phys* 1998;42:79–85.

58. Gallup DG, Talledo OE, Shah KJ, et al. Invasive squamous cell carcinoma of the vagina: a 14-year study. *Obstet Gynecol* 1987;69:782–785.

59. Chyle V, Zagars GK, Wheeler JA, et al. Definitive radiotherapy for carcinoma of the vagina: outcome and prognostic factors. *Int J Radiat Oncol Biol Phys* 1996;35:891–905.

60. Perez CA, Korba A, Sharma S. Dosimetric considerations in irradiation of carcinoma of the vagina. *Int J Radiat Oncol Biol Phys* 1977;2:639–649.

61. Frank SJ, Jhingran A, Levenback C, et al. Definitive radiation therapy for squamous cell carcinoma of the vagina. *Int J Radiat Oncol Biol Phys* 2005;62:138–147.

62. Eifel PJ, Moughan J, Erickson B, et al. Patterns of radiotherapy practice for patients with carcinoma of the uterine cervix: a patterns of care study. *Int J Radiat Oncol Biol Phys* 2004;60:1144–1153.

63. Chao KS, Williamson JF, Grigsby PW, et al. Uterosacral space involvement in locally advanced carcinoma of the uterine cervix. *Int J Radiat Oncol Biol Phys* 1998;40:397–403.

64. Tyagi N, Lewis JH, Yashar CM, et al. Daily online cone beam computed tomography to assess interfractional motion in patients with intact cervical cancer. *Int J Radiat Oncol Biol Phys* 2011;80:273–280.

65. Beadle BM, Jhingran A, Salehpour M, et al. Cervix regression and motion during the course of external beam chemoradiation for cervical cancer. *Int J Radiat Oncol Biol Phys* 2009;73:235–241.

66. Finlay MH, Ackerman I, Tirona RG, et al. Use of CT simulation for treatment of cervical cancer to assess the adequacy of lymph node coverage of conventional pelvic fields based on bony landmarks. *Int J Radiat Oncol Biol Phys* 2006;64:205–209.

67. Zunino S, Rosato O, Lucino S, et al. Anatomic study of the pelvis in carcinoma of the uterine cervix as related to the box technique. *Int J Radiat Oncol Biol Phys* 1999;44:53–59.

68. Grigsby P, Winter K, Komaki R, et al. Long-term follow-up of RTOG 88-05: twice-daily external irradiation

with brachytherapy for carcinoma of the cervix. *Int J Radiat Oncol Biol Phys* 2002;54:51–57.

69. MacLeod C, Bernshaw D, Leung S, et al. Accelerated hyperfractionated radiotherapy for locally advanced cervix cancer. *Int J Radiat Oncol Biol Phys* 1999;44:519–524.

70. Kavanagh BD, Gieschen HL, Schmidt-Ullrich RK, et al. A pilot study of concomitant boost accelerated superfractionated radiotherapy for stage III cancer of the uterine cervix. *Int J Radiat Oncol Biol Phys* 1997;38:561–568.

71. Carrascosa LA, Yashar CM, Parris KJ et al. Palliation of pelvic and head and neck cancer with paclitaxel and a novel radiotherapy regimen. *J Palliat Med* 2007;10:877–881.

72. Onsrud M, Hagen B, Strickert T et al. 10-Gy single-fraction pelvic irradiation for palliation and life prolongation in patients with cancer of the cervix and corpus uteri. *Gynecol Oncol* 2001;82:167–171.

73. Perez CA, Grigsby PW, Chao KS, et al. Tumor size, irradiation dose, and long-term outcome of carcinoma of uterine cervix. *Int J Radiat Oncol Biol Phys* 1998;41:307–317.

74. Wolfson AH, Abdel-Wahab M, Markoe AM, et al. A quantitative assessment of standard versus customized midline shield construction for invasive cervical carcinoma. *Int J Radiat Oncol Biol Phys* 1997;37:237–242.

75. McIntyre JF, Eifel PJ, Levenback C, et al. Ureteral stricture as a late complication of radiotherapy for stage IB carcinoma of the uterine cervix. *Cancer* 1995;75;836–843.

76. Roeske JC, Lujan A, Rotmensch J, et al. Intensity-modulated whole pelvic radiation therapy in patients with gynecologic malignancies. *Int J Radiat Oncol Biol Phys* 2000;48:1613.

77. Heron DE, Gerszten K, Selvaraj RN, et al. Conventional 3D conformal versus intensity-modulated radiotherapy for the adjuvant treatment of gynecologic malignancies: a comparative dosimetric study of dose-volume histograms. *Gynecol Oncol* 2003;91:39–45.

78. Chen Q, Izadifar N, King SM, et al. Comparison of IMRT with 3D CRT for gynecologic malignancies [abstract]. *Int J Radiat Oncol Biol Phys* 2001;51:332–333.

79. Ahamad A, D'Souza W, Salehpour M, et al. Intensity-modulated radiation therapy after hysterectomy: comparison with conventional treatment and sensitivity of the normal-tissue-sparing effect to margin size. *Int J Radiat Oncol Biol Phys* 2005;62:1117–1124.

80. Mell LK, Tiryaki H, Ahn KH, et al. Dosimetric comparison of bone marrow-sparing intensity-modulated radiotherapy versus conventional techniques for treatment of cervical cancer. *Int J Radiat Oncol Biol Phys* 2008;71:1504–1510.

81. Adli M, Mayr NA, Kaiser HS, et al. Does prone positioning reduce small bowel dose in pelvic radiation with intensity-modulated radiotherapy for gynecologic cancer? *Int J Radiat Oncol Biol Phys* 2003;57:230–238.

82. *International Commission on Radiation Units and Measurements.* ICRU *Report Number 50: prescribing, recording and reporting photon beam therapy.* Washington, DC:ICRU,1993.

83. Simpson DR, Lawson JD, Nath SK, et al. Utilization of advanced imaging technologies for target delineation in radiation oncology. *J Am Coll Radiol* 2009;6:876–883.

84. Grigsby PW. 18 F-FDG PET-guided target delineation for external beam radiotherapy and intracavitary brachytherapy planning in a patient with stage IIB cervical cancer (Case Study). In: Mundt AJ, Roeske JC, eds. *Image-guided radiation therapy: a clinical perspective.* Shelton, CT:People's Medical Publishing House, 2011:436–439.

85. Miller TR, Grigsby PW. Measurement of tumor volume by PET to evaluate prognosis in patients with advanced cervical cancer treated by radiation therapy. *Int J Radiat Oncol Biol Phys* 2002;53:353–359.

86. Mell LK, Kochanski JD, Roeske JC, et al. Dosimetric predictors of acute hematologic toxicity in cervical cancer patients treated with concurrent cisplatin and intensity-modulated pelvic radiotherapy. *Int J Radiat Oncol Biol Phys* 2006;66:1356–1365.

87. Small W Jr, Mell LK, Anderson P, et al. Consensus guidelines for delineation of clinical target volume for intensity-modulated pelvic radiotherapy in postoperative treatment of endometrial and cervical cancer. *Int J Radiat Oncol Biol Phys* 2008;71:428–434.

88. Taylor A, Rockall AG, Reznek RH, et al. Mapping pelvic lymph nodes: guidelines for delineation in intensity-modulated radiotherapy. *Int J Radiat Oncol Biol Phys* 2005;63:1604–1612.

89. Lim K, Small W, Portelance L, et al. Consensus guidelines for delineation of clinical target volume for intensity-modulated pelvic radiotherapy for the definitive treatment of cervical cancer. *Int J Radiat Oncol Biol Phys* 2011;79:348–355.

90. D'Souza WD, Ahamad AA, Iyer RB, et al. Feasibility of dose escalation using intensity-modulated radiotherapy in posthysterectomy cervical carcinoma. *Int J Radiat Oncol Biol Phys* 2005;61:1062–1070.

91. Mutic S, Malyapa RS, Grigsby PW, et al. PET-guided IMRT for cervical carcinoma with positive para-aortic lymph nodes-a dose-escalation treatment planning study. *Int J Radiat Oncol Biol Phys* 2003;55:28–35.

92. Low DA, Grigsby PW, Dempsey JF, et al. Applicator-guided intensity modulated radiation therapy. *Int J Radiat Oncol Biol Phys* 2002;52:1400–1406.

93. Roeske JC, Mundt AJ. A feasibility study of IMRT for the treatment of cervical cancer patients unable to receive intracavitary brachytherapy. *Med Phys* 2000;27:1382–1384.

94. Chan P, Milosevic M, Paterson J, et al. Cervical cancer not suitable for brachytherapy: case study. In: Mundt AJ, Roeske JC, eds. *Intensity modulated radiation therapy: a clinical perspective.* Hamilton, Canada: BC Decker, 2005:518–522.

95. Kidd EA, Siegel BA, Dehdashti F, et al. Clinical outcomes of definitive intensity-modulated radiation therapy with fluorodeoxyglucose-positron emission tomography simulation in patients with locally advanced cervical cancer. *Int J Radiat Oncol Biol Phys* 2010;77:1085–1091.

96. Mundt AJ, Lujan AE, Rotmensch J, et al. Intensity modulated whole pelvic radiation therapy in women with gynecologic malignancies. *Int J Radiat Oncol Biol Phys* 2002;52:1330–1337.

97. Roeske JC, Bonta D, Lujan AE, et al. A dosimetric analysis of acute gastrointestinal toxicity in women receiving intensity-modulated whole-pelvic radiation therapy. *Radiother Oncol* 2003;69:201–207.

98. Rose BS, Aydogan B, Liang Y, et al. Normal tissue complication probability modeling of acute hematologic toxicity in cervical cancer patients treated with chemoradiotherapy. *Int J Radiat Oncol Biol Phys* 2010;78:912–919.

99. Simpson DR, Song WY, Rose BS, et al. Normal tissue complication probability analysis of acute gastrointestinal toxicity in cervical cancer patients undergoing intensity modulated radiation therapy and concurrent cisplatin [abstract]. *Int J Radiat Oncol Biol Phys* 2010;78:S141–142.

100. Hasselle MD, Rose BS, Kochanski JD, et al. Clinical Outcomes of intensity-modulated pelvic radiation therapy for carcinoma of the cervix. *Int J Radiat Oncol Biol Phys* 2011;80:1436–1445.

101. Liang Y, Messer K, Rose BS, et al. Impact of bone marrow radiation dose on acute hematologic toxicity in cervical cancer: principal component analysis on high dimensional data. *Int J Radiat Oncol Biol Phys* 2010;78:912–919.

102. Mundt AJ, Mell LK, Roeske JC. Preliminary analysis of chronic gastrointestinal toxicity in patients with gynecologic malignancies treated with intensity modulated whole pelvic radiation therapy. *Int J Radiat Oncol Biol Phys* 2003;56:1354–1360.

103. Brixey C, Roeske JC, Lujan AE, et al. Impact of intensity modulated whole pelvic radiation therapy on acute hematologic toxicity in women with gynecologic malignancies. *Int J Radiat Oncol Biol Phys* 2002;54:1388–1396.

104. Beriwal S, Jain SK, Heron DE, et al. Clinical outcome with adjuvant treatment of endometrial carcinoma using intensity-modulated radiation therapy. *Gynecol Oncol* 2006;102:195–199.

105. Portelance L, Winter K, Jhingran A, et al. Post-operative pelvic intensity modulated radiation therapy (IMRT) with chemotherapy for patients with cervical carcinoma/RTOG 0418 phase II study. *Int J Radiat Oncol Biol Phys* 2009;75:S640–S641.

106. Jhingran A, Winter K, Portelance L, et al. A phase II study of intensity modulated radiation therapy (IMRT) to the pelvic for post-operative patients with endometrial carcinoma (RTOG 0418). *Int J Radiat Oncol Biol Phys* 2008;72:S16–S17.

107. International Radiotherapy Technologies and Oncology Consortium (IRTOC). International evaluation of radiotherapy technology effectiveness in cervical cancer (INTERTECC): a phase II/III clinical trial of IMRT with concurrent cisplatin for stage I-IVA cervical carcinoma. Available from http://radonc.ucsd.edu/irtoc/intertecc/intertecc1001.asp.

108. Portelance L, Chao KS, Grigsby PW, et al. Intensity-modulated radiation therapy (IMRT) reduces small bowel, rectum, and bladder doses in patients with cervical cancer receiving pelvic and para-aortic irradiation. *Int J Radiat Oncol Biol Phys* 2001;51:261–266.

109. Lian J, Mackenzie M, Joseph K, et al. Assessment of extended-field radiotherapy for stage IIIC endome-trial cancer using three-dimensional conformal radiotherapy, intensity-modulated radiotherapy, and helical tomotherapy. *Int J Radiat Oncol Biol Phys* 2008;70:935–943.

110. Hermesse J, Devillers M, Deneufbourg JM, et al. Can intensity-modulated radiation therapy of the paraaortic region overcome the problems of critical organ tolerance? *Strahlenther Onkol* 2005;181:185–190.

111. Ahmed RS, Kim RY, Duan J, et al. IMRT dose escalation for positive para-aortic lymph nodes in patients with locally advanced cervical cancer while reducing dose to bone marrow and other organs at risk. *Int J Radiat Oncol Biol Phys* 2004;60:505–512.

112. Salama JK, Mundt AJ, Roeske J, et al. Preliminary outcome and toxicity report of extended-field, intensity-modulated radiation therapy for gynecologic malignancies. *Int J Radiat Oncol Biol Phys* 2006;65:1170–1176.

113. Gerszten K, Colonello K, Heron DE, et al. Feasibility of concurrent cisplatin and extended field radiation therapy (EFRT) using intensity-modulated radiotherapy (IMRT) for carcinoma of the cervix. *Gynecol Oncol* 2006;102:182--188.

114. Du XL, Sheng XG, Jiang T, et al. Intensity-modulated radiation therapy versus para-aortic field radiotherapy to treat para-aortic lymph node metastasis in cervical cancer: prospective study. *Croat Med J* 2010;51:229–236.

115. Moran MS, Castrucci WA, Ahmad M, et al. Clinical utility of the modified segmental boost technique for treatment of the pelvis and inguinal nodes. *Int J Radiat Oncol Biol Phys* 2010;76:1026–1036.

116. Koh WJ, Chiu M, Stelzer KJ, et al. Femoral vessel depth and the implications for groin node radiation. *Int J Radiat Oncol Biol Phys* 1993;27:969–974.

117. Petereit DG, Mehta MP, Buchler DA, et al. Inguinofemoral radiation of N0,N1 vulvar cancer may be equivalent to lymphadenectomy if proper radiation technique is used. *Int J Radiat Oncol Biol Phys* 1993;27:963–967.

118. Dusenbery KE, Carlson JW, LaPorte RM, et al. Radical vulvectomy with postoperative irradiation for vulvar cancer: therapeutic implications of a central block. *Int J Radiat Oncol Biol Phys* 1994;29:989--998.

119. Beriwal S, Heron DE, Kim H, et al. Intensity-modulated radiotherapy for the treatment of vulvar carcinoma: a comparative dosimetric study with early clinical outcome. *Int J Radiat Oncol Biol Phys* 2006;64:1395–1400.

120. Ahmad M, Song H, Moran M, et al. IMRT of whole pelvis and inguinal nodes: Evaluation of dose distributions produced by an inverse treatment planning system. *Int J Radiat Oncol Biol Phys* 2004;60(Suppl):S484–S485.

121. Beriwal S, Coon D, Heron DE, et al. Preoperative intensity-modulated radiotherapy and chemotherapy for locally advanced vulvar carcinoma. *Gynecol Oncol* 2008;109:291–295.

122. Dembo AJ, Van Dyk J, Japp B, et al. Whole abdominal irradiation by a moving-strip technique for patients with ovarian cancer. *Int J Radiat Oncol Biol Phys* 1979;5:1933–1942.

123. Martinez A, Schray MF, Howes AE, et al. Postoperative radiation therapy for epithelial ovarian cancer: the curative role based on a 24-year experience. *J Clin Oncol* 1985;3:901–911.

124. Randall ME, Barrett RJ, Spirtos NM, et al. Chemotherapy, early surgical reassessment, and hyperfractionated abdominal radiotherapy in stage III ovarian cancer: results of a gynecologic oncology group study. *Int J Radiat Oncol Biol Phys* 1996;34:139–147.

125. Hong L, Alektiar K, Chui C, et al. IMRT of large fields: whole-abdomen irradiation. *Int J Radiat Oncol Biol Phys* 2002;54:278–289.

126. Duthoy W, De Gersem W, Vergote K, et al. Whole abdominopelvic radiotherapy (WAPRT) using intensity-modulated arc therapy (IMAT): first clinical experience. *Int J Radiat Oncol Biol Phys* 2003;57:1019–1032.

127. Wong E, D'Souza DP, Chen JZ, et al. Intensity-modulated arc therapy for treatment of high-risk endometrial malignancies. *Int J Radiat Oncol Biol Phys* 2005;61:830–841.

128. Pan H, Simpson DR, Mell LK, et al. A survey of stereotactic body radiotherapy use in the United States. *Cancer* 2011 (in press).

129. Choi CW, Cho CK, Yoo SY, et al. Image-guided stereotactic body radiation therapy in patients with isolated para-aortic lymph node metastases from uterine cervical and corpus cancer. *Int J Radiat Oncol Biol Phys* 2009;74:147–153.

130. Mollà M, Escude L, Nouet P, et al. Fractionated stereotactic radiotherapy boost for gynecologic tumors: an alternative to brachytherapy? *Int J Radiat Oncol Biol Phys* 2005;62:118–124.

131. Jorcano S, Molla M, Escude L, et al. Hypofractionated extracranial stereotactic radiotherapy boost for gynecologic tumors: a promising alternative to high-dose rate brachytherapy. *Technol Cancer Res Treat* 2010;9:509–514.

132. Tod MC, Meredith WJ. A dosage system for use in the treatment of cancer of the uterine cervix. *Br J Radiol* 1938;11:809–813.

133. Henscke UK. "Afterloading" applicator for radiation therapy of carcinoma of the uterus. *Radiology* 1960;74:834–836.

134. Heyman J, Reuterwall O, Benner S, et al. The Radium-hemmet experience with radiotherapy in cancer of the corpus of the uterus. *Acta Radiol* 1941;22:11–98.

135. Coon D, Beriwal S, Heron DE, et al. High-dose-rate Rotte "Y" applicator brachytherapy for definitive treatment of medically inoperable endometrial cancer: 10-year results. *Int J Radiat Oncol Biol Phys* 2008;71:779–783.

136. Perez CA, Slessinger E, Grigsby PW. Design of an afterloading vaginal applicator (MIRALVA). *Int J Radiat Oncol Biol Phys* 1990;18:1503–1508.

137. International commission on radiation units. ICRU Report 38. Dose and volume specifications for reporting intracavitary therapy in gynecology. Bethesda, MD: ICRU, 1985:1–16.

138. Eifel PJ. High-dose-rate brachytherapy for carcinoma of the cervix: high tech or high risk? *Int J Radiat Oncol Biol Phys* 1992;24:383–386.

139. Hareyama M, Sakata K, Oouchi A, et al. High-dose-rate versus low-dose-rate intracavitary therapy for carcinoma of the uterine cervix: a randomized trial. *Cancer* 2002;94:117–124

140. Lertsanguansinchai P, Lertbutsayanukul C, Shotelersuk K, et al. Phase III randomized trial comparing LDR and HDR brachytherapy in treatment of cervical carcinoma. *Int J Radiat Oncol Biol Phys* 2004;59:1424–1431.

141. De Brabandere M, Mousa AG, Nulens A, et al. Potential of dose optimisation in MRI-based PDR brachytherapy of cervix carcinoma. *Radiother Oncol* 2008;88:217–226.

142. Rath GK, Sharma DN, Julka PK, et al. Pulsed-dose-rate intracavitary brachytherapy for cervical carcinoma: the AIIMS experience. *Am J Clin Oncol* 2010;33:238–241.

143. Dooley WC, Thropay JP, Schreiber GJ, et al. Use of electronic brachytherapy to delivery postsurgical adjuvant radiation therapy for endometrial cancer: a retrospective multicenter study. *Onco Targets Ther* 2010;3:197–203.

144. Lee LJ, Sadow CA, Russell A, et al. Correlation of point B and lymph node dose in 3D-planned high-dose-rate cervical cancer brachytherapy. *Int J Radiat Oncol Biol Phys* 2009;75:803–809.

145. Nag S, Erickson B, Thomadsen B, et al. The American Brachytherapy Society recommendations for high-dose-rate brachytherapy for carcinoma of the cervix. *Int J Radiat Oncol Biol Phys* 2009;48:201–211.

146. Stitt JA, Fowler JF, Thomadsen BR et al., High dose rate intracavitary brachytherapy for carcinoma of the cervix: The Madison System: I. Clinical and radiobiological considerations. *Int J Radiat Oncol Biol Phys* 1992;24:383–386.

147. Maruyama Y, Nagell JR Jr, Wrede DE, et al. Approaches to optimization of dose in radiation therapy of cervix carcinoma. *Radiology* 1976;120:389–398.

148. Nag S, Erickson B, Parikh S, et al. The American Brachytherapy Society recommendations for high-dose-rate brachytherapy for carcinoma of the endometrium. *Int J Radiat Oncol Biol Phys* 2000;48:779–790.

149. Patil VM, Patel FD, Chakraborty S, et al. Can point doses predict volumetric dose to rectum and bladder: a CT-based planning study in high dose rate intracavitary brachytherapy of cervical carcinoma? *Br J Radiol* 2011;84:441–448.

150. Rotmensch J, Connell PP, Yamada D, Waggoner SE, Mundt AJ. One versus two intracavitary brachytherapy applications in early-stage cervical cancer patients undergoing definitive radiation therapy. *Gynecol Oncol* 2000;78:32–38.

151. Petereit DG, Sarkaria JN, Chappell R, et al. The adverse effect of treatment prolongation in cervical carcinoma. *Int J Radiat Oncol Biol Phys* 1995;32:1301–1307.

152. Jamema SV, Kirisits C, Mahantshetty U, et al. Comparison of DVH parameters and loading patterns of standard loading, manual and inverse optimization for intracavitary brachytherapy on a subset of tandem/ovoid cases. *Radiother Oncol* 2010;97:501–506.

153. Nag S, Chao C, Erickson B, et al. The American Brachytherapy Society recommendations for low-dose-rate brachytherapy for carcinoma of the cervix. *Int J Radiat Oncol Biol Phys* 2002;52:33–48.

154. Hegemann S, Schäfer U, Lellé R, et al. Long-term results of radiotherapy in primary carcinoma of the vagina. *Strahlenther Onkol* 2009;185:184–189.

155. Mock U, Kucera H, Fellner C, et al. High-dose-rate (HDR) brachytherapy with or without external beam radiotherapy in the treatment of primary vaginal carcinoma: long-term results and side effects. *Int J Radiat Oncol Biol Phys* 2003;56:950–957.

156. Dimopoulos JC, Schard G, Berger D, et al. Systematic evaluation of MRI findings in different stages of treatment of cervical cancer: potential of MRI on delineation of target, pathoanatomic structures and organs at risk. *Int J Radiat Oncol Biol Phys* 2006;64:1380–1388.

157. Mitchell D, Snyder B, Coakley F, et al. Early invasive cervical cancer: tumor delineation by magnetic resonance imaging, computed tomography and clinical examination, verified by pathologic results, in the ACRIN6651/GOG 183 Intergroup Study. *J Clin Oncol* 2006;26:5687–5694.

158. Wachter-Gerstner N, Wachter S, Reinstadler E, et al. Bladder and rectum dose defined from MRI based treatment planning for cervix cancer brachytherapy: comparison of dose-volume histograms for organ contours and organ wall, comparison with ICRU rectum and bladder reference point. *Radiother Oncol* 2003;68:269–276.

159. Viswanathan AN, Dimopoulos J, Kirisits C, et al. Computed tomography versus magnetic resonance imaging-based contouring in cervical cancer brachytherapy: results of a prospective trial and preliminary guidelines for standardized contours. *Int J Radiat Oncol Biol Phys* 2007;68:491–498.

160. Eskander RN, Scanderbeg D, Saenz CC, et al. Comparison of computed tomography and magnetic resonance imaging in cervical cancer brachytherapy target and normal tissue contouring. *Int J Gynecol Cancer* 2010;20:47–53.

161. Haie-Meder C, Pötter R, Van Limbergen E, et al. Recommendations from Gynaecological (GYN) GEC-ESTRO Working Group (I): concepts and terms in 3D image based 3D treatment planning in cervix cancer brachytherapy with emphasis on MRI assessment of GTV and CTV. *Radiother Oncol* 2005;74:235–245.

162. Nag S, Cardenes H, Chang S, et al. Proposed guidelines for image-based intracavitary brachytherapy for cervical carcinoma: report from Image-Guided Brachytherapy Working Group. *Int J Radiat Oncol Biol Phys* 2004;60:1160–1172.

163. Koom WS, Sohn DK, Kim JY, et al. Computed tomography-based high-dose-rate intracavitary brachytherapy for uterine cervical cancer: preliminary demonstration of correlation between dose-volume parameters and rectal mucosal changes observed by flexible sigmoidoscopy. *Int J Radiat Oncol Biol Phys* 2007;68:1446–1454.

164. Pötter R, Dimopoulos J, Bachtiary B, et al. 3D conformal HDR-brachy- and external beam therapy plus simultaneous cisplatin for high-risk cervical cancer: clinical experience with 3 year follow-up. *Radiother Oncol* 2006;79:80–86.

165. Tanderup K, Georg D, Potter R, et al. Adaptive management of cervical cancer radiotherapy. *Semin Radiat Oncol* 2010;20:121–129.

166. Dimopoulos JC, Pötter R, Lang S, et al. Dose-effect relationship for local control of cervical cancer by magnetic resonance image-guided brachytherapy. *Radiother Oncol* 2009;93:311–315.

167. Pötter R, Dimopoulos J, Georg P, et al. Clinical impact of MRI assisted dose volume adaptation and dose escalation in brachytherapy of locally advanced cervix cancer. *Radiother Oncol* 2007;83:148–155.

168. Sturdza A, Dimopoulos J, Potter R. MR-guided target delineation in a patient with locally advanced cervical cancer undergoing brachytherapy (case study). In: Mundt AJ, Roeske JC, eds. *Image-guided radiation therapy: a clinical perspective.* Shelton, CT:People's Medical Publishing House, 2011:430–435.

169. Malyapa RS, Mutic S, Low DA, et al. Physiologic FDG-PET three-dimensional brachytherapy treatment planning for cervical cancer. *Int J Radiat Oncol Biol Phys* 2002;54:1140–1146.

170. Mutic S, Grigsby PW, Low DA, et al. PET-guided three-dimensional treatment planning of intracavitary gynecologic implants. *Int J Radiat Oncol Biol Phys* 2002;52:1104–1110.

171. Erickson B, Eifel P, Moughan J, et al. Patterns of brachytherapy practice for patients with carcinoma of the cervix (1996-1999): a patterns of care study. *Int J Radiat Oncol Biol Phys* 2005;63:1083–1092.

172. Martinez A, Edmundson GK, Cox RS, et al. Combination of external beam irradiation and multiple-site perineal applicator (MUPIT) for treatment of locally advanced or recurrent prostatic, anorectal, and gynecologic malignancies. *Int J Radiat Oncol Biol Phys* 1985;11:391–398.

173. Ampuero F, Doss LL, Khan M, et al. The Syed-Neblett interstitial template in locally advanced gynecological malignancies. *Int J Radiat Oncol Biol Phys* 1983;9:1897–1903.

174. Nag S, Yacoub S, Copeland LJ, et al. Interstitial brachytherapy for salvage treatment of vaginal recurrences in previously unirradiated endometrial cancer patients. *Int J Radiat Oncol Biol Phys* 2002;54:1153–1539.

175. Erickson B, Albano K, Gillin M. CT-guided interstitial implantation of gynecologic malignancies. *Int J Radiat Oncol Biol Phys* 1996;36:699–709.

176. Nag S, Martínez-Monge R, Ellis R, et al. The use of fluoroscopy to guide needle placement in interstitial gynecological brachytherapy. *Int J Radiat Oncol Biol Phys* 1998;40:415–420.

177. Erickson B, Albano K, Withnell J, et al. Modification of the Syed-Neblett template system to enable loading of the vaginal obturator. *Endocuriether Hyperthem Oncol* 1996;12:7–12.

178. Randall ME, Evans L, Greven KM, et al. Interstitial reirradiation for recurrent gynecologic malignancies: results and analysis of prognostic factors. *Gynecol Oncol* 1993;48:23–31.

179. Brabham JG, Cardenes HR. Permanent interstitial reirradiation with 198Au as salvage therapy for low volume recurrent gynecologic malignancies: a single institution experience. *Am J Clin Oncol* 2009;32:417–422.

180. Yoshida K, Yamazaki H, Takenaka T, et al. A dose-volume analysis of magnetic resonance imaging-aided high-dose-rate image-based interstitial brachytherapy for uterine cervical cancer. *Int J Radiat Oncol Biol Phys* 2010;77:765–777.

181. Demanes DJ, Rodriguez RR, Bendre DD, et al. High dose rate transperineal interstitial brachytherapy for cervical cancer: high pelvic control and low complication rates. *Int J Radiat Oncol Biol Phys* 1999;45:105–112.

182. Kasibhatla M, Clough RW, Montana GS, et al. Predictors of severe gastrointestinal toxicity after external

beam radiotherapy and interstitial brachytherapy for advanced recurrent gynecologic malignancies. *Int J Radiat Oncol Biol Phys* 2006;65:398–403.

183. Gupta AK, Vicini FA, Frazier AJ, et al. Iridium-192 transperineal interstitial brachytherapy for locally advanced or recurrent gynecological malignancies. *Int J Radiat Oncol Biol Phys* 1999;43:1055–1060.

184. Isohashi F, Yoshioka Y, Koizumi M, et al. High-dose-rate interstitial brachytherapy for previously untreated cervical cancer. *Brachytherapy* 2009;8:234–239.

185. Beriwal S, Bhatnagar A, Heron DE, et al. High-dose-rate interstitial brachytherapy for gynecologic malignancies. *Brachytherapy* 2006;5:218–222.

186. De Crevoisier R, Sanfilippo N, Gerbaulet N, et al. Exclusive radiotherapy for primary squamous cell carcinoma of the vagina. *Radiother Oncol* 2007;85:362–370.

187. Beriwal S, Heron DE, Mogus R, et al. High-dose-rate brachytherapy (HDRB) for primary or recurrent cancer in the vagina. *Radiat Oncol* 2008;3:7–11.

188. Tewari KS, Cappuccini F, Puthawala AA, et al. Primary invasive carcinoma of the vagina: treatment with interstitial brachytherapy. *Cancer* 2001;91:758–770.

189. Pohar S, Hoffstetter S, Peiffer D, et al. Effectiveness of brachytherapy in treating carcinoma of the vulva. *Int J Radiat Oncol Biol Phys* 1995;32:1455–1460.

190. Tewari K, Cappuccini F, Syed AM,et al. Interstitial brachytherapy in the treatment of advanced and recurrent vulvar cancer. *Am J Obstet Gynecol* 1999;181:91–98.

191. Tewari K, Cappuccini F, Brewster WR,et al. Interstitial brachytherapy for vaginal recurrence of endometrial cancer. *Gynecol Oncol* 1999;74:416–422.

192. Seeger AR,Windschall A, Lotter M,et al. The role of interstitial brachytherapy in the treatment of vaginal and vulvar malignancies. *Strahlenther Onkol* 2006;182:142–148.

193. Taylor A, Baily NA, Halpern SE,et al. Loculation as a contraindication to intracavitary 32P-chromic phosphate therapy. *J Nucl Med* 1975;16:318–319.

194. Sharma SC. Procedure for P-32 administration. *Med Dosim* 1988;13:83–86.

195. van de Bunt L, van der Heide UA, Ketelaars M, et al. Conventional, conformal, and intensity-modulated radiation therapy treatment planning of external beam radiotherapy for cervical cancer: The impact of tumor regression. *Int J Radiat Oncol Biol Phys* 2006;64:189–196.

196. Men C, Jia X, Jiang SB. GPU-based ultra-fast direct aperture optimization for online adaptive radiation therapy. *Phys Med Biol* 2010;55:4309–4319.

197. Men C, Romeijn HE, Jia X, et al. Ultrafast treatment plan optimization for volumetric modulated arc therapy (VMAT). *Med Phys* 2010;37:5787–5791.

198. Liang Y, Bydder M, Hoh C, et al. Correlation between increased bone marrow glucose metabolism and acute changes in fat fraction during pelvic radiation therapy. *Int J Radiat Oncol Biol Phys* 2010;78:S118–S119.

199. Higginson DS, Morris DE, Jones EL, et al. Stereotactic body radiotherapy (SBRT): Technological innovation and application in gynecologic oncology. *Gynecol Oncol* 2011;120:404–412.

200. Song WY, Huh SN, Liang Y, et al. Dosimetric comparison study between intensity modulated radiation therapy and three-dimensional conformal proton therapy for pelvic bone marrow sparing in the treatment of cervical cancer. *J Appl Clin Med Phys* 2010;11:3255.

PART A
Prostate

Daniel A. Hamstra ▪ Michael E. Ray

INTRODUCTION

Prostate cancer is the most common malignancy in men in the United States with an estimated >190,000 new cases in 2009 and the second leading cause of prostate cancer death with >27,000 men presumed to die of prostate cancer in 2009 (1). The paradox in these numbers is the fact that <1 in 6 men diagnosed with prostate cancer will actually die from the disease. Therefore, the clinical evaluation and management of prostate cancer has changed dramatically over the last 10 years not only to improve treatment but also to better identify those who may not require treatment. The proven prognostic indicators including stage, grade, and pretreatment prostate-specific antigen (PSA) continue to be used for predicting outcomes with various therapies, although additional factors, such as PSA kinetics, are being increasingly considered.

Modern radiotherapy techniques for prostate cancer include external photon and particle beam treatments, as well as low dose rate (LDR) and high-dose rate (HDR) brachytherapy radioisotope implantation. Long-term follow-up of a number of trials utilizing external beam radiation therapy (EBRT) (2,3) have identified improvements in biochemical control of prostate cancer with only modest change in toxicity and patient reported quality of life as compared to conventional dose RT (4). These increases in RT dose without unreasonable increases in toxicity have occurred largely through the adoption of improved treatment techniques (4,5). Two-dimensional (2D) treatment planning techniques have at this time been essentially supplanted by the use of three-dimensional (3D) image sets based upon computed tomography (CT) and/or magnetic resonance imaging (MRI). Inverse planning and intensity modulated radiation therapy (IMRT) have become commonly used techniques that have further enabled the delivery of highly conformal treatment to targeted structures while minimizing radiation exposure to

adjacent normal tissues (5). In addition, the use of image guidance (using such varied techniques as: ultrasound, implanted markers, cone beam CT, or electromagnetic guidance) to localize the prostate at the start of treatment and even during each delivered fraction has ushered in an era of image-guided radiation therapy (IGRT) (6).

Improvements in brachytherapy (both LDR and HDR) either alone or in conjunction with EBRT have also led to a number of ways to bring about intensification of local treatment with ionizing radiation. These may help in reducing the local failure component of prostate cancer; however, the distant metastatic rate, especially with large tumors and aggressive histology, is significant as well and it is still unclear how much an improvement locally intensified radiation provides on this front. In the past, prostate brachytherapy was done through an open surgical approach, and dosimetry was compromised by technical difficulty and lack of imaging techniques for accurate volume assessment and dose calculation. Today this procedure has been revolutionized by sophisticated preimplant or intraoperative treatment planning systems and the broad implementation of postimplant dosimetry. Generally, the implant is done through a template transperineally, with ultrasound for guidance. Iodine-125 (I-125), palladium-103 (Pd-103), and more recently cesium-131 (Cs-131) have been used for LDR permanent seed implants. There has also been increased use of automated iridium-192 (Ir-192) after loading units to deliver temporary HDR prostate implants.

STAGING AND RISK STRATIFICATION

Staging

Since the three most important prognostic indicators in prostate cancer are stage, grade, and pretreatment PSA, diagnostic evaluation is aimed at defining these factors. The clinical stage of the primary tumor is determined by digital rectal exam along with pertinent imaging studies. The American Joint Commission on Cancer (AJCC) clinical staging system for the primary tumor (T staging) is shown in Table 26.1 (7) The digital rectal exam was previously the main tool for detecting clinically localized prostate cancer, however, because of PSA screening and

TABLE 26.1	2010 American Joint Committee on Cancer (AJCC) Clinical Primary Tumor (T) Staging for Prostate Cancer (7th Edition)

TX	Primary tumor cannot be assessed
T0	No evidence of primary tumor
T1	Clinically inapparent tumor neither palpable nor apparent by imaging
T1a	Tumor incidental histologic finding in 5% or less of tissue resected
T1b	Tumor incidental histologic finding in >5% of tissue resected
T1c	Tumor identified by needle biopsy (e.g., because of elevated PSA)
T2	Tumor confined within the prostate[a]
T2a	Tumor involves one-half of one lobe or less
T2b	Tumor involves more than one-half of one lobe but not both lobes
T2c	Tumor involves both lobes
T3	Tumor extends through prostatic capsule[b]
T3a	Extracapsular extension (unilateral or bilateral)
T3b	Tumor invades the seminal vesicle(s)
T4	Tumor is fixed or invades adjacent structures other than seminal vesicles: bladder, external sphincter, rectum, levator muscles, and/or pelvic wall

[a]Tumor found in one or both lobes by needle biopsy, but not palpable or reliably visible on imaging, is classified at T1 c.
[b]Invasion into prostatic apex or into (but not beyond) the prostatic capsule is not classified as T3, but as T2.

heightened patient awareness, the majority of tumors are being diagnosed at earlier stages of disease and T1c (nonpalpable disease only identified due to an elevated PSA) now represents the most common clinical stage.

Unfortunately, digital rectal examination and transrectal ultrasound do a poor job of predicting disease extent at the time of biopsy or treatment. Therefore, there has been increasing interest in obtaining more accurate staging information using more sophisticated imaging modalities. Although often obtained, the utility of a staging CT scan is limited in most patients. CT scans accurately predict local tumor extent only 65% of the time (8). CT scanning is rarely able to detect involvement of metastatic lymph nodes (9), although the addition of fine needle aspiration may increase sensitivity (10). Staging CT scans are not recommended in patients with low-risk features such as early clinical stage, low PSA and Gleason score (GS) (11). Recent improvements in MRI have shown promise in enhancing clinical staging; although, in randomized trials MRI did not add value for prostate screening as compared to ultra-sound and DRE (12). Nevertheless, once cancer has been identified, endorectal coil MRI may have a role in predicting local extension of disease beyond the prostate capsule or into seminal vesicles with sensitivity and specificity of 65% and 100% in one study of low to intermediate risk patients undergoing prostatectomy (13). Newer MRI sequences such as diffusion weighted MRI or dynamic contrast MRI have also shown promise in limited evaluation although their role has not gained common acceptance (14). Since the most common distant metastatic site for prostate cancer is the skeleton, radioisotopic bone scan has been advocated as part of the staging workup. With the trend toward earlier diagnosis, the necessity of ordering this study has been questioned in many patients. In one study, the incidence of an abnormal

bone scan was closely related to stage, GS and PSA, and was <1% among patients with clinical stage T2b or less, GS 7 or less, and PSA of 50 ng/mL or less (15). Therefore, this study need not be routinely ordered but rather applied only to patients at significant risk for disseminated disease.

Pathologic Evaluation

Given that PSA screening has led to more limited tumor stage coupled with the intrinsic limitations in clinical and radiological staging, histologic tumor grade and pretreatment PSA level have taken a profound role in patient evaluation and treatment selection. The Gleason system is based on the morphologic architecture of prostate cancer and is the method most often used for grading the aggressiveness of prostate cancer histologically (16). Based on the growth pattern and degree of differentiation, prostate cancer is graded on a scale from 1 (most differentiated) to 5 (least differentiated). The GS is the sum of the two most prevalent Gleason grades observed within a tissue sample and ranges from 2 through 10, with 2 the most indolent and 10 the most malignant. In conventional clinical practice, the GS is broken down into three main partitions: well differentiated (GS 2–6), moderately differentiated (Gleason 7), and poorly differentiated (Gleason 8–10). In addition, in contemporary clinical practice a GS of <6 is rarely encountered on needle biopsies due to a prevailing change in Gleason grading by pathologist which has led to a shift in GSs over time with higher GSs being more prevalent in the PSA era even as other clinical risk features have declined (17).

The serum PSA test is one of the most commonly ordered laboratory tests performed by thousands of clinical laboratories; however, there are a variety of manufacturers with commercially available serum PSA assays. The values for serum PSA are reported in nanograms per milliliter with conventionally most labs reporting the lowest detectable value in the range of 0.1 to 0.2 ng/mL. However, there can be variation in reported thresholds and even levels between different laboratories using different assays. In addition, newer techniques have led to the development of ultra-sensitive or super-sensitive PSA tests that can detect PSA at one to two orders of magnitude lower level, which may be useful to detect recurrence (or predict a lower risk of recurrence) after a radical prostatectomy (RP). The utility of an "undetectable PSA" following RP using such novel PSA evaluations are still being determined (18).

Risk Stratification

Prostate cancer has a very heterogeneous natural history, as a result clinical factors are typically utilized to segment patients into risk groups that can be utilized to help describe the natural history of the disease as well as to select treatment regimens. The new AJCC Cancer Staging System (7th edition) includes a prognostic risk group system based upon T-stage, PSA, and GS (7) (Table 26.1); however, the most commonly utilized method for risk stratification at this time is the similar NCCN risk grouping (see Table 26.2) (19). The NCCN stratification system has been applied across large groups of patients treated with diverse treatment regiments and breaks patients into 5 categories based upon risk of recurrence: very low, low, intermediate, high, and very high (although most typically only low, intermediate, and high-risk groups have been utilized). However, it suffers in that there can be broad diversity of risk and as a result clinical outcome within the intermediate (20) and high-risk groups (21). Therefore, a number of additional means to risk stratify patients have been developed which are predominantly based upon pretreatment clinical factors. A large group of surgically treated patients has been used to devise look-up tables to predict extracapsular tumor extension, seminal vesicle involvement, and lymph node metastasis based on a combination of grade, stage, and pretreatment PSA level (11), and this data has been updated with a more contemporary cohort (22). Additional nomograms developed for predicting individualized outcomes after surgery or radiation therapy (RT) have also been developed (23,24). Indeed at last count well over 130 different algorithms or nomograms had been developed and reported upon to predict clinical outcome and other events (recurrence, metastasis, benefit from salvage radiation, etc.) (25). The exact role and discriminatory power of each of these tools are still being evaluated.

The clinical assessment of risk for local, regional, and distant disease is important for prediction of ultimate outcome and individualized counseling of patients regarding appropriate treatment strategies. Using the risk groups and/or nomograms described above, many practitioners utilize risk stratification schemes that group patients with clinically localized disease into low-, intermediate-, and high-risk categories. These groupings can be used to formulate appropriate treatment schemes for individual

TABLE 26.2	Prostate Cancer Recurrence Risk Group By NCCN Criteria (2010 Version)
Clinically localized	
Very Low	T1 a AND Gleason score < = 6 AND PSA <10 AND Fewer than 3 biopsy cores positive with < = 50% cancer in each core AND PSA density < 0.15 ng/mL/g
Low Risk	T1-T2a AND Gleason score 2–6 AND PSA < 10 ng/mL
Intermediate Risk	T2b-T2c OR Gleason score 7 OR PSA 10–20 ng/ml
High Risk	T3a OR Gleason 8–10 OR PSA > 20 ng/mL
Locally Advanced/ Very High Risk	T3b-T4
Metastatic	
	Any T, N1 OR Any T, Any N, M1

patients such as the one used at the University of Michigan for EBRT: as shown in Table 26.3. For radiation oncologists, it is important for the design of appropriate target volumes and selecting appropriate delivery methods and doses to be used for the administration of effective RT. In particular, the risk of seminal vesicle and pelvic lymph node involvement has a large impact on these decisions as does the use and duration of androgen deprivation therapy (ADT).

TABLE 26.3	A Risk Stratification System for Clinically Localized Prostate Cancer with 3D Conformal or Intensity Modulated External Beam Radiation Therapy Treatment Guidelines utilized at the University of Michigan
GROUP 1	Low risk (PSA ≤ 10 and Gleason ≤ 6 and Tstage ≤ T2a)
CTV =	Prostate
PTV expansion =	0.5 cm[a]
Dose/Fraction =	79.2/1.8 Gy
GROUP 2	Intermediate Risk (T2b/c, Gleason 7, PSA 10–20)
CTV =	Prostate + proximal 1 cm of seminal vesicle
PTV expansion =	0.5 cm
Dose/Fraction =	79.2/1.8
GROUP 3	High Intermediate Risk
3 or 4 of the following: T2b/c, Gleason 4 + 3 = 7, PSA 10–20, >50% cores positive	
RT dose and volumes the same as for GROUP 2	
Androgen Deprivation Therapy:	
6 months of ADT: 2 months before, 2 months during, and 2 months after RT.	
GROUP 4	High Risk (PSA ≥ 20 or Gleason ≥ 8 or Tstage ≥ T3)
Phase 1:	
CTV1 =	Prostate + full seminal vesicle
CTV2 =	Pelvic lymph nodes
PTV1 expansion =	0.5 cm (match and adjust to prostate)
PTV2 expansion =	1.0 cm
Dose/Fraction	45.0/1.8 Gy
Phase 2:	
CTV =	Prostate + proximal seminal vesicle[b]
PTV expansion =	0.5 cm
Dose/Fraction =	34.2/1.8 Gy
Total Dose =	79.2/1.8 Gy
Androgen Deprivation Therapy:	
24–36 months of ADT: 2 months before, 2 months during, and 20–32 months after RT	

[a]0.5 cm PTV expansion utilized if delivered with IGRT. If non-IGRT then 1.0 cm PTV expansion.
[b]Unless SV grossly involved, then P + whole SV + 0.5 cm to 79.2 Gy.

TREATMENT OPTIONS

Watchful Waiting/Active Surveillance

For many men with prostate cancer the risk of clinical recurrence and/or death from prostate cancer may be small even without treatment. Therefore, the choice to observe without clinical intervention, particularly if patients are older or have an increased burden of comorbid illness, remains a viable option and may even be the optimal treatment plan. The largest trial to address this was the Scandinavian Prostate Cancer Group-4 Randomized Trial (26). In this study men with clinically localized prostate cancer (25% T1 and 75% T2) were randomized to RP versus observation (watchful waiting) and at 12 years there was a 5% difference in the risk of death from prostate cancer in favor of those who underwent treatment (18% vs. 13%, $p = 0.03$). However, the 12-year rate of all

cause mortality was not significantly different (22% vs. 18%, $p = 0.09$) There were, however, decreases in other clinically meaningful endpoints such as reduced metastasis with 19% of men in the treatment group and 26% of men in the watchful waiting group diagnosed with distant metastases at 12 years ($p = 0.006$). This trial pre-dated routine PSA screening and as such the majority of men had palpable disease on DRE and a median PSA >12. Therefore, the outcome with conservative therapy in the PSA era may have even smaller differences in clinical outcome which is supported by population-based analysis of prostate cancer outcomes in the USA (27).

An alternative to no active treatment (watchful waiting) for prostate cancer is to select patients for treatment based upon both initial clinical features as well as further clinical behavior in a process commonly referred to as "active surveillance." A number of institutions have reported on outcome from such series with that from the

University of Toronto being the largest and most mature (28). In the Canadian experience men, on average 70 years of age and mostly with NCCN low-risk disease, were managed with an initial expectant approach, and definitive intervention was offered to those patients with a PSA doubling time <3 years, GS progression (to 4 + 3 or greater), or unequivocal clinical progression. Overall after a median follow-up of 7 years 70% of men remained on surveillance with a 10-year rate of death due to prostate cancer of 2.8% and the risk of death due to other cause being more than sixfold greater at 18.6%. A randomized study in North America and Europe is now applying this concept of active surveillance.

Radical Prostatectomy

Nevertheless, for patients who elect treatment for their prostate cancer the best curative treatment for clinically localized carcinoma of the prostate has been a contentious topic for many years. The advent of the nerve-sparing RP in the early 1980s, increasing chances for retaining sexual potency, as well as more recent refinements in surgical techniques such as laparoscopic or robotic RP, have ensured that RP remains a popular treatment option. Laparoscopic prostatectomy techniques have decreased acute surgical morbidity, with decreased blood loss, shorter hospital stays, and more rapid postoperative recovery (29). However, some concerns have been raised over possible increased risk of positive surgical margins and need for salvage therapy (30), particularly among surgeons new to the technique (31). In addition, patients with clinical evidence of extra capsular (T3) disease or high-risk features such as high GS or PSA may be at increased risk of residual disease after nerve-sparing surgery. Prostatectomy results in a substantial risk of impotence, and at least some degree of urinary incontinence is common (32,33). Nerve sparing techniques may decrease these rates although most patients still report significant sexual dysfunction even following nerve sparing RP (33–35). Although there have not been adequate direct comparisons, it appears that disease cure rates with RP are comparable to those seen with RT for low and intermediate risk disease (36). More recently there is also increasing emphasis on the use of RP for patients with clinically high-risk disease as well, which may necessitate a higher rate of utilization of postoperative RT (37).

External Beam Radiation Therapy

Definitive Therapy

EBRT is commonly utilized to treat men with clinically localized or locally advanced prostate cancer. EBRT alone may be applied to any clinical stage—T1 to T4—but is also often used with adjunctive anti-androgen therapy for selected higher-risk patients. We will address issues in regard to radiation dose, volume, technique below, and here will focus on the combination of ADT with RT and the role of RT after RP.

ADT

For high-risk prostate cancer, there is level I evidence from randomized trials supporting an overall survival advantage with the combination of ADT and RT. The question of ADT added to RT was first evaluated in a series of randomized trials which revealed that for patients with locally advanced (T3–T4) or high-grade prostate cancer (Gleason 8–10) ADT when added to conventional dose EBRT increased biochemical control and decreased risks of metastasis, death from prostate cancer, and all cause mortality (38–42). Therefore, for patients with the highest risk disease the use of ADT for between 28 and 36 months along with conventional dose EBRT appears better than either EBRT alone or EBRT delivered with shorter duration ADT (4–6 months) (40,42). For example, on RTOG 92-02 the addition of 24 months adjuvant ADT in addition to 4 months neo-adjuvant ADT resulted in a an absolute 16% increase in biochemical control at 10 years ($p < 0.0001$) along with improvements in local control (10% improvement, $p < 0.0001$), metastasis (8% improvement, $p < 0.0001$), and disease-specific survival (5% improvement, $p = 0.004$). Overall survival, however, was not increased for all patients, but was significantly improved for those with Gleason 8 to 10 disease (32% vs. 45%, $p = 0.006$). More recently it was also demonstrated that for node-negative men with high-risk prostate cancer the addition of conventional dose RT dramatically increased disease outcome when combined with long-term ADT as compared to long-term ADT delivered alone (43). There was an absolute risk reduction of 50% for biochemical failure at 10 years (75% vs. 26%, $p < 0.0001$) with the addition of RT. More importantly, the cumulative incidence at 10 years for prostate cancer-specific mortality was 24% in the ADT alone group and 12% in the ADT plus RT group ($p < 0.0001$). While the cumulative incidence for overall mortality was 39% in the endocrine alone group and 30% in the endocrine plus RT group ($p = 0.004$).

The role of ADT in intermediate risk disease has been addressed in two recent randomized trials which would suggest a benefit to shorter course anti-androgen therapy (4–6 months) when treated with conventional dose RT of $<= 70$ Gy (44,45). The role for ADT in patients treated with higher dose RT (particularly if intermediate risk) is an area of active evaluation at this time. Finally, there does not appear to be meaningful benefit with the addition of short-term ADT in either cancer-specific or overall survival in men with clinical low-risk disease by NCCN risk criteria even when treated with RT dose < 70 Gy (45).

Adjuvant or Salvage EBRT

EBRT is also commonly utilized as either adjuvant or salvage therapy in the post-prostatectomy setting for patients with clinical high-risk features or with a rising PSA following RP. For adjuvant therapy there is now level I evidence from randomized trials supporting a decline in biochemical failure, metastasis, and prostate cancer-specific death with an improvement in overall survival with the use of adjuvant RT (ART) (46,47). The South West Oncology Group (SWOG) 8794 trial randomized men (stage pT3N0M0 disease or positive surgical margins) to observation or ART arms where the RT dose ranged from 60 to 64 Gy, with treatment portals including the prostatic fossa and paraprostatic tissues. With >12 years of follow-up the use of ART was associated with a 50% relative reduction in the risk of PSA recurrence in the ART group ($p < 0.001$). The use of ART yielded an absolute 10% improvement in metastasis-free survival at 10 years (71% vs. 61%, $p = 0.016$) and an 8% improvement in overall survival (66% vs. 74%, $p = 0.023$). Interestingly, the magnitude of benefit was similar for those with or without detectable PSA postoperatively although the utility of super-sensitive PSA remains to be determined (18). Two additional randomized trials support similar benefit in biochemical control of prostate cancer using ART although follow-up in these studies is insufficient to address more clinically meaningful end-points (48,49).

The role of salvage RT for patients with a rising PSA after RP has not been evaluated in randomized trials (although certainly a significant portion of patients on both the SWOG and EORTC trials had detectable PSA at the time of irradiation and as such would be consistent with salvage therapy). In general approximately 30% to 40% of patients given salvage RT will have long-term disease control (50,51). Preoperative, pathologic, and other clinical features have been utilized to construct a nomogram predicting the likelihood of PSA control (51) which was subsequently validated in a large multi-institutional data set (50). In addition, others have presented data supporting an improvement in prostate cancer-specific survival with the use of salvage RT particularly in those with the most rapidly rising PSA (52). No studies have directly compared ART (delivered 10–12 w after surgery) due to the presence of high-risk pathologic features even with undetectable PSA to salvage RT delivered at the time of rising PSA. However, a number of retrospective reviews have suggested an improved rate of biochemical control using ART as compared to salvage RT (53,54). In addition, the role of ADT concurrent with either ART or salvage RT has not been clearly established with some favoring its use (55) with others finding no benefit to concurrent ADT with RT in the salvage setting (52). Nevertheless, in Great Britain it has been assumed that salvage RT is the standard of care and a study has been undertaken test if ART is superior to salvage RT, and at the same time to evaluate the role of ADT concurrent with RT using a four arm dual-randomized trial (the Radiotherapy and Androgen Deprivation in Combination After Local Surgery (RADICALS) trial) (56).

Brachytherapy

Interstitial brachytherapy is a popular alternative to EBRT for delivery of RT to the intact prostate. Potential advantages of brachytherapy over EBRT include the convenience of undergoing a 1-day outpatient procedure, the lack of organ motion that can confound EBRT planning and delivery, and the use of low-energy isotopes with rapid dose fall-off outside the prostate, potentially minimizing treatment-related morbidity. Most commonly, LDR permanent interstitial radioisotopic implants are performed using I-125, Pd-103, or more recently, Cs-131 seeds which are placed transperineally via needles inserted through a template. HDR brachytherapy can also be used by similar needle placement of catheters that are used for remote afterloading of a high activity Ir-192 source. Multi-institutional and long-term data suggest that brachytherapy performs comparably to surgery or EBRT for low-risk patients (57–59). Brachytherapy may also be combined with a conventional course of EBRT to 45 to 50.4 Gy, particularly for patients with adverse risk features (60).

Since the incidence of urethral stricture can be high after transurethral prostatic resection (TURP), implant is usually not recommended for stage T1a and T1b tumors. Other relative contraindications to brachytherapy include large prostate size, a prominent median lobe, or significant preexisting obstructive urinary symptoms, as these may be associated with technical difficulty in performing an adequate implant or increased risks of complications. Patients with locally extensive tumors—clinical stages T3 and T4—are generally not suitable candidates for isotope therapy except possibly as a boost technique. Brachytherapy is also starting to have a role in salvage treatment after localized recurrence for patients treated with definitive RT although the results from this form of treatment at this time are very limited (61–65).

Other Treatments

Cryotherapy, or freezing the prostate by circulating liquid nitrogen through interstitial catheters, is also utilized as curative treatment for clinically localized disease. Early results reported high complication rates although with newer techniques the complication rates have declined. Nevertheless, sexual dysfunction remains with near 100% incidence (35). A Canadian randomized trial did compare short-term ADT followed by either EBRT (68–73.5 Gy) or cryotherapy in men with localized prostate cancer where most (80%) had NCCN high-risk disease (66). Sexual dysfunction was significantly greater in those treated with cryotherapy (67). There were no significant differences in clinical outcome between treatment arms although a number of treatment features were suboptimal for the RT group including: low RT dose (most ≤70 Gy) (68,69), no pelvic RT (70), and only a short course of ADT (40,42). Each of these factors has been demonstrated alone to increase the rate of biochemical control for men treated with EBRT for prostate cancer. In addition, early repeat cryotherapy was not considered a treatment failure so a modest number of patients were retreated after biopsy-proven residual disease in the cryotherapy arm. Nevertheless, cryotherapy may be an option for patients with biopsy-proven recurrence after previous RT(71).

Noncurative options for prostate cancer include watchful waiting and active surveillance (both covered above) as well as androgen-deprivation hormonal therapy. Types of hormonal therapies include: orchiectomy, luteinizing hormone-releasing hormone (LHRH) agonists (e.g., leuprolide, goserelin) or antagonists (e.g., abarelix, degarelix), nonsteroidal anti-androgens (e.g., flutamide, bicalutamide) and estrogens. These hormonal agents can be used as debulking and anti-metastatic measures; however, these treatments are not curative unless combined with effective local therapy (43). They are, however, usually the first-line and most effective therapies available for disseminated disease. New systemic innovations are on the horizon with the recent reporting of the first cytotoxic chemotherapy agents that demonstrated improved survival in men with metastatic, hormone-refractory prostate cancer (72,73). In addition, newer hormonal agents are being developed which have resulted in promising PSA-based responses even in men with what was considered hormone refractory prostate cancer (74–76). The roles of these and other newer agents both alone and when combined with RT remain to be seen.

TREATMENT PLANNING FOR EXTERNAL BEAM RADIATION THERAPY FOR DEFINITIVE PROSTATE TREATMENT

Target Volumes

Because prostate cancer is a multifocal disease and no current imaging modalities can reliably localize all areas of disease within the prostate, the prostate gland in its entirety is encompassed by the radiation prescription dose in current radiation oncology practice. The prostate is most commonly identified on a treatment planning CT; however, some have advocated for the use of MRI for treatment planning of the prostate (77). Although the prostate will always be treated, a clinical decision must be made as to whether the seminal vesicles and pelvic lymph nodes will be included. This decision depends on grossly demonstrated involvement of these structures or a substantial risk of being microscopically positive, as well as on institutional policy (see Table 26.3 for the criteria currently utilized at the University of Michigan).

The benefit of pelvic lymph node irradiation has been a controversial topic over many years (78); however, recent results from the Radiation Therapy Oncology Group clinical trial 94-13 provided insight (70,79). This trial included patients with an estimated likelihood of pelvic lymph node involvement of at least 15%. Patients were randomized to whole pelvic radiation versus prostate only radiation, as well as to short-term neoadjuvant and concurrent ADT versus adjuvant ADT starting at the completion of RT. No statistically significant differences were found in progression-free or overall survival between the two study questions that patients were randomized to:

neoadjuvant ADT versus adjuvant ADT and pelvic RT compared with prostate only RT. Nevertheless, a trend toward improved progression-free survival was found in favor of the pelvic and neoadjuvant ADT arm compared with the other three arms. In addition, when the size of the pelvic field was separately evaluated, it appeared that there was a direct benefit when using a whole pelvic field as compared to a mini-pelvic field or prostate only treatment with 7-year progression-free survival of 40%, 35%, and 27%, respectively ($p = 0.02$) (80). Two other studies have come to negative conclusions in regard to the benefit of pelvic RT; however, these have been criticized as either having such a low risk of pelvic lymph node involvement that a benefit was unlikely to be seen (81) or to have been performed with ineffectual treatments in the pre-PSA era when local control was so poor as to render pelvic RT meaningless (82). Current imaging technology, including CT, MRI, and lymphangiograms, has limited accuracy for detecting pelvic lymph node metastasis. Therefore, until improved methods for detecting pelvic lymph node metastases are developed, clinicians will be limited to using risk factor assessment and clinical judgment in deciding whether pelvic lymph nodes should be encompassed in the target volumes.

Likewise, seminal vesicle involvement is associated with a relatively high risk of lymph node disease and a worse clinical outcome (83). The clinical risk factors of stage, GS, and PSA can be related to risk of seminal vesicle involvement, similar to lymph node risk (84). To date no study documents improved local control or survival if seminal vesicles are electively irradiated for the risk of clinically undetected microscopic disease; however, intuitively it seems important to include these structures in higher risk patients, so that likely potential sites of local disease in its entirety is treated. Some authors have presented evidence that only the proximal portion of the seminal vesicles adjacent to the prostate needs to be included in the target volume (85). Including the seminal vesicles, lymph nodes, or both within the target volumes increases the field size and may likewise increase the acute side effects and long-term complications (70).

Pelvic Lymph Nodes

For treating of pelvic lymph nodes traditional 2D treatment techniques commonly utilized four fields from the anterior, posterior, right, and left lateral orientations covering the targeted anatomical areas: the prostate, the seminal vesicles, and the pelvic nodes. Accurate targeting is critically important if 3D conformal or IMRT-based treatment techniques are utilized to treat the pelvic lymph nodes, yet there is significant heterogeneity in how pelvic lymph nodes are contoured even amongst experience genitourinary radiation oncologists (86). A recent consensus definition was established to make pelvic nodal volumes more uniform (87). Based upon this consensus, the pelvic lymph node volumes to be irradiated include: distal common iliac, presacral lymph nodes (S(1)–S(3)), external iliac lymph nodes, internal iliac lymph nodes, and obturator lymph nodes. Lymph node CTVs include the vessels (artery and vein) and a 7-mm radial margin without extending into bowel, bladder, bone, and muscle. Volumes begin at the L5/S1 interspace and end at the superior aspect of the pubic bone (87). The treatment of presacral lymphatics is somewhat controversial as these nodes are infrequently problematic clinically, and are rarely an isolated site of recurrence if left untreated, and are not included in the standard pelvic lymph node dissection. Their inclusion in the radiation field necessitates that the posterior margin be expanded significantly, encompassing additional rectum and large bowel and unless using 3D conformal or IMRT techniques may result in increased irradiation of the rectum with increased risk of acute and long-term side effects. The role of RT in patients with known pelvic lymph node positive disease is less clear. However, as both RTOG 85-31 and the EORTC studies of high-risk prostate cancer allowed positive pelvic lymph nodes at diagnosis, treatment of patients with positive lymph nodes with both irradiation and ADT is a reasonable course of action.

Prostate and Seminal Vesicles

The prostate is situated behind the pubic symphysis at midline in the anteroposterior (AP) view and behind the femoral head and proximal femoral shaft in the lateral projection. The seminal vesicles are superior and usually slightly posterior to the prostate gland, attaching at the base. With reference to the bony pelvis, these structures are typically ~2 cm above the superior border of the pubis, although location can vary in any individual patient. The International Commission on Radiation Units and Measurements (ICRU) has defined volumes for treatment planning that take into account the extent of the known gross tumor, the areas of likely microscopic extension, and daily variations in patient setup and tumor position. These definitions of gross tumor volume (GTV), clinical target volume (CTV) and planning target volume (PTV) are given in Table 26.4 (88). Various institutions have adapted the ICRU definitions on tumor volumes for use in prostate cancer planning. In general, the prostate itself is considered the GTV. The GTV is then expanded by some amount to encompass potential microscopic extension of disease in the CTV. This may include all or some portion of the seminal vesicles, if they are at significant risk and are intended to be treated. Additional margin is added to the CTV to account for variation in daily treatment setup and organ motion to define the PTV.

The amount of margin added to the GTV to define the CTV and the PTV in this series of expansions has been the subject of extensive study and discussion. While it is important to make margins generous enough to consistently encompass gross and microscopic tumor by the prescribed dose, there is also compelling reason to keep the margins as small as possible near organs of limited toler-

TABLE 26.4 International Commission on Radiation Units and Measurements Designated Tumor Volumes and Definitions

Tumor volumes	
Gross tumor volume (GTV)	The palpable or visible extent of the tumor
Clinical target volume (CTV)	Gross tumor volume plus a margin for suspected subclinical disease
Planning target volume (PTV)	Clinical target volume plus a margin to account for variations in size, shape, and position relative to the treatment beam

ance, such as the rectum posteriorly, the bladder superiorly, and (possibly) the penile bulb inferiorly. In general, 0.5 to 1 cm is added around the prostate (and seminal vesicles) to ensure coverage of extracapsular microscopic tumor extension and to account for setup variability and organ motion. As an example, treatment guidelines for the recently closed RTOG clinical trial P0126 instruct that the GTV for intermediate-risk patients be defined as the prostate, the CTV be defined as the GTV plus the proximal 1 cm of the seminal vesicles, and the PTV be defined as the CTV plus a 0.5 to 1.0 cm margin depending on institutional policy. These volumes are then used for treatment planning using either 3D-CRT or IMRT techniques.

The PTV should be designed so that it covers the CTV with high probability for every treatment. Practitioners may adjust the size of the PTV depending on many factors that may influence the uncertainties in daily setup and prostate position including immobilization techniques, patient positioning, bladder and rectum filling, and others. Rigid immobilization devices such as the Alpha Cradle™ or thermoplastic body casts may increase setup accuracy. Rosenthal, et al. found that with immobilization only 1 of 10 patients had >0.5 cm variation in patient positioning for treatment, whereas 8 of 12 patients had more variation than this without immobilization (89). Improved positioning accuracy with rigid immobilization has been demonstrated in prospective randomized comparisons as well (90,91). Intra-rectal balloons may be expanded within the rectum to stabilize the prostate position, reducing the concerns over inter- and intra-fraction organ motion (92) (Fig. 26.1). However, use of these devices may be inconvenient for daily treatment and somewhat uncomfortable for the patient.

Instead of focusing on immobilization, many centers use daily imaging for prostate localization including daily CT (93), ultrasound (94), radiographic imaging of implanted radiopaque fiducial markers (95,96), or electro

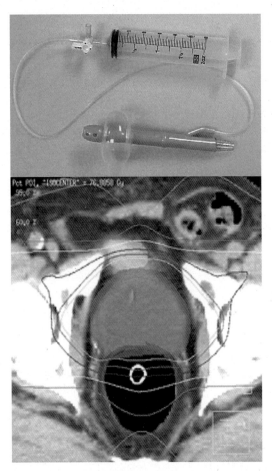

Figure 26.1. An intrarectal balloon device (*top panel*) can be used for stabilization of prostate position during external beam radiation therapy (*bottom panel*). Courtesy Dr. Mark Ritter.

magnetic transponders (97,98) (Fig. 26.2). Isocenter adjustments can then be made on a daily basis, ensuring adequate localization of the CTV at the start of treatment. These techniques fall under the category of a collection of adaptive RT practices termed IGRT (6). Using any of these IGRT techniques most authors have typically decreased

prostate CTV to PTV margins to 0.5 to 0.75 cm with posterior margins of ~0.5 cm.

Prostate movement and the margin necessary to compensate for it have been studied in great detail. Ten Haken, et al. (99) reported maximal superior, inferior, anterior, and posterior prostate movement of 1, 1.25, 2, and 0.75 cm, respectively. The overall average movement was 0.5 cm, most often in the anterior and superior direction, while the average left-to-right movement was <0.05 cm. Nevertheless, residual errors in prostate position of over 7 mm after pretreatment localization and adjustment of prostate position clearly demonstrate the influence of intra-treatment movement. In a limited trial using fluoroscopy, Dawson et al. demonstrated breathing-related movement of the prostate, the magnitude of which increased with the amplitude of the breathing cycle (deep breathing vs. shallow) which even varied in the same patients based upon prone or supine positioning with greater movement in those evaluated prone (100). Just as observed by others the magnitude of movement was greatest in the anterior–posterior and cranial-caudal directions while minimal lateral movement was seen (101,102). Using non-IGRT techniques.

Even with IGRT for localization of the prostate at the start of treatment residual errors in position during and at the end of each treatment can occur due to intra-treatment motion of the prostate (99,100). Noel et al. recently evaluated posttreatment prostate position following initial localization at the start of treatment and found poor sensitivity to identify prostate motion unless it was evaluated more than two times a minute (103). Nevertheless, despite this poor ability to detect prostate motion the overall frequency of significant prostate motion may not be high. Li et al. recently evaluated motion in 105 prostate patients treated with electromagnetic localization of the prostate and found displacement of the prostate by more than 3 or 5 mm in 13.4% and 1.8% of treatment fractions for the whole population (104). Some patients, however, may be more susceptible to prostate motion for when they identified the 7 patients with the greatest motion during

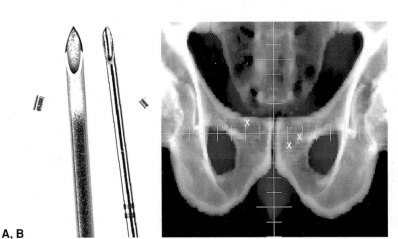

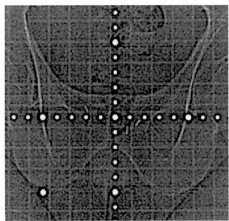

A, B   C

Figure 26.2. Gold fiducial marker seeds (**A**), can be implanted into the prostate. The position of the implanted markers, shown in a digitally reconstructed radiograph (DRR) (**B**), can be used for daily localization of the prostate, shown with the proper alignment of a daily portal image (**C**).

treatment there would have been excursion of more than 3 and 5 mm in 41% and 15% of fractions, respectively (105). The use of electromagnetic transponders (Calypso™ beacons) allows for real-time evaluation of prostate during treatment to account for prostatic motion. Given the above studies, it is likely that this technology does not add significantly to other IGRT methods for the majority of patients. However, in a poorly identified minority it may provide a significant improvement in PTV treatment and sparing of organs at risk (OAR). Using electromagnetic transponders, we have at present used the same PTV margins (0.5 cm in all directions); however, with interruption of treatment if the prostate moves >0.3 cm from isocenter (105,106). Some have suggested that significantly smaller PTV margins may be applied with the use of Calypso beacons(105,107); while others have suggested that rotational effects take a greater role with smaller PTVs and have cautioned for a more conservative approach to PTV margin reduction even with real-time prostate motion evaluation (104). A prospective Phase 2 study did assess PTV margins of 3 mm and suggested that there was a smaller decline in patient reported quality of life at the end of treatment as compared to a historical control group (108), but it remains to be determined if this will translate into any long-term benefits. In addition, it is unclear if this smaller margin was delivered without a decrease in clinical efficacy and if the differences observed were due to the smaller margin size or other differences in either technique or patient characteristics.

Treatment Planning

Once the process of defining the patient positioning and localization have been determined the process of treatment planning can commence. Most centers currently use forward planned, CT-based, 3D-CRT techniques, or inverse-planned IMRT. Although commonly utilized previously the added benefit of rectal, bladder, and/or urethral contrast when using CT-based planning is unclear. If the decision is made to treat the pelvic nodes, the classical superior bony landmarks in the AP view include the bottom of the L5 vertebral body to encompass the common, internal and external iliac nodes, midway through the sacroiliac joints to encompass the distal common, internal and external iliac lymph nodes or the bottom of the sacroiliac joints to encompass the internal and external iliac lymph nodes. The inferior margin is often set 1 cm below the ischial tuberosities inferiorly, and 1.5 to 2 cm to either side of the lateral bony pelvis laterally. In the lateral projection the anterior border is placed at the most anterior point of the pubis symphysis. The posterior border generally falls along the posterior ischium, although the field is usually shaped to bisect the rectum when filled with 20 to 30 mL barium GI contrast, administered via rectal tube. Retrograde urethrography may be performed using a small-gauge catheter to administer 5 to 10 mL of 30% Hypaque into the urethra with immediate penile clamping. The narrow point, or *beak,* in the contrast column

denotes the level where the urethra passes through the urogenital diaphragm (109,110). The most inferior aspect of the prostate gland is typically located 1 cm above the urethral apex, and the inferior field margin is placed 1 cm below the apex or beak, allowing a 2-cm inferior margin on the prostate.

In most practices, CT planning has now largely supplanted the setting of fields using 2D fluoroscopic techniques. CT images facilitate the identification and localization of both target and normal tissue structures (87). Lymph node regions follow the path of the common iliac artery and its bifurcation into the internal and external iliac arteries, and can usually be easily traced even without intravenous contrast administration. Compared with the estimated general localization provided by bony landmarks in 2D planning, the size, shape, and location of the prostate and particularly the seminal vesicles can be visualized and defined more precisely with CT planning. The seminal vesicles drape around the rectum in some patients, and standard blocking in 2D fields set using rectal contrast may not provide adequate coverage of these structures. Identification of the prostate apex on axial CT is sometime difficult and may be facilitated with MRI or with sagittal and coronal reconstruction of CT data sets (111). Normal tissue structures including the rectum, bladder, loops of small bowel, penile bulb, and even important anatomic anomalies such as pelvic or horseshoe kidneys can be readily identified and localized with CT planning.

Fluoroscopic or CT simulation for treatment planning may be performed with the patient either supine or prone, with or without customized immobilization as discussed above. External marks are placed on the patient or immobilization device, often chosen to designate a preliminary isocenter position. These locations may be delineated with radiopaque markers taped to the patient in the x, y, and z axes that can be referenced to the image set, facilitating the transposition of the isocenter from the treatment plan to the patient at the time of treatment. For CT-based planning, CT images are obtained at 1 to 5 mm intervals through the levels to be encompassed within the treatment fields. Target and normal structures can then be defined and expanded to create the relevant PTVs on axial CT images within specialized treatment planning software (Fig. 26.3).

The issues regarding immobilization technique, patient positioning, and image guidance were discussed above. Common choices for immobilization include the Alpha Cradle™, thermoplastic cast material similar to Aquaplast, and "vacuum lock" molds. The CT scan must be done with the patient in the planned treatment position in the immobilization device, with attention toward patient comfort and maximization of daily reproducibility. Alternatively, for ease of position adjustment, some practitioners utilize supine position without an immobilization device if daily prostate localization techniques are employed (see above). An advantage of the prone position is to shift the seminal vesicles forward, away from the

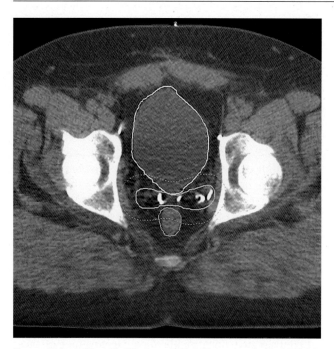

Figure 26.3. A "dumbbell"-shaped clinical target volume (CTV) is outlined to encompass the "prostate bed," between the bladder and rectum to facilitate treatment planning in the adjuvant or salvage situation after radical prostatectomy. Surgical clips are visible and also aid in defining the CTV.

rectum, potentially improving rectal sparing (112). On the other hand, prone positioning may be associated with more internal organ motion, including respiratory motion particularly in men with any degree of obesity (100). Roach et al. advocated nonuniform expansions around the prostate because of the variation in prostate movement depending on direction, the status of rectum and bladder filling as well as radiation tolerance of these two structures (113). The recommendations included anterior and inferior margins of 2 cm, lateral and superior margins of 1.5 cm, a posterior margin of 0.5 to 0.75 cm, and that CT planning be performed with the rectum empty and the bladder full. If bladder fullness is inconsistent from treatment to treatment, superior and inferior margins are more generous and accommodating, and this also helps to keep small bowel out of the field. If the rectum is empty when fields are planned, a rectum that is fuller during treatment only pushes the prostate further into the field, and 2 cm anterior margins should still provide adequate coverage of the CTV. However, with the use of image-guided therapy smaller margins may be appropriate (6).

Treatment Technique

Traditionally, a four-field technique is generally used to treat pelvic lymph nodes: anterior, posterior, right, and left lateral portals. Blocks can be drawn manually on simulation films or BEV digitally reconstructed radiographs (DRRs) from CT planning software. Construction of these blocked fields can be facilitated by reviewing the pelvic CT scan and entering lymph node volumes that track along

the course of the iliac vasculature (Fig. 26.4). Depending on the external contour, which can be done manually or automatically by CT scan, small angle wedges on the lateral fields may help to produce a more symmetrical dose distribution. In addition, IMRT is being utilized with greater frequency to treat pelvic lymph nodes in which case prostate, seminal vesicles, pelvic lymph nodes, and OAR must all be defined for appropriate treatment planning and optimization. Examples of recommended OAR tolerances are provided (Table 26.5) (87).

Two-dimensional planning to treat the prostate and seminal vesicles has classically used three fields (anterior, right, and left lateral fields), four fields (anterior, posterior, right, and left lateral fields), or even two bilateral 120° arc fields. With 2D planning, target volumes tend to be more generous and blocking more conservative to allow for the inaccuracies of manual transposition of PTVs to the simulation plain films. For CT-based planning, CT images are entered into a treatment planning software package. The lymph node regions, prostate, and seminal vesicles are outlined by the physician, and can be expanded by adding appropriate margins to establish the CTVs and PTVs. As noted previously, margins may vary between institutions and individual physicians and by the use of IGRT. Normal structures are also outlined including bladder, rectum, penile bulb, femoral heads, loops of small bowel or any other structures to which the physician may wish to limit dose. Treatment planning software packages allow manipulation of virtual 3D reconstructions of these volumes, allowing a variety of views for the planner, including "beam's eye view" (BEV) perspectives. These features are designed to allow the user to manipulate beam orientation (gantry, table, and collimator angles) and shaping (blocking or multileaf collimation) to encompass targets and avoid normal structures. For forward-planned 3D conformal treatment planning, a combination of beams is devised complete with beam modifiers such as wedges or compensators. High-energy beams such as 10 to 18 MV are customary for pelvic lymph node and prostate irradiation, and the beams should certainly be 6 MV or greater. The software allows rapid calculation of the dose that can be displayed on the overlying images in the form of isodose lines or surfaces (Fig 26.5). Additional tools including dose-volume histograms (DVHs) helps the clinician to compare treatment plans to determine the optimal plan for coverage of target volumes and avoidance of normal tissue structures (Fig. 26.6).

Forward planned 3D CRT beam arrangements for prostate cancer treatment may include the standard axial anterior, posterior, and lateral beams common to 2D prostate plans, but can also easily make use of oblique and nonaxial beam angles. Rotation of the collimator is commonly used to place the orientation of the multi-leaf collimator appropriately so as to maximize normal tissue blocking and target coverage. Segmental fields, physical wedges and dynamic wedge techniques can be used to improve target coverage and dose homogeneity. In addition to the classic

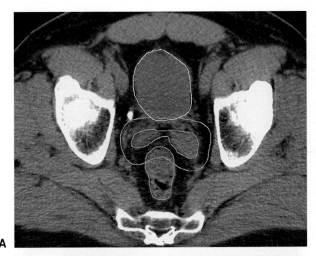

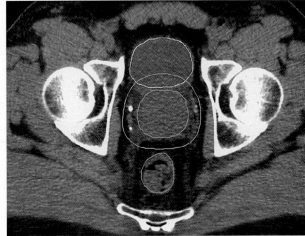

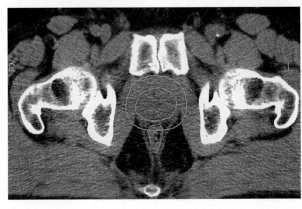

Figure 26.4. Three axial treatment planning computed tomography (CT) images are shown at the levels of the seminal vesicles (**A**), mid-prostate (**B**), and lower-prostate (**C**). The outlined clinical target volume (CTV) encompassing the seminal vesicles and the prostate is shown along with the planning target volume (PTV) expansion around the CTV. The normal bladder and rectum are also contoured.

four-field box technique, 3D CRT beam configurations include a six-field conformal technique (114) as well as a four-field variation using lateral and anterior obliques that eliminate the posterior-oblique beams. Marsh et al. have found that the four-field technique, using laterals and anterior–inferior obliques, often improves the rectal DVH

TABLE 26.5	**Dose Volume Histogram Constraints for Organs at Risk (87)**	
Structure	**Dose**	**Volume**
Rectum	2 data points	
	50 Gy	≤50%
	70 Gy	≤20%
Bladder	2 data points	
	55 Gy	≤50%
	70 Gy	≤30%
Femoral Heads	50 Gy	<5%
Small Bowel	52 Gy	0% at or above
Large Bowel	Same as rectum	
Penile Bulb	No constraints	
Iliac Crests	No constraints	

compared with axial plans (115) (Fig 26.7). This technique requires supine patient positioning to achieve table clearance for the anterior–inferior beams.

The application of IMRT technology to prostate cancer EBRT planning has enabled further improvements in normal tissue DVHs, mainly due to the ability of this technology to achieve convex dose distributions, reducing rectal dose (Fig. 26.8). The clinical significance of this advance toward reducing rectal toxicity remains undetermined although some groups have suggested that with the combination of IGRT and IMRT high dose EBRT can be delivered without increases in toxicity as compared to that observed in historical control groups treated to lower doses with less sophisticated techniques (5). For instance Zelefsky et al. noted an actuarial rate of grade 2 or greater rectal toxicity at 10 years of 13% in patients using 3D CRT and 5% using IMRT ($p < 0.0001$) (116) Of note IMRT patients received higher doses of RT than 3D conformal patients, but IGRT was also used with much greater frequency in the IMRT group as well. The inverse planning process starts with the contouring of target and normal tissue volumes on an axial CT image set—just as for 3D CRT planning. However, instead of inputting a candidate beam arrangement into the planning software and calculating a dose distribution for that plan, the IMRT software package uses an optimization algorithm to find a beam "solution" that maximizes a set of "cost functions." Typically,

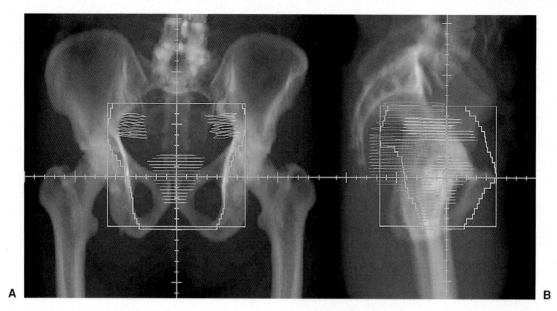

Figure 26.5. Digitally reconstructed radiograph (DRR) images are shown demonstrating typical anterior (**A**) and lateral (**B**) treatment fields encompassing the prostate, seminal vesicles, and regional pelvic nodes.

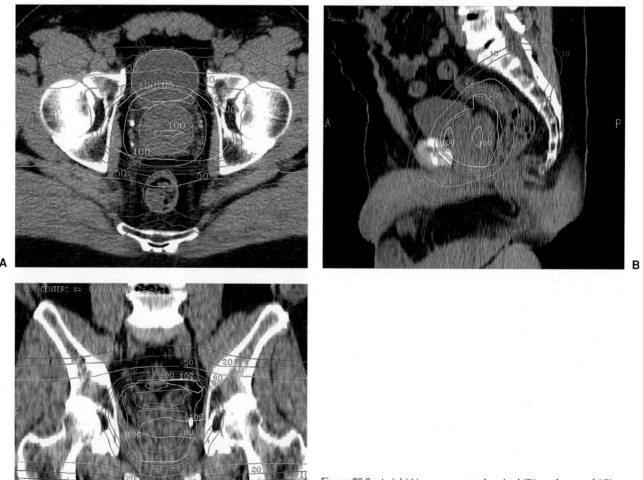

Figure 26.6. Axial (**A**), reconstructed sagittal (**B**), and coronal (**C**) computed tomography (CT) images are shown with contoured normal tissue structures (bladder and rectum) and target volumes (prostate and seminal vesicles). Isodose lines conforming to the planning target volume (PTV) are overlaid, depicting the dose distribution of a three-dimensional (3D) conformal radiation treatment plan.

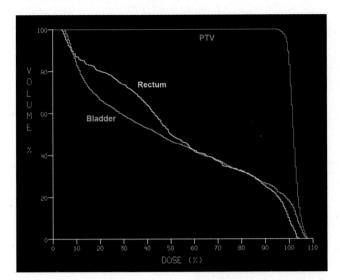

Figure 26.7. A typical dose-volume histogram (DVH) plot is shown for bladder, rectum and planning target volume (PTV) from a three-dimensional (3D) conformal radiation treatment plan.

the process begins with a certain number of axial beam angles for the algorithm to utilize. Each beam is subdivided into square "beamlets" that represent the incremental movement of multileaf collimator leafs across the field in 1 cm or less increments. The algorithm "modulates" the fluence through each of these beamlets in an iterative process, evaluating and comparing each candidate plan to identify a better one. Each plan is evaluated for dose coverage of target volumes, as well as dose avoidance for normal tissue structures. Target coverage and normal tissue structure sparing is prioritized based on clinical judgment, and a cost for achieving or failing to achieve each objective is assigned. The algorithm will iterate until it identifies a plan that best achieves the stated objectives. Once the optimization algorithm produces a plan, a formal dose calculation is performed, and a quality assurance procedure is followed to ensure that the delivered dose will be within a desired level of accuracy. For the prostate, where the target shape and volume are relatively consistent from patient to

patient, a template can be established to make the treatment planning process more efficient. Examples of typical dose constraints for rectum, bladder, femoral heads, and both large and small bowel are given in Table 26.5. The sparing of the penile bulb is controversial as different authors have come to differing conclusions about the utility of sparing the penile bulb in preserving sexual function (117). However, it is clear that if a penile bulb dose constraint is observed that it should not be at the cost of decreasing dose to the PTV. An example of an IMRT plan as well as dose volume histograms for both an IMRT plan and a 3D-CRT plan are given in Figure 26.9.

The sharp dose gradients that can be created using highly conformal techniques such as IMRT create a significant risk of missing the target due to inter- and intra-fraction setup uncertainty and organ motion. Therefore, highly conformal therapy should be combined with IGRT to ensure the accuracy of treatment and to minimize marginal misses due to setup error or changes in prostate position.

Dose and Fractionation

As advances in treatment techniques have allowed more conformal treatment of the target volumes with decreased dose to normal tissues, improved outcomes have been documented with increased doses to the prostate. However, the optimal treatment doses for various risk categories of prostate cancer remain unknown. With traditional 2D treatment techniques, doses of 45 to 50 Gy to the pelvis, 55 to 65 Gy to the seminal vesicles and 65 to 72 Gy to the prostate were typical. With the advent of 3D CRT, IMRT, and other highly conformal techniques, doses have been escalated without significant increases in acute side effects or late complications (118–120). In a landmark trial, the MD Anderson Cancer Center compared 70 to 78 Gy using 3D CRT techniques and found that patients receiving the higher dose had significant improved biochemical failure-free survival, particularly those patients with a pretreatment PSA above 10 ng/mL or with higher-risk clinical features (Table 26.6) (121). Toxicity; however,

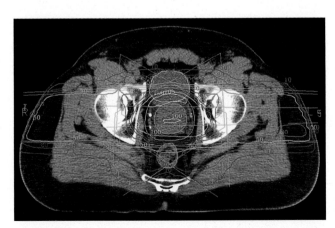

Figure 26.8. An axial computed tomography (CT) image with isodose lines is shown from a three-dimensional (3D) conformal radiation treatment plan utilizing a four-field technique with lateral and anterior inferior oblique beams.

TABLE 26.6	Long-Term Follow-up of the MD Anderson Dose Escalation Trial: Biochemcial Freedom from Recurrence (Phoenix Definition) at 8 Years (121)		
	70 Gy	**78 Gy**	*p*-value
Overall	59%	78%	< 0.004
PSA			
≤10	66%	78%	>0.2
>10	39%	78%	<0.001
Risk Group			
Low	63%	88%	< 0.04
Intermediate	76%	86%	> 0.3
High	26%	63%	< 0.004

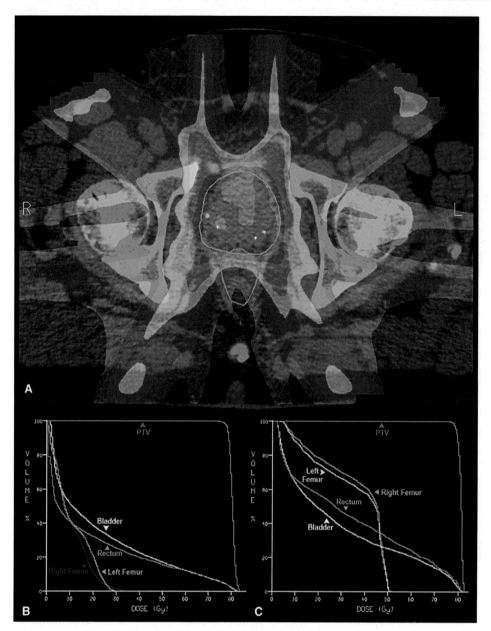

Figure 26.9. An axial computed tomography image is shown from a seven-field intensity modulated radiation therapy (IMRT) plan (**A**). The dose distribution is demonstrated using a dose "color-wash" and depicts the concave dose distribution achieved for the rectum. This results in the improved normal tissue dose volume histogram (DVH) for the IMRT plan (**B**) as compared with a four-field, three-dimensional (3D) conformal treatment plan DVH for the same patient (**C**).

was increased as a function of the volume of rectum treated to higher doses. Another significant randomized trial of dose escalation used a combination of external beam photon radiotherapy with a proton beam boost. Zietman et al. have reported that for mostly low-intermediate risk prostate cancer patients receiving 79.2 Gy had a 15% absolute reduction in the risk of biochemical recurrence at 10-years as compared to those receiving 70.2 Gy (32.4% vs. 16.7%) (2). Given the lack of biologic difference between protons and photons there is no reason to presume that these results are unique to the use of a proton boost. Using this technique, although there was a slight increase in mild acute rectal toxicity, there was no significant difference in clinically substantial toxicity rates or patient reported quality of life (122). These randomized trials as well as others (123,124), combined with

many retrospective studies, give strong evidence that dose escalation above 70 Gy may significantly improve prostate cancer biochemical cure rates. However, at present, dose escalated radiation has not resulted in clear differences in rates of metastasis, prostate cancer-specific death, or overall survival. Encouragingly, when dose-escalation is performed using conformal techniques toxicity rates seem to be acceptable (4,33,124). The potential interaction between dose-escalation and hormonal therapy in terms of disease control and toxicity has not yet been thoroughly explored although both the Dutch and British dose escalation studies included patients with short-term ADT; therefore, it is clear that dose escalation may still provide a benefit even in the setting of ADT use (123,124).

Most treatments have used conventional fraction sizes of 1.8 to 2.0 Gy/day. The use of a smaller number of treatments delivered at a higher daily dose (hypofraction-ation) has been suggested as a means to improve prostate cancer control and decrease overall cost and treatment time, while still achieving acceptable long-term rates of toxicity. Recent reports have supported modest hypofrac-tionation with daily fractions of 2.5 to 3.1 Gy (125–129) as being efficacious without increased risks of toxicity. Nevertheless, the impact of hypofractionation on late tox-icity has not been clearly established at this time and most practitioners await long-term results before adopting these shorter regimens. Evidence supporting this more cautious approach comes from the RTOG 94-08 dose escalation study, which was a sequential phase II trial that evaluated increasing doses between 70 and 79.2 Gy in fractions of 1.8 or 2.0 Gy. Interestingly, the rate of late rectal toxicity was higher in those treated with 78 Gy in daily fractions of 2 Gy than in any of the other arms including those receiving 79.2 Gy in daily fractions of 1.8 Gy (130).

A number of reports have retrospectively analyzed bio-chemical control of prostate cancer using EBRT, LDR, or HDR brachytherapy, or the combination of these modali-ties (131–134). Based on α/β corrections that take into account different radiation fraction sizes, it has been sug-gested that the α/β for prostate cancer is not actually in the range of 10 Gy (as commonly used for most tumor cells) but in the range of 1.2 to 3.0 Gy. If these hypotheses are indeed true then treating prostate cancer with larger frac-tion sizes, but to an appropriate total lower dose would result in an increase in the therapeutic ratio. Thus, by using larger radiation fraction sizes, one might decrease overall treatment dose, time, and cost with a similar rate of late toxicity and an increase in expected biologic effi-cacy for prostate cancer. Extreme hypofractionation with doses in excess of 6 to 7 Gy delivered in four to five frac-tions has been reported from a number of limited single institutions experiences (135–137). At present, however, follow-up on these studies is short and the use of extreme hypofractionation or stereotactic radiotherapy for pros-tate cancer should be considered experimental and is most appropriately utilized as part of prospective clinical trials (138). Larger phase 2 studies evaluating these techniques as well as randomized trials comparing these differing regimens to conventional fractionation schedules are at present on-going.

TREATMENT PLANNING FOR ADJUVANT OR SALVAGE EBRT

Treatment Volumes

There is now compelling evidence showing the benefit of adjuvant radiation therapy (ART) after RP. Nevertheless, the balance between ART as opposed to salvage RT remains to be determined. In addition, the optimal dose and volume for ART or salvage RT is unknown. It is, how-ever, clear from both the EORTC and SWOG ART studies that local failure after RP in patients with high-risk patho-logic features is high occurring at 5 years in as many as 15% to 22% of patients which was decreased to 5% to 8% with the use of early ART (48,139). The randomized trials of ART in general utilized large fields and 2D treatment techniques, therefore, there was not a need to precisely define target volume (47–49). Recently, consensus guide-lines have been published defining recommended ana-tomic boundaries of the CTV for RT delivered in the postoperative setting (140–143). The definition of treat-ment volumes for ART or salvage RT for patients who have undergone previous RP is difficult as there is usually no palpable or visible disease on imaging to constitute a GTV. The vesicourethral anastomosis (VUA), periurethral, and perivesicular tissues should all be treated as these are the most common sites of recurrence following RP (144–146). Some practitioners utilize pelvic or "mini-pelvic" fields, encompassing lymph node regions (as described above). Most typically, however, only residual microscopic disease within the "prostate bed" is targeted with the CTV. This can be accomplished using CT planning, and con-touring an elongated "dumbbell-shaped" volume encom-passing the plane between the posterior bladder and anterior rectum (Fig. 26.3). Surgical clips remaining from prostatectomy as well as preoperative staging and postoperative pathology report information, which may be valuable in constructing the CTV.

The VUA can frequently be identified in relationship to the urinary diaphragm on a CT scan sagittal reconstruc-tion; alternatively, either ultrasound or MRI may aid in this process. Given the prior location of the prostate at the level of the pubic symphysis, the region extending anteri-orly to posteriorly from the pubic symphysis to the rectum should be included in the CTV. The most recent consensus guidelines are only to include the seminal vesicles if they were pathologically involved at the time of the surgical resection. If not including the seminal vesicles the superior border should be either at or 5 mm above the cut of the vas deferens, or alternatively, at the level of the most supe-rior surgical clip. In addition, ~1.5 cm of posterior bladder and bladder wall are also included to account for the shift-ing of the bladder into the space previously occupied by the prostate. The inferior border should be ~10 mm below the VUA; however, if there is concern that the initial pros-tate tumor may have been apical then the inferior border of the CTV should end immediately superior to the penile bulb (141).

TREATMENT TECHNIQUE

Several IGRT methods have been developed to provide consistent localization of the prostate bed and reduce daily setup error, including Calypso™ beacon localiza-tion (147), daily portal imaging with implanted gold seed fiducials (148), ultrasound (149), and daily cone-beam imaging or kilovoltage imaging (150). The use of IGRT in the postoperative setting is not as clearly established as that in the definitive setting although the fundamental principles and rationale remain the same. These techniques are useful in detecting the location of the VUA, which in turn depends on variability in rectal and bladder distention. Similarly, the use of IMRT in the postoperative setting has not been well studied at present. Given the somewhat poorly defined treatment volume that includes a large portion of bladder and rectum as well as the typically utilized RT doses of <70 Gy the benefit of IMRT may be limited. However, use of both IGRT and IMRT may allow dose escalation in the postoperative setting which some have suggested will correlate with improvements in outcome just as it has in the definitive RT setting (151).

RT DOSE

To date, there have been few studies investigating the role of dose escalation in the adjuvant or salvage setting. Valicenti et al. suggested that doses of RT in excess of 64.8 Gy were associated with improved outcomes (152). In addition, Ost et al. reported on the clinical outcome and safety of ART in 104 patients treated with IMRT and median dose of 74 Gy (153). The 3- and 5-year actuarial biochemical relapse-free survival (bRFS) was 93%, a 20% gain as compared to the bRFS rate seen in the randomized trials with doses of 60 to 64 Gy. These results are limited by the study's retrospective nature, the short follow-up, and the impact of stage migration as compared to the randomized ART trials which enrolled patients from the late 1980s to early 1990s. Despite the higher dose, acute and late toxicities were rare, with only 4% of patients experiencing late grade 3 toxicities (all GU). These toxicity results are similar to that reported from a multi-institutional analysis using more conventional doses of radiation (154). It is possible that the use of IMRT allowed dose distributions that partially spared the posterior and lateral rectal walls, thus minimizing late rectal toxicity. King et al. recently evaluated a series of retrospective reviews to assess the impact of RT dose on outcome in the adjuvant and salvage setting (151). The authors found that the dose–response relationships were suggestive of a larger burden of disease for salvage patients with a detectable PSA and approximately one-tenth of this disease burden for adjuvant patients. They estimated an increase in the bRFS rate of ~3%/Gy over the range of 60 to 70 Gy. Of note, this is similar to the 2% to 3% improvement in bEFS observed per 1 Gy increase in radiation in the four randomized trials of dose escalation for definitive radiation of the prostate. At present, however, no prospective trials have directly compared different doses of EBRT in the adjuvant or salvage setting. Therefore, at present most practitioners will utilize RT doses of at least 64.8 Gy in the adjuvant and salvage setting with some considering doses even up to 66 to 70.2 Gy.

TREATMENT PLANNING FOR RADIOISOTOPIC IMPLANT

Target Volume

As discussed previously, candidates for implant must be chosen carefully, since extracapsular areas, seminal vesicles, and pelvic nodes are not treated with implant techniques. Classically, patients with stages T1c, T2a, GS no higher than 6, and PSA no higher than 10 are appropriate candidates for implant alone. Some argue that patients with small T2b tumors, GS of 7, and PSAs up to 15, can be treated with implant alone as well (155). Men with larger, higher-grade tumors with higher PSA levels have a substantial risk of having disease outside the prostate. These patients may be best treated by a combination of external beam and implant or external beam alone. Therefore, just as in planning treatment for external beam therapy, a decision must be made as to whether seminal vesicles and pelvic nodes will be externally irradiated. The target volumes and treatment techniques to encompass these structures are described in the previous section. The prostate gland itself, with minimal margin, is the target for radioisotopic implant. Advances in brachytherapy techniques have made it a popular, effective, and safe treatment for localized prostate cancer; however, for the treating physician, it does require specialized training and experience.

Localization and Treatment Technique

The present era of low-energy permanent radioisotopic implantation for prostate cancer traces its origins to Scardino and Carlton at Baylor College of Medicine in the 1960s and Whitemore and Harris at Memorial Sloan-Kettering Cancer Center in the 1970s, where an open, retropubic approach was used to perform implants using freehand placement of needles containing gold or iodine radioisotopes (156,157). Unfortunately, this technique was associated with inhomogeneous dose distribution, inexact dosimetry, and disappointing local control and disease-free survival, and by the mid-1980s, the retropubic technique was largely abandoned in favor of a transperineal approach (158).

Soon thereafter ultrasonography and a transperineal implant approach using a rigid template guidance system was developed (159). Two ultrasound-based planning approaches are generally used, either a preplan designed with the prostate in treatment position, or an intraoperative plan approach. With the preplanned technique, transverse transrectal ultrasound images are recorded at increments from the base to the apex of the prostate gland using a stepping device attached to the ultrasound probe and the patient in the dorsal lithotomy position. The physician may evaluate the pubic arch during this procedure to determine any potential for bone interference with needle insertion. The ultrasound software projects the template grid over each successive prostate image. Typically, seven to nine images are displayed at 5-mm increments, and the prostate volume is contoured by the physician on each image. The prostate itself or the prostate with a margin of 2 to 5 mm around the prostate may be defined as the PTV. Various software packages can be used for planning of a 3D implant volume, determining the number of needles, their placement according to template coordinates, and the number of seeds inserted per needle, prior to the actual implant.

With intraoperative planning, all these steps are performed in one setting in the operating suite, tailoring the plan to the individual. Without a preplan, there may be a risk of ordering too few or too many seeds; however, the intraoperative planning approach has the significant advantage in that the planning images are of the patient under anesthesia, minimizing discrepancies between the planning images and the actual anatomy and geometry. Furthermore, some treatment planning software packages now allow the users to register the location of sources as they are implanted and recalculate dosimetry in "real-time," allowing further adjustments and refinements to be made in the treatment plan to accommodate inaccuracies in needle placement and intraoperative prostate shift and swelling.

Seeds are usually spaced 0.5 to 1 cm apart in the transverse (right to left), anterior–posterior, and the superior–inferior planes. Computer-generated isodose curves predict the delivered dose, assuming the implant is completed as planned (Fig. 26.10). During the implant process each needle is guided to its predetermined position with the template placed against the perineum by the use of an on-screen template grid system and direct ultrasound

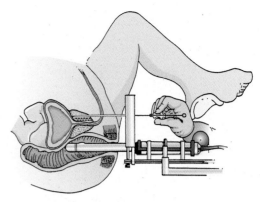

Figure 26.11. Transperineal prostate brachytherapy with transrectal ultrasound visualization and seed placement via needle insertion using template guidance.

visualization (Fig. 26.11). The specified number of radio-active seeds is implanted from the base to the apex of the gland as each needle is withdrawn, using either individual seeds—seeds linked together with custom-assembled spacers—or fixed-space seeds embedded within a polymer strand cut to the desired length. After completion of the seed placement, cystoscopy or fluoroscopy may be utilized to assess for inadvertent seed localization within the bladder or urethra and a Foley catheter may be placed. After anesthesia recovery and proper assessment of exposure rates outside the patient, most patients can safely be released to home and return for subsequent postimplant dosimetry studies.

A postimplant CT scan and dosimetry should be done on each patient to evaluate implant quality, thereby detecting any consistent underdosing or inhomogeneities. The positions of all seeds are identified, the target and normal tissues are contoured (prostate, urethra, bladder, rectum, bowel, penile bulb), and dose distributions are calculated (Fig. 26.12). This allows calculation of various dose–volume metrics, such as the D_{90} and D_{100}, the doses that cover 90% and 100% of the prostate volume respectively, as well as the V_{100}, the volume of the prostate receiving at least 100% of the prescribed dose. The reporting of these metrics is important in the medical literature to enable comparisons between treatment results, and also for individual prostate seed brachytherapy programs to enable ongoing assessment of implant quality and correlation with disease and toxicity outcomes. This enables any necessary adjustments to treatment techniques and procedures. Postimplant bleeding and edema can have significant effects on prostate volume. Given that this is a dynamic process, it can have significant implications for postimplant CT dosimetry. Practitioners may have varying preferences for the time interval between the implant procedure and when to perform postimplant dosimetry imaging, but it is important that implant programs remain consistent in their planning and dosimetry procedures to apply their dosimetry lessons toward quality improvement.

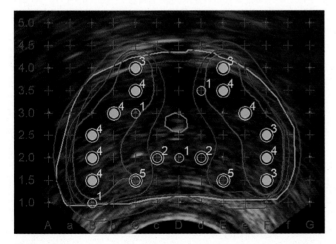

Figure 26.10. A typical preoperative or intraoperative prostate ultrasound is shown with the central urethra, prostate (clinical target volume) and prostate + 2 mm (planning target volume) contours. The loading positions and number of intended I-125 seeds to be implanted in each position are indicated at specific template coordinates, and the 290 Gy, 217.5 Gy, and 145 Gy isodose lines are shown. Courtesy of Dr. Vrinda Narayana.

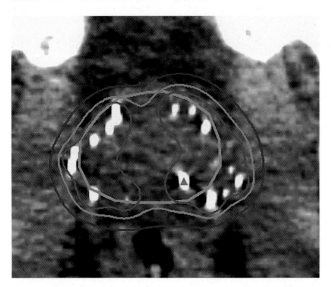

Figure 26.12. An axial computed tomography image is shown in a postimplant patient. Based upon the positions of the seeds and the contour of the prostate clinical and planning target volumes, one can assess the adequacy of the dose distribution, as shown by the overlaid 290, 217.5, and 145 Gray isodose lines. Courtesy of Dr. Vrinda Narayana.

Isotopes and Dose

Several isotopes have been used for prostate LDR—permanent interstitial prostate brachytherapy (Table 26.7). The most extensive experience with permanent interstitial, LDR implants has been with iodine-125 (I-125), which has been used for >40 years. Some radiobiologic evidence raised concerns that the dose-rate of ~8 cGy/h from I-125 was too low for prostate cancer doubling times, so palladium-103 (Pd-103), with a higher dose rate near 20 cGy/h, has been advocated (160). Since the energy of Pd-103 is still low and similar to that of I-125, 21 versus 28 keV, this isotope retains the advantage of delivering a relatively low dose to surrounding organs and minimal exposure to medical personnel. Clinical comparisons between the two isotopes have revealed no significant difference in biochemical control (161,162). More recently, Cesium-131 has been FDA-approved for permanent prostate brachytherapy.

Cs-131 has an energy (29 keV) similar to I-125, but a shorter half-life (9.7 days). Although early experience with this isotope has been positive, the follow-up is short, and there is no data to suggest superiority over I-125 or Pd-103 (163). Although given the shorter half-life of Pd-103 and Cs-131, these two isotopes due appear associated with greater short-term urinary toxicity with the potential to also have earlier resolution of urinary irritative and obstructive symptoms.

The American Association of Physics and Medicine (AAPM) Task Group 43 (TG-43), published in 1995, altered the dose calculation algorithm used for I-125, and its recommendations have been broadly implemented (164). As a result, prescription doses previously described as being 160 Gy have been lowered to 145 Gy as calculated under TG-43 with no change in implant activity, distribution, or geometry. This has consequently divided the prostate brachytherapy dosimetry literature into "pre-TG-43" and "TG-43" eras, an important consideration for clinicians' interpretation of older I-125 publications. Similarly, the dose for Pd-103 implant was 115 Gy before the National Institute of Standards and Technology 1999 Guidelines (NISTG-99) and 125 Gy afterwards (165).

Analysis of matched peripheral dose calculations within the Memorial Sloan-Kettering Cancer Center I-125 implant experience found that the 5-, 10-, and 15-year local relapse-free survival was 78%, 56%, and 30% among patients receiving doses of at least 140 Gy (126 Gy by TG-43), compared with 64%, 38%, and 21% among those receiving <140 Gy (126 Gy by TG-43) (158). Using modern transperineal prostate brachytherapy techniques with CT-based postimplant dosimetry, Stock et al. reported that patients receiving a D_{90} 140 Gy (using TG-43 criteria) had a 92% rate of 4-year biochemical control compared with only 68% for patients receiving a D_{90} < 140 Gy (166). Wallner demonstrated that both dose and volume of normal urethral and rectal tissue are related to toxicity from prostate implants (167). Based on these experiences and others, the American Brachytherapy Society has published guidelines for transperineal permanent brachytherapy for prostate cancer, recommending prescription doses

TABLE 26.7	Isotopes Used for Interstitial Prostate Implant			
Isotope	Implant	T½ days	Time to 90% of dose (days)	Energy (keV)
Iodine-125	LDR	60.0	204	28
Cesium-131	LDR	9.7	33	30
Palladium-103	LDR	17.0	58	21
Iridium-192	HDR	74.0	–	380

of 145 Gy (TG-43) for I-125 and 125 Gy for Pd-103 (after NISTG-99) as monotherapy (168). For combination therapy, an EBRT dose of 40 to 50 Gy should be combined with 100 to 110 Gy (TG-43) I-125 or 90 to 100 Gy (NISTG-99) Pd-103 implantation. For Cs-131, an experienced group of users has developed consensus recommendations for prostate implantation which includes a monotherapy prescription dose of 115 Gy and a boost prescription dose of 85 Gy, with special attention to urethral and rectal dosing (163).

Use of HDR iridium-192 (Ir-192) brachytherapy has become increasingly popular at many centers either as monotherapy or as a boost in combination with EBRT. As with LDR brachytherapy, the HDR technique employs transrectal ultrasound-guided transperineal placement of needles and catheters via a template, which is fixed to the perineum. Real-time, ultrasound-based dose planning software may be utilized. Planning may be accomplished using CT, ultrasound, or MRI images taken with the catheters in place. Targets and normal structures are contoured, and dwell times for source positions can be calculated to optimize delivery of the desired dose to the PTV while minimizing normal tissue dose. The hollow catheters can then be loaded by remote afterloading Ir-192 HDR unit either in single or in multiple insertions. Treatment is hypofractionated, generally using two or more large fractions delivered at dose rates of ~100 Gy/h. This HDR, which approximates that delivered with a linear accelerator during EBRT, is the main theoretical advantage of HDR brachytherapy and may result in a superior radiobiological effect compared with LDR brachytherapy, particularly for disease with adverse risk features (169).

Although several centers (169,170) and multi-institutional experience (171) have been published on HDR brachytherapy, no randomized trials have yet compared outcomes of HDR monotherapy with other primary treatment modalities. The follow-up is still insufficient to establish the role of HDR monotherapy for treatment of men with localized disease. HDR brachytherapy is more commonly utilized as a boost in combination with EBRT. A variety of dose and fractionation schedules have been reported. As one example, the most recent RTOG study for intermediate risk patients prescribed 45 Gy of conventional EBRT followed by an HDR prostate boost dose of 19 Gy given in two 9.5 Gy fractions with a minimum 6 hour interfraction time interval (171).

PROGNOSIS

The likelihood of biochemical, local, and distant failure as well as disease-specific survival after RT for prostate cancer is related to tumor stage, grade, and pretreatment PSA level (24,172–176). As discussed above, additional factors also contribute to long-term prognosis including: radiation dose, the use of adjunctive androgen ablative therapy,

and PSA kinetics. Posttreatment factors such as PSA nadir also have predictive value in estimating biochemical and distant failure (177). Provider experience and treatment volume have also been demonstrated to influence the likelihood of recurrence and the need for salvage hormonal therapy for both brachytherapy (178) and external beam radiation (117).

At a recent RTOG symposium in Phoenix, numerous candidate definitions of biochemical failure were evaluated, and a definition was endorsed of the posttreatment nadir PSA plus 2 ng/mL as being the threshold for defining clinically meaningful biochemical failure after primary EBRT for prostate cancer (179). The Phoenix definition was initially only defined for those receiving EBRT or brachytherapy with at most short-term androgen therapy (179,180). However, others have suggested that it is applicable to those treated with EBRT along with long-term ADT (181). Biochemical failure by the Phoenix definition has been demonstrated to correlate with patient survival although the risk of death from prostate cancer following biochemical failure is dependent upon both the clinical features of the cancer as well as patient age (182,183), and as a result it is not a reasonable surrogate for patient survival in most patients. Following biochemical failure patient risk group, the time to PSA failure (184,185) and the PSA kinetics during failure may help further elucidate those patients at high risk of distant metastasis and prostate cancer-specific mortality (185,186).

Long-term follow-up of the MD Anderson randomized trial of 70 versus 78 Gy (without ADT) revealed 8-year freedom from biochemical failure using the Phoenix definition of 88%, 86%, and 63% for low, intermediate, and high-risk prostate cancer, respectively (Table 26.7) (121). Radiation dose did appear to predict for improved outcome as well with freedom from biochemical or clinical failure at 8 years greater in the 78 Gy arm as compared to the 70 Gy arm (78% vs. 59%, $p = 0.004$). Distant metastasis had only been observed in a small number of patients; however, freedom from distant metastasis after 70 Gy versus 78 Gy was 95% versus 99% with a trend toward statistical significance ($p < 0.06$). The difference in metastasis as a function of radiation dose was greater in those in the high-risk group (83% vs. 96%, $p < 0.04$). With a median of 8 years of follow-up there were few deaths due to prostate cancer, as a result to date there was no difference in either prostate cancer-specific or overall survival (121).

Brachytherapy outcomes have also improved significantly with enhanced techniques, and multi-institutional and randomized trial data are now becoming available in the literature which should provide more generalizable experiences as opposed to single-institutional case series which are more prone to selection, individual practitioner experience/technique, and other biases. RTOG 98-05 examined LDR monotherapy for patients with low-risk prostate cancer treated at 27 different institutions with I-125 LDR monotherapy to 145 Gy (59). At 5 years, the biochemical failure-free survival rates exceeded 90%, which was comparable with other published brachytherapy series and with surgical or EBRT outcomes. Recently, a small Italian randomized trial comparing RP with LDR brachytherapy for low-risk patients showed no differences in 5-year bRFS rates between these two treatment modalities (187). Brachytherapy patients were noted to have persistent increased genitourinary irritative side effects, but superior urinary continence and erectile function compared with RP patients. RTOG study 00-19 examined combined EBRT with LDR brachytherapy boost for patients with intermediate risk features treated at over 20 different institutions (188). Treatment was delivered with combined conventionally fractionated 3D conformal EBRT to 45 Gy with LDR brachytherapy boost 2 to 6 weeks later to 108 Gy. At 4 years, biochemical recurrence rates were 14% to 19%, comparable with results achieved with dose-escalated EBRT. However, incidence of grade 3 or higher genitourinary or gastrointestinal toxicity was 15%, higher than that observed in contemporary studies of patients treated with brachytherapy or EBRT alone. RTOG study 03-21 examined combined EBRT with HDR brachytherapy boost for patients with a slightly higher intermediate risk group of patients (171). Treatment was delivered with EBRT to 45 Gy and two 9.5 Gy HDR boost fractions (total 19 Gy boost) within an overall treatment time of <8 weeks. At 29 months, the estimated rate of grade 3 through 5 genitourinary and gastrointestinal adverse events was 2.4%, demonstrating the feasibility of EBRT/HDR treatment in the multi-institutional setting and an acceptable level of adverse events. Finally, a prospective (but not randomized) study for intermediate to high-risk patients utilized ~9 months ADT with either 76 Gy EBRT as compared to 45 Gy EBRT with 18 Gy HDR boost given in two fractions and demonstrated a small but not statistically significant difference in 5-year bRFS between treatment arms, but lower rates of late grade 2 rectal toxicity in the HDR-treated patients (13% vs. 3%, $p < 0.005$) (189).

CONCLUSION

Significant advances have been made in the treatment of prostate cancer with RT over the last 10 years that have resulted in improvements in disease control with decreased risks of toxicity and series adverse impacts upon long-term patient quality of life. However, these advances have depended upon closer detail to the process of planning and delivery of RT to the prostate. The optimal selection of radiation modalities either alone or in combination and the timing and duration of ADT in this setting remain to be established. Nevertheless, the results to data suggest that RT is an attractive and viable treatment option for men with prostate cancer.

REFERENCES

1. Jemal A, Siegel R, Xu J, et al. Cancer statistics, 2010. *CA Cancer J Clin* 2010;60:277–300.
2. Zietman AL, Bae K, Slater JD, et al. Randomized trial comparing conventional-dose with high-dose conformal radiation therapy in early-stage adenocarcinoma of the prostate: long-term results from proton radiation oncology group/American college of radiology 95–09. *J Clin Oncol* 2010;28:1106–1111.
3. Kuban DA, Levy LB, Cheung MR, et al. Long-term failure patterns and survival in a randomized dose-escalation trial for prostate cancer. Who dies of disease? *Int J Radiat Oncol Biol Phys* 2011;79(5):1310–1317.
4. Talcott JA, Rossi C, Shipley WU, et al. Patient-reported long-term outcomes after conventional and high-dose combined proton and photon radiation for early prostate cancer. *JAMA* 2010;303:1046–1053.
5. Cahlon O, Hunt M, Zelefsky MJ. Intensity-modulated radiation therapy: supportive data for prostate cancer. *Semin Radiat Oncol* 2008;18:48–57.
6. Kupelian PA, Langen KM, Willoughby TR, et al. Image-guided radiotherapy for localized prostate cancer: treating a moving target. *Semin Radiat Oncol* 2008;18:58–66.
7. Edge SB, Byrd DR, Compton CC, et al. *AJCC cancer staging manual*, 7th ed. New York, NY: Springer, 2010.
8. Hricak H, Dooms GC, Jeffrey RB, et al. Prostatic carcinoma: staging by clinical assessment, CT, and MR imaging. *Radiology* 1987;162:331–336.
9. Lee N, Newhouse JH, Olsson CA, et al. Which patients with newly diagnosed prostate cancer need a computed tomography scan of the abdomen and pelvis? An analysis based on 588 patients. *Urology* 1999;54:490–494.
10. Van Poppel H, Ameye F, Oyen R, et al. Accuracy of combined computerized tomography and fine needle aspiration cytology in lymph node staging of localized prostatic carcinoma. *J Urol* 1994;151:1310–1314.
11. Partin AW, Kattan MW, Subong EN, et al. Combination of prostate-specific antigen, clinical stage, and Gleason score to predict pathological stage of localized prostate cancer. A multi-institutional update. *JAMA* 1997;277:1445–1451.
12. Rifkin MD, Zerhouni EA, Gatsonis CA, et al. Comparison of magnetic resonance imaging and ultrasonography in staging early prostate cancer. Results of a multi-institutional cooperative trial. *N Engl J Med* 1990;323:621–626.
13. D'Amico AV, Schnall M, Whittington R, et al. Endorectal coil magnetic resonance imaging identifies locally advanced prostate cancer in select patients with clinically localized disease. *Urology* 1998;51:449–454.
14. Gibbs P, Pickles MD, Turnbull LW. Diffusion imaging of the prostate at 3.0 tesla. *Invest Radiol* 2006;41:185–188.
15. Lee N, Fawaaz R, Olsson CA, et al. Which patients with newly diagnosed prostate cancer need a radionuclide bone scan? An analysis based on 631 patients. *Int J Radiat Oncol Biol Phys* 2000;48:1443–1446.
16. Gleason DF, Mellinger GT. Prediction of prognosis for prostatic adenocarcinoma by combined histological grading and clinical staging. *J Urol* 1974;111:58–64.

17. Chism DB, Hanlon AL, Troncoso P, et al. The Gleason score shift: score four and seven years ago. *Int J Radiat Oncol Biol Phys* 2003;56:1241–1247.

18. Eisenberg ML, Davies BJ, Cooperberg MR, et al. Prognostic implications of an undetectable ultrasensitive prostate-specific antigen level after radical prostatectomy. *Eur Urol* 2010;57(4):622–629.

19. Prostate Cancer, 2010. Available from http://www.nccn.org/professionals/physician_gls/PDF/prostate.pdf. Accessed 4/1/2010.

20. Chism DB, Hanlon AL, Horwitz EM, et al. A comparison of the single and double factor high-risk models for risk assignment of prostate cancer treated with 3D conformal radiotherapy. *Int J Radiat Oncol Biol Phys* 2004;59:380–385.

21. Nguyen PL, Chen MH, Catalona WJ, et al. Predicting prostate cancer mortality among men with intermediate to high-risk disease and multiple unfavorable risk factors. *Int J Radiat Oncol Biol Phys* 2009;73:659–664.

22. Partin AW, Mangold LA, Lamm DM, et al. Contemporary update of prostate cancer staging nomograms (Partin Tables) for the new millennium. *Urology* 2001;58:843–848.

23. Kattan MW, Eastham JA, Stapleton AM, et al. A preoperative nomogram for disease recurrence following radical prostatectomy for prostate cancer. *J Natl Cancer Inst* 1998;90:766–771.

24. Kattan MW, Zelefsky MJ, Kupelian PA, et al. Pretreatment nomogram for predicting the outcome of three-dimensional conformal radiotherapy in prostate cancer. *J Clin Oncol* 2000;18:3352–3359.

25. Lin GA, Aaronson DS, Knight SJ, et al. Patient decision aids for prostate cancer treatment: a systematic review of the literature. *CA Cancer J Clin* 2009;59:379–390.

26. Bill-Axelson A, Holmberg L, Filen F, et al. Radical prostatectomy versus watchful waiting in localized prostate cancer: the Scandinavian prostate cancer group-4 randomized trial. *J Natl Cancer Inst* 2008;100:1144–1154.

27. Lu-Yao GL, Albertsen PC, Moore DF, et al. Outcomes of localized prostate cancer following conservative management. *JAMA* 2009;302:1202–1209.

28. Klotz L, Zhang L, Lam A, et al. Clinical results of long-term follow-up of a large, active surveillance cohort with localized prostate cancer. *J Clin Oncol* 2010;28:126–131.

29. Trabulsi EJ, Guillonneau B. Laparoscopic radical prostatectomy. *J Urol* 2005;173:1072–1079.

30. Hu JC, Wang Q, Pashos CL, et al. Utilization and outcomes of minimally invasive radical prostatectomy. *J Clin Oncol* 2008;26:2278–2284.

31. Vickers AJ, Savage CJ, Hruza M, et al. The surgical learning curve for laparoscopic radical prostatectomy: a retrospective cohort study. *Lancet Oncol* 2009;10:475–480.

32. Stanford JL, Feng Z, Hamilton AS, et al. Urinary and sexual function after radical prostatectomy for clinically localized prostate cancer: the Prostate Cancer Outcomes Study. *JAMA* 2000;283:354–360.

33. Sanda MG, Dunn RL, Michalski J, et al. Quality of life and satisfaction with outcome among prostate-cancer survivors. *N Engl J Med* 2008;358:1250–1261.

34. Talcott JA, Rieker P, Propert KJ, et al. Patient-reported impotence and incontinence after nerve-sparing radical prostatectomy. *J Natl Cancer Inst* 1997;89:1117–1123.

35. Malcolm JB, Fabrizio MD, Barone BB, et al. Quality of life after open or robotic prostatectomy, cryoablation or brachytherapy for localized prostate cancer. *J Urol* 2010;183:1822–1828.

36. D'Amico AV, Whittington R, Malkowicz SB, et al. Biochemical outcome after radical prostatectomy, external beam radiation therapy, or interstitial radiation therapy for clinically localized prostate cancer. *JAMA* 1998;280:969–974.

37. Yossepowitch O, Eggener SE, Serio AM, et al. Secondary therapy, metastatic progression, and cancer-specific mortality in men with clinically high-risk prostate cancer treated with radical prostatectomy. *Eur Urol* 2008;53:950–959.

38. Bolla M, Gonzalez D, Warde P, et al. Improved survival in patients with locally advanced prostate cancer treated with radiotherapy and goserelin. *N Engl J Med* 1997;337:295–300.

39. Pilepich MV, Winter K, John MJ, et al. Phase III radiation therapy oncology group (RTOG) trial 86–10 of androgen deprivation adjuvant to definitive radiotherapy in locally advanced carcinoma of the prostate. *Int J Radiat Oncol Biol Phys* 2001;50:1243–1252.

40. Hanks GE, Pajak TF, Porter A, et al. Phase III trial of long-term adjuvant androgen deprivation after neoadjuvant hormonal cytoreduction and radiotherapy in locally advanced carcinoma of the prostate: the Radiation Therapy Oncology Group Protocol 92–02. *J Clin Oncol* 2003;21:3972–3978.

41. Lawton CA, Winter K, Grignon D, et al. Androgen suppression plus radiation versus radiation alone for patients with stage D1/pathologic node-positive adenocarcinoma of the prostate: updated results based on national prospective randomized trial Radiation Therapy Oncology Group 85–31. *J Clin Oncol* 2005;23:800–807.

42. Bolla M, de Reijke TM, Van Tienhoven G, et al. Duration of androgen suppression in the treatment of prostate cancer. *N Engl J Med* 2009;360:2516–2527.

43. Widmark A, Klepp O, Solberg A, et al. Endocrine treatment, with or without radiotherapy, in locally advanced prostate cancer (SPCG-7/SFUO-3): an open randomised phase III trial. *Lancet* 2009;373:301–308.

44. D'Amico AV, Chen MH, Renshaw AA, et al. Androgen suppression and radiation vs. radiation alone for prostate cancer: a randomized trial. *JAMA* 2008;299:289–295.

45. McGowan DG, Hunt D, Jones CU, et al. Short-term endocrine therapy prior to and during radiation therapy improves overall survival in patients with T1b-T2b adenocarcinoma of the prostate and PSA < 20: initial results of RTOG 94–08. In: ASTRO 2009 Annual Meeting, November 1–5, 2009, Chicago, IL, 2009.

46. Thompson IM Jr, Tangen CM, Paradelo J, et al. Adjuvant radiotherapy for pathologically advanced prostate cancer: a randomized clinical trial. *JAMA* 2006;296:2329–2335.

47. Thompson IM, Tangen CM, Paradelo J, et al. Adjuvant radiotherapy for pathological T3N0M0 prostate cancer significantly reduces risk of metastases and improves survival: long-term followup of a randomized clinical trial. *J Urol* 2009;181:956–962.

48. Bolla M, van Poppel H, Collette L, et al. Postoperative radiotherapy after radical prostatectomy: a randomised controlled trial (EORTC trial 22911). *Lancet* 2005;366:572–578.

49. Wiegel T, Bottke D, Steiner U, et al. Phase III postoperative adjuvant radiotherapy after radical prostatectomy compared with radical prostatectomy alone in pT3 prostate cancer with postoperative undetectable prostate-specific antigen: ARO 96–02/AUO AP 09/95. *J Clin Oncol* 2009;27:2924–2930.

50. Stephenson AJ, Scardino PT, Kattan MW, et al. Predicting the outcome of salvage radiation therapy for recurrent prostate cancer after radical prostatectomy. *J Clin Oncol* 2007;25:2035–2041.

51. Stephenson AJ, Shariat SF, Zelefsky MJ, et al. Salvage radiotherapy for recurrent prostate cancer after radical prostatectomy. *JAMA* 2004;291:1325–1332.

52. Trock BJ, Han M, Freedland SJ, et al. Prostate cancer-specific survival following salvage radiotherapy vs. observation in men with biochemical recurrence after radical prostatectomy. *JAMA* 2008;299:2760–2769.

53. Trabulsi EJ, Valicenti RK, Hanlon AL, et al. A multi-institutional matched-control analysis of adjuvant and salvage postoperative radiation therapy for pT3–4N0 prostate cancer. *Urology* 2008;72:1298–1302; discussion 302–304.

54. Cozzarini C, Bolognesi A, Ceresoli GL, et al. Role of postoperative radiotherapy after pelvic lymphadenectomy and radical retropubic prostatectomy: a single institute experience of 415 patients. *Int J Radiat Oncol Biol Phys* 2004;59:674–683.

55. King CR, Presti JC Jr, Gill H, et al. Radiotherapy after radical prostatectomy: does transient androgen suppression improve outcomes? *Int J Radiat Oncol Biol Phys* 2004;59:341–347.

56. Parker C, Sydes MR, Catton C, et al. Radiotherapy and androgen deprivation in combination after local surgery (RADICALS): a new Medical Research Council/National Cancer Institute of Canada phase III trial of adjuvant treatment after radical prostatectomy. *BJU Int* 2007;99:1376–1379.

57. Zelefsky MJ, Kuban DA, Levy LB, et al. Multi-institutional analysis of long-term outcome for stages T1-T2 prostate cancer treated with permanent seed implantation. *Int J Radiat Oncol Biol Phys* 2007;67:327–333.

58. Shapiro EY, Rais-Bahrami S, Morgenstern C, et al. Long-term outcomes in younger men following permanent prostate brachytherapy. *J Urol* 2009;181:1665–1671; discussion 71.

59. Lawton CA, DeSilvio M, Lee WR, et al. Results of a phase II trial of transrectal ultrasound-guided permanent radioactive implantation of the prostate for definitive management of localized adenocarcinoma of the prostate (radiation therapy oncology group 98–05). *Int J Radiat Oncol Biol Phys* 2007;67:39–47.

60. Zelefsky MJ, Nedelka MA, Arican ZL, et al. Combined brachytherapy with external beam radiotherapy for localized prostate cancer: reduced morbidity with an intraoperative brachytherapy planning technique and supplemental intensity-modulated radiation therapy. *Brachytherapy* 2008;7:1–6.

61. Burri RJ, Stone NN, Unger P, et al. Long-term outcome and toxicity of salvage brachytherapy for local failure after initial radiotherapy for prostate cancer. *Int J Radiat Oncol Biol Phys* 2010;77(5):1338–1344.

62. Nguyen PL, Chen RC, Clark JA, et al. Patient-reported quality of life after salvage brachytherapy for radio-recurrent prostate cancer: a prospective Phase II study. *Brachytherapy* 2009;8:345–352.

63. Jabbari S, Hsu IC, Kawakami J, et al. High-dose-rate brachytherapy for localized prostate adenocarcinoma post abdominoperineal resection of the rectum and pelvic irradiation: technique and experience. *Brachytherapy* 2009;8:339–344.

64. Tharp M, Hardacre M, Bennett R, et al. Prostate high-dose-rate brachytherapy as salvage treatment of local failure after previous external or permanent seed irradiation for prostate cancer. *Brachytherapy* 2008;7:231–236.

65. Lee HK, Adams MT, Motta J. Salvage prostate brachytherapy for localized prostate cancer failure after external beam radiation therapy. *Brachytherapy* 2008;7:17–21.

66. Donnelly BJ, Saliken JC, Brasher PM, et al. A randomized trial of external beam radiotherapy versus cryoablation in patients with localized prostate cancer. *Cancer* 2010;116:323–330.

67. Robinson JW, Donnelly BJ, Siever JE, et al. A randomized trial of external beam radiotherapy versus cryoablation in patients with localized prostate cancer: quality of life outcomes. *Cancer* 2009;115:4695–4704.

68. Pollack A, Zagars GK, Smith LG, et al. Preliminary results of a randomized radiotherapy dose-escalation study comparing 70 Gy with 78 Gy for prostate cancer. *J Clin Oncol* 2000;18:3904–3911.

69. Zietman AL, DeSilvio ML, Slater JD, et al. Comparison of conventional-dose vs. high-dose conformal radiation therapy in clinically localized adenocarcinoma of the prostate: a randomized controlled trial. *JAMA* 2005;294:1233–1239.

70. Lawton CA, DeSilvio M, Roach M 3rd, et al. An update of the phase III trial comparing whole pelvic to prostate only radiotherapy and neoadjuvant to adjuvant total androgen suppression: updated analysis of RTOG 94–13, with emphasis on unexpected hormone/radiation interactions. *Int J Radiat Oncol Biol Phys* 2007;69:646–655.

71. de la Taille A, Hayek O, Benson MC, et al. Salvage cryotherapy for recurrent prostate cancer after radiation therapy: the Columbia experience. *Urology* 2000;55:79–84.

72. Petrylak DP, Tangen CM, Hussain MH, et al. Docetaxel and estramustine compared with mitoxantrone and prednisone for advanced refractory prostate cancer. *N Engl J Med* 2004;351:1513–1520.

73. Tannock IF, de Wit R, Berry WR, et al. Docetaxel plus prednisone or mitoxantrone plus prednisone for advanced prostate cancer. *N Engl J Med* 2004;351:1502–1512.

74. Attard G, Reid AH, A'Hern R, et al. Selective inhibition of CYP17 with abiraterone acetate is highly active in the treatment of castration-resistant prostate cancer. *J Clin Oncol* 2009;27:3742–3748.

75. Attard G, Reid AH, Yap TA, et al. Phase I clinical trial of a selective inhibitor of CYP17, abiraterone acetate, confirms that castration-resistant prostate cancer commonly remains hormone driven. *J Clin Oncol* 2008;26: 4563–4571.

76. Tran C, Ouk S, Clegg NJ, et al. Development of a second-generation antiandrogen for treatment of advanced prostate cancer. *Science* (New York, NY) 2009;324:787–790.

77. McLaughlin PW, Troyer S, Berri S, et al. Functional anatomy of the prostate: implications for treatment planning. *Int J Radiat Oncol Biol Phys* 2005;63: 479–491.

78. Wang D, Lawton C. Pelvic lymph node irradiation for prostate cancer: who, why, and when? *Semin Radiat Oncol* 2008;18:35–40.

79. Roach M 3rd, DeSilvio M, Lawton C, et al. Phase III trial comparing whole-pelvic versus prostate-only radiotherapy and neoadjuvant versus adjuvant combined androgen suppression: radiation Therapy Oncology Group 9413. *J Clin Oncol* 2003;21:1904–1911.

80. Roach M 3rd, DeSilvio M, Valicenti R, et al. Whole-pelvis, "mini-pelvis," or prostate-only external beam radiotherapy after neoadjuvant and concurrent hormonal therapy in patients treated in the Radiation Therapy Oncology Group 9413 trial. *Int J Radiat Oncol Biol Phys* 2006;66:647–653.

81. Pommier P, Chabaud S, Lagrange JL, et al. Is there a role for pelvic irradiation in localized prostate adenocarcinoma? Preliminary results of GETUG-01. *J Clin Oncol* 2007;25:5366–5373.

82. Asbell SO, Krall JM, Pilepich MV, et al. Elective pelvic irradiation in stage A2, B carcinoma of the prostate: analysis of RTOG 77-06. *Int J Radiat Oncol Biol Phys* 1988;15:1307–1316.

83. Mukamel E, deKernion JB, Hannah J, et al. The incidence and significance of seminal vesicle invasion in patients with adenocarcinoma of the prostate. *Cancer* 1987;59:1535–1538.

84. Diaz A, Roach M 3rd, Marquez C, et al. Indications for and the significance of seminal vesicle irradiation during 3D conformal radiotherapy for localized prostate cancer. *Int J Radiat Oncol Biol Phys* 1994;30:323–329.

85. Kestin L, Goldstein N, Vicini F, et al. Treatment of prostate cancer with radiotherapy: should the entire seminal vesicles be included in the clinical target volume? *Int J Radiat Oncol Biol Phys* 2002;54:686–697.

86. Lawton CA, Michalski J, El-Naqa I, et al. Variation in the definition of clinical target volumes for pelvic nodal conformal radiation therapy for prostate cancer. *Int J Radiat Oncol Biol Phys* 2009;74:377–382.

87. Lawton CA, Michalski J, El-Naqa I, et al. RTOG GU Radiation oncology specialists reach consensus on pelvic lymph node volumes for high-risk prostate cancer. *Int J Radiat Oncol Biol Phys* 2009;74:383–387.

88. Intenational Commission on Radiation Units and Measurements. *Definitions of terms and concepts. Report 50: prescribing, recording, and reporting radiation therapy.* Bethesda, MD: ICRU, 1993.

89. Rosenthal SA, Roach M 3rd, Goldsmith BJ, et al. Immobilization improves the reproducibility of patient positioning during six-field conformal radiation therapy for prostate carcinoma. *Int J Radiat Oncol Biol Phys* 1993;27:921–926.

90. Kneebone A, Gebski V, Hogendoorn N, et al. A randomized trial evaluating rigid immobilization for pelvic irradiation. *Int J Radiat Oncol Biol Phys* 2003;56:1105–1111.

91. Malone S, Szanto J, Perry G, et al. A prospective comparison of three systems of patient immobilization for prostate radiotherapy. *Int J Radiat Oncol Biol Phys* 2000;48:657–665.

92. Wachter S, Gerstner N, Dorner D, et al. The influence of a rectal balloon tube as internal immobilization device on variations of volumes and dose-volume histograms during treatment course of conformal radiotherapy for prostate cancer. *Int J Radiat Oncol Biol Phys* 2002;52:91–100.

93. Lattanzi J, McNeely S, Hanlon A, et al. Daily CT localization for correcting portal errors in the treatment of prostate cancer. *Int J Radiat Oncol Biol Phys* 1998;41:1079–1086.

94. Lattanzi J, McNeeley S, Pinover W, et al. A comparison of daily CT localization to a daily ultrasound-based system in prostate cancer. *Int J Radiat Oncol Biol Phys* 1999;43:719–725.

95. Sandler HM, Bree RL, McLaughlin PW, et al. Localization of the prostatic apex for radiation therapy using implanted markers. *Int J Radiat Oncol Biol Phys* 1993;27:915–919.

96. Vigneault E, Pouliot J, Laverdiere J, et al. Electronic portal imaging device detection of radioopaque markers for the evaluation of prostate position during megavoltage irradiation: a clinical study. *Int J Radiat Oncol Biol Phys* 1997;37:205–212.

97. Litzenberg DW, Willoughby TR, Balter JM, et al. Positional stability of electromagnetic transponders used for prostate localization and continuous, real-time tracking. *Int J Radiat Oncol Biol Phys* 2007;68:1199–1206.

98. Willoughby TR, Kupelian PA, Pouliot J, et al. Target localization and real-time tracking using the Calypso 4D localization system in patients with localized prostate cancer. *Int J Radiat Oncol Biol Phys* 2006;65:528–534.

99. Ten Haken RK, Forman JD, Heimburger DK, et al. Treatment planning issues related to prostate movement in response to differential filling of the rectum and bladder. *Int J Radiat Oncol Biol Phys* 1991;20:1317–1324.

100. Dawson LA, Litzenberg DW, Brock KK, et al. A comparison of ventilatory prostate movement in four treatment positions. *Int J Radiat Oncol Biol Phys* 2000;48:319–323.

101. Litzenberg D, Dawson LA, Sandler H, et al. Daily prostate targeting using implanted radiopaque markers. *Int J Radiat Oncol Biol Phys* 2002;52:699–703.

102. Bayley AJ, Catton CN, Haycocks T, et al. A randomized trial of supine vs. prone positioning in patients undergoing escalated dose conformal radiotherapy for prostate cancer. *Radiother Oncol* 2004;70:37–44.

103. Noel C, Parikh PJ, Roy M, et al. Prediction of intrafraction prostate motion: accuracy of pre- and posttreatment imaging and intermittent imaging. *Int J Radiat Oncol Biol Phys* 2009;73(3):692–698.

104. Li JS, Jin L, Pollack A, et al. Gains from real-time tracking of prostate motion during external beam radiation therapy. *Int J Radiat Oncol Biol Phys* 2009;75:1613–1620.

105. Litzenberg DW, Balter JM, Hadley SW, et al. Influence of intrafraction motion on margins for prostate radiotherapy. *Int J Radiat Oncol Biol Phys* 2006;65:548–553.

106. Malinowski KT, Noel C, Roy M, et al. Efficient use of continuous, real-time prostate localization. *Phys Med Biol* 2008;53:4959–4970.

107. Li HS, Chetty IJ, Enke CA, et al. Dosimetric consequences of intrafraction prostate motion. *Int J Radiat Oncol Biol Phys* 2008;71:801–812.

108. Sandler HM, Liu PY, Dunn RL, et al. Reduction in patient-reported acute morbidity in prostate cancer patients treated with 81-Gy Intensity-modulated radiotherapy using reduced planning target volume margins and electromagnetic tracking: assessing the impact of margin reduction study. *Urology* 2010;75(5):1004–1008.

109. Roach M 3rd, Pickett B, Holland J, et al. The role of the urethrogram during simulation for localized prostate cancer. *Int J Radiat Oncol Biol Phys* 1993;25:299–307.

110. Schild SE, Wong W. The role of retrograde urethrography in the planning of prostate cancer radiotherapy. *Med Dosim* 1997;22:83–86.

111. McLaughlin PW, Evans C, Feng M, et al. Radiographic and anatomic basis for prostate contouring errors and methods to improve prostate contouring accuracy. *Int J Radiat Oncol Biol Phys;*76:369–378.

112. Zelefsky MJ, Happersett L, Leibel SA, et al. The effect of treatment positioning on normal tissue dose in patients with prostate cancer treated with three-dimensional conformal radiotherapy. *Int J Radiat Oncol Biol Phys* 1997;37:13–19.

113. Roach M 3rd, Pickett B, Rosenthal SA, et al. Defining treatment margins for six field conformal irradiation of localized prostate cancer. *Int J Radiat Oncol Biol Phys* 1994;28:267–275.

114. Ten Haken RK, Perez-Tamayo C, Tesser RJ, et al. Boost treatment of the prostate using shaped, fixed fields. *Int J Radiat Oncol Biol Phys* 1989;16:193–200.

115. Marsh LH, Ten Haken RK, Sandler HM. A customized non-axial external beam technique for treatment of prostate carcinomas. *Med Dosim* 1992;17:123–127.

116. Zelefsky MJ, Levin EJ, Hunt M, et al. Incidence of late rectal and urinary toxicities after three-dimensional conformal radiotherapy and intensity-modulated radiotherapy for localized prostate cancer. *Int J Radiat Oncol Biol Phys* 2008;70:1124–1129.

117. Roach M 3rd, Nam J, Gagliardi G, et al. Radiation dose-volume effects and the penile bulb. *Int J Radiat Oncol Biol Phys;*76:S130–S134.

118. Dearnaley DP, Khoo VS, Norman AR, et al. Comparison of radiation side-effects of conformal and conventional radiotherapy in prostate cancer: a randomised trial. *Lancet* 1999;353:267–272.

119. Sandler HM, McLaughlin PW, Ten Haken RK, et al. Three dimensional conformal radiotherapy for the treatment of prostate cancer: low risk of chronic rectal morbidity observed in a large series of patients. *Int J Radiat Oncol Biol Phys* 1995;33:797–801.

120. Ryu JK, Winter K, Michalski JM, et al. Interim report of toxicity from 3D conformal radiation therapy (3D-CRT) for prostate cancer on 3DOG/RTOG 9406, level III (79.2 Gy). *Int J Radiat Oncol Biol Phys* 2002;54:1036–1046.

121. Kuban DA, Tucker SL, Dong L, et al. Long-term results of the M. D. Anderson randomized dose-escalation trial for prostate cancer. *Int J Radiat Oncol Biol Phys* 2008;70:67–74.

122. Talcott JA, Rossi C, Shipley WU, et al. Patient-reported long-term outcomes after conventional and high-dose combined proton and photon radiation for early prostate cancer. *JAMA* 2010;303:1046–1053.

123. Peeters ST, Heemsbergen WD, Koper PC, et al. Dose-response in radiotherapy for localized prostate cancer: results of the Dutch multicenter randomized phase III trial comparing 68 Gy of radiotherapy with 78 Gy. *J Clin Oncol* 2006;24:1990–1996.

124. Dearnaley DP, Sydes MR, Graham JD, et al. Escalated-dose versus standard-dose conformal radiotherapy in prostate cancer: first results from the MRC RT01 randomised controlled trial. *Lancet Oncol* 2007;8:475–487.

125. Kupelian PA, Willoughby TR, Reddy CA, et al. Hypofractionated intensity-modulated radiotherapy (70 Gy at 2.5 Gy per fraction) for localized prostate cancer: Cleveland Clinic experience. *Int J Radiat Oncol Biol Phys* 2007;68:1424–1430.

126. Arcangeli G, Saracino B, Gomellini S, et al. A prospective phase III randomized trial of hypofractionation versus conventional fractionation in patients with high-risk prostate cancer. *Int J Radiat Oncol Biol Phys* 2010;78(1):11–18.

127. Marzi S, Saracino B, Petrongari MG, et al. Modeling of alpha/beta for late rectal toxicity from a randomized phase II study: conventional versus hypofractionated scheme for localized prostate cancer. *J Exp Clin Cancer Res* 2009;28:117.

128. Lukka H, Hayter C, Julian JA, et al. Randomized trial comparing two fractionation schedules for patients with localized prostate cancer. *J Clin Oncol* 2005;23:6132–6138.

129. Yeoh EE, Fraser RJ, McGowan RE, et al. Evidence for efficacy without increased toxicity of hypofractionated radiotherapy for prostate carcinoma: early results of a Phase III randomized trial. *Int J Radiat Oncol Biol Phys* 2003;55:943–955.

130. Michalski JM, Bae K, Roach M, et al. Long-term toxicity following 3D conformal radiation therapy for prostate cancer from the RTOG 9406 phase I/II dose escalation study. *Int J Radiat Oncol Biol Phys;*76:14–22.

131. Miles EF, Lee WR. Hypofractionation for prostate cancer: a critical review. *Semin Radiat Oncol* 2008;18:41–47.

132. Fowler JF. The radiobiology of prostate cancer including new aspects of fractionated radiotherapy. *Acta Oncol (Stockholm, Sweden)* 2005;44:265–276.

133. Ritter M. Rationale, conduct, and outcome using hypofractionated radiotherapy in prostate cancer. *Semin Radiat Oncol* 2008;18:249–256.

134. Proust-Lima C, Taylor JM, Secher S, et al. Confirmation of a low alpha/beta ratio for prostate cancer treated by external beam radiation therapy alone using a

post-treatment repeated-measures model for PSA dynamics. *Int J Radiat Oncol Biol Phys* 2011;79(1): 195–201.

135. Madsen BL, Hsi RA, Pham HT, et al. Stereotactic hypofractionated accurate radiotherapy of the prostate (SHARP), 33.5 Gy in five fractions for localized disease: first clinical trial results. *Int J Radiat Oncol Biol Phys* 2007;67:1099–1105.

136. King CR, Brooks JD, Gill H, et al. Stereotactic body radiotherapy for localized prostate cancer: interim results of a prospective phase II clinical trial. *Int J Radiat Oncol Biol Phys* 2009;73(4):1043–1048.

137. Tang C, Loblaw DA, Cheung P, et al. *Condensing external beam radiotherapy to five fractions for low risk localized prostate cancer: Early results of pHART3*. In: 2008 Genitourinary Cancers Symposia, San Francisco, CA, 2008.

138. Buyyounouski MK, Price RA Jr, Harris EE, et al. Stereotactic body radiotherapy for primary management of early-stage, low- to intermediate-risk prostate cancer: report of the American Society for Therapeutic Radiology and Oncology Emerging Technology Committee. *Int J Radiat Oncol Biol Phys* 2010;76:1297–1304.

139. Swanson GP, Hussey MA, Tangen CM, et al. Predominant treatment failure in postprostatectomy patients is local: analysis of patterns of treatment failure in SWOG 8794. *J Clin Oncol* 2007;25:2225–2229.

140. Poortmans P, Bossi A, Vandeputte K, et al. Guidelines for target volume definition in post-operative radiotherapy for prostate cancer, on behalf of the EORTC Radiation Oncology Group. *Radiother Oncol* 2007;84:121–127.

141. Michalski JM, Lawton C, El Naqa I, et al. Development of RTOG consensus guidelines for the definition of the clinical target volume for postoperative conformal radiation therapy for prostate cancer. *Int J Radiat Oncol Biol Phys* 2010;76(2):361–368.

142. Wiltshire KL, Brock KK, Haider MA, et al. Anatomic boundaries of the clinical target volume (prostate bed) after radical prostatectomy. *Int J Radiat Oncol Biol Phys* 2007;69:1090–1099.

143. Sidhom MA, Kneebone AB, Lehman M, et al. Postprostatectomy radiation therapy: consensus guidelines of the Australian and New Zealand Radiation Oncology Genito-Urinary Group. *Radiother Oncol* 2008;88: 10–19.

144. Miralbell R, Vees H, Lozano J, et al. Endorectal MRI assessment of local relapse after surgery for prostate cancer: A model to define treatment field guidelines for adjuvant radiotherapy in patients at high risk for local failure. *Int J Radiat Oncol Biol Phys* 2007;67:356–361.

145. Silverman JM, Krebs TL. MR imaging evaluation with a transrectal surface coil of local recurrence of prostatic cancer in men who have undergone radical prostatectomy. *AJR Am J Roentgenol* 1997;168:379–385.

146. Sella T, Schwartz LH, Swindle PW, et al. Suspected local recurrence after radical prostatectomy: endorectal coil MR imaging. *Radiology* 2004;231:379–385.

147. Wang K, Wu X, Bossart E, et al. The uncertainties in target localization for prostate and prostate-bed radiotherapy with Calypso 4D. *Int J Radiat Oncol Biol Phys* 2009;75:S594.

148. Schiffner DC, Gottschalk AR, Lometti M, et al. Daily electronic portal imaging of implanted gold seed

fiducials in patients undergoing radiotherapy after radical prostatectomy. *Int J Radiat Oncol Biol Phys* 2007; 67:610–619.

149. Chinnaiyan P, Tomee W, Patel R, et al. 3D-ultrasound guided radiation therapy in the post-prostatectomy setting. *Technol Cancer Res Treat* 2003;2:455–458.

150. Nath SK, Sandhu AP, Rose BS, et al. Toxicity analysis of postoperative image-guided intensity-modulated radiotherapy for prostate cancer. *Int J Radiat Oncol Biol Phys* 2010;78(2):435–441.

151. King CR, Kapp DS. Radiotherapy after prostatectomy: is the evidence for dose escalation out there? *Int J Radiat Oncol Biol Phys* 2008;71:346–350.

152. Valicenti RK, Gomella LG, Ismail M, et al. Durable efficacy of early postoperative radiation therapy for high-risk pT3N0 prostate cancer: the importance of radiation dose. *Urology* 1998;52:1034–1040.

153. Ost P, Fonteyne V, Villeirs G, et al. Adjuvant high-dose intensity-modulated radiotherapy after radical prostatectomy for prostate cancer: clinical results in 104 patients. *Eur Urol* 2009;56:669–675.

154. Feng M, Hanlon AL, Pisansky TM, et al. Predictive factors for late genitourinary and gastrointestinal toxicity in patients with prostate cancer treated with adjuvant or salvage radiotherapy. *Int J Radiat Oncol Biol Phys* 2007;68:1417–1423.

155. Papagikos MA, Rossi PJ, Urbanic JJ, et al. A simple model predicts freedom from biochemical recurrence after low-dose rate prostate brachytherapy alone. *Am J Clin Oncol* 2007;30:199–204.

156. Scardino P, Carlton C. Combined interstitial and external irradiation for prostatic cancer. In: Javadpour N, ed. *Principles and management of urologic cancer*. Baltimore, MD: William and Wilkins, 1983:392–408.

157. Whitmore WF Jr., Hilaris B, Grabstald H. Retropubic implantation to iodine 125 in the treatment of prostatic cancer. *J Urol* 1972;108:918–920.

158. Zelefsky MJ, Whitmore WF Jr. Long-term results of retropubic permanent 125iodine implantation of the prostate for clinically localized prostatic cancer. *J Urol* 1997;158:23–29; discussion 9–30.

159. Blasko JC, Grimm PD, Ragde H. Brachytherapy and Organ Preservation in the Management of Carcinoma of the Prostate. *Semin Radiat Oncol* 1993;3:240–249.

160. Ling CC. Permanent implants using Au-198, Pd-103 and I-125: radiobiological considerations based on the linear quadratic model. *Int J Radiat Oncol Biol Phys* 1992;23:81–87.

161. Wallner K, Merrick G, True L, et al. 125I versus 103 Pd for low-risk prostate cancer: preliminary PSA outcomes from a prospective randomized multicenter trial. *Int J Radiat Oncol Biol Phys* 2003;57:1297–1303.

162. Peschel RE, Colberg JW, Chen Z, et al. Iodine 125 versus palladium 103 implants for prostate cancer: clinical outcomes and complications. *Cancer J* 2004;10: 170–174.

163. Bice WS, Prestidge BR, Kurtzman SM, et al. Recommendations for permanent prostate brachytherapy with (131)Cs: a consensus report from the Cesium Advisory Group. *Brachytherapy* 2008;7:290–296.

164. Nath R, Anderson LL, Luxton G, et al. Dosimetry of interstitial brachytherapy sources: recommendations of

the AAPM Radiation Therapy Committee Task Group No. 43. American Association of Physicists in Medicine. *Med Phys* 1995;22:209–234.

165. Williamson JF, Coursey BM, DeWerd LA, et al. Recommendations of the American Association of Physicists in Medicine on 103 Pd interstitial source calibration and dosimetry: implications for dose specification and prescription. *Med Phys* 2000;27:634–642.

166. Stock RG, Stone NN, Tabert A, et al. A dose-response study for I-125 prostate implants. *Int J Radiat Oncol Biol Phys* 1998;41:101–108.

167. Wallner K, Roy J, Harrison L. Dosimetry guidelines to minimize urethral and rectal morbidity following transperineal I-125 prostate brachytherapy. *Int J Radiat Oncol Biol Phys* 1995;32:465–471.

168. Nag S, Beyer D, Friedland J, et al. American Brachytherapy Society (ABS) recommendations for transperineal permanent brachytherapy of prostate cancer. *Int J Radiat Oncol Biol Phys* 1999;44:789–799.

169. Martinez AA, Gustafson G, Gonzalez J, et al. Dose escalation using conformal high-dose-rate brachytherapy improves outcome in unfavorable prostate cancer. *Int J Radiat Oncol Biol Phys* 2002;53:316–327.

170. Pisansky TM, Gold DG, Furutani KM, et al. High-dose-rate brachytherapy in the curative treatment of patients with localized prostate cancer. *Mayo Clin Proc* 2008;83:1364–1372.

171. Hsu IC, Kyounghwa B, Shinohara K, et al. Phase II trial of combined high-dose-rate brachytherapy and external beam radiotherapy for adenocarcinoma of the prostate: preliminary results of RTOG 0321. *Int J Radiat Oncol Biol Phys* 2010;78(3):751–758.

172. D'Amico AV, Whittington R, Malkowicz SB, et al. Pretreatment nomogram for prostate-specific antigen recurrence after radical prostatectomy or external-beam radiation therapy for clinically localized prostate cancer. *J Clin Oncol* 1999;17:168–172.

173. Shipley WU, Thames HD, Sandler HM, et al. Radiation therapy for clinically localized prostate cancer: a multi-institutional pooled analysis. *JAMA* 1999;281:1598–1604.

174. Kuban DA, Thames HD, Levy LB, et al. Long-term multi-institutional analysis of stage T1-T2 prostate cancer treated with radiotherapy in the PSA era. *Int J Radiat Oncol Biol Phys* 2003;57:915–928.

175. Kattan MW, Zelefsky MJ, Kupelian PA, et al. Pretreatment nomogram that predicts 5-year probability of metastasis following three-dimensional conformal radiation therapy for localized prostate cancer. *J Clin Oncol* 2003;21:4568–4571.

176. Kattan MW, Potters L, Blasko JC, et al. Pretreatment nomogram for predicting freedom from recurrence after permanent prostate brachytherapy in prostate cancer. *Urology* 2001;58:393–399.

177. Ray ME, Levy LB, Horwitz EM, et al. Nadir prostate-specific antigen within 12 months after radiotherapy predicts biochemical and distant failure. *Urology* 2006;68:1257–1262.

178. Chen AB, D'Amico AV, Neville BA, et al. Provider case volume and outcomes following prostate brachytherapy. *J Urol* 2009;181:113–118; discussion 8.

179. Roach M 3rd, Hanks G, Thames H Jr, et al. Defining biochemical failure following radiotherapy with or without hormonal therapy in men with clinically localized prostate cancer: recommendations of the RTOG-ASTRO Phoenix Consensus Conference. *Int J Radiat Oncol Biol Phys* 2006;65:965–974.

180. Kuban DA, Levy LB, Potters L, et al. Comparison of biochemical failure definitions for permanent prostate brachytherapy. *Int J Radiat Oncol Biol Phys* 2006;65:1487–1493.

181. Pickles T, Kim-Sing C, Morris WJ, et al. Evaluation of the Houston biochemical relapse definition in men treated with prolonged neoadjuvant and adjuvant androgen ablation and assessment of follow-up lead-time bias. *Int J Radiat Oncol Biol Phys* 2003;57:11–18.

182. Kwan W, Pickles T, Duncan G, et al. PSA failure and the risk of death in prostate cancer patients treated with radiotherapy. *Int J Radiat Oncol Biol Phys* 2004;60:1040–1046.

183. Abramowitz MC, Li T, Buyyounouski MK, et al. The Phoenix definition of biochemical failure predicts for overall survival in patients with prostate cancer. *Canc* 2008;112:55–60.

184. Buyyounouski MK, Hanlon AL, Horwitz EM, et al. Interval to biochemical failure highly prognostic for distant metastasis and prostate cancer-specific mortality after radiotherapy. *Int J Radiat Oncol Biol Phys* 2008;70:59–66.

185. Denham JW, Steigler A, Wilcox C, et al. Time to biochemical failure and prostate-specific antigen doubling time as surrogates for prostate cancer-specific mortality: evidence from the TROG 96.01 randomised controlled trial. *Lancet Oncol* 2008;9:1058–1068.

186. D'Amico AV, Moul JW, Carroll PR, et al. Surrogate end point for prostate cancer-specific mortality after radical prostatectomy or radiation therapy. *J Natl Canc Inst* 2003;95:1376–1383.

187. Giberti C, Chiono L, Gallo F, et al. Radical retropubic prostatectomy versus brachytherapy for low-risk prostatic cancer: a prospective study. *World J Urol* 2009;27:607–612.

188. Lee WR, DeSilvio M, Lawton C, et al. A phase II study of external beam radiotherapy combined with permanent source brachytherapy for intermediate-risk, clinically localized adenocarcinoma of the prostate: preliminary results of RTOG P-0019. *Int J Radiat Oncol Biol Phys* 2006;64:804–809.

189. Guix B, Bartrina J, Tello J, et al. Dose escalation by high-dose 3D-conformal radiotherapy (HD-3D-CRT) or low-dose 3D-conformal radiotherapy plus HDR brachytherapy (LD-3D-CRT+HDR-B) for intermediate- or high-risk prostate cancer: Early results of a prospective comparative trial. *J Clin Oncol* 2009;27(Suppl): abstr 5118.

PART B
Bladder

Daniel A. Hamstra ■ Michael E. Ray

INTRODUCTION

Bladder cancer is a common urinary tract malignancy, with ~70,000 new cases per year in the United States, predominantly in the 50- to 70-year age group (1). These malignancies are most commonly transitional cell carcinoma (TCC) urothelial tumors, with other histologies such as squamous, adenocarcinomas, and small-cell cancers identified at lower frequencies. Progressive extension of disease into the muscle wall and surrounding tissue correlates well with prognosis. Patients diagnosed with noninvasive TCC bladder cancers may have indolent, albeit frequently recurrent, disease. In contrast, patients with muscle-invasive bladder cancers may have a narrow window of opportunity for cure that requires aggressive treatment. Surgery has been the mainstay of treatment; however, appropriate selection and radiation treatment (often with chemotherapy) can lead to outcomes similar to radical surgery with a high-likelihood of conserving a functional bladder.

Risk Straification

For bladder cancer, the depth of invasion by the primary tumor is the most important prognostic variable for progression and overall survival. At initial presentation, 75% of bladder cancers are found to be superficial or limited to the mucosal surface (2). Superficial tumors are often managed with local treatment such as transurethral resection of bladder tumor (TURBT), possibly followed by intravesical instillation of therapeutic agents such as mitomycin C or bacillus Calmette-Guerin (BCG). Recurrence rates are high, following initial treatment of superficial bladder tumors, particularly if there is associated carcinoma *in situ* (CIS). However, many recurrences are superficial and can again be managed with TURBT. Other patients will ultimately develop invasive disease and require more radical treatment.

Thus, multiple factors must be considered when planning appropriate therapy for bladder tumors. Treatment for superficial disease is considerably different from that for muscle-invading tumors. Invasive disease may be managed with a combination of modalities. In addition to depth of invasion, the tumor's biological aggressiveness and the overall condition of the patient must be evaluated when deciding on the appropriate treatment approach. For selected patients, multimodal treatment strategies for muscle-invasive tumors combine bladder-sparing transurethral surgery, chemotherapy, and radiation therapy.

The use of radiotherapy for multimodality management of bladder tumors requires careful attention when defining the target volume and location of surrounding structures so that effective treatment can be delivered while minimizing radiation effects on normal tissues. Maintaining the level of local control found in patients treated with radical cystectomy while preserving the bladder and its function is obviously advantageous to the patient. As efforts to improve local therapy continue, it must be remembered that ~50% of patients undergoing definitive local therapy for muscle-invading tumors will develop distant metastases and die of their disease (3). As a result, achieving significant improvement in the overall survival from muscle-invasive bladder cancer will require advances in systemic therapies.

DIAGNOSTIC STUDIES AND STAGING

The most common presenting symptom of bladder cancer is painless, gross, or microscopic hematuria, occurring in 70% to 80% of cases. Irritative symptoms alone, including urinary urgency, frequency, and dysuria may occur in 30% of patients, particularly among patients with CIS. Symptoms such as pelvic pain or lower-extremity edema may suggest advanced disease. The diagnostic workup is essential not only for identifying prognostic factors but also for precise determination of disease extent, which is crucial in the planning of radiotherapy. This is true especially when attempting to plan boost volumes, which may not necessarily encompass the entire bladder. Because of the high incidence of metastatic disease, this aspect must also be evaluated.

In conjunction with a thorough history and physical examination, routine laboratory studies include a complete blood count, serum chemistry screen, and urinalysis with urine cytology. Additional urologic evaluation should include cystoscopy with transurethral biopsy. This initial procedure may be accompanied by fulguration or TURBT. Bimanual examination under anesthesia at the time of cystoscopy allows for the evaluation of possible disease extension as evidenced by bladder fixation or a palpable mass. Appropriate imaging studies include a chest x-ray study as well as contrast-enhanced computed tomography (CT) of the abdomen and pelvis to evaluate possible metastatic spread in addition to local extent of disease. Radioisotopic bone scan should be obtained in patients with large, muscle-invasive tumors or when clinical findings raise the suspicion of osseous metastasis.

The standard staging system utilized is the tumor, nodal, and metastasis (TNM) staging system of the American

| TABLE 26.8 | 2010 American Joint Committee on Cancer (AJCC) TNM Staging System for Bladder Cancer |

Primary tumor (T)

TX	Primary tumor cannot be assessed
T0	No evidence of primary tumor
Ta	Noninvasive papillary carcinoma
Tis	Carcinoma *in situ:* "flat tumor"
T1	Tumor invades subepithelial connective tissue
T2	Tumor invades muscularis propria
	T2a Tumor invades superficial muscularis propria (inner half)
	T2b Tumor invades deep muscularis propria (outer half)
T3	Tumor invades perivesical tissue
	T3a Microscopically
	T3b Macroscopically (extravesical mass)
T4	Tumor invades any of the following: prostatic stroma, seminal vesicles, uterus, vagina, pelvic wall, or abdominal wall
	T4a Tumor invades prostatic stroma, uterus, and/or vagina
	T4b Tumor invades pelvic wall and/or abdominal wall

Regional lymph nodes (N)

Nx	Regional lymph nodes cannot be assessed
N0	No regional lymph node metastasis
N1	Single regional lymph node metastasis in the true pelvis (hypogastric, obturator, external iliac, or presacral lymph node)
N2	Multiple regional lymph nodes metastases in the true pelvis (hypogastric, obturator, external iliac, or presacral lymph node)
N3	Lymph node metastasis to the common iliac nodes

Distant metastasis (M)

Mx	Distant metastasis cannot be assessed
M0	No distant metastasis
M1	Distant metastasis

Stage grouping

Stage 0a	Ta	N0	M0
Stage 0is	Tis	N0	M0
Stage I	T1	N0	M0
Stage II	T2a-T2b	N0	M0
Stage III	T3a-T4a	N0	M0
Stage IV	T4b	N0	M0
Any T	N1-N3	M0	
Any T	Any N	M1	

Joint Committee on Cancer (AJCC) (Table 26.8) (4). The system is based on sub-dividing patients into groups by the extent of local tumor invasion and the presence or absence of nodal or distant metastases. In this system T-staging, based upon the depth of invasion of the primary tumor (T), conveys important prognostic information. The most useful assessment is whether the tumor is organ-confined (≤T2) or nonorgan-confined (≥T3). However, the utility of available methods for determining the degree of muscle invasiveness preoperatively is modest with accuracy at most 70% even with the combination of cystoscopic evaluation and TURBT when compared to pathologic examination following cystectomy. Determination of the extent of muscle invasion at biopsy also requires adequate sampling of the bladder wall muscle. In addition to depth of invasion, other factors to be determined at the time of staging include the size and location of the lesion, the presence of CIS, the histologic type, and the degree of differentiation. The majority (90%) of bladder cancers in the United States are transitional cell malignancies, and for these by consensus definition, the degree of differentiation is limited to low-grade and high-grade. With rare exception, muscle-invasive (T2 or greater) urothelial cancer is high-grade. Given the high incidence of multicentric

TABLE 26.9	Approximate 5-year Relapse-Free and Overall Survival After Radical Cystectomy for Bladder Cancer by Stage (5)	
Stage	RFS (%)	OS (%)
Ta-T1 N0	80–90	75–85
T2-T3a N0	75–90	65–75
T3b-T4 N0	50–60	40–50
Node+	30–40	20–30

disease examination of specimens taken from clinically uninvolved areas of the bladder is also recommended.

TREATMENT OPTIONS

The standard treatment for muscle-invasive bladder cancer in the United States is radical cystectomy with a pelvic lymph node dissection. This results in a high rate of local control for patients with organ-confined disease, but the development of distant metastasis is common, which incited the use of adjuvant systemic chemotherapy (Table 26.9). A variety of approaches have been explored as supplements or even alternatives to cystectomy. Multimodality organ-preservation strategies similar to those used in treatment of laryngeal, breast, anal, and extremity malignancies have also been developed for bladder cancer. Almost all possible combinations of surgery, radiotherapy, and/or chemotherapy, as well as single-modality treatments have been utilized. The patient's ability to tolerate therapy and the institution's policy play large roles in deciding what form definitive treatment will take.

Non-bladder Sparing Treatment Approaches

Radical cystectomy involves *en bloc* removal of the bladder, prostate, seminal vesicles, and proximal urethra in males. In females, it involves removal of the bladder, urethra, uterus, fallopian tubes, ovaries, and anterior vaginal wall. Local control rates approach 90% for organ-confined disease and node-negative disease, and relapse-free and overall survival range from 30% to 90%, depending on the extent of disease (5). Radical surgery requires urinary diversion or construction of some form of continent reservoir, having significant impact on patients' urinary function and quality of life.

The goal of adjuvant chemotherapy is to enhance survival by targeting occult micrometastatic disease. Neoadjuvant chemotherapy using cisplatin-based regimens such as CMV (cisplatin, methotrexate, vinblastine) or MVAC (methotrexate, vinblastine, adriamycin, cisplatin) followed by cystectomy has been shown to result in significant downstaging of tumors and to improve survival. In a meta-analysis of 11 randomized trials, platinum-based combination chemotherapy showed a significant benefit to overall survival ($p < 0.0003$) with a 5% absolute improvement in survival at 5 years. Interestingly, although most patients did undergo cystectomy, the beneficial effect was observed irrespective of the type of local treatment (6). Therefore, platinum-based combination chemotherapy constitutes the current standard of care for patients with muscle-invasive/locally advanced operable bladder cancer (7). The response to neoadjuvant chemotherapy is prognostic for outcome; however, local therapy is still indicated because even with a complete response to multiagent chemotherapy at time of posttherapy cystoscopy, as many as 60% of patients may still harbor persistent cancer in the cystectomy specimen (8).

Preoperative radiotherapy followed by cystectomy has been investigated using a wide range of doses and fractionation schemes (9). Irradiation in this setting was utilized to decrease the likelihood of metastatic spread at the time of surgery and eradicate microscopic local and regional disease extension that might be missed by surgical resection alone. In a randomized trial, Cole et al. found that for patients with T3b disease, there was a decreased risk of pelvic recurrence with preoperative RT to doses near 50 Gy (10). However, no similar local control benefits were seen for patients with T2, T3a, or T4 disease. There was no statistically significant difference in distant metastasis or survival. Because of the lack of a survival benefit, as well as surgical considerations such as trying to create continent reservoirs in areas of irradiated tissues, preoperative radiotherapy for bladder cancer has fallen out of favor.

Postoperative radiotherapy may be delivered for patients at high risk of local recurrence after surgical resection. This is particularly important for patients with either extra-bladder extension or lymph-node-positive disease where local and/or pelvic recurrence may be as high as 30% and with positive margins this may approach 60% to 70% (11). Therefore, although no randomized trials have evaluated postoperative radiation therapy in this setting, retrospective studies have suggested improved outcomes with acceptable toxicity (12).

Bladder-Sparing Approaches

Non-Muscle-Invasive Disease

Bladder conserving surgery using TURBT alone may be appropriate treatment for selected early stage patients (13), particularly for patients who are poor candidates for aggressive interventions. TURBT is also a critical component of multimodality treatment strategies for more advanced disease, and the completeness of resection is an important predictor of local control and survival (14). Nevertheless, for noninvasive disease, recurrence after TURBT alone is common, particularly for high-grade lesions (15). Recurrence rates can be decreased by the use of intravesical BCG, resulting in 70% to 80% 5-year survival for T1 tumors (16,17). With progression from T1 to muscle-invasive disease, radical cystectomy has been the

TABLE 26.10	**Radiation Therapy Oncology Group (RTOG) Protocols for Invasive Bladder Cancer (1985–2009) (28,42)**			
Protocol	Induction treatment	Number of patients	Complete response (%)	5-Year survival (%)
85–12	TURBT, XRT + Cis	42	66	52
88–02	TURBT, MCV, XRT + Cis	91	75	51
89–03	TURBT, +/− MCV, XRT + Cis	123	59	49
95–06	TURBT, 5-FU, XRT + Cis	34	67	NA
97–06	TURBT, XRT (BID) + Cis + adj MCV	52	74	NA
99–06	TURBT, Tax, XRT + Cis; adj Cis + Gem	84	81	56

standard recommendation; however, some would argue that at this point, organ-preserving therapy with radiation and chemotherapy may also be an option (18,19).

Muscle-Invasive Disease

Radiotherapy alone for muscle-invasive bladder cancer has resulted in 5-year local control rates around 50% and overall survival rates of 20% to 40% (20–25); however, these retrospective studies likely involved patients with multiple medical comorbidities and occult extravesical disease. The highest rates of success with bladder preservation are obtained with solitary T2 or early T3 tumors <6 cm, no tumor-associated hydronephrosis, a visibly complete TURBT, a lack of extensive CIS, adequate renal function for administration of cisplatin concurrently with radiation, and those who can be treated with adequate radiation dose (64–68 Gy). For patients who are not candidates for cystectomy or chemotherapy, definitive irradiation remains a satisfactory option although as expected results are worse in these patients.

The modern bladder-sparing approaches select patients who are good candidates and who respond favorably to induction trimodality therapy using TURBT, chemotherapy, and radiotherapy. In North America, a bladder-sparing treatment approach has evolved out of studies pioneered at the Massachusetts General Hospital and continued under the Radiation Therapy Oncology Group (RTOG) (26–28). These protocols include maximal TURBT followed by concurrent chemotherapy and radiotherapy. A variety of chemotherapeutic agents (cisplatin, 5-fluorouracil, paclitaxel, etc.) and radiation fractionation schedules have been studied. Typical initial treatment is to bladder and pelvic lymph nodes to 40 to 45 Gy in fractions of 1.8 to 2.0 Gy with boost(s) to the bladder and bladder tumor to a total dose of 64 to 64.8 Gy. Concurrent chemotherapy is most often delivered with cisplatin or for patients judged unsuitable for cisplatin, paclitaxel, or oral capectiabine concurrent with radiation therapy have been utilized (29,30).

For patients treated with selected bladder preservation therapy following several weeks of treatment, cystoscopic biopsy and urine cytology evaluation of disease response is performed, and patients with a complete response receive consolidative chemoradiotherapy while patients without complete response undergo cystectomy. Patients with early cystectomy for lack of appropriate response do not appear to have worse outcomes than those with a good response, who are able to go on to bladder preservation. The available data suggest that using modern trimodality bladder-sparing treatment for appropriately selected patients, complete response rates from 60% to 80% are achievable with 5-year survival rates of 50% to 60% (Table 26.10) (26,27,31–34). These results are comparable with cystectomy series. Following completion of treatment, careful surveillance is crucial for patients undergoing bladder preserving treatment, as they are at risk for both superficial and invasive recurrences that must be appropriately managed (35). However, overall functional outcomes after selective bladder preservation are excellent. A recent analysis of late toxicity for 157 patients treated on 4 RTOG protocols revealed that there were no grade 4 toxicities or treatment-related deaths. Further, only 7% of patients experienced late grade 3+ pelvic toxicity (6% GU and 2% GI), and the grade 3 toxicities resolved in all but one patient. Overall quality of life after combined modality therapy is excellent for the majority of patients with only ~30% requiring a cystectomy (36). In addition, for those with a retained bladder, >75% are able to retain normal urinary function by urodynamic studies, and >85% with no bothersome urinary side effects (37).

TREATMENT PLANNING

Target Volume

Initial treatment fields for bladder cancer usually include the entire bladder and the regional nodes. Encompassing the bladder, which can vary in size from day to day, as well as the external, internal, and common iliac nodes of the pelvis results in a relatively large treatment area. Some

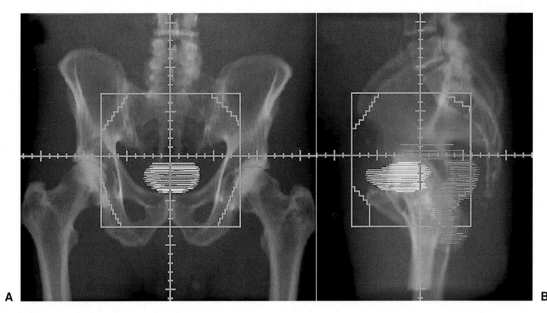

Figure 26.13. Digitally reconstructed radiographs (DRRs) demonstrating typical anterior (**A**) and lateral (**B**) fields encompassing the bladder and regional nodes.

treatment protocols have opted instead for "small" or "mini" pelvic fields, which do not extend as far superiorly to encompass the common iliac nodes. Smaller boost volumes may encompass the entire or partial bladder volume with a 2-cm margin.

Simulation and Planning

As with other sites, the goal of simulation and planning is to design treatment portals to encompass the chosen tumor volume while minimizing the amount of normal tissue irradiated. Although with the adoption of CT-based planning, three-dimensional (3D)-conformal therapy is commonly utilized, given the significant uncertainty about bladder size, position, and motion, intensity-modulated radiation therapy has not typically been used for the treatment of bladder cancer. For simulation, patients are placed in a supine position. Previously, fluoroscopic techniques were used; although in current clinical practice CT-based planning is most often utilized (Fig. 26.13). On CT, the soft tissue anatomy is quite visible even in the absence of contrast material. The bladder is usually easily contoured on CT, and often the tumor, including extravesical tumor extension is discernable as well. Contouring of the iliac vasculature, rectum, femoral heads, and small bowel also facilitates target coverage and normal tissue avoidance and allows 3D dose calculations for assessment of dose volume histograms.

A planning CT is obtained with the patient in the supine position. The bladder is voided prior to simulation, and a pelvic immobilization device is recommended. Use of bladder or rectal contrast and a foley catheter while critical fluoroscopic simulation are less necessary for CT-based planning and are considered optional. The use of cystoscopically placed bladder fiducials prior to simulation

is also optional, but may be utilized to localize the GTV for a planned boost.

Pelvic Fields

To treat the initial field pelvic fields a four-field box is most often utilized with minimum 10 MV photons (Fig. 26.14). The initial treatment to the pelvis (CTV1) will include the entire bladder, prostate and prostatic urethra (in men), and the regional lymph nodes. Given potential differences in location, size, and movement of the different components of the CTV, a PTV of at least 1.5 to 2.0 cm is practical. There is some disagreement concerning the superior border of the treatment fields. It was previously common to treat superiorly all the way to the distal common iliac vessels; however, with the introduction of combined treatment with systemic chemotherapy,

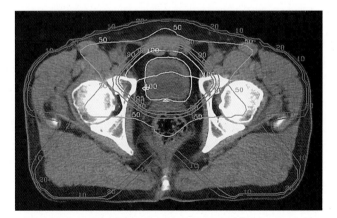

Figure 26.14. An axial slice from a computed tomography (CT) scan is shown demonstrating the dose distribution from a three-dimensional (3D) conformal treatment plan encompassing the bladder.

the superior border is now most often placed at the mid-sacrum (the anterior aspect of S2–S3 junction) with the inferior margin to just below the obturator foramen. The anterior–posterior opposed fields should extend 1.5 to 2.0 cm laterally beyond the medial aspect of the pelvic bones to encompass the iliac lymph nodes. Customized blocks are used on the inferior lateral edges of these fields to reduce exposure of the femoral heads. The parallel-opposed lateral fields will extend at least 2.5 cm anteriorly to the bladder boundary, as defined on CT, although care should be taken to avoid fall-off anteriorly and <2.5 cm may be required in some patients. The posterior margin should also be 2.5 cm beyond the bladder or any visible tumor mass. Inferiorly on the lateral fields, corner blocks should be used to shield the soft tissue inferior to the pubic symphysis anteriorly and the anal canal posteriorly. Superiorly on the lateral fields, a corner block should be placed anteriorly to shield bowel anterior to the external iliac lymph nodal chain. The fields should be adjusted to cover unusual anatomical variations, such as a bladder diverticulum, cystocele, or herniation into the anterior abdominal wall.

Whole Bladder Field

Following treatment to the whole pelvis a boost to the whole bladder is delivered. The whole bladder (CTV2) encompasses the entire bladder plus any bladder-associated masses visible on CT or other imaging modality (e.g., MRI, PET). A PTV margin of 2 cm is appropriate with the fields shaped so that the minimum dose to the PTV is no less than 95% of the isocentric dose. This should recapitulate a field similar to the 2.5 cm block margin commonly utilized using 2D planning.

Tumor Boost

The Tumor Boost (CTV3) encompasses the GTV, which includes any bladder-associated masses defined by CT or other imaging modality (e.g., MRI, PET) and cystoscopy. Close coordination with urology is vital to accurately define a final boost volume based upon the disease observed at cystoscopy. Like the whole bladder treatment, a PTV margin of 2 cm (or block margin of 2.5 cm) with the dose prescribed such that the PTV receives no less than 95% of the prescription dose.

Treatment Technique

When planning initial external radiation treatment to the bladder alone or to the bladder plus pelvic lymph nodes, a four-field box technique is typically preferred. This arrangement consists of parallel opposed anterior and posterior fields in addition to right and left lateral fields. Weighting of the fields and wedges should be utilized taking into account the planned boost technique in order to limit dose to normal tissues. For instance, an attempt

should be made to limit cumulative dose to the femoral head and neck from the entire course of therapy, including the initial large fields and final boost, to 40 to 50 Gy. The four-field box technique may deliver a higher dose than desired to the rectum. As the bladder is an anterior structure, with much of the organ located anterior to the mid-plane, unequal weighting in favor of the anterior field often decreases the volume of rectum unnecessarily included in the high-dose volume. Unequal weighting of the anterior field or a marked curvature of the patient's transverse external contour may create a high-dose area within the anterior portion of the treatment volume, which can be compensated for with wedges on the lateral fields.

Definitive radiotherapy for bladder cancer, whether given alone or in combination with chemotherapy, requires that a higher dose be delivered to the known tumor volume following elective nodal irradiation. After initial treatment of the pelvic field, the boost may be delivered by a variety of techniques. Often, a simple cone-down of the four-field technique can be utilized. However, if the tumor extends laterally from the bladder, parallel opposed anterior and posterior fields may be preferable for the boost dose, as this method allows for exclusion of uninvolved segments of the bladder from the high-dose area. In contrast to the lateral boost technique, little additional dose is delivered to the femoral heads, and the initial whole-pelvis treatment can be delivered with a standard four-field arrangement. With tumors confined to the trigone area or posterior bladder wall, two parallel opposed lateral fields may be used. Although this technique offers the advantage of sparing portions of the rectum and bladder, it also requires delivery of the entire boost through the femoral heads. Careful attention must therefore be given to the total cumulative dose to these structures. Preferentially weighting the anterior and posterior fields during the four-field technique allows the entire boost dose to be delivered through the lateral fields while maintaining the total dose to the femoral heads below 40 to 50 Gy. CT-planning with 3D conformal planning techniques may achieve tumor coverage with superior normal tissue avoidance. Regardless of the boost technique selected, in addition to the boost plan, a composite dose plan combining the initial whole-pelvis treatment with the final boost should be reviewed to ensure that the tolerance dose to critical structures such as the rectum, small intestine, uninvolved bladder, and femoral heads is not exceeded. As with any pelvic irradiation, high photon energies are desirable (minimum 6 MV, preferably 10 or 15 MV).

Since the bladder is a distensible structure, one must actively decide whether to treat with it empty or full. When the desired treatments are limited to the bladder only, treatment planning and therapy should be given with an empty bladder. The patient is asked to void prior to daily treatment, and it may be useful to assess postvoid residual volumes at the time of simulation. This minimizes the bladder volume and, therefore, the field size, which results in a smaller treatment volume. Conversely, when treatment of the bladder and its lymph node drainage to include the whole pelvis is planned, consideration should be given to treating the patient with a full bladder, which may displace small intestine from the pelvis, decreasing the risk of radiation enteritis. For treating the tumor only during the boost phase of treatment, distending the bladder may help to decrease the dose to areas outside the target volume. It is essential that the treatment technique duplicates simulation in this regard. Treatment of the patient in a prone position with a "belly board" may also be used to minimize the amount of small bowel within the field, particularly if using a lateral technique for the boost.

DOSAGE AND FRACTIONATION

Patients treated with radiotherapy alone typically receive 1.8 to 2 Gy fractions, one fraction per day, 5 days per week, with all fields treated daily. This conventional fractionation may also be used in conjunction with systemic chemotherapy. This regimen is well tolerated, and severe complications are uncommon, regardless of whether chemotherapy is given (38). Mild acute effects, including transient dysuria and diarrhea, which are to be expected, occur with greater frequency when chemotherapy is given. Typical whole-pelvis radiotherapy consists of 45 to 50 Gy over 4 to 5 weeks. This is typically followed by a boost(s) of 10 to 20 Gy. The total dose to the tumor is based on several factors, including disease stage, whether or not combined-modality treatment is planned, patient tolerance, and the likelihood of surgical salvage. The typical dose to the entire bladder is 55.8 to 60 Gy, and if a boost dose confined to the tumor is delivered, the total tumor dose is about 64 to 64.8 Gy. Patients who are medically unsuitable for surgery should be considered for more aggressive radiotherapy in an effort to control the disease. The potential benefit of treatment with higher doses must be carefully weighed against the increased risk of complications involving the bladder and surrounding tissues. Hyperfractionated and accelerated fractionation schemes have also been studied with and without chemotherapy (39–41).

PROGNOSIS

Survival from bladder cancer is largely determined by distant metastasis; therefore, current treatment approaches are increasingly focused on enhancing systemic therapy. Radical cystectomy remains the standard treatment for muscle-invasive bladder cancer. It provides excellent rates of local control, and 5-year survival that ranges from 30% to 90% depending on the extent of disease and risk for distant metastasis (Table 26.9). Multimodality treatment

using TURBT, chemotherapy, and radiotherapy provides high rates of complete disease response, and survival that is comparable to radical cystectomy (Table 26.10). Furthermore, 60% to 70% of patients treated with multimodality, bladder-preserving treatment strategies are able to retain their native bladder, offering the potential of superior long-term bladder function and patient quality of life.

REFERENCES

1. Jemal A, Siegel R, Xu J, et al. Cancer statistics, 2010. *CA Cancer J Clin* 2010;60:277–300.
2. Montie J, Smith DC, Sandler HM. *Carcinoma of the bladder.* In: Abeloff MD, Armitage JO, Lichter AS, et al., eds. Clinical oncology. Philadelphia, PA: Elsevier, 2004: 2059–2084.
3. Waehre H, Ous S, Klevmark B, et al. A bladder cancer multi-institutional experience with total cystectomy for muscle-invasive bladder cancer. *Cancer* 1993;72: 3044–3051.
4. Greene F, Page D, Fleming I, et al. *AJCC cancer staging manual*, 6th ed. New York: Springer, 2002.
5. Stein JP, Lieskovsky G, Cote R, et al. Radical cystectomy in the treatment of invasive bladder cancer: long-term results in 1,054 patients. *J Clin Oncol* 2001;19:666–675.
6. Neoadjuvant chemotherapy in invasive bladder cancer: update of a systematic review and meta-analysis of individual patient data advanced bladder cancer (ABC) meta-analysis collaboration. *Eur Urol* 2005;48:202–205; discussion 205–206.
7. Sonpavde G, Petrylak DP. Perioperative chemotherapy for bladder cancer. *Crit Rev Oncol Hematol* 2006;57(2):133–144.
8. deVere White RW, Lara PN Jr, Goldman B, et al. A sequential treatment approach to myoinvasive urothelial cancer: a phase II Southwest Oncology Group trial (S0219). *J Urol* 2009;181:2476–2480; discussion 2480–2481.
9. Crawford ED, Das S, Smith JA Jr. Preoperative radiation therapy in the treatment of bladder cancer. *Urol Clin North Am* 1987;14:781–787.
10. Cole CJ, Pollack A, Zagars GK, et al. Local control of muscle-invasive bladder cancer: preoperative radiotherapy and cystectomy versus cystectomy alone. *Int J Radiat Oncol Biol Phys* 1995;32:331–340.
11. Herr HW, Faulkner JR, Grossman HB, et al. Surgical factors influence bladder cancer outcomes: a cooperative group report. *J Clin Oncol* 2004;22:2781–2789.
12. Cozzarini C, Pellegrini D, Fallini M, et al. Reappraisal of the role of adjuvant radiotherapy in muscle-invasive transitional cell carcinoma of the bladder (abstract). *Int J Radiat Oncol Biol Phys* 1999;45:221.
13. Herr HW. Conservative management of muscle-infiltrating bladder cancer: prospective experience. *J Urol* 1987;138:1162–1163.
14. Dunst J, Sauer R, Schrott KM, et al. Organ-sparing treatment of advanced bladder cancer: a 10-year experience. *Int J Radiat Oncol Biol Phys* 1994;30:261–266.
15. Herr HW, Jakse G, Sheinfeld J. The T1 bladder tumor. *Semin Urol* 1990;8:254–261.

16. Herr HW. Tumour progression and survival in patients with T1 G3 bladder tumours: 15-year outcome. *Br J Urol* 1997;80:762–765.

17. Brake M, Loertzer H, Horsch R, et al. Long-term results of intravesical bacillus Calmette-Guerin therapy for stage T1 superficial bladder cancer. *Urology* 2000;55:673–678.

18. Wo JY, Shipley WU, Dahl DM, et al. The results of concurrent chemo-radiotherapy for recurrence after treatment with bacillus Calmette-Guerin for non-muscle-invasive bladder cancer: is immediate cystectomy always necessary? *BJU Int* 2009;104:179–183.

19. Weiss C, Wolze C, Engehausen DG, et al. Radiochemotherapy after transurethral resection for high-risk T1 bladder cancer: an alternative to intravesical therapy or early cystectomy? *J Clin Oncol* 2006;24:2318–2324.

20. Gospodarowicz MK, Hawkins NV, Rawlings GA, et al. Radical radiotherapy for muscle invasive transitional cell carcinoma of the bladder: failure analysis. *J Urol* 1989;142:1448–1453; discussion 1453–1454.

21. Duncan W, Quilty PM. The results of a series of 963 patients with transitional cell carcinoma of the urinary bladder primarily treated by radical megavoltage X-ray therapy. *Radiother Oncol* 1986;7:299–310.

22. Pollack A, Zagars GZ. Radiotherapy for stage T3b transitional cell carcinoma of the bladder. *Semin Urol Oncol* 1996;14:86–95.

23. De Neve W, Lybeert ML, Goor C, et al. Radiotherapy for T2 and T3 carcinoma of the bladder: the influence of overall treatment time. *Radiother Oncol* 1995;36:183–188.

24. Gospodarowicz MK, Quilty PM, Scalliet P, et al. The place of radiation therapy as definitive treatment of bladder cancer. *Int J Urol* 1995;2(Suppl 2):41–48.

25. Mameghan H, Fisher R, Mameghan J, et al. Analysis of failure following definitive radiotherapy for invasive transitional cell carcinoma of the bladder. *Int J Radiat Oncol Biol Phys* 1995;31:247–254.

26. Shipley WU, Kaufman DS, Tester WJ, et al. Overview of bladder cancer trials in the Radiation Therapy Oncology Group. *Cancer* 2003;97:2115–2119.

27. Shipley WU, Kaufman DS, Heney NM, et al. An update of combined modality therapy for patients with muscle invading bladder cancer using selective bladder preservation or cystectomy. *J Urol* 1999;162:445–450; discussion 450–451.

28. Kaufman DS, Winter KA, Shipley WU, et al. Phase I-II RTOG study (99–06) of patients with muscle-invasive bladder cancer undergoing transurethral surgery, paclitaxel, cisplatin, and twice-daily radiotherapy followed by selective bladder preservation or radical cystectomy and adjuvant chemotherapy. *Urology* 2009;73:833–837.

29. Muller AC, Diestelhorst A, Kuhnt T, et al. Organ-sparing treatment of advanced bladder cancer: paclitaxel as a radiosensitizer. *Strahlenther Onkol* 2007;183:177–183.

30. Patel B, Forman J, Fontana J, et al. A single institution experience with concurrent capecitabine and radiation therapy in weak and/or elderly patients with urothelial cancer. *Int J Radiat Oncol Biol Phys* 2005;62:1332–1338.

31. Rodel C, Grabenbauer GG, Kuhn R, et al. Combined-modality treatment and selective organ preservation in invasive bladder cancer: long-term results. *J Clin Oncol* 2002;20:3061–3071.

32. Shipley WU, Kaufman DS, Zehr E, et al. Selective bladder preservation by combined modality protocol treatment: long-term outcomes of 190 patients with invasive bladder cancer. *Urology* 2002;60:62–67; discussion 67–68.

33. Given RW, Parsons JT, McCarley D, et al. Bladder-sparing multimodality treatment of muscle-invasive bladder cancer: a five-year follow-up. *Urology* 1995;46:499–504; discussion 504–505.

34. Housset M, Maulard C, Chretien Y, et al. Combined radiation and chemotherapy for invasive transitional-cell carcinoma of the bladder: a prospective study. *J Clin Oncol* 1993;11:2150–2157.

35. Zietman AL, Grocela J, Zehr E, et al. Selective bladder conservation using transurethral resection, chemotherapy, and radiation: management and consequences of Ta, T1, and Tis recurrence within the retained bladder. *Urology* 2001;58:380–385.

36. Lagrange JL, Bascoul-Mollevi C, Geoffrois L, et al. Quality of life assessment after concurrent chemoradiation for invasive bladder cancer: results of a multicenter prospective study (GETUG 97–015). *Int J Radiat Oncol Biol Phys* 2011;79(1):172–178.

37. Zietman AL, Sacco D, Skowronski U, et al. Organ conservation in invasive bladder cancer by transurethral resection, chemotherapy and radiation: results of a urodynamic and quality of life study on long-term survivors. *J Urol* 2003;170:1772–1776.

38. Efstathiou JA, Bae K, Shipley WU, et al. Late pelvic toxicity after bladder-sparing therapy in patients with invasive bladder cancer: RTOG 89–03, 95–06, 97–06, 99–06. *J Clin Oncol* 2009;27:4055–4061.

39. Cole DJ, Durrant KR, Roberts JT, et al. A pilot study of accelerated fractionation in the radiotherapy of invasive carcinoma of the bladder. *Br J Radiol* 1992;65:792–798.

40. Zietman AL, Shipley WU, Kaufman DS, et al. A phase I/II trial of transurethral surgery combined with concurrent cisplatin, 5-fluorouracil and twice daily radiation followed by selective bladder preservation in operable patients with muscle invading bladder cancer. *J Urol* 1998;160:1673–1677.

41. Danesi DT, Arcangeli G, Cruciani E, et al. Conservative treatment of invasive bladder carcinoma by transurethral resection, protracted intravenous infusion chemotherapy, and hyperfractionated radiotherapy: long term results. *Cancer* 2004;101:2540–2548.

42. Fernando SA, Sandler HM. Organ preservation in muscle-invasive bladder cancer. *Oncology (Williston Park)* 2005;19:334–339;discussion 339–340,345,349,350–353.

PART C
Testis

Daniel A. Hamstra ■ Michael E. Ray

INTRODUCTION

Testicular cancer is an uncommon tumor, accounting for 1% of all malignancies and <0.2% of all deaths due to cancer in American men with approximately 8,500 new cases in the year 2010 (1). Despite this, it is the most common malignancy found in men between the ages of 15 and 35 (2). Germ cell tumors, which account for 95% of testicular tumors, for the purposes of therapeutic management are commonly divided into two broad groups: pure seminomas, which account for nearly two-thirds, and all others, which are grouped as nonseminomatous tumors and make up the remaining third (3). Members of this latter group may have a single cell type or be composed of multiple elements, including a component of seminoma.

Germ cell tumors are now among the most curable malignancies with overall cure rates near 95% or even higher (4). This is largely due to the development of platinum-based chemotherapy. Prior to this introduction, germ cell tumors accounted for 11% of all cancer deaths in men aged 25 to 34 and the 5-year survival was 64%. In contrast, it is estimated that in 2010 there were only 380 deaths in men due to germ cell tumor in the United States (1). With the development of effective systemic chemotherapy, the role of radiotherapy in the treatment of nonseminomatous germ cell tumors has greatly diminished. Platinum-based multiagent chemotherapy has become the rule for advanced seminomatous disease as well, but radiotherapy following inguinal orchiectomy remains important in the treatment of patients with early-stage pure seminoma. Therefore, the focus of this section is to detail the role of radiotherapy in the treatment of early stage (stages I and II) seminomatous germ cell tumors.

Pure seminoma is a remarkably radiosensitive tumor, with orchiectomy and radiation effecting cure in the majority of patients presenting with localized or regional nodal disease (5–12). The high rate of expected cure and relatively young age at presentation of this group of patients place responsibility on the physician to carefully plan therapy that maximizes the probability for cure while minimizing the risk of adverse side effects and long-term complications. In contrast to malignant neoplasms of many other sites, in which the aim of treatment is palliation of symptoms or limited prolongation of life, the goal of modern therapy in even advanced germ cell tumors is cure and even cure at the cost of the least long-term harm to the patient (13).

DIAGNOSTIC STUDIES

The classical presentation is a painless testicular swelling or mass in the scrotum (14). Localized discomfort or pain may be present in the scrotum, low back, or abdomen. Symptoms outside the scrotum raise the question of pelvic, retroperitoneal, or more widespread metastasis. Associated gynecomastia may also be present. Clinical history should include query of testicular maldescent, as well as any inguinal or scrotal surgery. Cryptorchidism increases the risk of malignant transformation in testicular tissue by approximately fourfold relative to a normal testis (15), and a history of testicular maldescent can be found in approximately 10% of patients with testicular cancer. The risk of malignancy is further increased if the testis is intra-abdominal. Physical examination should include careful bimanual examination of both testes with special attention to any areas of induration. Transillumination or ultrasonography is used to distinguish cystic masses such as a hydrocele or spermatocele from solid masses more suspicious for malignancy.

A high-resolution computed tomographic scan of the abdomen should be obtained for patients with a suspected testicular neoplasm to exclude liver or infradiaphragmatic lymph node metastases. A chest x-ray film should also be obtained, and if any abnormalities are found, a chest computed tomography (CT) is warranted to detect possible pulmonary or mediastinal metastases. Bipedal lymphangiogram has largely been replaced by high-resolution CT for evaluating the status of the retroperitoneal lymph nodes, although bipedal lymphangiogram may have greater sensitivity for detecting small-volume retroperitoneal disease (16).

A complete blood cell count and serum chemistry screen with lactate dehydrogenase, liver function studies, and blood urea nitrogen as well as urinalysis are recommended. In patients who are suspected of having a testicular neoplasm, pretreatment serum α-fetoprotein (AFP) and serum β-human chorionic gonadotropin (β-HCG) titers should be obtained. These serum markers aid the clinician in distinguishing between pure seminoma and other germ cell tumors and are very useful in monitoring treatment response. AFP or β-HCG levels may be elevated in up to 90% of nonseminomatous germ cell tumors. A modest elevation of β-HCG may be found in 15% to 20% of patients with pure seminoma, whereas an elevated AFP raises the suspicion of mixed tumor. The latter should be treated as nonseminomatous disease even if histologic evaluation does not support this finding. Elevation of these markers after treatment raises concern for residual or recurrent disease.

Prior to initiating treatment, it is important to discuss and offer semen cryopreservation to men with suspected testicular cancer. It is important to note that many of these men will have impaired spermatogenesis at baseline, and sperm counts may further deteriorate after orchiectomy (17).

All patients with a suspected testicular tumor should undergo radical inguinal orchiectomy with high ligation of the vessels and spermatic cord to establish a definitive diagnosis and local control of disease. Transscrotal biopsy or orchiectomy is avoided out of concern for seeding tumor into the scrotum, although studies have not conclusively demonstrated increased recurrence risks or the necessity for additional local therapy after scrotal violation (18). Retroperitoneal lymph node dissection is not used in the primary treatment of pure seminomas but is used selectively in nonseminomatous germ cell tumors.

Several staging systems have been proposed for testicular cancer. A consensus model has been adopted by the International Germ Cell Cancer Collaborative Group (IGCCG) (13) in which testicular seminoma patients are segregated into either "good prognosis" if there are no nonpulmonary visceral metastases or "intermediate prognosis" if there are nonpulmonary visceral metastases. The American Joint Commission on Cancer (AJCC) staging system incorporates information on the primary tumor (T), regional lymph nodes (N), presence or absence of distant metastases (M), as well as serum tumor markers (S) to establish prognostic stage groupings (Table 26.11) (19).

TREATMENT OPTIONS

The treatment for testicular germ cell tumors should begin with radical inguinal orchiectomy for diagnosis as well as therapy for the primary tumor. From this point, treatment depends on the histopathological diagnosis of pure seminoma versus nonseminomatous disease and staging information.

Stage I Seminoma

The postorchiectomy options for stage I seminoma include active surveillance, radiotherapy, and single-agent chemotherapy (20). In one series, approximately 20% of men who undergo surveillance will develop recurrent stage II or stage III disease; however, active surveillance remains a viable option because chemotherapy salvage rates are excellent, and survival is not compromised if recurrence is detected early (21). Appropriate candidates for surveillance are highly motivated men with small (≤4 cm) stage I disease without rete testis invasion (22). In one series, patients with small primary tumors without rete testis invasion had 5-year relapse-free survival rates of 88%, whereas those with both high-risk features this was 69% and those with only one feature had an intermediary risk (22). Advantages of surveillance include avoidance of the cost and short-term

side effects of either abdominal radiotherapy or chemotherapy, but the main benefit is the avoidance of late effects and secondary malignancies of these treatments, which are an important consideration in treating these often young patients (23). Patients who consider surveillance must be reliable and must agree to adhere closely to clinical and radiographic surveillance, including frequent clinic visits, physical examinations, serum tumor markers levels, and chest and abdominal imaging.

Postorchiectomy radiotherapy to the infradiaphragmatic nodes is an acceptable standard curative therapy for patients with pathologically confirmed, stage I pure seminoma. Traditional fields encompassed both para-aortic (PA) and ipsilateral pelvic nodes; however, a randomized trial for appropriately selected patients compared PA only radiation to a dog-leg (DL) field that included the ipsilateral pelvic nodes and demonstrated no difference in 3-year relapse-free survival at 96% for PA and 97% for DL (24). The use of PA treatment was associated with less acute toxicity and improved sperm count over the first 18 months. Because of the marked radiosensitivity of seminoma and out of desire to reduce late effects, delivered radiation doses continue to decrease without compromising disease cure rates. A randomized trial compared 30 Gy with 20 Gy (with most patients receiving PA only RT) the 5-year relapse-free survival was 97% for the 30 Gy arm and 96.4% in the 20 Gy arm (25). Perhaps due to improvements in supportive care, patients treated with 30 Gy had only modestly worse nausea and leucopenia than those treated with 20 Gy. However, those treated with the lower dose did report less fatigue and a greater ability to continue to work. This radiosensitivity, the orderly metastatic spread to draining lymph nodes, and the infrequency of hematogenous metastases at the time of presentation combine to make seminoma a highly curable disease with low rates of associated morbidity.

Single-agent carboplatin chemotherapy has also been investigated as adjuvant postorchiectomy treatment in men with stage I seminoma, based on the activity of cisplatin-based combination chemotherapy in more advanced disease. A randomized study comparing postorchiectomy radiotherapy with a single course of carboplatin chemotherapy found no difference in recurrence-free survival between the two arms which at 3-years was 96% in those treated with RT and 95% in those treated with carboplatin (26). Interestingly, in those given RT relapses tended to occur in the pelvic nodes or supradiaphragmatic, whereas in those treated with carboplatin relapses were most common in the PA nodes. In addition, following chemotherapy there was a lower rate of secondary germ cell tumors in the contralateral testicle when compared with those treated with RT. In another trial, patients were prospectively allocated such that those with no high-risk features (size >4 cm or rete testis invasion) were allocated to surveillance, whereas those with one or more high-risk features received two cycles of carboplatin. Relapses were observed in six patients (6.0%) on surveillance and in seven patients (3.3%) treated with carboplatin (0.8% of tumors >4 cm,

TABLE 26.11	2010 American Joint Committee on Cancer (AJCC) TNM Staging System for Testicular Cancer

Primary Tumor (pT)

pTX[a] Primary tumor cannot be assessed

pT0 No evidence of primary tumor (e.g., histologic scar in testis)

pTis Intratubular germ cell neoplasia (carcinoma *in situ*)

pT1 Tumor limited to the testis and epididymis without vascular/lymphatic invasion; tumor may invade into the tunica albuginea but not the tunica vaginalis

pT2 Tumor limited to the testis and epididymis with vascular/lymphatic invasion, or tumor extending through the tunica albuginea with involvement of the tunica vaginalis

pT3 Tumor invades the spermatic cord with or without vascular/lymphatic invasion

pT4 Tumor invades the scrotum with or without vascular/lymphatic invasion

Regional Lymph Nodes (N)

Clinical

NX Regional lymph nodes cannot be assessed

N0 No regional lymph node metastasis

N1 Metastasis with a lymph node mass 2 cm or less in greatest dimension; or multiple lymph nodes, none >2 cm in greatest dimension

N2 Metastasis with a lymph node mass, >2 cm but not >5 cm in greatest dimension; or multiple lymph nodes, any one mass >2 cm but not >5 cm in greatest dimension

N3 Metastasis with a lymph node mass >5 cm in greatest dimension

Distant Metastasis (M)

M0 No distant metastasis

M1 Distant metastasis

M1a Nonregional nodal or pulmonary metastasis

M1b Distant metastasis other than to nonregional lymph nodes and lungs

Serum Tumor Markers (S)

SX Marker studies not available or not performed

S0 Marker study levels within normal limits

S1 LDH < 1.5 × normal and hCG (mIu/mL) <5,000 and AFP (ng/mL) <1,000

S2 LDH 1.5–10 × normal or hCG (mIu/mL) 5,000–50,000 or AFP (ng/mL) 1,000–10,000

S3 LDH > 10 × normal or hCG (mIu/mL) >50,000 or AFP (ng/mL) >10,000

Stage Grouping

Stage 0	Tis	N0	M0	S0
Stage I	pT1–4	N0	M0	SX
Stage IA	pT1	N0	M0	S0
Stage IB	pT2–4	N0	M0	S0
Stage IS	Any pT/TX	N0	M0	S1–3 (measured postorchiectomy)
Stage II	Any pT/TX	N1–3	M0	SX
Stage IIA	Any pT/TX	N1	M0	S0–1
Stage IIB	Any pT/TX	N2	M0	S0–1
Stage IIC	Any pT/TX	N3	M0	S0–1
Stage III	Any pT/TX	Any N	M1	SX
Stage IIIA	Any pT/TX	Any N	M1a	S0–1
Stage IIIB	Any pT/TX	N1–3	M0	S2
	Any pT/TX	Any N	M1a	S2
Stage IIIC	Any pT/TX	N1–3	M0	S3
	Any pT/TX	Any N	M1a	S3
	Any pT/TX	Any N	M1b	Any S

[a]Except for pTis and pT4, extent of primary tumor is classified by radical orchiectomy. TX may be used for other categories in the absence of radical orchiectomy.

LDH, lactate dehydrogenase; hCG, human chorionic gonadotropin; AFP, α-fetoprotein.

9.1% of those involving the rete testis, and 6.0% of patients with both risk criteria) (27). Similarly, another risk-adapted trial utilized two cycles of cisplatinum/etoposide in those with high-risk state I seminoma and reported excellent disease-free survival, although the benefit of this more toxic chemotherapy regimen as compared with single-agent carboplatin or RT is less clear (28). Longer follow-up of these trials are warranted; nevertheless, 10-year data from single institutions due appear to support single-agent carboplatin as an acceptable treatment regimen (29).

Stage II and Relapsed Seminoma

The standard postorchiectomy treatment for patients with nonbulky stage II seminoma is radiotherapy, although platinum-based chemotherapy is an alternative (20). Surveillance is not appropriate and retroperitoneal lymph node dissection is rarely used because of the tumors' sensitivity to chemotherapy and radiotherapy. Bulky PA or pelvic disease should be treated initially with systemic chemotherapy, reserving radiation for treatment of residual or recurrent disease.

For patients with infradiaphragmatic lymph node metastasis measuring <5 cm in greatest dimension (stages IIA and IIB), radiotherapy to the PA and ipsilateral pelvic nodal regions is appropriate treatment (30). Treatment of PA nodes only and use of very low-radiotherapy doses, as applied to selected stage I patients, are not appropriate for stage II disease. Typical treatments have been to a DL field to 25 to 30 Gy with a boost to sites of gross disease to doses between 34 and 36 Gy. Multiple series have suggested 5-year relapse-free survival rates for stage II seminoma treated with RT of 85% to 95% with better results in stage IIA than IIB. Many patients who fail, however, can be successfully salvaged with platinum-based chemotherapy; therefore, disease specific and overall survival remains above 90% even in the presence of infradiaphragmatic lymph node metastasis (31). Chemotherapy is also being evaluated as an alternative to radiotherapy for patients with nonbulky stage II disease, with a recent study using three to four cycles of combination platinum-based chemotherapy yielding 5-year relapse-free survival of 90% in a cohort of men with stage IIA/B seminoma (32). Alternatively, others have utilized a single cycle of carboplatin followed by RT to the PA field only which may minimize the toxicity associated with multiple cycles of combination platinum-based chemotherapy while also yielding results that appear superior to RT alone in this small group of patients (33,34).

Patients with bulky or relapsed stage II disease have up to a 50% risk of mediastinal or supraclavicular relapse when only the PA and ipsilateral pelvic lymph nodes are irradiated following orchiectomy (31). Because of this, stage IIC patients (lymph node metastases 5 cm in greatest dimension) should be treated with platinum-based chemotherapy, which can achieve cure rates approaching 90% even in the presence of bulky disease (35). Previously, elective irradiation of the mediastinal and left supraclavicular nodal areas was commonly used to decrease the likelihood of recurrence in these sites. Although recurrence was decreased, there was no proven survival benefit. Mediastinal and supraclavicular irradiation has been largely abandoned because of concerns over increased late cardiac and secondary cancer mortality (36) and the availability of highly effective salvage chemotherapy regimens.

A high proportion of men treated with chemotherapy for bulky retroperitoneal seminoma will have a persistent mass after treatment (37). Many of these masses do not harbor viable disease and will resolve over time. PET scans may be the best method to assess for residual viable disease in residual masses (38). The use of radiotherapy or surgical resection for residual disease is a controversial issue, especially with regard to improving outcome (39).

TREATMENT PLANNING

Target Volume

Seminomas metastasize in a predictable pattern, following the lymphatic drainage from the testicle, along the spermatic vein (within the spermatic cord), through the inguinal canal, to the PA nodes, to the mediastinal and supraclavicular nodes, and then to distant sites. The right and left testicles differ slightly in their lymphatic drainage. The right testicular lymphatic trunks terminate in the sentinel nodes along the inferior vena cava and common iliac vein. The left testicular lymphatic trunks travel along the spermatic vein to drain into the lateral aortic nodes at the left renal vein pedicle. Right testicular lymphatics may cross over directly to the left PA nodes, but left testicular lymphatics generally cross to the right only after extensive involvement of the first station nodes. Tumor may spread in a retrograde fashion to nodes surrounding the vena cava and aorta. Further extension may occur via the thoracic duct to the left supraclavicular region or by the transdiaphragmatic lymphatics to the mediastinum. Although the primary drainage is to the retroperitoneal area, some lymphatic channels may also drain to the iliac lymph nodes. Normal lymphatic drainage may be altered if the patient has had an orchiopexy, herniorrhaphy, or other surgical procedures in the pelvis or inguinal region. Early tumor involvement of the epididymis increases the risk of external iliac nodal involvement.

The tunica albuginea surrounding the testicle normally provides a barrier to the spread of tumor into the scrotum. Transscrotal orchiectomy or needle biopsy compromises this barrier, placing the scrotum at risk. Prior scrotal surgery, scrotal involvement by tumor, and massive retroperitoneal metastasis resulting in retrograde lymphatic spread all create the opportunity for inguinal lymph node metastasis.

Clinical studies show that the most common site of lymph node metastasis is the infradiaphragmatic PA area (40,41). Therefore, traditional radiotherapy fields have encompassed the PA nodes and ipsilateral pelvic nodes (42,43). Under usual circumstances, pelvic nodal involvement occurs in only 2% to 3% of patients. A randomized trial has shown that the ipsilateral pelvic nodes may be safely excluded with a low risk of pelvic recurrence (24). In stage II patients, the PA and ipsilateral pelvic nodes should be treated, and if the PA disease is bulky, consideration may be given to including the contralateral pelvic nodes. Although in the past inguinal nodes and the orchiectomy incision have been treated, more recent information indicates that this is unnecessary, even if the inguinal area has been violated by surgery. Surveillance studies have shown an extremely low risk of relapse at these sites (18); therefore, adding the hemiscrotum and inguinal nodal region to the treatment portal is normally not required and should be avoided if possible because of the resulting significant dose to the remaining testicle. Patients with a history of inguinal or pelvic surgery were also thought to be at risk for altered lymphatic drainage, and it has been recommended that the treatment fields be altered to include the pelvic nodes (44). Several authors challenge this practice, however, since recurrence rates in surveillance studies are extremely low (43,45).

Localization

Simulation for seminoma is carried out with the patient supine. Simulation may be conducted using fluoroscopic methods, setting fields clinically using bony landmarks, or using computed tomographic simulation, using bony landmarks and other soft tissue anatomic information. Use of intravenous contrast may aid in identifying the vascular pathways and gross lymphadenopathy on CT in stage II patients, as well as identifying the position of the kidneys if using fluoroscopic simulation. Computed tomographic scanning is very useful for localization of the kidneys so that they can be excluded from the treatment field.

Field borders are generally determined according to bony landmarks to encompass the lymph node drainage sites at risk for microscopic metastasis (stage I) as well as any known gross disease (stage II). Radiation treatment planning for early-stage seminoma, in contrast to that of prostate or bladder, usually does not require an elaborate technique, as the tumor is relatively radiosensitive and the total dose is quite low. Specialized immobilization devices are generally not necessary.

Treatment Technique

Postorchiectomy radiation to the PA region, with or without coverage of the ipsilateral hemipelvic region, is the standard treatment technique for patients with stage I seminoma. PA with ipsilateral hemipelvic radiation is standard for nonbulky stage II disease. For PA only fields, the superior border may be placed at the interspace above the tenth, eleventh, or twelfth thoracic vertebra, as long as

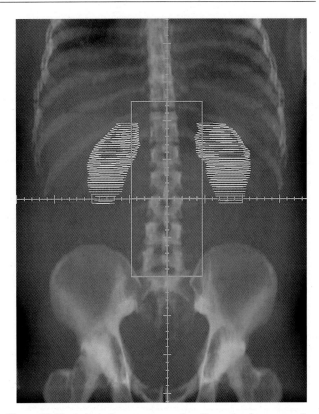

Figure 26.15. A digitally reconstructed radiograph of a rectangular, 9-cm wide, para-aortic field extending from the eleventh thoracic vertebra through the fifth lumbar vertebra is shown with the positions of both kidneys indicated.

the renal hila are well covered (Fig. 26.15). The inferior border is at the interspace between the fifth lumbar vertebra and the sacrum. The PA field is usually 9 to 12 cm wide, and lateral field borders should include the PA lymph nodes as visualized by either CT or lymphangiogram, in addition to the ipsilateral renal hilum. For inclusion of the ipsilateral hemipelvis, a "hockey stick" or "dogleg" is added to the PA field, in which the inferior border may be place near the top of the acetabulum (Fig. 26.16). The ipsilateral pelvic nodes are encompassed with 2-cm margins. Fields are shaped by customized blocks or multileaf collimation appropriately shielding the kidneys. Similar anterior and posterior fields are treated daily, preferably using high-energy photons. Dose is typically calculated to midplane. It is not necessary to include the orchiectomy scar in the treatment portal. If bulky abdominal disease is present, the field width is increased to include the involved nodes with at least a 2-cm margin. After the initial lower dose, the areas of known gross disease are boosted to a total of 34 to 36 Gy. When fields are large and portions of the kidneys are included, it is important not to exceed normal tissue tolerance. This can be accomplished by appropriate half-value layer shielding posteriorly, if major portions of both kidneys are within the treatment field, and by carefully shaping the boost field if possible. If it is not possible to adequately treat the required lymph node regions without sparing of the

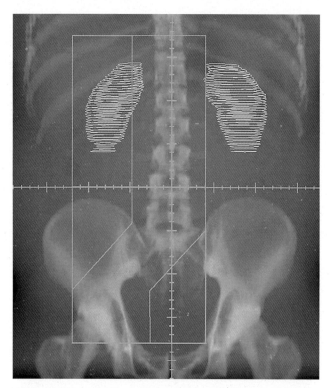

Figure 26.16. A digitally reconstructed radiograph of a treatment field encompassing the para-aortic and ipsilateral pelvic nodal regions. This field is commonly referred to as a "dogleg" field or a "hockey stick" field.

kidneys (such as in patients with a horseshoe kidney), strong consideration should be given to surveillance or chemotherapy as treatment options.

If the pelvis is to be treated, shielding should be used to reduce dose to the remaining testis during simulation and treatment. This can be done with a commercial lead clamshell device. With proper care the dose to the intact testicle can be reduced to <1% to 2% of the prescribed dose, which should preserve normal testicular function (46). This is an important issue in this young patient population when preservation of fertility is desired. When only PA nodes are treated, testicular dose is much reduced; however, some authors suggest that shielding is still advisable (47).

DOSAGE AND FRACTIONATION

Because of the exquisite sensitivity of seminoma to radiation, even relatively bulky disease can be controlled with modest doses. Trends toward use of lower doses and smaller fields are motivated by the desire to reduce risks of late effects and secondary malignancies. A recent randomized study supported the use of 20 Gy in 10 fractions as adequate treatment of typical low risk, stage I seminoma (25). For stage II disease, 25 to 30 Gy is given to PA and ipsilateral pelvic regions with a planned boost through coned-down portals to the areas of gross disease plus a

1.5- to 2.0-cm margin for an additional 5 to 10 Gy, bringing the dose to any gross disease to 35 Gy or more. The total dose may vary somewhat depending on the bulk of disease. More protracted fractionation schemes, such as 25 Gy in 20 fractions, do not appear to reduce treatment efficacy, and they minimize the risk of acute and late gastrointestinal complications.

PROGNOSIS

Successful treatment of germ cell tumors offers the potential for many years of productive life following treatment. Treatment results vary significantly with tumor histology and disease stage (Table 26.12). Pure seminoma, even when metastatic to retroperitoneal nodes, can be cured in the majority of patients. Stage I seminoma is associated with a 15% to 20% risk of relapse when treated with orchiectomy alone; however, virtually all recurrences can be successfully salvaged, and disease-specific survival approaches 100% (21,40,41). For stage I disease treated with inguinal orchiectomy and infradiaphragmatic radiation approaches, relapse rates are approximately 3% to 4% (5–12,24–26,30,35,42,43,45). Virtually all recurrences will be outside the irradiated area, and again, nearly all recurrences are successfully salvaged, most by systemic chemotherapy.

Relapse rates for stage II patients depend on the bulk of disease and are higher than for stage I disease but are still only in the range of 5% to 15%. Nonetheless, due to excellent salvage options postorchiectomy radiotherapy results in disease-specific survival rates above 90% (5,7, 11,12,30,48,49). Patients with bulky disease treated with cisplatin-based chemotherapy still have excellent survival rates, with long-term survival possible even in advanced metastatic disease (20,50).

Because of the success in treating testicular cancer, increased attention is paid to the long-term sequelae resulting from treatment, particularly impaired fertility,

TABLE 26.12	Outcome Following Primary Radiation Therapy for Early Stage Seminoma and Chemotherapy for Bulky or Advanced Stage Seminoma (13,20)	
Stage	**Postorchiectomy treatment**	**5-y progression-free survival (%)**
I	Radiotherapy	95–100
IIA, IIB	Radiotherapy	85–95
IIC and III (M1a)	Chemotherapy	~80
III (M1b)	Chemotherapy	~70

secondary malignancies, and cardiac disease. Men with seminoma commonly have impaired spermatogenesis at baseline; however, use of proper radiotherapy techniques is critical to minimize dose to the remaining testicle and preserve fertility. Second malignancies are increasingly recognized as a significant problem after radiotherapy and/or chemotherapy for testicular cancer, perhaps occurring in close to 20% of patients treated for testicular cancer (51). Current trends toward increased use of surveillance in selected patients and avoidance of mediastinal irradiation should decrease the rates of these serious late effects. In addition, the adoption of smaller volumes and lower doses of RT is predicted to significantly reduce the risk of second malignancy following RT without compromising long-term survival (52).

The relatively indolent course, predictable patterns of early progression, and marked sensitivity to both radiation and chemotherapy make seminoma one of the most curable malignancies. Testicular germ cell tumors have become a model for a curable cancer, with cure being the goal of treatment while optimizing the risks of late effects even in advanced disease. Clinical outcome and survival for nonseminomatous disease is slightly less than that expected for seminoma, but with cisplatin-based treatment, it is still quite good.

REFERENCES

1. Jemal A, Siegel R, Xu J, et al. Cancer statistics, 2010. *CA Cancer J Clin* 2010;60:277–300.
2. Jemal A, Murray T, Ward E, et al. Cancer statistics, 2005. *CA Cancer J Clin* 2005;55:10–30.
3. Ulbright T, Amin M, Young R. Tumors of the testis, adnexa, spermatic cord, and scrotum. In: Rosai J, Sobin H, eds. *Atlas of tumor pathology*, 3rd ed. Washington, DC: Armed Forces Institute of Pathology, 1999.
4. Ries L, Eisner M, Kosary C. *SEER Cancer Statistics Review, 1975–2001*. Bethesda, MD: National Cancer Institute, 2004.
5. Bayens YC, Helle PA, Van Putten WL, et al. Orchidectomy followed by radiotherapy in 176 stage I and II testicular seminoma patients: benefits of a 10-year follow-up study. *Radiother Oncol* 1992;25:97–102.
6. van Rooy EM, Sagerman RH. Long-term evaluation of postorchiectomy irradiation for stage I seminoma. *Radiology* 1994;191:857–861.
7. Bamberg M, Schmidberger H, Meisner C, et al. Radiotherapy for stages I and IIA/B testicular seminoma. *Int J Cancer* 1999;83:823–827.
8. Bauman GS, Venkatesan VM, Ago CT, et al. Postoperative radiotherapy for Stage I/II seminoma: results for 212 patients. *Int J Radiat Oncol Biol Phys* 1998;42:313–317.
9. Coleman JM, Coleman RE, Turner AR, et al. The management and clinical course of testicular seminoma: 15 years' experience at a single institution. *Clin Oncol (R Coll Radiol)* 1998;10:237–241.
10. Giacchetti S, Raoul Y, Wibault P, et al. Treatment of stage I testis seminoma by radiotherapy: long-term results—a 30-year experience. *Int J Radiat Oncol Biol Phys* 1993;27:3–9.
11. Lai PP, Bernstein MJ, Kim H, et al. Radiation therapy for stage I and IIA testicular seminoma. *Int J Radiat Oncol Biol Phys* 1994;28:373–379.
12. Dosmann MA, Zagars GK. Post-orchiectomy radiotherapy for stages I and II testicular seminoma. *Int J Radiat Oncol Biol Phys* 1993;26:381–390.
13. International Germ Cell Consensus Classification: a prognostic factor-based staging system for metastatic germ cell cancers. International Germ Cell Cancer Collaborative Group. *J Clin Oncol* 1997;15:594–603.
14. Bosl GJ, Motzer RJ. Testicular germ-cell cancer. *N Engl J Med* 1997;337:242–253.
15. Aetiology of testicular cancer: association with congenital abnormalities, age at puberty, infertility, and exercise. United Kingdom Testicular Cancer Study Group. *BMJ* 1994;308:1393–1399.
16. Marks LB, Shipley WU, Walker TG, et al. Role of lymphangiography in staging testicular seminoma. *Urology* 1991;38:264–266.
17. Petersen PM, Skakkebaek NE, Vistisen K, et al. Semen quality and reproductive hormones before orchiectomy in men with testicular cancer. *J Clin Oncol* 1999;17:941–947.
18. Capelouto CC, Clark PE, Ransil BJ, et al. A review of scrotal violation in testicular cancer: is adjuvant local therapy necessary? *J Urol* 1995;153:981–985.
19. Greene F, Page D, Fleming I, et al. *AJCC cancer staging manual*, 6th ed. New York: Springer, 2002.
20. Schmoll HJ, Souchon R, Krege S, et al. European consensus on diagnosis and treatment of germ cell cancer: a report of the European Germ Cell Cancer Consensus Group (EGCCCG). *Ann Oncol* 2004;15:1377–1399.
21. Warde P, Jewett MA. Surveillance for stage I testicular seminoma. Is it a good option? *Urol Clin North Am* 1998;25:425–433.
22. Warde P, Specht L, Horwich A, et al. Prognostic factors for relapse in stage I seminoma managed by surveillance: a pooled analysis. *J Clin Oncol* 2002;20:4448–4452.
23. Fossa SD, Oldenburg J, Dahl AA. Short- and long-term morbidity after treatment for testicular cancer. *BJU Int* 2009;104:1418–1422.
24. Fossa SD, Horwich A, Russell JM, et al. Optimal planning target volume for stage I testicular seminoma: a Medical Research Council randomized trial. Medical Research Council Testicular Tumor Working Group. *J Clin Oncol* 1999;17:1146.
25. Jones WG, Fossa SD, Mead GM, et al. Randomized trial of 30 versus 20 Gy in the adjuvant treatment of stage I testicular seminoma: a report on Medical Research Council Trial TE18, European Organisation for the Research and Treatment of Cancer Trial 30942 (ISRCTN18525328). *J Clin Oncol* 2005;23:1200–1208.
26. Oliver RT, Mason MD, Mead GM, et al. Radiotherapy versus single-dose carboplatin in adjuvant treatment of stage I seminoma: a randomised trial. *Lancet* 2005;366:293–300.
27. Aparicio J, Germa JR, Garcia del Muro X, et al. Risk-adapted management for patients with clinical stage I seminoma: the Second Spanish Germ Cell Cancer Cooperative Group study. *J Clin Oncol* 2005;23:8717–8723.

28. Bamias A, Aravantinos G, Deliveliotis C, et al. Two cycles of etoposide/cisplatin cured all patients with stage I testicular seminoma: risk-adapted protocol of the Hellenic Cooperative Oncology Group. *Urology* 2007;70:1179–1183.

29. Powles T, Robinson D, Shamash J, et al. The long-term risks of adjuvant carboplatin treatment for stage I seminoma of the testis. *Ann Oncol* 2008;19:443–447.

30. Classen J, Schmidberger H, Meisner C, et al. Radiotherapy for stages IIA/B testicular seminoma: final report of a prospective multicenter clinical trial. *J Clin Oncol* 2003;21:1101–1106.

31. Warde P, Gospodarowicz M, Panzarella T, et al. Management of stage II seminoma. *J Clin Oncol* 1998;16:290–294.

32. Garcia-del-Muro X, Maroto P, Guma J, et al. Chemotherapy as an alternative to radiotherapy in the treatment of stage IIA and IIB testicular seminoma: a Spanish Germ Cell Cancer Group Study. *J Clin Oncol* 2008;26:5416–5421.

33. Gilbert DC, Vanas NJ, Beesley S, et al. Treating IIA/B seminoma with combination carboplatin and radiotherapy. *J Clin Oncol* 2009;27:2101–2102; author reply 2102–2103.

34. Patterson H, Norman AR, Mitra SS, et al. Combination carboplatin and radiotherapy in the management of stage II testicular seminoma: comparison with radiotherapy treatment alone. *Radiother Oncol* 2001;59:5–11.

35. Gospodarwicz MK, Sturgeon JF, Jewett MA. Early stage and advanced seminoma: role of radiation therapy, surgery, and chemotherapy. *Semin Oncol* 1998;25:160–173.

36. Zagars GK, Ballo MT, Lee AK, et al. Mortality after cure of testicular seminoma. *J Clin Oncol* 2004;22:640–647.

37. Peckham MJ, Hendry WF. Clinical stage II non-seminomatous germ cell testicular tumours. Results of management by primary chemotherapy. *Br J Urol* 1985;57:763–768.

38. De Santis M, Bokemeyer C, Becherer A, et al. Predictive impact of 2-18 fluoro-2-deoxy-D-glucose positron emission tomography for residual postchemotherapy masses in patients with bulky seminoma. *J Clin Oncol* 2001;19:3740–3744.

39. Duchesne GM, Stenning SP, Aass N, et al. Radiotherapy after chemotherapy for metastatic seminoma—a diminishing role. MRC Testicular Tumour Working Party. *Eur J Cancer* 1997;33:829–835.

40. von der Maase H, Specht L, Jacobsen GK, et al. Surveillance following orchidectomy for stage I seminoma of the testis. *Eur J Cancer* 1993;29A:1931–1934.

41. Warde PR, Gospodarowicz MK, Goodman PJ, et al. Results of a policy of surveillance in stage I testicular seminoma. *Int J Radiat Oncol Biol Phys* 1993;27:11–15.

42. Dosoretz DE, Shipley WU, Blitzer PH, et al. Megavoltage irradiation for pure testicular seminoma: results and patterns of failure. *Cancer* 1981;48:2184–2190.

43. Fossa SD, Aass N, Kaalhus O. Radiotherapy for testicular seminoma stage I: treatment results and long-term post-irradiation morbidity in 365 patients. *Int J Radiat Oncol Biol Phys* 1989;16:383–388.

44. Marks LB, Anscher MS, Shipley WU. Radiation therapy for testicular seminoma: controversies in the management of early-stage disease. *Oncology (Williston Park)* 1992;6:43–48; discussion 51–52.

45. Warde P, Gospodarowicz MK, Panzarella T, et al. Stage I testicular seminoma: results of adjuvant irradiation and surveillance. *J Clin Oncol* 1995;13:2255–2262.

46. Fraass BA, Kinsella TJ, Harrington FS, et al. Peripheral dose to the testes: the design and clinical use of a practical and effective gonadal shield. *Int J Radiat Oncol Biol Phys* 1985;11:609–615.

47. Bieri S, Rouzaud M, Miralbell R. Seminoma of the testis: is scrotal shielding necessary when radiotherapy is limited to the para-aortic nodes? *Radiother Oncol* 1999;50:349–353.

48. Vallis KA, Howard GC, Duncan W, et al. Radiotherapy for stages I and II testicular seminoma: results and morbidity in 238 patients. *Br J Radiol* 1995;68:400–405.

49. Whipple GL, Sagerman RH, van Rooy EM. Long-term evaluation of postorchiectomy radiotherapy for stage II seminoma. *Am J Clin Oncol* 1997;20:196–201.

50. Mencel PJ, Motzer RJ, Mazumdar M, et al. Advanced seminoma: treatment results, survival, and prognostic factors in 142 patients. *J Clin Oncol* 1994;12:120–126.

51. Travis LB, Curtis RE, Storm H, et al. Risk of second malignant neoplasms among long-term survivors of testicular cancer. *J Natl Cancer Inst* 1997;89:1429–1439.

52. Zwahlen DR, Martin JM, Millar JL, et al. Effect of radiotherapy volume and dose on secondary cancer risk in stage I testicular seminoma. *Int J Radiat Oncol Biol Phys* 2008;70:853–858.

CHAPTER 27

The Lymphomas

Joachim Yahalom

INTRODUCTION

Lymphomas are malignant neoplasms arising in the lymphatic system, most commonly in lymph nodes. Yet, lymphomas may appear in any organ of the body where lymphocytes are present or may travel into. Lymphomas that arise outside the lymph nodes are called *extranodal* lymphomas. We recognize two main groups of lymphomas: The Hodgkin's lymphomas (HL) and the non-Hodgkin's lymphomas (NHL). The HL includes two categories: lymphocyte-predominant Hodgkin's lymphomas (LPHL) and classical HL. The NHL is a more heterogeneous group that includes many entities with different characteristics and prognosis. This chapter will address general principles of radiation treatment of NHL, rather than each individual lymphoma or organ-specific involvement. The standard approaches for management of HL and NHL are outlined in the annually updated guidelines of the U.S. National Comprehensive Cancer Network (NCCN) (1,2).

In general, the lymphomas are among the most radiosensitive malignancies, and indeed, ionizing radiation is a highly effective modality for the treatment of both HL and NHL. The dramatic effects of radiation alone in reducing large lesions and even eliminating HL lesions were reported more than 100 years ago, soon after the discovery of x-rays by Wilhelm Conard Roentgen. Yet, during the first half of the twentieth century, due to technical constraints and/or poor methods of delivering radiation, all lymphomas remained incurable; radiation was used mostly for palliation and responses were brief. As x-ray technology improved in the 1940s and the concept of irradiating beyond the involved area was adopted, patients with early stage HL and NHL could be cured with radiation alone—the only effective curative modality that was available for lymphomas until the late 1960s.

Before the advent of effective chemotherapy, attempts were made to cure even advanced HL and NHL by maximizing the use of radiation alone. Optimizing the selection of patients and tailoring the radiation fields were associated with aggressive staging efforts that included using staging laparotomy and splenectomy for HL and even NHL. Moreover, the dependency on radiotherapy (RT) as the primary modality required wide extension of the radiation field as well as raising the dose to normal tissue tolerance levels. Although this mega-RT led to the cure of many patients, it

was also associated with late development of complications and increased the mortality of cured patients beyond what was expected of the normal population. This was the price of successfully pioneering radiation therapy as a curative modality before the availability of effective chemotherapy.

The emergence of more effective and less toxic chemotherapy over the last three decades led to considerable changes in the use of RT in the management of lymphomas. First, in several types of NHL and in classical HL, chemotherapy has become the primary modality with RT used for consolidation and reduction of the risk of relapse. Yet, in some lymphomas, mostly in early stage low-grade lymphomas where chemotherapy is less effective, radiation alone remained the primary standard of care.

Radiation alone is currently the treatment of choice for early stage follicular lymphoma, mucosa-associated lymphoid tissue (MALT) lymphoma, and LPHL. The role of RT in consolidation following chemotherapy is well established in early stage "classic" HL, whereas in advanced-stage HL following programs of brief chemotherapy or following incomplete response. RT also plays an important role in high-dose therapy programs for salvage of HL and NHL. In early stage "aggressive" NHL, consolidation with RT is also the standard of care.

RT is also an excellent palliative modality that provides long-term local control and clinical benefit even for lymphomas in advanced stage such as mantle cell lymphoma (MCL), small lymphocytic lymphoma, advanced-stage MALT lymphoma, and follicular lymphoma. These specific types of lymphoma are highly sensitive to radiation and very low doses may be adequate for local control. The indications for using RT for treating lymphomas are summarized in Table 27.1.

BASICS OF STAGING AND PROGNOSTIC GROUPS

The staging system (3) for both HL and NHL is detailed in Table 27.2. The assignment of stage is based on the following:

- The number of involved sites
- Whether lymph nodes are involved on both sides of the diaphragm and whether this involvement is bulky (particularly in the mediastinum)

TABLE 27.1	**Indications for Radiotherapy in the Treatment of Lymphomas**

Radiation alone—potentially curative
- Hodgkin's lymphoma—lymphocyte predominance
  Stage I–II
- Hodgkin's lymphoma—classical[a]
  Stage IA–IIA (nonbulky)
- Follicular lymphoma
  Stage I–II
  Stage III (rarely used)
- Extranodal marginal zone (MALT) lymphoma
  Stage IE–IIE
- Nodal marginal zone lymphoma
  Stage I–II
- Mycosis fungoides
  Stage IA, IB, IIA
- Anaplastic large cell lymphoma of skin
  Stage IE

Radiation is part of a combined-modality treatment—potentially curable
- Hodgkin's lymphoma—classical
  Stage I–II (favorable and unfavorable)
- Hodgkin's lymphoma
  Advanced stage[b]
- Diffuse large B cell lymphoma
  Stage I–II
- Primary mediastinal lymphoma
  Stage I–II
- Peripheral T cell lymphoma
  Stage I–II
- Extranodal natural killer/T cell lymphoma–nasal type
- Primary central nervous system lymphoma
- In high-dose therapy programs for Hodgkin's lymphoma, diffuse large B cell lymphoma, follicular lymphoma, and mantle cell lymphoma

Radiation is effective for palliation and local control—highly sensitive
- Follicular lymphoma
- Mantle cell lymphoma
- Small lymphocytic lymphoma/chronic lymphocytic leukemia
- Marginal zone lymphoma
- Mycosis fungoides

Radiation is effective for palliation and local control—moderately sensitive
- Diffuse large cell lymphoma

[a]Combined modality is treatment of choice.
[b]For bulky sites, incomplete response, and as part of brief chemotherapy program (e.g., Stanford V).
MALT, mucosa associated lymphoid tissue.

- Whether there is contiguous extranodal involvement (E sites) or disseminated extranodal disease
- Whether typical systemic symptoms (B symptoms) are present

In defining the stage of the disease, it is important to note how the information was obtained, because this fact reflects on the remaining uncertainties in the evaluation of the extent of disease. Clinical staging refers to information that has been obtained by initial biopsy, history, physical examination, and laboratory and radiographic studies only. A pathologic stage is determined by more extensive surgical assessment of potentially involved sites, for example, by surgical staging laparotomy and splenectomy.

TABLE 27.2	The Cotswald's Modification of the Ann Arbor Staging for Hodgkin's Lymphomas and Non-Hodgkin's Lymphomas

Stage description

Stage I Involvement of a single lymph node region or lymphoid structure (e.g., spleen, thymus, Waldeyer's ring)

Stage II Involvement of two or more lymph node regions on the same side of the diaphragm (i.e., the mediastinum is a single site, hilar lymph nodes are lateralized). The number of anatomic sites should be indicated by a subscript (e.g., II_2)

Stage III Involvement of lymph node regions or structures on both sides of the diaphragm:
III_1: With or without involvement of splenic, hilar, celiac, or portal nodes
III_2: With involvement of para-aortic, iliac, or mesenteric nodes

Stage IV Involvement of extranodal site(s) beyond that designated E

Designations applicable to any disease stage

A   No symptoms

B   Presence of either fever, drenching sweats, or weight loss

X   Bulky disease:
>1/3 the width of the mediastinum
>10 cm maximal dimension of nodal mass

E   Involvement of a single extranodal site, contiguous or proximal to a known nodal site

CS Clinical stage

PS Pathologic stage

Prognostic Factors for Early Stage Hodgkin's Lymphomas

In practice, most experts categorize HL as either early stage (stages I–II) or advanced stage (stages III–IV). In the early stage category, it is important to distinguish between favorable early stage and unfavorable early stage. To be considered as unfavorable early stage, one or more of the following should be present: B symptoms, bulky disease, or involvement of more than three sites.

INDICATIONS FOR RADIOTHERAPY

Hodgkin's Lymphoma

It is important to distinguish between the two well-defined entities of HL, classical HL, and the less common nodular LPHL. The radiation approach to each entity is different. Most patients with LPHL are potentially curable with radiation alone, whereas combined-modality therapy is the standard approach for most patients with classical HL.

Lymphocyte-Predominant Hodgkin's Lymphoma

Most (>75%) patients with LPHL present at an early stage; the disease is commonly limited to one peripheral site (neck, axilla, or groin) and involvement of the mediastinum is extremely rare. The treatment recommendations for LPHL differ markedly from those for classic HL. Involved or regional field radiation alone is the standard

treatment for all early stage LPHL. It should be emphasized that even if regional radiation fields are selected, the uninvolved mediastinum should not be irradiated, thereby avoiding the site most prone for radiation-related short- and long-term side effects. Although there has not been a study that compared extended-field RT (commonly used in the past) with involved-field radiotherapy (IFRT), retrospective data suggest that IFRT is adequate (4). The radiation dose recommended is between 30 and 36 Gy with an optional additional boost of 4 Gy to a (rare) bulky site. In most cases, chemotherapy is not indicated.

Classical Hodgkin's Lymphoma

Early Stage (Favorable and Unfavorable). Over the last two decades, the treatment of early stage classical HL has drastically changed. Combined-modality therapy consisting of short-course chemotherapy (most often doxorubicin [Adriamycin], bleomycin, vinblastine, dacarbazine [ABVD]) consolidated by reduced-dose radiation carefully directed only to the involved lymph node(s) site successfully replaced radiation alone as the treatment of choice (1,5). Although no longer the primary treatment, RT limited to smaller volumes, administered to a reduced dose with improved targeting, which is achieved with new imaging technology and supported by modern delivery systems, remains an important component of effective treatment programs for HL.

In the early 1960s, the implementation of a new concept—irradiating all involved and uninvolved lymph nodes—was termed *radical RT* (6). Radical RT soon cured an increasing number of patients with HL, a disease that was then considered incurable. Radiotherapists used the newly available linear accelerators to treat enormous fields termed *total lymphoid irradiation* (*TLI*). TLI spared little other than brain, limbs, and some of the lungs, liver, and kidneys. Bulky sites were covered with large radiation field margins, and occasionally, even the lungs and the liver were intentionally irradiated. Mechlorethamine, vincristine (Oncovin), procarbazine, and prednisone (MOPP) chemotherapy was used for consolidation or salvage. The giant radiation field size compensated for lack of good imaging information. The dose was also maximized (the standard dose at Stanford was 44 Gy), and often treatment was given in a technique that delivered even higher doses anteriorly, to the heart and breast.

Although the above approaches are not used anymore, it should be appreciated that, thanks to those pioneering efforts, tens of thousands of young patients who were treated during the 1960s, 1970s, and 1980s survive today, free of HL. Indeed, some succumbed to the early and to the then unknown, late treatment-related toxicities, such as leukemia and lung cancer related to MOPP and other chemotherapy regimens (7), or developed breast, lung, other solid tumors, and coronary heart disease related to radiation.

Through a series of randomized trials, the following treatment principles have been established: ABVD is better than MOPP and is less toxic (8); combined modality is more effective and less toxic than radical radiation alone (9); when combined with chemotherapy, the radiation field could be minimized to include only the involved site (IFRT) (10) and the radiation dose can be reduced from over 40 to 30 Gy and possibly even lower (11), and only four cycles of ABVD are sufficient in early stage (and probably only two cycles in favorable disease) when used with mini-RT (12).

The conversion from large multisite radiation fields to a smaller and better-defined radiation field also allowed for accurate conformal radiation therapy. The large fields of the past limited the radiation technique to two simple opposed anterior and posterior fields. The conversion to smaller and better-defined radiation volumes allowed the utilization of more conformal radiation therapy, based on better imaging, computerized planning programs, and when indicated, advanced tools such as intensity-modulated radiotherapy (IMRT). Modern breakthroughs in RT technology can now be implemented in HL to increase accuracy even further, avoid normal organs irradiation, and thereby improve the therapeutic ratio.

Advanced-Stage Hodgkin's Lymphoma. The role of consolidation RT after induction chemotherapy depends on several factors: The response to chemotherapy (complete, uncertain, or partial), the presence of bulky disease before chemotherapy, and the type and length of the chemotherapy program. Patients who had no bulky disease, have received the full course of chemotherapy (e.g., ABVD X 6–8), and obtained an unquestionable complete response (CR) are unlikely to benefit from additional RT (13). IFRT should be added in patients with advanced-

stage HL who present with bulky disease or to patients who remain in an uncertain or incomplete remission after chemotherapy. When advanced-stage HL is treated with the new highly effective and less toxic treatment program of Stanford V, it is imperative to follow the brief chemotherapy program with IFRT to sites originally >5 cm or to a clinically involved spleen. When RT was fully or partially omitted on this program, the results were inferior (14).

Salvage Programs for Refractory and Relapsed Hodgkin's Lymphoma. High-dose therapy supported by autologous stem cell transplantation (ASCT) has become a standard salvage treatment for patients who relapsed or remained refractory to chemotherapy or to combined-modality therapy. Many of the patients who enter these programs have not received prior RT or had a relapse at sites outside the original radiation field. These patients could benefit from integrating RT into the salvage regimen.

At Memorial Sloan-Kettering Cancer Center (MSKCC), a program that integrated RT into the high-dose regimen for salvage of Hodgkin's disease (HD) was developed almost 20 years ago, and modified every several years. Accelerated hyperfractionated irradiation (b.i.d. fractions of 1.8 Gy each) is scheduled to start after the completion of reinduction chemotherapy and stem cell collection and before the high-dose chemotherapy and stem cell transplantation. Patients who had not been previously irradiated received IFRT (18 Gy in 5 days) to sites of initially bulky (>5 cm) disease and/or residual clinical abnormalities followed by TLI of 18 Gy (1.8 Gy per fraction, b.i.d.) within an additional 5 days. Patients who had prior RT, received only IFRT (when feasible) to a maximal dose of 36 Gy. This treatment strategy has been in place since 1985, with over 350 patients treated so far. The program has been very effective in salvaging both relapsed and chemotherapy-refractory patients, has a low toxic profile with no mortality for the last 10 years, and compares favorably with programs that do not use RT as critical part of the regimen (15,16).

NON-HODGKIN'S LYMPHOMA ENTITIES THAT ARE COMMONLY TREATED WITH RADIOTHERAPY

Follicular Lymphoma

Approximately 20% of patients with low-grade follicular lymphomas present in localized stages (I–II). The standard treatment for these patients is regional RT or IFRT. The reports of patients with stage I and II low-grade follicular lymphoma from Stanford with long-term follow-up indicated that a substantial number of patients in this category have, indeed, been "cured" by RT (17). The median follow-up was 7.7 years and observation has been maintained for up to 31 years. The median survival after RT was 14 years. The actuarial survival rates at 5, 10, 15, and 20 years were 82%, 64%, 44%, and 35%, respectively. Freedom from relapse (FFR) at 5, 10, 15, and 20 years was 55%, 44%, 40%, and 37%, respectively. Only 5 of 47 patients who reached 10 years without a relapse developed a late recurrence. There was no significant FFR difference between stages I and II or between nodal or extranodal disease. The survival of patients irradiated after the age of 60 was significantly shorter than the survival of younger patients, but the decrease of survival in this age group was strongly affected by death from other causes.

Most relapses in early stage patients occur in unirradiated sites during the first 5 to 6 years following therapy (18). In the Stanford series, administration of RT to nodal sites on both sides of the diaphragm was associated with a significantly better FFR compared with more localized treatment but did not translate into a clear survival benefit (17). A similar experience was reported from M.D. Anderson (19). In the absence of a clear survival benefit for TLI in this setting, the common involvement of mesenteric nodes that may require whole abdominal irradiation, and considering the fact that almost half of the patients will eventually require chemotherapy for relapse, involved or regional field irradiation is currently employed for these patients.

The optimal radiation dose for indolent lymphoma has not been determined in a prospective study. However, most current RT series for stages I and II indolent lymphomas usually employ 30 to 40 Gy, and in-field recurrences have been uncommon. Data from the Princess Margaret Hospital showed in-field disease control in 78% of patients treated with doses of <25 Gy and 91% control with doses >25 Gy (20). At M.D. Anderson, excellent local control was achieved with 30 Gy to lesions <3 cm (19). Fuks correlated the relapse rate in regional areas of follicular lymphoma with the radiation dose delivered to these sites and showed 63% relapse in areas receiving <27.5 Gy, 27% relapse with a dose range of 30 to 35 Gy, 12% and 6% relapse rate for 40 and 44 Gy, respectively (21). A dose of 30 to 36 Gy (in 1.8 Gy daily fractions) to involved sites (40 Gy, if bulky) and 24 to 36 Gy to uninvolved adjacent sites is currently recommended.

Extranodal Marginal Zone Lymphoma of Mucosa-Associated Lymphoid Tissue

The most common organ involved with MALT lymphoma is the stomach. Gastric MALT lymphoma (GML) is often associated with the presence of *Helicobacter pylori* in the stomach and the antibiotic eradication of this pathogen leads to regression of GML in many patients. Yet, approximately 30% to 50% of patients with *H. pylori*-positive GML will show persistent or progressing lymphoma even after eradication of *H. pylori* with antibiotic therapy and even in complete responders, almost 15% will relapse within 3 years, suggesting that about half of the patients with GML will eventually be considered for additional therapies (22). Most of those will still have disease limited to the stomach. In these patients and in those that present

with no evidence of *H. pylori* infection IFRT with relatively low radiation dose is the treatment of choice (2).

Several institutions reported excellent results using IFRT of the stomach in *H. pylori*-independent GML patients who either failed antibiotic therapy or had no evidence of *H. pylori* infection (23–26). The recent update of the MSKCC experience included 51 patients with GML (stage I-39; stage II-10; stage IV-2) who were either *H. pylori*-negative (30 patients) or remained with persistent lymphoma after antibiotic therapies and adequate observation (21 patients) (27). All patients were treated with radiation to the stomach and perigastric nodes; the median total dose was 30 Gy in 4 weeks. All patients had regular follow-up endoscopic evaluations and biopsies. Forty-nine of fifty-one (96%) patients obtained a biopsy-proven CR. Of the three patients who relapsed, two were salvaged. Three patients died of other malignancies; all second tumors developed outside the radiation field. At a median follow-up of 4 years, freedom from treatment failure, overall survival (OS), and cause-specific survival were 89%, 83%, and 100%, respectively. Treatment was well tolerated, with no significant acute or chronic side effects. The experience from Toronto and Boston, using the same radiation approach, was equally successful (28–30) supporting the approach that modest dose IFRT is the treatment of choice for patients with persistent GML who have exhausted the antibiotic therapy approach or are unlikely to respond to it (*H. pylori*-negative patients) (31,32). The techniques for treatment of gastric lymphoma have been recently published (33).

MALT lymphomas (ML) have also been described in various nongastric sites, such as salivary glands, skin, orbit, conjunctiva, lung, thyroid, larynx, breast, kidney, liver, bladder, prostate, urethra, small intestine, rectum, pancreas, and even in the intracranial dura (32).

The optimal management of non-GMLs has not yet been clearly established. Retrospective series included patients treated with surgery, RT, and chemotherapy, alone or in combination. Marginal zone lymphomas are exquisitely sensitive to relatively low doses of radiation. Specifically, ML in sites such as salivary glands, ocular, conjunctiva, thyroid, breast, and bladder have been successfully eradicated with IFRT encompassing the involved organ alone with a dose of 24 to 36 Gy (28,30). Even unusual sites (such as larynx, base of skull, urethra, and prostate) not easily amenable to surgery have been well controlled by IFRT.

Radiation Therapy for Relapsed and Refractory Low-Grade Lymphomas

While chemotherapy and antibody therapy are the primary treatments for advanced-stage low-grade lymphomas, the very high sensitivity of these lymphomas to radiation should not be ignored. Even extremely low doses of radiation can provide long-standing local control and effective palliation. Several European groups showed that patients with low-grade lymphoma and persistent or relapsed disease following several regimens of chemotherapy, responded to only two treatments of 2 Gy each (a total of 4 Gy). Using this schedule, a Dutch group reported in 109 patients (304 symptomatic sites), mostly with follicular lymphoma, an overall response rate of 92% and a CR rate of 61% (34,35). The 2-year actuarial freedom from local progression (FFLP) rate was 56%. Similarly, a French team reported an objective response of 81% of the sites, with 57% attaining a complete remission. The 2-year actuarial FFLP rate was 56% (36).

Mantle Cell Lymphoma

Although MCL presents in stage IV in most patients and is treated primarily with chemotherapy, its exquisite sensitivity to radiation should not be ignored. A British Columbia Cancer Center study indicated that patients with MCL stages I to II benefited significantly from localized RT alone or RT combined with chemotherapy. The 5-year progression-free survival (PFS) was 68% for those receiving RT compared with 11% in patients not receiving RT ($p = 0.002$), 6-year OS was 71% and 25%, respectively ($p = 0.13$) (37). At MSKCC, low-dose RT was used for local control and palliation of 38 sites in 21 patients previously treated with chemotherapy. Local control with radiation was achieved in all sites and a CR was achieved in 64% of the sites. Ninety-four percent of symptomatic patients obtained pain control with RT. Local progression occurred in 34% of the patients at a median time to progression of 10 months. Because only a low dose of radiation is required (15–30 Gy) in MCL, large nodal sites may be treated with only minor side effects and without jeopardizing other future therapeutic options.

Diffuse Large B Cell Lymphoma

Early Stage

In the past, radiation alone was considered an appropriate treatment for patients with localized (stage I–II) diffuse large B cell lymphoma (DLBCL). Young patients with low-bulk stage I DLBCL obtained 10 years survival rate of 87%, but other patients have relapsed at a rate >50%.

Until the 1980s, most patients with early stage aggressive lymphoma were treated with RT alone (18). In clinically staged patients, the use of regional or extended-field irra-

diation for stage I disease resulted in a cure rate of ~50%. The survival of similarly treated stage II patients was only 20% (38). Most of the relapses in patients treated with RT alone were extranodal or occurred outside the irradiated field. More restrictive selection of patients (stage I only), utilizing staging laparotomy and treatment with extensive fields of radiation, yielded a 10-year relapse-free survival rate of 90% to 100% (39). Still, even staging laparotomy and TLI yielded unsatisfactory survival rates of 35% to 55% in patients with pathologic stage II disease (40).

The present standard of care for early stage DLBCL is a short course of doxorubicin-based chemotherapy (usually cyclophosphamide, doxorubicin, vincristine, and prednisone [CHOP]), followed by IFRT. Two prospective studies (by Eastern Cooperative Oncology Group [ECOG] and Southwest Oncology Group [SWOG]) have demonstrated that the combination is more effective and less toxic compared with a longer course of chemotherapy alone (Table 27.3). The ECOG study involved patients with bulky or extranodal stage I and II intermediate-grade NHL (according to the Working Formulation) (14). All patients received eight cycles of CHOP chemotherapy. Patients who attained only a partial response following chemotherapy received IFRT of 40 Gy, and 28% converted to complete-response status. Patients with CR (61%) following chemotherapy alone were randomly assigned either to receive RT of 30 Gy to site pretreatment involvement or to observation alone. The recent 15-year update showed a statistically significant advantage to the adjuvant RT arm. The patients who received adjuvant RT attained a better failure-free survival rate than those receiving CHOP alone (54% vs. 39%; $p = 0.06$) (14). Overall survival that included all courses of death in this aging population was better in the irradiated group (60% vs. 44%) but the difference was not statistically significant. Cause-specific survival was not reported.

The SWOG study enrolled patients with stage I and nonbulky stage II aggressive NHL. The patients were randomly assigned to receive either eight cycles of CHOP chemotherapy alone or three cycles of CHOP, followed by an IFRT of 40 Gy (with an optional boost of up to 55 Gy). At a median follow-up of 4 years, the PFS rate was significantly greater for the short-course CHOP plus RT group: 77% compared with 66% in the group receiving eight cycles of CHOP with no RT. The combined-modality

TABLE 27.3	**Role of Radiotherapy in Stage I to II Aggressive Lymphomas: Randomized Studies**			
	Progression-free survival (%)			
Reference	**Patients _n_**	**CHOP%**	**CHOP-RT%**	**_p_ value**
Horning et al. (14)	345	39	54	0.06
Miller et al. (41)	401	66	77	0.01

CHOP, cyclophosphamide, doxorubicin, vincristine, and prednisone; RT, radiotherapy.

treatment also resulted in a superior OS rate (87% vs. 75%; $p = 0.01$). In addition, reversible toxicity occurring during therapy also favored the combined-modality arm (41). Recent analysis of the SWOG data suggested that patients with early stage modified high International Prognostic Index (IPI) had inferior survival and may require more than three cycles of chemotherapy (42).

The results of both randomized studies confirm the importance of adjuvant radiation therapy to the involved field in patients who attained a CR following short (three cycles) or long (eight cycles) chemotherapy. A relatively low dose of 30 Gy was adequate for patients who attained a CR in the ECOG study (using eight cycles of CHOP), whereas a higher dose (40–55 Gy) was used in the short chemotherapy arm of the SWOG study. Consolidation with a dose of 30 to 36 Gy for patients who have attained an unquestionable CR following three to six cycles of chemotherapy is currently advocated. This is based on our excellent local control data with dose range and also that of others (43,44). Yet, other groups advocate doses in the range of 39 to 51 Gy for lymphomas >3.5 cm (45). A higher dose (40–50 Gy) is advised for uncertain complete responses. For evaluating response, obtaining positron emission tomography–computed tomography (PET–CT) scans before and after chemotherapy is recommended, because a positive PET scan following chemotherapy may indicate an incomplete response that mandates a more aggressive approach.

Advanced Stage

The standard treatment for patients with advanced-stage (III or IV) aggressive lymphoma is combination chemotherapy, and rituximab-CHOP (R-CHOP) is the most commonly used combination (42). In North America, radiation therapy as consolidation to even bulky sites or incomplete responders is rarely being considered, although supported by retrospective studies (46). Surprisingly, the data regarding the irrelevance of RT in these situations are scanty and/or indirect, at best (47).

Unfortunately, although the superiority of combined modality over chemotherapy alone has been established for early stages of NHL in the United States, the concept and the feasibility have not been tested in trials for advanced-stage NHL. It is of interest that recent randomized studies from other countries suggest that RT, particularly if administered to areas of originally bulky disease, may significantly improve the relapse-free survival and OS of patients who attained a CR with chemotherapy (48–51).

Investigators from Mexico City conducted two consecutive randomized studies with a similar design. In the first study, 218 patients with stage IV diffuse large cell lymphoma (DLCL) were included. Following chemotherapy, 155 patients (71%) achieved a CR. Of the complete responders, 88 patients (56%) originally presented with bulky disease (>10 cm) and therefore were prospectively randomized to observation or to receive IFRT at a dose of 40 to 50 Gy. At 5 years, 72% of 43 patients randomized to receive RT were alive and disease-free as compared with only 35% of the

45 patients who were not irradiated ($p < 0.01$). Most of the relapses occurred in the original site. Overall survival also improved for the irradiated patients (81% vs. 55%; $p < 0.01$) (48). In the more recent study, 341 patients with aggressive DLCL and the presence of nodal bulky disease (tumor mass >10 cm) in pathologically proved CR after intensive chemotherapy were randomized to receive RT (involved fields, 40 Gy) or not. The 5-year event-free survival (EFS) and OS in radiated patients were 82% and 87%, respectively. Both EFS and OS were significantly better in the control group: EFS—55% ($p < 0.001$) and OS—66% ($p < 0.01$), respectively. RT was well tolerated, acute toxicity was mild, and late toxicity has not appeared so far (51).

These data support the notion that although intermediate-grade NHL is a systemic disease, all stages should primarily be treated with chemotherapy and RT to bulky or residual disease may improve the outcome of the treatment program. Although more studies should address the potential benefit of radiation therapy in advanced-stage disease, the above data provide an adequate basis to justify the combined-modality approach in selected cases.

Primary Mediastinal Lymphoma

In most patients the disease is bulky and limited to the mediastinum. Consolidation with IFRT of the mediastinum after a complete, uncertain, or partial response with chemotherapy is a standard approach in most centers (52,53). Several large retrospective studies have indicated the superiority of the combined-modality approach in primary mediastinal lymphoma over chemotherapy alone (54). Yet, prospective randomized studies evaluating the contribution of RT in mediastinal lymphoma have not been reported.

RADIATION FIELDS: PRINCIPLES AND DESIGN

In the past, the design of radiation fields attempted to include multiple involved and uninvolved lymph node sites. The large fields known as *mantle, inverted Y*, and "TLI" were synonymous with the radiation treatment of HL and NHL. These fields should rarely be used nowadays. The involved field, or its slightly larger version—the regional field, encompasses a significantly smaller but adequate volume when RT is used as consolidation after chemotherapy in HL. Even when radiation is used as the only treatment in LPHL, the field should be limited to the involved site or sites and immediately adjacent lymph node groups. Further, even more limited radiation fields restricted to the originally involved lymph node are currently under study by several European groups.

The many terminologies given to radiation field variations in HL have caused significant confusion and difficulties in comparing treatment programs. Although the final determination of the field may vary from patient to patient and depends on many clinical, anatomic, and normal

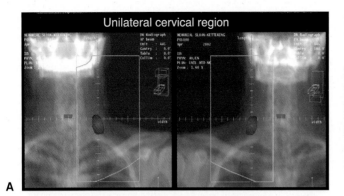

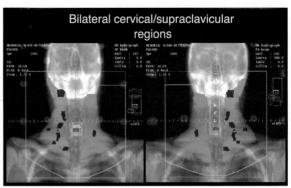

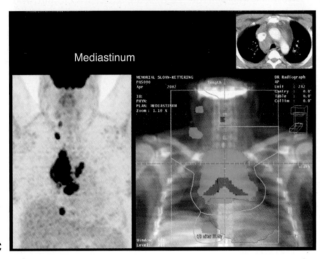

Figure 27.1. Involved-field radiotherapy (IFRT). **A:** Stage I Hodgkin's lymphomas (HL) involving the right neck. **B:** Stage II HL involving the right neck and the left lower neck. **C:** Stage IIX HL with involvement of the right neck, bulky mediastinum, right hilum, and right cardiophrenic area.

tissue tolerance considerations, general definitions and guidelines are available and should be followed.

The following are definitions of types of radiation fields used in HL.

Involved Field

This field is limited to the site of the clinically involved lymph node group. For extranodal sites, the field includes the organ alone (if no evidence for lymph node involvement). The "grouping" of lymph nodes is not clearly defined and involved field borders for common presentation of HL will be discussed in the subsequent text (Fig. 27.1A–C).

Regional Field

This field includes the involved lymph node group field plus at least one adjacent clinically uninvolved group. For extranodal disease, it includes the involved organ plus the clinically uninvolved lymph nodes region (Fig. 27.2).

Extended Field

This field includes *multiple* involved and uninvolved lymph node groups. If the multiple sites are limited to one side of the diaphragm, the upper field is called the *mantle* field. The extended field includes all lymph node sites below the diaphragm (with or without the spleen and is called after its shape—*inverted Y* [Fig. 27.3A,B]).

When the radiation treatment includes all lymph nodes on both sides of the diaphragm, these large fields are combined, and the resulting field is called *TLI* or *total nodal irradiation (TNI)*; if the pelvic lymph nodes are excluded the field is called *subtotal lymphoid irradiation (STLI)* (Fig. 27.4).

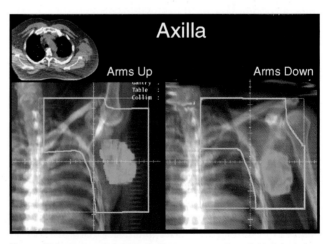

Figure 27.2. Regional field radiotherapy. Stage I Hodgkin's lymphomas (HL) involving the left axilla.

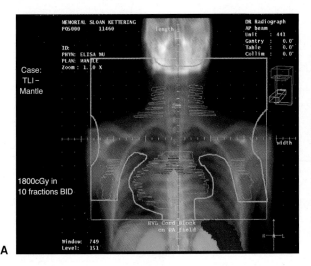
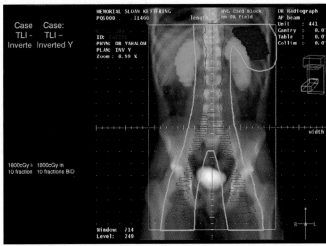

Figure 27.3. Extended field. **A:** Mantle field. **B:** Inverted Y. TLI, total lymphoid irradiation.

Involved Lymph Node(s) Field

This is the most limited radiation field that has just recently been introduced. The clinical treated volume (CTV) includes only the originally involved lymph node(s) volume (prechemotherapy) with the addition of 1 cm margin to create planned treatment volume (PTV).

Considerations in Designing Involved-Field Radiotherapy

Although it is understood that the involved field should address an area smaller than the classical extended fields

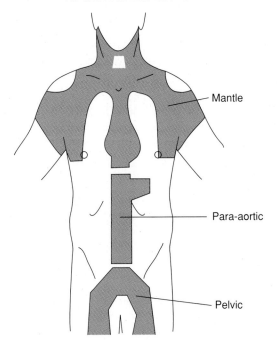

HD and NHL: Extended fields

Mantle

Para-aortic

Pelvic

Figure 27.4. Total lymphoid irradiation (TLI). HD, Hodgkin's disease; NHL, non-Hodgkin's lymphomas.

of mantle or inverted Y, it is not entirely clear how small the field should remain. Should only the area of the enlarged lymph node (with margins) be irradiated? Should a region of lymph nodes be addressed? And if yes, what are the borders of this region? Many use the lymph node region diagram that was adopted for staging purposes at the Rye symposium (1966) to define a region of lymph nodes. However, this diagram was not developed for individual radiation field design and strangely enough the chart distinguishes between a mediastinal and a hilar region, has a separate infraclavicular lymph region, and does not provide borders of the individual sites. Other questions relate to the change in size (or complete resolution) of the lymph node after chemotherapy. Should the prechemotherapy volume be irradiated? Or should we spare the tissues (such as lung) that are no longer involved by the disease by irradiating the postchemotherapy residual abnormality alone?

There are no definitive answers to the above questions and it is often the individual clinical situation that affects the field design. At the same time, uniform general guidelines are important for assuring a high standard of treatment and are essential for collaborative group studies.

Suggested guidelines for delineating the involved field to nodal sites areas follows: (55)

1. IFRT is the treatment of a region, not of an individual lymph node.
2. The main involved-field nodal regions are neck (unilateral), mediastinum (including the hilar regions bilaterally), axilla (including the supraclavicular (SCL) and infraclavicular lymph nodes), spleen, para-aortic lymph nodes, and inguinal nodes (including the femoral and iliac).
3. In general, the fields include the involved prechemotherapy sites and volume, with an important exception that involves the transverse diameter of the mediastinal and para-aortic lymph nodes. For the field width of these sites, it is recommended to use the reduced

postchemotherapy diameter. In these areas, the regression of the lymph nodes is easily depicted by CT scanning and the critical normal tissue is saved by reducing the irradiated volume.

4. The SCL lymph nodes are considered part of the cervical region and whether involved alone or with other cervical nodes, the whole neck is unilaterally treated. Only if the SCL involvement is an extension of mediastinal disease and the other neck areas are not involved (based on CT scanning with contrast and gallium/PET imaging, when appropriate) the upper neck (above the larynx) is spared. This is to save the salivary glands when the risk for the area is low.

5. All borders should be easy to outline (most are bony landmarks) and to plan with a two-dimensional (2D) standard simulation unit. CT scan data are required for outlining the mediastinal and para-aortic region and will also help in designing the axillary field.

6. Prechemotherapy and postchemotherapy information (both CT and PET scans) regarding lymph node localization and size is critical and should be available at the time of planning the field.

Involved Field Guidelines for Common Nodal Sites

Unilateral Cervical/Supraclavicular Region

Involvement at any cervical level, with or without involvement of the SCL nodes:

Arm position: Akimbo or at sides. *Upper Border*: 1 to 2 cm above the lower tip of the mastoid process and midpoint through the chin. *Lower Border*: 2 cm below the bottom of the clavicle. *Lateral Border*: To include the medial two-thirds of the clavicle. *Medial Border*: (a) If the SCL nodes are not involved, the border is placed at the ipsilateral transverse processes except when medial nodes close to the vertebral bodies are seen on the initial staging neck CT scan. For medial nodes, the entire vertebral body is included. (b) When the SCL nodes are involved, the border should be placed at the contralateral transverse processes. For stage I patients, the larynx and vertebral bodies above the larynx can be blocked (assuming no medial cervical nodes). *Blocks*: A posterior cervical cord block is required only if cord dose exceeds 40 Gy. Mid-neck calculations should be performed to determine the maximum cord dose, especially when the central axis is in the mediastinum. A laryngeal block should be used unless lymph nodes were present in that location. In that case, the block should be added at 20 Gy.

Bilateral Cervical/Supraclavicular Region

Both cervical and SCL regions should be treated as described in the preceding text regardless of the extent of disease on each side. Posterior cervical cord and larynx blocks should be used as described in the preceding text. Use a posterior mouth block if treating the patient supine to block the upper field divergence through the mouth.

Mediastinum

Involvement of the mediastinum and/or the hilar nodes: In HL, this field also includes the medial SCL nodes even if they are not clinically involved. In NHL, the volume is limited to the mediastinum.

Arms position: Akimbo or at sides. The arms-up position is optional if the axillary nodes are involved. *Upper Border*: C5–6 interspace. If SCL nodes are also involved, the upper border should be placed at the top of the larynx and the lateral border should be adjusted as described in the section on treating neck nodes. *Lower Border*: The lower of: (a) 5 cm below the carina or (b) 2 cm below the *prechemotherapy* inferior border. *Lateral Border*: The *postchemotherapy* volume with 1.5 cm margin. *Hilar Area*: To be included with 1 cm margin unless initially involved, in which case the margin should be 1.5 cm.

Mediastinum with Involvement of the Cervical Nodes

When both cervical regions are involved, the field is a mantle without the axilla using the guidelines described in the preceding text. If only one cervical chain is involved, the vertebral bodies, contralateral upper neck, and larynx can be blocked as previously described. Because of the increased dose to the neck (the isocenter is in the upper mediastinum), the neck above the lower border of the larynx should be shielded at 30.6 Gy. If paracardiac nodes are involved, the whole heart should be treated to 14.4 Gy and the initially involved nodes should be treated to 30.6 Gy.

Axillary Region

The ipsilateral axillary, infraclavicular, and SCL areas are treated when the axilla is involved. Whenever possible, CT scan-based planning should be used for this region. *Arms position*: Arms akimbo or arms up. *Upper Border*: C5–6 interspace. *Lower Border*: The lower of the two: (a) the tip of the scapula or (b) 2 cm below the lowest axillary node. *Medial Border*: Ipsilateral cervical transverse process. Include the vertebral bodies only if the SCLs are involved. *Lateral Border*: Flash axilla.

Spleen

The spleen is treated only if abnormal imaging is suggestive of involvement. The *postchemotherapy* volume is treated with 1.5-cm margins.

Abdomen (Para-aortic Nodes)

Upper Border: Top of T11 and at least 2 cm above prechemotherapy volume. *Lower Border*: Bottom of L4 and at least 2 cm below prechemotherapy volume. *Lateral Borders*: The edge of the transverse processes and at least 2 cm from the postchemotherapy volume.

Inguinal/Femoral/External Iliac Region

These ipsilateral lymph node groups are treated together if any of the nodes are involved.

Upper Border: Middle of the sacroiliac joint. *Lower Border:* 5 cm below the lesser trochanter. *Lateral Border:* The greater trochanter and 2 cm lateral to initially involved nodes. *Medial Border:* Medial border of the obturator foramen with at least 2 cm medial to involved nodes. If common iliac nodes are involved, the field should extend to the L4–5 interspace and at least 2 cm above the initially involved nodal border.

Involved-Fields Radiotherapy of Extranodal Sites

In most cases, the whole involved organ is the target and draining lymph nodes are not included unless involved. The optimal plan is 3D conformal and CT scan-simulation based. The margins for the PTV depend on the quality of imaging and the reliability of immobilization, and most importantly, should account for organ motion during respiration. Typically, organs in the head and neck require margins of 1 cm and organs in the mediastinum, abdomen, and pelvis require margins of 2 cm.

NEW ASPECTS OF RADIATION FIELD DESIGN AND DELIVERY

As the notion of treating large sites of involved and uninvolved areas has changed in favor of treating only the involved lymph node group or extranodal organ, new options of more conformal RT have opened up. The old extensive radiation fields like mantle or inverted Y included multiple sites at various depths (from the body surface) and each site had different limitations of access and tolerance of normal tissue. The only way to include these sites in one radiation field (and therefore avoid over-laps and gaps when radiation fields were matched) was to treat the whole field from only two opposed directions: anterior and posterior. This technique assured the inclusion of most lymph nodes in one field, yet it also resulted in the exposure of large volumes of normal organs (e.g., heart, lungs, breasts, and spinal cord) to the full prescribed radiation dose.

The RT of the involved field alone, as is practiced today, avoids this shortcoming in most cases by allowing the use of three-dimensional conformal radiotherapy (3DCRT). For example, 3DCRT of an anterior mediastinal mass could avoid radiation of the spine and much of the heart and lung tissue located behind the mass.

The change in the lymphoma RT paradigm coincided with the substantial improvement in imaging and treatment planning technology, which have revolutionized the field of RT over the last 15 years. The integration of fast high-resolution computerized tomography into the simulation and planning systems of radiation oncology has changed how treatment volumes and relationship to normal critical structures are determined and planned. In the recent past, tumor volume determinations have been made with fluoroscopy-based simulators that produced less than optimal chest x-ray films that obviously resulted in a need to include wide "safety margins" that detracted from accuracy and sparing of critical organs. The most modern simulators are, in fact, high-resolution CT scanners with capabilities and software that allow accurate conformal treatment planning with detailed information on the dose-volume delivered to normal structures in each individual optional plan and the homogeneity of dose delivered to the target. More recently, these simulators are also integrated with a PET scanner that provides additional tumor volume information for consideration during radiation planning (Fig. 27.5).

IMRT is the most advanced planning and radiation delivery mode and is mainly used for small volume cancers that require high radiation doses (e.g., prostate and head

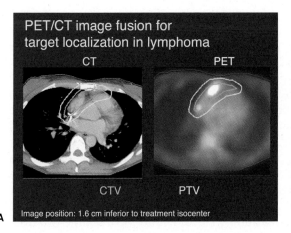 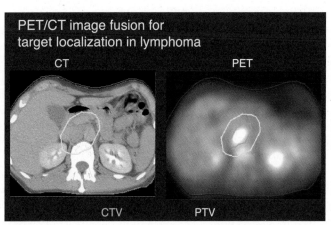

Figure 27.5. A, B: Fusion of positron emission tomography (PET) and computed tomography (CT) scans for target contouring. CTV, clinical target volume; PTV, planned treatment volume.

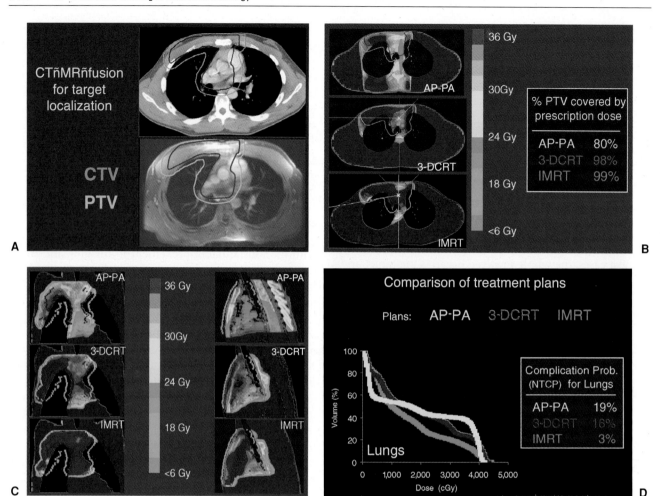

Figure 27.6. A–D: Magnetic resonance imaging–computed tomography (MRI–CT) scans fusion and intensity-modulated radiation therapy (IMRT) for extensive Hodgkin's lymphomas (HL), involving the mediastinum and the chest wall compared to anteroposterior/posteroanterior (AP/PA) and three-dimensional conformal radiotherapy (3DCRT) beam arrangement. CTV, clinical target volume; PTV, planned treatment volume.

neck cancers) or are adjacent to critical organs. IMRT allows for accurately enveloping the tumor with either a homogenous radiation dose ("sculpting") or delivering higher doses to predetermined areas in the tumor volume ("painting"). The end result of this new modality is highly accurate treatment with maximal sparing of normal tissues. In the RT of lymphoma, there are several clinical situations where IMRT provides a benefit: Treatment of very large or complicated tumor volumes in the mediastinum and abdomen, head, and neck lymphomas. IMRT also allows reirradiation of sites before high-dose salvage programs, which will otherwise be prohibited by normal tissue tolerance, particularly of the spinal cord (56) (Figs. 27.6 and 27.7).

SIDE EFFECTS AND COMPLICATIONS OF RADIOTHERAPY OF LYMPHOMAS

Side effects of RT depend on the irradiated volume, the dose administered, and the technique employed. They

are also influenced by the extent and type of prior chemotherapy, if any, and by the patient's age. Most of the information that we use today to estimate risk of RT is derived from strategies that used radiation alone. The sizes of the fields and configuration, doses, and technology have all drastically changed over the last decade. It is therefore probably misleading to judge current RT for lymphomas and inform patients solely on the basis of different past practice of using RT in treating lymphomas.

It is of interest that most of the data of long-term complications associated with RT and particularly second solid tumors and coronary heart disease were reported from databases of patients with HL treated more than 25 years ago. We have very little information on patients with NHL treated with combined modality or with radiation alone and their potential long-term complications. The difference between the two diseases with regard to increased risk reported may be a result of differences in the age-group treated, length of follow-up,

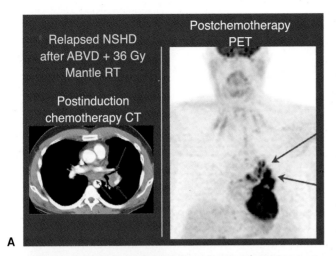

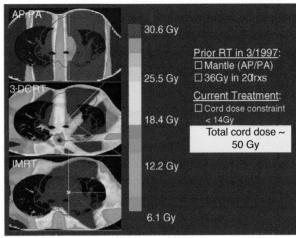

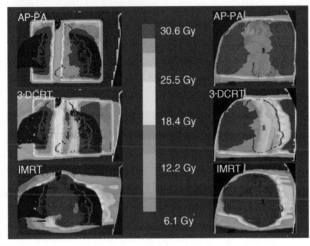

Figure 27.7. A–C: Reirradiation of a relapsed mediastinal mass using intensity-modulated radiation therapy (IMRT) to avoid the spinal cord. ABVD, adriamycin (doxorubicin), bleomycin, vinblastine, dacarbazine; NSHD, nodular sclerosis Hodgkin's disease; RT, radiotherapy; PET, positron emission tomography; CT, computed tomography; AP/PA, anteroposterior/posteroanterior.

and smaller volumes of RT fields used in NHL. It is also important to note that we have very limited long-term follow-up data on patients with HL or patients with NHL who were treated with chemotherapy alone. Yet, increased incidence of lung cancer following treatment with chemotherapy alone was reported for both HL and NHL (7,57,58).

Acute Effects

Radiation, in general, may cause fatigue and areas of the irradiated skin may develop mild sun-exposure like dermatitis. The acute side effects of irradiating the full neck include mouth dryness, change in taste, and pharyngitis. These side effects are usually mild and transient. The main potential side effects of subdiaphragmatic irradiation are loss of appetite, nausea, and increased bowel movements. These reactions are usually mild and can be minimized with standard antiemetic medications.

Irradiation of more than one field, particularly after chemotherapy, can cause myelosuppression, which may necessitate short treatment interruption and very rarely the administration of granulocyte-colony stimulating factor (G-CSF).

Early Side Effects

Lhermitte's sign: <5% of patients may note an electric shock sensation radiating down the backs of both legs when the head is flexed (Lhermitte's sign) 6 weeks to 3 months after mantle-field RT. Possibly secondary to transient demyelinization of the spinal cord, Lhermitte's sign resolves spontaneously after a few months and is not associated with late or permanent spinal cord damage.

Pneumonitis and pericarditis: During the same period, radiation pneumonitis and/or acute pericarditis may occur in <5% of patients; these side effects occur more often in those who have extensive mediastinal disease. Both inflammatory processes have become rare with modern radiation techniques.

Late Side Effects

Subclinical Hypothyroidism

Irradiation of the neck and/or upper mediastinal can induce subclinical hypothyroidism in approximately one-third of patients. This condition is detected by the elevation of the thyroid-stimulating hormone (TSH). Thyroid replacement with levothyroxine (T4) is recommended, even in asymptomatic patients, to prevent overt hypothyroidism and decrease the risk of benign thyroid nodules.

Infertility

Only irradiation of the pelvic field may have deleterious effects on fertility. In most patients, this problem can be avoided by appropriate gonadal shielding. In women, the ovaries can be moved into a shielded area laterally or inferomedially near the uterine cervix. Irradiation outside the pelvis does not increase the risk of sterility.

Secondary Malignancies

Patients with HD who were cured with RT and/or chemotherapy have an increased risk of secondary solid tumors (most commonly, lung, breast, and stomach cancers, as well as melanoma) and NHL, 10 or more years after treatment. Unlike MOPP and similar chemotherapy combinations or etoposide, RT for HD is not leukemogenic.

Lung Cancer. Patients who are smokers should be strongly encouraged to quit the habit because the increase in lung cancer that occurs after irradiation or chemotherapy has been detected mostly in smokers.

Breast Cancer. For women whose HD was successfully treated at a young age, the main long-term concern is the increased risk of breast cancer. During the last decade, multiple studies have documented and characterized the risk of breast cancer after HD, and have established the fact that the increase in risk of breast cancer is undoubtedly associated with the use of radiation. The magnitude of the risk is not completely clear and different methods of risk reporting and data are found in the literature with relative risk (RR) ratios from 2 to 450. Unfortunately, RR, absolute risk, and actuarial risks are often cited without detailing specifics that could have influenced the findings (i.e., length of follow-up for the group and for the individuals; age group, age incidence, and actuarial risk of the malignancy in an untreated population; and quality of follow-up, which may result in event overestimation). According to the largest long-term follow-up study of second neoplasms in survivors of HD, which included data from 16 cancer registries of >35,000 patients, the RR for breast cancer in women was 2 and the absolute excess risk (AER) was 10.5.

The increase in risk of breast cancer is inversely related to the patient's age at HD treatment; no increased risk has been found in women irradiated after 30 years of age. It is also inversely related to the radiation dose to the breast and the volume of breast tissue exposed. Travis et al., in a recent study from 13 centers in 7 countries, reported a large case-control study that included 105 women who developed breast cancer within a cohort of more than 3,800 1-year female survivors of HD, diagnosed at age 30 or less. Unique to this study is the use of patients who received a very low radiation dose (<4 Gy) or no radiation to the breast area where breast cancer developed. This approach allowed isolating treatment factors and analyz-

ing the radiation dose and chemotherapy dose–risk relationships. For all patients who received RT alone (≥4 Gy), the RR of breast cancer is 3.2 and increases to 8 in the highest radiation dose group. The results reported by Travis et al. clearly demonstrate the influence of radiation dose on the risk of breast cancer. Within the range of doses to which the breast was exposed in past years, more radiation translates into a higher risk of developing breast cancer. This information, as well as data from earlier publications showing a significantly lower risk of second tumors when radiation was reduced from 40 to 20 Gy, support the notion that "lower is better" as long as the radiation dose used augments HD cure rate.

RT alone had been the standard treatment and primary curative modality for HD through the 1970s and early 1980s. Irradiating all lymph node regions, regardless of clinical involvement with HD, has been standard practice, and relatively high doses (over 40 Gy) have been used. Consequently, a substantial amount of breast tissue has been exposed to either the full-prescribed dose or to an attenuated dose (at field margins or under the lung shields) in almost all women irradiated for HD. Most breast exposure in the "mantle" era resulted from the radiation of the axillae (65% of tumors in this study developed in the outer part of the breast), and to a lesser extent from wide mediastinal and hilar irradiation. Approximately, two-thirds of women with early stage HD do not require radiation of the axillae, and additional protection to the upper and medial aspects of the breast could be provided by further reducing field size using careful CT scan-based planning that usually allows for smaller mediastinal volumes, especially postchemotherapy, exposed to radiation with the risk of breast cancer. During the last decade, reduction in field size has been the most important change in radiation therapy of HD. Reduction in the volume of exposed breast tissue together with dose reduction (from over 40 Gy to a dose in the range of 20–30 Gy) is likely to dramatically change the long-term risk profile of young male and female patients cured of HD. Emerging data from trials using smaller fields and lower doses support the expectation that the modern application of "mini-RT" will be associated with a significantly lower risk of breast cancer as well as other solid tumors and cardiac sequela. Yet, longer follow-up of studies that employ smaller fields and lower doses is necessary.

Breast cancer is curable in its early stages, and early detection has a significant impact on survival. Breast examination should be part of the routine follow-up for women cured of HD, and routine mammography should begin ~8 years after treatment.

Coronary Artery Disease

An increased risk of coronary artery disease has recently been reported among patients who have received mediastinal irradiation. To reduce this hazard, patients should be monitored and advised about other established coronary disease risk factors, such as smoking, hyperlipidemia, hypertension, and poor dietary and exercise habits. There are data supporting the notion that reduced fields and lower doses to the mediastinum have reduced the risk of heart disease in irradiated patients.

Effects on Bone and Muscle Growth

In children, high-dose irradiation will affect bone and muscle growth and may result in deformities. Current treatment programs for pediatric HD are chemotherapy based; RT is limited to low doses.

SUMMARY

Radiation therapy is an invaluable tool for the curative treatment of HL and many types of NHL. RT can also provide important palliation for many patients who failed chemotherapy. The standard field in most situations is the involved field, not the extended fields of the radiation alone era. Like most cancer treatments, radiation may have long-term side effects, particularly second solid tumors. These risks are related to the volume of normal tissue irradiated and to the radiation dose delivered. Since the use of RT has drastically changed over the last two decades, the radiation fields are markedly smaller, the doses are lower, and the enhanced technology of planning and delivery has improved the identification of the appropriate target and the precision of delivery, resulting in reduced short- and long-term risks to normal structures. Radiation when used smartly can reduce the amount of chemotherapy and length of treatment and its optimal integration in treatment programs for lymphomas should continue to be pursued.

REFERENCES

1. Hoppe RT. *NCCN physician guidelines: Hodgkin disease.* Volume 1. 2006. Available from www.nccn.org.
2. Zelenetz AD. *NCCN physician guidelines: non-Hodgkin lymphoma.* Volume 1. 2005. Available from www.nccn.org.
3. Lister TA, Crowther D, Sutcliffe SB, et al. Report of a committee convened to discuss the evaluation and staging of patients with Hodgkin's disease: cotswolds meeting. *J Clin Oncol* 1989;7:1630–1636.
4. Schlembach PJ, Wilder RB, Jones D, et al. Radiotherapy alone for lymphocyte-predominant Hodgkin's disease. *Cancer J* 2002;8:377–383.
5. Diehl V, Thomas RK, Re D. Part II: Hodgkin's lymphoma—diagnosis and treatment. *Lancet Oncol* 2004;5:19–26.
6. Kaplan H. The radical radiotherapy of Hodgkin's disease. *Radiology* 1962;78:553–561.
7. Travis LB, Gospodarowicz M, Curtis RE, et al. Lung cancer following chemotherapy and radiotherapy for Hodgkin's disease. *J Natl Cancer Inst* 2002;94:182–192.
8. Canellos GP, Anderson JR, Propert KJ, et al. Chemotherapy of advanced Hodgkin's disease with MOPP, ABVD, or MOPP alternating with ABVD. *N Engl J Med* 1992;327:1478–1484.
9. Press OW, LeBlanc M, Lichter AS, et al. Phase III randomized intergroup trial of subtotal lymphoid irradiation versus doxorubicin, vinblastine, and subtotal lymphoid irradiation for stage IA to IIA Hodgkin's disease. *J Clin Oncol* 2001;19:4238–4244.
10. Bonadonna G, Bonfante V, Viviani S, et al. ABVD plus subtotal nodal versus involved-field radiotherapy in early-stage Hodgkin's disease: long-term results. *J Clin Oncol* 2004;22:2835–2841.
11. Loeffler M, Diehl V, Pfreundschuh M, et al. Dose-response relationship of complementary radiotherapy following four cycles of combination chemotherapy in intermediate-stage Hodgkin's disease. *J Clin Oncol* 1997;15:2275–2287.
12. Diehl V, Brillant C, Engert A, et al. HD10: investigating reduction of combined modality treatment intensity in early stage Hodgkin's lymphoma. Interim analysis of a randomized trial of the German Hodgkin Study Group (GHSG). *J Clin Oncol* 2005;21(Suppl 1):Abstract # 6506.
13. Aleman BM, Raemaekers JM, Tirelli U, et al. Involved-field radiotherapy for advanced Hodgkin's lymphoma. *N Engl J Med* 2003;348:2396–2406.
14. Horning SJ, Weller E, Kim K, et al. Chemotherapy with or without radiotherapy in limited-stage diffuse aggressive non-Hodgkin's lymphoma: Eastern Cooperative Oncology Group study 1484. *J Clin Oncol* 2004;22:3032–3038.
15. Moskowitz CH, Nimer SD, Zelenetz AD, et al. A 2-step comprehensive high-dose chemoradiotherapy second-line program for relapsed and refractory Hodgkin disease: analysis by intent to treat and development of a prognostic model. *Blood* 2001;97:616–623.
16. Moskowitz CH, Kewalramani T, Nimer SD, et al. Effectiveness of high dose chemoradiotherapy and autologous stem cell transplantation for patients with biopsy-proven primary refractory Hodgkin's disease. *Br J Haematol* 2004;124:645–652.
17. Mac Manus MP, Hoppe RT. Is radiotherapy curative for stage I and II low-grade follicular lymphoma? Results of a long-term follow-up study of patients treated at Stanford University. *J Clin Oncol* 1996;14:1282–1290.
18. Sutcliffe SB, Gospodarowicz MK, Bush RS, et al. Role of radiation therapy in localized non-Hodgkin's lymphoma. *Radiother Oncol* 1985;4:211–223.
19. Wilder RB, Jones D, Tucker SL, et al. Long-term results with radiotherapy for Stage I-II follicular lymphomas. *Int J Radiat Oncol Biol Phys* 2001;51:1219–1227.
20. Bush RS, Gospodarowicz M, Sturgeon J, et al. Radiation therapy of localized non-Hodgkin's lymphoma. *Cancer Treat Rep* 1977;61:1129–1136.
21. Fuks Z, Kaplan H. Recurrence rates following radiation therapy of nodular and diffuse malignant lymphomas. *Radiology* 1973;108:675–679.
22. Bertoni F, Conconi A, Capella C, et al. Molecular follow-up in gastric mucosa-associated lymphoid tissue lymphomas: early analysis of the LY03 cooperative trial. *Blood* 2002;99:2541–2544.
23. Fisher RI, Dahlberg S, Nathwani BN, et al. A clinical analysis of two indolent lymphoma entities: mantle cell

lymphoma and marginal zone lymphoma (including the mucosa-associated lymphoid tissue and monocytoid B-cell subcategories): a Southwest Oncology Group study. *Blood* 1995;85:1075–1082.

24. Coiffier B, Salles G. Does surgery belong to medical history for gastric lymphomas? *Ann Oncol* 1997;8:419–421.

25. Wotherspoon AC, Doglioni C, Isaacson PG. Low-grade gastric B-cell lymphoma of mucosa-associated lymphoid tissue (MALT): a multifocal disease. *Histopathology* 1992;20:29–34.

26. Schechter NR, Portlock CS, Yahalom J. Treatment of mucosa-associated lymphoid tissue lymphoma of the stomach with radiation alone. *J Clin Oncol* 1998;16:1916–1921.

27. Yahalom J, Portlock C, Gonzales M, et al. H. Pylori-independent MALT lymphoma of the stomach: excellent outcome with radiation alone. *Blood* 2002;100:160a.

28. Tsang RW, Gospodarowicz MK, Pintilie M, et al. Stage I and II MALT lymphoma: results of treatment with radiotherapy. *Int J Radiat Oncol Biol Phys* 2001;50:1258–1264.

29. Fung CY, Grossbard ML, Linggood RM, et al. Mucosa-associated lymphoid tissue lymphoma of the stomach: long term outcome after local treatment. *Cancer* 1999;85:9–17.

30. Hitchcock S, Ng AK, Fisher DC, et al. Treatment outcome of mucosa-associated lymphoid tissue/marginal zone non-Hodgkin's lymphoma. *Int J Radiat Oncol Biol Phys* 2002;52:1058–1066.

31. Gospodarowicz MK, Pintilie M, Tsang R, et al. Primary gastric lymphoma: brief overview of the recent Princess Margaret Hospital experience. *Recent Results Cancer Res* 2000;156:108–115.

32. Yahalom J. MALT lymphomas: a radiation oncology viewpoint. *Ann Hematol* 2001;80:B100–B105.

33. Dell Bianca C, Hunt M, Furhang E, et al. Radiation treatment planning techniques for lymphoma of the stomach. *Int J Radiat Oncol Biol Phys* 2005;62:745–751.

34. Haas RL, Poortmans P, de Jong D, et al. High response rates and lasting remissions after low-dose involved field radiotherapy in indolent lymphomas. *J Clin Oncol* 2003;21:2474–2480.

35. Haas RL, Girinsky T. HOVON 47/EORTC 20013: chlorambucil vs 2 × 2 Gy involved field radiotherapy in stage III/IV previously untreated follicular lymphoma patients. *Ann Hematol* 2003;82:458–462.

36. Girinsky T, Guillot-Vals D, Koscielny S, et al. A high and sustained response rate in refractory or relapsing low-grade lymphoma masses after low-dose radiation: analysis of predictive parameters of response to treatment. *Int J Radiat Oncol Biol Phys* 2001;51:148–155.

37. Leitch HA, Gascoyne RD, Chhanabhai M, et al. Limited-stage mantle-cell lymphoma. *Ann Oncol* 2003;14:1555–1561.

38. Yahalom J. Radiation therapy in the treatment of lymphoma. *Curr Opin Oncol* 1999;11:370–374.

39. Levitt SH, Lee CK, Bloomfield CD, et al. The role of radiation therapy in the treatment of early stage large cell lymphoma. *Hematol Oncol* 1985;3:33–37.

40. Hallahan DE, Farah R, Vokes EE, et al. The patterns of failure in patients with pathological stage I and II diffuse histiocytic lymphoma treated with radiation therapy alone. *Int J Radiat Oncol Biol Phys* 1989;17:767–771.

41. Miller TP, Dahlberg S, Cassady JR, et al. Chemotherapy alone compared with chemotherapy plus radiotherapy for localized intermediate- and high-grade non-Hodgkin's lymphoma. *N Engl J Med* 1998;339:21–26.

42. Fisher RI, Miller TP, O'Connor OA. Diffuse aggressive lymphoma. *Hematology (Am Soc Hematol Educ Program)* 2004;221–236.

43. Kamath SS, Marcus RB Jr, Lynch JW, et al. The impact of radiotherapy dose and other treatment-related and clinical factors on in-field control in stage I and II non-Hodgkin's lymphoma. *Int J Radiat Oncol Biol Phys* 1999;44:563–568.

44. Roy I, Yahalom J. Excellent local control with involved-field radiotherapy following CHOP chemotherapy: analysis of 145 patients with early-stage intermediate-grade non-Hodgkin's lymphoma. *Int J Radiat Oncol Biol Phys* 2001;51:562a–563a.

45. Wilder RB, Tucker SL, Ha CS, et al. Dose-response analysis for radiotherapy delivered to patients with intermediate-grade and large-cell immunoblastic lymphomas that have completely responded to CHOP-based induction chemotherapy. *Int J Radiat Oncol Biol Phys* 2001;49:17–22.

46. Schlembach PJ, Wilder RB, Tucker SL, et al. Impact of involved field radiotherapy after CHOP-based chemotherapy on stage III-IV, intermediate grade and large-cell immunoblastic lymphomas. *Int J Radiat Oncol Biol Phys* 2000;48:1107–1110.

47. Shipp MA, Klatt MM, Yeap B, et al. Patterns of relapse in large-cell lymphoma patients with bulk disease: implications for the use of adjuvant radiation therapy. *J Clin Oncol* 1989;7:613–618.

48. Aviles A, Delgado S, Nambo MJ, et al. Adjuvant radiotherapy to sites of previous bulky disease in patients stage IV diffuse large cell lymphoma. *Int J Radiat Oncol Biol Phys* 1994;30:799–803.

49. Ferreri AJ, Dell'Oro S, Reni M, et al. Consolidation radiotherapy to bulky or semibulky lesions in the management of stage III-IV diffuse large B cell lymphomas. *Oncology* 2000;58:219–226.

50. Fouillard L, Laporte JP, Labopin M, et al. Autologous stem-cell transplantation for non-Hodgkin's lymphomas: the role of graft purging and radiotherapy posttransplantation–results of a retrospective analysis on 120 patients autografted in a single institution. *J Clin Oncol* 1998;16:2803–2816.

51. Aviles A, Fernandezb R, Perez F, et al. Adjuvant radiotherapy in stage IV diffuse large cell lymphoma improves outcome. *Leuk Lymphoma* 2004;45:1385–1389.

52. Aviles A, Garcia EL, Fernandez R, et al. Combined therapy in the treatment of primary mediastinal B-cell lymphoma: conventional versus escalated chemotherapy. *Ann Hematol* 2002;81:368–373.

53. Zinzani PL, Martelli M, Bertini M, et al. Induction chemotherapy strategies for primary mediastinal large B-cell lymphoma with sclerosis: a retrospective multinational study on 426 previously untreated patients. *Haematologica* 2002;87:1258–1264.

54. Todeschini G, Secchi S, Morra E, et al. Primary mediastinal large B-cell lymphoma (PMLBCL): long-term results from a retrospective multicentre Italian experience in 138 patients treated with CHOP or MACOP-B/VACOP-B. *Br J Cancer* 2004;90:372–376.

55. Yahalom J, Mauch P. The involved field is back: issues in delineating the radiation field in Hodgkin's disease. *Ann Oncol* 2002;13(Suppl 1):79–83.

56. Goodman KA, Toner S, Hunt M, et al. Intensity modulated radiation therapy in the treatment of lymphoma involving the mediastinum. *Int J Radiat Oncol Biol Phys* 2005;62:198–206.

57. Andre M, Mounier N, Leleu X, et al. Second cancers and late toxicities after treatment of aggressive non-Hodgkin lymphoma with the ACVBP regimen: a GELA cohort study on 2837 patients. *Blood* 2004;103:1222–1228.

58. Travis LB, Curtis RE, Glimelius B, et al. Second cancers among long-term survivors of non-Hodgkin's lymphoma. *J Natl Cancer Inst* 1993;85:1932–1937.

CHAPTER 28

Cancers of the Head and Neck

Jonathan J. Beitler ■ Robert J. Amdur ■ William M. Mendenhall

INTRODUCTION

In the United States, the predominant risk factors contributing to the development of squamous cell cancers of the head and neck are related to lifestyle. Smoking and alcohol abuse are habits that disproportionately affect the poor. The least wealthy and the least educated patients are often ill-equipped to handle the impact of the cancer and the toxicities of treatment. Health care providers must address the disease as well as the socioeconomic needs of these patients. Therapy needs to be individualized, the patients educated, and the importance of both lifestyle change and good nutrition cannot be overemphasized. It has been estimated that if a patient continues to smoke during treatment, not only are the acute toxicities (and possibly the late complications) enhanced, but the response rates are lower (45% vs. 74%) as is 2-year survival (39% vs. 66%) (1).

In the Western world we have seen a tripling of the rate of oropharyngeal cancer, and this human papillomavirus (HPV)-related disease affects patients who are younger, and often neither tobacco smokers nor alcohol drinkers. From 1970 to 2002 the incidence of tonsil cancer increased 2.6-fold in men and 3.5-fold in women in a study from Stockholm (2). Using the national registry of Sweden, and looking at other smoking-related cancers such as lung and oral cavity cancers as reference, illustrates that the increase is not related to cigarette smoking (3). Looking at SEER data, the incidence of HPV-unrelated cancer was stable from 1973 to 1982 and significantly decreased from 1983 to 2004 (4). For individual HPV-related sites within the oropharynx, from 1973 to 2004 the annual percentage increase in base of tongue cancers and tonsil cancers was 1.27% and 0.6%, respectively, whereas the incidence of cancer was stable for other oropharyngeal sites. More recently, 85% of the tonsillar cancers biopsied between 2002 and 2007 in the county of Stockholm had HPV DNA recovered from their biopsy (5). The proportion of HPV-positive tonsil cancers nearly doubled each decade from 1970 until 2007 and from 2006 to 2007 the proportion of tonsil cancers with HPV DNA was 93%. With such a high proportion of these cancers being virally related, the role of prophylactic vaccination is being discussed (6).

The natural history of most head and neck cancers is an orderly and relatively predictable pattern of spread. Cancers tend to spread both locally and regionally, with regional disease being dependent on the anatomic location and extent of the primary tumor. As the affected neck nodes increase in size and exhibit extracapsular extension, the propensity for hematogenous dissemination increases; but distant metastases are a relatively uncommon pattern, and most patients presenting with head and neck cancer have the opportunity for cure.

WORKUP

After the history and physical examination, a biopsy, a detailed physical examination of the head and neck (including an endoscopic examination), and imaging are the work-up requirements. Computed tomography (CT) with intravenous contrast is the main imaging modality, although for nasopharyngeal cancer and advanced laryngeal cancers MRI will be more useful (7). Some patients with advanced disease of the head and neck may benefit from positron emission tomography (PET)/CT scanning to suggest the location of an occult primary, to provide functional data about lymphadenopathy and detect distant metastases. However, PET may underestimate the extent of local-regional disease that is apparent in the CT scan. Despite increasingly sophisticated imaging, the cancer-directed physical examination remains essential.

IMMOBILIZATION

To assure setup reproducibility, optimum immobilization is essential. Often optimum immobilization is achieved by letting the patients obtain a comfortable position. Even without the changes in contour expected when a massive neck node resolves during treatment, through cancer- and treatment-related loss of muscle mass, patients may have difficulty maintaining certain positions. Consider the low-neck match. When matching two lateral field edges with an anterior field edge, inhomogeneity at the match line is an appropriate concern. In the past, particularly when primary disease was likely to extend inferior to the lateral fields, the patient was put in an uncomfortable treatment position to lower the shoulders so that the entire primary tumor could be encompassed by the lateral beams. Experience has suggested that achieving difficult treatment positions can be a transient victory. Proper positioning may be maintained during the simulation and early in the treatment, but as muscles become weaker, reproducibility diminishes (8). In the era when many treatments for head and neck can be performed with intensity-modulating radiation therapy (IMRT), extensive lowering of the shoulders may be eliminated in many cases. As much immobilization as practical is endorsed and we use aquaplast casts to include the shoulders for immobilization. An important point to be noted is that the patient and not the cast is being treated, and marking the cast is a good first step in setting up the patient, but image-guided radiation therapy (IGRT) allows our therapists to concentrate on the bony anatomy expeditiously. Particularly in the head and neck, IGRT has been a big step forward in increasing treatment accuracy. We are exploring the role of weekly, cone-beam CT scanning during radiation.

The bite block is commonly used for treating the oral tongue and the device needs to be used carefully. An effective tongue blade can push the tongue inferiorly and allow for mucosal sparing of the hard palate. The concern is that the bite blocks that most patients can tolerate are narrower than the tongue, and that the lateral aspects of the tongue could possibly extend above the tongue depressor, sometimes resulting in an insufficient margin. This is particularly important in the treatment of oral tongue cancers because the predominant site of involvement is the lateral aspect of the oral tongue.

GENERAL TREATMENT GUIDELINES

In the era of IMRT, the danger lies in specifying too small a target volume. This new technology affords us the opportunity to limit doses to the parotid glands and other important normal structures, but it should not be used in cases where it is likely to reduce the probability of cure. The guidelines for the initial treatment volume are to treat the gross and subclinical disease with expansion to a planning target volume (PTV) that makes sense for both the patients and the local expertise of the therapists. Typical PTV expansions range from 3 to 10 mm.

INTENSITY-MODULATING RADIATION THERAPY—PRACTICAL TIPS

Apart from early glottic cancers and situations where ipsilateral portals are indicated (e.g., lateralized tonsillar carcinoma), many patients with head and neck cancer may benefit from properly delivered IMRT if doses to uninvolved normal organs, such as the larynx and parotid(s), can be minimized. Although keeping the parotids below a median dose of 26 Gy does not absolutely prevent xerostomia, it reduces its severity. Patients should not have false expectations that they will have normal salivary flow after external radiation delivered with IMRT,

but they should be assured that IMRT is a technique that may meaningfully improve their quality of life (9).

Treatment-planning CT is performed with 2- to 3-mm cuts; target volumes are identified on all cuts. Issues with matching the low supraclavicular field with the IMRT fields suggest the need to scan the entire supraclavicular region, so that a sensible treatment technique decision can be made. Treating the entire supraclavicular field within the IMRT fields eliminates the matching problem, but must be weighed against increasing the dose to the uninvolved larynx (10).

Intravenous contrast at the time of the CT simulation aids in delineating the primary tumor and the nodal disease, and enhances the visualization of the normal structures. Normal structures that need to be outlined include both parotid glands, the spinal cord, the brain stem, and, when relevant, the larynx, the submandibular glands, the thyroid glands, the lacrimal glands, the retina, the lenses, the optic nerves, the optic chiasm, the inner and middle ears, and the lips. When required by the RTOG, the brachial plexus needs to be outlined. Because few plans meet the brachial plexus constraints suggested by the RTOG protocols (11), do not underdose the CTV or GTV because of those constraints. Thus, outside of protocols, this contour is generally optional.

The parotid glands can be visualized by location and texture. The anatomic description by Netter (12) is as follows:

The parotid gland, the largest of the salivary glands, is roughly a three-sided wedge, which is fitted in below and in front of the external ear. The triangular superficial surface of the wedge is practically subcutaneous, with one side of the triangle almost as high as the zygomatic arch and the opposing angle at the level of the angle of the mandible. The anteromedial side of the wedge abuts against and overlaps the ramus of the mandible and the related masseter and internal pterygoid muscles. The posteromedial side of the wedge turns toward the external auditory canal, the mastoid process, and the sternocleidomastoid and digastric muscles.

The deep lobe of the parotid points toward, but does not reach, the carotid artery, wraps around the ramus of the mandible, and extends between the styloglossus and internal pterygoid muscles anteriorly and the posterior belly of the digastric and the stylohyoid muscles posteriorly. The CT appearance is somewhat akin to roughly ground glass.

The International Commission on Radiation Units (ICRU) Report 62 introduced the concepts of organ at risk volume (ORV) and the planning organ at risk volume (PRV). The spinal cord and other normal structures should be outlined and a 3-mm PRV margin should be added to the ORV for additional safety. At the University of Florida, all IMRT dose-volume histogram (DVH) displays are based on the PTVs and PRVs.

Conflicts between PRVs and PTVs are common and certain common sense rules have been developed. When dealing with overlaps of the spinal cord and the brain stem with the PTV, the PTV is more important than the PRV,

TABLE 28.1	University of Florida Dose Constraints for Head and Neck Intensity-Modulating Radiation Therapy
Nomenclature	
"Constraints" are what you require the plan to produce. "Objectives" are what you enter into the planning system to trick it to produce a plan that meets your constraints.	
PTVs and PRVs	
All plans are judged on expanded volumes—meaning PTVs and PRVs. Dose–volume data related to the ORV, CTV, or GTV are not displayed or analyzed.	
Dose Constraints to PTV and PRV	
All uncontoured tissue is defined as a PRV called *Skin-PTV*. There are no firm constraints for Skin-PTV. The objective is: 0% volume receives >4,950 cGy with a 1.5 weighting in all cases.	
PTV coverage	≥95% of the PTV receives the prescription dose, and 99% of the PTV receives ≥93% of the prescription dose
Hot spot in high-risk PTV[a]	20% of the high-risk PTV receives ≥110% of the prescription dose[a]
Brain stem	5,500 cGy to 0.1 cc
Spinal cord	5,000 cGy to 0.1 cc
Optic nerve	5,500 cGy to 0.1 cc
Optic chiasm	5,500 cGy to 0.1 cc
Lens (ant chamber)	1,200 cGy to 0.1 cc
Retina (posterior globe)	5,000 cGy to 0.1 cc
Contralateral parotid	mean ≤26 Gy

[a]The hot spot is not constrained in PTVs that surround the high-risk PTV.
PTV, planning target volume; PRV, planning organ at risk volume; ORV, organ at risk volume; CTV, clinical target volume; GTV, gross tumor volume.

but the ORV is most important. Practically speaking, this means that the plan will spare the spinal cord or the brain stem when the 3-mm PTV expansion would overdose the spinal cord or the brain stem.

When the conflict is between the PTV and the parotid, submandibular, and lacrimal glands, and the mandible, oral cavity and the skin, the PTV is more important than the PRV or the ORV. Conflicts regarding the PTV and the visual structures need to be individualized. There are two main schools of thought on this: (1) Reduce the dose to part of the tumor to keep normal tissues below selected threshold doses, and (2) accept higher doses to the normal tissues to adequately treat the entire tumor. The latter approach is followed.

Tables 28.1 and 28.2 show normal tissue guidelines. Although IMRT may be used in patients with positive bilateral neck nodes, it is often difficult to adequately treat the neck and meaningfully spare one or both parotid glands.

Contouring Target Volumes

The gross primary and nodal disease as well as the high-risk subclinical disease sites are outlined by the physicians on the treatment-planning CT scan on the basis of physical and radiographic findings. At the University of Florida, these volumes are referred to as CTV 7200. Areas that have a 10% or greater risk of subclinical disease are contoured and labeled as CTV 4950. High-risk subclinical disease areas are contoured as a CTV 5400. The clinical target volumes (CTVs) are expanded by 3 mm with treatment-planning software to develop the PTVs, but special expansions for mobile structures, such as the oral tongue, may be necessary because of their potential for movement.

TABLE 28.2	Parotid and Submandibular Gland: Same With or Without Concomitant Chemotherapy
Both neck N0	Ipsilateral and contralateral glands: Mean dose ≤26 Gy
Ipsilateral neck N+; contralateral neck N0	No constraint on ipsilateral gland. Contralateral gland: Mean dose ≤26 Gy
Both necks N+	Individualized

TREATMENT OF THE NECK WITH INTENSITY-MODULATING RADIATION THERAPY

The likelihood of subclinical disease metastatic to the regional lymph nodes varies with the location and extent of the primary tumor. If clinically positive nodes are present, the risk of subclinical disease in the remaining cervical lymphatics also depends on the location and extent of the involved nodes. The definition of lymph node levels is depicted in Table 28.3. The clinically negative neck (or clinically negative regions of a node positive neck) are irradiated electively if the risk of subclinical disease exceeds 10%. The algorithm employed to determine which regions of the neck are to be treated is shown in Tables 28.4–28.6. Patients with well-lateralized T1-T2 N0-N2b tonsillar carcinomas are usually treated with ipsilateral field arrangements and the contralateral neck is not irradiated.

TABLE 28.3	Imaging-Based Nodal Classification
Level I	The submental and submandibular nodes. They lie above the hyoid bone, below the mylohyoid muscle, and anterior to the back of the submandibular gland.
Level IA	The submental nodes. They lie between the medial margins of the anterior bellies of the digastric muscles.
Level IB	The submandibular nodes. On each side, they lie lateral to the level IA nodes and anterior to the back of each submandibular gland.
Level II	The upper internal jugular nodes. They extend from the skull base to the level of the bottom of the body of the hyoid bone. They are posterior to the back of the submandibular gland and anterior to the back of the sternocleidomastoid muscle.
Level IIA	A level II node that lies either anterior, medial, lateral, or posterior to the internal jugular vein. If posterior to the vein, the node is inseparable from the vein.
Level IIB	A level II node that lies posterior to the internal vein and has a fat plane separating it and the vein.
Level III	The middle jugular nodes. They extend from the level of the bottom of the body of the hyoid bone to the level of the bottom of the cricoid arch. They lie anterior to the back of the sternocleidomastoid muscle.
Level IV	The low jugular nodes. They extend from the level of the bottom of the cricoid arch to the level of the clavicle. They lie anterior to a line connecting the back of the sternocleidomastoid muscle and the posterolateral margin of the anterior scalene muscle. They are also lateral to the carotid arteries.
Level V	The nodes in the posterior triangles. They lie posterior to the back of the sternocleidomastoid muscle from the skull base to the level of the bottom of the cricoid arch and posterior to a line connecting the back of the sternocleidomastoid muscle and the posterolateral margin of the anterior scalene muscle from the level of the bottom of the cricoid arch to the level of the clavicle. They also lie anterior to the anterior edge of the trapezius muscle.
Level VA	Upper level V nodes extend the skull base to the level of the bottom of the cricoid arch.
Level VB	Lower level V nodes extend from the level of the bottom of the cricoid arch to the level of the clavicle, as seen on each axial scan.
Level VI	The upper visceral nodes. They lie between the carotid arteries from the level of the bottom of the body of the hyoid bone to the level of the top of the manubrium.
Level VII	The superior mediastinal nodes. They lie between the carotid arteries below the level of the top of the manubrium and above the level of the innominate vein.
Supraclavicular nodes	They lie at, or caudal to, the level of the clavicle and lateral to the carotid artery on each side of the neck, as seen on each axial scan.
Retropharyngeal nodes	Within 2 cm of the skull base, they lie medial to the internal carotid arteries.

Source: From Som PM, Curtin HD, Mancuso AA. An imaging-based classification for the cervical nodes designed as an adjunct to recent clinically based nodal classifications. *Arch Otolaryngol Head Neck Surg* 1999;125:388–396 and Imaging-based nodal classification for evaluation of neck metastatic adenopathy. *AJR AM J Roentgenol* 2000;174:837–844 (6,7).

TABLE 28.4 N0 Bilaterally

Primary site	IA	IB IP	IB C	II IP	II C	III IP	III C	IV IP	IV C	V IP	V C	VI	Retropharyngeal IP	Retropharyngeal C
Nasopharynx	—	—	—	R	R	R	R	R	R	R	R	—	R	R
Soft palate	—	—	—	R	R	R	R	R	R	—	—	—	R	—
Anterior tonsillar pillar	—	—	—	R	R if near midline	R	R if near midline	R	R if near midline	—	—	—	—	—
Tonsil	—	—	—	R	R if near midline	R	R if near midline	R	R if near midline	—	—	—	—	—
Base of tongue	—	—	—	R	R	R	R	R	R	—	—	—	—	—
Pharyngeal wall	—	—	—	R	R	R	R	R	R	—	—	Only if esophagus or apex PS + but spare larynx	R	R
Pyriform sinus	—	—	—	R	R	R	R	R	R	—	—	Only if apex + but spare larynx	R	Only if to midline
Postcricoid	—	—	—	R	R	R	R	R	R	—	—	Only if esophagus or apex PS +	R	R
Larynx	—	—	—	R	R	R	R	R	R	—	—	Only if subglottic +	—	—

IP, ipsilateral neck; C, contralateral; apex PS, apex of pyriform sinus; R, radiotherapy to nodes.
Source: Image borrowed with permission from the University of Florida Department of Radiation Oncology treatment planning guidelines and from Mendenhall WM, Amdur RJ, Palta Jr. Head and neck cancer. In: Levitt SH, Purdy JA, Perez CA, Vijayakumar S, eds. *Technical basis of radiation therapy: practical clinical applications (medical radiology/radiation oncology)*, 4th ed. New York, NY: Springer-Verlag. 2006.

TABLE 28.5 **N1, N2 A, N2B, or Unilateral N3**

Primary site	IA	IB		II[a]		III		IV		V		VI	Retropharyngeal	
		IP	C	IP	C	IP	C	IP	C	IP	C		IP	C
Nasopharynx	—	½[b]	—	R	R	R	R	R	R	R	—	—	R	R
Soft palate	—	½[b]	—	R	R	R	R	R	R	R	—	—	R	—
Anterior tonsillar pillar	—	½[b]	—	R	R	R	R	R	R	R	—	—	R	—
Tonsil	—	½[b]	—	R	R	R	R	R	R	R	—	—	R	—
Base of tongue	—	½[b]	—	R	R	R	R	R	R	R	—	—	R	—
Pharyngeal wall	—	½[b]	—	R	R	R	R	R	R	R	—	Only if esophagus or apex PS + but spare larynx	R	R
Pyriform sinus	—	½[b]	—	R	R	R	R	R	R	R	—	Only if apex PS + but spare larynx	R	Only if to midline
Postcricoid	—	½[b]	—	R	R	R	R	R	R	R	—	R	R	R
Larynx	—	½[b]	—	R	R	R	R	R	R	R	—	R	R	Only if to midline

IP, ipsilateral neck; C, contralateral neck; apex PS, apex of pyriform sinus; R, radiotherapy to nodes.

[a]Cover jugular foramen if positive nodes are found in level II, V, and retropharyngeal.

[b]In the absence of high-volume level II disease, we usually cover only the posterior ½ of level Ib: 1 cm anterior to the submandibular gland.

Source: Image borrowed with permission from the University of Florida Department of Radiation Oncology treatment planning guidelines and from Mendenhall WM, Amdur RJ, Palta Jr. Head and neck cancer. In: Levitt SH, Purdy JA, Perez CA, Vijayakumar S, eds. *Technical basis of radiation therapy: practical clinical applications (medical radiology/radiation oncology),* 4th ed. New York, NY: Springer-Verlag, 2006.

TABLE 28.6 **N2 C (Bilateral Neck Nodes)**

| Primary Site | Node levels and laterality |||||||||||| Retropharyngeal ||
| | IA | IB || II[a] || III || IV || V || VI | | |
		IP	C	IP	C	IP	C	IP	C	IP	C		IP	C
Nasopharynx	—	½[b]	—	R	R	R	R	R	R	R	R	—	R	R
Soft palate	—	½[b]	—	R	R	R	R	R	R	R	R	—	R	R
Anterior tonsillar pillar	—	½[b]	—	R	R	R	R	R	R	R	R	—	R	R
Tonsil	—	½[b]	—	R	R	R	R	R	R	R	R	—	R	R
Base of tongue	—	½[b]	—	R	R	R	R	R	R	R	R	—	R	R
Pharyngeal wall	—	½[b]	—	R	R	R	R	R	R	R	R	Yes but spare larynx	R	R
Pyriform sinus	—	½[b]	—	R	R	R	R	R	R	R	R	Yes but spare larynx	R	R
Postcricoid	—	½[b]	—	R	R	R	R	R	R	R	R	R	R	R
Larynx	—	½[b]	—	R	R	R	R	R	R	R	R	R	R	R

IP, ipsilateral neck; C, contralateral; apex PS, apex of pyriform sinus; R, radiotherapy to nodes.

[a] Cover jugular foramen if positive nodes are found in level II, V, or retropharyngeal.

[b] In the absence of high-volume level II disease, we usually cover only the posterior ½ of level Ib: 1 cm anterior to the submandibular gland.

Source: Image borrowed with permission from the University of Florida Department of Radiation Oncology treatment planning guidelines and from Mendenhall WM, Amdur RJ, Palta Jr. Head and neck cancer. In: Levitt SH, Purdy JA, Perez CA, Vijayakumar S, eds. *Technical basis of radiation therapy: practical clinical applications (medical radiology/radiation oncology),* 4th ed. New York, NY: Springer-Verlag, 2006.

Intensity-Modulating Radiation Therapy— Dose Guidelines

At the University of Florida, the concomitant boost schedule is used for most patients who are treated with definitive IMRT. All PTVs receive 54 Gy in 30 once-daily (q.d.) fractions. During the last 12 days, the CTV 7200 receives an additional 18 Gy in 12 twice-daily (b.i.d.) fractions with a 6-hour interfraction interval. Therefore, 72 Gy is delivered in 42 fractions over 30 treatment days when treatment is delivered 5 days a week. The initial plan delivers ~49.5 Gy at 1.65 Gy/day in 30 fractions to intermediate-risk volumes. Plan optimization goals are to deliver the prescription dose to 95% or more of the PTV and to ensure that 99% of the PTV receives 93% or more of the prescription dosage to reduce the risk of injuring the visual apparatus.

Patients with lesions involving the skull base (e.g., nasopharynx; skin cancer with clinical perineural invasion) are treated with hyperfractionated IMRT to 74.4 Gy in 62 b.i.d. fractions to reduce the risk of injury to the visual apparatus.

Whereas RTOG 90–03 showed the superiority of hyperfractionated radiation over standard radiation when the patient was not receiving concurrent chemotherapy, RTOG 0129 added 100 mg/m^2 of Cisplatinum on days 1 and 22 and randomized 721 eligible patients with locally advanced head and neck cancers to 72 Gy in 42 fractions delivered over 6 weeks versus 70 Gy in 35 (plus a third cycle of Cisplatinum). There was no difference in overall survival, local-regional failure, distant metastases, late toxicities, or feeding tube dependencies (13). One conclusion could be that in the setting of concurrent chemotherapy, hyperfractionation does not add benefit for these patients. Of course, in the era of IMRT, we are generally doing simultaneous in-field boosting as our high value targets are treated to higher daily doses than our intermediate or lower risk target volumes.

ORAL CAVITY

Most lesions of the oral cavity are treated surgically, but because the need for postoperative radiation therapy (RT) is common, the radiation oncologist should endeavor to examine the patient preoperatively. Despite the widespread use of postoperative RT, there are no randomized data that supports its use. Postoperative RT of the primary site is based on positive margins, bone invasion, invasion of the soft tissues of neck, perineural invasion, and endothelial-lined space invasion. Looser et al. reported that a margin of 5 mm or less is equivalent in impact to a positive margin (14). Indications for postoperative RT related to the neck include extracapsular extension and multiple positive nodes. In a multivariate analysis of patients treated with postoperative RT for oral cavity cancers, independent significant risk factors for local-regional failure

were positive margins, vascular invasion, perineural invasion, extracapsular extension, and stage T3-T4 lesion (15). Only extracapsular extension and perineural invasion adversely impacted cause-specific survival. At the University of Florida, patients with negative margins receive 60 Gy in 30 fractions over 6 weeks. Patients with positive margins receive 66 Gy in 33 q.d. fractions or 74.4 Gy in 62 b.i.d. fractions with concomitant cisplatin (16). The larynx should be spared when treating the oral cavity and this can be done by placing the field junction between the primary fields and the low-neck field at the thyroid notch or 2 cm below the most inferior extent of the primary tumor. A tapered 1- to 2-cm wide midline block is placed in the anterior low-neck field and extends from the junction superiorly to the bottom of the cricoid cartilage inferiorly. IMRT can also be used to constrain the larynx within the context of the planning process.

Lips

For lip cancers, functional and cosmetic results are critical. Surgery can lead to microstomia as well as drooling and difficulty in eating due to lack of sensory and/or motor control. Therefore, RT is often preferred for oral commissure, upper lip, and larger lower lip cancers. Depending on the T-stage, the primary tumor (gross tumor volume [GTV]) is treated with a 1.5- to 2-cm margin, therefore defining the CTV.

Local treatment can be performed with brachytherapy, orthovoltage x-rays, or even photons, but most patients will receive definitive electron RT for the primary tumor (Fig. 28.1). The total RT dose usually varies from 60 to 70 Gy depending on the extent of the tumor and fractionation schedule. For electron RT, it is necessary to add an additional 1 cm to the lateral margins of the CTV for the PTV to account for beam constriction. One to 0.5 cm of bolus is used to ensure an adequate surface dose and the electron energy necessary to deliver 90% of the dose to a depth of 5 to 10 mm beneath the estimated deepest extent of the disease is selected. A lead shield is placed beneath the lip to reduce exit dose to the oral cavity and the mouth is kept open to move the uninvolved upper or lower lip out of the field.

As stated earlier, disease involving the oral commissure is best treated with definitive RT owing to the functional consequences of surgery. Local treatment fields should be generous and the regional nodes may require elective RT. Although patients with T1 N0 or T2 N0 lip cancers have a low regional failure rate of 4.8% (17), those with commissure involvement and/or T3/T4 primaries have significantly (18) higher rates of positive nodes and require regional treatment. Generally, the ipsilateral submandibular nodes should be the first echelon nodes followed by the level IIA nodes. The facial nodes are at relatively slight risk (19), but may be targeted. Other risk factors for nodal disease include recurrent disease, poor differentiation, and involvement of the "wet" mucosa.

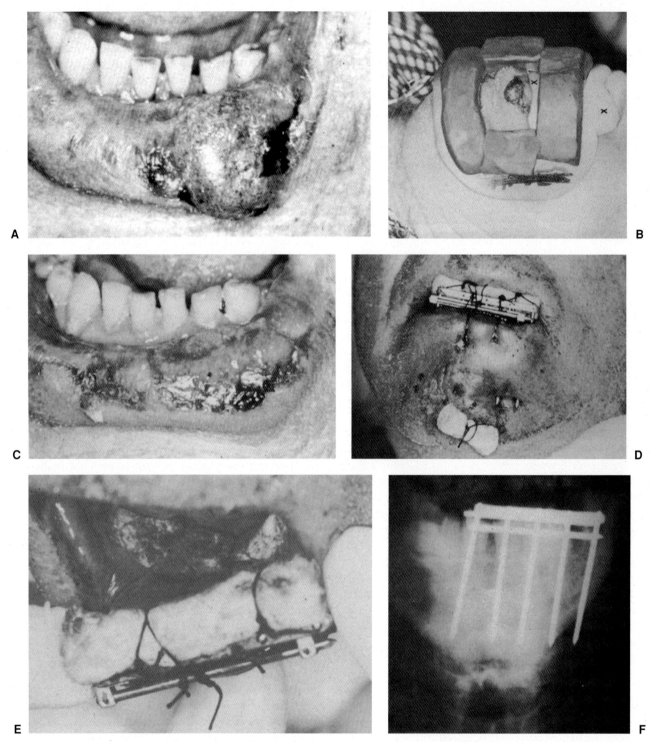

Figure 28.1. A 67-year-old man had T2 N0 squamous cell carcinoma of the lower lip. **A:** Lesion measured 3.0 × 2.0 × 1.5 cm. Radiation therapy was elected because of functional deficit likely to result from the excision of the large lesion. **B:** Lead mask, 2 mm thick, designed to outline portal. Lead putty was added to the shield to reduce transit irradiation to <1%. A separate lead shield covered with beeswax was inserted behind lower lip. The patient received 30 Gy in 2 weeks, 3 Gy per fraction, 250 kV (0.5 mm Cu). **C:** By the time of completion of 30 Gy, he had brisk mucositis of lip and approximately 60% to 70% regression of obvious tumor. **D:** Single-plane radium needle implant with double crossing. The pack was tied to the top of the bar to displace upper lip away from radiation, and the chin pack anchored the gingivolabial pack in place (see **E**). **E:** A gauze pack (*arrows*) sewn into gingivolabial gutter to displace radium from mandible, teeth, and gums. **F** and **G:** Anteroposterior and lateral views of implant. Implant added 35 Gy at 0.5 cm. **H:** 2.5 weeks after implantation. Note superficial ulceration. **I:** 22 months after treatment. No evidence of disease, and lip was completely healed. Nine-year follow-up revealed no evidence of disease. *Source:* From Million RR, Cassisi NJ, Mancuso AA. Oral cavity. In: Million RR, Cassisi NJ, eds. *Management of head and neck cancer: a multidisciplinary approach,* 2nd ed. Philadelphia, PA: JB Lippincott Co, 1994:321–400, Fig. 16.7, pp. 330–331. (*continued*)

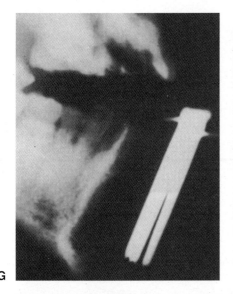

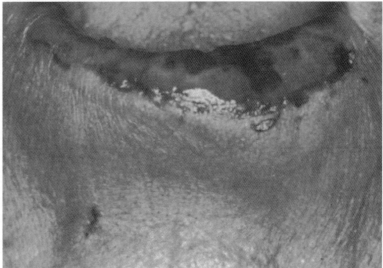

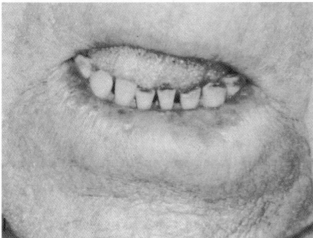

Figure 28.1. (*Continued*)

Buccal Mucosa and Gingiva

These are generally surgical diseases. Much buccal mucosa can be resected with manageable functional outcomes and postoperative RT need only be considered for the indications previously described. Generally, the level IB, IIA, and the superior level III nodes are electively treated when necessary (20).

Gingival cancers are usually treated with surgical resection followed by postoperative RT, if indicated. Even with clinically negative nodes, elective neck dissection revealed occult disease in 27% of 52 patients studied (20). Levels IB, IIA, III, and IV are the primary lymphatic routes of spread with contralateral disease becoming a problem for midline lesions and those with bulky ipsilateral cervical disease.

Floor of Mouth

Postoperative Irradiation

Although sometimes grouped with oral tongue cancers, floor of mouth cancers tend to have fewer local failures

than oral tongue malignancies (21). These patients are usually treated surgically and it is important to appreciate that the risk of bilateral cervical disease may be high. Careful preoperative examination of the extent of local spread is critical and the final CTV is probably best defined as the original GTV plus 1.5 cm. The initial primary field should cover the entire floor of mouth, the adjacent gingiva, and the adjacent tongue (Figs. 28.2 and 28.3). Fields should be even more generous if the mylohyoid muscles, which form the inferior border of the oral cavity, have been violated. When treating floor of mouth cancers, the lips can usually be shielded. This is a situation where an intraoral device can displace the hard palate away from the floor of mouth and thereby decrease the mucosal reaction and save the upper teeth.

In the absence of clinically positive regional nodes, most of the floor of mouth cancers should have level IB, IIA, and III electively dissected. As long as the disease is not far advanced, 1 cm of skin and subcutaneous tissue in the submental region can be shielded. If the tumor is <2 mm in thickness and has no ominous features, elective nodal treatment can be withheld (22).

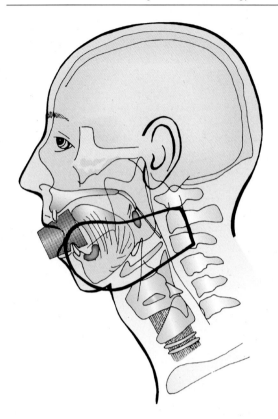

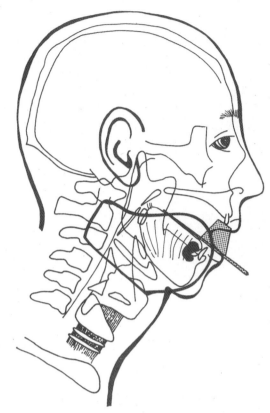

Figure 28.2. Portal for irradiation of limited anterior floor of mouth carcinoma (no tongue invasion; N0 or N1 neck disease) by parallel-opposed cobalt 60 (^{60}Co), 4-MV x-ray, or 6-MV x-ray fields. Two notches on a cork ensure that it is held in the same position between upper and lower incisors during every treatment session; tip of tongue is displaced from treatment field. Anterior border of field covers full thickness of mandibular arch. Lower field edge is at the thyroid cartilage, ensuring adequate coverage of submandibular (level I) lymph nodes. Subdigastric lymph (level II) nodes are covered adequately by including the entire width of vertebral bodies posteriorly. The superior border is shaped so that the oropharynx, much of the oral cavity, and parotid glands are out of portal. The minimum tumor dose is specified at primary site (i.e., not along central axis of portal). *Source:* From Parsons JT, Mendenhall WM, Million RR. Radiotherapy of tumors of the oral cavity. In: Thawley SE, Panje WR, Batsakis JG, Lindberg RD, eds. *Comprehensive management of head and neck tumors,* 2nd ed. Philadelphia, PA: WB Saunders Co, 1999: 861–875, Fig. 35.8, p. 704; Fig. 16.16 in Levitt 2nd ed.

Figure 28.3. The treatment portal for carcinoma of the floor of mouth with tongue invasion. Tongue is depressed into floor of mouth with tongue blade and cork. *Source:* From Parsons JT, Mendenhall WM, Million RR. Radiotherapy of tumors of the oral cavity. In: Thawley SE, Panje WR, Batsakis JG, Lindberg RD, eds. *Comprehensive management of head and neck tumors,* 2nd ed. Philadelphia, PA: WB Saunders Co, 1999, 861–875, Fig. 35.9, p. 704.

Dose-fractionation schedules vary with the margins: Negative, 60 Gy in 30 q.d. fractions; close or positive margins, 66 Gy in 33 q.d. fractions or 74.4 Gy in 62 b.i.d. fractions. Concomitant chemotherapy should be considered for those with positive margins and/or extracapsular extension.

Definitive Radiation of the Floor of Mouth

For cases when surgery is not possible, brachytherapy or an intraoral cone RT are used to obtain optimal local control rates. When patients are treated with definitive RT, a stainless steel marker can be inserted into the floor of the mouth at the posterior tumor border. After local anesthesia has been administered, the metal marker can be accurately placed with a cooperative patient. This confirms that the entire extent of mucosal spread, which can be difficult to delineate on CT scan, is properly treated.

An intraoral cone (if available) is optimal if the patient is edentulous, has a small, anterior, superficial lesion, and has a low alveolar ridge. The very smallest lesions might be treated solely by cone RT (50 Gy/3 weeks or 60 Gy/4 weeks, given doses), but larger lesions require 20 to 25 Gy at 2.5 to 3 Gy per fraction in addition to 45 to 50 Gy external-beam RT. In this latter instance, intraoral cone irradiation precedes external-beam RT because the lesion can be well delineated and the mouth is not sore, therefore facilitating cone placement.

For lesions thicker than 1 cm and not abutting the gingiva, interstitial brachytherapy is preferred. This can be done up-front or, if adequately marked with both metal and tattoos, after external-beam RT. At the University of Florida, a pre-loaded, custom-designed implant device for cesium has been in use since 1976 (Fig. 28.4). Interstitial brachytherapy can also be performed with high dose-rate (HDR) iridium catheters. A submental approach is used; the catheters are secured to the surface of the floor of the mouth with two buttons separated by half-moon spacers that are secured with sutures

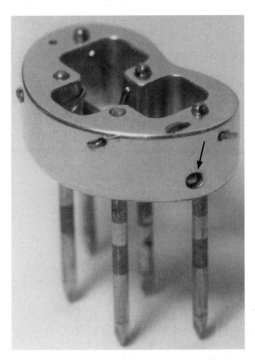

Figure 28.4. Custom-made implant device for stage T1-T2 cancers of the floor of the mouth. Note single crossing needle (*arrow*) through the center. Devices machined from nylon also are available. Cesium needles usually are used (2.0 cm active length, 3.2 cm actual length). Intensity of needles is adjusted so that dose-rate is approximately 0.4 Gy/h to area of gross disease. To ensure adequate surface dose, height of implant device (9 mm) is such that the active ends of the needles extend above the mucosal surface. Crossing needle is also 3 mm above mucosal surface (i.e., at active ends of needles). *Source:* From Marcus RB Jr, Million RR, Mitchell TP. A preloaded, custom-designed implantation device for stage T1-T2 carcinoma of the floor of mouth. *Int J Radiat Oncol Biol Phys* 1980;6:111–112, Fig. 2, p. 112; Fig. 16–18 in Levitt 2nd ed.

so as not to be aspirated or swallowed. Likewise, the catheters are secured to the neck with a third stainless steel button that is sutured to the skin. A typical treatment course is 20 Gy in 10 b.i.d. fractions and more specific details are discussed in the section on oral tongue cancer. Custom-made lead shielding of the nearby teeth, gingiva, and mandible are generally necessary, as is a feeding tube. If the plan is to treat with external-beam RT first followed by brachytherapy, the borders of the tumor need to be carefully tattooed and good photographs or a tumor diagrams need to be obtained. One should not inject the ink under pressure (i.e., using a syringe) because the ink will disperse widely.

Oral Tongue

Oral tongue cancers most often arise from the lateral aspect of the tongue. The choice of therapy usually depends upon the functional result. Most patients with tongue cancer treated at the University of Florida and at Emory University undergo surgery.

Size for size, oral tongue cancers are more difficult to control than base of tongue tumors, probably because they

are less radiosensitive. Compression of the overall treatment time is critical and, for this reason, brachytherapy is an integral part of the treatment if patients are treated with definitive RT. A typical dose-fractionation schedule is 30 Gy in 10 q.d. fractions to the primary tumor and upper neck followed by 35 to 40 Gy with a brachytherapy boost.

Conventional treatment can be designed to exclude portions of the parotid glands in the node negative patient. During the pretherapy evaluation, if gold crowns are appreciated, a fluoride tray (without the fluoride) will decrease the effect of secondary electrons that can cause an increased mucosal reaction. For small, well-lateralized lesions with no evidence of adenopathy, ipsilateral nodal and primary treatment may be feasible (Fig. 28.5).

The pattern of lymphatic spread for oral tongue cancer is such that nodal disease may spread to level III or IV with the ability to bypass level II. Therefore, most patients with node negative oral tongue cancers should have levels IB, IIA, III, and IV electively treated.

Because these are large fields and the patients are apt to present with weight loss, special attention to the nutritional needs of these patients is important. Inserting a pretherapy feeding tube in a patient who will likely require one prevents treatment breaks and may not increase the long-term risk of dysphagia so long as the patient continues to take some nutrition orally (23).

Treatment includes external-beam RT for the lymphatic disease as well as the primary tumor, with a boost to the latter with brachytherapy. For patients who will receive brachytherapy, a lead shield to protect the contiguous gingiva, teeth, and mandible should be part of the treatment preparations. Accordingly, most patients will not only undergo a dental consultation, but the prosthodontist will also take impressions to build a wax-covered, lead, mandibular shield. Without a lead shield, a 10% incidence of osteoradionecrosis has been associated with an HDR (>50 cGy/h using the Paris System) and a large reference volume (>25,000 mm^3 (24). These patients need an elective tracheostomy and feeding tube inserted prior to catheter insertion. Patient-controlled anesthesia is also helpful.

To perform the brachytherapy, the tongue cancer is carefully measured in the clinic and again under anesthesia. Because clinical understaging is common, the implantation is planned to cover a PTV at least 1 cm beyond the GTV. Prior to treatment, permanent metal markers are inserted to radiographically delineate the original borders of the tongue tumor, and draw detailed tumor diagrams (photographs can also be helpful). The marker can be inserted in the clinic or in the operating room.

With a heavy silk suture, the tongue is manipulated so that the target volume does not overlie the patient's mandible. The catheters are inserted submentally in parallel rows; a number 15 surgical scalpel is useful in penetrating the skin prior to catheter insertion. Depending on the circumstances, the lead shield may be sutured in place immediately before or after the inserting the catheters.

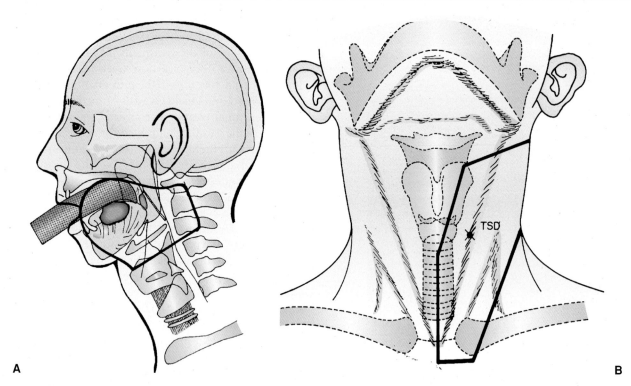

A

B

Figure 28.5. Superficial lateralized squamous cell carcinoma of the oral tongue; N0 neck. **A:** Single ipsilateral field encompasses submandibular (level I) and subdigastric (level II) lymph nodes; the entire width of vertebral body is included to ensure adequate posterior coverage of level II lymph nodes. Stainless steel pins inserted into most anterior and posterior aspects of lesion aid in localizing cancer on treatment-planning (simulation) radiograph and confirm coverage by interstitial implant. The larynx is excluded from the radiation field. Anterior submental skin and subcutaneous tissues are shielded when possible. The upper border is shaped to exclude most of the parotid gland. Intraoral lead block (*stippled area*) shields the contralateral mucosa and is coated with beeswax to prevent high-dose effect on adjacent mucosa from scattered low-energy electrons from the metal surface. The usual preinterstitial tumor dose is 30 Gy over 10 fractions with cobalt 60 (^{60}Co). For larger lesions that extend near midline, treatment is by parallel-opposed portals without intraoral lead block. **B:** For patients with clinically negative necks, only the ipsilateral low-neck field is irradiated. TSD, tumor-to-source distance. *Source:* From Parsons JT, Mendenhall WM, Million RR. Radiotherapy of tumors of the oral cavity. In: Thawley SE, Panje WR, Batsakis JG, Lindberg RD, eds. *Comprehensive management of head and neck tumors,* 2nd ed. Philadelphia, PA: WB Saunders, 1999:861–875, Figure 35.17A and B, p. 714.

The distance between the catheters varies from 1.0 to 1.5 cm. Rather than differentially loading the source closest to the surface (25), it is preferable to extend the catheter 1 cm above the dorsum of the tongue. To protect the palate from mechanical trauma and to ensure that the implant covers any exophytic disease above the surface of the tongue, two "half-moon" spacers and a metal button are used. Metal buttons are inserted so that the top button is positioned with the flat side abutting the palate. Buttons and spacers are secured with long (15 in.) 00 silk sutures and brought out through the mouth. The implant is designed to treat the area 1 cm above the surface of the tongue. The inferior portion of the catheter is secured using metal buttons gently crimped around the catheter and sutured to the skin. After the metal buttons have been crimped, methylmethacrylate ("bone cement") is applied to glue the catheters to the metal buttons. Since adopting this technique, our catheters have not inadvertently slipped.

After the desired dose has been delivered, the catheters are removed by gentle traction on the submental end of the catheter, and then the exposed catheter is amputated

flush with the submental skin. Next, the catheters are pulled out through the mouth. The dental shield is removed and the mouth is irrigated.

Hard Palate

Hard palate RT often entails treating an adenoid cystic carcinoma, which is a cancer known for its perineural pattern of spread.

At the University of Florida and at Emory University, patients with adenoid cystic cancers undergo resection of the primary tumor when medically and surgically feasible (26). Postoperative RT to the primary site of the disease is recommended for practically all patients except the rare patient with a Grade 1 T1 N0 cancer with a widely negative margin. Patients with lymphadenopathy receive neck dissection with regional RT.

For advanced unresectable tumors, neutron therapy may be considered. Alternatively, patients may be treated with photon and/or proton RT. Although there is no convincing evidence that chemotherapy benefits the patient with adenoid cystic carcinoma, 85% of patients with this disease stain positively for the epidermal growth factor receptor (27) and this may influence the selection of systemic therapy.

Treating the named cranial nerves is key to adequately treating adenoid cystic carcinomas. The perineural spread occurs by way of the greater and lesser palatine foramen. The greater palatine canal originates in the posterolateral aspect of the hard palate, abutting the pterygoid plate anteriorly and the pterygoid fossa. The nerves travel superiorly just lateral to the nasal cavity to the pterygopalatine fossa and through the foramen rotundum to the cavernous sinus.

OROPHARYNX

Essentially all cancers of the oropharynx will be treated with definitive RT combined with concurrent chemotherapy for patients with unfavorable American Joint Committee on Cancer (AJCC) Stage III or IV cancers (28). Patients treated conventionally usually receive 74.4 to 76.8 Gy at 1.2 Gy per fraction administered b.i.d or 70 to 72 Gy using daily treatments. Those treated with IMRT at the University of Florida receive 72 Gy in 42 fractions using the concomitant boost technique. Unless the larynx is involved or is in close proximity to the tumor, it is excluded from the portals used to treat the primary tumor. The patients are generally at high risk for both upper and lower neck disease, and the entire neck is irradiated except for those with well-lateralized tonsillar cancers when only the ipsilateral neck is treated. Planned neck dissection is usually added for patients with >5% risk of residual disease based on a CT scan obtained 1 month post-RT.

Base of Tongue

Base of tongue cancer has a high propensity for regional adenopathy. In the patient with clinically negative nodes, the risk of subclinical nodal disease is probably at least 50% (29) and levels IB, II, III, IV, and V as well as the retropharyngeal nodes should be treated. Conventional parallel-opposed portals used to treat a base of tongue cancer are depicted in Figure 28.6. Alternatively, the patient may be treated with IMRT. The low neck is treated with an anterior field with a tapered midline larynx block.

Base of tongue cancer is highly infiltrative and clinical understaging is common. The initial anterior border for the primary cancer should be 2 cm anterior to the tumor as defined by physical examination and radiographic evaluation. The superior border should include the soft palate (2 cm superior to the hard palate-soft palate junction), and the inferior border should include a 2-cm margin on the vallecula (the inferior border is usually at the thyroid notch).

There are no randomized data comparing the efficacy of a brachytherapy boost versus external beam alone. If brachytherapy is chosen, it is often done "up-front" to

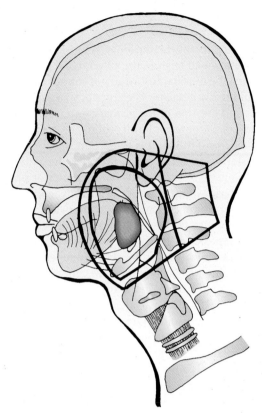

Figure 28.6. Radiation treatment technique for carcinoma of the base of the tongue. Superiorly, the portal treats the jugular and spinal accessory (level V) lymph nodes to the base of skull. Posterior border is behind spinous process of C2. Inferior border is at or just below thyroid notch, depending on extent of the disease. Anteroinferiorly, skin and subcutaneous tissues of submentum are shielded, except in case of advanced disease. The portals are usually reduced off of the spinal cord at approximately 45 Gy and a second reduction occurs at 60 Gy. The portals are usually equally weighted 3:2 toward the side of the lesion, if it is lateralized. *Source:* From Parsons JT, Mendenhall WM, Million RR. Radiotherapy of tumors of the oropharynx. In: Thawley SE, Panje WR, Batsakis JG, Lindberg RD, eds. *Comprehensive management of head and neck tumors,* 2nd ed. Philadelphia, PA: WB Saunders, 1999:861–875, Fig. 42.1, p. 866.

allow for better target delineation. Patients treated at both the University of Florida and Emory University receive external-beam with chemotherapy rather than brachytherapy plus external beam and chemotherapy for initial treatment.

Brachytherapy requires a preprocedure tracheotomy because, as a rule, the tongue swells massively after the implant. The implant is performed with the tracheostomy balloon inflated during the procedure and using the submental approach (as used for the oral tongue). Placing the inferior row of catheters posterior to the tumor is crucial. Generally, the catheters are inserted midweek, and 10 b.i.d. treatments of 2 Gy per fraction are prescribed during the following week. Because there is a 10% risk of lingual artery bleeding, the catheters need to be removed in the operating room under general anesthesia. Inspecting the catheters and buttons at the time of removal is necessary to assure that they are all accounted for.

Tonsil

The minimum treatment volume for early tonsillar cancers includes the retromolar trigone, the anterior and posterior tonsillar pillars, the tonsillar fossa and portions of the base of tongue, and the soft palate. The anterior margin varies with the size and location of the primary tumor but, even for small cancers, the anterior border should be at the level of the first or second molar. It is important to appreciate that the posterior tonsillar pillar includes the palatopharyngeous muscle, which inserts on the posterior pharyngeal wall inferior to the level of the pharyngoepiglottic fold. If the posterior tonsillar pillar is involved, it is necessary to include the attachment to the pharyngeal wall. Both the anterior and posterior pillars originate on the soft palate and therefore the initial field must have a superior border generous enough to include those attachments (2 cm superior to the junction of the hard and soft palate).

For the T1-T2/N0-N2 well-lateralized tonsil lesions with no tongue invasion and no significant extension onto the soft palate, ipsilateral treatment with a wedge pair can preserve contralateral salivary flow. For more advanced disease treated with conventional RT, parallel-opposed portals with either a 3:2 or 1:1 weighting are generally used. When trismus is present, it is necessary to include the pterygoid plates up to the base of skull.

Because T1 and T2 lesions of the anterior tonsillar pillar treated by definitive RT have a higher failure rate than tonsillar fossa lesions, treatment can consist of external-beam RT (45 Gy) combined with an intraoral cone or iridium boost of 20 to 30 Gy (30). When performing interstitial implantation of the tonsillar region, one must pay careful attention to the location of the nearby carotid artery.

Soft Palate

Cancers of the soft palate are relatively infrequent and can be treated conventionally using a parallel-opposed technique (Fig. 28.7). Early, discrete lesions can be boosted with an intraoral cone, which delivers a high dose to a limited volume in a relatively short time. T1 and T2 lesions enjoy a 90% 5-year local control rate (31). Because the risk of lymphadenopathy is appreciable, patients benefit from irradiating levels IB, IIA, III, IV, and V as well as the retropharyngeal nodes. If a boost is to be delivered by intraoral cone, the boost is done before the external-beam RT to allow for more accurate target volume delineation.

NASOPHARYNX

Patterns of Spread

Nasopharyngeal cancers usually originate from the superior and lateral walls of the nasopharynx; they frequently occlude the Eustachian tube orifice and can spread anteriorly to the nasal cavity, inferiorly to the oropharynx, and

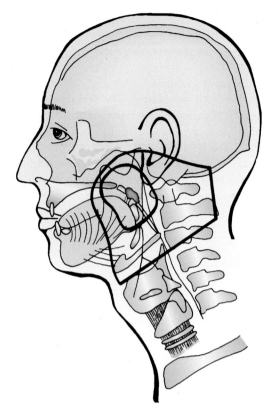

Figure 28.7. Initial and reduced lateral fields for treatment of carcinoma of the soft palate. Usual technique involves parallel-opposed portals. The minimum treatment volume for early-stage disease includes entire soft palate and adjacent pillars. The timing and the extent of field reductions after 50 Gy depend on the status of the neck as well as the extent of the primary lesion. If the primary lesion extends to midline or if clinically positive lymph nodes are present, both sides of the lower neck are irradiated. *Source:* From Parsons JT, Mendenhall WM, Moore GJ, Million RR. Tumors of the pharynx: treatment of tumors of the oropharynx—radiotherapy. In: Thawley SE, Panje WR, Batsakis JG, Lindberg RD, eds. *Comprehensive management of head and neck tumors,* 2nd ed. Philadelphia, PA: WB Saunders, 1998:861–875, Fig. 42.3.

both superiorly and laterally. Inferior extension to the oropharynx through the pharyngeal walls and the tonsillar pillars occurs in up to one-third of patients. The soft palate is involved secondarily in advanced cases but is rarely an initial site of the disease. MRI and CT may be complementary imaging modalities for nasopharyngeal cancers.

Anterior extension to the nasal cavity is relatively common and can be detected by a fiber-optic examination. It is important to evaluate both sides of the nasal cavity to detect nasal cavity involvement. Anterior extension can involve the posterior ethmoid sinuses and, less commonly, the maxillary sinus.

Superior extension is also common and base of skull involvement occurs radiographically in 31% to 59% of cases (32,33). The foramen lacerum opens directly into the middle cranial fossa and is a common route of invasion, as is the posterior petroclinoid fissure. Tumors that invade the skull frequently involve the cavernous sinus within which lies the vertical segment of the carotid artery. Occasionally, overzealous imagers will note erosion of the carotid artery and recommend that intravascular procedures be considered to preclude disruption before RT. In our experience, this has not been necessary. Approximately 1 cm lateral to the foramen lacerum is the foramen ovale, which is the point of egress of the mandibular nerve (V3). Taking a transverse section through the nasopharynx at the level of the foramen lacerum (from inferior to superior), one will find cranial nerves V3, V2, VI, IV, and III. The involvement of these nerves has been referred to as the petrosphenoidal syndrome with V3, V2, and VI being most frequently involved and diplopia being the most common cranial nerve finding.

Another cranial nerve syndrome involves IX, X, XI, and XII and indicates lateral extension through the parapharyngeal space. The sinus of Morgagni is a defect in the lateral superior wall of the nasopharynx and allows for egress of the Eustachian tube and the levator veli palatini muscle as well as advanced nasopharyngeal cancers. The tumor sometimes extends to the poststyloid parapharyngeal space and whether this is primary tumor extension or lateral spread of retropharyngeal adenopathy may be difficult to discern. Cranial nerve IX to XII invasion can cause hemiparesis of the superior constrictor muscle (CN IX) and soft palate (CN X), loss of taste (CN IX), and numbness of the soft palate, pharynx, and larynx (CN X).

Nasopharyngeal cancer has an extremely high risk of lymphadenopathy and, even in the clinically N0 situation, levels IB, IIA, IIB, III, IV, V, and the retropharyngeal nodes are irradiated bilaterally. Concurrent chemotherapy and RT (34–37) is the standard of care for advanced lesions; the role of induction and/or maintenance chemotherapy is investigational.

Treatment Techniques

Temporal lobe necrosis is a potential complication (38) and has been attributed to both technique and fractionation schedule. In addition to considering the dose to the temporal lobe, the optic chiasm, cornea, retina, and optic nerve doses must be considered.

The target volume is the primary cancer with a 2- to 3-cm margin, the base of skull, and the retropharyngeal and cervical lymph nodes in both sides of the neck. Bilateral cervical disease is present in >50% of these patients. Margins around the primary tumor are individualized on the basis of its size and local extent. One must take care to shield the brain stem and the optic nerves whenever possible. The optic nerves exit the orbits just beneath the anterior clinoids, and the brain stem lies immediately posterior to the clivus. Patients are treated with hyperfractionated RT to 74.4 Gy in 62 twice-daily fractions to reduce the risk of optic neuropathy and central nervous system (CNS) injury. The interfraction interval is at least 6 hours. Because of the proximity of the brain stem and spinal cord, doses of this magnitude are difficult to deliver when the primary cancer

extends laterally into the poststyloid parapharyngeal space. CT-based three-dimensional planning with beam's eye view to visualize the spatial relationship between the tumor and CNS has improved the ability to irradiate these cases with high doses without exceeding the tolerance of the adjacent normal tissues. DVHs can be used to analyze which of several options best localizes the dose to the target and restricts the dose to critical structures. IMRT is particularly useful to adequately irradiate the tumor when there is posterolateral spread of the primary tumor and most patients with nasopharyngeal cancers are treated with this technique.

When using conventional treatment, most nasopharyngeal cancers can be irradiated with a series of shrinking fields to deliver a high dose to the primary cancer and to limit the dose to critical structures (Fig. 28.8). The field is reduced to protect the spinal cord after 40 to 45 Gy in 4 weeks and to boost the primary cancer and retropharyngeal lymph nodes after 60 Gy. Patients are treated with 6-MV rays. The inferior margin of the upper lateral fields is placed at the level of the hyoid bone or thyroid notch to protect as much of the larynx as possible. After the spinal cord is shielded, the posterior neck is irradiated with 9 to 10 MeV electrons to a minimum dose of 70 Gy for involved lymph nodes and 50 Gy for subclinical disease. The low neck is treated with an anterior field with a 1.5- to 2-cm wide midline shield that extends from the superior junction to the bottom of the cricoid cartilage.

If persistent disease is suspected, brachytherapy may be used to boost the nasopharynx. With intraluminal appliances, the nasopharynx is irradiated for an additional 10 Gy to a depth of 1 cm by placing afterloading catheters through each nostril. Before proceeding with intracavitary RT with manual or remote afterloading, it is important to be sure that the catheters abut the tumor on the roof of the nasopharynx. Too often the catheters fall downward and prevent satisfactory delivery of dose to the depth of the tumor in the vault of the nasopharynx.

LARYNX

Supraglottic Larynx

Most cancers of the supraglottic larynx can be treated with definitive RT or a supraglottic laryngectomy as long as the patient has acceptable pulmonary function and no medical contraindications to surgery. A transverse supraglottic laryngectomy has a low recurrence rate in properly selected patients. Patients with clinically positive nodes may be treated with supraglottic laryngectomy, bilateral neck dissection, and postoperative RT or definitive RT followed by a neck dissection if the nodes have incompletely regressed. Avoiding a bilateral neck dissection after definitive RT is desirable. Patients treated with a supraglottic laryngectomy receive 55.8 Gy in 31 fractions plus a boost to the involved neck, if postoperative

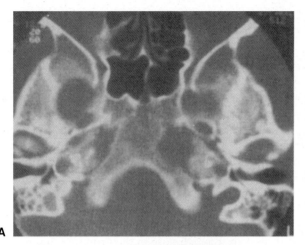

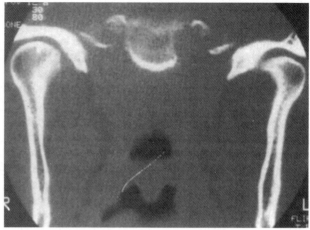

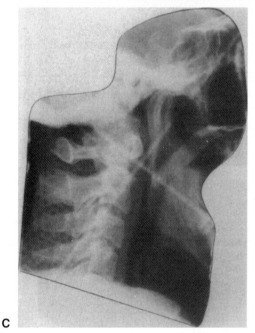

Figure 28.8. Radiation treatment technique for carcinoma of the nasopharynx. Axial (**A**) and coronal (**B**) computed tomographs of patient with T4 N2 squamous cell carcinoma of nasopharynx. Note bone destruction at petroclival junction. **C:** Beam angled 5 degrees posteriorly to avoid exit irradiation through posterior pole of contralateral eye. Because of the destruction of the base of the skull, the superior border of treatment volume is above pituitary fossa; in less advanced presentations, the superior border often passes through anterior and posterior clinoid processes, thereby placing the optic nerve in penumbra or out of radiation beam. Lymph nodes are included up to the jugular foramen or approximately 2 cm above the tip of the mastoid. Posteriorly, the level V chain is irradiated; in the presence of large or multiple lymph nodes, posterior coverage can be more generous. Inferior border excludes larynx, except in the rare circumstance of tumor extension down the lateral pharyngeal wall into the hypopharynx. Submandibular (level I) lymph nodes are at risk in patients with extensive lymph node metastases. The anterior border is designed to shield the segment of the posterior mandible while still encompassing tonsillar area. The portals include the posterior 2 cm of the nasal cavity. If necessary, the portal may be bowed anteriorly to cover more of the nasal cavity. (From Levitt 3rd ed., Fig. 16.12A, B, C.)

RT is indicated. Those treated with definitive RT receive 74.4 Gy in 62 b.i.d. fractions. If IMRT is used, the concomitant boost technique (72 Gy in 42 fractions over 6 weeks) is employed. It is desirable to avoid the Pearson near-total laryngectomy because of variable functional outcomes (39–41).

T1, T2, and low-volume T3 supraglottic cancers have good control rates with RT alone (42). Retrospective data has suggested that T3 tumors with volumes of <6 cm³ have 83% local control with RT alone (43,44). Unfavorable T3 and T4 tumors are often treated with laryngectomy and adjuvant RT; patients who receive definitive RT also receive concomitant chemotherapy.

If the neck is clinically negative and the tumor does not extend beyond the larynx, only the levels II, III, and IV nodes are treated. If the base of tongue or pyriform sinus is involved or if neck disease is extensive, the primary portal includes the entire jugular chain, spinal accessory chain (level V), and retropharyngeal nodes. In all situations, the low neck is treated with an anterior en face portal, the size

and shape of which varies according to the N stage and laterality of the disease.

The treatment volume is similar to that shown in Figure 28.9, with the exception that the beam generally is not allowed to "fall off" over the anterior skin surface, except in thin patients, in those with very bulky lymphadenopathy that extends anteriorly, or in those who have lesions involving the infrahyoid epiglottis near the anterior commissure. Shielding even a few millimeters of the anterior skin, subcutaneous tissues, and lymphatic vessels reduces the likelihood of desquamation (particularly in patients who receive concomitant chemotherapy) and may lessen the risk of serious laryngeal edema.

The inferior border of the portal is adjusted according to the extent of the disease. For a false cord or infrahyoid epiglottic cancer, the bottom of the cricoid cartilage is usually chosen. For an epiglottic tip cancer, the lower border may be placed at or above the level of the true cords, depending on the extent and growth pattern (infiltrative vs. exophytic) of the disease.

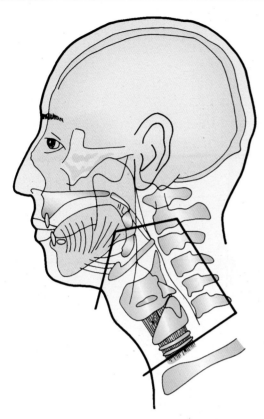

Figure 28.9. Radiation treatment technique for carcinoma of the glottic larynx, stage T3-T4 N0. Patient is treated supine, and field is shaped with Lipowitz's metal. Anteriorly, the field is allowed to fall off. The entire pre-epiglottic space is included by encompassing the hyoid bone and the epiglottis. The superior border (just above angle of mandible) includes jugulodigastric (level II) lymph nodes. Posteriorly, portion of spinal cord must be included within the field to ensure adequate coverage of midjugular (level III) lymph nodes; spinal accessory (level V) lymph nodes themselves are at low risk of involvement. The lower border is slanted (1) to facilitate matching with the low-neck field and (2) to reduce the length of the spinal cord in the high-dose field. The inferior border is placed at the bottom of cricoid cartilage if the patient has no subglottic spread; in the presence of subglottic extension, the inferior border must be lowered according to the disease extent. *Source:* From Parsons JT, Mendenhall WM, Mancuso AA, et al. Twice-a-day radiotherapy for T3 squamous cell carcinoma of the glottic larynx. *Head Neck* 1989;11(2):123, Fig. 1, p. 124; Fig. 16.2 in Levitt 2nd ed. p. 271.

Glottic Larynx

Treating early glottic larynx with definitive RT produces high rates of cure (45) owing to the relatively small tumor volumes when these patients present and the low likelihood of regional metastases. A recent randomized trial has shown that patients treated at 2 Gy per fraction once daily have inferior local control rates compared with those treated at 2.25 Gy per fraction once-daily (46).

Tis

As a treatment modality, transoral laser excision is more convenient than RT; the problem is that voice quality worsens as the extent of resection increases.

Proper selection for transoral laser excision requires an experienced team. The lamina propria sits beneath the basement membrane and has three distinct layers. The most superficial layer is Reinke's space and is filled with a loose gelatinous tissue that allows motion between the overlying mucosa and the underlying intermediate and deep layers of the lamina propria, which together form the vocal ligament. When Reinke's space is functioning, the mucosal waves travel across the glottis unimpeded. When videostroboscopic laryngoscopy reveals that the mucosal wave is unaffected, the patient with microinvasive cancer who does not have anterior commissure involvement may be best served by transoral laser excision performed with a narrow margin. Generally, when patients have anterior commissure involvement when the mucosal wave is impaired, or when the patient is not a good medical candidate, RT is an excellent choice for carcinomas *in situ* (Tis). Treatment for Tis is identical to that offered for T1 disease and consists of 63 Gy in 28 q.d. fractions.

Stage T1-T2

Because the risk of subclinical disease in the cervical lymphatics is remote, the portals are limited to the primary lesion (Fig. 28.10) (45). Although a common practice is to treat early vocal cord cancer with a standard field size (e.g., 6 × 6 cm), our preference is to design the portal to fit the specific lesion. The patient is treated in the supine position with the neck extended and the head immobilized in an aquaplast mask. The physician at the treatment machine checks the field each day according to palpable anatomic landmarks. This practice allows the treatment volume to be kept at a minimum while virtually eliminating the risk of geographic miss. Overall treatment time as well as total dose is critical in obtaining maximum control rates (45,47); failure to use the smallest field size consistent with adequate coverage of the tumor usually means that either the total dose or the dose per fraction must be compromised to limit acute reactions and/or late effects. The patient is treated with parallel-opposed 6-MV x-ray fields weighted 3:2 to the side of the tumor if it is lateralized. An anterior boost field is usually employed to deliver approximately 5% to 10% of the total dose to reduce the high-dose distribution laterally. ⁶⁰Co or 4-MV x-ray beams are ideal but are not available in most radiation oncology facilities; therefore, most patients are treated with 6-MV x-rays. The typical borders for a T1 N0 cancer are the middle of the thyroid notch, the bottom of the cricoid cartilage, 1 cm posterior to the thyroid ala, and 1.5 cm anterior to the skin of the anterior neck. The portals may be modified depending on the precise extent of the tumor.

CT helps determine tumor extent and therefore portal design in patients with large T2 cancers. It is useful in detecting subglottic spread, which may be submucosal and difficult to detect by direct laryngoscopy. T1 and early T2 cancers are often superficial and unappreciated on the planning CT. The dose-fractionation schedule is 63 Gy in 28 once-daily fractions for T1-T2 a cancers and 65.25 Gy

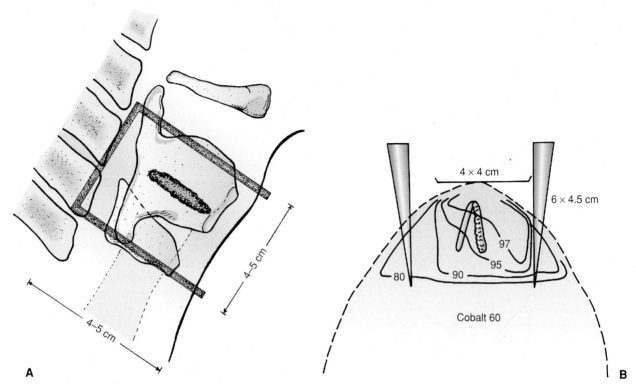

Figure 28.10. Radiation treatment technique for carcinoma of the glottic larynx, stage T1-T2. **A:** For T1 cancer, superior border of field usually is at mid-thyroid notch (height of notch typically is approximately 1.0 cm or slightly more in male adults). If ventricle or false vocal cords are minimally involved, top of the notch (which corresponds to cephalad portion of thyroid lamina as palpated just off midline) is often selected; more advanced lesions call for greater superior coverage. If only the anterior one-half of the vocal cord is involved, the posterior border is placed at the back of the midportion of the thyroid lamina. If the posterior portion of the cord is involved, border is 1.0 cm behind the lamina. If the anterior face of the arytenoid is also involved, posterior border is placed 1.5 cm behind cartilage. If no subglottic extension is detected, inferior border of the irradiation portal is at the bottom of the cricoid arch as palpated at midline. If computed tomography (CT) demonstrates subglottic extension, portal is adjusted accordingly. Anteriorly, beam falls off (by 1.5 cm) over patient's skin. **B:** Three-field technique (two lateral wedge fields and an anterior open field). Lateral fields are differentially weighted to involved side. Anterior field, which usually measures 4 × 4 cm, is centered approximately 0.5 cm lateral to midline in patients with one cord involved and typically delivers approximately 5% of total tumor dose (usually on last two treatment days) after treatment from lateral portals is completed. The anterior portal is essentially the reduced portal that centers high dose to the tumor. The isodose line at which the dose is specified is that which covers gross disease. By appropriate field weightings, encompassing the tumor within 95% to 97% of maximum isodose line is virtually always possible. *Source:* Part **A** from Million RR, Cassisi NJ, Mancuso AA. Larynx. In: Million RR, Cassisi NJ, eds. *Management of head and neck cancer: a multidisciplinary approach,* 2nd ed. Philadelphia, PA: JB Lippincott Co, 1994:431–497, Fig. 18–21, p. 464. Part **B** from Levitt 2nd ed., Fig 16.1C, p. 270.

in 29 fractions for T2b tumors (45). The prescribed dose is the minimum target dose (MTD). The maximum dose in the irradiated volume is typically <103%.

Owing to the paucity of lymphatic spread, early glottic cancers would seem reasonable candidates for carotid sparing techniques using IMRT. Studies have suggested that neck radiation increases the risk of stroke and other cerebrovascular events, and differences appear statistically significant but small. A Surveillance, Epidemiology and End Results (SEER) study found that the incidence of cerebrovascular events in head and neck cancer patients treated with radiation alone versus surgery alone was 35% versus 26%; yet, there was no increase in events in patients treated with surgery and adjuvant radiotherapy (25%) (48). Head and neck cancer patients may be at increased risk for stroke prior to any treatment, and IMRT allows carotid sparing. The risk of stroke may be dependent on

the length of carotid irradiated. The question is whether the risk of local failure is worth the theoretical risk of decreased dose to a small portion of the carotid artery (49). There is no conclusive data.

Stage T3–Favorable T4

The initial portals for T3-T4 N0 true vocal cord cancer are shown in Figure 28.9 (50). Patients selected for definitive RT have favorable low-volume cancers without significant cartilage destruction (42). Because of a 20% to 25% risk of subclinical involvement of the jugulodigastric (level II) or midjugular (level III) lymph nodes, these areas are electively treated with 45.6 to 50 Gy MTD. A small low-neck portal treats the low jugular (level IV) lymph nodes with 50 Gy given dose (at D_{max}) over 5 weeks. Primary fields are then reduced, and the treatment is continued to the final tumor dose with fields that are usually slightly larger than those described for early vocal cord cancer. Most patients currently receive 74.4 Gy MTD at 1.2 Gy b.i.d. with a minimum 6-hour interfraction interval. One must take care not to underdose a tumor that extends anteriorly through the cricothyroid membrane for patients with favorable T4 tumors who are treated with 6-MV x-rays. Patients with high-volume unfavorable tumors are usually not treated with RT alone or combined with concomitant chemotherapy because of a relatively low probability of cure with a functional larynx (51), but our understanding of advanced laryngeal cancer continues to evolve (52,53).

HYPOPHARYNX

Posterior pharyngeal tumors are often not completely resectable because of prevertebral fascia involvement and are usually treated with definitive RT, often combined with concomitant chemotherapy. Most patients with pyriform sinus cancers have advanced (unfavorable T2-T4) lesions and are not candidates for laryngeal preservation and are therefore treated with surgery and postoperative RT. The dose-fractionation schedules for postoperative RT have been previously described.

Pyriform Sinus

The pyriform sinus lies posteriorly within the pharynx and extends from the pharyngoepiglottic fold superiorly to the apex, which is located between the superior and inferior borders of the cricoid cartilage. Because the apex is situated below the level of the vocal cords, invasion by tumor can readily produce vocal cord paralysis. Because of this proximity, pyriform sinus RT unfortunately entails treating the larynx with its attendant morbidity. Patients with T1 and low-volume (<6 cc) T2 cancers are usually treated with definitive RT with 87% local control (54); concomitant chemotherapy is used for those with N2-N3 neck disease. Patients receive 74.4 Gy in 62 b.i.d. fractions or, if IMRT is employed, 72 Gy in 42 fractions using the concomitant boost technique. Portals for treating early and moderately advanced pyriform sinus cancers are shown in Figure 28.11. Bilateral level IIA, IIB, III, IV, and V neck nodes require treatment, even in the clinically N0 situation. Note that anterior skin "fall off" of lateral parallel-opposed treatment is rarely necessary for treating pyriform sinus cancers. Generally, if the anterior skin is at risk, the patient is not a good candidate for laryngeal preservation. Patients with unfavorable T2-T4 cancers are

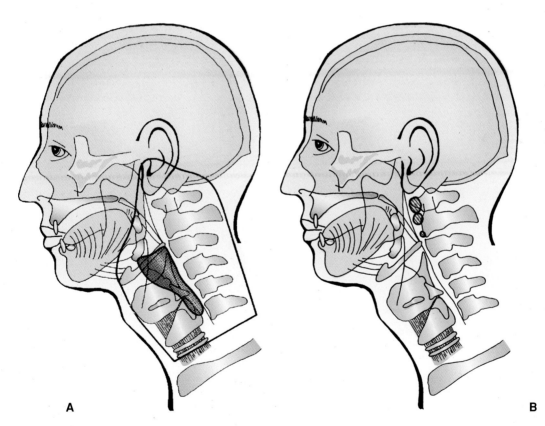

Figure 28.11. **A:** Portals used for initial treatment volume in a patient with carcinoma (*stippled area*) of pyriform sinus. Superiorly, portal covers lymph nodes at the base of the skull, then sweeps anteroinferiorly to cover posterior tongue base and level II lymph nodes. Anteriorly, at least 1 cm of skin and subcutaneous tissues (as viewed from lateral projection) is usually spared. Inferior border is 2 to 3 cm below the bottom of the cricoid cartilage and is slanted to facilitate matching with the low-neck portal and to avoid irradiating shoulders. The posterior field edge usually encompasses the spinous process of the C2 vertebral body. As treatment progresses, several field reductions are made (to shield spinal cord and to limit volume of mucosa that receives high-dose irradiation). **B:** The location of lateral retropharyngeal lymph nodes in relation to C1–2 vertebral bodies. (From Levitt 3rd ed., Fig. 17.3A and B.)

usually treated with total laryngectomy, partial or total pharyngectomy, neck dissection, and postoperative RT.

Pharyngeal Wall

The preferred treatment for essentially all patients with pharyngeal wall carcinomas is definitive RT. The radiation oncologist treating with lateral fields has a problem with adequately

treating the tumor and limiting the dose to the spinal cord. Once spinal cord tolerance has been reached, even if a half-beam block is used to "sharpen" the beam edge, placing the posterior beam edge anywhere within the vertebral body will risk underdosage to the posterior pharyngeal wall. Placing the beam edge at the posterior extent of the vertebral body, directly adjacent to the anterior surface of the spinal cord, has produced improved cure rates (Fig. 28.12) (55). For tumors

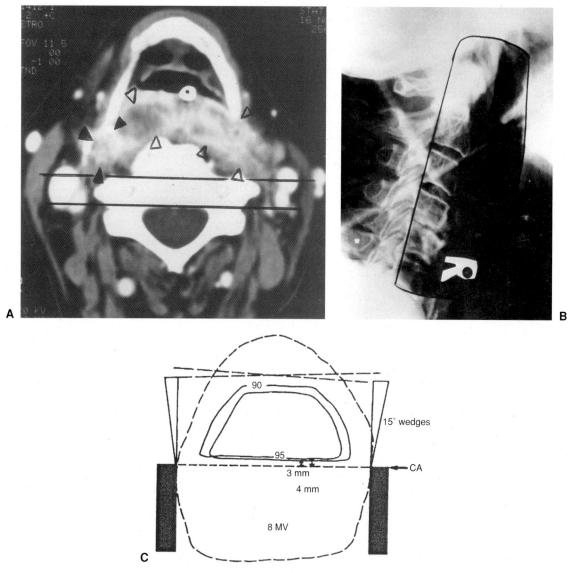

Figure 28.12. Radiation treatment techniques for carcinoma of the posterior pharyngeal wall. **A:** Computed tomogram of T3 posterior pharyngeal wall cancer (*arrowheads*). Horizontal lines represent two possible placements of posterior field edge. If field edge bisects vertebral body when spinal cord is shielded, part of cancer will be in penumbra or altogether outside irradiated volume. Entire width of the vertebral body is always treated in patients with posterior pharyngeal wall tumors. **B:** Simulation film shows first field reduction (to shield spinal cord) for a patient with T3 N0 cancer. Note that with reduced portals, little of the larynx remains within treatment volume. Only the epiglottis and part of arytenoids and aryepiglottic folds cannot be excluded. **C:** Isodose plots for reduced portals. In our practice, 6-MV x-rays are ideal energy. Because of the characteristics of high-energy (e.g., 20 MV) x-rays near field edge, isodose distributions are constricted compared to low-energy beams (43). Result is reduced dosage to cancer near posterior field edge, which is undesirable in treatment of posterior pharyngeal wall cancer. Central axis is placed at posterior field edge to provide nondivergent posterior field edge. Wedges are used to reduce dose anteriorly and to pull isodose distribution slightly posteriorly. *Source:* Parts **A** and **B** from Mendenhall WM, Hinerman RW, Amdur RJ, et al. Squamous cell carcinoma of the pharyngeal wall treated with irradiation. *Radiother Oncol* 1988;11:205, Fig. 3B and C, p. 210. Part **C** from Levitt 2nd ed., Fig. 16.4.

Now.

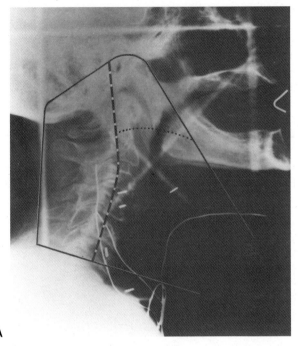
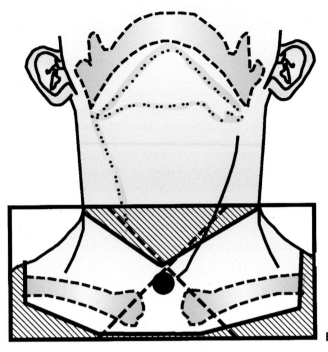

Figure 28.13. **A:** Typical postoperative simulation film of a patient with advanced-stage cancer of the laryngopharynx. *Dashed line,* initial field reduction (after 50 Gy, to shield spinal cord); *dotted line,* final reduction (after 60 Gy). Wires mark surgical scars and stoma. Slanting line used on lower border reduces length of the spinal cord treated by the primary field, allows better caudal coverage of mucosal surfaces while simultaneously bypassing shoulders, and facilitates matching with low-neck field. **B:** Low-neck field. Beam is vertical (0 degree). Rectangle (*solid line*) represents light field. *Dashed line,* central axis; *shaded areas,* blocked portions of field (stacked lead blocks). The superior border of the neck field is the inferior border of the primary field. The actual line is treated only with the primary field. The upper border of the low-neck field assumes V shape. At the midline of the patient, apex of V generally is at or close to central axis, so portion of beam that irradiates the spinal cord is nondivergent. At the junction of the three fields, a short (2–3 cm) segment of the spinal cord remains untreated through any of the fields. *Source:* From Amdur RJ, Parsons JT, Mendenhall WM et al. Postoperative irradiation for squamous cell carcinoma of the head and neck: an analysis of treatment results and complications. *Int J Radiat Oncol Biol Phys* 1989;16:25–36, Fig. 1, p. 27; Fig. 16.5 in Levitt 2nd ed.

that are wrapped around the vertebral body, IMRT is the technique of choice. Essentially all patients at the University of Florida are treated with external-beam RT alone or combined with chemotherapy. Patients treated with conventional RT receive 74.4 to 76.8 Gy in 1.2 Gy fractions administered b.i.d. Those treated with IMRT receive 72 Gy in 42 fractions using the concomitant boost technique.

Another method to boost the posterior pharyngeal wall bed is interstitial brachytherapy. Catheters are placed transversely in the plane anterior to the vertebral bodies and sutured in place with chromic. Because of the increased density of the vertebral body and the relatively thin target volume, this technique can safely deliver tumoricidal doses keeping the spinal cord below tolerance.

As in pyriform sinus cancers, levels II, III, IV, and V as well as the retropharyngeal nodes are at risk and the upper margin of the initial field should include the jugular foramen at the base of skull. Like esophageal cancers, "skip" lesions are possible and the inferior border needs to be generous.

Postoperative Irradiation of Laryngeal and Hypopharyngeal Tumors

When the larynx has been removed, the primary tumor bed and upper neck can be treated with lateral parallel-opposed portals (Fig. 28.13) (56). The inferior border of the lateral fields is usually at the top of the tracheal stoma. Techniques with either anterior or anterior and posterior portals have the disadvantages of underdosage of lymph nodes in the upper neck and unnecessarily irradiate a large volume of brain in the posterior cranial fossa. The field is reduced after ~45 Gy MTD, so that the spinal cord is no longer in the treatment field; the dose to high-risk areas behind the plane of the spinal cord may be boosted with 8- to 10-MV electrons.

The low-neck portal, which usually includes the stoma, is treated as shown in Figure 28.13 and receives 50 Gy in 25 fractions specified at D_{max} (the dose at maximum buildup) (56). Patients with subglottic extension and/or involvement of the apex of the pyriform sinus receive a 10 Gy boost in 5 fractions to the stoma with 12-MV electrons. Petrolatum gauze bolus can be placed on all scars and over drain sites. All scars, suture holes, and drain sites are treated with generous (2–3 cm) margins.

UNKNOWN PRIMARY

One of the advances in head and neck cancer within the last 10 to 15 years has been the realization that most patients who present with an unknown primary cell carcinoma of the head and neck have tumors arising in the tonsillar fossa or tongue base (57–59). Classically, treating the possible primary sites for the patient who presents with upper cervical node squamous cell cancer included treating the nasopharynx, oropharynx, larynx, and hypopharynx. Because of advances in imaging and the availability of fiber-optic endoscopes, the vast majority of nasopharyngeal, laryngeal, and hypopharyngeal tumors can be detected at presentation.

It can be argued that if the cervical disease has been adequately treated by surgery, the patient can be observed with a 25% to 50% chance of the primary being discovered (60,61).

The problem with this approach is that the head and neck cancer patient is often unreliable in follow-up. PET scanning to detect small, subclinical primary sites has been disappointing (62–64). In one study, 18-fluorodeoxyglucose-positron emission tomography (FDG-PET) imaging for patients with unknown primary cancers and cervical disease correctly detected the location of the primary tumor in one patient (8%) and was falsely positive in 6 (46%) of 13 patients (62).

Currently, patients presenting with the involvement of the level II lymph nodes receive RT to the oropharynx, through parallel-opposed portals (Fig. 28.14), and low-neck

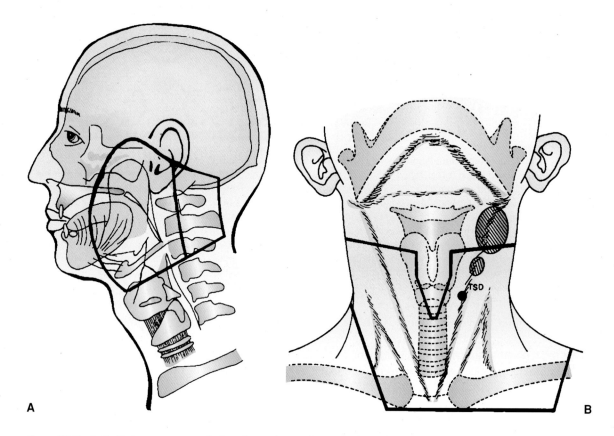

A **B**

Figure 28.14. **A:** Radiation treatment technique for carcinoma from an unknown primary site. Superiorly, the portal treats the nasopharynx and the jugular and spinal accessory lymph nodes to the base of the skull. The posterior border is behind the spinous process of C2. The inferior border is at the thyroid notch. Anteroinferiorly, the skin and subcutaneous tissues of the submentum are shielded, except in the case of advanced neck disease. The anterior tongue margin is set so as to obtain a 2-cm margin on the base of the tongue and tonsillar fossa, as well as the nasopharynx. One portal reduction is shown. **B:** Fields for bilateral lower neck radiotherapy. The larynx shield should be carefully designed. Because the internal jugular vein lymph nodes lie adjacent to the posterolateral margin of the thyroid cartilage, the shield cannot cover the entire thyroid cartilage without producing a low-dose area in these nodes. A common error in the treatment of the lower neck is to extend the low-neck portal laterally out to the shoulders, encompassing lateral supraclavicular lymph nodes that are at negligible risk while partially shielding the high-risk level III and IV lymph nodes with a large, rectangular block extending infraclavicularly, the medial supraclavicular nodal coverage could be compromised. The inferior extent of the shield is at the cricoid cartilage or first or second tracheal ring; with a rectangular laryngeal block. The inferior extent of the shield is at the midline as the lower neck is approached. Lateral borders of the low-neck portals are set to cover only the lymph nodes in the root of the neck when the risk of low-neck disease on that side is small (i.e., stage N0 or N1 disease). If there are clinically positive lymph nodes in the lower neck, or if major disease is present in the upper neck, the lateral border of the low-neck field is widened on that side to cover the entire supraclavicular region out to the junction of the trapezius muscle with the clavicle. TSD, tumor-to-source distance. *Source:* Part **A** from Mendenhall WM, Mancuso AA, Amdur RJ, et al. Squamous cell carcinoma metastatic to the neck from an unknown head and neck primary site. Am J Otolaryngol 2001; 22:261–267, Fig. 1. Part **B** from Million RR, Cassisi NJ, Stringer SP, et al. Management of the neck for squamous cell carcinoma. In: Million RR, Cassisi NJ, eds. *Management of head and neck cancer: a multidisciplinary approach,* 2nd ed. Philadelphia, PA: JB Lippincott Co, 1994:75–142.

RT to the level of the clavicles through an anterior field. Alternatively, IMRT may be employed if the patient presents with unilateral adenopathy. The retropharyngeal nodes are included and the portals are enlarged to a modest degree to include the nasopharynx in the unlikely event that the primary site is located there. The oropharynx receives 64.8 Gy in 36 q.d. fractions; the low neck receives 50 Gy in 25 q.d. fractions. Gross nodal disease is boosted to approximately 70 Gy. The portals are extended to include the supraglottis and the hypopharynx if the presentation is primarily in the level III nodes. Sparing a midline strip of skin on the neck is important to avoid lymphedema. When a solitary lymph node without extracapsular extension is involved and the neck has not been violated with an open biopsy, treatment with neck dissection and observation is preferred to avoid RT-related morbidity and because the chance of cure is not compromised if the patient is closely followed. A preauricular lymph node(s) containing squamous cell carcinoma typically represents metastasis from a skin cancer and is treated by a combination of parotidectomy and RT or RT alone, if surgery is not feasible. The ipsilateral low neck is treated with a separate anterior field. Low-neck presentation almost always arises from a primary site below the clavicles and the treatment is palliative.

Boost Technique for Large or Fixed Lymph Nodes

Some patients have small or unknown primary lesions that require only 60 to 65 Gy, but have a large, fixed nodal mass (e.g., 7–8 cm or more in size) that requires a higher dose (e.g., 70–80 Gy) even when neck dissection is planned (43). In many treatment centers, the common practice is to treat the neck node with electrons after irradiating the primary lesion. Use of anterior and posterior parallel-opposed wedged portals with 6-MV x-rays is preferred, to spare the mucosal surfaces and to avoid the excessive skin reaction and fibrosis produced by high-energy electrons (Fig. 28.15). Only the large mass, and not the entire neck, receives the high-dose boost, even if there are other involved lymph nodes in the neck. Neck dissection usually is performed 6 weeks after RT, unless the nodal mass completely regresses on the basis of both a physical examination and CT performed 3 to 4 weeks after completing RT. It is believed that wound healing after neck dissection is less likely to be a problem when the patient has been irradiated with photons rather than electrons.

When there is residual disease at the time of neck dissection, brachytherapy afterloading may be used. The problem is often disease involving the carotid sheath, and

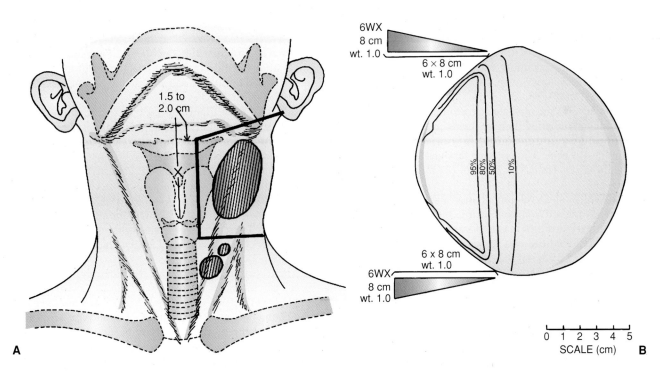

Figure 28.15. Photon portals for boosting dose to neck node after completion of treatment to primary lesion by lateral portals. **A:** Parallel-opposed anterior and posterior neck portals with wedges. Medial border is usually 1.5 to 2.0 cm from midline. Technique spares much of normal mucosa and the cervical spinal cord from high-dose irradiation and is particularly useful in a patient with a small primary cancer (e.g., T1) that requires a dose of 60 Gy and a large neck node (e.g., N3 a) that requires a high dose (e.g., 70–75 Gy). **B:** Dose distribution produced by anterior and posterior portals with equally weighted cobalt 60 (^{60}Co) wedge pair. Portals may be differentially weighted or high-energy x-rays may be used to produce a variety of dose distributions. *Source:* **A** from Parsons JT, Million RR. Treatment of tumors of the oropharynx: radiation therapy. In: Thawley SE, Panje WR, eds. Comprehensive management of head and neck tumors, Vol. 1. Philadelphia, PA: WB Saunders & Co: 1987, Fig. 15–37, p. 230. **B** from Million RR, Cassisi NJ, Mancuso AA. The unknown primary. In: Million RR, Cassisi NJ, eds. *Management of head and neck cancer: a multidisciplinary approach,* 2nd ed. Philadelphia, PA: JB Lippincott Co, 1994:311–320, Fig. 15.4D, p. 318; Fig. 16–37 in Levitt 2nd ed.

a single-plane implant is used with catheters crossing and lying on top of the carotid artery. The dose is 20 Gy in 10 b.i.d. fractions and the treatment has been well tolerated (65).

REFERENCES

1. Browman GP, et al. Influence of cigarette smoking on the efficacy of radiation therapy in head and neck cancer. *N Engl J Med* 1993;328(3):159–163.
2. Hammarstedt L, et al. Human papillomavirus as a risk factor for the increase in incidence of tonsillar cancer. *Int J Cancer* 2006;119(11):2620–2623.
3. Hammarstedt L, et al. The incidence of tonsillar cancer in Sweden is increasing. *Acta Otolaryngol* 2007;127(9): 988–992.
4. Chaturvedi AK, et al. Incidence trends for human papillomavirus-related and -unrelated oral squamous cell carcinomas in the United States. *J Clin Oncol* 2008;26(4):612–619.
5. Nasman A, et al. Incidence of human papillomavirus (HPV) positive tonsillar carcinoma in Stockholm, Sweden: an epidemic of viral-induced carcinoma? *Int J Cancer* 2009;125(2):362–366.
6. Chaturvedi AK. Beyond cervical cancer: burden of other HPV-related cancers among men and women. *J Adolesc Health* 2010;46(4 Suppl):S20–S26.
7. Beitler JJ, et al. Prognostic accuracy of computed tomography findings for patients with laryngeal cancer undergoing laryngectomy. *J Clin Oncol* 2010;28(14):2318–2322.
8. Garg MK, Yaparpalvi R, Beitler JJ. loss of cervical spinal curvature during radiotherapy for head-and-neck cancers: the neck moves, too. *Int J Radiat Oncol Biol Phys* 2004;58(1):185–188.
9. Pacholke HD, et al. Late xerostomia after intensity-modulated radiation therapy versus conventional radiotherapy. *Am J Clin Oncol* 2005;28(4):351–358.
10. Amdur RJ, et al. Unnecessary laryngeal irradiation in the IMRT era. *Head Neck* 2004;26(3):257–263; discussion 263–264.
11. Hall WH, et al. Development and validation of a standardized method for contouring the brachial plexus: preliminary dosimetric analysis among patients treated with IMRT for head-and-neck cancer. *Int J Radiat Oncol Biol Phys* 2008;72(5):1362–1367.
12. Netter FH. Ciba Pharmaceutical Products Inc., and CIBA-GEIGY Corporation, The Ciba collection of medical illustrations: a compilation of pathological and anatomical paintings. Summit, NJ: Ciba Pharmaceutical Products. 8 v. in 13, 1959.
13. Ang KK, et al. Human papillomavirus and survival of patients with oropharyngeal cancer. *N Engl J Med* 2010; 363(1):24–35.
14. Looser KG, Shah JP, Strong EW. The significance of "positive" margins in surgically resected epidermoid carcinoma. *Head Neck Surg* 1978;1:107–111.
15. Hinerman RW, et al. Postoperative irradiation for squamous cell carcinoma of the oral cavity: 35-year experience. *Head Neck* 2004;26(11):984–994.
16. Cooper JS, et al. Postoperative concurrent radiotherapy and chemotherapy for high-risk squamous-cell carcinoma of the head and neck. *N Engl J Med* 2004;350(19):1937–1944.
17. Petrovich Z, et al. Carcinoma of the lip and selected sites of the head and neck skin. A clinical study of 896 patients. *Radiother Oncol* 1987;8:11–17.
18. Vartanian JG, et al. Predictive factors and distribution of lymph node metastasis in lip cancer patients and their implications on the treatment of the neck. *Oral Oncol* 2004;40(2):223–227.
19. Tart RP, et al. Facial lymph nodes: normal and abnormal CT appearance. *Radiology* 1993;188(3):695–700.
20. Shah JP, Candela FC, Poddar AK. The patterns of cervical lymph node metastases from squamous carcinoma of the oral cavity. *Cancer* 1990;66(1):109–113.
21. Zelefsky MJ, et al. Postoperative radiotherapy for oral cavity cancers: impact of anatomic subsite on treatment outcome. *Head Neck* 1990;12(6):470–475.
22. Spiro RH, et al. Predictive value of tumor thickness in squamous carcinoma confined to the tongue and floor of the mouth. *Am J Surg* 1986;152(4):345–350.
23. Al-Othman MO, et al. Does feeding tube placement predict for long-term swallowing disability after radiotherapy for head and neck cancer? *Head Neck* 2003;25(9):741–747.
24. Lozza L, et al. Analysis of risk factors for mandibular bone radionecrosis after exclusive low dose-rate brachytherapy for oral cancer. *Radiother Oncol* 1997;44(2):143–147.
25. Schmidt-Ullrich R, et al. Interstitial Ir-192 implants of the oral cavity: the planning and construction of volume implants. *Int J Radiat Oncol Biol Phys* 1991;20:1079–1085.
26. Mendenhall WM, et al. Radiotherapy alone or combined with surgery for adenoid cystic carcinoma of the head and neck. *Head Neck* 2004;26(2):154–162.
27. Vered M, Braunstein E, Buchner A. Immunohistochemical study of epidermal growth factor receptor in adenoid cystic carcinoma of salivary gland origin. *Head Neck* 2002;24(7):632–636.
28. Calais G, et al. Randomized trial of radiation therapy versus concomitant chemotherapy and radiation therapy for advanced-stage oropharynx carcinoma. *J Natl Cancer Inst* 1999;91(24):2081–2086.
29. Candela FC, Kothari K, Shah JP. Patterns of cervical node metastases from squamous carcinoma of the oropharynx and hypopharynx. *Head Neck* 1990;12(3):197–203.
30. Mazeron JJ, et al. Interstitial radiation therapy for squamous cell carcinoma of the tonsillar region: the Creteil experience (1971–81). *Int J Radiat Oncol Biol Phys* 1986; 12:895–900.
31. Chera BS, et al. Definitive radiation therapy for squamous cell carcinoma of the soft palate. *Head Neck* 2008;30(8): 1114–1119.
32. Cheung YK, et al. Evaluation of skull base erosion in nasopharyngeal carcinoma: comparison of plain radiography and computed tomography. *Oncology* 1994;51(1): 42–46.
33. Ng SH, et al. Nasopharyngeal carcinoma: MRI and CT assessment. *Neuroradiology* 1997;39(10):741–746.
34. Al-Sarraf M, et al. Chemoradiotherapy versus radiotherapy in patients with advanced nasopharynx cancer: phase III randomized intergroup study 0099. *J Clin Oncol* 1998;16:1310–1317.
35. Chan AT, et al. Overall survival after concurrent cisplatin-radiotherapy compared with radiotherapy alone in locoregionally advanced nasopharyngeal carcinoma. *J Natl Cancer Inst* 2005;97(7):536–539.

36. Lin JC, et al. Phase III study of concurrent chemoradiotherapy versus radiotherapy alone for advanced nasopharyngeal carcinoma: positive effect on overall and progression-free survival. *J Clin Oncol* 2003;21(4):631–637.

37. Wee J, et al. Randomized trial of radiotherapy versus concurrent chemoradiotherapy followed by adjuvant chemotherapy in patients with American Joint Committee on Cancer/International Union against cancer stage III and IV nasopharyngeal cancer of the endemic variety. *J Clin Oncol* 2005;23(27):6730–6738.

38. Leung SF, Kreel L, Tsao SY. Asymptomatic temporal lobe injury after radiotherapy for nasopharyngeal carcinoma: incidence and determinants. *Br J Radiol* 1992;65(776):710–714.

39. Hoasjoe DK, et al. A comparative acoustic analysis of voice production by near-total laryngectomy and normal laryngeal speakers. *J Otolaryngol* 1992;21(1):39–43.

40. Keith RL, Leeper HA, Doyle PC. Microanalytic acoustical voice characteristics of near-total laryngectomy. *Otolaryngol Head Neck Surg* 1995;113(6):689–694.

41. Tang P, Qi Y, Tu G. Near-total laryngectomy in the treatment of advanced laryngeal and hypopharyngeal carcinoma. *Zhonghua Er Bi Yan Hou Ke Za Zhi* 1994;29(1):10–12.

42. Mendenhall WM, et al. Parameters that predict local control after definitive radiotherapy for squamous cell carcinoma of the head and neck. *Head Neck* 2003;25(7):535–542.

43. Freeman DE, et al. Irradiation alone for supraglottic larynx carcinoma: can CT findings predict treatment results? *Int J Radiat Oncol Biol Phys* 1990;19(2):485–490.

44. Mancuso AA, et al. Preradiotherapy computed tomography as a predictor of local control in supraglottic carcinoma. *J Clin Oncol* 1999;17(2):631–637.

45. Mendenhall WM, et al. T1-T2N0 squamous cell carcinoma of the glottic larynx treated with radiation therapy. *J Clin Oncol* 2001;19(20):4029–4036.

46. Yamazaki H, et al. Radiotherapy for early glottic carcinoma (T1N0M0): results of prospective randomized study of radiation fraction size and overall treatment time. *Int J Radiat Oncol Biol Phys* 2006;64(1):77–82.

47. Mendenhall WM, et al. Management of T1-T2 glottic carcinomas. *Cancer* 2004;100(9):1786–1792.

48. Smith GL, et al. Cerebrovascular disease risk in older head and neck cancer patients after radiotherapy. *J Clin Oncol* 2008;26(31):5119–5125.

49. Chera BS, et al. Carotid-sparing intensity-modulated radiotherapy for early-stage squamous cell carcinoma of the true vocal cord. *Int J Radiat Oncol Biol Phys* 2010; 77(5):1380–1385.

50. Parsons JT, et al. Twice-a-day radiotherapy for T3 squamous cell carcinoma of the glottic larynx. *Head Neck* 1989; 11(2):123–128.

51. Mendenhall WM, et al. Altered fractionation and/ or adjuvant chemotherapy in definitive irradiation of squamous cell carcinoma of the head and neck. *Laryngoscope* 2003;113(3):546–551.

52. Wolf GT. Routine computed tomography scanning for tumor staging in advanced laryngeal cancer: implications for treatment selection. *J Clin Oncol* 2010;28(14):2315–2317.

53. Chen SA, et al. Patterns of extralaryngeal spread of laryngeal cancer: thyroid cartilage penetration occurs in a minority of patients with extralaryngeal spread of laryngeal squamous cell cancers. *Cancer* 2011 Apr 26. doi: 10.1002/cncr.26130. [Epub ahead of print].

54. Rabbani A, et al. Definitive radiotherapy for T1-T2 squamous cell carcinoma of pyriform sinus. *Int J Radiat Oncol Biol Phys* 2008;72(2):351–355.

55. Fein DA, et al. Pharyngeal wall carcinoma treated with radiotherapy: impact of treatment technique and fractionation. *Int J Radiat Oncol Biol Phys* 1993;26(5): 751–757.

56. Amdur RJ, et al. Postoperative irradiation for squamous cell carcinoma of the head and neck: an analysis of treatment results and complications. *Int J Radiat Oncol Biol Phys* 1989;16:25–36.

57. Koch WM, et al. Oncologic rationale for bilateral tonsillectomy in head and neck squamous cell carcinoma of unknown primary source. *Otolaryngol Head Neck Surg* 2001;124(3):331–333.

58. Lapeyre M, et al. Cervical lymph node metastasis from an unknown primary: is a tonsillectomy necessary? *Int J Radiat Oncol Biol Phys* 1997;39(2):291–296.

59. Righi PD, Sofferman RA. Screening unilateral tonsillectomy in the unknown primary. *Laryngoscope* 1995;105 (5 Pt 1):548–550.

60. Iganej S, et al. Metastatic squamous cell carcinoma of the neck from an unknown primary: management options and patterns of relapse. *Head Neck* 2002;24(3): 236–246.

61. Wang RC, et al. Unknown primary squamous cell carcinoma metastatic to the neck. *Arch Otolaryngol Head Neck Surg* 1990;116(12):1388–1393.

62. Greven KM, et al. Occult primary tumors of the head and neck: lack of benefit from positron emission tomography imaging with 2-[F-18]fluoro-2-deoxy-D-glucose. *Cancer* 1999;86(1):114–118.

63. Keys H, Bundy B, Stehman F. Adjuvant hysterectomy after radiation therapy reduces detection of local recurrence in "bulky" stage IB cervical cancer without improving survival: Results of a prospective randomized GOG study. *Cancer J Sci Am* 1997;3:117.

64. McGuirt WF, et al. PET scanning in head and neck oncology: a review. *Head Neck* 1998;20(3):208–215.

65. Beitler JJ, Garg M, Owen RP, Yaparpalvi R, Smith RV. High dose rate brachytherapy plus neck dissection for nodal disease. *Head & Neck* 2008;30(7):933–938.

Cancers of the Skin, Including Mycosis Fungoides

Kenneth R. Stevens, Jr

INTRODUCTION

The superiority and justification for radiotherapy for these common cancers of the skin is in its ability to cure while preserving normal tissues, ensuring a superior aesthetic and functional outcome. To achieve this type of outcome, radiation therapy planning and implementation must be tailored to the anatomic site, tumor volume, histology, previous treatment, patient's age, and socioeconomic constraints. The treatment planning and implementation are usually straightforward, because the cancer can be directly visualized, palpated, and observed directly during each treatment setup. The treatment volume is rarely more than a superficial thin slab requiring a single direct beam collimated by a simple field-defining device placed on or near the skin.

The steps in planning irradiation for cancer of the skin are as follows:

1. Define the extent and size of the cancer.
2. Delineate the surface area and depth to be encompassed in the target volume.
3. Select the beam type, energy, daily fraction size, and total dose.
4. Tailor the field-defining device, allowing for margins, as discussed later.
5. Tailor the device for blocking beam exit when appropriate.
6. Tailor the bolus when appropriate.
7. Tailor the technique for patient immobilization and for reproducing the precise placement of the field-defining device each day.
8. Determine the machine position and setting for the irradiation.
9. Document the setup with photographs of gross lesion, lesion with shields in place, and finally with machine and shields in place.

Extent and Size of Cancer

Despite the fact that these cancers can be seen and palpated before planning treatment and on each day at treatment setup, geographic miss is the most common cause of failure. Most of these cancers are on the face or neck, are detected early, grow slowly, and present with a small tumor volume. The gross dimensions are usually readily determined by examination with a good light to aid inspection for edema or swelling, and by palpation to determine the extent of induration and fixation. A magnifying glass is useful to define the lateral extent of the gross tumor margins. For the occasional suspicion of invasion into a bone, such as the maxilla, or into deep soft tissue, such as the orbit, investigations with computed tomography (CT) scan, magnetic resonance imaging (MRI), or bone scan should be considered. Most lesions are <5 cm in diameter and <1 cm thick. Occult extension of cancer beyond these gross margins is generally limited to a few millimeters, but this varies, especially for cancers with clinically indistinct margins or high histologic grade, for sclerosing basal cell carcinomas, for recurrent cancer following surgery or irradiation, and for lesions >5 to 6 cm in diameter. In a prospective analysis of 117 previously untreated basal cell carcinomas, Wolf and Zitelli (1) reported that for cancers 2 cm in diameter, preoperative lateral surgical margins of 2, 3, and 4 mm produced local control rates of 75%, 85%, and 95%, respectively. Choo et al. (2) measured the lateral extent of nonmelanoma skin cancers at the time of resection, and determined that a margin of 10 mm was required to provide a 95% chance of obtaining clear resection margins. The microscopic tumor extent was positively correlated with the size of the tumor. Liu et al. (3) suggest that the deep margin of the tumor is more often underestimated by the surgeon than the lateral margins, and microscopically assessed inadequate deep margins are more likely to be followed by recurrence than "inadequate" lateral margins. Tumors at or near the naso-malar crease may extend deep into it. Occult extension may be well over 1 cm for cancers of high histologic grade, recurrent cancers, cancers with indistinct gross margins, and sclerosing basal cell carcinomas.

Delineation of the Target Volume

The facts cited earlier, together with the extensive clinical experience with x-ray and electron beam techniques, guides selection of the width of margins around the grossly defined lesion to be encompassed in the target volume. Incorporated in this decision should be an appreciation of the fact that for small fields, x-ray beams have better flatness and sharper penumbra than the electron beams. In practice, with an x-ray beam, 1-cm lateral margins around lesions 2 cm in diameter produce control rates >90%. Lateral margins up to 2 cm should be considered for lesions 6 cm or greater in diameter and for all lesions at high risk for occult extension as described earlier. A review of isodose curves reveals that lateral margins for fields irradiated with electron beams should be wider compared to orthovoltage beams for similar-sized cancers, but these margins have been less well defined. If a lesion is 2 cm in diameter and a 1-cm margin is to be given a minimum of 90% of D_{max}, the lateral margin for the electron beam field needs to be almost 1.5 cm. This requirement for a larger field size with the electron beam can be a major disadvantage in treating lesions of the eyelids and canthi. Lateral margins of 2 cm or even more should be considered for larger lesions (7–8 cm diameter), infiltrating lesions, and lesions at high risk for occult extension. Measurement and review of each treatment machine's central axis percent depth dose and cross-sectional isodose curves, based on the type of radiation, energy, and field size should be routine.

The deep edge of gross cancer infiltration can be assessed to some degree with bidigital palpation for cancers of the eyelid, ala nasi, pinna, and skin of lips and cheeks. Judgment of depth of infiltration for lesions of the scalp, forehead, malar eminence, canthi (which may invade orbital tissues), and preauricular regions includes an assessment of fixation to deep tissues. Because these clinical judgments are imprecise, the depth selected to be encompassed within the high-dose volume must be generous. With either the electron or x-ray beam, the full thickness of the eyelid, pinna, and ala nasi is usually carried to the high dose. For lesions ~4 cm in diameter and with minimal infiltration at other sites, a beam is selected to ensure that a deep margin of at least 1 cm is encompassed by the 80% to 90% isodose curve. The depth of larger infiltrating lesions may be assessed from clinical findings, and when appropriate, by CT scan or MRI. For infiltrative lesions at high risk for deep or occult extension, a deep margin up to 2 cm is encompassed by the 80% to 90% isodose curve. This may be difficult to achieve with a superficial or orthovoltage beam. Hence, an electron beam or mixed beam may be preferable. Caution should be exercised in planning and treating skin cancers over the calvarium, and consideration should be given to the dose to the brain cortex.

The replacement of x-ray simulators with CT scan-based treatment planning has added to the complexity of treatment planning for treating small superficial skin cancers. The use of CT scan-based treatment planning for small skin lesions may introduce more errors than if a simpler technique of using a transparency to determine the field size and shape is used.

Skin Cancer of the Head and Neck with Perineural Invasion

Perineural invasion occurs in 2% to 6% of cutaneous basal and squamous cell carcinomas of the head and neck and is associated with midface location, recurrent tumors, high histologic grade, and increasing tumor size (4). The cranial nerves most commonly involved are the trigeminal and facial nerves. Cranial nerve involvement portends a worse prognosis, with tumor extension and recurrence along the cranial nerves and to adjacent lymph nodes. Surgical resection should be considered if the tumor is considered to be completely resectable. University of Florida investigators recommend elective regional irradiation of first-echelon lymph nodes for patients with clinical perineural invasion and for those with squamous cell carcinoma with microcscopic perineural invasion. Patients with involvement of named branches of cranial nerves should have radiation volumes that include the involved cranial nerve to the base of the skull (4,5). Planning for these volumes requires careful clinical examination, detailed CT and MRI imaging, and 3D conformal radiation treatment planning and delivery.

University of Michigan investigators have detailed the pathways of recurrent tumor for skin squamous cell carcinomas involving the trigeminal and facial cranial nerves (6). They identified the auriculo-temporal nerve and the greater superficial petrosal nerves as the pathways of tumor spreading between those nerves. They recommend that for tumors involving cranial nerve VII, the auriculo-temporal nerve and V3 are at risk; and for tumors involving V2, the greater superficial petrosal and cranial nerve VII are at risk. These at-risk volumes should be included in the planned radiation volume when these nerves are involved.

Beam Type, Energy, Quality, and Other Factors

Clinical factors bearing on beam selection include diameter, depth, shape, and anatomic site of the target volume. Anatomic site is important in beam selection insofar as it relates to the presence of underlying critical tissues, ability to block the exit beam, adjacent critical tissue encompassed, and any cartilage or bone in the target volume. The increased availability of electron beams has resulted in a decrease in the availability of orthovoltage machines. In addition to the differences in dose drop-off at the field's lateral edges, the following differences between x-ray and electron beams are important in treating cancer of the skin:

1. The depth dose of an electron beam drops off sharply beyond the therapeutic range, depending on the beam energy (Table 29.1). This can be a major advantage in sparing tissues deep to the cancer.
2. Electron beams <12 MeV are associated with skin sparing, which requires the use of bolus material 0.5 to 1 cm thick (Table 29.1 and Fig. 29.1). This added thickness must, of course, be included in beam selection and in depth dose calculation.
3. The electron-beam low-percentage isodose curves expand laterally quite rapidly as they pass through tissues, especially for low-energy beams. Curves of

TABLE 29.1	Range of Depth of 90% Isodose Lines of Electron Beams		
Electron beam (MeV)	Minimum depth (cm)	Maximum depth (cm)	Depth of 5.0% dose (cm)
6	0.6 to 1.0	1.7	3.0
9	0.4 to 1.0	2.7	4.5
12	0 (skin surface)	3.5	6.0
16	0 (skin surface)	4.5	9.0
20	0 (skin surface)	5.5	12.0

Electron-beam depth-dose data depend greatly on the collimation system employed by the accelerator. These data must be measured specifically for the given machine (Field size 8 cm², source-to-surface distance = 100 cm).

high-percentage isodose levels and of high-energy beams tend to constrict, especially for small fields. Bolus contributes to the risk of placing this constriction near the margins of the cancers. Sharply narrowed portions of an irregularly shaped large electron field shows strikingly different surface doses and isodose curves from those of the remainder of the volume. Systematic review of the relevant isodose curves is essential.

4. The relative biologic effectiveness (RBE) of the electron beam is 10% to 20% less than that of the superficial or orthovoltage beam. Because, virtually all publications have quoted optimal doses for orthovoltage beams, systematic correction is necessary when the electron beam is used. For equivalent effect, electron beam dose should be 10% to 20% greater than orthovoltage dose.

5. The absorption of electron beams in bone resembles that of orthovoltage beams rather than that of megavoltage beams. This lack of bone sparing is sometimes an important consideration.

6. Surface and depth doses with both types of beams vary substantially with the spectrum of technical factors (field size, energy, and collimation) selected in tailoring irradiation to the volume requiring treatment. Each new set of factors requires an assessment of dose rate and dose distribution.

With a few exceptions as cited in examples given later, the control rates and the aesthetic and functional results of irradiation of lesions of similar size and location should be similar whether treated with orthovoltage photon beams or electron beams. When differences in outcome have been reported, they sometimes suggest superior control rates with orthovoltage photon beams (3). The most likely explanation for this type of difference relates to the direct transfer of x-ray beam techniques and radiation dose to the use of electron beams in the early days without taking into full consideration of all these differences.

For large fields >8 to 10 cm in diameter, electron beams produce a more homogeneous dose distribution across the surface of the lesion, but decreased dose near the edges must be respected. Also, dose deep to the cancer must be kept to a minimum, such as brain cortex dose when irradiating a cancer of the scalp, where the rapid drop-off in dose at a known depth is a significant advantage of the electron beam. The flexibility and ease of setup, along with the relatively sharp field lateral edges, especially for smaller cancers, are advantages of the x-ray beams. The approximate range of the depth of the 90% isodose line for electron beam energies are shown in Table 29.1. The depth and shape of the isodose lines should be determined for each treatment machine at various energies and field sizes.

Electronic and Radiosotope Brachytherapy

There has been recent interest in using low-energy photons in new electronic and radioisotope brachytherapy devices and techniques. These devices have been initially used in locally irradiating intracavitary locations such as

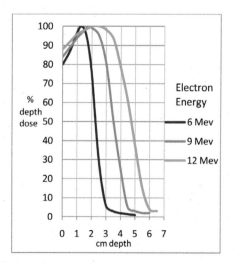

Figure 29.1. Isodose curves for 6-, 9-, and 12-MeV electrons, 8 × 8-cm field, showing greater skin sparing for lower energy electron beams.

breast operative sites (7). Their use is expanding to include irradiation of small skin cancers. These devices may be useful in treating small superficial skin cancers that have a diameter of <5 cm and a thickness of <3 or 4 mm. Circular treatment cones are 10, 20, 35, and 50 mm in diameter. The target/source to skin distance is 2 to 3 cm, resulting in a rapid decrease in radiation dose with increasing depth from the cone applicator and skin surface. The percent depth doses for a 50-keV beam at these treatment distances are approximately 58% to 66% at 4 mm depth, and 51% to 60% at 5 mm depth. Some treatment cones use a step filter to provide a flatter isodose curve. There is limited clinical information regarding the efficacy of these devices for treatment of skin cancers at this time.

Field-Defining Devices

When a lead or lead alloy (Cerrobend) cutout is used, the metal must be thick enough to allow transmission of not >5% of the maximum dose (Table 29.2) (8). The following techniques may be used to design the metal cutouts. The outline of the treatment field, which includes consideration of the characteristics of the treatment beam and of occult tumor spread, is marked on the skin with a ballpoint pen or skin-marking ink. This outline is transferred to the surface of the lead as follows:

1. Overlay the skin surface with a clear plastic sheet that readily conforms to undulations of the surface.
2. Trace the field outline on the plastic.
3. Overlay the lead with the plastic. Then with the point of a knife punch the outline through the plastic onto the surface of the lead. Another technique is to draw the field outline on the skin with a ballpoint pen. Overlay

TABLE 29.2	Minimum Cerrobend Thickness to Block 95% of Electron Treatment Beam (10 × 10 cm Field Size)
Electron energy (MeV)	**Cerrobend thickness (mm)**
6	2.3
9	4.4
12	8.5
16	18.0
20	25.0

The thickness of lead required for *electron beam* blocking is approximately given by ($E/2$) mm Pb, where E is the incident electron energy; for example, blocking of an 6-MeV electron beam requires lead at least 3-mm thick. *Source:* From Purdy JA, Choi MC, Feldman A. Lipowitz metal shielding thickness for dose reduction of 6–20 MeV electrons. *Med Phys* 1980;7:251–253.

clear adhesive tape on the skin. The tape will pick up the ink outline. Place the clear adhesive tape with outline on lead sheet and proceed with the next step.

4. Cut out the lead sheet target field outline with a knife and smooth the edges of the cutout. Rubbing the edge of the cutout with cloth or paper can remove small burrs. Shape the lead to the patient's contour. Thin lead can be shaped with the fingers. For thicker lead or for shaping to sharply undulating surfaces, such as the medial canthus, the lead can be pressed or hammered lightly to conform to a plaster cast of a face used specifically for this purpose. The hammering must not appreciably thin the lead. Occasionally, it may be necessary to make a plaster cast of the region to shape the lead cutout.

5. When an electron beam field is defined with a lead cutout placed directly on the skin, the substantial thickness of the cutout requires that it be constructed of multiple layers of thin lead, thick lead cut with a saw, or a shield molded from Cerrobend. With such a surface shield, a zone of increased dose develops just deep into the edge of the cutout (9). The magnitude of this dose increases with beam energy. At lower energies this effect is commonly disregarded. Concern for this effect, the need for bolus, and the ease of block construction encourage the practice of fixing the field-defining device for the electron beam on the end of an electron cone several centimeters from the skin.

6. When a Cerrobend tailored block is used to define the field of an electron beam, the treatment field outline on the patient is overlaid with a fine metal wire taped in place. The block is constructed from a simulation film or CT scan taken with the patient in the treatment position and with the geometry of the treatment setup in mind. The tailored block is mounted on a cone at a fixed distance from the skin (5–10 cm is common). The thickness of lead required for electron beam blocking is approximately given by ($E/2$) mm of lead, where E is the incident electron energy in MeV. This means that the field-defining device for electron beams must be substantially thicker than for superficial x-ray beams and that the usual eye shield for an x-ray beam is not adequate for the electron beam commonly used in its place (10,11). For further details of the electron beam's characteristics and shielding, see Khan (12). When bolus is used, it must be placed on the skin and not placed in an electron cone at some distance from the skin surface (see section on "Bolus").

Electron Output Correction Factor

It is very important to critically double-check the output factors for small electron fields. Microchambers, thermoluminescent dosimeters (TLDs), or film dosimetry should be used to confirm the proper output factor. Output factors for electron fields smaller than 3 cm in diameter can be erroneous. The output factor for radiation fields of

2 to 3 cm in diameter in our institution is ~0.90 cGy/MU at 100 source-to-surface distance (SSD). Significant errors in dosage can occur if the output factor is not correct. Output factors that are significantly greater or less than 0.90 should be critically reviewed and double-checked.

Exit Beam Blocking

Often, normal tissues deep to the treatment volume can be spared by blocking a part or the entire exit beam. The ability to do this varies with anatomic site, extent of cancer, and the patient's tolerance to the blocking device. Usually with an x-ray beam, a tailored lead shield ~1 mm thick can be encased in paraffin or dental compound to block, at least, a part of the exit beam and to diminish electron backscatter. When an electron beam exit shield is to be used, some caution is appropriate. Backscatter from the lead can be substantial (30–70% of depth dose at that level). Encasing the shield in dental acrylic or wax of 3 mm thick generally reduces the scatter to an acceptable level for beam energies up to 12 MeV. Finally, the eye shields commonly used with orthovoltage beams are of 2-mm thick lead. This is insufficient for commonly used electron beams, inasmuch as the scatter and transmitted dose can be sufficient to produce cataracts (10,11). In addition, thicker lead eye shields and shields encased in dental acrylic or wax are difficult to insert. For these reasons, x-ray beams are usually preferred for cancers around the eyes.

Bolus

A scattering material such as bolus must be used with 6 and 9 MeV electron beams to ensure that the dose on the skin surface is the maximum tissue dose and to even out irregular contours so as to present a flat surface normal to the electron beam. Superflab (Mick Radio-Nuclear Instruments) is our choice for bolus material, because it is nearly tissue equivalent, transparent, and easy to shape. It is available in 3-, 5-, and 10-mm thickness. This bolus, of course, blurs or masks the outline of the treatment field. For this reason, it is helpful during the treatment setup to align the patient and machine as for irradiation but with a gap to permit bolus placement. The correctness of the position of the treatment field should be visually confirmed. The bolus is then slipped into place. The minimum thickness of bolus to achieve maximum dose at the surface varies with the energy of the electron beam (Table 29.1). Although 5- and 10-mm thick boluses are commonly used for 6- and 9-MeV electrons, based on the percent depth-dose data, an 8-mm thick bolus (combination of 5- and 3-mm thickness) may be more appropriate. When treating to the 90% line, bolus may not be necessary for electron beams of 12 MeV or greater. When it is used, bolus should always be placed on the skin surface. When bolus is located at a distance above the skin, it will cause a scattering of radiation laterally from the designed radiation treatment area.

Selected Aspects of Treatment Setup

Because the lateral radiation margins are often narrow, the importance of effective patient immobilization and precision in cutout positioning cannot be overemphasized. Immobilization techniques used for irradiating head and neck cancers are used for skin cancers of the face and neck. The surface of the treatment field should be as nearly perpendicular to the treatment beam axis as is practical. With an orthovoltage photon beam, dose inhomogeneities because of irregular surface contours can usually be diminished to acceptable levels by increasing the SSD. Lead cutout positioning and fixation are facilitated if the shield conforms closely to the contours of the region and the tape fixes the cutout to the patient. When the cutout can be fixed to the skin, the treatment beam breadth should exceed that of the cutout area by ~1 cm, minimizing the effect of patient movement. Of course, the width of the lead must exceed that of the treatment beam.

Frequent clinical physician visualization of the treatment setup is very important to confirm that the treatment field is properly aligned relative to the tumor.

The techniques used in the irradiation of skin cancers of the lip, ala nasi, temporal skin and external ear, and medial orbital canthus with spread to the eyelid are illustrated in the four patient examples discussed later. The techniques used to irradiate squamous and basal cell cancer of the skin in sites other than the face, that is, unexposed skin, vulva, penis, anus, and the like, are the modifications of the techniques described.

Fractionation Schedules

A spectrum of fractionation schedules and total doses for irradiation of skin cancer have been advocated. The two most commonly used are those of Mendenhall et al. (Table 29.3) and of Solan et al. (Table 29.4). Local control by both schedules is excellent. Comparable electron doses should be 10% to 20% greater than orthovoltage doses. The more protracted schedules are designed to minimize fibrosis, telangiectasia, and necrosis. Such schedules are especially useful for large lesions and for all lesions of the canthi, eyelids, nose, and ears. Schedules using higher daily doses, fewer fractions, and fewer fractions per week may be considered for smaller lesions (usually in other sites) or when the number of patients' visits must be limited.

The published data are not always clear regarding whether the radiation doses are D_{max} doses, or whether they are calculated to a 90% or an 80% isodose line.

Clinical judgment and experience are necessary to give the appropriate radiation dose. The lesion at the completion of treatment should show evidence of significant regression, and a moist reaction and surface crusting may be present. In the author's own experience over 40 years, some tumors are controlled with lesser doses and some

TABLE 29.3			Recommended Orthovoltage Dose and Fractionation Schedule
Total dose (Gy)	No. of fractions	Duration of treatment	Comments
40	10	2 weeks	Less satisfactory cosmetic results but used when treatment course must be short or for <1.0-cm lesion away from nose, ear, or eyelids
30	5	1 week	
20	1	1 day	
45	15	3 weeks	Moderate size (5 × 5) lesion away from nose, ears, or lids
50	20	4 weeks	<1.5-cm thin lesion of nose, ears, eyelids, or canthi
55	30	6 weeks	Moderate-size (5 × 5 cm) lesion of nose, ear, canthi, or eyelid
60	33	7 weeks	Large lesion with minimal or suspected involvement of bone or cartilage
65	36	7 weeks	Large lesion recurrent or with cartilage or bone involved

Electron beam doses should be 10–20% greater for equivalent effect.
Fractions given 5 days a week unless indicated otherwise.
Source: Reprinted from Mendenhall WM, Million RR, Mancuso AM, et al. Carcinoma of the skin. In: Million RR, Cassisi NJ, eds. Management of head and neck cancer. Philadelphia, PA: JB Lippincott Co., 1994:672, with permission.

require higher doses. Hence, it is very important for the physician to visually examine the tumor on a periodic basis, especially near the estimated time of completion of treatment, because it may be appropriate to decrease or increase the originally prescribed radiation dose, based on the clinical examination.

Examples of Treated Patients

Case 1: Squamous cell carcinoma of lip Figures 29.2 through 29.6.

An 87-year-old woman had a destructive squamous cell carcinoma of the right side of her upper lip. Because of

TABLE 29.4		Recommended Orthovoltage Dose and Fractionation	
Area size	Total dose (Gy)	No. of fractions	Duration of treatment (days)
Small areas (<5 × 5 cm²) (Less satisfactory cosmetic results with large dose/ fraction)	20	1–2	1–2
	30	5	5–7
	40	10–16	16–20
Larger areas	45	15–18	21–30
	50	20–25	28–35
	60	20–30	28–40

Electron beam doses should be 10–20% greater for equivalent effect.
Source: Reprinted from Solan MJ, Brady LW, Binnick SA. Skin. In: Perez CA, Brady LW, eds. *Principles of radiation oncology.* Philadelphia, PA: JB Lippincott Co., 1992:486, with permission.

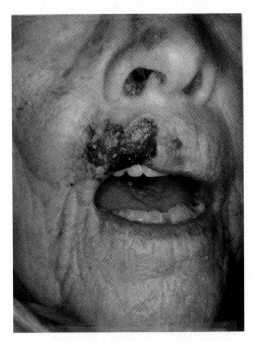

Figure 29.2. An 87-year-old woman with squamous cell carcinoma of right side of upper lip. Prior to irradiation.

her age and difficulty in arranging transportation, she was treated with 300 cGy/day to the 90% line, three fractions per week with 6-MeV electrons, with 5 mm of gel bolus over the lip and a lead shield between the upper lip and the upper alveolar ridge. Following eight fractions, she was given a 13-day break because of an intense radiation reaction on the surface of the tumor and the surrounding skin, and then she returned for an additional eight fractions. Her tumor was subsequently totally controlled with good cosmetic result with a total dose of 4,800 cGy in 16 fractions over 42 elapsed days.

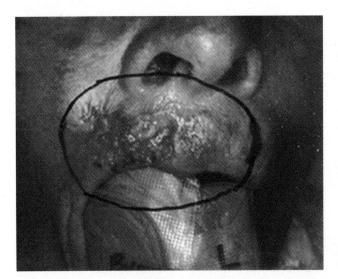

Figure 29.3. At time of fourth radiation treatment with 6-MeV electrons, 5-mm gel bolus on the skin, black line is edge of radiation field as defined by Cerrobend cutout, treated at 300 cGy per day to 90% line, three fractions per week. A lead shield enclosed in a folded glove is placed between the upper lip and the upper alveolar ridge.

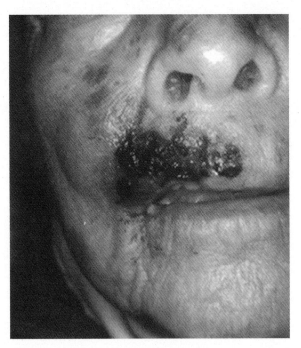

Figure 29.4. At seventh radiation fraction, 2,100 cGy to 90% line. Following the eighth treatment (2,400 cGy) she was given a 13-day break in her treatments because of the intense symptomatic radiation reaction over the surface of the tumor.

Case 2: Squamous cell carcinoma of the left ala nasi Figures 29.7 through 29.11.

This 79-year-old man had a very large ulcerated 4 × 4 × 3.5-cm squamous carcinoma that involved and distorted the left ala nasi blocking the left nostril (Figs. 29.7 through 29.11). The treatment planning CT scan and the

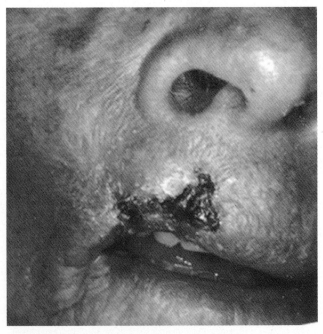

Figure 29.5. At completion of radiation treatments, 4,800 cGy in 16 fractions, 3 fractions per week, over 42 elapsed days. Eight fractions followed by a 13-day break, followed by eight more fractions.

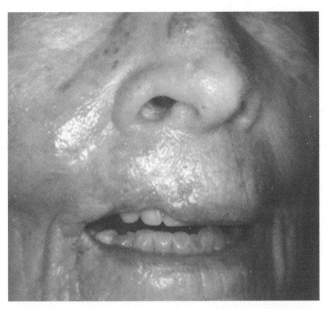

Figure 29.6. Six weeks following completion of irradiation. No evidence of tumor. There is slight deformity of the right side of the upper lip because of prior destruction from the tumor. Considering the original tumor appearance, this is a very good functional and cosmetic result.

radiation treatments were performed with the patient immobilized in a thermoplastic mask. The CT scan showed the depth of the tumor involvement. He was initially treated with a combination of 12-MeV electrons (70% weighting) and 16-MeV electrons (30% weighting). The shaped left anterior oblique field (Cerrobend cutout in electron cone) included a 1-cm peripheral margin. He received a total of 5,100 cGy to the 90% line in 17 frac-

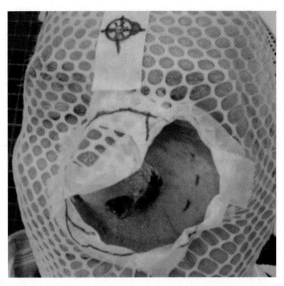

Figure 29.8. Photo taken at 3,000 cGy, original field is marked in *black ink* and reduced field is marked in *red ink;* treatment continued to total of 4,800 cGy.

tions over 30 days, treating 4 days/week. The final 1,800 cGy was given with a reduced field size and with 12-MeV electrons because the tumor depth had decreased by that time. No bolus was used because the 90% isodose line (green line) of the 12- and 16-MeV electron beams was at the tumor surface.

Cancer of the ala nasi commonly invades and destroys the underlying cartilage. Laterally, the lesion may extend

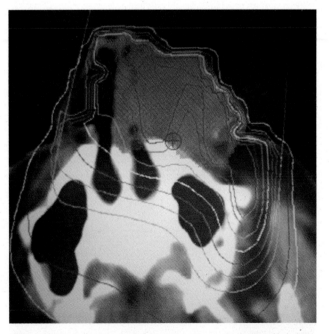

Figure 29.9. Isodose lines of treatment with combination of left anterior oblique 12- and 16-MeV electrons, treatment prescription calculated to green 90% line, which surrounded tumor volume and also included tumor surface, no bolus was used. Colors and percent isodose lines: *red* 105%, *blue* 100%, *green* 90%, *yellow* 80%, *magenta* 70%, *light blue* 60%, *orange* 50%, *purple* 30%, *light yellow* 20%.

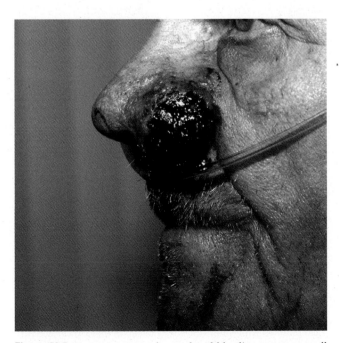

Figure 29.7. 4 × 4 × 3.5 cm ulcerated and bleeding squamous cell carcinoma of left ala nasi, prior to treatment.

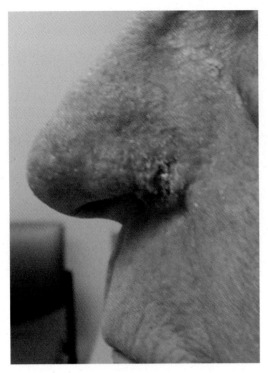

Figure 29.10. Two weeks following the completion of 4,800 cGy.

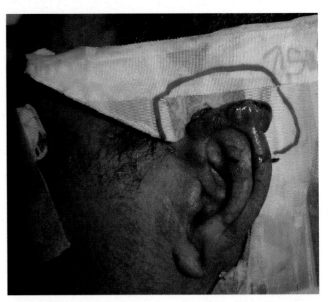

Figure 29.12. Nodular exophytic basal cell carcinoma of dorsum of left external ear, lead shield behind ear to shield scalp and brain, purple line is field outline from lead shield cutout in 9-MeV electron cone, 1-cm gel bolus placed directly over tumor. Prior to treatment.

to the embryonic fusion planes of the nasolabial fold. This permits deep infiltration. Although not used in this patient, exit beam shields of lead, coated with paraffin, and then slipped into the left nostril or anterior to the upper gum may be used. When the tumor is close to the orbits, extra eye shields are used.

Case 3: Sclerosing basal cell carcinoma of anterior left temple and exophytic nodular basal cell carcinoma of left external ear in same patient Figures 29.12 through 29.15.

The skin of the pinna is thin and is loosely attached to an easily denuded cartilage. Irradiation is designed to minimize the risk of cartilage (connective tissue) necrosis,

yet eradicate the cancer. Usually, the margins of the cancer at this site are readily defined. A 1-cm cancer-free lateral margin and the full thickness of the pinna are included in the target volume. The electron beam and the x-ray beam are equally effective for this site.

This 75-year-old man had two basal cell carcinomas: a flat sclerosing tumor of the anterior temple skin and a separate thick exophytic nodular tumor on the dorsum of the left external ear (Figs. 29.12 through 29.15). A tracing on plastic was made of each tumor with a 5- to 10-mm margin around each tumor and lead cutouts were used to define the radiation fields. His head was

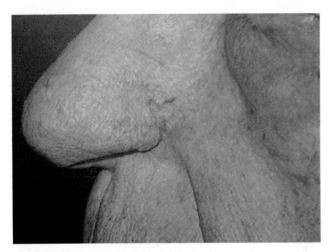

Figure 29.11. Two months following the completion of radiation treatment, no visible tumor, slight skin distortion, excellent cosmetic result considering initial tumor appearance.

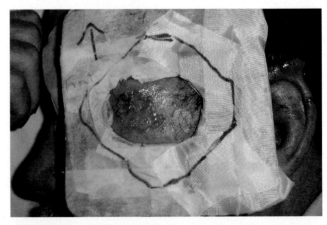

Figure 29.13. Infiltrating sclerosing basal cell carcinoma in anterior left temple area. This tumor was separate from the external ear tumor. Field outlined with 3-mm-thick lead shield on the skin surface with 1-cm-thick gel bolus placed on top of the lead shield. Treated with 6-MeV electrons. Prior to treatment.

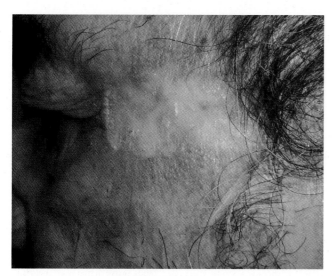

Figure 29.14. Five weeks following 5,000 cGy at 250 cGy/day, 20 fractions in 27 overall days for sclerosing basal cell carcinoma, complete response.

placed in a lateral position with the left side up. For the treatment of pinna tumor, an exit beam shield of 3-mm thick lead was cut to fit the junction of the posterior surface of the pinna with the scalp; this was to shield the underlying scalp and brain. A field-defining cutout of 10-mm-thick lead was placed in the end of a 9-MeV electron cone, and a 1-cm-thick gel bolus was placed on the tumor surface. The anterior temple skin tumor was treated with 6-MeV electrons with a 1-cm bolus, with a separate lead eye shield. Both tumors were treated at 250 cGy/day, 5 days/week, to the 100% dose. The anterior tumor received 5,000 cGy. At that dose, there was still an evident tumor on the external ear. After a 6-day break in treatments, the ear tumor received three additional treatments, then after an additional 5-day break, three more

treatments were given, for a total of 6,500 cGy in 26 treatments over 42 elapsed days. This patient illustrates the importance of monitoring the tumor response and adjusting the dose accordingly.

When the external auditory canal is in the electron beam, a tissue-equivalent plug or warm water filling the canal significantly reduces dose to the drum and the middle ear (13). Caccialanza et al. reported complete remission in 97% of skin carcinomas of the pinna treated with orthovoltage, with 88% of patients having good or acceptable cosmetic results (14).

Case 4: Basal cell carcinoma of the left medial canthus and bridge of nose with extension into the left lower eyelid.

Cancers near the eye may invade the bone or soft tissues of the orbit. When there is any question of deep invasion, imaging studies through this level may provide useful information. Such invasion was not present in this patient. Gross margins were otherwise readily determined. The relatively small size of the treatment field, together with the problems of dose distribution and use of a lead eye shield of appropriate thickness for the electron beam, made the x-ray beam preferable (10,11,15,17). The contour across the treatment field was irregular. (The bridge of the nose was ~1.5–2 cm anterior to the canthus.) The resulting variation in surface dose was decreased by increasing SSD of the x-ray beam to 50 cm rather than the usual 20 to 30 cm.

A 200-keV x-ray beam of half-value layer (HVL) 1-mm copper at 50-cm SSD is appropriate. The field diameter, allowing at least 1 cm of lateral margin around the lesion, was 4.5 cm. A lead cutout of 1-mm thick was constructed and shaped. Before it was taped in place, an eye shield of 2-mm-thick lead was inserted on the surface of the anesthetized left eye (Fig. 29.16). The closed right eye was covered with an additional 1-mm-thick shield to block radiation that might be transmitted to the

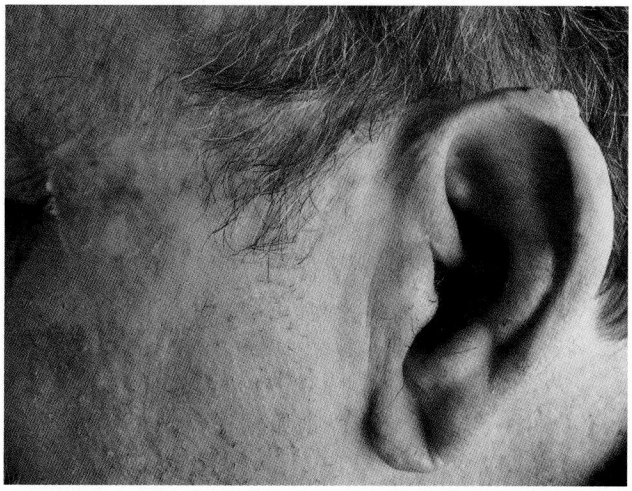

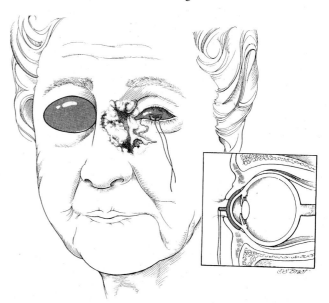

Figure 29.15. Three months following the completion of 6,500 cGy to nodular basal cell carcinoma of external ear. No evidence of cancer; there is a residual soft pliable skin irregularity on the superior edge of the ear at the former cancer site.

Figure 29.16. An internal (Gougelman) eye shield is in place in the anesthetized left eye. An external eye shield covers the right eye.

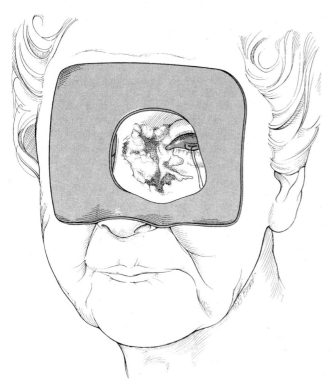

Figure 29.17. A lead cutout and the eye shields are in place.

right lens through the lead of the cutout. The lead cutout was then taped in place (Fig. 29.17). After each treatment, an eye patch is worn until sensation returns to the cornea.

Fractionation and total dose schedules, chosen to produce minimum fibrosis, telangiectasia, and edema of eyelids and adjacent skin, were 54 Gy given in 27 fractions. Obviously, larger and more deeply infiltrating lesions require consideration of electron beam techniques, some requiring 12- to 22-MeV electron beams (11). In such patients, loss of vision or even of the eye may be unavoidable if the cancer is to be cured.

Clinical Observation of Radiation Response

The total radiation dose ultimately delivered may vary from the planned prescribed dose. It is important for the radiation oncologist to closely observe the reaction of the surface of the tumor and the surface of the surrounding normal skin, particularly toward the end of the planned time of completion of the irradiation. The author's own experience has taught the importance of observing and appropriately modifying the radiation treatment schedule based on the appearance of the reaction. There should be erythema and superficial ulceration and crusting of the tumor surface. The desired radiation response may require a break in the treatments, and either a reduction or an increase in the number of planned treatments and ultimate total radiation dose, to achieve the desired result of tumor control with absence of normal tissue necrosis.

MELANOMA OF THE SKIN

Radiotherapy Indications

Surgical resection is the most common treatment of cutaneous melanoma, and primary irradiation is rarely used in the treatment of primary melanoma. However, adjuvant irradiation has significant potential in decreasing local-regional recurrences. University of Texas M.D. Anderson Cancer Center investigators have reported the use of adjuvant irradiation following regional nodal dissection (18,19). Features that are at high risk for regional recurrence following surgery are extracapsular extension, multiple involved node, or large or matted nodes.

Australian investigators reported that following neck dissection and parotidectomy for metastatic melanoma, the nodal recurrence rate was 18% with adjuvant irradiation and 40% without it (20). The Trans Tasman Radiation Oncology Group (Australia and New Zealand) irradiated (48 Gy in 20 daily fractions) the regional lymph nodal basin in 234 patients with regional lymph node or extra-nodal soft tissue in the lymph node basin involvement (21). They treated the head and neck, axillary and supraclavicular, and ilio-inguinal nodal basins. They reported that as the first site of relapse, regional in-field relapse occurred in 6.8% of patients, and regional control rate was 91% at 5 years. They found that patients with more than two involved nodes had a significantly worse outcome in terms of distant relapse, overall survival, and progression-free survival, but their regional control was comparable to patients with one or two involved nodes.

Radiation Therapy Technique

The technique developed at University of Texas M.D. Anderson Cancer Center utilizes irradiation to cover the primary site, nodal operative site, and regional lymph nodes using shaped electron beams. Appropriate electron energies of 9 to 16 MeV are used. They use a dose and fractionation irradiation schedule of 30 Gy in five fractions (6 Gy per fraction) delivered over 2.5 weeks, Monday and Thursday, or Tuesday and Friday. Dose is calculated at D_{max}. The central nervous system (brain and spinal cord) must be spared and should be treated to a maximum of 24 Gy in four fractions (18,19).

This radiotherapy technique has also been extended to treat metastatic nodal disease of the axilla and inguinal regions.

MERKEL CELL CARCINOMA

Merkel cell carcinoma is a rare cutaneous malignancy with a roughly 25% mortality rate and a high propensity of regional and distant tumor spread. Boyer et al. compared Mohs surgery with and without postoperative irradiation. None of the 20 irradiated patients had local recurrence, whereas 4 of the 25 nonirradiated patients had marginal or in-transit metastases (22). Mortier et al. reported tumor control in nine patients with inoperable Merkel cell carcinoma treated primarily with irradiation (23). Longo and Nghiem have confirmed the value of irradiation as primary and adjuvant treatment (24).

Medina-Franco et al. reviewed 18 series containing 926 patients with stages I to II disease. The local control rate was 89% with irradiation and 47% without irradiation (25).

A review of the literature and of the University of Florida experience by Mendenhall et al. (26) and by McAfee et al. (27) reports that "The optimal treatment for patients with Merkel cell carcinoma remains unclear. The primary tumor may either be widely excised or treated with radiation therapy. Because of the risk of in-transit metastases, margins should be generous. Our preference is to use surgery unless it would result in a suboptimal functional or cosmetic result. Postoperative radiation therapy is added if margins are close or positive and in cases where it is not possible to obtain wide margins because of the location of the tumor. In practice, almost all of the patients treated at the authors' institution receive radiation therapy after surgery." Because of the high incidence of nodal metastases, the regional lymphatics should be electively treated in all patients with apparently localized disease, either with surgery or irradiation. If nodal disease is found at surgery, postoperative irradiation should be given. The radiation doses are similar for squamous cell carcinomas of the head and neck: primary tumor—negative margins, 60 Gy in 30 fractions over 6 weeks; microscopically positive margins, 66 Gy in 33 fractions over 6.5 weeks; gross disease, 70 Gy in 35 fractions over 7 weeks. Elective irradiation of subclinical disease in a nonresected neck would be 50 Gy in 25 fractions over 5 weeks. Radiation fields should be generous around the primary site because of the propensity of cutaneous in-transit tumor spread. Some patients have extensive regional tumor involvement that makes it difficult to encompass all the tumors within the irradiated volume. The author has observed that radiation fields are frequently too small for the ultimate spread of Merkel cell carcinoma—"For some patients, you can't treat a radiation field big enough."

MYCOSIS FUNGOIDES

Mycosis fungoides is an indolent low-grade T-cell lymphoma, which involves the skin. Patients usually have a gradual progression from scaly flat lesions to erythematous plaques to tumors and ulceration. In its early stages, it may be misdiagnosed as psoriasis, eczema, or dermatitis. Microscopically, there is a band-like infiltrate of atypical lymphoid cells in the upper dermis. The Pautrier microabscess of mycosis fungoides cells in the upper dermis is pathognomonic of this condition. Lymphadenopathy may occur, and is more frequent in more advanced involvement of the skin. Some patients present with generalized erythroderma. Sezary syndrome is defined as having mycosis fungoides with >10% of the blood lymphocytes being malignant convoluted atypical mononuclear mycosis fungoides cells.

Radiation Therapy Indications

Because of the variable nature of progression of this condition, the therapy should be chosen so that the results of treatment are not worse than the disease. Early mycosis fungoides can be effectively treated with psoralen-UVA (PUVA) therapy, topical nitrogen mustard, or with topical steroids. For small lesions, placing a topical steroid ointment on a bandage pad placed directly over the cutaneous lesion can be locally effective. These treatment techniques can be used either before or following the more aggressive treatment technique of total-skin electron irradiation.

Radiation Treatment Techniques

Radiation therapy using limited field-size orthovoltage or electron irradiation is highly effective in the local control of a limited number of localized lesions. Custom lead or Cerrobend blocking is used to define the radiation field. A total dose of 2,000 to 3,000 cGy at 250 to 300 cGy per daily fractions is usually effective in long-term control of such local involvement. It is appropriate to use this technique either before or following a course of total-skin electron treatment.

When >20% to 30% of the skin surface is involved, then total-skin electron irradiation is the optimal treatment. Total-skin electron irradiation is a time-consuming treatment, which requires experienced radiation oncology physicians, medical physicists, medical dosimetrists, and radiation therapists to properly plan and deliver. This is a very specialized radiation treatment, which requires knowledge and use of the proper positioning of the patient's trunk and extremities to optimally expose all skin surfaces to the electron beam. Significant medical physics and medical dosimetry effort is required in the preparation and delivery of the optimal radiation therapy technique.

The Stanford 6-position technique has become the standard for total-skin electron treatment. This technique entails treating the patient in six different body positions over 2 days. On the first day, the anterior, left posterior, and right posterior orientation of the body is exposed to the electron beam. On the second day, the posterior, left anterior, and right anterior orientation of the body is exposed to the electron beam. These body positions are then repeated on alternate days. Every 2 days, the patient is treated in all six positions. For each position treatment, the linear accelerator gantry is rotated upward or downward to cover the entire body surface. The specific gantry angle will be dependent on the distance from the radiation source to the patient. We have used an SSD of 320 cm and gantry angles that are oriented 15 degrees upward and downward from a horizontal axis. Examples of the

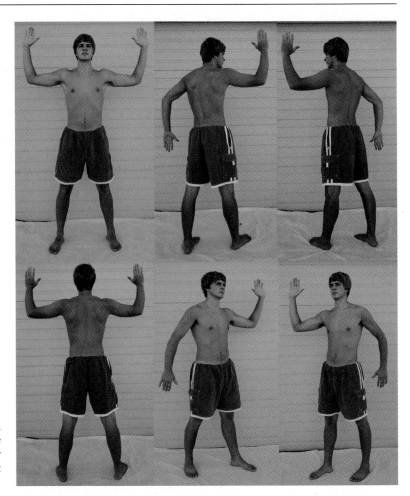

Figure 29.18. Patient positions for treatment of total skin for mycosis fungoides; upper figure positions are treated on odd-numbered treatment days, and lower figure positions are treated on even-numbered treatment days.

patient's positions are illustrated in Figure 29.18, and are described by Smith and Wilson (28).

The patient stands in a Formica-covered wood frame, which helps maintain the proper patient position. The bottom of the frame is 15 cm above the floor, and has a plastic-covered base that shows outlines of the foot position for each of the six body positions. Multiple TLDs are placed on the patient's skin surface for a full course of all six body positions. These TLD measurements are used to measure the actual skin dose. The use of TLDs for this purpose is well described by Antolak et al. (29). We have placed TLDs in the following locations: head apex, anterior and posterior right and left side of head, shoulders, biceps, forearms, hips, thighs and calves, middle of groin, and dorsal right and left feet. On the first day of treatment, all six positions are treated with TLDs in place. Based on the TLDs reading, the daily MUs for three position treatments per day are determined. For potentially underdosed areas, such as infra-mammary folds, 2D dose mapping using radiochromic film has been used to understand surface dose heterogeneity (30).

The high dose-rate total-skin 6-MeV electron mode is selected on the linear accelerator. Although some authors

have described the use of plastic compensators in front of the patient, the author's institution has not used them, and appropriate skin reactions and results have occurred. Patients may wear cotton examination gowns for modesty during treatment, although some institutions treat patients in the nude.

A combined skin dose of 100 cGy per daily fraction is given 4 to 5 days/week, for a total of ~34 to 36 Gy for the whole course of the treatment.

Guidelines for total-skin electron radiation in the management of mycosis fungoides have been developed by the European Organization for Research and Treatment of Cancer (EORTC) Cutaneous Lymphoma Project Group (31). These guidelines are: optimal treatment distance should be between 3 and 8 m; distribution of dose in air should be within 10% across the entire vertical and lateral dimensions; short treatment distances may necessitate the use of beam-scattering devices but these produce greater bremsstrahlung or x-ray contamination; photon contamination at the level of the bone marrow must be <0.7 Gy for a full course of treatment to avoid hematologic sequelae; the 80% isodose surface should be at least 4 mm deep to the skin surface along the primary beam axis; the primary goal is to administer at least 26 Gy at a depth of 4 mm in truncal skin, for an effective electron energy of 4 to 5.5 MeV, the skin surface dose is ~31 to 36 Gy, and patch treatments to underdosed skin surfaces (perineum, soles of feet, scalp, and behind pendulous tissue) should be utilized. The consensus statement recommends a minimum dose of 26 Gy at a depth of 4 mm for all skin surfaces. However, caution should be exercised in giving >20 Gy to the soles of the feet because of the limited tolerance of the skin of the sole.

Treatments are generally started with the use of internal eye shields to protect the patient's corneas and lens when the eyes are within the electron beam. These shields can be removed when the patient is facing away from the radiation beam, and that helps the patient maintain their body position. Because of the increased backscatter dose from the internal shield to the eyelid, the internal eye shields are replaced with external eye shields during the later portion of the treatment course. During the course of treatment, the fingers, hands, and feet may show evidence of a more intense reaction and those thinner areas of the body may be shielded with lead or by placing the hands and fingers behind the upright supports of the treatment frame in which the patient stands. The importance of careful clinical judgment and the appropriate use of individualized shielding are well described by Hoppe (32).

The typical response to radiation is a gradual decrease in the size and symptoms (pruritus) that can start within a few days of starting the treatments. Even large tumors or deeply ulcerated tumors will eventually resolve and be replaced with normal skin. In some patients, additional boost treatments with orthovoltage or electron radiation may be necessary to areas of the body that have not had full exposure to the electron irradiation, or to localized lesions that have not totally responded to treatment. A 5-mm-thick gel bolus should be used on the skin surface when treating small areas with 6-MeV electrons at approximately 100-cm SSD. Patients with Sezary syndrome may have a rapid, dramatic, and durable response to irradiation. The author has treated a patient who was initially bedridden with extensive erythema of the skin with Sezary syndrome. She was unable to move and required treatment in a reclining position when treatment was started on her. She rapidly responded, was able to continue the treatment in a more conventional standing position, and was alive and well without symptoms for >5 years.

Some patients may be candidates for a second course of total-skin electron irradiation for recurrent mycosis fungoides. Stanford University authors have described giving a mean dose of 23 Gy for the second course, with all patients having at least a partial response and 40% of patients having a complete response to the second treatment course (33).

Some patients with multiple recurrent skin lesions require many subsequent treatments to provide palliation of symptomatic lesions. This disease can be frustrating for the patient and treating physician because of its tendency to recur. One can sometimes run out of ways to effectively treat patients with multiply recurrent lesions.

REFERENCES

1. Wolf DJ, Zitelli JA. Surgical margins for basal cell carcinoma. *Arch Dermatol* 1987;123:340–344.
2. Choo R, Woo T, Assaad D, et al. What is the microscopic tumor extent beyond clinically delineated gross tumor boundary in nonmelanoma skin cancers? *Int J Radiat Oncol Biol Phys* 2005;62:1096–1099.
3. Liu FF, Maki E, Warde P, et al. A management approach to incompletely excised basal cell carcinomas of the skin. *Int J Radiat Oncol Biol Phys* 1997;20:423–428.
4. Mendenhall WM, Amdur RJ, Hinerman RW, et al. Skin cancer of the head and neck with perineural invasion. *Am J of Clin Oncol* 2007;30:93–96.
5. Garcia-Serra A, Hinerman RW, Mendenhall WM, et al. Carcinoma of the skin with perineural invasion. *Head Neck* 2003;25:1027–1033.
6. Gluck I, Ibrahim M, Popovtzer A, et al. Skin cancer of the head and neck with perineural invasion: defining the clinical target volumes based on the pattern of failure. *Int J Radiat Oncol Biol Phys* 2009;74:38–46.
7. Park CC, Yom SS, Podgorsk MB, et al. American Society for Therapeutic Radiology and Oncology (ASTRO) Emerging Technology Committee report of electronic brachytherapy. *Int J Radiat Oncol Biol Phys* 2010;76:963–972.
8. Purdy JA, Choi MC, Feldman A. Lipowitz metal shielding thickness for dose reduction of 6–20 Mev electrons. *Med Phys* 1980;7:251–253.
9. Pohlit W, Manegold KH. Electron-beam dose distribution in inhomogeneous media. In: Kramer S, Suntharalingam N, Zinninger GF, eds. *High energy photons and electrons.* New York: John Wiley & Sons, 1977:243.
10. Shiu AS, Tung SS, Gastorf RJ, et al. Dosimetric evaluation of lead and tungsten eye shields in electron beam treatment. *Int J Radiat Oncol Biol Phys* 1997;35:599–604.
11. Amdur RJ, Kalbaugh KJ, Ewald LM, et al. Radiation therapy for skin cancer near the eye: kilovoltage x-rays versus electrons. *Int J Radiat Oncol Biol Phys* 1992;23:769–779.
12. Khan FM. Electron beam therapy. In: *The physics of radiation therapy,* 4th ed. Baltimore, MD: Wolters Kluwer Lippincott Williams & Wilkins, 2010:264–314.
13. Morrison WH, Wong PF, Starkschall G, et al. Water bolus for electron irradiation of the ear canal. *Int J Radiat Oncol Biol Phys* 1995;33:479–483.
14. Caccialanza M, Piccinno R, Kolesnikova L, et al. Radiotherapy of skin carcinomas of the pinna: a study of 115 lesions in 108 patients. *Int J Dermatol* 2005;44:513–517.
15. Million RR. Radiotherapy for carcinoma of the eyelid. *Int J Radiat Oncol Biol Phys* 1996;34:507.
16. Lovett RD, Perez CA, Shaprio SJ, et al. External irradiation of epithelial skin cancer. *Int J Radiat Oncol Biol Phys* 1990;19:235–242.
17. Schlienger P, Brunin F, Desjardins L, et al. External radiotherapy for carcinoma of the eyelid: report of 850 cases treated. *Int J Radiat Oncol Biol Phys* 1997;34:277–287.
18. Ballo MT, Ang KK. Radiation therapy for malignant melanoma. *Surg Clin N Am* 2003;83:323–342.

19. Ballo MT, Ang KK. Radiotherapy for cutaneous malignant melanoma: rationale and indications. *Oncology* 2004;18:99–107.

20. O'Brien CJ, Petersen-Schaefer K, Stevens GN. Adjuvant radiotherapy following neck dissection and parotidectomy for metastatic malignant melanoma. *Head Neck* 1997;19:589–594.

21. Burmeister BH, Smithers BM, Baumann K, et al. A prospective phase II study of adjuvant postoperative radiation therapy following nodal surgery in malignant melanoma—Trans Tasman Radiation Oncology Group (TROG) study 96.06. *Radiother Oncol* 2006;81: 136–142.

22. Boyer JD, Zitelli JA, Brodland DG, et al. Local control of primary Merkel cell carcinoma: review of 45 cases treated with Mohs micrographic surgery with and without adjuvant radiation. *J Am Acad Dermatol* 2002;47:885–892.

23. Mortier L, Mirabel X, Fournier C, et al. Radiotherapy alone for primary Merkel cell carcinoma. *Arch Dermatol* 2003;139:1587–1590.

24. Longo MI, Nghiem JP. Merkel cell carcinoma treatment with radiation. *Arch Dermatol* 2003;139:1641–1643.

25. Medina-Franco H, Urist MM, Fiveash J, et al. Multimodality treatment of Merkel cell carcinoma: case series and literature review of 1024 cases. *Ann Surg Oncol* 2001; 8:204–208.

26. Mendenhall WM, Mendenhall CM, Mendenhall NP. Merkel cell carcinoma. *Laryngoscope* 2004;114:906–910.

27. McAfee WJ, Morris CG, Mendenhall CM, et al. Merkel cell carcinoma. Treatment and outcomes. *Cancer* 2005; 104:1761–1764.

28. Smith BD, Wilson LD. Management of mycosis fungoides: Part 2. Treatment. *Oncology* 2003;17:1419–1428.

29. Antolak JA, Cundiff JH, Ha CS. Utilization of thermoluminescent dosimetry in total skin electron beam radiotherapy of mycosis fungoides. *Int J Radiat Oncol Biol Phys* 1998;40:101–108.

30. Gamble LA, Farrell TJ, Jones GW, et al. Two-dimensional mapping of underdosed areas using radiochromic film for patients undergoing total skin electron beam radiotherapy. *Int J Radiat Oncol Biol Phys* 2005;62:920–924.

31. Jones GW, Kacinski BM, Wilson LD, et al. Total skin electron radiation in the management of mycosis fungoides: consensus of the European Organization for Research and Treatment of Cancer (EORTC) Cutaneous Lymphoma Project Group. *J Am Acad Dermatol* 2002;47:364–370.

32. Hoppe RT. Mycosis fungoides: radiation therapy. *Dermatol Ther* 2003;16:347–354.

33. Becker M, Hoppe RT, Knox SJ. Multiple courses of high-dose total skin electron beam therapy in the management of mycosis fungoides. *Int J Radiat Oncol Biol Phys* 1995; 32:1445–1449.

CHAPTER 30

Breast Cancer

Benjamin T. Gielda ■ Katherine L. Griem ■ Adam Dickler

INTRODUCTION

Radiotherapy plays an integral role in the management of many patients with breast cancer whether they present with localized or disseminated disease. Treatment of breast cancer patients with radiotherapy requires knowledge of the anatomy of the breast and regional nodes as well as the treatment techniques available to encompass these volumes. This chapter discusses the management of clinically localized disease and describes the pertinent anatomy as well as the epidemiology and staging of breast cancer. We review the indications for irradiation of the intact breast and for irradiation in the postmastectomy setting, and we describe treatment techniques, volumes, and dose for these clinical situations.

ANATOMY

Located within the superficial fascia of the anterior thoracic wall, the breast is composed of 15 to 20 segments of glandular tissue. Fibrous connective tissues connect the segments with adipose tissue abundantly interspersed between the segments. These segments compose the parenchyma and converge at the nipple in a radial fashion. Subcutaneous connective tissues surround the gland and extend as septa between the segments, providing structural support for the glandular elements. The deep layer of superficial fascia lies on the posterior surface of the breast adjacent to and at points fusing with the deep pectoral fascia of the chest wall. The retromammary bursa lies between the deep layer of superficial fascia and the deep pectoral fascia. It contains loose areolar tissue that allows for mobility of the breast over the chest wall. Fibrous bands of connective tissue attached between parenchyma extend from the deep pectoral fascia and attach to the superficial fascia (dermis of the skin). These ligaments, which are known as Cooper's ligaments, insert perpendicular to the superficial fascial layers of the skin and permit mobility of the breast while also giving structural support.

The mature breast of the woman lies between the second rib superiorly and extends to the inframammary fold at the level of the sixth or seventh rib in the vertical axis. In the horizontal axis, it extends from the lateral edge of the sternum to the anterior or midaxillary line. The posterior surface rests on the deep pectoralis fascia, serratus anterior, external oblique abdominal muscles, and the upper rectus sheath. Breast tissue also projects into the axilla as the axillary tail of Spence, which may be very prominent. The upper half of the breast, the upper outer quadrant in particular, contains the greatest volume of glandular tissue.

The stroma and subcutaneous tissue of the breast contain fat, connective tissue, blood vessels, nerves, and lymphatics. The glands of the breast, derived from modified sweat glands of the epidermis, lie in the subcutaneous tissues. Each of the 15 to 20 segments of branched tubuloalveolar glands has collecting ducts draining them that are 2 mm in diameter and that terminate in subareolar lactiferous sinuses, which are 5 to 8 mm in diameter. Between 5 and 10 major collecting ducts open at the nipple.

Blood Supply

The breast receives its principal blood supply from the internal mammary (IM) and lateral thoracic arteries. The medial and central portions of the breast, ~60%, are supplied by the anterior perforating branches of the IM artery. The remaining portion, the upper outer quadrant, is supplied by the lateral thoracic artery. Minor contributions to the arterial supply of the breast are supplied by subscapular and thoracodorsal arteries, the lateral branches of the third, fourth, and fifth intercostal arteries, and the pectoral branch of the thoracoacromial artery (Fig. 30.1*A* and B).

Lymphatic Drainage

The most common sites of regional lymph node involvement in breast cancer are the axillary, IM, and supraclavicular regions. An understanding of the distribution and likelihood of involvement of the specific nodal groups is vital for treatment planning. More than 75% of lymph from the breast passes to the axillary nodes (Fig. 30.2), with the remainder flowing into parasternal lymphatics. The axillary nodes are thus the major site of regional metastases from breast carcinoma, and ~40% of patients have histopathologic evidence of spread to the axillary nodes at presentation.

Physical examination of the axilla has both high false-positive and high false-negative rates in terms of determining axillary nodal involvement. Palpable axillary lymph nodes

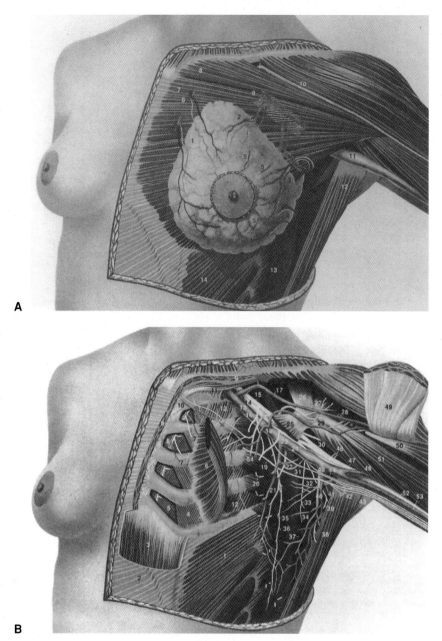

Figure 30.1. A: Breast anatomy: relationships of blood vessels and muscle groups. *1.* Perforating branches from internal mammary artery and vein. *2.* Pectoral branches from thoracoacromial artery and vein. *3.* External mammary branch from lateral thoracic artery and vein. *4.* Branches from subcapsular and thoracodorsal arteries and veins. *5.* Lateral branches of third, fourth, and fifth intercostal arteries and veins. *6.* Internal mammary artery and veins. *7.* Sternocostal head of pectoralis major muscle. *8.* Clavicular head of pectoralis major muscle. *9.* Axillary artery and vein. *10.* Cephalic vein. *11.* Axillary sheath. *12.* Latissimus dorsi muscle. *13.* Serratus anterior muscle. *14.* External abdominal oblique muscle. **B:** Chest wall and vascular anatomy. *1.* External abdominal oblique muscle. *2.* Rectus sheath. *3.* Rectus abdominis muscle. *4.* Internal intercostal muscle. *5.* Transverse thoracic muscle. *6.* Pectoralis minor muscle. *7.* Perforating branches from internal mammary artery and vein. *8.* Internal mammary artery and vein. *9.* Cut edge of pectoralis major muscle. *10.* Sternoclavicular branch of thoracoacromial artery and vein. *11.* Subclavius muscle and Halsted's ligament. *12.* External intercostal muscle. *13.* Axillary vein. *14.* Axillary artery. *15.* Lateral cord of brachial plexus. *16.* Lateral pectoral nerve (from the lateral cord). *17.* Cephalic vein. *18.* Thoracoacromial vein. *19.* Intercostobrachial nerve. *20.* Lateral cutaneous nerve. *21.* Lateral thoracic artery and vein. *22.* Scapular branches of lateral thoracic artery and vein. *23.* Medial pectoral nerve (from medial cord). *24.* Ulnar nerve. *25.* Pectoralis minor muscle. *26.* Coracoclavicular ligament. *27.* Coracoacromial ligament. *28.* Cut edge of deltoid muscle. *29.* Acromial and humeral branches of thoracoacromial artery and vein. *30.* Musculocutaneous nerve. *31.* Medial cutaneous nerve of arm. *32.* Subscapular nerve. *33.* Lower subscapular nerve. *34.* Teres major muscle. *35.* Long thoracic nerve. *36.* Serratus anterior muscle. *37.* Latissimus dorsi muscle. *38.* Latissimus dorsi muscle. *39.* Thoracodorsal nerve. *40.* Thoracodorsal artery and vein. *41.* Scapular circumflex artery and vein. *42.* Branching of intercostobrachial nerve. *43.* Teres major muscle. *44.* Medial cutaneous nerve of foramen. *45.* Subscapular artery and vein. *46.* Posterior humeral circumflex artery vein. *47.* Median nerve. *48.* Coracobrachialis muscle. *49.* Pectoralis major muscle. *50.* Biceps brachii muscle, long head. *51.* Biceps brachii muscle, short head. *52.* Brachial artery. *53.* Basilic vein. *54.* Pectoral branch of thoracoacromial artery and vein. *Source:* Reprinted from Osborne MP. Breast development and anatomy. In: Harris JR, Lippmann ME, Morrow M, Hellman S, eds. *Diseases of the breast.* Philadelphia, PA: Lippincott-Raven, 1996, with permission.

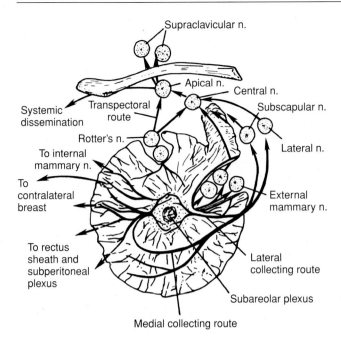

Figure 30.2. Schematic drawing of the breast identifying the position of lymph nodes relative to the breast and illustrating route of lymphatic drainage. *Arrows*, Routes of lymphatic drainage. *Source:* Reprinted from Romrell LJ, Bland KI. Anatomy of the breast, axilla, chest wall, and related metastatic sites. In: Bland KI, Copeland EM, eds. *The breast: comprehensive management of benign and malignant disease.* Madison, WI: WB Saunders, 1991:531–593, with permission.

are found to have evidence of metastatic disease in only 75% of patients. However, if enlarged axillary nodes are not palpated, metastatic disease is detected in ~30% of the patients (1). This is important because the extent of axillary nodal involvement is the single most important

prognostic factor in breast cancer. The 10-year survival of patients treated with radical mastectomy found to have negative axillary nodes is 65% to 80%, and with positive axillary nodes, 10-year survival is 25% to 48%. The prognosis is inversely related to the number of involved nodes (2).

The anatomical arrangement of the axillary lymph nodes has several classifications. Pickren (3) has the most detailed studies of the pathologic anatomy of tumor spread. These groups include the following: (a) The axillary vein group (lateral group), which consists of four to six nodes medial or posterior to the vein (Fig. 30.3), receives most of the lymph drainage from the upper extremity. (b) The external mammary group, which contains five to six nodes along the lower border of the pectoralis minor, receives the majority of lymphatic drainage from the lateral breast. (c) The scapular group consists of five to seven nodes from the posterior wall of the axilla at the lateral border of the scapula. These nodes receive lymph from the lower posterior neck, posterior trunk, and posterior shoulder. (d) The central group consists of three or four large groups in the fat of the axilla posterior to the pectoralis minor muscle. This group not only receives lymph from the three preceding groups, but may also receive lymphatics directly from the breast. (e) The subclavicular group consists of 6 to 12 nodal groups posterior and superior to the upper border of the pectoralis minor. This group receives lymph from all groups of axillary nodes and unites with vessels from the subclavicular nodes to form the subclavian trunk. (f) The interpectoral (Rotter's) group consists of one to four nodes interposed between the pectoralis major and inner muscles. Lymph from these nodes passes directly into the central and subclavicular groups.

Figure 30.3. Schematic drawing of the major lymph node groups associated with the lymphatic drainage of the breast. Roman numerals indicate three groups of lymph nodes defined by their location relative to the pectoralis minor. *I.* Lateral to the pectoralis minor. *II.* Deep to the muscle. *III.* Medial to the muscle. *Arrows.* The general direction of lymph flow. *Source:* Reprinted from Romrell LJ, Bland KI. Anatomy of the breast, axilla, chest wall, and related metastatic sites. In: Bland KI, Copeland EM, eds. *The breast: comprehensive management of benign and malignant disease.* Madison, WI: WB Saunders, 1991:531–593, with permission.

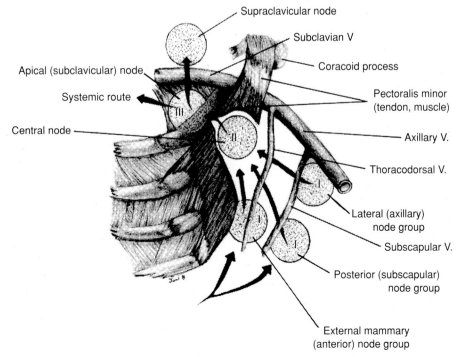

TABLE 30.1	Internal Mammary (IM) Node Involvement in Relation to Site of Primary Tumor

	UIQ	LIQ	Central	UOQ	LOQ
Total	248	61	216	382	93
IM nodes (+)	67 (27%)	20 (33%)	70 (32%)	54 (14%)	12 (13%)

U, upper; I, inner; Q, quadrant; L, lower, O, outer.
Source: Reprinted from Handley R. Carcinoma of the breast. *Ann R Coll Surg Engl* 1975;57:59–66, with permission.

An alternative and more commonly used method of determining pathological anatomy and metastatic progression is to divide the axillary nodal groups into three levels (Fig. 30.3). These levels are related to their position relative to the pectoralis minor muscle that inserts at the coracoid process. Level I lymph nodes lie lateral to the lateral border of the pectoralis minor muscle, level II nodes lie behind the pectoralis minor muscle, and level III nodes lie medial to the medial border of the pectoralis minor muscle.

The second major site of regional metastases for breast carcinoma is the IM lymph node chain. These nodes lie close to the IM vessels in extrapleural fat and are distributed in the intercostal spaces. The distribution of nodes in the intercostal space is as follows: first space, 97%; second space, 98%; third space, 82%; fourth space, 9%; fifth space, 12%; and sixth space, 62% (4). Initial studies by Handley (5) reported the results of IM node biopsies in 1,000 patients in 1975 and illustrated that IM node involvement is more common for inner-quadrant or central lesions than for outer-quadrant lesions (Table 30.1). Even in patients with inner or central lesions, the axilla is more commonly involved than the IM nodes: 42% versus 28%. Involvement of the IM nodes also correlates with tumor size. IM nodes are involved in 19% of patients with tumors smaller than 5 cm and 37% of patients with tumors larger than 5 cm. Injection studies with radiolabeled colloid demonstrate that drainage of lymph to the IM chain may be observed after injection of any quadrant of the breast.

The primary route of supraclavicular node involvement is through the axillary nodes. The significance of this nodal involvement was first shown by Halsted (6), who performed supraclavicular nodal dissection in 119 patients. Only 2 of the 44 women with positive supraclavicular nodes had no evidence of disease at 5 years. Thus, supraclavicular nodal involvement represents a late stage of axillary involvement and carries a grave prognosis. Supraclavicular lymph nodal involvement is classified as regional lymph node involvement rather than a site of metastatic disease in the most recent edition of American Joint Commission on Cancer (AJCC) Staging Handbook (7).

Local Involvement

The primary site of breast cancer is described by the quadrant of the breast that contains the carcinoma. In one series of 696 patients (8), 48% of the tumors were in the upper outer quadrant, 17% in the central region, 15% in the upper inner quadrant, 11% in the lower outer quadrant, and 6% in the lower inner quadrant. The frequency of a quadrant's involvement is related to the proportion of breast tissue in that region. The relationship between the tumor location and prognosis was examined by the National Surgical Adjuvant Breast Project. Survival was found to be related to the pathological status of the lymph nodes but not to the primary tumor location (9) (Table 30.2).

The spread of cancer through the breast has been described by Haagensen (10). This spread occurs by direct infiltration into the breast parenchyma, along mammary ducts, and through the lymphatics. Direct infiltration occurs by projections having a characteristic stellate appearance. If the cancer is left untreated, involvement of skin and underlying fascia of the pectoralis muscle is

TABLE 30.2	Five-Year Recurrence Rate According to Tumor Location and Nodal Status

	Negative nodes (# pts)	Positive nodes (# pts)
UIQ	25.0% (75)	59.0% (37)
UOQ	17.0 (208)	63.0 (239)
LOQ	26.0 (46)	70.0 (44)
LIQ	22.0 (23)	55.0 (22)
Total	20.3 (497)	66.1 (508)
Overall	43.5% (1005)	

U, upper; I, inner; Q, quadrant; L, lower, O, outer.
Source: Reprinted from Fisher B, Slack N, Ausman R. Location of breast carcinoma and prognosis. *Surg Gynecol Obstet* 1969;129: 705–716, with permission.

common. Intraductal components, which are frequently observed, may include more than one segment of the breast. It is not clear whether this is spread of the primary cancer or a field cancerization that results in transformation of the ductal lining. Because of lymphatic spread vertically to the plexus of the pectoralis fascia and spread to the central subareolar region, cancer beyond the palpable mass may be present in the breast.

EPIDEMIOLOGY

It is estimated that 192,730 new cases of invasive breast cancer and 62,280 cases of *in situ* disease will be diagnosed in the United States during 2009. Breast cancer will account for about 27% of all new cancers in women. Approximately 40,170 women will die of breast cancer, making breast cancer second only to lung cancer with respect to female cancer mortality (11). The cumulative lifetime estimated risk of developing breast cancer is one in eight for U.S. women (11). The factors that increase the risk of developing breast cancer include family history, reproductive history, exposure to radiation and hormones, age over 50, nulliparity, and first child after age 30. Even so, ~70% of women who develop breast cancer will do so without identifiable risk factors. Age-adjusted mortality rates in the United States have declined by ~3% per year since 1989, possibly due to improved screening and treatment (12). A similar trend has been observed in the United Kingdom where the overall breast cancer mortality rate has fallen 36% since 1989 (13).

Many studies have found a link between the incidence of breast cancer and the age at menarche, menopause, and first pregnancy. An early age at menarche has been associated with an increased risk of developing premenopausal and postmenopausal breast cancer. Later onset of menarche, which is associated with a delay in the beginning of regular cycles, suggests a 20% decrease in breast cancer risk for every year delayed (14). Recent evidence demonstrates that early menarche, while altering the incidence of all major histological subtypes of breast cancer, may increase the risk of lobular carcinoma the most (15).

Another risk factor for breast cancer is age at menopause. The risk of breast cancer increases by about 3% per each year in delay of age at menopause, and this risk extends to all histologic subtypes (15,16). This information led to the general acceptance that it is the total duration of estrogen exposure and its resultant effect on cell division that affects the risk of breast cancer.

Breast cancer risk is also affected by other factors that influence hormonal exposure, including parity and age at birth of the first child. Nulliparous women are at greater risk for developing breast cancer than parous women. This risk is modulated by age at first full-term pregnancy, as women who have their first pregnancy after the age of 30 have a twofold to fivefold higher risk of developing breast

cancer than women whose first pregnancy is before age 20. An abortion of any kind does not have the protective effect of a full-term pregnancy and may even increase the risk of cancer (17). During an incomplete pregnancy, the breast is exposed only to high levels of estrogen and is thus unable to undergo the complete differentiation that results from a term pregnancy.

The association between oral contraceptive use and breast cancer is complex. In the United States, the trend has been that the duration of contraceptive use has increased, and age at first use of oral contraceptive pills has decreased. Most studies have shown no significant increase in the breast cancer risk with long durations of use (16,18). Several studies have shown a transiently increased risk of breast cancer with current or recent use (<10 years since last use) in women younger than age 45 (19,20).

Multiple sources suggest that postmenopausal hormone replacement may be associated with an increased risk of breast cancer, with the degree of risk related to the duration of use (21–23). To date, the effect of this increased incidence on mortality has not been determined, but in general, cancers developing in the setting of estrogen replacement have a relatively favorable prognosis (24). There is little information regarding the use of low-dose therapy over a short time. Thus, the risk versus benefits should be considered on an individual basis prior to the initiation of therapy.

Women who have a strong family history of breast cancer demonstrate an increased risk of breast cancer. The risk is increased 1.5 to 3 times if a first-degree relative has breast cancer; the risk is greater if the affected relative developed their breast cancer prior to menopause (25). Only 5% to 10% of breast cancer patients have a family history consistent with hereditary carcinoma. Hereditary breast carcinoma has been linked to the BRCA 1 gene located on the long arm of chromosome 17 (17q21). Carriers of BRCA 1 mutation have 36% to 56% lifetime risk of developing a breast carcinoma and are also at increased risk for developing ovarian cancer (26). BRCA 1 accounts for approximately 40% to 50% of hereditary breast cancers. An additional gene, BRCA 2 accounts for a portion but not all of the additional cases of hereditary breast cancer (27).

There is clear evidence that exposure to ionizing radiation of any source, especially during and after puberty, increases the risk of breast cancer, and that the degree of risk is dose dependent (28–31). Land et al. (32) reviewed studies of exposed populations and concluded that the risk of radiation-induced breast cancer increased linearly according to dose and the age at exposure. There is a long latent period between exposure and the development of breast carcinoma; therefore exposure after age 40 causes only a minimal increase in risk. It should be stressed that the benefit to women from screening mammography outweighs any increased risk of breast cancer.

The currently available data do not support a significant causal effect between manmade chemical exposure and breast cancer. In addition, active and passive smoking have not been shown to increase the overall rates of breast cancer (33). A large review of >100 studies did not show a significant association between breast cancer and specific occupations (34).

Staging

The current staging system in widespread use is a joint system developed by the American Joint Committee on Cancer (AJCC) and Union for International Centre Cancer (UICC). This staging system uses the TNM system of staging and information obtained before surgery or post-surgical pathologic results. The seventh edition of the staging system is presented in Table 30.3 (7).

TREATMENT

Postmastectomy Radiotherapy

Randomized studies, from British Columbia and the Danish Breast Cancer Cooperative Group, have shown a benefit in high risk patients from the addition of radiotherapy to modified radical mastectomy combined with cyclophosphamide, methotrexate, and 5-fluorouracil (CMF) chemotherapy (35,36). These studies included patients who were node positive and premenopausal. The addition of radiotherapy to chemotherapy improved local recurrence, disease free survival, and overall survival. The benefit of radiation in combination with Tamoxifen has also been shown in high risk postmenopausal patients (37). The Early Breast Cancer Trialists' Collaborative Group performed a meta-analysis analyzing 8,500 women with node positive breast cancer receiving mastectomy and axillary clearance. Radiotherapy was associated with an absolute improvement of 17% in locoregional control at 5 years, that subsequently translated into an absolute overall survival benefit of 4.4% at 15 years (38).

Indications

The rationale for postmastectomy radiotherapy is to prevent recurrence of cancer in the chest wall, skin, mastectomy scar, and the regional nodes, including the axillary, supraclavicular, and IM nodes. Available evidence suggests that prevention of local failure has a positive impact on survival (38). Prevention of recurrence is an important end point. Local recurrence is often symptomatic; these recurrences can ulcerate and be a source of bleeding as well as pain and infection. Furthermore, regional recurrence, particularly in the axilla and supraclavicular regions, can be symptomatic and cause significant pain from brachial plexus involvement. Local and regional recurrences are difficult to control once they occur. In one series (39), two-thirds of patients who failed locally after mastectomy died with uncontrolled locally

recurrent breast cancer. Finally, local recurrences may have the ability to seed distant recurrence; prevention may decrease the likelihood of the development of metastatic disease (40).

Careful selection of patients for postmastectomy irradiation is critical, given the potential morbidity of treatment. Following publication of the British Columbia and Danish randomized trials, consensus criteria were formulated recommending postmastectomy radiotherapy for patients with four or more involved lymph nodes and tumors larger than 5 cm (41,42). Other frequently used indications drawn from prospective and retrospective experiences include involved nodal ratio >0.20, invasion of pectoral fascia, lymph-vascular space invasion, positive margins, involvement of the skin or nipple, gross multicentric disease, and gross extracapsular lymph node spread (35,37,43–45) Further analysis of the Danish Trials demonstrated a benefit in patients with one to three positive nodes as well, but radiotherapy in this subset remains controversial (46).

The use of neoadjuvant chemotherapy has increased in recent years. Indications for postmastectomy radiotherapy in patients treated with neoadjuvant chemotherapy are less clear secondary to the lack of randomized prospective data. Recent consensus guidelines based on large retrospective experiences recommend postmastectomy radiotherapy for patients presenting with stage III disease or with lymph node involvement at the time of resection (47).

Simulation Technique

Treatment of the chest wall and regional nodes is traditionally accomplished by matching a supraclavicular field to tangents treating the chest wall. Careful treatment planning is necessary to avoid excessive irradiation of normal tissue while encompassing the areas at risk without overlap. Several methods to achieve an ideal match between the caudal edge of an anterior supraclavicular port and the cephalad edge of two opposed tangential fields have been described. The supraclavicular port is usually treated with a half-beam technique to achieve a nondivergent edge, and some form of mounted or hanging block, couch rotation, and/or collimator angulation is used on the tangential fields to achieve a match (48–51). A simulation technique for comprehensive postmastectomy irradiation using a conventional simulator, requiring only an asymmetric collimator on the treatment machine and breast tilt board, has been previously described in detail (52,53). Below is presented the CT adaptation of the three field technique used at Rush University Medical Center.

Three-Field Single Isocenter

The patient is placed supine with both arms above the head. Raising both arms is desirable should it become

| TABLE | 30.3 | **AJCC Staging for Breast Cancer** |

T	Tumor
TX	Primary tumor cannot be assessed
T0	No evidence of primary tumor
Tis	Carcinoma *in situ*
Tis	Ductal carcinoma *in situ* (DCIS)
Tis	Lobular carcinoma *in situ* (LCIS)
Tis	(Paget's) Paget's disease of the nipple NOT associated with invasive carcinoma and/or carcinoma in situ (DCIS and/or LCIS) in the underlying breast parenchyma. Carcinomas in the breast parenchyma associated with Paget's disease are categorized based on the size and characteristics of the parenchymal disease, although the presence of Paget's disease should still be noted
T1	Tumor ≤20 mm in greatest dimension
T1mi	Tumor ≤1 mm in greatest dimension
T1a	Tumor >1 mm but ≤5 mm in greatest dimension
T1b	Tumor >5 mm but ≤10 mm in greatest dimension
T1c	Tumor >10 mm but ≤20 mm in greatest dimension
T2	Tumor >20 mm but ≤50 mm in greatest dimension
T3	Tumor >50 mm in greatest dimension
T4	Tumor of any size with direct extension to the chest wall and/or to the skin (ulceration or skin nodules). *Note:* Invasion of the dermis alone does not qualify as T4
T4a	Extension to the chest wall, not including only pectoralis muscle adherence/invasion
T4b	Ulceration and/or ipsilateral satellite nodules and/or edema (including peau d'orange) of the skin, which do not meet the criteria for inflammatory carcinoma
T4c	Both T4a and T4b
T4d	Inflammatory carcinoma
N (nodes)	**Tumor**
Clinical	
NX	Regional lymph nodes cannot be assessed (e.g., previously removed)
N0	No regional lymph node metastases
N1	Metastases to movable ipsilateral level I, II axillary lymph node(s)
N2	Metastases in ipsilateral level I, II axillary lymph nodes that are clinically fixed or matted; or in clinically detected[a] ipsilateral internal mammary nodes in the *absence* of clinically evident axillary lymph node metastases
N2a	Metastases in ipsilateral level I, II axillary lymph nodes fixed to one another (matted) or to other structures
N2b	Metastases only in clinically detected[a] ipsilateral internal mammary nodes and in the *absence* of clinically evident level I, II axillary lymph node metastases
N3	Metastases in ipsilateral infraclavicular (level III axillary) lymph node(s) with or without level I, II axillary lymph node involvement; or in clinically detected[a] ipsilateral internal mammary lymph node(s) with clinically evident level I, II axillary lymph node metastases; or metastases in ipsilateral supraclavicular lymph node(s) with or without axillary or internal mammary lymph node involvement
N3a	Metastases in ipsilateral infraclavicular lymph node(s)
N3b	Metastases in ipsilateral internal mammary lymph node(s) and axillary lymph node(s)
N3c	Metastases in ipsilateral supraclavicular lymph node(s)

(continued)

| TABLE 30.3 | **AJCC Staging for Breast Cancer (*Continued*)** |

M (distant metastasis)	Tumor
M0	No clinical or radiographic evidence of distant metastases
cM0(i+)	No clinical or radiographic evidence of distant metastases, but deposits of molecularly or microscopically detected tumor cells in circulating blood, bone marrow, or other nonregional nodal tissue that are no larger than 0.2 mm in a patient without symptoms or signs of metastases
M1	Distant detectable metastases as determined by classic clinical and radiographic means and/or histologically proven larger than 0.2 mm

Pathologic classification of breast cancer	Tumor
pN0(i−)	No regional lymph node metastases histologically, negative IHC
pN0(i+)	Malignant cells in regional lymph node(s) not >0.2 mm (detected by H&E or IHC including ITC)
pN0(mol−)	No regional lymph node metastases histologically, negative molecular findings (RT-PCR)
pN0(mol+)	Positive molecular findings (RT-PCR),[b] but no regional lymph node metastases detected by histology or IHC
pN1	Micrometastases; or metastases in one to three axillary lymph nodes; and/or in internal mammary nodes with metastases detected by sentinel lymph node biopsy but not clinically detected[c]
pN1mi	Micrometastases (>0.2 mm and/or >200 cells, but none >2.0 mm)
pN1a	Metastases in one to three axillary lymph nodes, at least one metastasis >2.0 mm
pN1b	Metastases in internal mammary nodes with micrometastases or macrometastases detected by sentinel lymph node biopsy but not clinically detected[c]
pN1c	Metastases in one to three axillary lymph nodes and in internal mammary lymph nodes with micrometastases or macrometastases detected by sentinel lymph node biopsy but not clinically detected
pN2	Metastases in four to nine axillary lymph nodes; or in clinically detected[d] internal mammary lymph nodes in the *absence* of axillary lymph node metastases
pN2a	Metastases in four to nine axillary lymph nodes (at least one tumor deposit >2.0 mm)
pN2b	Metastases in clinically detected[d] internal mammary lymph nodes in the *absence* of axillary lymph node metastases
pN3	Metastases in ten or more axillary lymph nodes; or in infraclavicular (level III axillary) lymph nodes; or in clinically detected[d] ipsilateral internal mammary lymph nodes in the *presence* of one or more positive level I, II axillary lymph nodes; or in more than three axillary lymph nodes and in internal mammary lymph nodes with micrometastases or macrometastases detected by sentinel lymph node biopsy but not clinically detected[c]; or in ipsilateral supraclavicular lymph nodes
pN3a	Metastases in ten or more axillary lymph nodes (at least one tumor deposit >2.0 mm); or metastases to the infraclavicular (level III axillary lymph) nodes
pN3b	Metastases in clinically detected[d] ipsilateral internal mammary lymph nodes in the *presence* of one or more positive axillary lymph nodes; or in more than three axillary lymph nodes and in internal mammary lymph nodes with micrometastases or macrometastases detected by sentinel lymph node biopsy but not clinically detected[c]
pN3c	Metastases in ipsilateral supraclavicular lymph nodes

[a]Classification is based on axillary lymph node dissection with or without sentinel lymph node biopsy. Classification based solely on sentinel lymph node biopsy without subsequent axillary lymph node dissection is designated (sn) for "sentinel node," for example, pN0(sn).
[b]RT-PCR: reverse transcriptase/polymerase chain reaction.
[c]"Not clinically detected" is defined as not detected by imaging studies (excluding lymphoscintigraphy) or not detected by clinical examination.
[d]"Clinically detected" is defined as detected by imaging studies (excluding lymphoscintigraphy) or by clinical examination and having characteristics highly suspicious for malignancy or a presumed pathologic macrometastasis based on fine needle aspiration biopsy with cytologic examination.
From Edge SB, Byrd DR, and Compton CC, et al, *AJCC Cancer Staging Manual*, 7th edition. New York, Springer, 2010, pp 371–373.

necessary to use intensity-modulated radiation therapy (IMRT). We attempt to make the chest as parallel to the simulation table as possible, using the breast board as necessary. The clinical boundaries of the intended treatment field, mastectomy scar, and drain sites are marked with radioopaque wire. The medial border splits the sternum and connects the center of the xiphoid process with the center of the thoracic inlet. The lateral border is defined by the mid-axillary line. The superior border is the inferior edge of the clavicular head. The inferior border is placed 1 to 2 cm below the location of the inframammary fold. The contralateral breast, if present, is typically used to aid in placing the inferior border. An IV is placed in the contralateral upper extremity if there is no contraindication to IV contrast.

Scout images are obtained to verify patient setup. Axial 3-mm CT slices are acquired from the angle of the mandible through the entire thorax, taking care to include the aforementioned inferior border plus at least 4 cm. IV contrast is infused to improve nodal basin delineation. A four-dimensional (4D) simulation is performed to assess motion of the chest wall. A more thorough discussion of respiratory motion follows later in this chapter. Breath-holding techniques or gating, also discussed later, may be used if available, particularly in the setting of left-sided cancers.

Following acquisition, the scan is manipulated using the simulator software. Contours are placed on the CT slices containing the superior and inferior wires respectively. The CT slice midway between the superior and inferior wires is selected. A line is drawn between the medial and lateral wires on this slice. The distance of the line is measured and a point is placed at the midpoint of the line. This point represents the psuedoisocenter. Opposed tangents are created with a shared central axis that intersects the psuedoisocenter, the medial wire, and the lateral wire. The superior and inferior jaws are set to their respective clinically defined wires. The x, y, and z coordinates of the pseudoisocenter are recorded. The CT scan is then advanced to the slice containing the superior wire. This slice defines the match plane. The true isocenter is placed on this slice containing the superior wire, with the same x and y coordinates as the psuedoisocenter. The tangent fields are tagged to the true isocenter; the superior jaw is set to zero, and the inferior jaw is opened to the inferior wire. The tangents are now a quarter beam encompassing the intended chest wall, with a nondivergent superior edge. A supraclavicular field is created and tagged to the true isocenter. The supraclavicular inferior jaw is set to zero, the superior jaw is set to the level of the cricoid cartilage, the medial jaw is set to the vertebral bodies, and the lateral jaw is set to cover either the level III axillary nodes and supraclavicular nodes or the whole axilla, depending on the clinical situation. The single isocenter is marked on the patient, and the images are transferred to the treatment planning system.

One limitation of this technique is that the useful field size of the tangents is limited to 20×20 cm^2, but this rarely poses a problem. The superior border can be adjusted after scan acquisition to modify the size of the fields, as long as the modification does not result in excessive lung dose from the larger supraclavicular field.

Volumes

In the past, breast cancer was treated using clinical landmarks. However, as treatment techniques have grown increasingly sophisticated, it has become necessary to precisely delineate target volumes. Unfortunately, there is significant interobserver variability with respect to contouring the chest wall and regional nodes in the setting of postmastectomy radiotherapy, even among experts (54). One method to ensure consistency entails designating the chest wall encompassed by clinically defined ports as the clinical target volume. This method can be expected to reliably reproduce the results achieved in historical trials. However, this approach may not take optimal advantage of modern radiation delivery and availability of three-dimensional (3D) imaging techniques. Hence, a clinician can manually delineate chest wall target volumes. The RTOG has published guidelines for the delineation of the chest wall and draining nodal regions, shown in Table 30.4 (55).

The target volumes for postmastectomy radiotherapy generally include the chest wall and supraclavicular, axillary, and IM nodes (Fig. 30.4). The necessity of treating the IM nodes continues to be a point of controversy. A recent EORTC trial demonstrated no difference in overall survival of patients with stage I and II breast cancer treated with mastectomy and postoperative radiotherapy with or without treatment of the IM nodes (56). On the other hand, the major trials demonstrating the benefit of postmastectomy radiotherapy routinely included the IM nodes (35–37). The decision to include these nodes in the target volume remains a question of balancing recurrence risk with morbidity that must be decided on an individual patient basis. Some clinicians may choose to exclude the IM nodes in patients thought to be at low risk for involvement due to a lateral location of their tumor or in whom cardiotoxicity is a concern (e.g., patients with left-sided tumors, those who have had anthracycline chemotherapy, and/or those receiving trastuzumab).

In the setting of postmastectomy radiotherapy the clinician can define a CTV (either manually or using clinically defined radiotherapy ports) that includes the entire at risk chest wall, axillary lymph nodes, supraclavicular lymph nodes, and IM nodes (Fig. 30.4A and B). Organs at risk (OAR) should be defined including contralateral breast, ipsilateral lung, whole heart, and spinal cord. The physician may consider contouring additional structures including the contralateral lung if an IMRT technique is to be utilized.

Planning

Chest Wall Irradiation

The entire at-risk ipsilateral chest wall should be treated with an adequate dose of radiation. When 3D techniques are

TABLE 30.4	The RTOG Consensus Guidelines for Delineation of Chest Wall, Breast, and Nodal Targets				
	Cranial	**Caudal**	**Medial**	**Lateral**	**Posterior**
Breast	Clinical reference + second rib insertion	Clinical reference + loss of CT apparent breast tissue	Sternal-rib junction	Clinical reference + mid-axillary line, excluding lattisimus dorsi	Excludes chest wall muscles, pectoral muscles, and ribs
Breast and chest wall	Same	Same	Same	Same	Same
Chest wall	Inferior border clavicular head	Clinical reference + loss of CT apparent contralateral breast	Same	Same	Pleural interface. Includes chest wall muscles, pectoral muscles, and ribs

	Cranial	**Caudal**	**Medial**	**Lateral**	**Anterior**	**Posterior**
Supraclavicular	Inferior aspect cricoid cartilage	Junction of brachioceph.-axillary vns./caudal edge clavicle head	Excludes thyroid and trachea	Cranial: lateral edge of SCM m. Caudal: junction 1st rib-clavicle	Sternocleido mastoid (SCM) muscle (m.)	Anterior aspect of the scalene
Level I axilla	Axillary vessels cross lateral aspect of pec minor	Pectoralis (Pec.) major muscle insert into ribs	Lateral border of Pec. minor m.	Medial border of lat. dorsi m.	Posterior surface Pec. Major m.	Anterior surface of subscapularis
Level II axilla	Axillary vessels cross medial aspect of pec minor	Axillary vessels cross lateral edge of Pec. Minor m.	Medial border of Pec. Minor m.	Lateral border of Pec. Minor m.	Anterior surface Pec. Minor m.	Ribs and intercostal muscles
Level III axilla	Pec minor insertion on cricoid	Axillary vessels cross medial edge of Pec. Minor m.	Thoracic inlet	Medial border of Pec. Minor m.	Posterior surface Pec. Major m.	Ribs and intercostal muscles
Internal mammary	Superior aspect of medial first rib	Cranial aspect of the fourth rib				

used, the chest wall is typically encompassed within tangential photon fields (Fig. 30.5). The tangent fields may be modified to encompass the mastectomy scar, and sometimes to include drain sites. When drain sites fall outside the tangents they can be boosted to full dose using supplementary electron fields. If the ipsilateral IM chain is to be included in the treatment volume, great care must be taken to minimize dose to the underlying heart and lung. The IM chain lies beside the sternum, generally in the first through the third intercostal spaces, although the depth may vary (Fig. 30.6).

Various methods of encompassing the IM chain within the chest wall fields have been described including extended tangent fields, partially wide tangent fields, and matching electron and photon fields. These techniques of treating the IM lymph nodes were compared in a dosimetric evaluation. It was found that the partially wide tangent technique provided optimal target volume coverage, reduced normal tissue doses, and produced a high degree of target volume homogeneity (57). Subsequent investigators agreed that partially wide tangents achieve the optimal blend of target

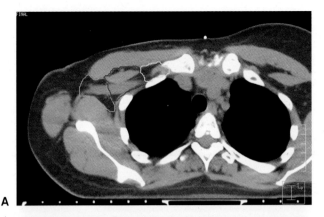

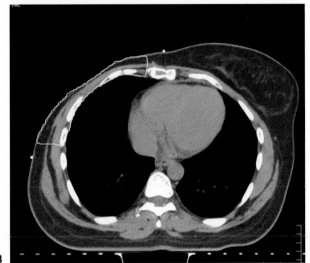

Figure 30.4. A: Axial slice demonstrating contours of the axillary levels I (*orange*), II (*blue*), and III (*yellow*). **B:** A representative contour of the chest wall target (*yellow*).

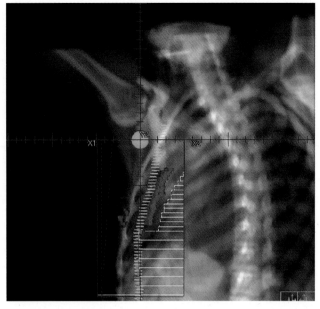

Figure 30.5. The digital reconstructed radiograph of a medial tangent in the setting of postmastectomy, three field, mono-isocentric radiotherapy. The *green sphere* is the true isocenter. The *red sphere* is the psuedoisocenter. The aquamarine wireframe is the medial wire used to guide posterior blocking of the tangent port except where the internal mammary (IM) nodes, shown in *magenta*, are included. Drain sites are *blue* and included in the field.

coverage and normal tissue sparing (58). Physicians may also consider using an IMRT technique.

Dose to the chest wall and IM nodes is typically 45 to 50.4 Gy in 25 to 28 fractions. Partially wide tangents are the preferred 3D technique used by the authors. The medial wire is visualized and used to guide blocking (59). Dose is prescribed to a point 1.5 cm into the chest wall located on the orthogonal to the posterior border of the tangents at the level of the psuedoisocenter. Enhanced dynamic wedges are used to improve homogeneity and are preferred for their decreased scatter relative to physical wedges. Alternatively, forward planning can be used to improve homogeneity. In most patients chest wall bolus is applied every other day to generate a brisk skin reaction is recommended. Daily bolus is considered for patients with inflammatory disease.

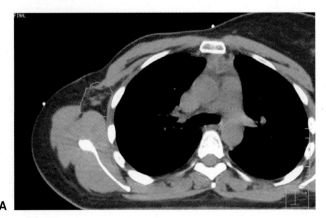

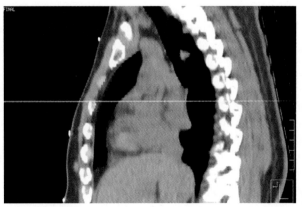

Figure 30.6. A: The internal mammary (IM) nodes, in *magenta*, coursing along the lateral aspect of the sternum. The inferior aspect of the level one axilla is shown in *orange*. **B:** The internal mammary (IM) nodes are contoured from the inferior aspect of the first rib to the superior aspect of the fourth rib.

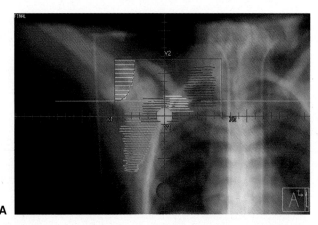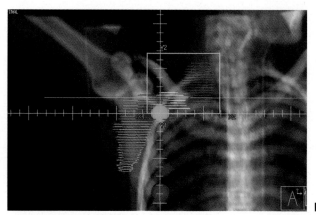

Figure 30.7. A: The digital reconstructed radiograph of the supraclavicular field in the same patient with field borders set to treat the whole axilla. **B:** The supraclavicular field with lateral borders set to the coracoid process for treating only level III and the supraclavicular nodes. Level I is *orange*, II is *blue*, III is *yellow*, and the supraclavicular nodes are *red*.

Supraclavicular/Axillary Field

The supraclavicular and axillary nodes are usually encompassed with a single anterior oblique photon field angled slightly away from the spinal cord. Dose should be prescribed to adequately encompass the nodal volumes within the prescription dose as seen on CT planning.

Conventional field borders are set at the time of simulation and then modified as necessary based on CT information. If possible, avoidance of flash on the skin of the supraclavicular region may decrease acute skin reaction (Fig. 30.7). Avoidance of flash may also preserve a strip of skin, thereby decreasing the likelihood of developing lymphedema. A humeral head block is added to block the humeral head and acromioclavicular joint.

A dose of 45 to 50.4 Gy is delivered in 25 to 28 fractions. In patients with clinically evident supraclavicular disease, an additional boost may be delivered using conformal techniques, bringing total dose to 54 to 60 Gy, taking care to respect the tolerance of the brachial plexus.

Posterior Axillary Field

With the use of CT planning, it can be determined whether nodal structures are adequately encompassed with a minimum dose of 4,500 cGy through the supraclavicular/axillary field without excessive doses to normal lung or the creation of suboptimal dose distributions. If coverage is suboptimal, dose can be supplemented with a posterior axillary field. The field is set up opposed to the supraclavicular/axillary field.

Conventional field borders for the posterior axillary field are as follows: superiorly, the clavicle; inferiorly, blocked to match the superior edge of the chest wall portal; medially, including 2 cm of lung; and laterally, medial border of the humeral head (Fig. 30.8).

Breast Conservation

Supine Irradiation of the Intact Breast

Breast conservation, consisting of lumpectomy/partial mastectomy followed by postoperative radiotherapy, has been validated in large randomized trials as a standard of care in the treatment of early stage breast cancer and carcinoma *in situ* (60,61). Moderate doses of radiation are delivered to the entirety of the breast in an attempt to eradicate microscopic foci of disease and minimize risk of local recurrence.

Patient Selection

A patient may be considered a candidate for breast conversation if she is motivated to preserve the breast, and she does not have an absolute contraindication. The contraindications to breast preservation include prior irradiation of the index breast, multicentric disease, extensive microcalcifications, persistent positive margins, active collagen

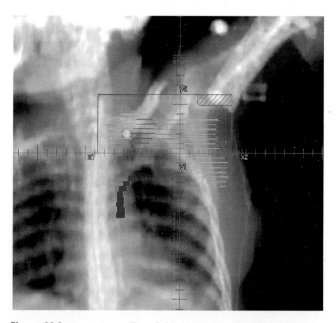

Figure 30.8. Posterior axillary field simulation film illustrating the field. Superiorly, the clavicle; inferiorly, blocked to match the superior edge of the chest wall portal; medially, includes 2 cm of lung and lateral-medial border of the humeral head.

vascular disease (62), and pregnancy that cannot be delivered prior to the start of radiotherapy. The ratio of tumor size to breast size and the resultant cosmesis may be a relative contraindication. Patients whose tumors contain an extensive intraductal component may be appropriate candidates provided that the margins of resection are negative, either initially or after reexcision. Youth (age below 35) is not a contraindication to conservative management, but particular attention should be paid to the contralateral breast dose. Other patient-related factors, such as extremes of breast size and pendulous breasts, also do not by themselves contraindicate conservative treatment.

Supine Simulation Technique

The technique for performing CT simulation to deliver tangential irradiation to the intact breast is similar to that described above in the postmastectomy setting.

The patient is placed supine on a breast board with both arms raised overhead. The clinical boundaries of the breast are marked with fiducial wire. These boundaries are similar to those described above with the exception that all boundaries must have 1- to 2-cm margin on palpable breast tissue. Fiducial wire is placed over the lumpectomy scar. Axial CT slices are acquired from 4 cm above the superior border to 4 cm below the inferior border. The slice midway between the superior and inferior borders is selected; the isocenter is placed at midseparation between the medial and lateral wires on this slice. Opposed tangents are placed with parallel central axes passing through the medial and lateral wires. The isocenter is marked on the patient. Ideally, there should be 1 to 3 cm of lung visible on the simulation digitally reconstructed radiograph in the field anterior to the central axis. A study from the Harvard Joint Center for Radiation Therapy found the best predictor of the percentage of ipsilateral lung volume treated by the tangential fields to be the demagnified perpendicular distance from the posterior field edge to the

posterior part of the anterior chest wall at the central axis, or the central axis distance (CAD). A CAD of 1.5 cm predicted that about 6% of the ipsilateral lung would be treated; a CAD of 2.5 cm, about 16%, and a CAD of 3.5 cm, about 26% (63). With CT planning, lung volumes can be more accurately determined, but a CAD of 1 to 3 cm serves as a useful guideline.

Three-Field Technique

The indications for irradiation of a third field are controversial but include greater than four lymph nodes involved, or significant extracapsular extension. The three-field technique used at Rush University Medical Center is described in the section on "Postmastectomy Radiotherapy." Figure 30.9 illustrates the patient position for setup, and the fields are outlined.

Prone Irradiation of the Intact Breast

The recognition that large breasted women may experience more severe acute dermatitis and worse cosmesis when treated in the setting of breast conservation with supine breast radiotherapy led to exploration of alternative treatment techniques (64). Breast radiotherapy in the prone position was proposed as a means to improve outcomes in this group of patients (65,66). Prone radiotherapy improves dose homogeneity according to some authors, and also improves lung dose in virtually all patients, while exerting a variable effect on cardiac dose (67–72).

Patient Selection for Prone Treatment

There are no cooperative group trials evaluating the efficacy or safety of prone breast radiotherapy. The published experience to date has been limited to single institution series treating patients with early stage disease (70,71). Local regional control and toxicity have been excellent in these carefully selected patients. The prone position is

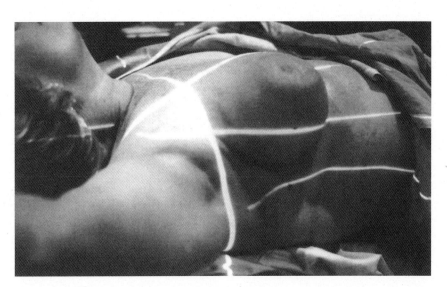

Figure 30.9. Patient positioning and treatment fields for treating the intact breast using a three-field isocentric technique.

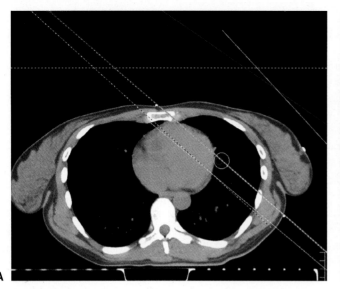
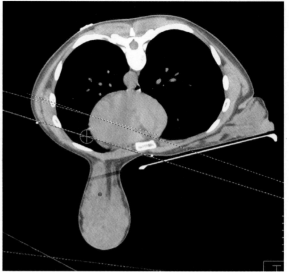

Figure 30.10. (A) Supine and (B) prone tangents are shown for the same patient. The parallel central axes of the tangents denote the block field edge on this slice. The prone position significantly spares the lung in the majority of patients.

considered by the authors in patients with large/pendulous breasts, and/or unacceptably high volumes of lung included in conventional supine tangents (Fig. 30.10).

Prone CT Simulation Techniques

The Rush technique for prone simulation is presented here. The patient is seated upright with both arms overhead. Radioopaque markers are placed to delineate the medial, lateral, superior, and inferior borders of the breast. The clinical boundaries are identical to those used in the supine position, but making allowances for differences in tissue position based on gravity. The wires are secured with adhesive, and then the patient lies prone on a prone breast board. Care is taken to suspend the breast in the center of the table cutout. Allowing the breast to contact table surfaces can lead to undesirable bolus effect. Axial CT slices encompassing the entire breast are acquired. The procedure for placing the isocenter and setting the tangents is the same as described above in the setting of two-field supine breast RT. Additional leveling marks are placed on the patient and the patient is indexed to the breast board to facilitate daily setup.

Prone setup can be subject to significant interfraction variability (73). These variations could potentially be clinically significant, particularly if IMRT is being used. Daily imaging can assist in verifying positioning. Indexing and leveling marks are important to minimize patient roll.

Intact Breast Volume: Prone and Supine

Similar issues exist in the intact breast setting with respect to volume definition as described above. The clinician may choose to manually designate a CTV including all ipsilateral breast tissue, or can designate tissue that is within the clinically defined field as CTV. The lumpectomy cavity is contoured, using clips as guidance if present. The cavity can be expanded by a clinician determined margin of 0.5 to 1.5 cm to form the CTV, taking care to trim the CTV off the skin and ribs. An institution specific margin is then added to create the boost PTV. Tangent fields must always be checked to ensure they include the entirety of the boost PTV. Boost treatment is discussed in a separate section below. OARs to be contoured include the ipsilateral lung, entire heart, and contralateral breast.

Intact Breast Planning: Prone and Supine

A dose of 45 to 50 Gy is delivered over 5 to 5.5 weeks at 180 to 200 cGy per fraction, depending on breast size, comorbidity, and chemotherapy agents delivered prior to RT or concurrently. The dose is prescribed to a point 1.5 cm from the isocenter into the breast if a half-beam tangential technique is used. Dynamic wedges are used as compensators on the tangent fields. Similar to the postmastectomy setting, the chest wall contour is used to guide creation of blocking. Both the medial and the lateral fields are treated each day. In some patients, an accelerated fractionation schedule delivering 42.5 Gy in 16 fractions is delivered (74,75). This schedule is typically restricted to patients with smaller breast size who have not received adjuvant chemotherapy. Patients treated prone requiring a boost are simulated again supine to deliver a supine boost.

Boost

In the treatment of the intact breast, a boost is defined as a supplemental dose of radiation delivered to the tumor bed. There are several rationales for the use of a boost following conservative surgery. Most local recurrences are at or near the primary site and may be encompassed in a boost field. The morbidity of a boost of moderate size and dose is small whether delivered by electron beam or interstitial implant (76).

Bartelink et al. reported the results of the EORTC trial, which randomized patients after whole-breast radiation to either no further treatment or a 16 Gy boost to the tumor bed. In this study, the boost could be given with electrons, tangential photon fields, or an iridium-192 (Ir-192) implant. The 10-year cumulative rates of local recurrence were 10.2% versus 6.2% in favor of the arm that received the tumor bed boost ($p < 0.001$) (77).

Electron beam radiation is the most widely used modality for delivering a tumor bed boost. Treatment with electrons provides a method for delivering dose to a localized area while limiting the dose to adjacent tissue. The design of an accurate boost field and volume requires careful consideration. Previous studies have shown that coverage of the tumor bed can be inadequate 20% to 80% of the time when methods utilizing the lumpectomy scar rather than CT are used to plan the tumor bed boost (78–80). The lumpectomy cavity is a dynamic entity. Recent evidence demonstrates that the majority of lumpectomy cavities may shrink by >50% during a course of standard 5 to 6 week whole-breast radiotherapy (81–83). In patients undergoing postoperative radiotherapy in the absence of chemotherapy, resimulating the patient after tangential irradiation could help minimize the volume of radiated tissue during the boost. In patients undergoing chemotherapy first, further cavity shrinkage during treatment is negligible, obviating the need for resimulation. We recommend using the CT scan to define the tumor bed. A typical boost volume encompasses the lumpectomy cavity plus a 1- to 2-cm margin within the 90% isodose line. The energies chosen are typically in the range of 9 to 12 MeV. If coverage with electrons is suboptimal, the tumor bed can also be boosted using photon fields or an interstitial implant. Interstitial implants require technical expertise not available at many institutions.

Dose Volume Constraints and Treatment Planning Considerations in Breast Radiotherapy

An awareness of dose to normal tissues, particularly the heart and the lung, is crucial to minimize morbidity in the setting of postmastectomy and intact breast radiotherapy. A correlation can be drawn between the volume of lung receiving 20 Gy (V20) and the risk of subsequent toxicity. In a dosimetric study performed by Lind et al., it was found that no cases of clinical or radiological pulmonary complications were seen with an ipsilateral lung V20 of 29% or below (84). Similar studies have been performed in the treatment of lung cancer, reporting no cases of high-grade pneumonitis in patients with a V20 below 32% (total lung volume) (85). Other authors have also noted a link between the development of pulmonary toxicity and the volume of lung irradiated (86,87). Overall, pulmonary toxicity from postoperative breast irradiation is uncommon, particularly in the setting of breast conservation. Limiting the central lung distance to <3 cm and minimizing the volume of lung exposed to 20 Gy appears to minimize the risk (86,88).

A significant association between irradiation for breast cancer and cardiac mortality has been noted by multiple authors, particularly in the setting of left-sided cancers (38,89–95). Studies employing functional imaging demonstrate a connection between dose, cardiac volume irradiated, and myocardial perfusion defects (96,97). However, the dose-volume relationships between various elements of the heart and overall outcome remain unclear. The patient groups demonstrating the highest risk of cardiac mortality in the meta-analyses mentioned above were treated using outdated techniques, and determination of dose-volume relationships for patients treated during the pre-CT era is difficult.

Contemporary analyses report little risk of excess cardiac morbidity with postoperative irradiation using modern technique (98,99). Nevertheless, identification of patients at higher risk of cardiac morbidity is important. Patients with highly unfavorable cardiac anatomy have been defined as those with a cardiac contact distance of >5 cm in the axial plane at the level of the right hemidiaphragm, and/or 2 cm in the sagittal plane at the midpoint of the left hemithorax (100). Maximum heart distance (Fig. 30.11), or the maximum amount of heart present anterior to the posterior border of the tangent field, has also been shown by multiple authors to be a reliable surrogate for cardiac dose (101–104). If CT planning is not available, limiting maximum heart distance to <1 cm appears to effectively minimize the risk of late cardiac mortality (101,102,105). When dose-volume histogram (DVH) information is available, recent analysis of the available data suggests that limiting <10% of the heart to 25 Gy by conventional fractionation results in a <1% risk of cardiac mortality (106).

Several breathing maneuvers have been investigated in an attempt to minimize the amount of myocardium included in the radiation port. Lu et al. demonstrated that treatment during deep inspiration breath hold was both feasible and capable of substantially decreasing the maximum heart distance within tangent ports (107). Subsequent dosimetric reports echoed these findings, while reporting a variable effect on lung dose (108–114). Gated delivery has also been investigated, which appears to offer improved sparing versus free breathing, but of less magnitude than the sparing achievable with breath-holding techniques (115). NTCP estimates of cardiac mortality suggest that use of breath-holding techniques could reduce the risk of cardiac toxicity. In one planning study Korreman et al. predicted a cardiac mortality rate of 4.8% with standard free breathing delivery compared to only 0.5% with gated delivery and 0.1% with deep inspiration breath hold (116). Other authors have noted a similar theoretical decrease in cardiac risk (117), but it remains to be seen whether a clinical benefit will result from implementation of breathing adapted radiotherapy. In the meantime, awareness of cardiac dose is important, and the use of available means to decrease cardiac dose is advised.

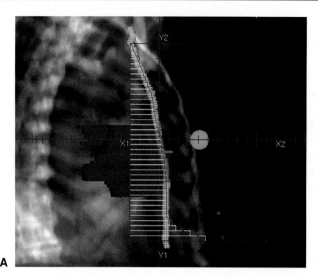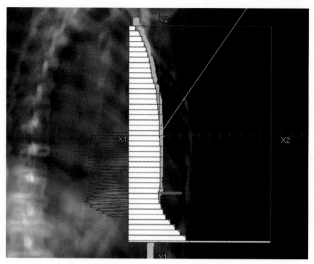

Figure 30.11. **A:** The aquamarine wireframe represents the medial wire; note how it delineates the chest wall and is used to create tangent field blocking. The *maroon contour* represents the cardiac ventricles. The *blue bar* demonstrates maximum heart distance, in this case <1 cm. **B:** This patient has less favorable cardiac anatomy, with a maximum heart distance >2 cm.

The effect of breathing motion on target coverage is an area under intense study. Available evidence suggests that respiratory motion tends to blur the beam penumbra without compromising target coverage, while introducing greater than expected heterogeneity (118,119). There are several methods of dealing with respiratory motion. Motion can be removed using breath-holding techniques, minimized using gated treatment delivery, minimized using physical compression, or compensated through modifications of the leaf sequence or treatment planning process (109,115,120). At Rush University Medical Center, the 4D average, or average intensity projection, is used for planning IMRT, thereby taking into account the relative position of tissue throughout the respiratory cycle (121,122). To date, none of these techniques has acquired universal acceptance. In patients where beamlet IMRT is likely to be used, minimizing respiratory motion or using 4D data to assess chest wall motion may be considered.

Intensity Modulated Radiation Therapy

IMRT has several meanings within the context of breast radiotherapy including anything from inverse planned, multifield, full fluence IMRT, to "field in field" treatment with multiple "segmental" portals treated through the same gantry angle to create an aggregate intensity modulation (123). IMRT offers the potential to improve target volume coverage, produce a more homogenous plan, and decrease the dose to normal organs compared to conventional or nonintensity-modulated CT planning methods (103,124–130). The use of IMRT has been shown to significantly reduce acute skin toxicity in the setting of intact breast radiation (131–134). Longer follow-up is necessary to determine if similar gains in late toxicity result from the use of IMRT.

The optimal implementation of IMRT remains undefined. In most clinical situations, treatment through tangential beam angles is preferred to treatment utilizing other beam angles, but questions remain regarding how to best use IMRT from tangential angles. One published comparison of five different planning techniques demonstrated that a hybrid plan consisting of conventional open fields plus IMRT tangents achieved a better dose distribution in less time than exclusively IMRT tangents or field in field techniques (135). Subsequent investigators have supported the superiority of combining open tangent fields with direct aperture optimized full fluence tangents (136,137). Not only was coverage more homogeneous, but also planning time was faster than that achieved using iterative forward planning with segmental IMRT.

IMRT also offers the ability to simultaneously treat two volumes concurrently. Several institutions have initiated protocols using a simultaneous integrated boost (SIB) to concurrently treat the whole breast and the tumor bed boost. This shortens the overall treatment time and potentially leads to improved quality of life (QOL) for patients undergoing radiation treatment for breast cancer. Early experience suggests a favorable toxicity profile and good local control at 3 years (138). Long term follow-up is necessary to assess impact on local control and cardiac morbidity.

Outside of an IRB approved protocol, we do not routinely utilize inverse planned IMRT to treat patients with breast cancer. Segmental IMRT, with a limited number of control points, is frequently employed when inadequate dose distributions are obtained using conventional dynamic wedges. Inverse planned IMRT is typically reserved for the patients whose plans are found to have suboptimal coverage, unacceptable inhomogeneity, and/or unacceptable doses to OARs.

Partial Breast Irradiation

With a substantial number of women being diagnosed with breast cancer at an early stage and being cured of their disease,

QOL issues become increasingly important. Breast conservation has become an accepted treatment, but the 6 to 7 weeks of postoperative radiotherapy poses a significant burden for many women. At present, only 10% to 40% of women eligible for breast conservation actually undergo this form of treatment (139). There has been a considerable amount of research exploring ways to decrease the treatment time and, as a result, improve the QOL for patients undergoing external beam radiation for the treatment of breast cancer.

APBI has been proposed as a means to meet the above objectives. APBI treats only the lumpectomy cavity with a 1- to 2-cm margin rather than the whole breast and can usually be completed in 1 week or less. The rationale for treating only the tumor bed comes from large retrospective studies, which have shown that failure outside of the lumpectomy bed is infrequent in certain subsets of patients with early-stage breast cancer. Also, failure outside the lumpectomy bed does not appear to be affected significantly by whole-breast radiation (140,141).

There are several methods for delivering APBI, including multiple interstitial catheters, balloon brachytherapy, and external beam APBI. Multi-catheter-based APBI is the method with the longest reported experience. Several institutions, including William Beaumont Hospital, have reported favorable cosmesis and rates of local control with reported follow-up approaching 8 years (142–144). A prospective randomized trial comparing APBI using either electron beam irradiation or interstitial catheter brachytherapy against conventional whole-breast irradiation has also been published. Similar rates of local control were achieved across methods, and interstitial brachytherapy achieved the best cosmesis (145). Unfortunately, multi-catheter-based APBI requires much expertise and is not offered at many institutions across the United States.

To make APBI more accessible and reproducible, the MammoSite brachytherapy device was developed. The MammoSite device consists of a silicone balloon connected to a catheter (Fig. 30.12). The catheter contains an inflation channel and a port for passage of the high-dose rate (HDR) brachytherapy source. The balloon is inflated with

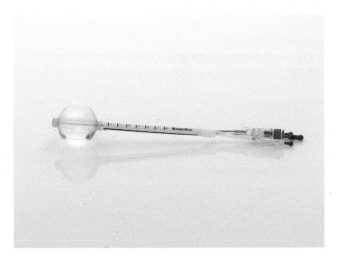

Figure 30.12. The MammoSite Catheter. (Reprinted with Permission, from Cytyc, Inc.)

saline solution mixed with a small amount of radiographic contrast to aid in visualization. An Ir-192 source, connected to a computer-controlled HDR remote afterloader, is inserted into the balloon to deliver the prescribed dose of radiation.

Early results regarding the cosmesis and complication rates with the use of the MammoSite Brachytherapy applicator have been favorable. Benitez et al. reported the 63-month results of the 43 patients treated in a prospective trial testing the safety of the device for FDA approval. As many as 81.3% of the patients achieved good or excellent cosmetic results at last follow-up. No instances of adverse sequelae requiring intervention were reported, and the rate of local failure was 0% (146). The single institution results for 30 patients treated at Rush University Medical Center were reported. Ninety-three percent of the patients achieved an excellent or good cosmetic outcome. The rate of infections was 13%; however, this has subsequently decreased with the routine use of antibiotics and more meticulous catheter care (147). Nelson et al. recently reported 4-year follow-up for the Mammosite registry trial including 1,440 patients. The 3-year actuarial rate of local recurrence was 2.15% and 91% of patients achieved good to excellent cosmetic results at 48 months follow-up (148).

An additional method of APBI utilizes external beam radiation. External beam based APBI eliminates the need for an extra invasive procedure. However, data on EBRT APBI is limited. Feasibility studies from New York University, University of Southern California, and William Beaumont Hospital have generated considerable interest (149–151). Initial clinical experience has also been encouraging, at least in part. One published series of 94 patients treated prospectively with 3D conformal APBI and median follow-up of 4.2 years reported an in-breast failure rate of 1.1% (152). Toxicity results were also encouraging; 88% of patients achieved good to excellent cosmetic results at 36 months (152). The recently published initial results of RTOG 0319 have also been encouraging (153). The role of IMRT in APBI has been evaluated and reported (154). In contrast to the excellent cosmetic results reported by others, a recent publication noted that 22% of patients treated using IMRT-based accelerated APBI developed unacceptable cosmesis (155). All patients but one experiencing unacceptable cosmesis were treated within the dosimetric constraints imposed by B-39, highlighting the need for caution in treating patients off protocol.

The continuing NSABP B-39/RTOG 0314 trial randomizes patients between whole-breast external beam radiation and APBI (Fig. 30.13). The APBI arm consists of interstitial brachytherapy, MammoSite brachytherapy, or 3D conformal partial breast irradiation. The results of this trial will not be available for several years. Until these results become available, it is important to limit APBI to patients who are at a low risk for failure outside the area of the lumpectomy cavity. Chen et al. demonstrated the importance of proper patient selection in their report on

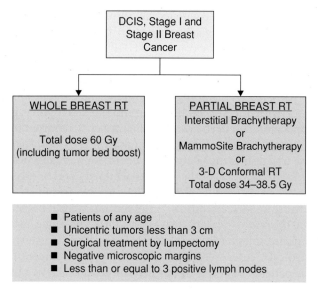

- Patients of any age
- Unicentric tumors less than 3 cm
- Surgical treatment by lumpectomy
- Negative microscopic margins
- Less than or equal to 3 positive lymph nodes

Figure 30.13. Schema and eligibility for NSABP/RTOG 0314.

70 patients treated with APBI using the Mammosite device. There were four local failures in this cohort, of which two were outside of ABS and/or ASBS criteria (156). The American Brachytherapy Society (ABS) and the American Society of Breast Surgeons (ASBS) have published conservative patient selection criteria in an attempt to select patients who would be at a minimal risk for recurrence after treatment with APBI (157,158). The ABS and ASBS selection criteria are listed in Table 30.5.

Dose and Volume of Treatment

The MammoSite breast brachytherapy applicator is our preferred method to deliver APBI. A dose of 340 cGy per fraction is delivered twice a day for 5 days. We allow a minimum of 6 hours between fractions. Dose is prescribed to a PTV located 1.0 cm from the balloon surface in 3D with the skin and chest wall as limiting structures. Dose is prescribed using a six-prescription point, multiple dwell

position technique, which has been previously described in a publication by our institution (159). This technique involves placing six prescription points 1 cm from the balloon surface. Four points are in a plane transverse to the balloon axis perpendicular to the catheter and two points are placed along the axis of the catheter (Fig. 30.14). Other optimization techniques have been described elsewhere (160).

After the catheter is placed, a CT scan is then used to assess the quality of the implant (Figs. 30.15). It is recommended that the distance from the balloon surface to the skin be at least 7 mm. Conformance of the balloon to the cavity is assessed. If >10% of the PTV is composed of air or fluid, conformance is considered inadequate. In addition, the symmetry of the balloon in relation to the catheter should be assessed. Implants in which the catheter lumen is placed asymmetrically can lead to underdosage of tissue around the cavity.

Future Directions in Accelerated Partial Breast Irradiation

The success and simplicity of balloon-based brachytherapy has led to the development of additional balloon devices. The Contura applicator, by Seno Rx, the SAVI device, by Cianna, and the multi-lumen MammoSite catheter are second-generation balloon brachytherapy devices that offer multiple lumens for the Ir-192 source in various configurations. These devices have been compared dosimetrically to the Mammosite device; the multiple lumen devices demonstrate similar target coverage but improved organ sparing versus the single lumen catheter (161,162). Initial clinical experience with the Contura applicator has yielded toxicity equivalent to that expected from the Mammosite experience (163). The additional flexibility in dose afforded by a multi-lumen design may allow a greater percentage of patients to be eligible for APBI secondary to the ability to achieve acceptable dose levels at the skin or chest wall when distance is <7 mm; however, longer follow-up is necessary with these devices to ensure equivalence to the Mammosite device.

TABLE 30.5	The American Brachytherapy Society (ABS) and American Society of Breast Surgeons (ASBS) Patient Selection Criteria for Partial Breast Irradiation	
	ABS recommendations	**ASBS recommendations**
Age	≥50 years	≥50 years
Histology	Unifocal, invasive ductal carcinoma	Invasive ductal carcinoma or DCIS
Tumor size	≤3 cm	≤3 cm
Surgical margins	Negative microscopic surgical margins of excision	Negative microscopic surgical margins of excision
Nodal status	N0	N0

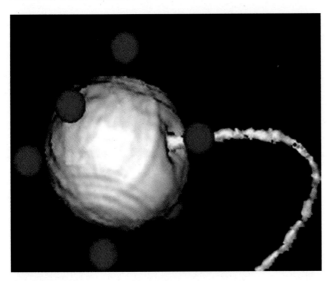

Figure 30.14. Schematic showing the six prescription point, multiple dwell position technique (Rush technique).

Electronic brachytherapy has recently been applied to the treatment of APBI in a fashion analogous to the Ir-192-based balloon brachytherapy devices. Xoft Inc. manufactures the Axxent x-ray source, a miniature generator of 50 kV rays. The source is delivered into the lumpectomy cavity through a balloon applicator. Similar to the procedure with Ir-192-based applicators, treatment with Xoft is prescribed to a surface 1 cm from the balloon surface. Preliminary studies have investigated the role of Xoft to deliver intraoperative radiotherapy in the setting of breast cancer (164). The dosimetric characteristics of the Xoft device in comparison to Mammosite have been described (165). The lower energy of the Xoft source in comparison to Ir-192 has many important implications. Strengths of this device include more rapid dose falloff beyond the prescription

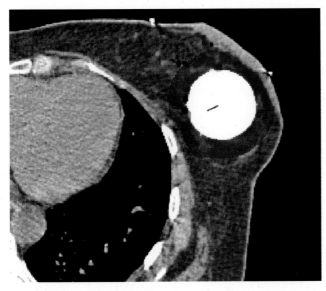

Figure 30.15. CT slice showing MammoSite balloon and PTV.

line resulting in lower dose to the heart, ipsilateral lung, and lower integral dose. On the other hand, dose inside the prescription line is considerably higher with the Xoft device, and the lower energy photons used are more susceptible to photoelectric interaction, potentially leading to excess dose deposition near high-Z materials (bone). These characteristics may ultimately impact rates of fat necrosis, rib, and skin toxicity (166). Clinical experience is necessary to fully characterize the toxicity profile of this device. Because of the energy differences, extrapolation of Mammosite dose-volume constraints should only be undertaken with caution, if at all.

Zeiss Inc. manufactures the Intrabeam device. The Intrabeam device has been adapted to deliver intraoperative breast radiotherapy. To date, Intrabeam has been used in lieu of a boost in a single small trial, with excellent rates of local control (167). The TARGIT trial is currently underway comparing a single 20 Gy fraction of intraoperative radiotherapy using the Intrabeam device to conventional whole-breast radiotherapy. Patient selection is critical when using Intrabeam either as an up-front boost or as definitive postoperative treatment since it requires the delivery of radiotherapy prior to final pathologic assessment of margin status.

REFERENCES

1. Buclossi P, Veronesi U, Zingo L, et al. Enlarged mastectomy for breast cancer: review of 1213 cases. *Am J Roentgenol Radium Ther Nucl Med* 1971;111:119–122.
2. Nemoto T, Vana J, Bedwani R. Management and survival of female breast cancer. *Cancer* 1980;45:2917–2924.
3. Pickren JW. Lymph node metastases in carcinoma of the female mammary gland. *Bull Roswell Park Memorial Inst* 1956;1:79.
4. Stibbe EP. The internal mammary lymphatic glands. *J Anat* 1918;52:257.
5. Handley R. Carcinoma of the breast. *Ann R Coll Surg Engl* 1975;57:59–66.
6. Halsted W. The results of radical operations for the cure of carcinoma of the breast. *Ann Surg* 1907;46:1–19.
7. American Joint Committee on Cancer. *AJCC cancer staging handbook*, 7th ed. New York: Springer, 2010.
8. Spratt J, Donegan W. *Cancer of the breast*. Philadelphia, PA: WB Saunders, 1967.
9. Fisher B, Slack N, Ausman R. Location of breast carcinoma and prognosis. *Surg Gynecol Obstet* 1969;129:705–716.
10. Haagensen C. *Diseases of the breast*, 2nd ed. Philadelphia, PA: WB Saunders, 1971.
11. Jamel A, Siegel R, Ward E, et al. Cancer statistics, 2009. *CA Cancer J Clin* 2009;59(4):225–249.
12. Wingo PA, Cardinez CJ, Landis SH, et al. Long-term trends in cancer mortality in the United States, 1930–1998. *Cancer* 2003;97:3133–3275.
13. Mayor S. UK deaths from breast cancer fall to lowest figure for 40 years. *BMJ* 2009;28:338.
14. Kelsey JL, Gammon MD, John EM. Reproductive factors and breast cancer. *Epidemiol Rev* 1993;15:36–47.

15. Reeves GK, Pirie K, Green J, et al. Reproductive factors and specific histological types of breast cancer: prospective study and meta-analysis. *Br J Cancer* 2009; 100(3):538–544.

16. Collaborative group on hormonal factors in breast cancer. Breast cancer and hormonal contraceptives: collaborative research analysis of individual data on 53,297 women with breast cancer and 100,239 women without breast cancer from 54 epidemiological causes. *Lancet* 1996;347:1713–1727.

17. Pike M, Henderson B, Casagrande J, Oral contraceptive use and early abortion as risk factors for breast cancer in young women. *Br J Cancer* 1981;43:720–776.

18. Vessey M, Painter R. Oral contraceptive use and cancer. Findings from a large cohort study, 1968–2004. *Br J Cancer* 2006;95:385–389.

19. Kumle M, Weiderpass E, Braaten T, et al. Use of oral contraceptives and breast cancer risk: the Norwegian-Swedish women's lifestyle and health cohort study. *Cancer Epidemiol Biomarkes Prev* 2002;11:1375–1381.

20. Kay CR, Hannaford PC. Breast cancer and the pill. A further report from the Royal College of General Practitioners' oral contraception study. *Br J Cancer* 1988;58: 675–680.

21. Collaborative group on Hormonal Factors in Breast Cancer. Breast cancer and hormone replacement therapy: collaborative reanalysis of data from 51 epidemiological studies of 52705 women with breast cancer and 108411 women without breast cancer. *Lancet* 1997;350: 1047–1059.

22. Beral V, Million Women Study Collaborators. Breast Cancer and hormone-replacement therapy in the Million Women Study. *Lancet* 2003;362(9382):419–427.

23. Rossouw JE, Anderson GL, Prentice RL, et al. Risks and benefits of estrogen plus progestin in healthy postmenopausal women: principal results from the Women's Health Initiative randomized controlled trial. *JAMA* 2002;288;321–333.

24. Henderson I. What can a woman do about her risk of dying of breast cancer? Curr Probl Cancer 1990;14: 166–230.

25. Ottman R, King M, Pike M, et al. Practical guide for estimating risk of familial breast cancer. *Lancet* 1983;2: 556–558.

26. Nicoletto MO, Donach M, De Nicolo A. BRCA-1 and BRCA-2 mutations as prognostic factors in clinical practice and genetic counseling. *Cancer Treat Rev* 2004; 27:295.

27. Carter RF. BRCA1, BRCA2, and breast cancer: a concise clinical review. *Clin Invest Med* 2001;27:295.

28. Tokunaga M, Land C, Yamamoto T, et al. Incidence of female breast cancer among atomic bomb survivors, Hiroshima and Nagasaki, 1950–1980. *Radiat Res* 1987; 112:243–272.

29. Miller A, Howe G, Sherman G, et al. Mortality from breast cancer after irradiation during fluoroscopic examinations in patients being treated for tuberculosis. *N Engl J Med* 1989;321:1285–1289.

30. Hildreth N, Shore L, Dvoretsky P. The risk of breast cancer after irradiation of the thymus in infancy. *N Engl J Med* 1989;321:146–151.

31. Hancock SL, Tucker MA, Hoppe RT. Breast cancer after treatment of Hodgkin's disease. *J Natl Cancer Inst* 1993;85:25–31.

32. Land CE, Boice JD Jr, Shore RE, et al. Breast cancer risk from low-dose exposure to ionizing radiation. *J Natl Cancer Inst* 1980;65:353–376.

33. Baron JA, Newcomb PA, Longnecker MP, et al. Cigarette smoking and breast cancer. *Cancer Epidemiol Biomarkers Prev* 1996;5:399–403.

34. Goldberg M, Labreche F. Occupational risk factors for female breast cancer: a review. *Occup Environ Med* 1996;53:145–146.

35. Overgaard M, Hansen P, Overgaard J, et al. Postoperative radiotherapy in high-risk premenopausal women with breast cancer who receive adjuvant chemotherapy. *N Engl J Med* 1997;337:949–955.

36. Ragaz J, Jackson SM, LE N, et al. Adjuvant radiotherapy and chemotherapy in node-positive premenopausal women with breast cancer the overall survival of breast cancer patients in the presence of adjuvant chemotherapy? N Engl J Med 1997;337:956–962.

37. Overgaard M, Jensen MB, Obergaard J, et al. Postoperative radiotherapy in high-risk postmenopausal patients given adjuvant tamoxifen: Danish breast cancer cooperative group DBCG 82c randomized trial. *Lancet* 1999; 353:1641–1648.

38. Clarke M, Collins R, Darby S, et al. Effects of radiotherapy and of differences in the extent of surgery for early breast cancer on local recurrence and 15-year survival: an overview of the randomized trials. *Lancet* 2005; 366(9503):2087–2106.

39. Aberizk WJ, Silver B, Henderson IC, et al. The use of radiotherapy for treatment of isolated regional recurrence of breast cancer after mastectomy. *Cancer* 1986; 58:1214–1218.

40. Nielsen HM, Overgaard M, Grau C, et al. Study of failure pattern among high-risk breast cancer patients with or without postmastectomy radiotherapy in addition to adjuvant systemic therapy: long-term results from the Danish Breast Cancer Cooperative Group DBCG 82 b and c randomized studies. *J Clin Oncol* 2006;24(15): 2268–2275.

41. Recht A, Edge SB, Solin LJ, et al. Postmastectomy radiotherapy: clinical practice guidelines of the American Society of Clinical Oncology. *J Clin Oncol* 2001;19; 1539–1569.

42. Harris JR, Halpin-Murphy P, McNeese M, et al. Consensus statement on postmastectomy radiation therapy. *Int J Radiat Oncol Biol Phys* 1999;44:989–990.

43. Katz A, Strom EA, Buchholz TA, et al. The influence of pathologic tumor characteristics on locoregional recurrence rates following mastectomy. *Int J Radiat Biol Phys* 2001;50:735–742.

44. Truong PT, Woodward WA, Thames HD, et al. The ratio of positive to excised nodes identifies high-risk subsets and reduces inter-institutional differences in locoregional recurrence risk estimates in breast cancer patients with 1–3 positive nodes: an analysis of prospective data from British Columbia and the M. D. Anderson Cancer Center. *Int J Radiat Oncol Biol Phys* 2007;68(1):59–65.

45. Katz A, Buchholz TA, Thames H, et al. Recursive partitioning analysis of locoregional recurrence patterns following mastectomy: Implications for adjuvant irradiation. *Int J Radiat Oncol Biol Phys* 2001;50:397–403.

46. Overgaard M, Nielsen HM, Overgaard J. Is the benefit of postmastectomy irradiation limited to patients with four or more positive nodes, as recommended in international consensus reports? A subgroup analysis of the DBCG 82 b&c randomized trials. *Radiother Oncol* 2007; 82(3):247–253.

47. Buchholz TA, Lehman CD, Harris JR, et al. Statement of the science concerning locoregional treatments after preoperative chemotherapy for breast cancer: a National Cancer Institute conference. *J Clin Oncol* 2008;26:791–797.

48. Siddon RL, Tonneson GL, Svensson GK. Three-field technique for breast treatment using a rotatable half-beam block. *Int J Radiat Oncol Biol Phys* 1981;7:1473–1477.

49. Chu JCH, Solin LJ, Hwang CC, et al. A nondivergent three field matching technique for breast irradiation. *Int J Radiat Oncol Biol Phys* 1990;19:1037–1040.

50. Lichter AS, Fraass BA, van de Geijn J. A technique for field matching in primary breast irradiation. *Int J Radiat Oncol Biol Phys* 1983;9:263–270.

51. Svensson GK, Bjarngard BE, Larsen RD. A modified three-field technique for breast treatment. *Int J Radiat Oncol Biol Phys* 1980;6:689–694.

52. Hartsell WF, Kelly CA, Schneider L, et al. A single isocenter three-field breast irradiation technique using an empiric simulation and asymmetric collimator. *Med Dosim* 1994;19:169–173.

53. Khan FM. *Treatment planning in radiation oncology,* 2nd ed. Philadelphia, PA. Lippincott Williams & Wilkins, 2007:391–409.

54. Li XA, Tai A, Arthur DW, et al. Variability of target and normal structure delineation for breast cancer radiotherapy: an RTOG Multi-Institutional and Multiobserver Study. *Int J Radiat Oncol Biol Phys* 2009;73(3): 944–951.

55. RTOG Breast Contouring Atlas. Available from http://www.rtog.org/pdf_file2.html?pdf_document=BreastCancerAtlas.pdf. Accessed March 18, 2010.

56. Romestaing P, Belot A, Hennequin C, et al. Ten-year results of a randomized trial of internal mammary chain irradiation after mastectomy. *Int J Radiat Oncol Biol Phys* 2009;75(3 Suppl 1):S1 (abstract).

57. Arthur D, Arnfield M, Warwicke L, et al. Internal mammary node coverage: an investigation of presently accepted techniques. *Int J Radiat Biol Phys* 2000;48: 139–146.

58. Pierce LJ, Butler JB, Martel MK, et al. Postmastectomy radiotherapy of the chest wall: dosimetric comparison of common techniques. *Int J Radiat Oncol Biol Phys* 2002;52(5):1220–1230.

59. Hartsell WF, Murthy AK, Kiel KD, et al. Technique for breast irradiation using custom blocks conforming to the chest wall contour. *Int J Radiat Oncol Biol Phys* 1990;19:189–195.

60. Fisher B, Anderson S, Bryant J, et al. Twenty-year follow-up of a randomized trial comparing total mastectomy, lumpectomy, and lumpectomy plus irradiation for the treatment of invasive breast cancer. *N Engl J Med* 2002; 347(16):1233–1241.

61. Fisher B, Land S, Mamounas E, et al. Prevention of invasive breast cancer in women with ductal carcinoma in situ: an update of the National Surgical Adjuvant Breast and Bowel Project experience. *Semin Oncol* 2001;28(4): 400–418.

62. Fleck RS, McNeese M, Ellerbroek NA, et al. Consequences of breast irradiation in patients with pre-existing collagen vascular diseases. *Int J Radiat Oncol Biol Phys* 1989;17:829–833.

63. Bornstein BA, Cheng CW, Rhodes L, et al. Can simulation measurements be used to predict the volume of lung within the radiation therapy treatment field in breast cancer patients? *Int J Radiat Oncol Biol Phys* 1990;18:181–187.

64. Gray JR, McCormick B, Cox L, et al. Primary breast irradiation in large-breasted or heavy women: analysis of cosmetic outcome. *Int J Radiat Oncol Biol Phys* 1991;21:347–354.

65. Merchant TE, McCormick B. Prone position breast irradiation. *Int J Radiat Oncol Biol Phys* 1994;30(1): 197–203.

66. Zierhut D, Flentje M, Frank C, et al. Conservative treatment of breast cancer: modified irradiation technique for women with large breasts. *Radiother Oncol* 1994; 31(3):256–261.

67. DeWyngaert JK, Jozsef G, Mitchell J, et al. Accelerated intensity-modulated radiotherapy to breast in prone position: dosimetric results. *Int J Radiat Oncol Biol Phys* 2007;68(4):1251–1259.

68. Griem KL, Fetherston P, Kuznetsova M, et al. Three-dimensional photon dosimetry: a comparison of treatment of the intact breast in the supine and prone position. *Int J Radiat Oncol Biol Phys* 2003;57(3): 891–899.

69. Kurtman C, Nalça Andrieu M, Hiçsönmez A, et al. Three-dimensional conformal breast irradiation in the prone position. *Braz J Med Biol Res* 2003;36(10): 1441–1446.

70. Croog VJ, Wu AJ, McCormick B, et al. Accelerated whole breast irradiation with intensity-modulated radiotherapy to the prone breast. *Int J Radiat Oncol Biol Phys* 2009;73(1):88–93.

71. Formenti SC, Gidea-Addeo D, Goldberg JD, et al. Phase I-II trial of prone accelerated intensity modulated radiation therapy to the breast to optimally spare normal tissue. *J Clin Oncol* 2007;25(16):2236–2242.

72. Varga Z, Hideghéty K, Mezö T, et al. Individual positioning: a comparative study of adjuvant breast radiotherapy in the prone versus supine position. *Int J Radiat Oncol Biol Phys* 2009;75(1):94–100.

73. Mitchell J, Formenti SC, Dewyngaert JK. Interfraction and intrafraction setup variability for prone breast radiation therapy. *Int J Radiat Oncol Biol Phys* 2010;76(5): 1571–1577.

74. Whelan T, MacKenzie R, Julian J, et al. Randomized trial of breast irradiation schedules after lumpectomy for women with lymph-node negative breast cancer. *J Natl Cancer Inst* 2002;94:1143–1150.

75. Whelan TJ, Pignol JP, Levine MN, et al. Long-term results of hypofractionated radiation therapy for breast cancer. *N Engl J Med* 2010;362(6):513–520.

76. De la Rochefordiere A, Abner A, Silver B, et al. Are cosmetic results following conservative surgery and radiation therapy for early breast dependent on technique? *Int J Radiat Oncol Biol Phys* 1992;23:925.

77. Bartelink H, Horiot JC, Poortmans PM, et al. Impact of a higher radiation dose on local control and survival in breast-conserving therapy of early breast cancer: 10-year results of the randomized boost versus no boost EORTC 22881–10882 trial. *J Clin Oncol* 2007;25(22): 3259–3565.

78. Denham JW, Sillar Rw, Clarke D. Boost dosage to the excision site following conservative surgery for breast cancer: it's easy to miss. *Clin Oncol* 1991;3:257–261.

79. Hunter MA, McFall TA, Hehr KA. Breast conserving surgery for primary breast Cancer: necessity for surgical clips to define the tumor bed for radiation planning. *Radiology* 1996;200:281–282.

80. Benda RK, Yasuda G, Sethi A, et al. Breast boost: are we missing the target? Cancer 2003;97:905–909.

81. Prendergast B, Indelicato DJ, Grobmyer SR, et al. The dynamic tumor bed: volumetric changes in the lumpectomy cavity during breast-conserving therapy. *Int J Radiat Oncol Biol Phys* 2009;74(3):695–701.

82. Tersteeg RJ, Roesink JM, Albregts M, et al. Changes in excision cavity volume: prediction of the reduction in absolute volume during breast irradiation. *Int J Radiat Oncol Biol Phys* 2009;74(4):1181–1185.

83. Strauss JB, Gielda BT, Chen SS, et al. Variation in post-surgical lumpectomy cavity volume with delay in initiation of breast irradiation because of chemotherapy. *Int J Radiat Oncol Biol Phys* 2010;77(3):831–835.

84. Lind P, Wennberg B, Gagliardi G, et al. Pulmonary complications following different radiotherapy techniques for breast cancer, and the association to irradiated lung volume and doses. *Breast Cancer Res Treat* 2001;68: 199–210.

85. Graham MV, Purdy JA, Emami B, et al. Clinical dose-volume histogram analysis for pneumonitis after 3D treatment for non-small cell lung cancer (NSCLC). *Int J Radiat Oncol Biol Phys* 1999;45:323–329.

86. Krengli M, Sacco M, Loi G, et al. Pulmonary changes after radiotherapy for conservative treatment of breast cancer: a prospective study. *Int J Radiat Oncol Biol Phys* 2008;70:1460–1467.

87. Kimsey FC, Mendenhall NP, Ewald LM, et al. Is radiation treatment volume a predictor for acute or late effects on pulmonary function? A prospective study of patients treated with breast-conserving surgery and post-operative irradiation. *Cancer* 1994;73:2549–2555.

88. Lingos L, Recht A, Vicini F, et al. Radiation pneumonitis in breast cancer patients treated with conservative surgery and radiation therapy. *Int J Radiat Oncol Biol Phys* 1991;21:355–360.

89. Haybittle JL, Brinkley D, Houghton J, et al. Postoperative radiotherapy and late mortality: evidence from the Cancer Research Campaign trial for early breast cancer. *Br Med J* 1989;298:1611–1614.

90. Cuzick J, Stewart H, Rutqvist L, et al. Cause-specific mortality in long-term survivors of breast cancer who participated in trials of radiotherapy. *J Clin Oncol* 1994;12:447–453.

91. Jones JM, Ribeiro GG. Mortality patterns over 34 years of breast cancer patients in a clinical trial of post-operative radiotherapy. *Clin Radiol* 1989;40:204–208.

92. Rutqvist LE, Lax I, Fornander T, et al. Cardiovascular mortality in a randomized trial of adjuvant radiation therapy versus surgery alone in primary breast cancer. *Int J Radiat Oncol Biol Phys* 1992;22:887–896.

93. Gyenes G, Fornander T, Carlens P, et al. Morbidity of ischemic heart disease in early breast cancer 15–20 years after adjuvant radiotherapy. *Int J Radiat Oncol Biol Phys* 1994;28:1235–1241.

94. Paszat LF, Mackillop WJ, Groome PA, et al. Mortality from myocardial infarction following postlumpectomy radiotherapy for breast cancer: a population-based study in Ontario, Canada. *Int J Radiat Oncol Biol Phys* 1999;43:755–761.

95. Darby SC, McGale P, Taylor CW, et al. Long-term mortality from heart disease and lung cancer after radiotherapy for early breast cancer: prospective cohort study of about 300 000 women in US SEER cancer registries. Lancet Oncol 2005;6:557–565.

96. Lind PA, Pagnanelli R, Marks LB, et al. Myocardial perfusion changes in patients irradiated for left-sided breast cancer and correlation with coronary artery distribution. *Int J Radiat Oncol Biol Phys* 2003;55:914–920.

97. Gyenes G, Fornander T, Carlens P, et al. Myocardial damage in breast cancer patients treated with adjuvant radiotherapy: a prospective study. *J Radiother Oncol* 1996;36:899–905.

98. Giordano SH, Kuo YF, Freeman JL, et al. Risk of cardiac death after adjuvant radiotherapy for breast cancer. *J Natl Cancer Inst* 2005;97:419–424.

99. Hojris I, Overgaard M, Christensen JJ, et al. Morbidity and mortality of ischemic heart disease in high-risk breast-cancer after adjuvant postmastectomy systemic treatment with or without radiotherapy: analysis of DBCG 82b and 82c randomized trails. *Lancet* 1999;354: 1425–1430.

100. Hiatt JR, Evans SB, Price LL, et al. Dose-modeling study to compare external beam techniques from protocol NSABP B-39/RTOG 0413 for patients with highly unfavorable cardiac anatomy. *Int J Radiat Oncol Biol Phys* 2006;65(5):1368–1374.

101. Hurkmans CW, Borger JH, Bos LJ, et al. Cardiac and lung complication probabilities after breast cancer irradiation. *Radiother Oncol* 2000;55:145–151.

102. Hurkmans CW, Cho BC, Damen E, et al. Reduction of cardiac and lung complication probabilities after breast irradiation using conformal radiotherapy with or without intensity modulation. *Radiother Oncol* 2002;62: 163–171.

103. Coon AB, Dickler A, Kirk MC, et al. Tomotherapy and multifield intensity-modulated radiotherapy planning reduce cardiac doses in left-sided breast cancer patients with unfavorable cardiac anatomy. *Int J Radiat Oncol Biol Phys* 2010;78(1):104–110.

104. Taylor CW, McGale P, Povall JM, et al. Estimating cardiac exposure from breast cancer radiotherapy in clinical practice. *Int J Radiat Oncol Biol Phys* 2009;73: 1061–1068.

105. Gagliardi G, Lax I, Rutqvist LE. Partial irradiation of the heart. *Semin Radiat Oncol* 2001;11:224–233.

106. Gagliardi G, Constine LS, Moiseenko V, et al. Radiation dose–volume effects in the heart. *Int J Radiat Oncol Biol Phys* 2010;76(3 Suppl 1):S77–S85.

107. Lu HM, Cash E, Chen MH, et al. Reduction of cardiac volume in left-breast treatment fields by respiratory maneuvers: a CT study. *Int J Radiat Oncol Biol Phys* 2000;47(4):895–904.

108. Sixel KE, Aznar MC, Ung YC. Deep inspiration breath hold to reduce irradiated heart volume in breast cancer patients. *Int J Radiat Oncol Biol Phys* 2001;49(1):199–204.

109. Remouchamps VM, Vicini FA, Sharpe MB, et al. Significant reductions in heart and lung doses using deep inspiration breath hold with active breathing control and intensity-modulated radiation therapy for patients treated with locoregional breast irradiation. *Int J Radiat Oncol Biol Phys* 2003;55(2):392–406.

110. Pedersen AN, Korreman S, Nyström H, et al. Breathing adapted radiotherapy of breast cancer: reduction of cardiac and pulmonary doses using voluntary inspiration breath-hold. *Radiother Oncol* 2004;72(1):53–60.

111. Krauss DJ, Kestin LL, Raff G, et al. MRI-based volumetric assessment of cardiac anatomy and dose reduction via active breathing control during irradiation for left-sided breast cancer. *Int J Radiat Oncol Biol Phys* 2005;61(4):1243–1250.

112. Stranzl H, Zurl B. Postoperative irradiation of left-sided breast cancer patients and cardiac toxicity. Does deep inspiration breath-hold (DIBH) technique protect the heart? *Strahlenther Onkol* 2008;184(7):354–358.

113. Nemoto K, Oguchi M, Nakajima M, et al. Cardiac-sparing radiotherapy for the left breast cancer with deep breath-holding. *Jpn J Radiol* 2009;27(7):259–263.

114. Stranzl H, Zurl B, Langsenlehner T, et al. Wide tangential fields including the internal mammary lymph nodes in patients with left-sided breast cancer. Influence of respiratory-controlled radiotherapy (4D-CT) on cardiac exposure. *Strahlenther Onkol* 2009;185(3):155–160.

115. Korreman SS, Pedersen AN, Nøttrup TJ, et al. Breathing adapted radiotherapy for breast cancer: comparison of free breathing gating with the breath-hold technique. *Radiother Oncol* 2005;76(3):311–318.

116. Korreman SS, Pedersen AN, Aarup LR, et al. Reduction of cardiac and pulmonary complication probabilities after breathing adapted radiotherapy for breast cancer. *Int J Radiat Oncol Biol Phys* 2006;65(5):1375–1380.

117. Lohr F, El-Haddad M, Dobler B, et al. Potential effect of robust and simple IMRT approach for left-sided breast cancer on cardiac mortality. *Int J Radiat Oncol Biol Phys* 2009;74(1):73–80.

118. Ding C, Li X, Huq MS, et al. The effect of respiratory cycle and radiation beam-on timing on the dose distribution of free-breathing breast treatment using dynamic IMRT. *Med Phys* 2007;34(9):3500–3509.

119. Richter A, Sweeney R, Baier K, et al. Effect of breathing motion in radiotherapy of breast cancer: 4D dose calculation and motion tracking via EPID. *Strahlenther Onkol* 2009;185(7):425–430.

120. Keall PJ, Joshi S, Vedam SS, et al. Four-dimensional radiotherapy planning for dynamic MLC-based respiratory motion tracking. *Med Phys* 2005;32:942–951.

121. Ehler ED, Tomé WA. Lung 4D-IMRT treatment planning: an evaluation of three methods applied to four-dimensional data sets. *Radiother Oncol* 2008;88(3):319–325.

122. Kang Y, Zhang X, Chang JY, et al. 4D Proton treatment planning strategy for mobile lung tumors. *Int J Radiat Oncol Biol Phys* 2007;67:906–914.

123. Fraass BA, Kessler ML, McShan DL, et al. Optimization and clinical use of multisegment intensity-modulated radiation therapy for high-dose conformal therapy. *Semin Radiat Oncol* 1999;9:60–77.

124. Vicini FA, Sharpe M, Kestin L, et al. Optimizing breast cancer treatment efficacy with intensity-modulated radiotherapy. *Int J Radiat Oncol Biol Phys* 2002;54:1336–1344.

125. Chui CS, Hong L, McCormick B. Intensity-modulated radiotherapy technique for three-field breast treatment. *Int J Radiat Oncol Biol Phys* 2005;62(4):1217–1223.

126. Borghero YO, Salehpour M, McNeese MD, et al. Multileaf field-in-field forward-planned intensity-modulated dose compensation for whole-breast irradiation is associated with reduced contralateral breast dose: a phantom model comparison. *Radiother Oncol* 2007;82(3):324–328.

127. Lo YC, Yasuda G, Fitzgerald TJ, et al. Intensity modulation for breast treatment using static multi-leaf collimaters. *Int J Radiat Oncol Biol Phys* 2000;46:187–194.

128. Li JG, Williams SS, Goffinet DR, et al. Breast-conserving radiation therapy using combined electron and intensity-modulated radiotherapy technique. *Radiother Oncol* 2000;56:65–71.

129. Krueger EA, Fraass BA, Pierce LJ. Clinical aspects of intensity modulated radiotherapy in the treatment of breast cancer. *Semin Radiat Oncol* 2002;12:250–259.

130. Cho BC, Hurkmans CW, Damen EM, et al. Intensity modulated vs. non-intensity modulated in the treatment of left breast and upper internal mammary lymph node chain: a comparative planning study. *Radiother Oncol* 2002:62:127–136.

131. Pignol JP, Olivotto I, Rakovitch E, et al. A multicenter randomized trial of breast intensity-modulated radiation therapy to reduce acute radiation dermatitis. *J Clin Oncol* 2008;26:2085–2092.

132. Donovan E, Bleakley N, Denholm E, et al. Randomised trial of standard 2D radiotherapy (RT) versus intensity modulated radiotherapy (IMRT) in patients prescribed breast radiotherapy. *Radiother Oncol* 2007;82:254–264.

133. Harsolia A, Kestin L, Grills I, et al. Intensity-modulated radiotherapy results in significant decrease in clinical toxicities compared with conventional wedge-based breast radiotherapy. *Int J Radiat Oncol Biol Phys* 2007;68(5):1375–1380.

134. Freedman GM, Anderson PR, Li J, et al. Intensity modulated radiation therapy (IMRT) decreases acute skin toxicity for women receiving radiation for breast cancer. *Am J Clin Oncol* 2006;29(1):66–70.

135. Mayo CS, Urie MM, Fitzgerald TJ. Hybrid IMRT plans—concurrently treating conventional and IMRT beams for improved breast irradiation and reduced planning time. *Int J Radiat Oncol Biol Phys* 2005;61:922–932.

136. Descovich M, Fowble B, Bevan A, et al. Comparison between hybrid direct aperture optimized intensity-modulated radiotherapy and forward planning intensity-modulated radiotherapy for whole breast irradiation. *Int J Radiat Oncol Biol Phys* 2010;76(1):91–99.

137. Ahunbay EE, Chen GP, Thatcher S, et al. Direct aperture optimization-based intensity-modulated radiotherapy for whole breast irradiation. *Int J Radiat Oncol Biol Phys* 2007;67(4):1248–1258.

138. McDonald MW, Karen D. Godette KD, et al. Three-year outcomes of breast intensity-modulated radiation therapy with simultaneous integrated boost. *Int J Radiat Oncol Biol Phys* 2010;77(2):523–530.

139. Morrow M, White J, Moughan J, et al. Factors predicting the use of breast-conserving therapy in stage I and II breast carcinoma. *J Clin Oncol* 2001;19:2254–2262.

140. Fisher B, Anderson S, Redmond CK, et al. Reanalysis and results after 12 years of follow-up in a randomized clinical trial comparing total mastectomy with or without irradiation in the treatment of breast cancer. *N Engl J Med* 1995;333:1465–1461.

141. Jacobsen JA, Danforth DN, Cowan CK, et al. Ten-year results of a comparison of conservative surgery with mastectomy in the treatment of stage I and II breast cancer. *N Engl J Med* 1995;332:907–911.

142. Vicini FA, Kestin L, Chen P, et al. Limited-field radiation therapy in the management of early-stage breast cancer. *J Natl Cancer Inst* 2003;95:1205–1210.

143. Arthur DW, Koo D, Zwicker RD, et al. Partial breast brachytherapy after lumpectomy: low-dose-rate and high-dose-rate experience. *Int J Radiat Oncol Biol Phys* 2003;56:681–689.

144. Kuske RR, Winter K, Arthur DW, et al. A phase II trial of brachytherapy alone following lumpectomy for stage I or II breast cancer: initial outcomes of RTOG 95–17. *Proc Am Soc Clin Oncol* 2004;23:18 (abstract).

145. Polgar C, Fodor J, Major T, et al. Breast-conserving treatment with partial or whole breast irradiation for low-risk invasive breast carcinoma-5-year results of a randomized trial. *Int J Radiat Oncol Biol Phys* 2007;69:694–702.

146. Benitez PR, Keisch ME, Vicini F, et al. Five-year results: the initial clinical trial of MammoSite balloon brachytherapy for partial breast irradiation in early-stage breast cancer. *Am J Surg* 2007;194:456–462.

147. Dickler A, Kirk M, Choo J, et al. Cosmetic outcome and incidence of infection with the MammoSite breast brachytherapy applicator. *Breast J* 2005;11:306–310.

148. Nelson JC, Beitsch PD, Vicini FA, et al. Four year clinical update from the American Society of Breast Surgeons MammoSite Brachytherapy Trial. *Am J Surg* 2000;198(1):83–91.

149. Formenti SC, Rosenstein B, Skinner KA, et al. T1 stage breast cancer: adjuvant hypofractionated conformal radiation therapy to tumor bed in selected postmenopausal breast cancer patients—pilot feasibility study. *Radiology* 2002;222:171–178.

150. Formenti SC, Truong MT, Goldberg JD, et al. Prone accelerated partial breast radiation (p-apbi) after breast conserving surgery: preliminary clinical results and dose volume histogram (DVH) analysis. *Int J Radiat Oncol Biol Phys* 2004;60:493–504.

151. Vicini FA, Remouchamps V, Wallace M, et al. Ongoing clinical experience utilizing 3D conformal external beam radiotherapy to deliver partial-breast irradiation in patients with early-stage breast cancer treated with breast-conserving therapy. *Int J Radiat Oncol Biol Phys* 2003;57:1247–1253.

152. Chen PY, Wallace M, Mitchell C, et al. Four-year efficacy, cosmesis, and toxicity using three-dimensional conformal external beam radiation therapy to deliver accelerated partial breast irradiation. *Int J Radiat Oncol Biol Phys* 2010;76(4):991–997.

153. Vicini F, Winter K, Wong J, et al. Initial efficacy results of RTOG 0319: three-dimensional conformal radiation therapy (3D-CRT) confined to the region of the lumpectomy cavity for stage I/II breast carcinoma. *Int J Radiat Oncol Biol Phys* 2010;77(4):1120–1127.

154. Lacombe MA, McMahon J, Al-Najjar WD, et al. Accelerated partial breast irradiation using intensity modulated radiotherapy. *Int J Radiat Oncol Biol Phys* 2004;60(1 Suppl):S273–S274.

155. Jagsi R, Ben-David MA, Moran JM, et al. Unacceptable cosmesis in a protocol investigating intensity-modulated radiotherapy with active breathing control for accelerated partial-breast irradiation. *Int J Radiat Oncol Biol Phys* 2010;76(1):71–78.

156. Chen S, Dickler A, Kirk M, et al. Patterns of failure after MammoSite brachytherapy partial breast irradiation: a detailed analysis. *Int J Radiat Oncol Biol Phys* 2007;69(1):25–31.

157. Consensus statement for accelerated partial breast irradiation. The American Society of Breast Surgeons, October 7, 2008. Available from http://www.breastsurgeons.org/statements/PDF_Statements/APBI_statement_revised_100708.pdf. Accessed March 23, 2010.

158. Keish M, Arthur D, Patel R, et al. American Brachytherapy Society Breast Brachytherapy Task Group. American Brachytherapy Society, February 2007. Available from http://www.americanbrachytherapy.org/resources/abs_breast_brachytherapy_taskgroup.pdf. Accessed March 28, 2010.

159. Dickler A, Kirk M, Choo J, et al. Treatment Volume and dose optimization of the mammosite breast brachytherapy applicator. *Int J Radiat Oncol Biol Phys* 2004;59:469–474.

160. Strauss JB, Dickler A. Accelerated partial breast irradiation utilizing balloon brachytherapy techniques. *Radiother Oncol* 2009;91(2):157–165.

161. Foo M, Rogers K, Raulerson S, et al. Comparative dosimetry of 3 single-entry, afterloading brachytherapy applicators for partial breast irradiation: SAVI, Contura and MammoSite. *Int J Radiat Oncol Biol Phys* 2008;72(1 Suppl 1):S512.

162. Dickler A, Seif N, Kirk MC, et al. A dosimetric comparison of MammoSite and ClearPath high-dose-rate breast brachytherapy devices. *Brachytherapy* 2009;8(1):14–18.

163. Brown S, McLaughlin M, Pope K, et al. Initial radiation experience evaluating early tolerance and toxicities in patients undergoing accelerated partial breast irradiation using the Contura Multi-Lumen Balloon

breast brachytherapy catheter. *Brachytherapy* 2009;8(2): 227–233.

164. Dickler A, Ivanov O, Francescatti D. Intraoperative radiation therapy in the treatment of early-stage breast cancer utilizing Xoft Axxent electronic brachytherapy. *World J Surg Oncol* 2009;7:24.

165. Dickler A, Kirk MC, Seif N, et al. A dosimetric comparison of MammoSite high-dose-rate brachytherapy and Xoft Axxent electronic brachytherapy. *Brachytherapy* 2007;6(2):164–168.

166. Chen SS, Strauss JB, Shah AP, et al. Radiation recall reaction with docetaxel administration after accelerated partial breast irradiation with electronic brachytherapy. *Brachytherapy* 2009;8(3):331–334.

167. Kraus-Tiefenbacher U, Bauer L, Kehrer T, et al. Intraoperative radiotherapy (IORT) as a boost in patients with early-stage breast cancer—acute toxicity. *Onkologie* 2006;29:77–82.

CHAPTER 31

Cancers of the Central Nervous System

Lucien A. Nedzi ■ Kevin S. Choe ■ Arnold Pompos ■ Ezequiel Ramirez

INTRODUCTION

The central nervous system (CNS) comprises the brain, the spinal cord, and their coverings. Patients with benign lesions may live out their natural lifespan, whereas the survival of those with malignant tumors is frequently measured in weeks to months. The optimal radiation therapy treatment technique should maximize the therapeutic benefit and minimize the potential toxicities, especially for long-term survivors.

NATURAL HISTORY

Anatomy of the Brain

Knowledge of the basic topographic and functional anatomy of the brain is critical for tumor localization and delineation of regions that need to be spared during treatment. Generally, the brain consists of three major divisions: The cerebrum, cerebellum, and brainstem. The cerebral hemispheres and midline structures are supratentorial, and the cerebellum and lower brainstem are infratentorial. The longitudinal cerebral fissure divides the cerebrum into two hemispheres. Each hemisphere is divided by the major sulci into six lobes: Frontal, parietal, occipital and temporal, and the midline central and limbic lobes. The central sulcus (of Rolando) separates the frontal lobe from the parietal lobe. The parietal-occipital fissure separates the parietal lobe from the occipital lobe. The lateral fissure (of Sylvius) defines the temporal lobe boundaries. The cerebral hemispheres are connected by the corpus callosum, beneath which are located the midline structures (third ventricle, pineal body, and midbrain) and the deep paramedian structures (lateral ventricles, caudate nucleus, lentiform nucleus, thalamus, and hypothalamus).

There are three historic approaches to defining the functional anatomy of the cerebral hemispheres. Brodmann's schema numbers 52 areas of structural specialization to provide both anatomic and functional "road map" of the brain by which tumor location can be described (1,2). Another approach is a regional (lobe) division of function. The occipital lobe is primarily involved with vision and its dependent functions. The temporal lobe processes sound, vestibular sensations, sights, smells, and

other perceptions into complex "experiences" important for memory. Wernicke's area is located on the posterior portion of the superior temporal gyrus and plays a critical role in receptive speech. The parietal lobe, specifically the postcentral gyrus, is involved in somatosensory function, sensory integration (body image), and Gnostic (perceptive) functions. The frontal lobe is associated with higher level cognitive functions, such as reasoning and judgment. The frontal lobe contains the primary motor cortex (precentral gyrus) and Broca's area (inferior third of the frontal gyrus), which is important in expressive speech. The limbic lobe mediates memories, drives, and stimuli. It affects visceral functions central to emotional expression, including sexual drive. Finally, the central lobe (insula) is important in visceral sensation and motility. The most modern method to describe functional neuroanatomy is through various techniques of functional mapping. Classic mapping utilizes microelectrode stimulation of the cortical surface directly. Newer noninvasive techniques such as functional magnetic resonance imaging (fMRI), positron emission tomography (PET), and magnetoencephalography (MEG) are increasingly being integrated into clinical practice (3–5). Together, these procedures allow for precise mapping of function in an individual and can accurately predict deficits related to injury of a given area by tumor or therapy.

Epidemiology of Primary Central Nervous System Tumors

Annually, an estimated 63,000 new cases of primary nonmalignant and malignant CNS tumors are diagnosed in the United States with an estimated 13,000 deaths (6,7). The incidence of all primary nonmalignant and malignant brain and CNS tumors is 18.71 cases per 100,000 person-years. In the United States, the rate is slightly higher in females (19.88 per 100,000 person-years) than males (17.44 per 100,000 person-years) (7). The incidence rates are higher in more developed countries than in less-developed countries (8). The incidence rate of childhood primary nonmalignant and malignant brain and CNS tumors is 4.7 cases per 100,000 person-years. The rate is (4.75 per 100,000 person-years in males and 4.66 per 100,000 person-years in females) (7).

Most of the primary CNS tumors are located within the frontal, temporal, parietal, and occipital lobes of the brain.

Sixty-one percent of gliomas occur in the frontal, temporal, parietal, and occipital lobes. Tumors in other locations in the cerebrum account for another 3%. Of all tumors, 2%, 4%, and 2% are found in the ventricles, cerebellum, and brainstem, respectively. The pituitary and pineal gland account for ~7% of tumors. Tumors of the meninges represent 24% of all tumors (7).

The overall incidence of primary spinal cord tumors is approximately 10% to 19% of all primary brain tumors (9). Schwannomas and meningiomas account for ~60% of primary spinal tumors, with schwannomas being slightly more frequent; both types occur primarily in adults. Most primary spinal gliomas are ependymomas with a predilection for the cauda equina. The frequency of individual spinal cord tumors is quite different from that of their histopathologic counterparts in the brain. Gliomas constitute 46% of primary intracranial tumors but only 23% of spinal tumors. The incidence ratios of intracranial to intraspinal astrocytomas, ependymomas, and meningiomas are approximately 10:1, 3:1, and 18:1, respectively (10). Finally, the incidence ratio of intracranial to intraspinal tumors is higher up to four times in pediatric patients than in adults.

Table 31.1 shows the current WHO pathologic classification system of common primary CNS tumors (11). The most frequently reported histology is meningioma, which accounts for over 29% of all tumors, followed closely by glioblastoma and astrocytoma. The predominately benign nerve sheath tumors account for 8% of all tumors, of which 54% are acoustic neuromas. Pituitary tumors compose 6% of these lesions. Tumors of the glial cell origin represent about a half of all tumors. These include astrocytomas, glioblastomas, oligodendrocytomas, ependymomas, mixed gliomas, and neuroepithelial tumors. Astrocytomas and glioblastomas account for three-quarters of gliomas—the majority being glioblastomas (7). The most common spinal cord intramedullary tumors are those that are derived from glial precursors (astrocytes, ependymocytes, and oligodendrocytes) (12).

Epidemiology of Tumors Metastatic to the Central Nervous System

Metastatic brain tumors are the most common intracranial neoplasms in adults and it is about 10 times more common than primary intracranial tumors. In two cohorts of patients diagnosed with colorectal, lung, breast, or kidney carcinoma or melanoma, brain metastases were diagnosed in 8.5% to 9.6% (13,14). The cumulative incidence was estimated between 16% and 20% in patients with lung carcinoma, 7% in patients with renal carcinoma, 7% in patients with melanoma, 5% in patients with breast carcinoma, and 1% to 2% in patients with colorectal carcinoma.

With the exception of a primary paraspinal or neuraxis tumor, spinal cord tumors occur most often in the setting of disseminated disease from a distant primary tumor site. The spine is overall the most common site of bony metastases, with a reported incidence of 40% in patients with cancer (15). Of those patients with spine metastases, 10% to 20% develop malignant spinal cord compression (MSCC), accounting for 14,100 to 28,200 cases annually (16,17,18). MSCC from epidural metastases occurs in 5% to 10% of all patients with cancer and in up to 40% of patients with preexisting nonspinal bone metastases (15,19,20,21). MSCC may involve the spinal cord at any level, and symptoms depend on the location of the compression. The incidence of MSCC by vertebral levels is 10% to 16% cervical, 35% to 40% in T1 to 6, 44% to 55% in T7 to 12, and 20% in the lumbar spine (22,23,24). In 10% to 38% of cases, metastatic lesions present initially at multiple, noncontiguous levels (22,25,26).

The histology of MSCC follows the incidence patterns of primary malignancies, with the most common histologic diagnoses (i.e., breast, lung, and prostate) accounting for approximately half of all cases (6,15). Approximately 25% of all patients with MSCC have breast cancer, 15% have lung cancer, and 10% have prostate carcinomas. Overall, 5.5% of patients with breast cancer, 2.6% of patients with lung cancer, 7.2% of patients with prostate cancer, and 0.8% of patients with colorectal cancer experience a MSCC (17). Other commonly reported histologic diagnoses in adults include, in the order of cumulative incidence, multiple myeloma, nasopharynx, renal cell, melanoma, small cell lung, lymphoma, and cervix (15,17,27).

WORKUP AND STAGING

For both benign and malignant CNS tumors, magnetic resonance imaging (MRI) is the gold standard for imaging (28). The preferred slice thickness of MRI is ≤5 mm with ≤2.5 mm slice sampling. T1-weighted images with contrast provide excellent visualization of contrast-enhancing tumors, such as meningiomas, glioblastoma multiforme, and brain metastases. T2-weighted images generally demonstrate areas of edema, and T1-weighted fluid-attenuated inversion recovery (FLAIR) images better delineate infiltration by low- or high-grade gliomas. MRI registration with the treatment-planning computed tomography (CT) scan is therefore essential for target delineation. Additional imaging studies can reflect the biologic characteristics of CNS tumors, such as tumor metabolism, proliferation, oxygenation, blood flow, and the function of surrounding normal brain; these include MRI spectroscopy, fMRI, PET scans, and single photon emission tomography (SPECT) scans (29,30,31). After radiation therapy, PET scans and MRI spectroscopy assist in differentiating active tumor versus radionecrosis.

MRI of the entire neural axis along with cerebrospinal fluid (CSF) cytology is required for staging of tumors with a high propensity for spread within the CNS by involvement of the CSF, leptomeninges, or spinal cord. These tumors include medulloblastomas, primitive neuroectodermal tumors (PNETs), anaplastic ependymomas, choroid

| TABLE 31.1 | WHO Grades of CNS Tumours |

Astrocytic tumours	I	II	III	IV
Subependymal giant cell astrocytoma	•			
Pilocytic astrocytoma	•			
Pilomyxoid astrocytoma		•		
Diffuse astrocytoma		•		
Pleomorphic xanthoastrocytoma		•		
Anaplastic astrocytoma			•	
Glioblastoma				•
Giant cell glioblastoma				•
Gliosarcoma				•

Oligodendroglial tumours	I	II	III	IV
Oligodendroglioma		•		
Anaplastic oligodendroglioma			•	

Oligoastrocytic tumours	I	II	III	IV
Oligoastrocytoma		•		
Anaplastic oligoastrocytoma			•	

Ependymal tumours	I	II	III	IV
Subependymoma	•			
Myxopapillary ependymoma	•			
Ependymoma		•		
Anaplastic ependymoma			•	

Choroid plexus tumours	I	II	III	IV
Choroid plexus papilloma	•			
Atypical choroid plexus papilloma		•		
Choroid plexus carcinoma			•	

Other neuroepithelial tumours	I	II	III	IV
Angiocentric glioma	•			
Chordoid glioma of the third ventricle		•		

Neuronal and mixed neuronal-glial tumours	I	II	III	IV
Gangliocytoma	•			
Ganglioglioma	•			
Anaplastic ganglioglioma			•	
Desmoplastic infantile astrocytoma and ganglioglioma	•			
Dysembryoplastic neuroepithelial tumour	•			

	I	II	III	IV
Central neurocytoma		•		
Extraventricular neurocytoma		•		
Cerebellar liponeurocytoma		•		
Paraganglioma of the spinal cord	•			
Papillary glioneuronal tumour	•			
Rosette-forming glioneuronal tumour of the fourth ventricle	•			

Pineal tumours	I	II	III	IV
Pineocytoma	•			
Pineal parenchymal tumour of intermediate differentiation		•	•	
Pineoblastoma				•
Papillary tumour of the pineal region		•	•	

Embryonal tumours	I	II	III	IV
Medulloblastoma				•
CNS primitive neuroectodermal tumour (PNET)				•
Atypical teratoid / rhabdoid tumour				•

Tumours of the cranial and paraspinal nerves	I	II	III	IV
Schwannoma	•			
Neurofibroma	•			
Perineurioma	•	•	•	
Malignant peripheral nerve sheath tumour (MPNST)		•	•	•

Meningeal tumours	I	II	III	IV
Meningioma	•			
Atypical meningioma		•		
Anaplastic / malignant meningioma			•	
Haemangiopericytoma		•		
Anaplastic haemangiopericytoma			•	
Haemangioblastoma	•			

Tumours of the sellar region	I	II	III	IV
Craniopharyngioma	•			
Granular cell tumour of the neurohypophysis	•			
Pituicytoma	•			
Spindle cell oncocytoma of the adenohypophysis	•			

plexus carcinomas, pineoblastomas, germ cell tumors, and lymphomas.

In patients who present for urgent symptom management, CT scan can be obtained rapidly, providing information on ventricular obstruction, hemorrhage, or edema. Owing to the risk of herniation and death, lumbar puncture should be avoided, if at all possible, until the intracranial pressure has normalized. The most important modality in the workup of suspected MSCC is gadolinium enhanced MRI of the entire spinal axis. In the initial evaluation of a patient with suspected metastatic spinal cord compression, it is critical to image the entire spine, as 25% of these patients have spinal cord compression verified at multiple levels by MRI, and approximately two-thirds of these have involvement of different regions of the spine (32). In addition, a sensory level present on patient evaluation may be two or more levels different from the actual lesion on MRI in 28% of patients, and four or more levels distant in 21% of patients (32).

GENERAL MANAGEMENT

Multimodality therapy for CNS tumors may consist of medical therapy, surgical resection, radiation therapy, or some combination of the above.

Medical Therapy

Medical treatment generally consists of steroids with or without mannitol (33). Patients who present with emergent symptoms are typically treated with dexamethasone. Response to therapy is usually noted within 12 to 18 hours of administration with over 80% of patients showing dramatic improvement by 3 to 4 days after initiation of therapy (34,35). A common regimen in patients receiving radiation therapy is high dose dexamethasone (10–25 mg IV or po) followed by maintenance on oral steroids (4–6 mg three or four times a day), with tapering initiated upon stabilization of symptoms and initiation of therapy, usually over 1 to 2 months (33,36,37). In the setting of MSCC from solid tumors, dexamethasone has been shown to improve rates of surviving with intact gait function (38,39). Side effects of intermediate- to long-term steroid use may include: hyperglycemia, insomnia, emotional lability, thrush, gastric irritation, ulceration and possibly perforation, proximal muscle wasting, weight gain and adiposity (moon facies, buffalo hump, and centripetal obesity), osteoporotic compression fractures, arthralgias with withdrawal, and aseptic necrosis of the hip joints (40). Some of these side effects persist even after steroid withdrawal. Owing to the incidence of steroid-induced complications with dosing longer than 21 days in duration, higher doses and longer tapering schedules should be based on the physician's assessment of symptom severity and response (39,41,42). Patients should be instructed during tapering to note signs of worsening headaches and/

or existing neurological deficits. They should be instructed to resume a higher steroid dose should such symptoms occur and consult their physician. Asymptomatic patients generally do not require corticosteroids and routine use of corticosteroids during radiation therapy in asymptomatic patients should be avoided. Select patients with MSCC may not receive steroids during treatment if they are at high risk of complications due to underlying medical comorbidities, such as peptic ulcer disease, uncontrolled diabetes, or other medical problems that may cause severe or life-threatening problems if exacerbated by steroids (43). Dexamethasone and mannitol drugs decrease peritumoral brain edema by different mechanisms of action and mannitol is therefore often used in steroid refractory patients (44). A common regimen of mannitol is a 20% to 25% solution given intravenously over ~30 minutes dosed at 0.5 to 2.0 g/kg (45).

Stabilization of the patient in status epilepticus to perform imaging and make management decisions is critical (46). After securing the airway and stabilizing the patient, seizure activity must be terminated as rapidly as possible, especially as failure to control seizures can potentially lead to physical injuries, airway compromise, secondary brain hypoxia/injury, or coma (45,46). Rapid onset/short acting benzodiazepines and phenytoin are commonly used. Recommended initial regimens include 0.1 mg/kg at 2 mg/min of lorazepam or diazepam at 0.2 mg/kg at 5 mg/min. Phenytoin infusion of 15 to 20 mg/kg at <50 mg/min in adults is indicated for seizure activity refractory to benzodiazepines or after truncation of seizures with diazepam (46). There is no clear evidence to support the prophylactic use of anticonvulsants in patients diagnosed with a brain tumor in the absence of documented seizures (47,48).

Surgical Therapy

Surgical resection and/or placement of a shunt are often required for emergent management of brain tumors causing life-threatening hydrocephalus, mass effect, or profound neurologic impairment. This may relieve symptoms enough that other treatment modalities can be initiated. Symptoms are usually related to mass effect, so resection or debulking are often the only logical choices if medical therapy fails to provide improvement in neurologic symptoms. Rapid surgical decompression is the treatment of choice for such problems when surgery can be safely performed based on patient performance status or tumor location. If no neurosurgical team is available, transfer of the patient should be initiated while medical measures are undertaken to stabilize the patient.

Many patients with spinal cord compression are not candidates for laminectomy and are treated with steroids and radiation therapy. Most series in the literature show no difference in outcomes when comparing laminectomy-treated patients to those managed with radiation therapy alone (15,24,49,50). However, a randomized trial evaluating the benefit of adding surgical decompression to the radiotherapeutic management of symptomatic metastatic spinal cord compression showed that patients who underwent decompressive surgery had a significantly improved median time of gait retention and ability to regain gait function albeit without affecting overall survival (51). Therefore, all patients presenting with MSCC of short duration should be evaluated by an experienced neurosurgeon for emergent decompression before initiating radiation therapy.

Radiation Therapy

Definitive Radiation Therapy

Radiation therapy plays a primary role in the management of most malignant and many benign primary CNS tumors. Table 31.2 provides a referenced overview of the most common primary CNS tumors with International Commission on Radiation and Measurement Units (ICRU) definitions of treatment volumes for initial and (when applicable) boost fields, general dosing guidelines, and outcome endpoints. More detailed descriptions are provided for selected indications later in this chapter.

Palliative Radiation Therapy

Because 60% to 70% of patients who present brain metastases have multiple lesions, radiotherapy is the primary modality for palliation in this setting (52,53). Many patients treated with medical therapy and radiation experience an improvement in their performance status. Radiation therapy dosing schedules for the treatment of emergent patients should take into account their initial response to steroids, the extent of extracranial disease, the primary diagnosis, and its anticipated response to systemic therapy.

Two randomized trials comparing radiotherapy with or without surgical resection in the management of a solitary brain metastasis have documented a survival advantage with the addition of surgery over radiation alone (54,55). However, a third randomized trial was negative (56). There is no level I evidence demonstrating any survival benefit from operating on patients with multiple metastases. However, patients with severe neurologic symptoms from one or more dominant metastases who are unresponsive to medical therapy may benefit from a craniotomy. An improvement in the patient's performance status can then be followed by external-beam radiation therapy. Acute leukemic brain infiltration is a rare, potentially fatal presentation treated with whole-brain radiation therapy.

Patients with malignant glioma who require emergent treatment are typically treated with surgical debulking and steroid therapy. Patients with a poor performance status who are unable to undergo surgical debulking may be treated with a short course of whole-brain radiation similar to that used for brain metastases.

For metastatic MSCC, there are no randomized trials comparing radiotherapy over best supportive care or medical therapy alone. Every published series of radiotherapy for MSCC has shown that it is effective in relieving pain and maintaining or improving neurologic function. Morbidity is generally low and well tolerated even by patients with a poor performance status. Approximately 89% of patients who are ambulatory before radiation therapy retain gait function, although an average of 39% of patients with paralysis and only 10% of paraplegic patients will remain ambulatory (17).

GENERAL CONCEPTS OF RADIATION THERAPY

Workup and Staging

Multimodality Imaging for Simulation, Treatment Planning, and Dose Delivery

The success of modern radiation therapy, besides the introduction of new irradiation technologies, can also partially be attributed to the development and availability of various novel imaging techniques that help to (i) better delineate targets and regions of avoidance, (ii) assess the motion of target and critical structures throughout breathing cycles, (iii) better understand the dosimetrically relevant composition of the tissue in the path of the radiation, (iv) lower the setup uncertainty of the patient, (v) verify the location of the target during dose delivery, and (vi) assess the location of the deposited dose.

A high-resolution CT scan acquired at the time of treatment planning simulation provides a three-dimensional (3D) voxel grid of the patient. In each elementary voxel, the CT software calculates the linear attenuation coefficient of the matter contained in it. Based on this, each voxel gets assigned a shade of gray (for visualization purposes of the tissue) and a CT number also called Hounsfield Unit, which later is translated into physical density in the treatment planning software (for dose calculation purposes). Since the CT modality has poor soft tissue contrast, iodine-based contrast agents are often injected into the blood to better visualize vessels or tumors. Images with sub-millimeter voxel dimensions can be acquired with only a minute or two scanning time.

MRI is a complementary imaging modality to CT. Since it does not involve ionizing radiation and has very good soft tissue contrast, it is one of the most widely used imaging modalities in management of CNS tumors. Its signal is based on relaxation properties of proton spins in a strong external magnetic field. The patient body is again subdivided into voxels, and based on their signal strength received during imaging a shade of gray is assigned to them and the image is reconstructed. Numerous ways (called sequences) have been researched and developed (i) to disturb the spin lattice of patients' protons in the applied external magnetic field and (ii) to detect their relaxation properties. The two most commonly known techniques are the T1- and T2-weighted sequence, where T1 and T2 are the longitudinal and transverse relaxation times of proton spins, respectively. Generally speaking, the shorter the voxel's T1, the

| TABLE | 31.2 | **World Health Organization Classification of Tumors of the Nervous System** |

Tumors of neuroepithelial tissue

Astrocytic tumors
Diffuse astrocytoma
Fibrillary astrocytoma
Protoplasmatic astrocytoma
Gemistocytic astrocytoma
Anaplastic astrocytoma
Glioblastoma
Giant cell glioblastoma
Gliosarcoma
Pilocytic astrocytoma
Pleomorphic xanthoastrocytoma
Subependymal giant cell astrocytoma

Oligodendroglial tumors
Oligodendroglioma
Anaplastic oligodendroglioma

Mixed gliomas
Oligoastrocytoma
Anaplastic oligoastrocytoma

Ependymal tumors
Ependymoma
Cellular
Papillary
Clear cell
Tanycytic
Anaplastic ependymoma
Myxopapillary ependymoma
Subependymoma

Choroid plexus tumors
Choroid plexus papilloma
Choroid plexus carcinoma

Glial tumors of uncertain origin
Astroblastoma
Gliomatosis cerebri
Chordoid glioma of the third ventricle

Neuronal and mixed neuronal-glial tumors
Gangliocytoma
Dysplastic gangliocytoma of cerebellum (Lhermitte-Duclos)
Desmoplastic infantile astrocytoma/ganglioglioma
Dysembryoplastic neuroepithelial tumor
Ganglioglioma
Anaplastic ganglioglioma
Central neurocytoma
Cerebellar liponeurocytoma
Paraganglioma of the filum terminale

Neuroblastic tumors
Olfactory neuroblastoma (Esthesioneuroblastoma)
Olfactory neuroepithelioma
Neuroblastomas of the adrenal gland and sympathetic
  nervous system

Pineal parenchymal tumors
Pineocytoma
Pineoblastoma
Pineal parenchymal tumor of intermediate differentiation

Embryonal tumors
Medulloepithelioma
Ependymoblastoma
Medulloblastoma
Desmoplastic medulloblastoma
Large cell medulloblastoma
Medullomyoblastoma
Melanotic medulloblastoma
Supratentorial primitive neuroectodermal tumor
Neuroblastoma
Ganglioneuroblastoma
Atypical teratoid/Rhabdoid tumor

Tumors of peripheral nerves

Schwannoma (neurilemmoma, neurinoma)
Cellular
Plexiform
Melanotic

Neurofibroma
Plexiform

Perineurioma
Intraneural perineurioma
Soft tissue perineurioma

Malignant peripheral nerve sheath tumor
Epithelioid
MPNST with divergent mesenchymal and/or epithelial
  differentiation
Melanotic
Melanotic psammomatous

Tumors of the meninges

Tumors of meningothelial cells
Meningioma
Meningothelial
Fibrous (fibroblastic)
Transitional (mixed)
Psammomatous
Angiomatous
Microcystic
Secretory
Lymphoplasmacyte-rich
Metaplastic
Clear cell
Chordoid
Atypical
Papillary
Rhabdoid
Anaplastic meningioma

(continued)

TABLE 31.2	World Health Organization Classification of Tumors of the Nervous System (*Continued*)

Tumors of the meninges (*continued*)

Mesenchymal, nonmeningothelial tumors
Lipoma
Angiolipoma
Hibernoma
Liposarcoma (intracranial)
Solitary fibrous tumor
Fibrosarcoma
Malignant fibrous histiocytoma
Leiomyoma
Leiomyosarcoma
Rhabdomyoma
Rhabdomyosarcoma
Chondroma
Chondrosarcoma
Osteoma
Osteosarcoma
Osteochondroma
Hemangioma
Epithelioid hemangioendothelioma
Hemangiopericytoma
Angiosarcoma
Kaposi's sarcoma

Primary melanocytic lesions
Diffuse melanocytosis
Melanocytoma

Malignant melanoma
Meningeal melanomatosis

Tumors of uncertain histogenesis
Hemangioblastoma

Lymphomas and hematopoietic neoplasms
Malignant lymphomas
Plasmacytoma
Granulocytic sarcoma

Germ cell tumors
Germinoma
Embryonal carcinoma
Yolk sac tumor
Choriocarcinoma
Teratoma
Mature
Immature
Teratoma with malignant
    transformation
Mixed germ cell tumors

Tumors of the sellar region
Craniopharyngioma
Adamantinomatous
Papillary
Granular cell tumor

PNET, primitive neuroectodermal tumor; MPNS, malignant peripheral nerve sheath tumor.

more signal it produces and it appears brighter on the scan. On the other hand, the longer the T2, the longer the signal is acquired, making the signal-producing tissue brighter. Water in the bulk phase (e.g., CSF) has long T1 and T2 relaxation times; therefore, it appears dark on T1-weighted but bright on T2-weighted acquisitions. Gadolinium-based contrast agents, which lower T1 relaxation times, are often utilized to enhance brain tumor appearance. The mechanism of their action is that the tumor compromises the brain blood barrier, making the membranes more permeable and letting the contrast agents in. The contrast agent lowers the T1 time making the tumor brighter on T1-weighted images than it was before the contrast administration. Vasogenic edema associated with brain tumors appears bright on T2-weighted images. If fine structures (cranial nerves, inner ear) need to be visualized, that is, extremely high spatial resolution is needed, the constructive interference steady state (CISS, called also FIESTA) sequence is utilized. If hyper-intense abnormalities obscured by CSF within ventricles are needed to be seen, a specialized MRI technique called FLAIR can be utilized to null signal from the CSF.

Magnetic resonance spectroscopy (MRS) measures the levels of various metabolites in body tissues. It can be tuned to recognize metabolites of tumors. The level of these metabolites can be spatially overlaid with MRI images allowing a better differentiation of tumor from normal tissue. It is often difficult to decide what margins to add to the GTV in order to keep as much healthy tissue as possible intact, or in order to avoid irradiating functionally critical parts of the brain. In these cases, Diffusion MRI and fMRI provide vital information.

The diffusion tensor imaging enables visualization of neural fiber directions to examine the connectivity of different regions in the brain and potentially avoid hot spots and high doses to be placed at critical regions. fMRI measures signal changes in the brain that are due to changing neural activity. The measurement is done through the mechanism called blood-oxygen-level dependent (BOLD) effect, which is based on the fact that increased neural activity requires enhanced oxygen levels. Deoxygenated hemoglobin attenuates the MRI signal, while the oxygenated one enhances it leading to a T2 signal increase that is related to the neural activity.

After the desired MRI scans were acquired, they are carefully co-registered with CT images in the treatment planning software with the help of specially designed mutual information seeking algorithms combined with human eye. This co-registration allows delineation of the region of interest on the scan that is most suitable for it and ensures its proper placement into the framework of the treatment planning CT.

Another very important functional imaging technique in cancer management is the PET. It uses a radioactive fluorine-18 (F-18) marked fluorodeoxyglucose (FDG), called FDG-PET tracer. It is a glucose analog that is taken up by glucose-using cells.

The FDG is trapped in any cell, which takes it up, until it decays. This results in intense radiolabeling of tissues with high glucose uptake, such as the brain, the liver, and most cancers. Despite a high background coming from normal gray matter, brain PET scans are very useful in prediction of biologic behavior and aggressiveness of the tumors and differentiating recurrent tumor from treatment-related changes (e.g., radiation necrosis and postsurgical changes). The PET scanners have as well the ability to obtain CT scans while the patient is in the same positions. The two image sets are then co-registered allowing a precise 3D localization of the PET signal in the body. Research has been done and the first such machine has already been build, in which PET images are taken simultaneously with MRI scans (57).

It is often needed to asses the magnitude of tissue displacement throughout patients breathing cycle. Even though dosimetrically no significant displacement of CNS tumors is usually observed during the breathing cycle, other organs through which radiation will propagate to reach the tumor might significantly change their location and geometry, for example lung or kidney in irradiation of spinal lesions.

Fluoroscopic imaging is helpful and motion margins can be determined. A more elaborate method to determine the actual volume the tumor spans during breathing is via 4D CT (the fourth dimension being the time). In this technique, the breathing cycle is subdivided into bins of temporal phases and the whole region of interest is imaged in each of these phase bins. In the treatment planning systems, the information about the structure of interest contained in each of these bins is combined resulting to a total volume it spans.

After an acceptable treatment plan has been created, the patient is placed into the treatment position and the technicians proceed with patient position verification. The simplest image modality to do this is the radiographic film. Port films are compared to digitally reconstructed radiograms from the TPS and setup corrections are made if necessary. Electronic devices such as electronic portal imaging device (EPID) substituted the film with an electronic screen. In both of these cases, it is the megavoltage photon beam that is used to create the patient image. The Compton interaction is responsible for image creation and the resulting tissue contrast is very low making it difficult to interpret the images. As technology advanced, it introduced in-room imaging with kilovoltage photon beam in which the portion of photoelectric interactions significantly increase, resulting in a very substantial increase in tissue contrast therefore image quality as well. Modern irradiators have on gantry mounted x-ray sources and imaging panels. These allow them to acquire CT type image sets, called cone beam CT, or 4D cone beam CT. As a result, a 3D (4D) information at the time of the patient setup is compared with the 3D (4D) image sets on which the treatment plans have been generated. Necessary shifts or breathing control can be applied to best match the treatment planning conditions.

Currently, substantial research effort is being devoted to the development of imaging techniques that would allow monitoring the tumor position during radiation delivery, for example a fast MRI scanner coupled with a linear accelerator. For CNS tumors, this is of marginal or academic interest only given their fairly stable spatial position.

It is interesting to mention, that one of the advantages of using heavy charged particles for treatment, such as carbon-12 nuclei is the tiny amount of produced carbon 10 and carbon 11. These isotopes are positron emitters. Their concentration is proportional to the amount of deposited dose. Scanning the patient with a CT coupled with PET scanner after the therapeutic dose was delivered, enabling us to directly verify the whereabouts of deposited dose in the patient body.

Volume Definition

Treatment-planning volumes are based on reports 50 and 62 of the ICRU (58,59). Gross tumor volume (GTV) represents grossly identifiable disease (58,59). For glioblastoma multiforme, this is T1-enhancing abnormality on MRI. If there is no postoperative residual enhancement, the GTV is defined as the tumor resection cavity. The clinical target volume (CTV) includes the subclinical microscopic tumor extent, seen as edema on T2-weighted MRI and often better visualized as FLAIR abnormality on MRI (58). Uniform expansion may result in an excessively large volume with unnecessary dose to normal surrounding tissues. The CTV may therefore be reduced around natural barriers to tumor growth, such as the skull, ventricles, and the longitudinal fissure. In addition, the CTV margin maybe limited in areas near critical organs.

The planning target volume (PTV) is also referred to as the "dosimetric margin." The dosimetric margin has two components (59). The internal margin accounts for variations in size, shape, and position of the CTV in relation to anatomic reference points. In the CNS, this is due mainly to physiologic variations, such as the possible changes in the mass effect from cerebral edema that may occur over the course of treatment. Set-up margin is added to take into account uncertainties in patient-to-beam positioning, and this may be reduced by utilizing appropriate immobilization devices, Dosimetric margins as low as 3 to 5 mm are acceptable with optimal immobilization devices.

TABLE 30.3	**Normal Tissue Tolerance of Intracranial Organs at Risk**[a]							

Organ →	TD5/5			TD50/5			
Volume →	1/3	2/3	3/3	1/3	2/3	3/3	Endpoint
Brain	6,000	5,000	4,500	7,500	6,500	6,000	Necrosis, infarction
Brainstem	6,000	5,300	5,000			6,500	Necrosis, infarction
Optic nerve			6,000				Blindness
Optic chiasm			5,400				Blindness
Eye (lens)			1,000				Cataracts
Eye (retina)			4,500				Blindness
Lacrimal gland			3,000				Dry eye syndrome
Ear (mid/external)	3,000	3,000	5,500	4,000	4,000	4,000	Acute serous otitis
	5,500	5,500	5,500	6,500	6,500	6,500	Chronic serous otitis
Pituitary			<4,500			6,000	Panhypopituitarism

[a]All doses are in cGy at conventional fractionation (86).

For treatment plans emphasizing homogenous dose delivery, the maximum dose to PTV should be generally less than 110% of the prescription dose, and 95% of the target should receive at least the prescription dose. Suggested margins and dose fractionation by histology are summarized in Table 31.2.

Organs at risk (OARs) are critical normal structures whose relative radiation sensitivity and proximity to the CTV may significantly influence the prescribed dose and the treatment-planning strategy. It is especially important to limit the risk of late toxicities by respecting the dose tolerances of normal structures when long-term survival is expected. The relationship between the planning organ at risk volume (PRV) and the OAR is analogous to that of the PTV and the CTV (59). For each OAR, when part of the organ or the whole organ are irradiated above the accepted tolerance level, the maximum dose should be reported (58). The volume receiving more than the maximum allowable dose should be evaluated using the corresponding dose–volume histogram (DVH).

In the dose range of 45 to 60 Gy generally used for CNS tumors, the probability of causing serious late toxicity is relatively low (Table 31.3) (60). Without compromising therapeutic dose to the target, attempts should be made to limit OAR dose as follows: Optic chiasm (54 Gy), optic nerves (60 Gy), optic globes including retina (50 Gy), brainstem to include midbrain, pons, and medulla (54 Gy), pituitary gland (50 Gy), and spinal cord (50 Gy). In pediatric patients, doses as low as 18 Gy have been implicated in neurocognitive deficits (61,62). A more detailed guideline to dose tolerances is provided in Table 31.3.

With conventionally fractionated radiotherapy (1.8–2.0 Gy per fraction, five fractions per week), the incidence of spinal cord myelopathy at 5 years is ~1% for doses in the range of 45 to 50.4 Gy, 5% for 57 to 61 Gy, and 50% for 68 to 73 Gy, regardless of the length or level of cord irradiated (63,64). The tolerance of the lumbosacral nerve roots appears to be somewhat higher than that of the spinal cord. Most series report a 0% complication rate if patients are treated to doses of 70 Gy (or equivalent) as long as fraction sizes are kept at or below 2 Gy (65,66,67).

Intensity-Modulated Radiation Therapy

Intensity-modulated radiation therapy (IMRT) is an advanced form of the 3D CRT. While CRT delivers an irregularly shaped beam of uniform intensity, IMRT modulates the intensity of the photon beam across the treated area by delivering multiple subfields (segments) each of irregular shape and of different photon intensities. There are four major advantages of utilizing IMRT for CNS tumors: (i) shape dose around concave PTVs (such as with some meningiomas); (ii) improve homogeneity of the delivered dose to complex-shaped PTVs; (iii) permit a simultaneous integrated plan using two or more PTV dose levels (such as for glioblastoma multiforme); and (iv) improve dose homogeneity to target in the regions where large variations of external contours exist (such as in case of posterior fossa lesions or spinal cord meningiomas).

These advantages of IMRT technique are achieved through so called inverse planning during which dosimetric objectives are set for tumor coverage and for OAR avoidance. An optimization algorithm is then employed to find the optimal photon fluence for each of the employed beams that meets the predetermined dosimetric objectives. After the optimal photon fluence has been found, another optimization algorithm is employed to determine the optimal way (i.e., the shape, the number, and the intensity of segments) to deliver the calculated fluence. In order to fully utilize the power of IMRT, the irradiated tissue should be as static as possible during delivery, the dosimetric objectives for planning should not be unrealistic and great care should be given to contour targets, and OARs which include lenses, eye globes, optic nerves, chiasm, brainstem, temporal lobes, pituitary gland, inner ears, general brain parenchyma, and spinal cord.

Great immobilization can help to reduce the necessary margins when creating PTVs. IMRT, however, is not a tool to reduce margins. Margins should be set based on a realistic assessment of setup uncertainties and the quality of immobilization. Due to a relatively static nature of CNS lesions, IMRT is a great tool for their irradiation.

Unrealistic desired objectives lead to suboptimal plans. It is less than optimal to try to cover the PTV with a homogeneous dose of 80 Gy and at the same time try to constrain the maximum dose to the adjacent, say 1 mm distant chiasm to 40 Gy. The software will substantially increase the needed monitor units and will try to come up with a huge number of very tiny area segments, which might not be deliverable due to machine limitations. Good IMRT plans can achieve better than 5%/mm dose gradient while still preserving good target dose uniformity.

It is desirable to use the appropriate imaging modality for contouring, since the accuracy of contours is crucial for inverse planning. MRI offers good soft tissue contrast much needed for delineation of CNS tumors. If combined with contrast agents that are able to penetrate tumor tissue and co-registered with the planning CT, it makes it an excellent tumor visualization method. If some tissue is not contoured and objectives are not set for it, the software might create unacceptable hot spots in it. This leads to a need for a very careful and close examination of the calculated treatment plan. It is not enough to look at DVHs since small hot spots in a critical organ could be overlooked. Rather, the whole 3D distribution needs a careful review and appropriateness of the maximum and minimum doses must be assessed.

Since the IMRT plan is a delicate collection of small segments often having high photon intensities, the quality of the delivery is very sensitive to tissue motion. Even small disposition of the target can result in a large dose being deposited to unwanted regions. The high conformality of the dose to the target, that is, very sharp dose fall off can actually be a disadvantage of IMRT if the tumor edges are poorly defined hence part of the target can be missed.

SIMULATION PROCEDURES

Positioning

When simulating CNS tumor patients, patient positioning becomes very important and appropriate position devices should be used to aid in reproducibility and setup. The head, neck, and body should be positioned such that the setup marks are in locatable and reproducible positions. Marks on steeply sloping surfaces, ears, nose, lips, and chin should be avoided whenever possible. In general, the head should be positioned with the patient on a pituitary head board for posteriorly located tumors (e.g., occipital lobes or posterior fossa). For patients requiring craniospinal irradiation, it is ideal to have the patient supine with the chin slightly extended such that the exit of the PA spine field does not exit through the patient's oral cavity. CT scan simulation, 3D treatment planning and IMRT allow for different head and neck positions in most situations as noncoplanar beams can be used to avoid entry and exit dose to OARs.

Immobilization

There exist a variety of commercially available head immobilization devices, most of which use thermoplastic or other materials, such as expandable foam or plastic beads in a vacuum bag. They are adaptable for flexion or extension when the patient is in the supine position. Variability of setup should not be >2 or 3 mm with a thermoplastic mask. To obtain more accurate and/or rigid head positioning and immobilization, a modified stereotactic aquaplast mask with reinforcement strips may be used to help insure reproducibility and setup.

Once the patient is placed in the appropriate positioning device, they are scanned, typically using between 2 and 3 mm slice thicknesses. The clinician decides at the time of simulation where the isocenter should be placed. After completion of treatment planning in virtual reality (see subsequent text), verification films should be taken before treatment; these should include orthogonal radiographs to verify the isocenter, and films of any custom-shaped portal fields. Isocenter films (with or without portal images) are usually obtained weekly to verify accuracy of the treatment setup.

Generally, special custom immobilization devices are used for patients with spinal cord tumors to ensure setup reproducibility, especially with craniospinal irradiation patients since the match lines or areas where fields abut is of importance. Regardless of the immobilization device chosen, it must be designed to fit the physical dimensions of the CT scan or MRI and constructed of materials that are compatible with the imaging modalities to prevent image artifact or distortion.

Simulation

In this chapter, the reader may assume that patients are simulated in the supine position using 3D CT scan-based planning, unless otherwise stated. The primary body planes are transverse, sagittal, and coronal, with body axes anterior, posterior, right, left, superior, and inferior. Isocentric treatment machines rotate 360 degrees around a transverse plane of the patient's body, and treating in a coronal or sagittal plane requires the treatment couch to be rotated.

For CT scan simulation involving the brain, the patient is placed in the positioning device and scanned and isocenter is placed in CT or reference markers can be used if necessary and marked on the thermoplastic mask. For intracranial disease, a single-field or opposed-beam two-field arrangements are usually not considered acceptable, as they deliver excessive dose to normal tissues in the beam paths. The exception is a short course of palliative radiation therapy to the whole brain or cervical spinal cord using an opposed lateral beam arrangement. An optimum beam arrangement typically consists of four to six noncoplanar beams. For tumors involving both hemispheres of the brain, the ideal beam arrangement is six noncoplanar beams; two on the right and left sides of the patient (entering anterior to shoulder and posterior to shoulder), and two superior obliques. When applicable, the contralateral uninvolved hemisphere of the brain should be spared as much as possible. In these cases, for patients with right-sided lesions, for example, the contralateral beams will not be utilized. Beam exit through the thyroid gland should also be avoided.

Typically, a homogenous dose distribution within the target volume is desirable, with not >5% to 10% inhomogeneity in the irradiated volume. When IMRT is used, a practical timesaving approach uses the beam arrangement of an optimized noncoplanar 3D plan as a starting point. This can significantly shorten the treatment-planning effort and allows for greater freedom of optimization than a coplanar (i.e., two-dimensional) plan.

Beam arrangements suggested in this chapter are described by the standard 3D naming system summarized in Table 31.4 (68). Beams entering the patient's body are always named relative to the patient, based on the plane and the axis closest to its entry and angle of deviation, therefore literally spelling out the correct gantry and couch positions to be used for treatment. Most lesions can be treated well with higher energy beams 10 to 18 MV photons. For more lateralized tumors, it is ideal to not include contralateral beams if possible. Differential weighting of beams and the use of wedges or compensators (static beams or modulated) is assumed and will not be described in detail. An overview of suggested beam arrangements (as described in the sections in the subsequent text) is provided in Table 31.5. These should not be taken as definitive recommendations but rather as generalized conceptual approaches.

Specific Examples of Treatment Techniques

Whole Brain Radiation Therapy

Whole brain radiation therapy evolved in the early days of radiation therapy when precise anatomic definition of tumor was limited to plain radiography. Nonetheless, the benefits were apparent. In the first randomized clinical trial in brain tumors in the United States, 60 Gy whole brain radiotherapy increased survival in patients with glioblastoma multiforme over steroids alone (69). With the advent of CT and MRI, more focal radiation techniques for brain tumors became the standard. Still, there are important clinical settings in which the brain and/or meninges are the target for which whole brain radiation therapy is an essential component of therapy. These clinical situations with examples are reviewed below.

Acute Leukemia

A known sanctuary site from leukemic chemotherapy is the CNS. After failures in the CNS and eyes were noted, CNS penetrating therapy such as intrathecal drugs and radiation therapy became an important component of treatment of leukemia (70). While the doses of radiotherapy are low, in the 12 to 18 Gy range, the target remains the entire brain, cranial meninges down to the level of C2, and the posterior retina and optic nerves. An example of a C2-whole brain field for cranial prophylaxis is shown in Figure 31.1A. Opposed lateral fields in an aquaplast mask with a 2 to 3 degree posterior cant on the fields can help spare exit through the contralateral lens. The anterior border is set at the fleshy canthus of the eye, which corresponds to the anatomic equator of the eye. Radio-opaque markers placed on the fleshy canthus are very helpful for conventional simulation For a CT simulation, the anterior border is placed at the posterior border of the lens, and the gantry angle is adjusted to make the beam nondivergent across the posterior aspect of both lenses. It is very important to note that the block be placed to insure that the entire posterior globe be included in the fields. At least a 1-cm margin should be included on the middle cranial and base of skull meninges. One centimeter of flash should be provided over the convexity, and the soft tissue of the posterior neck should be shielded with a minimum 1-cm margin on the intracranial contents.

Brain Metastases

The radiation therapy oncology group (RTOG) conducted a number of trials in the early 1980s on whole brain

TABLE 31.4	Beam Gantry and Couch Angles for Six Field Brain Set up on Pituitary Board for a Varian™ Accelerator

Field	Gantry (Degrees)	Couch (Degrees)
RPO	0	245
RIO	15	270
LPO	0	115
LIO	245	90
IO	90	30
SO	90	340

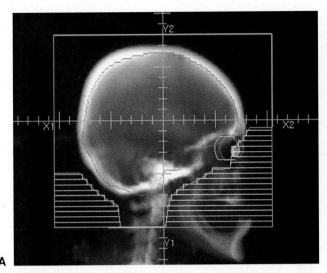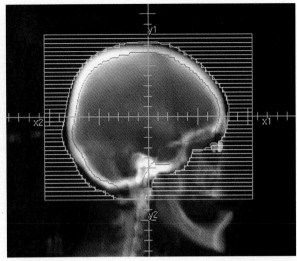

A **B**

Figure 31.1. Sample whole brain radiotherapy fields illustrating blocking for C2-whole brain fields (**A**) that would be appropriate for leukemic prophylaxis and whole brain fields with a scalp block (**B**) that would be appropriate for whole brain radiotherapy of metastatic disease.

radiotherapy for brain metastases (71). These trials conclusively established a survival benefit for whole brain radiation therapy compared to steroids alone. More recently, whole brain radiotherapy with a stereotactic boost showed a survival and neurological function benefit in selected patients with brain metastases (72). A Japanese randomized trial between stereotactic radiosurgery (SRS) and whole brain radiation showed equivalent survival, but suggested a local control benefit to whole brain RT (73). The addition of whole brain radiation therapy to SRS in favorable patients with brain metastases remains controversial and there is an ongoing ACOSOG trial to answer this question.

Traditionally, an open flashing rectangular field with the inferior border collimated to a line connecting the superior orbital rim with the mastoid tip was used. Increasingly, MLC blocking techniques with CT simulation have become common, allowing relatively easy target definition and blocking. The target in whole brain radiation is the brain parenchyma. While posterior fossa metastases may have a higher association with leptomeningeal spread, there is no evidence that including the cranial meninges prevents this pattern of failure. Figure 31.1B illustrates a whole brain field that includes the brain parenchyma with a 1-cm block margin. This typically blocks the lenses of the eyes, but occasionally adjustment of the leaves over the lenses is necessary. The advantage of including a "scalp block" is to avoid the tangent effect of the beam over the vertex scalp that often leads to a characteristic "reverse mohawk" bald patch among surviving patients. Inhomogeneities across the superior thinned parts of the head can also be reduced with simple field-within-a-field techniques.

Whole brain radiation is now known to cause mild-to-moderate executive function and memory deficits over time in adults (74). The more significant deleterious effects in children are well known. It has been observed that the hippocampus rarely (<5%) harbors metastatic disease and <10% of brain metastases occur within a 5-mm margin of the hippocampus (75). One intriguing technique to reduce the effect on memory is hippocampal sparing with IMRT for delivering whole brain radiation. The additional advantage of an IMRT technique is that patients with a limited number of metastasis can be "boosted" using a simultaneous integrated plan to deliver a selective higher radiation dose to gross tumor. Whether this technique reduces neurocognitive deficits and improves control remains to be demonstrated.

Craniospinal Irradiation

Certain neoplasms will require treatment to the entire craniospinal axis. This may include medulloblastomas and PNETs, high-grade ependymomas, some germ cell tumors, pineoblastomas, disseminated CNS lymphoma, and leptomeningeal carcinomatosis or gliomatosis. Several positioning variations are used in clinical practice often in an immobilization cast to ensure daily positional reproducibility (76). Patients are ideally treated in the supine position with the neck extended to avoid beams exiting the oral cavity. Conventional methods utilize field "feathering" to reduce hot or cold spots caused by imperfect fields matching between cranial and spine fields. This method feathered each junction on a weekly basis with the cranial fields' inferior border decreasing between 5 and 10 mm. The intracranial contents and upper one or two segments of the cervical cord are treated through opposed lateral fields, usually positioned so that the isocenter is at midline with the beam axes passing through the lateral canthi to minimize divergence into the contralateral eye. The collimator and couch are rotated to create a straight line through the inferior portion of the brain fields that removes the possibility of overlap with the posterior spine field. This can be visualized with the treatment planning systems simulation software (see subsequent text).

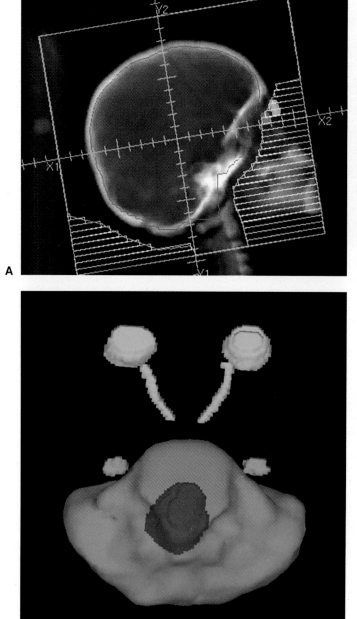

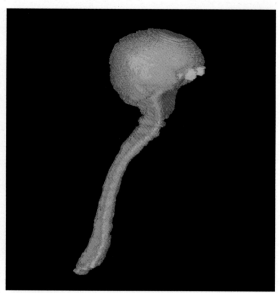

Figure 31.2. Sample whole brain field with angled collimator for craniospinal radiotherapy of medulloblastoma (**A**). **B** represents the prescription dose cloud for craniospinal radiation of medulloblastoma. Note no loss of dose at the junction between brain and spine fields on account of a daily 3-feathered junction using the independent jaw. **C** illustrates the isodose cloud for an IMRT medulloblastoma posterior fossa boost specifically avoiding the cochlea (shown in green). The optic pathway is shown in aqua and the primary tumor is shown in pink.

Customized blocks protect the normal head and neck tissues from the primary radiation beam; as mentioned above, care must be taken not to underdose the cribriform plate. Figure 31.2A represents a typical cranial field with blocks for the lenses and collimator angled to match the divergence of the PA spine field. The inferior border of the initial "short" field is placed around C2–3, leaving adequate room for subsequent shifts in the match with the upper spine field, a technique commonly referred to as "feathering the gap."

Depending on length, the spine is treated through one or two posterior fields. It is customary practice to maximize the field length of the upper spinal field (40 cm at 100 cm source–skin distance [SSD]) and minimize the length of the lower spinal field, therefore simplifying planning for junction shifts (see in subsequent text). If 40 cm or less of length covers the spine inclusive of the end of the thecal sac (typically near the level of S3, this should be confirmed by MRI), a lower spine field is not necessary. All fields' central axes remain fixed; it is only the fields' lengths, which are changed. Therefore, the caudal border of the lower PA spine field should be set inferior to S3 by a length equal to the two-field shifts, and then blocked back to S3 using asymmetric collimators.

Matching the upper border of the spine field to the lower border of the cranial field requires strict attention to accuracy, as overlap (i.e., overdosing) in the upper cervical cord may have catastrophic outcomes for the patient. In one method, the collimator for the lateral cranial fields is angled to match the divergence of the upper border of the adjacent spinal field, and the treatment couch is angled so that the inferior border of the cranial field is perpendicular to the superior edge of the spinal field ("exact-match" technique). Both the rotation of the collimator and degree of couch rotation are calculated from Equation (Fig. 31.1), and typically range from 9 to 11 degrees. The drawback to this technique is that the couch rotation displaces the contralateral eye cephalad, so that it cannot be blocked without blocking frontal brain tissue. This technique may also result in underdosing of the temporal lobes and cribriform plate.

One method for craniospinal irradiation involves a 3D CT simulation of a patient in the supine position in a wooden box that encompasses the entire spinal canal. The patients cranium extends outside the end of the box to allow for positioning, utilizing an aquaplast mask (see photo). This method, referred to as "simulated dynamic feathering," feathers the gap daily as opposed to conventional methods where the fields are feathered after five fractions. The process is as follows:

Simulation

The patient is placed in the wooden box on top of a vac bag. The vac bag provides comfort as well as elevates the patient inside the box to allow for larger SSDs that will help encompass the entire spine in one field. An aquaplast mask is used to immobilize the cranium and extend the mandible as mentioned earlier. The patient is aligned with the spine as straight as possible and no rotation of the cranium before scanning. A scout is usually needed to confirm that the patient is aligned and no adjustments are needed. An isocenter is placed in the CT room for the cranium fields only and the mask is marked. The isocenter is usually placed midline and will serve as a reference point for the spine field. Ideally, the spine isocenter is placed such that the couch is moved as little as possible between brain and spine fields. Generally, after the cranium fields are treated, the couch is shifted in two directions: toward the gantry and raised to accommodate the extended SSD of the PA spine field.

Treatment Planning

The cranial fields are designed as well as the spine field for the initial beams. Collimator and couch are rotated to prevent the overlap between the brain and spine fields using the treatment planning system. The planning system allows visualization of beam divergence for all beams in the axial, sagittal, and coronal views. Once the initial fields have been designed, they are copied and labeled accordingly (Shift #1, 2, etc.). The cranial field's inferior border is increased by 5 mm and the spine fields' superior border is decreased to match the inferior border of the brain fields. A total of 1.5 cm shift is used for this technique, which requires 3 shifts 5 mm each shift. It is important to note that the spine field will not necessarily be 5 mm due to beam divergence as these fields are generally treated at extended SSD's (between 125 and 135 cm). The following shifts are created using the same process. The number of beams can be as many as 12 treated on a daily basis using the dynamic method; therefore, patient comfort is important as it contributes greatly to reproducibility. The number of shifts or junctions is physician dependent.

Plan optimization usually involves a forward planned field in field technique for the brain fields as well as for the spine field. However, it is possible to optimize the spine fields using inverse planning to cool off hot spots. The rationale for inverse planning the spine field is merely related to time. The control points needed for the spine field are generally higher than that of the brain fields. Figure 31.2B shows the dose cloud for such a craniospinal plan. Figure 31.2C shows the dose cloud for an IMRT-planned posterior fossa boost, sparing cochlea.

Documenting junction match requires placing wires on the inferior border of brain fields before imaging the spine field for each junction shift.

Partial Brain Radiation

The era of 3D CRT in the 1990s allowed substantial reduction of unnecessary radiation to normal brain. The anatomic location of the brain atop the head also maximized the benefits of noncoplanar beams, because vertex beam arrangements were available with a simple rotation of the treatment couch. While the wedge requirements of noncoplanar beam to produced homogeneous plans are more complicated, they are solvable (77). In spite of this, the compensation requirements of such noncoplanar arrangements are more easily handled with IMRT inverse planning. In addition, intensity modulation can produce concave dose distributions around critical adjacent structures such as the optic chiasm, brainstem and cochlea and thus provide more adequate dose sparing. IMRT also allows differential prescription of doses and simultaneously integrated boost plans that has made IMRT routine for contemporary partial brain irradiation.

At the University of Texas Southwestern Medical Center, we employ a standard set of six noncoplanar beams for our brain treatments. Table 31.1 lists the gantry and couch angles of the standard set. For lateralized tumors, the contralateral fields typically are omitted to reduce dose to the contralateral hemisphere. This results in a final set of four IMRT fields for lateralized tumors. In order to eliminate exit dose through the axial skeleton and thyroid, we simulate all patients on a pituitary board with flexed neck and use a reinforced aquaplast mask that covers over the chin to prevent the patient from slipping down on the board. We also build a vac-loc bag for the body and neck and shoulders to prevent the patient from sliding down the treatment table while on the pituitary board. The vac-loc bag is built-up to support the back of the neck and abuts the base of the head holder. We find that the "F" head holder often provides the greatest and most optimal neck

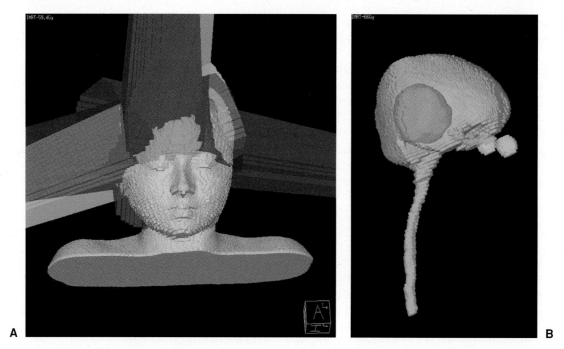

Figure 31.3. Sample non-coplanar field arrangement for a thalamic anaplastic astrocytoma (**A**) and isodose cloud (**B**) illustrating convex dose cloud avoiding the optic pathway.

flexion. The field arrangements in Table 31.1 would be appropriate even if a standard nonflexed neck position is selected. In this situation, the inferior and superior oblique fields need to be rotated superiorly to avoid the eyes and care should be exercised to ensure beams avoid exit through the thyroid and axial skeleton. The following are specific disease specific applications of this arrangement.

Low-Grade Glioma

Low-grade gliomas form a heterogeneous group of tumors that include the most favorable pilocytic astrocytoma and the fibrillary astrocytomas with a less favorable prognosis and propensity to degenerate into a higher grade histology. Doses are 45 to 54 Gy in standard fractions with a typical 1 cm clinical margin on the radiographically defined GTV. Higher radiation doses have been studied, but only resulted in increased toxicity with no survival benefit. Figure 31.3 presents the isodose distribution for a suprasellar pilocytic astrocytoma progressive on chemotherapy.

A helpful quantitative tool to evaluate brain plans is the conformity index. Born from radiosurgical planning, various conformity indices have been described. For an ideal plan, conformity indices approach 1. From a practical point of view, the indices have value in discriminating between generally acceptable treatment plans, since poorly conformal plans and plans that do not cover the target are usually quite apparent to the keen observer. The simplest conformity index is formed by dividing the target volume into the ICRU treatment volume:

Conformity Index = Treatment Volume/Target Volume

When the entire body is contoured in the planning system, the treatment volume is easily obtained from the DVH as the volume of the body receiving the prescription dose. A conformity index < 1.2 indicates a highly conformal plan and should be an important and achievable planning goal. Figure 31.4 presents a representative plan for a child with a cystic suprasellar pilocytic astrocytoma.

High-Grade Glioma

Most high-grade gliomas are glioblastomas. Although temozolomide with radiation prolongs median survival by about 2 months with a small number of 5-year survivors (ref), most patients invariably recur, requiring salvage therapy. While hypofractionated treatments and smaller treatment volumes are under investigation, the radiation standard remains 45 to 50 Gy to a clinical target including all surrounding postoperative flair signal plus a 2-cm margin along continuous white matter tracks within the brain with a boost to a clinical target including the enhancing tumor or postoperative cavity plus a 1 to 2 cm margin. It is important to adjust clinical targets along known anatomic white matter tracks to avoid unnecessary irradiation of the posterior fossa or contralateral brain, as both the tentorium and falx are effective barriers to spread of glial tumors. The standard boost dose remains 60 Gy. Higher doses, including a radiosurgical boost, have been studied, in randomized trials, but showed no survival benefit and only resulted in greater toxicity.

Figure 31.3A and B illustrates the filed arrangements and resulting dose cloud, respectively, for a thalamic anaplastic astrocytoma boost showing how concave IMRT dose distributions can be achieved that specifically avoid the optic chiasm. Figure 31.5 compares the isodose distributions and DVHs for two successive IMRT plans with first course to 45 Gy boost to 60 Gy and an integrated

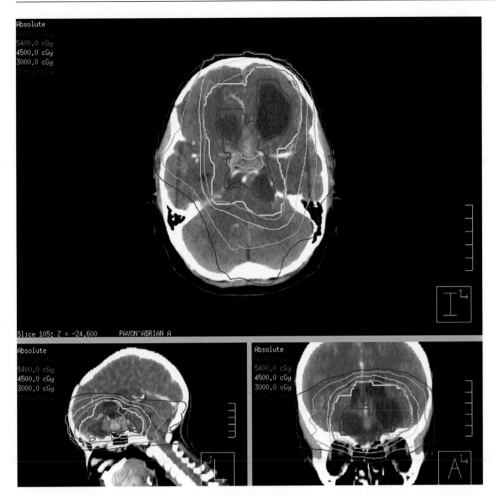

Figure 31.4. Sample IMRT dose distribution for a child with a suprasellar pilocytic astrocytoma.

boost plan, where the larger CTV received 50 Gy and the boost simultaneously received 60 Gy. The conformity index (see above) for the 60 Gy volume is better for the integrated boost plan (1.56 vs. 1.05), because the dose contribution from the first course treatment in not accounted in the boost plan. In addition, more brain overall is treated to a higher dose for the sequential plan as is seen from the separation of the brain DVH curves in Figure 31.6. Whether 50 Gy/30 fractions (1.67 Gy per fraction) or 45 Gy/25 fractions (1.80 Gy per fraction) are equivalent for microscopic disease has not been compared in a prospective trial, but they likely have similar biological effects.

Ependymoma

Ependymomas are uncommon primary glial CNS tumors that typically arise in the posterior fossa and cauda equina. Ependymomas in the cauda equine are most often low grade myxopapillary type and carry a relatively favorable prognosis. Radiation therapy is reserved for incompletely resected or recurrent tumors. Ependymomas account for 5% to 10% of childhood intracranial tumors, but occur as well in adults. Standard management involves complete surgical removal. Most authors agree that posterior fossa ependymomas should receive postoperative radiotherapy,

as recurrence rates remain high even after complete surgical removal in this location. The addition of radiotherapy for supratentorial ependymomas after complete surgical resection is controversial, as this appears to be a more favorable subsite. Figure 31.6 illustrates an IMRT dose cloud for a posterior fossa ependymoma specifically designed to spare adjacent cochlea and temporal lobes.

Meningiomas

Meningiomas are common CNS tumors, for which radiation therapy is a safe and effective treatment approach. Radiotherapy for meningiomas can be challenging because they often have irregular shapes and are located near critical structures. With the advent of IMRT, fractionated stereotactic radiotherapy (FSRT), and SRS, radiotherapeutic options in the management of meningiomas are now diverse. However, regardless of the treatment modality, careful treatment planning is central, since meningiomas are mostly benign tumors, and therefore the risk of serious late toxicities needs to be minimized.

Fusion of a contrast-enhanced MRI with the planning CT scan provides the optimal definition of the meningioma and adjacent OARs. For well-demarcated lesions, the GTV and CTV are identical. Stereotactic positioning may be useful to reduce the margin for PTV, which takes into account the error in tumor volume delineation, errors

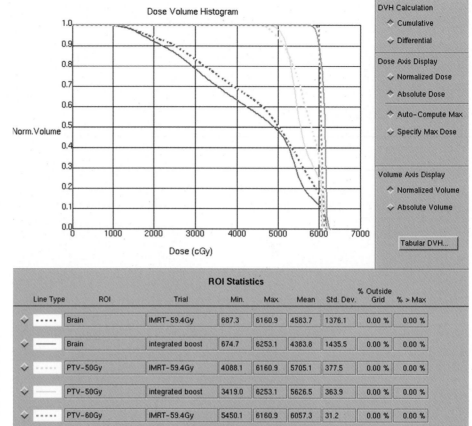

Line Type	ROI	Trial	Min.	Max.	Mean	Std. Dev.	% Outside Grid	% > Max
·····	Brain	IMRT–59.4Gy	687.3	6160.9	4583.7	1376.1	0.00 %	0.00 %
———	Brain	integrated boost	674.7	6253.1	4383.8	1435.5	0.00 %	0.00 %
·····	PTV–50Gy	IMRT–59.4Gy	4088.1	6160.9	5705.1	377.5	0.00 %	0.00 %
———	PTV–50Gy	integrated boost	3419.0	6253.1	5626.5	363.9	0.00 %	0.00 %
·····	PTV–60Gy	IMRT–59.4Gy	5450.1	6160.9	6057.3	31.2	0.00 %	0.00 %
———	PTV–60Gy	integrated boost	5661.9	6253.1	6117.8	75.9	0.00 %	0.00 %

Figure 31.5. Dose volume histogram comparing an IMRT integrated 59.4Gy high dose, 50Gy intermediate dose anaplastic astrocytoma plan (shown as the solid curve) with an IMRT 45Gy first course and 14.4Gy cone down composite (shown as the dashed curve).

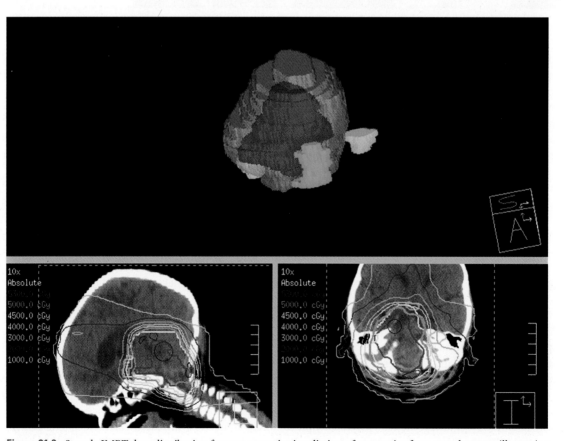

Figure 31.6. Sample IMRT dose distribution for post-operative irradiation of a posterior fossa ependymoma illustrating cochlear avoidance. The pre-operative tumor is shown in pink, the chiasm in green and the cochlea in aqua. The prescription isodose cloud is illustrated in orange.

inherent to image fusion, and for the variation in day-to-day setup. With invasive tumors, such as those involving the sphenoid or cavernous sinuses, there is greater uncertainty, which must be considered in determining the CTV.

The optimal beam arrangement is dictated by both the shape and location of the lesion. With a large convexity lesion, for example, a potential arrangement may be three coplanar beams angled at 120 degrees from one another ("Mercedes Star"), or a cruciform arrangement of four coplanar beams. The couch and gantry are then rotated so that each beam is shifted ~10 degrees inferiorly with respect to the patient (Fig. 31.2). These arrangements minimize the cross-sectional area of the lesion within the beam's eye view. Other suggestions for beam arrangements are presented in the subsequent text, based on the region of the brain. The use of IMRT may be useful for concave-shaped lesions. With superficially located lesions, 6-MV photons are typically utilized owing to the short buildup depth; for more deeply situated tumors, such as cavernous sinus lesions, higher energy beams may be considered.

Pituitary Tumors

Fusion of a contrast-enhanced MRI with a contrasted planning CT scan provides the optimum definition of the suprasellar optic apparatus and the extensiveness of the tumor. The GTV is the pituitary adenoma, including any of its extension into adjacent anatomic regions. Generally, the entire content of the sella and, if appropriate, extension into the sphenoid or cavernous sinuses are included in the CTV. With appropriate immobilization devices, CTV expansion of 0.5 cm, that is, 1.0 to 1.5 cm margin to block edge is adequate to create the PTV. Stereotactic positioning can reduce the PTV, with margins of 7 mm giving excellent dose distribution with minimal dose to surrounding tissues. OARs to be contoured include the optic globes, lenses, optic nerves, optic chiasm, brainstem, and temporal lobes.

The traditional three-field approach using wedged opposed laterals and an anterior or vertex beam superior to the eyes leads to unacceptably high doses to the temporal lobes. IMRT may be useful to further improve dose distribution, especially for irregularly shaped lesions. A selection of noncoplanar six beams suitable for IMRT for a pituitary tumor is give in Table 31.1. Beam energies of at least 6 MV should be used to spare surrounding structures, most notably the temporal lobes. Ten-megavolt photons provide a good balance between depth dose and penumbra width, although for stereotactic plans with small margins, 6-MV photons may be more advantageous.

Spinal Tumors

The most favorable field arrangement will be determined by the location and adjacent OARs, and it may be a single posteroanterior (PA) field, opposed-lateral fields, a PA field with opposed laterals, opposed anterior-posterior (AP/PA) fields, or oblique wedge-pair fields (78,79). In some circumstances, IMRT may be useful to spare esophagus, heart, lung, kidney, and bowel, especially when higher doses need to be delivered. Some metastatic lesions may be suitable for treatment in a single fraction with spinal radiosurgery using appropriate immobilization and image guidance tools. In the cervical region, an opposed-lateral beam approach minimizes the dose to the anterior neck. When palliating a tumor in the cervicothoracic region, a split beam approach facilitates the match with another treatment field. In this case, the central axis is placed just above the shoulders and opposed-lateral beams are used to treat the upper spine, and a PA field is used for the area of the spine below the central axis. Tumors in the thoracic region can be treated with opposed lateral beams, a three-field approach using a PA field and opposed lateral beams, a two-field approach using AP/PA beams, or a posterior beam prescribed to an appropriate depth. When treating with a single posterior beam, the depth prescription should take into account the dose to the spinal cord to prevent accidental overdosing. In the lumbar region, AP/PA or PA fields reduce the exposure to the kidneys. In the sacral region, opposed lateral beams with or without a posterior beam or a four-field approach using AP/PA and opposed lateral beams may be useful. Comparison of various treatment setups by means of DVHs is recommended.

Acknowledgments

The authors would like to acknowledge the contributions of Volker W. Stieber, Kevin P. McMullen, Allan DeGuzman, and Edward G. Shaw to the writing of this chapter in the previous edition of this book.

REFERENCES

1. Brodmann K. Beiträge zur histologischen Lokalisation der Großhirnrinde. VI: Die Cortexgliederung des Menschen. *J Psychol Neurol* 1908;10:231–246.
2. Brodmann K. Beiträge zur histologischen Lokalisation der Großhirnrinde. VI: Die Cortexgliederung des Menschen. *J Psychol Neurol* 1908;10:287–334.
3. Babiloni F, Mattia D, Babiloni C, et al. Multimodal integration of EEG, MEG and fMRI data for the solution of the neuroimage puzzle. *Magn Reson Imaging* 2004;22:1471–1476.
4. Barnes D, Egan G, O'Keefe G, et al. Characterization of dynamic 3-D PET imaging for functional brain mapping. *IEEE Trans Med Imaging* 1997;16:261–269.
5. Choi SJ, Kim JS, Kim JH, et al. [18F]3′-deoxy-3′-fluorothymidine PET for the diagnosis and grading of brain tumors. *Eur J Nucl Med Mol Imaging* 2005;32:653–659.
6. American CS. *Cancer facts and figures.* Atlanta: American Cancer Society, 2010.
7. CBTRUS. 2009–2010 CBTRUS Statistical Report: Primary Brain and Central Nervous System Tumors Diagnosed in the United States in 2004–2006. Hinsdale, IL: Central Brain Tumor Registry of the United States, 2010.

8. Ferlay J. *GLOBOCAN 2000 [electronic resource]: cancer incidence, mortality, and prevalence worldwide/WHO,* International Agency for Research on Cancer. Lyon: IARC Press, 2001.

9. Connolly E. Spinal cord tumors in adults. In: Youmans Y, ed. *Neurological surgery vol 5.* Philadelphia: WB Saunders, 1982:3196.

10. Sasanelli F. Primary intraspinal neoplasms in Rochester, Minnesota, 1935–1981. *Neuroepidemiology* 1983;2:156–163.

11. IARC. WHO Classification of tumours of the central nervous system. *Lyon: IARC,* 2007.

12. Preston-Martin S. Descriptive epidemiology of primary tumors of the spinal cord and spinal meninges in Los Angeles County, 1972–1985. *Neuroepidemiology* 1990;9:106–111.

13. Barnholtz-Sloan JS, Sloan AE, Davis FG, et al. Incidence proportions of brain metastases in patients diagnosed (1973 to 2001) in the Metropolitan Detroit Cancer Surveillance System. *J Clin Oncol* 2004;22:2865–2872.

14. Schouten LJ, Rutten J, Huveneers HA, et al. Incidence of brain metastases in a cohort of patients with carcinoma of the breast, colon, kidney, and lung and melanoma. *Cancer* 2002;94:2698–2705.

15. Byrne TN. Spinal cord compression from epidural metastases. *N Engl J Med* 1992;327:614–619.

16. Gerszten P. Current surgical management of metastatic spinal disease. *Oncology* 2000;14:1013–1024.

17. Loblaw DA, Laperriere NJ, Mackillop WJ. A population-based study of malignant spinal cord compression in Ontario. *Clin Oncol (R Coll Radiol)* 2003;15:211–217.

18. Schaberg J, Gainor BJ. A profile of metastatic carcinoma of the spine. *Spine (Phila Pa 1976)* 1985;10:19–20.

19. Bilsky MH, Lis E, Raizer J, et al. The diagnosis and treatment of metastatic spinal tumor. *Oncologist* 1999;4:459–469.

20. Healey JH, Brown HK. Complications of bone metastases: surgical management. *Cancer* 2000;88:2940–2951.

21. Wong DA, Fornasier VL, MacNab I. Spinal metastases: the obvious, the occult, and the impostors. *Spine (Phila Pa 1976)* 1990;15:1–4.

22. Gilbert RW, Kim JH, Posner JB. Epidural spinal cord compression from metastatic tumor: diagnosis and treatment. *Ann Neurol* 1978;3:40–51.

23. Patchell RA. A randomized trial of direct decompressive surgical resection in the treatment of spinal cord compression caused by metastasis. *J Clin Oncol* 2003;21(1):67–86.

24. Pigott KH, Baddeley H, Maher EJ. Pattern of disease in spinal cord compression on MRI scan and implications for treatment. *Clin Oncol (R Coll Radiol)* 1994;6:7–10.

25. O'Rourke T, George CB, Redmond J 3rd, et al. Spinal computed tomography and computed tomographic metrizamide myelography in the early diagnosis of metastatic disease. *J Clin Oncol* 1986;4:576–583.

26. Ruff RL, Lanska DJ. Epidural metastases in prospectively evaluated veterans with cancer and back pain. *Cancer* 1989;63:2234–2241.

27. Schiff D, Batchelor T, Wen PY. Neurologic emergencies in cancer patients. *Neurol Clin* 1998;16:449–483.

28. Ricci PE, Dungan DH. Imaging of low- and intermediate-grade gliomas. *Semin Radiat Oncol* 2001;11:103–112.

29. Munley M. Bioanatomic IMRT treatment planning with dose function histograms. *Int J Rad Oncol Biol Phys* 2002;54:126.

30. Nuutinen J, Sonninen P, Lehikoinen P, et al. Radiotherapy treatment planning and long-term follow-up with [(11)C]methionine PET in patients with low-grade astrocytoma. *Int J Radiat Oncol Biol Phys* 2000;48:43–52.

31. Pirzkall A, McKnight TR, Graves EE, et al. MR-spectroscopy guided target delineation for high-grade gliomas. *Int J Radiat Oncol Biol Phys* 2001;50:915–928.

32. Husband DJ, Grant KA, Romaniuk CS. MRI in the diagnosis and treatment of suspected malignant spinal cord compression. *Br J Radiol* 2001;74:15–23.

33. Sarin R, Murthy V. Medical decompressive therapy for primary and metastatic intracranial tumours. *Lancet Neurol* 2003;2:357–365.

34. French LA. The use of steroids in the treatment of cerebral edema. *Bull N Y Acad Med* 1966;42:301–311.

35. Long DM, Hartmann JF, French LA. The response of human cerebral edema to glucosteroid administration. An electron microscopic study. *Neurology* 1966;16:521–528.

36. Vecht CJ, Hovestadt A, Verbiest HB, et al. Dose-effect relationship of dexamethasone on Karnofsky performance in metastatic brain tumors: a randomized study of doses of 4, 8, and 16 mg per day. *Neurology* 1994;44:675–680.

37. Wolfson AH, Snodgrass SM, Schwade JG, et al. The role of steroids in the management of metastatic carcinoma to the brain. A pilot prospective trial. *Am J Clin Oncol* 1994;17:234–238.

38. Kalkanis SN, Eskandar EN, Carter BS, et al. Microvascular decompression surgery in the United States, 1996 to 2000: mortality rates, morbidity rates, and the effects of hospital and surgeon volumes. *Neurosurgery* 2003;52:1251–1261; discussion 1261–1262.

39. Sorensen S, Helweg-Larsen S, Mouridsen H, et al. Effect of high-dose dexamethasone in carcinomatous metastatic spinal cord compression treated with radiotherapy: a randomised trial. *Eur J Cancer* 1994;30A:22–27.

40. Bilsky MH. Intensive and postoperative care of intracranial tumors, 3rd ed. New York: Raven Press, 1993:309–329.

41. Heimdal K, Hirschberg H, Slettebo H, et al. High incidence of serious side effects of high-dose dexamethasone treatment in patients with epidural spinal cord compression. *J Neurooncol* 1992;12:141–144.

42. Weissman DE, Janjan NA, Erickson B, et al. Twice-daily tapering dexamethasone treatment during cranial radiation for newly diagnosed brain metastases. *J Neurooncol* 1991;11:235–239.

43. Maranzano E, Latini P, Beneventi S, et al. Radiotherapy without steroids in selected metastatic spinal cord compression patients. A phase II trial. *Am J Clin Oncol* 1996;19:179–183.

44. Bell BA, Smith MA, Kean DM, et al. Brain water measured by magnetic resonance imaging. Correlation with direct estimation and changes after mannitol and dexamethasone. *Lancet* 1987;1:66–69.

45. Quinn JA, DeAngelis LM. Neurologic emergencies in the cancer patient. *Semin Oncol* 2000;27:311–321.

46. Working Group on Status Epilepticus. Treatment of convulsive status epilepticus. Recommendations of the Epilepsy Foundation of America's Working Group on Status Epilepticus. *JAMA* 1993;270:854–859.

47. Forsyth PA, Weaver S, Fulton D, et al. Prophylactic anticonvulsants in patients with brain tumour. *Can J Neurol Sci* 2003;30:106–112.

48. Glantz MJ, Cole BF, Friedberg MH, et al. A randomized, blinded, placebo-controlled trial of divalproex sodium prophylaxis in adults with newly diagnosed brain tumors. *Neurology* 1996;46:985–991.

49. Loblaw DA, Laperriere NJ. Emergency treatment of malignant extradural spinal cord compression: an evidence-based guideline. *J Clin Oncol* 1998;16:1613–1624.

50. Young RF, Post EM, King GA. Treatment of spinal epidural metastases. Randomized prospective comparison of laminectomy and radiotherapy. *J Neurosurg* 1980;53:741–748.

51. Patchell RA, Tibbs PA, Regine WF, et al. Direct decompressive surgical resection in the treatment of spinal cord compression caused by metastatic cancer: a randomised trial. *Lancet* 2005;366:643–648.

52. Hazuka MB, Burleson WD, Stroud DN, et al. Multiple brain metastases are associated with poor survival in patients treated with surgery and radiotherapy. *J Clin Oncol* 1993;11:369–373.

53. Patchell RA. The management of brain metastases. *Cancer Treat Rev* 2003;29:533–540.

54. Patchell RA, Tibbs PA, Walsh JW, et al. A randomized trial of surgery in the treatment of single metastases to the brain. *N Engl J Med* 1990;322:494–500.

55. Vecht CJ, Haaxma-Reiche H, Noordijk EM, et al. Treatment of single brain metastasis: radiotherapy alone or combined with neurosurgery? *Ann Neurol* 1993;33:583–590.

56. Mintz AH, Kestle J, Rathbone MP, et al. A randomized trial to assess the efficacy of surgery in addition to radiotherapy in patients with a single cerebral metastasis. *Cancer* 1996;78:1470–1476.

57. A close look into the brain. Juelich Research Centre, 2009.

58. ICRU report 50. Prescribing, recording, and reporting photon beam therapy. International Commission on Radiation Units and Measurements, ICRU, Bethesda, 1993.

59. ICRU report 62. Prescribing, recording, and reporting photon beam therapy (Supplement to ICRU Report 50). International Commission on Radiation Units and Measurements, 1999.

60. Emami B, Lyman J, Brown A, et al. Tolerance of normal tissue to therapeutic irradiation. *Int J Radiat Oncol Biol Phys* 1991;21:109–122.

61. Jankovic M, Brouwers P, Valsecchi MG, et al. Association of 1800 cGy cranial irradiation with intellectual function in children with acute lymphoblastic leukaemia. ISPACC. International Study Group on Psychosocial Aspects of Childhood Cancer. *Lancet* 1994;344:224–227.

62. Silber JH, Radcliffe J, Peckham V, et al. Whole-brain irradiation and decline in intelligence: the influence of dose and age on IQ score. *J Clin Oncol* 1992;10:1390–1396.

63. Marcus RB Jr, Million RR. The incidence of myelitis after irradiation of the cervical spinal cord. *Int J Radiat Oncol Biol Phys* 1990;19:3–8.

64. Schultheiss TE, Kun LE, Ang KK, et al. Radiation response of the central nervous system. *Int J Radiat Oncol Biol Phys* 1995;31:1093–1112.

65. Fuller DB, Bloom JG. Radiotherapy for chordoma. *Int J Radiat Oncol Biol Phys* 1988;15:331–339.

66. Pieters RS, O'Farrell D, Fullerton B, et al. 2167 Cauda equina tolerance to radiation therapy. *Int J Radiat Oncol Biol Phys* 1996;36:359–359.

67. Schoenthaler R, Castro JR, Petti PL, et al. Charged particle irradiation of sacral chordomas. *Int J Radiat Oncol Biol Phys* 1993;26:291–298.

68. Jasper KR, Hummel SM, Laramore GE. 3D naming system. *Med Dosim* 2004;29:97–103.

69. Walker MD, Alexander E, Hunt WE, et al. Evaluation of BCNU and/or radiotherapy in the treatment of anaplastic gliomas. *J Neurosurg* 1978;49:333–343.

70. Aur RJ, Simone JV, Hustu HO, et al. A comparative study of central nervous system irradiation and intensive chemotherapy early in remission of childhood acute lymphocytic leukemia. *Cancer* 1972;29:381–391.

71. Borgelt B, Gelber R, Kramer S, et al. The palliation of brain metastases: final results of the first two studies by the Radiation Therapy Oncology Group. *Int J Radiat Oncol Biol Phys* 1980;6:1–9.

72. Andrews DW, Scott CB, Sperduto PW, et al. Whole brain radiation therapy with or without stereotactic radiosurgery boost for patients with one to three brain metastases: phase III results of the RTOG 9508 randomised trial. *Lancet* 2004;363:1665–1672.

73. Aoyama H, Shirato H, Tago M, et al. Stereotactic radiosurgery plus whole-brain radiation therapy vs stereotactic radiosurgery alone for treatment of brain metastases: a randomized controlled trial. *JAMA* 2006;295:2483–2491.

74. Aoyama H, Tago M, Kato N, et al. Neurocognitive function of patients with brain metastasis who received either whole brain radiotherapy plus stereotactic radiosurgery or radiosurgery alone. *Int J Radiat Oncol Biol Phys* 2007;68:1388–1395.

75. Gondi V, Tome WA, Marsh J, et al. Estimated risk of perihippocampal disease progression after hippocampal avoidance during whole-brain radiotherapy: Safety profile for RTOG 0933. *Radiother Oncol* 2010;95:327–331.

76. Shiu AS, Chang EL, Ye JS, et al. Near simultaneous computed tomography image-guided stereotactic spinal radiotherapy: an emerging paradigm for achieving true stereotaxy. *Int J Radiat Oncol Biol Phys* 2003;57:605–613.

77. Sherouse GW. A mathematical basis for selection of wedge angle and orientation. *Med Phys* 1993;20:1211–1218.

78. JM M. Spinal canal. In: Haperin EC, Perez CA, Brady LW, eds. *Principles and practice of radiation oncology,* 5th ed. Philadelphia, PA: Lippincott Williams & Wilkins, 2008:765–777.

79. Minehan KJ, Shaw EG, Scheithauer BW, et al. Spinal cord astrocytoma: pathological and treatment considerations. *J Neurosurg* 1995;83:590–595.

CHAPTER 32

Pediatric Malignancies

Jeffrey C. Buchsbaum ■ Lee T. Myers

INTRODUCTION

In addition to the psychosocial issues, which require increased understanding and involvement, radiotherapy (RT) for pediatric malignancies differs from adult treatment in three fundamental physical and biological respects. First, many pediatric tumors are radioresponsive and require relatively low doses, especially as chemotherapy is also used. Second, growing tissues are likely to suffer more damage from RT than their adult counterparts. Third, there are immobilization issues with babies and young children that are not major factors in adult RT.

Treatment planning in pediatric RT is intimately involved with all three issues. In particular, target volumes are out of necessity well defined, with narrow margins, and therefore immobilization is the key. Developments in radiation therapy over the past 15 years have provided multiple tools and techniques that are especially useful with the pediatric population. Virtual simulation with multimodality image fusion (positron emission tomography [PET], magnetic resonance imaging [MRI], and magnetic resonance spectroscopy [MRS]), simplifies the simulation process and improves our ability to localize the target. The use of biological and molecular markers may significantly help us define target volumes. Dynamic multileaf collimators (MLCs) and automatic sequencing of table, gantry, and collimator motions have significantly enhanced our ability to quickly deliver complex treatment plans, which spare normal tissues and cover the necessary target. The use of three-dimensional conformal radiotherapy (3DCRT), intensity-modulated radiotherapy (IMRT), and more recently image-guided radiotherapy (IGRT) have allowed us to tailor dose and minimize margins necessary to treat the disease. Stereotactic radiosurgery (SRS), both linac-based and with the gamma knife, has allowed us to treat brain lesions with high conformality. Developments in stereotactic body radiotherapy (SBRT) are helping us to treat extracranial lesions with increased precision, which has obvious benefits for the pediatric population. In situations where integral dose may be an issue or where organ motion may be problematic, both low-dose-rate and high-dose-rate brachytherapy continue to offer practical alternatives. Finally, because protons can provide a more conformal physical dose distribution than photons, they may be especially useful for treating smaller targets in smaller patients and in optimizing integral dose (1,2). It is important to understand that the physics and dosimetry of protons in a clinical environment is less well tested over time than photons (3), and we may not fully understand the physics of protons in areas such as the sinuses and moving organs. We do not fully understand the biology of the proton at the Bragg peak. We also do not fully understand the risks of one form of proton beam as compared to another form of proton beam delivery system (4).

An open, critical pediatric radiation oncology question is "what is the long-term role of low-dose radiation therapy" in the form of integral dose as it is delivered with IMRT. By integral dose, we generally refer to the effects of the low-dose radiation bath delivered to a relatively large volume of tissue usually outside of the planned treatment volume. Formally, it is the sum of all doses to the entire body volumetrically. In the pediatric population, this needs to be studied prospectively. Some presentations at the American Society for Therapeutic Radiology and Oncology (ASTRO; Denver, 2005 meeting) evaluated the varied dose to organs in a pediatric phantom from 3D conformal and IMRT techniques. The results of the study highlighted both expected and unexpected issues and pointed to a need to design linear accelerators (LINACS) with less leakage from the head. Since the time of presentation, head leakage issues have been addressed by the manufacturers to varying degrees. It is imperative that centers and manufacturers monitor their designs and implementations to minimize dose to patients that do not come from the beam.

Integral dose needs to be considered in the treatment planning of pediatric patients as we move to increasingly higher usage of IMRT and IGRT (5). At present, it is critical that clinicians, dosimetrists, and physicists carefully communicate about this issue as we move forward with complex IMRT-based technologies that may in the end cause more secondary malignancies. In general, the increased doses and anatomic conformality allowed by IMRT and IGRT are likely to be more beneficial (6) than the cost of increased integral dose, but this is not yet backed by long-term data of 20 or more years duration (7). Image guidance further confuses the issues as very large volumes of tissue are often receiving low doses of radiation on a daily basis.

After a short discussion of immobilization, anesthesia, and image guidance, the various diseases (essentially different from adult cancer) are discussed separately, as the issues concerned with each are diverse. Methods for treating and for treatment planning will be reviewed with special emphasis on new modalities and techniques. Tolerance of normal structures is not specifically covered here as it is beyond the scope and complexity of this chapter and it is well covered in *Pediatric Radiation Oncology* by Halperin, Constine, Tarbell, and Kun. The Children's Oncology Group (COG) is currently looking at exploring this topic in a prospective fashion. Current protocols place goal doses for normal anatomy (often with the chemotherapy lowering normal tolerance dosing to some degree). This has been recognized by the leadership in radiation oncology in COG as an area of critical importance.

If possible, children should be treated on protocols in the definitive setting. We are in an era of rapid technological change and we need to collect data on the new modalities of treatment. Some offer enormous promise but may hide enormous costs. In fact, our success in pediatric cancer has opened up a new horizon in pediatric radiation oncology—reirradiation. At present, there is little data in this realm, but the newest technologies will come to bear so as to minimize dose to tissue that has already seen some treatment in the past. Toxicity to wide margin re-treatment is high, so stereotactic body irradiation, proton therapy, and SRS will likely plan a role in this nascent field (8,9).

IMMOBILIZATION OF THE CHILD

Children resist immobilization. As mentioned earlier, tumor targeting with accurate dose delivery is even more important with children than with adults. Fields are smaller, margins are tighter, anatomy is smaller, and critical structures are more sensitive. This dichotomy becomes a major problem in the radiation oncology of pediatric cancers. Often, the more children are restrained, the more they struggle to move. Consequently, one should carefully and practically immobilize only the region of the anatomy that requires immobilization. In the process of developing immobilization, child life personnel can help to make the child more comfortable with the devices and concepts of immobilization. In some instances, they can allow the avoidance of anesthesia (Fig. 32.1).

Bite blocks, thermoplastic masks, and body casts are good methods of ensuring accurate and consistent setups and beam delivery. Bite blocks and thermal masks are particularly good for head immobilization. Body casts can be made with plaster of Paris strips, polyurethane molds (Alpha Cradle), or vacuum bags (Vac-Lok). It may simplify future setups to allow the child ample opportunity to play with and get accustomed to the immobilization device. Although virtual simulation significantly reduces the time necessary for a child to endure the simulation process, it may be useful to have the child repeat the setup to check immobilization and to gain some additional

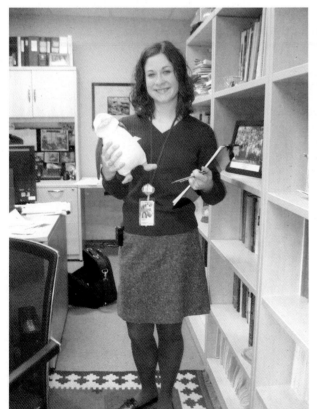

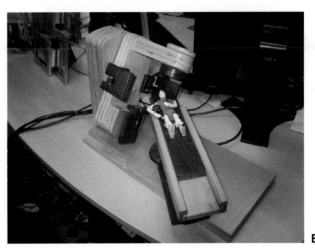

Figure 32.1. The use of child life experts allows the incorporation of teaching tools into the process of immobilization early, often weeks before a simulation day. This can often help a nervous child to be happy to use a mask like "his penguin's mask" and can sometimes avoid the use of anesthesia. It is critical to familiarize pediatric patients with the devices they will experience and the child life is very important in the overall process from consultation to the follow-up. The penguin's mask was custom-made by Jeffrey Buchsbaum and his team with pieces of Aquaplast material (**A**). A toy linac was designed by Jeffrey Buchsbaum for teaching purposes as well (**B**).

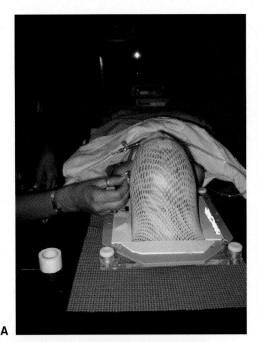
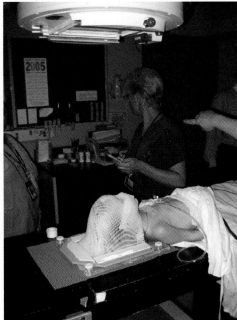
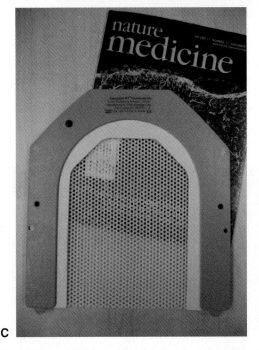
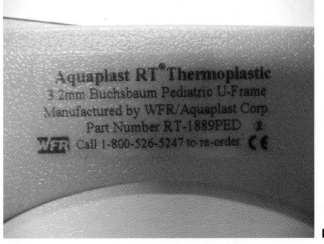

Figure 32.2. Pediatric simulation under anesthesia (**A** and **B**) with a prototype of a special mask for pediatric use with an insert that can be custom-ordered for skull size matching (note, the author Jeffrey Buchsbaum does not receive any funding/royalties from the sale of this device) (**C** and **D**). The patient was enrolled on COG ACNS0121.

comfort with their device. A dry run may help make the "real" simulation proceed more smoothly. If targeting and immobilization become problematic, sedation should be considered. The simulation process can be significantly lengthened when cooperation of an unsedated child is required. Figure 32.2 shows the setup and immobilization of a child. Ample room must be available for the anesthesiology team to setup and do their work. Immobilization devices should always be constructed for nonsedated

treatment because the need for anesthesia or sedation may decrease as the child adapts to the treatment process.

ANESTHESIA

Although modern, general anesthesia (GA) is essential for the treatment of babies and very young children, on a daily basis, it is time consuming and labor intensive, requiring expertise and special equipment for patient monitoring (which can be a problem in some RT departments and adult hospitals) as well as for administration of the anesthetic.

Fortney, Halperin, Hertz, and Schulman (10) have given an excellent description and discussion of the subject, where they review the need for and application of anesthesia in 512 patients under the age of 16. Anesthesia is generally necessary for children under 3 years of age and rarely required for children over 5 years of age.

With the advent of IMRT and IGRT, treatment times are increasing. In the cross section of risk, it is generally felt that time under the effects of GA should be minimized if at all possible. In the design of pediatric plans, elapsed time needs to be evaluated carefully along with the same constraints as adults. Segmentation efficiency of planning systems is critical and research in this area will be critical to help minimize toxicity to the population of patients described in this chapter who are under GA. An IMRT plan generated and treated is shown in Figure 32.3. In its

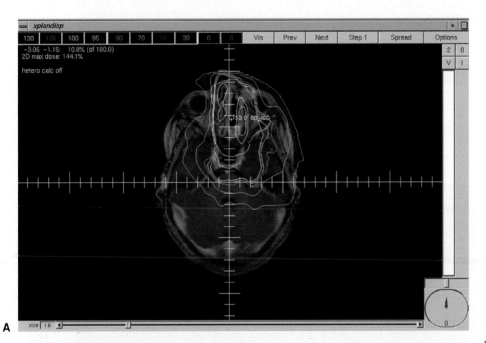

A

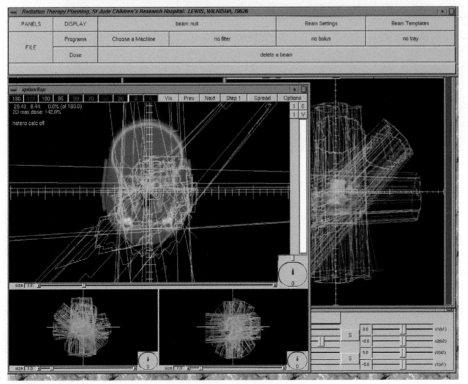

B

Figure 32.3. An intensity-modulated radiotherapy (IMRT) plan optimized for a recurrent chondrosarcoma not only for dose, but also for anesthesia exposure time (**A** and **B**). This plan could be completed within 15 minutes and used over eight noncoplanar beams, each of which was subsegmented via IMRT. The segmentation algorithm was written by Alf Siocchi, PhD. An example of newer planning software using noncoplanar partial arc therapy is shown for a supratentorial tumor (**C**). The treatment time for this newer technique was 3 minutes plus 3 minutes to make one table kick. Another example of this is shown for a low-grade salivary gland tumor in a fashion to further illustrate partial arcs that were selected to minimize integral dose and yield a plan that was superior to any static IMRT plan we could generate up to 13 beams (**D**). (Image supplied by Bruce Phillips while working with Jeffrey Buchsbaum.)

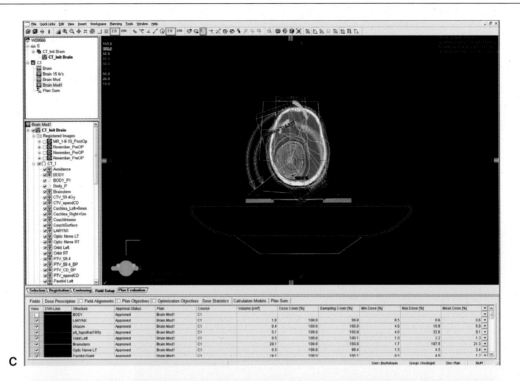

C

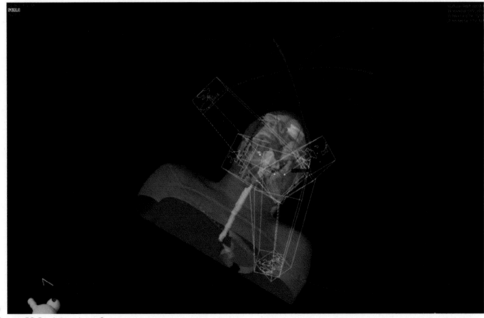

D

Figure 32.3. (*Continued*)

initial form, this plan would have taken 30 to 40 minutes to deliver a dose. After several days of optimization, the same dosimetry was achieved in a 15-minute time slot. Newer techniques can deliver this treatment in minutes using arc therapy, but at the possible cost of integral dose. One often needs to be clever and use small partial arcs to gain a dosimetric advantage without a huge integral dose penalty. The radiation oncology team must balance integral dose against time on the table, conformality, and critical structure sparing. In some cases, a few well-chosen beams that do not pass through critical structures may provide a better result.

IMAGE GUIDANCE

Although daily image guidance might significantly benefit the pediatric population, its use needs to be balanced against the long-term risks of increased radiation dose. In January 2008, the Alliance for Radiation Safety in Pediatric Imaging launched its Image Gently, Step Lightly campaign designed to reduce the radiation dose received by children during imaging procedures (11,12). In the past, children frequently underwent imaging procedures that were designed for adult patients, which generally delivered more radiation dose than was necessary to get the

TABLE 32.1 Imaging Doses from OBI (14)

Site	Dose per imaging session (cGy)		
	kV portal imaging	MV portal imaging	kV CBCT
Linac OBI			
Head/neck	0.1–0.3	2–8	0.1 (XVI) to 1.1 (OBI 1.3)
Pelvis	0.1–0.3	2–8	2.4 (XVI) to 5.4 (OBI 1.3)
			OBI 1.4 is lower (124)
SRS/SBRT			
CyberKnife	0.01–0.2	n/a	
Novalis Brainlab	0.0334–0.0551	n/a	

required information. This campaign suggests that imaging procedures be appropriately child-sized, frequently cutting the dose in half to get the same level of information. A major advantage of image guidance is that it allows margins to be reduced and smaller target volumes to be treated to therapeutic doses. Imaging volumes, however, are generally somewhat larger than target volumes. Frequent imaging may introduce a significant dose to a larger volume. It is important for the radiation oncologist to consider this dose when imaging protocols are established. Optimal techniques delivering minimal dose to the smallest overall volume should be planned. Table 32.1 shows some expected (13) doses for various imaging techniques to be considered and includes data from the AAPM Task Group 75 report (14). Since imaging doses significantly depend upon x-ray energy, technique, and where the dose is delivered, it is difficult to compare or combine therapy and imaging doses. Table 32.1 is provided for general guidance and pediatric imaging protocols should be carefully established.

Portal imaging practices within the COG were reviewed in a paper by Olch. They found that much could be done to reduce imaging dose to tissue outside the treatment volume. Their recommendations include: (1) use a single exposure when the area of interest is large enough to see reference anatomy, (2) minimize the additional area irradiated when a second exposure is necessary, (3) check record and verify parameters and light field shapes against treatment plan parameters and beam's eye view, (4) image during treatment when possible, (5) use kV imaging rather than MV imaging when possible, and (6) use the minimum number of monitor units possible to get a readable image. Imaging is thought to add 0.3% to 12% more lifetime risk of a cancer. Something to keep in mind is the effective dose while flying in the continental USA on a commercial flight has been estimated to be 0.0003 cSv/h (15). The effective dose of a CT of the head (adult) is felt to be 0.15 cSv or about 50 times flying for 10 hours (16). An adult CT of the chest is felt to be about 0.54 cSv or about 180 times the dose from flying 10

hours (17). The effective doses of an abdominal CT scan for an adult, a young adult, and a child are 0.39, 0.44, and 0.61 cSv, respectively, in the literature (18). Newer CT scanners and more attention to this issue have made the current exposures lower. It is advised that a department measure their equipment and review the sequences used for all patients in the simulator and on the machine so as to achieve doses that are "as low as reasonably achievable (ALARA)" (19–21).

LEUKEMIA

Clinical Overview

Acute lymphoblastic leukemia (ALL) is the most common cancer in children treated by the radiation oncologist, although the indications for radiation therapy have diminished in the past several years. Concerns about the long-term sequelae from radiation treatment and improvements in chemotherapeutic regimens have fueled the debate about the role of radiation therapy for ALL. Table 32.2 lists the indications.

Total body irradiation (TBI) is frequently given as part of the preparatory regimen for bone marrow transplanta-

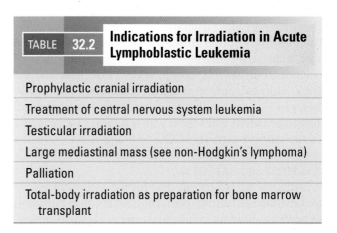

TABLE 32.2 Indications for Irradiation in Acute Lymphoblastic Leukemia

Prophylactic cranial irradiation

Treatment of central nervous system leukemia

Testicular irradiation

Large mediastinal mass (see non-Hodgkin's lymphoma)

Palliation

Total-body irradiation as preparation for bone marrow transplant

tion. Although it was originally given alone, TBI is much more effective when chemotherapy is also employed. Therefore, typical regimens consist of cyclophosphamide and TBI or cyclophosphamide and busulfan, as TBI is primarily employed for immunosuppression. TBI regimens are, therefore, part of allogeneic but not autologous transplantations. Although single-dose TBI can be employed, fractionated regimens are now generally used with or without lung shielding and electron boosts to the chest wall.

Prophylactic cranial irradiation (PCI) used to be routinely prescribed as part of the consolidation of remission in all patients following the experience at St. Jude's Hospital (22). Today, however, because of the potential late effects on pituitary (growth effects) and cerebral function (neurocognitive deficits), its use is quite variable among single institutions and cooperative groups. Improved long-term survival has caused additional concern about the development of secondary, radiation-induced malignancies (23). Although some use PCI in most patients, it has been virtually eliminated by others. Almost all centers have lowered the dose from 24 to 18 Gy at 1.5 Gy per fraction and lower doses are currently under investigation (24). However, all would agree that cranial irradiation—often craniospinal irradiation (CSI)—is indicated for overt central nervous system (CNS) leukemia (25,26). Currently, it is a standard of care to use cranial irradiation in patients that are CNS 3 (≥5 white blood cells [WBCs] per μL) and slow responders in high-risk populations. The current COG trial for high-risk ALL evaluates 12 Gy for slow early responders and 18 Gy for CNS 3 patients (COG trials AALL0232 and AALL0434). New data from St. Jude has been presented, which suggests that high-dose chemotherapy may be able to achieve equivalent cure, but without data regarding the long-term toxicity of chemotherapy or the salvagability of those patients, if they relapse.

Testicular irradiation is no longer given as prophylactic treatment, although it reduced the incidence of testicular relapse, because it had no influence on survival in one reported trial (27). Routine testicular biopsy on boys in remission at the end of therapy also used to be popular, with approximately a 10% to 15% yield (22). Approximately 60% to 70% of patients can be cured with intensive chemotherapy plus bilateral testicular irradiation to 24 Gy (27). All cases of overt testicular relapse must be treated with bilateral irradiation in addition to reinduction of chemotherapy, as relapses can occur in the contralateral testis. Although persistent disease sometimes occurs with 24 Gy in 12 fractions, this dose is generally recommended. Testicular radiation for those with testicular disease is part of the current high-risk COG trial and is given during consolidation at 24 Gy in 12 fractions (COG trials AALL0232 and AALL0434).

Palliative RT is very effective for the control of symptomatic masses causing pain, chloromas (most common in acute myeloblastic leukemia), and renal involvement.

More often than not this is performed just before death, and the total doses of 2 to 6 Gy are usually highly effective.

Lesions such as histiocytosis X often respond to very low doses of radiation therapy. One typical dose scheme used is 9 Gy in six fractions. This low-dose approach limits long-term toxicity and allows follow-up dosing to more historical doses such as 30 Gy while still staying within most toxicity thresholds, ultimately without causing growth and hormonal dysfunction. 3DCRT is often sufficient to give very good dose distribution without requiring long treatment times.

Treatment Planning

Central Nervous System Irradiation

Whole-brain irradiation is most often accomplished with opposed lateral fields. The patient is treated supine unless the spine is also to be treated. The field size is set to encompass the whole brain, with the helmet technique to exclude the anterior part of the eyes. The optic nerve is a site for relapse and must be included, as must the cribriform plate. This results in tight ports in the superior and posterior orbit. Setting the center of the field to the posterior orbit and blocking to protect the anterior portion of the orbit also eliminates beam divergence to the opposite eye. The radiation beam energy usually employed is 6-MV x-rays, although 4-MV or cobalt teletherapy can be used as effectively for most children. Lens dose can also be reduced by rotating the beam posteriorly ~5 degrees (28). Virtual simulation is crucial once the anatomy is contoured as patients are often asymmetrical.

If it is necessary to match the brain field with a spinal field, the patient is generally treated in the prone position, and the couch can be kicked for each lateral brain field to produce a nondivergent edge at the inferior border. This edge can be matched to the top of the spinal field with a small gap (0.5 cm or less). The angle of the couch kick is arctan (L/2 × SAD), where L is the length of the brain field and SAD is the source-to-axis distance of the treatment machine.

The spinal field in most children can be treated with a single (posteroanterior [PA]) field. Therefore, the match to the brain field becomes the prime issue. Rotating the couch to a 90 degree position and rotating the gantry to direct the upper edge of the spinal field straight up can achieve a long field with a good match. The gantry angle is given by the arctan mentioned earlier, where L is the length of the spinal field. Alternatively, if the spinal field is small, a half-beam block can be used.

If the spinal field and the brain field must be matched, it is wise to migrate the border of the match at least twice during the course of treatment. The benefit to migrating the match line is shown in Figure 32.4. Including three match line changes improves the dose uniformity by ~15%. An excellent discussion of craniospinal field matching techniques is given in Chapter 13 of *The Physics of*

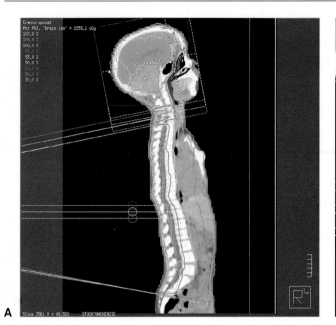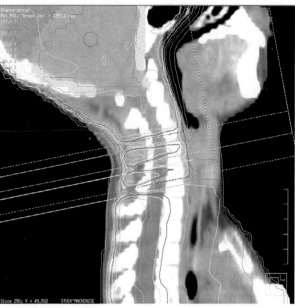

A

B

Figure 32.4. Craniospinal field matching with the traditional 3-day feathering technique. Spinal fields are treated at 130 cm source-to-surface distance (SSD) to allow a single spinal field. The match between the brain and the spine field has a 0.5-cm gap with no couch kick for the brain fields. Brain isocenter remains fixed. The spine isocenter is shifted by 1.5 cm each day, and the inferior border of the brain fields is also shifted to maintain the gap. The inferior border of the spinal field is decreased. **A:** The field arrangements on a sagittal projection. **B:** An enlarged image in the region of the gap.

Radiation Therapy (29). A review of the techniques used by Pediatric Oncology Group (POG) participants showed a surprising diversity in methods. Match line feathering was used by most institutions. Both prone and supine methods have been published, and one method that developed at the Cleveland Clinic avoids junction shifts by the use of wedges to "smear" the dose at the junction (30). The latter places an isocenter at the junction. Care must be employed to make the dose to junctioned areas equal, as unexpected dosimetry can result if the dose to adjacent areas is different (31).

Modern IMRT techniques allow the match to be optimized using either forward or inverse planning. The spinal field is designed to overlap with the brain field and the dose uniformity to the spine is set as an objective. The inverse planning engine will then derive optimal segmentation on the spinal field to optimize the field matching. This method allows the same fields to be treated each day with appropriate field segmentation, but may not necessarily provide the setup error tolerance of more conventional techniques.

Spinal cord irradiation has also been done with a single posterior electron-beam portal (32). In this technique the electron energy is chosen so that the 90% isodose line falls ~7 mm anterior to the anterior cord. Bolus is designed to treat uniformly to this depth. The concern with electron irradiation of the spine is the effects of dose inhomogeneity associated with the presence of higher density bone (33). Although the electron technique may work well with very young patients, it may underdose patients when the depth of the cord exceeds 6 cm. Combinations of photons

and electrons may sufficiently treat the cord and spare anterior structures. Careful planning that allows combinations of photons and electrons can determine optimal beam weighting to accomplish this treatment (34). The use of protons has enormous promise as it may allow the blunting of most of the gastrointestinal (GI) toxicity associated with CSI and decrease the integral dose of the child in the spinal regions significantly (35,36). Currently, most centers outside Switzerland have used passive scattering to shape fields and that has caused some concern due to neutron generation. The long-term effects of this are unknown, but there has not been a report of unusually high second malignancy in those treated with passively scattered protons. Scanning proton therapy eliminates neutron generation from materials placed in the primary beam.

Most treatment planning systems provide a sagittal view of dose along the craniospinal axis. When dose variations along the spinal cord exceed 10%, compensators or beam segmentation can be designed and used to provide a more uniform dose to the craniospinal axis. Some institutions prefer compensators and others use beam segmentation. This is an issue of spatial versus temporal intensity modulation. Either method works.

Testicular Irradiation

Irradiation of the testes in pediatrics is most often done with a single anteroposterior (AP) field set to the smallest field of the accelerator. If a photon beam is used, it can be angled in the superior–inferior direction treating the testes tangentially. If an electron beam is used, it is setup *en face* to treat the testes directly. The penis is taped to the abdomen and out of the treatment field. The patient is placed in a frog-leg position. The scrotal sack may be taped to minimize the size of the electron cone needed. In all cases, a taping technique is used to avoid applying adhesive to the scrotal sack and penis shaft. The testes should be centered in the field, and a bolus may be applied to bring the center of the testes to the depth of maximum dose. The field may be reduced as the testicular mass decreases in size during therapy and electron energy should be chosen to minimize dose beyond the target if possible. Testicular boost in high-risk ALL patients can be added as part of TBI in the form of two 2-Gy fractions and has been employed at St. Jude on PM fractions of days 3 and 4.

Local Recurrence or Site-Related Disease

Treatment of local, isolated disease, whether nodal or otherwise, is site specific. In most children, individual sites can be treated with a simple AP/PA technique, with appropriate blocks for critical structures. If the spinal column is in the fields, the entire width of the vertebral body should be included. Similar clinical issues need to be addressed case by case. Although 3DCRT or IMRT may play a role in dealing with site-related disease, this role still needs to be determined and may be very site specific. Often, the simpler AP/PA approach may be sufficient.

Total Body Irradiation

TBI in children is very similar to that in adults. Doses of 12 Gy over 3 to 4 days in six to eight fractions is sufficient for immunosuppression. Dose is prescribed to midplane, typically at the level of the umbilicus. Compensators or bolus materials are used to maintain a dose uniformity of better than ±10% (Fig. 32.5).

A variety of treatment techniques have been used successfully (37,38). The advantage of the bilateral technique is that the arms shield the heart and lungs. The disadvantage is the general need for bolus or specially designed compensators. The AP/PA technique is inherently simpler but often requires whole or partial blocks to shield the heart and lungs. In general, higher-energy beams also improve dose uniformity but often require a spoiler or bolus to increase skin dose. A popular regimen is 12 Gy in six to eight fractions over 3 to 4 days. Institutions around the country have individualized the delivery of TBI. Lung blocking is typically employed lowering the midplane lung dose to 8 to 10 Gy. Computed tomography (CT) data can be useful for accurate lung dosimetry and block design (thickness). The cross section of lung blocking is a clinical decision made using treatment ports in many centers. New delivery device technology, such as TomoTherapy, may prove useful for more complex and accurate lung blocking and dosimetry (39). Currently, the use of MLC dose compensation and the dosimetry of the use of arms to block the lungs in lateral techniques has been studied using 3D planning systems and is the focus of clinical research (40). It is advantageous to keep the dose rate under 10 cGy per minute to help decrease emesis. Large treatment rooms are generally necessary for larger patients and are an advantage even with smaller patients. In addition to dose rate, immobilization is important because treatment can last up to 40 minutes or more. Institutions use various methods of immobilization; discussion of the merits of each type of device or positioning tool goes beyond the scope of this chapter.

Small children and infants require smaller fields and have relatively little variation in thickness throughout their anatomy. In addition, they often provide much less scatter than adults. Therefore, they can often be treated at

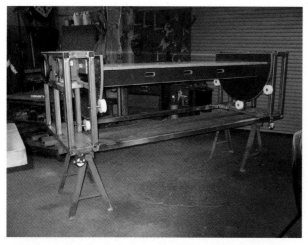
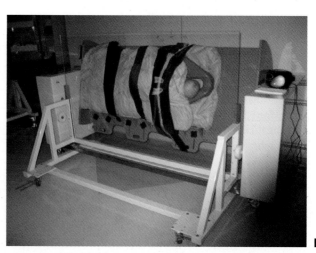

Figure 32.5. The total body irradiation (TBI) couch currently at use at Penn State and designed by Jeffrey Buchsbaum (inspired by the St. Jude device) is just one of many examples of immobilization devices used to simplify complex TBI procedure. In this case, 6-MV photon beams are used anteroposterior (AP) and posteroanterior (PA) and the patient is rotated on the table to allow treatment perpendicular to the beam's central ray. Commercial devices and simple institutional approaches are all in use and give very good dose distribution. The critical aspect of TBI is institutional comfort with a given device/position. It is shown under construction (**A**) and in use (**B**). It was designed to support 400 pounds.

an extended distance with a lower-energy beam. Consequently, many centers use a different TBI technique for children. Infants can be treated on the floor with the gantry at zero degrees, underneath a spoiler that may also support lung blocks. The infant can be flipped from the supine to the prone position to allow an AP/PA treatment.

Regardless of the technique, TBI should be set up as a special procedure with attention to the limitations of the room and equipment, as well as the nature of the patient. Most treatment planning systems do not permit treatment planning at the extended distances necessary for whole-body irradiation.

Individual patient dosimetry is important for monitoring the overall dose uniformity during treatment. Typically thermoluminescent dosimeters (TLDs) or diodes are used for the first or the first few treatments. Entrance and exit doses are measured at several points along the patient's anatomy. Adaptive RT was developed from the necessary improvements in TBI irradiation. Total dose or dose compensation can be adjusted as necessary. Subsequent measurements can be used to check setup reproducibility. It is not always possible to get a very homogeneous plan based on a child's anatomy. In these situations, it is often best to use lung dose and then normal tissue toxicity to guide treatment design. Compromises are almost always necessary in TBI.

LYMPHOMAS IN CHILDREN

Hodgkin's Disease

Clinical Overview

The disease process is essentially the same as in adults. For children, the concern is to provide the appropriate treatment for the minimum cost in late effects. Hodgkin's disease is predictably radioresponsive, chemoresponsive, and frequently curable by either modality, alone or in combination, allowing for choice in management. Since current long-term survival rates may approach 97%, concerns about long-term sequelae with radiation treatment, including radiation-induced second malignancies, are very real.

In the adult, total nodal irradiation up to 35 Gy may be used, but the potential sequelae are such that this is almost always inappropriate in children. Primary chemotherapy, usually followed by involved-field RT to a reduced dose (15–25 Gy), is often preferred. The disease is predictable in its propensity to relapse in unirradiated, initially involved sites, and therefore involved-field RT is used. Assuming complete remission has been obtained by chemotherapy, the reduced dose is appropriate on the reduced tumor burden. Occasionally, a child is treated with involved-field RT only (e.g., pathologically staged 1A midneck), but in that situation full-dose (25–40 Gy) RT must be employed. Adolescents who have passed through puberty may be treated as adults with extended fields to full doses. Overall results are comparable with those of adult therapy, but pediatric dosing is lower and is likely to lead to lower dose standards for adult Hodgkin's disease.

Treatment Planning

Involved-field RT in children requires precise staging and localization of involved nodes. Most treatments are done with an AP/PA technique to a reduced dose. The most common site is the neck and supraclavicular nodes.

For children past the age of puberty, extended-field RT can be used as in an adult. For supradiaphragmatic presentations, this usually includes a tailored mantle field followed by a para-aortic field treated to the level of L4. For subdiaphragmatic presentation, this usually includes para-aortic fields and inguinoiliac fields as an inverted Y.

The role of treatment planning in Hodgkin's disease has been reviewed (41). Particularly when wide-field irradiation is employed, it is important to calculate and carry doses to a number of points throughout the treatment field. The AP/PA technique, with appropriate custom blocking of critical structures, such as the lung, is preferred. Inhomogeneities should be included, especially in mantle fields. Dose compensators or beam segmentation should be used if the dose variation exceeds ±7.5% or per protocol guideline. The general practice in adults is not to have special immobilization devices, but these are frequently necessary with children. In the case of subdiaphragmatic presentations and the use of the inverted-Y technique, gonadal shields are not generally used, especially if the gonads are not close to the field. Nonetheless, for adolescents, the use of gonadal shielding is more likely to be advised, as the issues of parenting are critical. The use of TLDs or diodes as an *in vivo* dosimeter is advised in the treatment of children. Currently, early stage disease fields in favorable patients are shrinking. The general move is to use risk-adapted algorithms to determine treatment portal design. The extreme of this can be seen in the current series of studies in Europe (42–45). Hodgkin's disease is under intense study in terms of late effects on children, so dose and technique are likely to change in time so as to continue the high cure rates while hopefully decreasing toxicity (46).

The newest protocols coming out of COG for Hodgkin's now allow 3D conformal and IMRT treatment using photons and electrons. Radiation is delivered in a "risk adapted" fashion. The dose is still 21 Gy at 1.5 Gy per fraction. Current COG protocols require central review. All treatment plans are submitted electronically and must be reviewed prior to treatment.

Non-Hodgkin's Lymphoma

Clinical Overview

The spectrum of non-Hodgkin's lymphomas (NHL) in children is different from that of adult NHL. In childhood,

TABLE 32.3	Role of Radiotherapy in Childhood Non-Hodgkin's Lymphoma

Emergency radiotherapy
  Mediastinal masses
  Cranial nerve palsies

CNS irradiation
  Primary lymphomas (very rare)
  Established CNS disease

Localized disease

Bone lymphoma (uncertain value)

Transplantation (immunosuppression with total body irradiation)

CNS, central nervous system.

nodular histology is very rare and extranodal presentations are common. Management by RT alone has only historical interest, as the cure rate even in local disease is ~50%. With modern therapy, most patients are curable.

Simplistically, NHL is divided into lymphoblastic and nonlymphoblastic disease, with both forms being managed primarily with chemotherapy. For childhood lymphoblastic disease, leukemia-style regimens based on lymphosarcoma$_2$ leukemia$_2$ Leukemia$_2$ (LSA$_2$L$_2$) popularized by Norma Wollner at Memorial Sloan-Kettering (47) have been used successfully by (among others) the Children's Cancer Group (CCG) (48). This same study showed that for nonlymphoblastic disease an intermittent regimen of cyclophospha mide, vincristine, methotrexate, and prednisone (COMP) was superior to LSA$_2$L$_2$. Initially, all patients received local RT along with chemotherapy, but more recent results from the POG show that in 129 patients there was no difference in the pattern of relapse or survival (93%) for patients with local NHL treated with chemotherapy with or without (27 Gy) local RT (49).

Current indications for RT in childhood NHL are listed in Table 32.3. Emergency RT of symptomatic mediastinal masses (4.5–6 Gy in three fractions is often adequate) is sometimes required. Less commonly, it is used to reverse cranial nerve palsies. Primary CNS lymphoma is rare in children, but meningeal involvement in systemic disease is not. Many authors consider that CNS (cranial or craniospinal) irradiation is essential in the control of such CNS disease, as summarized by Donaldson (50). The results of cranial irradiation in CNS prophylaxis of NHL in children are not compelling (51).

Lymphoma of bone has traditionally been treated with involved-field RT (40–50 Gy) plus chemotherapy, but it is not certain that RT is necessary. The role of TBI for children with NHL is mainly immunosuppression before bone marrow transplantation.

Treatment Planning

Mediastinal masses are most often treated with a simple AP/PA technique. Although these are tailored fields, no special techniques are required because the cumulative dose is low. CNS treatment is discussed in the section on "Leukemia."

WILMS' TUMOR

Clinical Overview

Wilms' tumor of the kidney (nephroblastoma) is another neoplasm that is highly responsive to both radiation and chemotherapy. Even patients with advanced stage and unfavorable histology can often expect to be cured with aggressive chemotherapy, and the results of the National Wilms' Tumor Studies (NWTS) (52–54) have shown that patients with low-stage tumors can be managed with much less treatment. The disease staging system used in NWTS-5 is shown in Table 32.4. This staging system is still used for COG AREN532 and AREN533, the open studies at the time of submission of this chapter. Biologic criteria

TABLE 32.4	National Wilms' Tumor Studies (NWTS) 5 Staging System

Stage	Criteria
I	Tumor limited to the kidney and completely resected
II	Tumor extends beyond the kidney but is completely resected. Any tumor spillage confined to flank
III	Residual tumor confined to abdomen or lymph nodes in renal hilum or pelvis. May be tumor spread beyond the flank area
IV	Hematogenous metastatic disease to lung, liver, bone, or brain. Lymphatic metastasis outside abdomen or pelvis
V	Bilateral renal involvement at diagnosis

are far more significant in the current era, and the loss of heterozygosity in 1p and 16q is critical for risk stratification in the current COG set of protocols.

Patients are divided into risk groups: low, standard, and high. Radiation is indicated for local stage III disease, for metastastic disease sites (lung can avoid RT if there is a CR to chemo), and for any tumor treated with preoperative chemotherapy. Thus, on the current protocol, a child could have a favorable tumor by histology, stage II local disease, and lung metastases that respond completely to chemo, and avoid all radiation therapy. The precise doses per site of metastasis are complex and best evaluated via review of the appropriate protocol (55,56).

Treatment Planning

RT was historically delivered with an AP/PA technique. Fields are generally limited to the operative bed, which consists of the kidney outline and any associated tumor. The superior border of the fields should extend to the diaphragmatic dome only if there is a tumor present. Fields should overlap the entire vertebral body but exclude the other kidney unless there is bilateral involvement (57). New COG protocols provide normal tissue constraint doses. The new protocols allow 3DCRT and IMRT. Allowing IMRT on this protocol is a major departure from prior studies. Protons are not allowed on the current COG studies.

Indications for whole-abdomen radiation are given in Table 32.5. In the case of diffuse peritoneal disease, diffuse operative spillage, preoperative rupture, or multifocal gross disease, fields may extend from the diaphragmatic dome to the obturator foramen with the femoral head blocked. When whole-abdomen fields are treated, dose to the uninvolved kidney should be kept below 15 Gy. Because most patients receive only 10 Gy, this is often not an issue. This can be done with a kidney block on the posterior field at the start of treatment and an anterior block added when organ tolerance is approached. Typical dose fractions can be as high as 2 Gy or as low as 1.5 Gy for large treatment volumes. Figure 32.6 shows a typical treatment portal for a stage III operative-bed field. Figure 32.7 shows a typical whole-abdomen field.

When pulmonary metastases are present, bilateral lung irradiation may be concurrent with abdominal irradiation. Fields extend from the clavicles to approximately L1 (a lateral film or a CT data set will show the bases of the

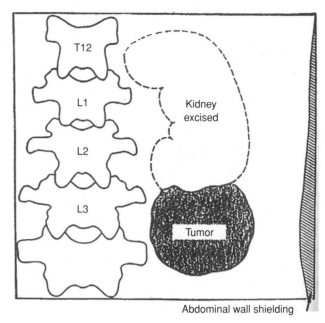

Figure 32.6. A typical treatment for a stage III Wilms' tumor patient's operative-bed field.

lungs), with the shoulders appropriately blocked. Mediastinal blocks are never used.

Historically, the issue of ovarian dose avoidance was addressed through surgical movement of the ovaries to the extent allowed by the ovarian ligament, oophoropexy. For unknown reasons, these surgeries were less successful in sparing ovarian function than first thought. One hypothesis for this is that the ovarian blood supply could not tolerate the degree of stress caused by these procedures. This could be studied in the future as a protocol question.

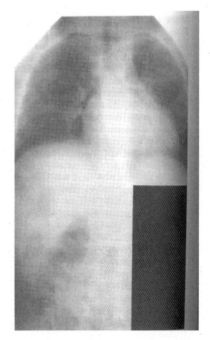

Figure 32.7. A typical whole abdominal external-beam radiotherapy (XRT) plan.

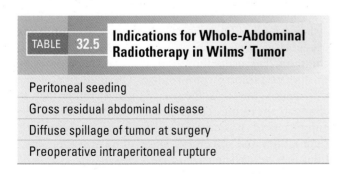

TABLE 32.5	Indications for Whole-Abdominal Radiotherapy in Wilms' Tumor
Peritoneal seeding	
Gross residual abdominal disease	
Diffuse spillage of tumor at surgery	
Preoperative intraperitoneal rupture	

NEUROBLASTOMA

Clinical Overview

Neuroblastoma remains an enigma, with prognosis depending not only on stage, age, and histology, but also on chromosomal observations, such as ploidy and N-myc amplification. The role of RT has diminished in recent years, as the good-prognosis tumors are often cured surgically and advanced disease usually indicates dissemination. More than half of patients with neuroblastoma present with demonstrable metastases at diagnosis. Several studies have indicated that there may be a role for radiation therapy with high-risk patients as part of a multimodality approach (58–61). Recent work has also demonstrated a role for intraoperative radiotherapy (IORT) using electrons to irradiate the tumor bed at the end of the surgical procedure (62,63). Benefit seems to be limited to cases where all gross disease is successfully removed. Table 32.6 lists the indications for irradiation in neuroblastoma.

The POG undertook a study for patients older than 1 year with stage C disease (histologically positive intracavitary nodes not adherent to primary tumor). These patients were randomized to receive wide-field irradiation to the regional lymph nodes or no RT. The dose was 24 to 30 Gy in 16 to 20 fractions. All patients received identical chemotherapy. Patients receiving combined-modality therapy had significantly higher incidence of complete remission and longer survival (24/33, or 73%) than those receiving chemotherapy alone (12/29, or 41%) (40). The benefit of RT does not seem be as relevant with infants (<1 year) (59).

In a very limited study, the use of IMRT was compared with the conventional AP/PA technique showing some limited benefit in terms of kidney dose (reduced 10–15%) for midline lesions (64). Care must be exercised so as to provide even dose to the vertebral bodies while also avoiding normal tissue. Conventional AP/PA treatment may actually be better for more lateralized lesions.

Proton therapy may also offer better coverage with lower morbidity because the improved physical dose distribution spares more normal tissue, especially the spine (65).

Bone marrow transplantation is frequently employed for patients older than 1 year who have disseminated disease at diagnosis (International stage IV, POG stage D) or who have relapsed. Various dose schedules are prescribed depending on the protocol.

Neuroblastoma frequently metastasizes to bone, and the orbit is a favored site. Total palliative dose may be as little as 10 Gy in 2-Gy fractions.

For a number of years metaiodobenzylguanidine (mIBG) has been used to treat refractory metastatic neuroblastoma in view of its initial use in scintigraphy of this disease. Experience in Germany of treatment in metastatic disease showed a number of responses (66). When incorporated into the initial treatment of advanced (stages III and IV) neuroblastoma, no significant improvement in survival was demonstrated (67).

Treatment Planning

Because of the limited role of RT in the treatment of neuroblastoma, there is little to say specifically relevant to the treatment planning for this disease. Irradiation of regional lymph nodes depends on disease presentation.

For abdominal presentations, the gross tumor volume (GTV) is defined as the volume of tumor before surgery and after induction chemotherapy as defined by CT or MRI. The clinical target volume (CTV) is defined as the GTV plus a 1- to 2-cm margin. If spine is defined in the CTV, it is generally extended to include complete vertebral bodies to minimize differential growth effects. The planning target volume (PTV) is the CTV plus a 0.5-cm margin.

IMRT planning typically will include at least seven beams, preferably coplanar to simplify treatment, oriented to minimize dose to critical structures. Noncoplanar beams may be required to avoid organs at risk and this is noted on the current protocol for high-risk disease. The dose objectives are: (a) to treat the entire CTV to 100% of the prescribed dose (typically 20 Gy), (b) to keep one-third of the ipsilateral kidney below 16 Gy (or less, often 10 Gy is attempted first), and (c) to keep two-thirds of the contralateral kidney below 16 Gy. Doses to the liver, spleen, and stomach should be calculated and kept reasonable. Dose will likely be raised in future studies to small volumes while at the same time immunotherapy is showing promise in advanced disease as well. Both approaches are being evaluated by COG at present.

Stage IV-S (POG stage D-S) is unusual in that the prognosis is often excellent, as spontaneous regression is common. The usual indication for RT is hepatomegaly causing respiratory compromise. The objective of the treatment is to reduce the size of the liver rather than to eliminate the tumor. The liver can be treated with a single anterior field; however, lateral fields mainly avoid the right kidney and spine (68). Doses of 6 Gy in three fractions may be sufficient.

TABLE 32.6	Indications for Irradiation in Neuroblastoma
Irradiation of positive regional lymph nodes
Total body irradiation
Symptomatic in stage 4-S
Palliation
Iodine 131, metaiodobenzylguanidine (mIBG) avid on scan
Per protocol, i.e., COG/SIOP study as appropriate, post-transplant residual regions, etc.

Children's Oncology Group.

RHABDOMYOSARCOMA

Clinical Overview

As rhabdomyosarcoma (RMS) is a malignant tumor of mesenchyme, it can arise at almost any site. The local treatment is therefore complicated by the tolerance of various developing normal tissues. It is unclear whether good prognosis is associated with favorable histology or favorable site because favorable sites often present with favorable histology. Figure 32.8 shows age at presentation, histology, and site of presentation. Favorable sites are orbit, paratesticular, vagina, vulva, uterus, and superficial head and neck. Unfavorable sites are bladder, prostate, extremities, parameningeal head and neck, trunk, retroperitoneal, perineal, and perianal. In general, favorable sites have higher incidence of embryonal histology, while unfavorable sites have higher incidence of alveolar histology. It is not clear whether histology or site drives the need for radiation therapy or more aggressive treatment. Favorable histologies in favorable sites may be cured with surgery and minimal chemotherapy. The ratio of male to female presentation is 3 to 2.

The Intergroup Rhabdomyosarcoma Study (IRS) has done much to define the treatment policies for this heterogeneous group of diseases. For the fourth study (IRS-4), the IRS grouping system based on the surgical findings (Table 32.7) is now used to determine the RT, and the tumor-node-metastasis (TNM) pretreatment staging classification (Table 32.8) is used for the chemotherapy.

In IRS-2, despite acceptable dose ranges of 40 to 45 Gy for children <6 years old with tumors 5 cm or less and 45 to 50 Gy for >5 cm in diameter (doses 5 Gy more for those 6 years and older), there was 30% local relapse in group III. This accounted for 48% of all relapses (69).

In IRS-3, the protocol doses for patients under 6 years were 41.4 Gy for tumors <5 cm and 45 Gy for tumors

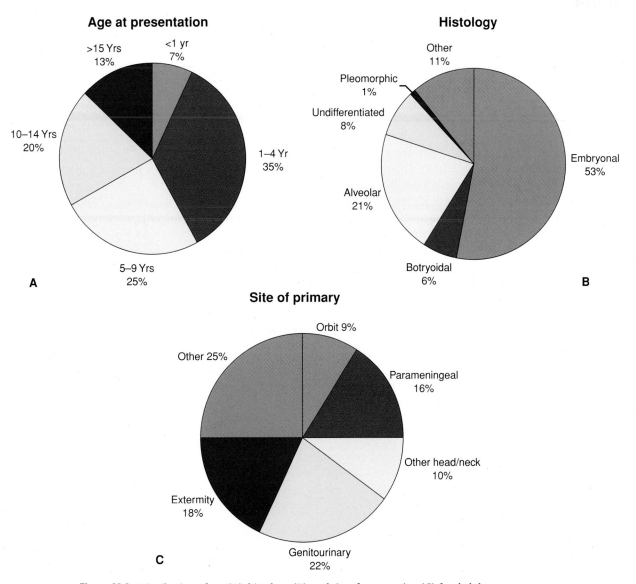

Figure 32.8. Distribution of age (**A**), histology (**B**), and site of presentation (**C**) for rhabdomyosarcoma.

TABLE 32.7	**The Intergroup Rhabdomyosarcoma Grouping System**
Group I	Localized disease, completely resected (regional nodes not involved; lymph node biopsy or dissection required except for head and neck lesions) a. Confined to muscle or organ of origin b. Contiguous involvement; infiltration outside the muscle or organ of origin, as through fascial planes
Group II	Total gross resection with evidence of regional spread a. Grossly resected tumor with microscopic residual disease b. Regional disease with involved nodes, completely resected with no microscopic residual c. Regional disease with involved nodes, grossly resected but with evidence of microscopic residual and/or histologic involvement of the most distal regional node (from the primary site) in the dissection
Group III	Incomplete resection with gross residual disease a. After biopsy alone b. After gross or major resection of the primary tumor (>50%)
Group IV	Distant metastatic disease present at onset (lung, liver, bones, bone marrow, brain and distant soft tissue and lymph nodes)

5 cm or more in greatest diameter. Doses were 45 and 50.4 Gy, respectively, for patients 6 years or older. The overall results of the protocol showed an event-free survival (EFS) advantage in group III patients over IRS-2 (70). Local control (LC) has been shown to be better for nonparameningeal head and neck RMS when doses >45 Gy are used. When tumor size exceeds 5 cm, LC improves for doses >47.5 Gy. For patients with high risk of meningeal impingement or intracranial extension, there appears to be an advantage to starting radiation therapy earlier. If there is no meningeal impingement, there does

not seem to be any effect from delaying treatment up to 10 weeks to allow chemotherapy before radiation therapy. Because modern imaging modalities have allowed us to better determine the extent of disease and adequately cover the tumor, the benefit of whole-brain radiation therapy (WBRT) has been greatly reduced (71–73).

In the review article by Schuck (74), 203 patients in clinical group 2 were analyzed to determine the benefit of radiation therapy. They found a benefit in 5-year LC, 83% versus 65%; EFS, 76% versus 58%; and overall survival,

TABLE 32.8	**Tumor-Node-Metastasis (TNM) Pretreatment Staging Classification for Intergroup Rhabdomyosarcoma Study 4**			
Stage	**Sites**	**T**	**N**	**M**
I	Orbit Head and neck (except parameningeal) Genitourinary (nonbladder, nonprostate)	T1, T2, a or b	N0, N1, NX	M0
II	Other sites	T1a, T2a	N0, NX	M0
III	Same as stage II	T1a, T2a T1b, T2b	N1 N0, N1, NX, M0	M0
IV	All	T1, T2, a or b	N0, N1	M1

T, tumor; 1, confined to anatomic site of origin; 2, extension; a, 5 cm in diameter; b, ≥5 cm in diameter; N, regional nodes; NX, clinical status unknown; N0, not clinically involved; N1, clinically involved; M, metastatic; M0, none; M1, present.

TABLE 32.9 **Radiotherapy in Intergroup Rhabdomyosarcoma Study 4**

TNM and site stage	IRS group		
	I	II	III
I	No radiotherapy	Conventional (41.4 Gy)	Conventional vs. hyperfractionated[a]
II	No radiotherapy	Conventional (41.4 Gy)	Conventional vs. hyperfractionated[a]
III	Conventional (41.4 Gy)	Conventional (41.4 Gy)	Conventional vs. hyperfractionated[a]
IV	Conventional (50.4 Gy)[b]	Conventional (50.4 Gy)[b]	Conventional (50.4 Gy)[b]

[a]50.4 Gy at 1.8 Gy daily vs. 59.4 Gy at 1.1 Gy b.i.d.
[b]If primary not resected.
TNM, tumor-node-metastasis; IRS, Intergroup Rhabdomyosarcoma Study.

84% versus 77% for patients treated with and without radiation therapy, respectively. No subgroup could be defined that would have equivalent outcome without radiation therapy.

IRS-4 was designed to test the benefits of further increasing the dose to 59.4 Gy using hyperfractionated radiation therapy twice-daily. This study failed to demonstrate an advantage to the higher radiation dose. The schema of IRSIV is shown in Table 32.9.

Treatment Planning

Because RMS has a variety of special presentations, it is necessary to approach each presentation systematically, according to the group. Because of the concerns about radiation therapy-related toxicities, especially in head and neck cancers, studies have been done comparing conventional RT techniques, 3DCRT, IMRT, and proton therapy. Proton therapy allows the best dose conformality with minimal dose to surrounding critical structures in some but not all cases. Both IMRT and 3DCRT are significantly better than conventional radiation therapy in reducing RT-related toxicities. How these various tools can best be used to treat RMS in its wide range of presentations continues to be investigated.

For many other presentations, it was originally thought that a large 5 cm margin was necessary to ensure LC and to prevent relapse. Current thinking is that a 2-cm margin on CT scan or MRI may be sufficient. For IMRT planning, the GTV is defined as the extent of disease at diagnosis (pre-chemotherapy volume). The CTV is the GTV plus 1 cm, and the PTV is the CTV plus 0.5 cm. Margins depend upon site, immobilization, and image-guided verification techniques. Therefore, tight margins may be reasonable for head and neck therapy, but inappropriate for other sites.

Figure 32.9 shows an IMRT treatment of an 11-year-old boy with an embryonal RMS of the maxillary sinus invading the lower half or the left orbit. The figure shows the initial fields treated to a dose of 36 Gy.

Figure 32.10 shows an IMRT treatment to the diaphragm of an 11-year-old girl with an embryonal sarcoma of the liver. This treatment was done post partial hepatectomy, with positive margins adjacent to the diaphragm. The treatment is shown to illustrate how IMRT planning allows sparing of sensitive and critical structures.

It is difficult to address all the special presentations of this disease other than to reemphasize the importance of early determination of the extent of the disease. Although 2-cm margins are probably adequate to treat most tumors and to shield normal structures and growth centers where possible, local recurrence for both IRS stages III and IV is the primary cause of failure in the treatment of this disease.

Pediatric Brachytherapy

Brachytherapy offers the advantage of delivering tumoricidal dose to a very limited volume. Therefore, it seems to be an excellent modality for many local childhood tumors, improving long-term control and reducing late morbidity. Genitourinary malignancies have been treated successfully with iridium 192 using a needle-template technique (75). Although most of these tumors were RMS, other sites and histologies have been examined (76,77). Brachytherapy may be useful in properly selected cases offering LC with little long-term morbidity.

EWING'S SARCOMA

Clinical Overview

The chemoresponsiveness of Ewing's sarcoma suggests that it may be relatively easy to cure. Unfortunately, metastases

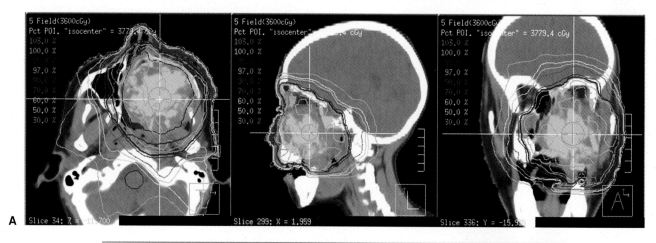

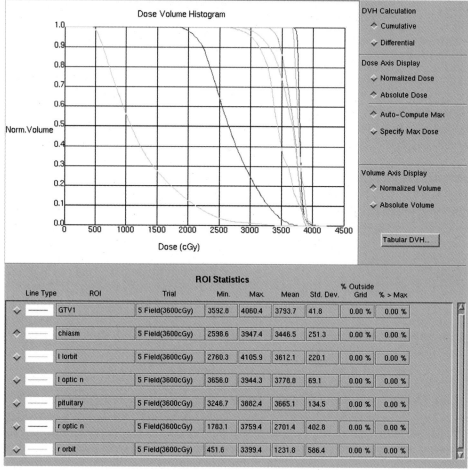

Figure 32.9. Intensity-modulated radiotherapy (IMRT) treatment for a 11-year-old boy with an embryonal rhabdomyosarcoma of the maxillary sinus invading the nasal septum and the lower half of the left orbit. The plan consists of five coplanar segmented beams. This was an initial IMRT treatment to a dose of 36 Gy that was followed by a reduced field plan to a total dose of 50 Gy.

remain the main cause of failure. The recent intergroup study, while showing that ifosfamide and etoposide improved results when added to vincristine, doxorubicin, cyclophosphamide, and actinomycin D (69% 3-year EFS), also showed that 65% of failures were systemic only (78). Prognosis is generally poorer for children that present with metastatic disease or with nonmetastatic disease, which presents in the pelvis.

Nevertheless, local management of Ewing's sarcoma is an important issue. Although early series suggested an advantage for surgically treated patients, it is clear that prognosis for both LC and survival depends on the size of the tumor (79). Smaller tumors in expendable bones (e.g., fibula, ribs) may be cured by either surgery or RT, although surgery is often preferred if the defect is minimal (80). Larger tumors are usually unresectable, although in some

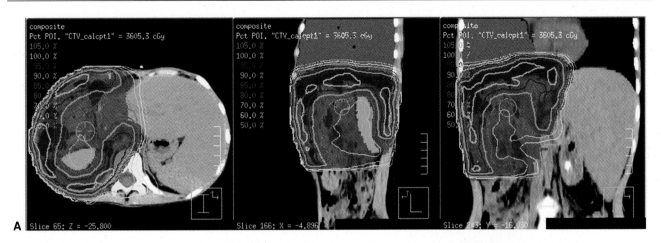

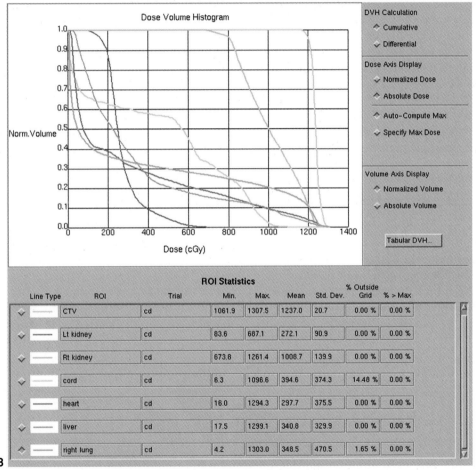

Figure 32.10. Intensity-modulated radiotherapy (IMRT) treatment for a 10-year-old girl with an embryonal sarcoma of the liver. The gross tumor was resected with a partial hepatectomy leaving positive margins adjacent to the diaphragm. This plan was designed to treat the entire diaphragm while sparing the surrounding critical structures. An automatic breathing control (ABC) device was used to minimize the effects of breathing motion. The child adapted well to the use of the device.

circumstances the optimum management includes debulking surgery plus RT (81). A review (82) of the Cooperative Ewing's Sarcoma Study (CESS) 81, CESS 86, and European Intergroup Cooperative Ewing's Sarcoma Study (EICESS) 92 trials showed that patients with responsive tumors after induction chemotherapy had good LC. Preoperative RT was indicated to avoid intralesional resection with comparable LC. After intralesional or marginal resec-

tions and when a wide resection had poor histologic response (>10% residual tumor cells in the resected specimen), postoperative RT may be indicated.

The original Intergroup Ewing's Sarcoma Study-1 (IESS-1) was unable to demonstrate a dose response at doses above 40 Gy (83). The earlier M.D. Anderson series showed a concerning number of second malignancies at doses above 60 Gy (84). The St. Jude study, with induction therapy of vincristine and doxorubicin (Adriamycin) followed by 35 Gy, showed a high incidence of local recurrence (85). The earlier POG study showed excellent (90%) LC with tailored portals (i.e., bony disease with a 5-cm margin plus soft-tissue extension) (86). The advent of the MRI has had a major effect on the definition of soft tissue and bone marrow extension.

Large tumors with major soft-tissue extension are relatively poorly managed; experience from the University of Florida suggests that hyperfractionated RT may offer some improvement in LC (87).

Treatment Planning

Ewing's sarcoma has a variety of presentations. In all cases, it is essential to determine the complete extent of disease using radiographs, T2-weighted MRI, and bone scans. It is important to have the extent of disease confirmed by a radiologist well trained in the particular imaging modality.

Although early POG protocols (88) suggested treating the entire bony disease with a 5-cm margin plus soft-tissue extension, the most recent POG study suggests tighter margins. In this study, the entire initial bony disease is treated with a 2-cm margin plus soft-tissue extension (tailored portal) as seen on T2-weighted MRI (89,90). This initial field is treated to 45 Gy in 1.8-Gy fractions. A reduced field is treated to 55.8 Gy. This boost field includes the soft-tissue component to the postchemotherapy volume with a 2-cm margin. There is no field reduction for the bony disease.

Large soft-tissue masses are treated with a 2-cm margin around the postchemotherapy soft-tissue tumor volume plus a 2-cm margin around the initial bony disease. In the case of a complete response to chemotherapy, the margin is reduced to 1 cm around the original abnormality. RT

may, under some circumstances, follow limb saving surgery when margins are suspect.

Presentations in the extremities are often treated with surgery or surgery combined with radiation and chemotherapy. When possible, treatment of the growth plates (epiphyses) should be avoided. In addition, uninvolved regions of the soft tissue should be left untreated to avoid interference with lymphatic flow and consequent limb edema.

BRAIN TUMORS

Brain tumors are the most common solid tumors in childhood. Supratentorial tumors tend to present with localizing signs, and infratentorial tumors frequently show evidence of raised intracranial pressure. The relative incidence of brain tumors in children is shown in Figure 32.11.

Supratentorial Tumors

Glioma

The current histologic classification divides astrocytoma into differentiated (so-called benign) anaplastic tumors (cellular, pleomorphic, mitotic figures, and perivascular cuffing) and glioblastoma multiforme (GBM), which requires evidence of tumor necrosis for diagnosis and is very rare in children. The World Health Organization (WHO) grading system classifies the juvenile pilocytic astrocytoma (JPA) as grade 1, differentiated astrocytoma as grade 2, anaplastic astrocytoma as grade 3, and GBM as grade 4.

JPA carries an excellent prognosis, however it is treated. Because it is most common in the diencephalon, RT is frequently employed. Differentiated astrocytomas that are

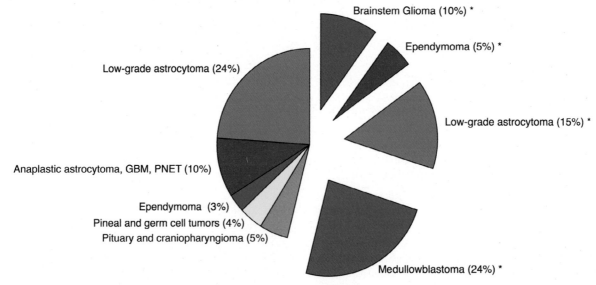

Figure 32.11. The distribution of brain-tumor histologies among pediatric patients. Approximately half of all pediatric tumors are brain tumors. GMB, glioblastoma multiforme; PNET, primitive neuroectodermal tumor. Infratentorial tumors are marked by an asterisk (*) in the figure.

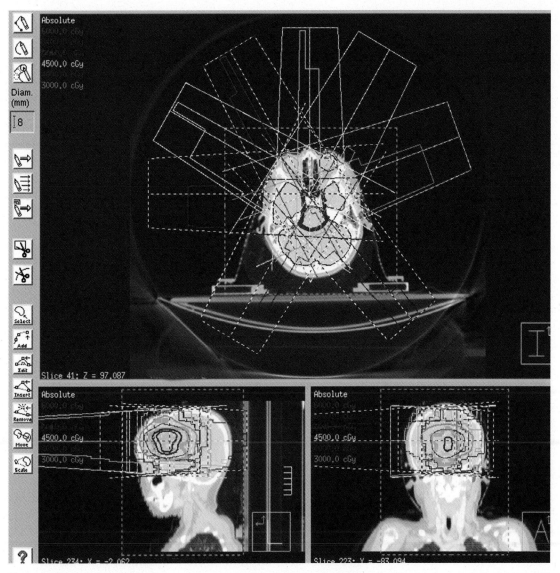

Figure 32.12. The plan shown represents an intensity-modulated radiotherapy (IMRT) plan for a patient with a World Health Organization (WHO) grade 2 lesion that was seen in consultation after two surgeries and 2 months of temozolomide. It was felt to be a higher grade tumor overall (WHO grade 3 or higher) on the basis of rapid progression and some magnetic resonance imaging (MRI) suggestions of necrosis.

completely excised are usually curable. However, they are usually only subtotally or partially removed, and therefore the question of postoperative irradiation or irradiation at recurrence is pertinent and is currently under investigation. The role of 3DCRT, IMRT, and proton techniques has been investigated in COG trial ACNS0221. Figure 32.12 shows an IMRT plan for a patient after two resections for a JPA and subsequent progression on temozolomide after 2 months and felt to be WHO grade 2. The tumor did not enhance with contrast, so the treatment in this case was designed to respect temporal lobes, visual pathways, and the cochleae. The patient's pituitary–hypothalamic axis was dysfunctional at the outset from the second surgery.

Anaplastic astrocytomas and GBM require aggressive management. A CCG study of RT alone versus RT plus lomustine (CCNU), vincristine, and prednisone showed an advantage for the patients treated with combined-modality therapy (91). Autologous bone marrow transplantation has been attempted with some success and also significant toxicity (92). Standard doses of RT are 50 to 60 Gy in 1.8 Gy to 2-Gy fractions to a 3-cm margin around the GTV as seen on the preoperative MRI and 1-cm margin on the boost to residual tumor. Stereotactic boosts are also under investigation.

Optic gliomas deserve special consideration. They are often associated with neurofibromatosis. Because of their usually indolent behavior, conservative therapy is sometimes appropriate. RT is highly effective at halting progression. Failure of chemotherapy to halt progression has raised the question of when to use radiation therapy, and, as such, it is now a question under investigation.

Other Supratentorial Tumors

The supratentorial primitive neuroectodermal tumor (PNET) is an aggressive infiltrative neoplasm that spreads widely throughout the CNS. It carries a poor prognosis despite aggressive CSI. CCG has had some preliminary promising data with RT and eight-in-one (vincristine, CCNU, procarbazine, hydroxyurea, cisplatin, cytarabine, dacarbazine, and methylprednisolone) chemotherapy. A 3-year progression-free survival of 49% was reported (93).

Pineal tumors include pineoblastoma (PNET of the pineal gland), and similar results to those for supratentorial PNET have been obtained with RT and eight-in-one chemotherapy or vincristine, CCNU, and prednisone. A 3-year progression-free survival of 70% is reported (94). Other pineal tumors include germ cell tumors, divided into germinomas (seminoma) and nongerminomatous (embryonal cell, choriocarcinoma) tumors. Frequently, the suprasellar region is also involved, giving rise to diabetes insipidus. Germinomas are easily cured by RT; but routine CSI is controversial (95). Germinomas are also chemoresponsive and have produced long-term survival with low-dose local RT and chemotherapy (96). Nongerminomatous germ cell tumors fare less well, but with aggressive platinum-containing chemotherapy and CSI, some cures have been obtained (97). The rare retinoblastoma case that involves the pineal gland is under investigation via COG trial ARET 0321 and receives CSI.

Treatment Planning

In general, treatment planning for pediatric brain tumors has evolved significantly over the past several years. Because of concerns about long-term sequelae, improvements in imaging for defining targets and treatment planning techniques are being used that minimize dose to normal brain yet effectively treat the tumor and regions of risk. 3DCRT and IMRT are more frequently used to treat the tumor and spare the surrounding brain. SRS and SRT are playing an increasing role in treating the boost volume (98,99). SRS or SRT is also often used to treat the postoperative tumor bed (100). SRT allows for more flexibility in fractionating the dose. Proton therapy is also being explored in an effort to further reduce the dose to normal brain and surrounding critical structures. For all these modalities, the treatment volumes and recommended radiation doses are comparable.

The GTV is the enhancement observed during the initial imaging study or at simulation. Frequently, this is the region of enhancement on a T1 MRI sequence with gadolinium enhancement (or as seen on a T2 or flair sequence for nonenhancing lesions). CTV is the GTV plus a 1-cm margin, while the PTV is the CTV plus a 0.5-cm margin. The general trend is to deliver at least 45 Gy to the whole brain at risk (wide-field irradiation), followed by a cone down to a more conformal boost volume.

For children between the ages of 2 and 5 years, typical doses are 50 to 54 Gy in 150- to 180-cGy fractions. Radiation should be delayed, if possible, for children under the age of 2 years, but for some tumors, such as in ependymoma, the radiation option may be better to use earlier. For children older than 5 years of age, the standard dose of 54 to 59.4 Gy is recommended in 150- to 180-cGy fractions.

As stated earlier, the role of WBRT has diminished, especially for children. For large lesions, such as diffuse gliomas outside the brainstem, opposed lateral fields may still provide appropriate coverage but come at a price. When the PTV can be made smaller, a three-field technique using wedges can provide a highly conformal dose distribution. A sagittal arc can further improve the dose conformality in many cases. Multiple, noncoplanar beams (5–14) can be used to further improve dose conformality. IMRT can further improve the dose conformality, but the increase in treatment time may not be warranted and counterproductive with pediatric patients.

SRT generally uses a hypofractionated treatment schedule, which may be highly preferred for children. Whether treated with conformal cone arcs, arcs with a micro-multileaf collimator (mMLC), conformal, mMLC fields with static fields, or IMRT with an mMLC, SRT offers precise, highly conformal dose distributions that spare the surrounding normal brain. The gamma knife is used for SRS and requires a fiducial frame mounted to the skull of the patient. Although treatment is a single day procedure, it can be a grueling process. The patient arrives in the morning and the frame is attached to the skull. The patient then goes for any necessary imaging studies then returns to the gamma knife suite. Images are transferred to the planning system and the planning process is started. Shots are added to the plan until the tumor is adequately covered by the 50% isodose line. CyberKnife (Fig. 32.13) therapy allows shorter anesthesia times, equivalent dose distributions, equal accuracy, and is, as such, a more pediatrics friendly SRS solution. Because of the beneficial physical dose distribution, protons are also being used to treat pediatric brain tumors (101).

Infratentorial Tumors

Infratentorial tumors include cerebellar astrocytomas, brainstem gliomas, medulloblastoma, and ependymoma.

Cerebellar Astrocytoma

Cerebellar astrocytomas are usually surgically curable (>80%) well-differentiated tumors. On recurrence, reexcision should be attempted, and if it is incomplete, irradiation (50–54 Gy) may be indicated, but there are few data supporting this (102). Anaplastic astrocytomas are rare in this location and should be treated like supratentorial anaplastic astrocytomas.

Brainstem Gliomas

Brainstem gliomas are usually deeply infiltrative, histologically aggressive on biopsy, and seldom curable. Children

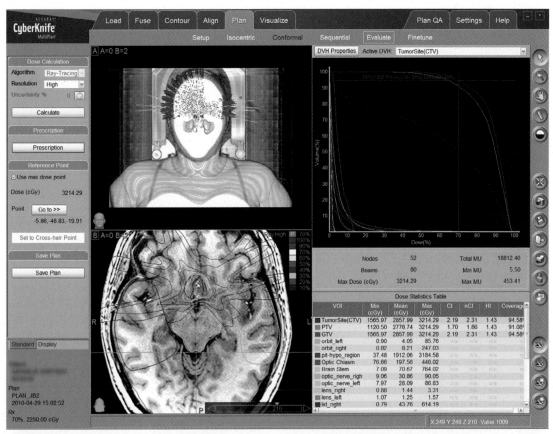

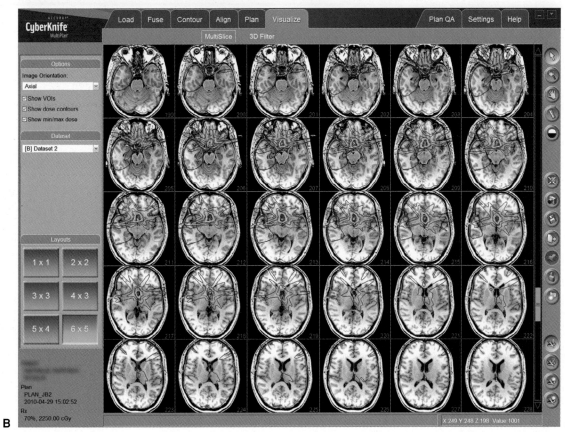

Figure 32.13. Cyberknife plan of a recurrent craniopharyngioma after a salvage surgery was able to remove all tumor within 10 mm of the chiasm. The patient had seen prior radiation and the new plan kept the chiasm dose to under 50 Gy when the current and prior plans were added together linearly (**A** and **B**).

with neurofibromatosis and those with exophytic tumors fare better. The standard dose of irradiation is 54 to 59.4 Gy (1.8-Gy fractions). POG 8495 studied four doses of hyperfractionated RT (66–75.6 Gy). There was no improvement with higher doses. The median time to progression was 7 months. There was a suggestion of higher complications of intralesional necrosis and skin reactions at 75.6 Gy, and it was therefore recommended to go no higher than 70.2 Gy (103).

Multiple national and institutional phase I studies are currently under way to study this disease with a large number of new agents. The typical radiation dose is 59.4 Gy at 1.8 Gy per fraction. Hyperfractionation has been abandoned at present.

Medulloblastoma

Medulloblastoma is a radioresponsive and chemoresponsive tumor that arises in the cerebellum and has all the histologic characteristics of a PNET. It is currently staged as high risk and low risk. High risk includes those with >1.5 cm³ of residual tumor postoperatively, high-grade

histology, or metastatic disease anywhere in the cranial–spinal axis (cerebrospinal fluid [CSF] or gross disease). What was once called anaplastic histology is now under investigation as a large percentage of these might be a new entity, atypical teratoid rhabdoid tumors (ATRT). These are treated on protocol with aggressive chemotherapy and craniospinal radiation. Standard risk is everything else (<1.5 cm³ residual, normal histology, and Chang staging M0).

CSI (54-Gy posterior fossa, 36-Gy neuraxis-standard dose RT) has been the yardstick for high-risk disease, with boosts to visible areas of metastatic disease to doses of 39.6 to 50.4 Gy. It is clear that high-stage tumors need chemotherapy in addition to standard-dose RT (104,105). When very young children fail to respond to chemotherapy or posterior fossa only radiation on protocol, CSI has shown efficacy but with toxicity relatively greater than that seen in older children (106,107) (Fig. 32.14).

The combined POG and CCG protocol for low-stage disease (POG 8631) compared standard dose with reduced-dose RT (54-Gy posterior fossa, 23.4-Gy neuraxis). The results were disappointing in that patients receiving

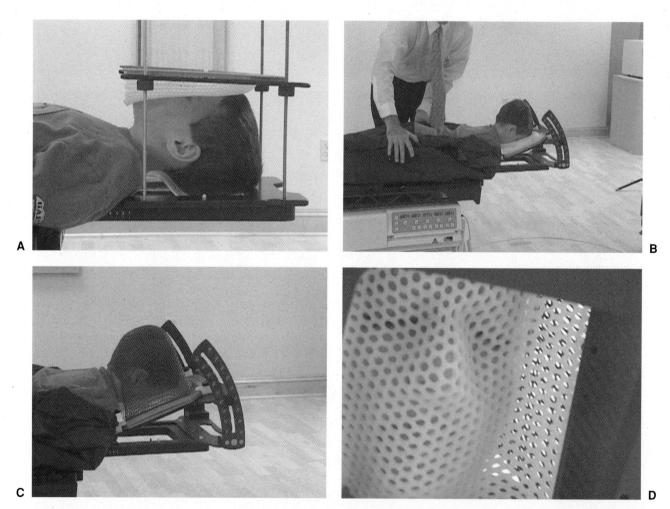

Figure 32.14. An example of a craniospinal immobilization device that takes many aspects of noncommercial devices the authors have used over the years and combines them. The device images are used with permission of the vendor (www.wfr-aquaplast.com). The device allows sedation of a prone patient. One makes the inferior half mask first (**A**), then moves the patient to the prone position (**B**), a posterior mask is made (**C**), and if needed an airway access region can easily be cut into the inferior half mask (**D**).

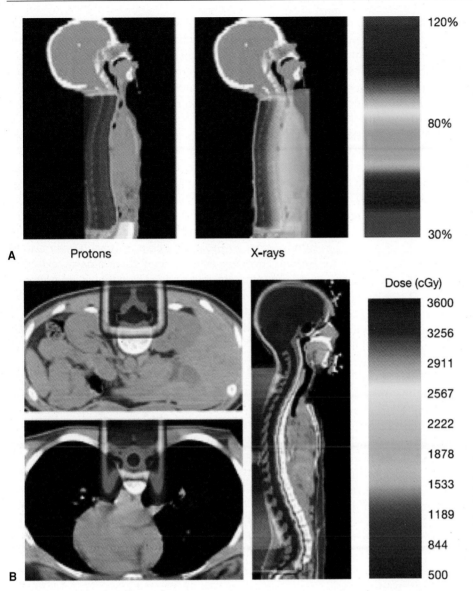

120%

80%

30%

A   Protons   X-rays

Dose (cGy)

3600
3256
2911
2567
2222
1878
1533
1189
844
500

B

Figure 32.15. Proton dosimetric plan of craniospinal irradiation (CSI) compared with photons. The difference between the abdominal doses (**A**). If a patient is fully grown, thecal sac targeting is also possible (**B**). (The image was provided by Torunn Yock, M.D., M.C.H. of Massachusetts General Hospital, Boston, MA, with permission.)

reduced-dose irradiation had a significantly higher incidence of isolated neuraxis relapse and a significantly lower 4-year recurrence-free survival (108). Improved, more intensive chemotherapy has allowed reduced-dose radiation therapy to assume a standard of care status. The volume of the posterior fossa boost is currently under study on the COG trial ACNS0331. It has been studied at St. Jude in trials SJMB96 (109) and SJMB03. ACNS0331 study is also studying reduction of the CSI dose from 23.4 to 18 Gy.

Protons allow improvement in craniospinal dosimetry (Fig. 32.15) as the abdomen can be avoided, significantly decreasing the toxicity of therapy (35,110). IMRT is felt to allow similar clinical toxicity reduction for the boost (6) and has been used for the entire CSI portion with less high dose delivered to the gut. Both techniques lack long-term data because they are so new, but it is likely that both will be included in all future protocols. Newer planning systems may allow the use of electrons to mimic some of the dosimetry advantages of protons (111). Indiana University and M.D. Anderson Cancer Center are currently doing

proton CSI in the supine position allowing for better setup reproducibility and safer airway management of these patients when they are treated with anesthesia.

Ependymoma

Although ependymoma may arise in other parts of the CSF pathway (112), it is most frequent in the fourth ventricle, and this discussion considers only that location.

The histology of ependymoma is quite varied, from benign to anaplastic (113). The standard treatment for fourth-ventricular ependymoma is RT to the posterior fossa, including the aqueduct and the upper cervical spine (114,115). In view of the nature of the tumor, which arises from the ependymal lining of the CSF pathways, craniospinal RT has been frequently practiced in the past, although it has always been controversial.

The initial POG study (POG 8532) gave 54 Gy to the posterior fossa for low-grade tumors. Isolated spinal failures did not occur. Local recurrences accounted for 90% of relapses, and late failures were reported.

A large, single institutional study, RT1, at St. Jude showed that conformal radiation therapy allowed superior control in completely resected ependymomas (116) and that intellectual development could be predicted by dosimetric parameters (117). The results of this study made up the data behind COG trial ACNS0121. In the St. Jude study, conformal radiation was used with automated treatment and with MLC and mMLC. In the COG trial, conformal radiation is required and the dose is 59.4 Gy to the tumor bed with no cone down performed unless one is over the cervical cord, where the cord dose is limited to 54 Gy. The new COG study is an extension of ACNS0121 with the primary goal being to ask a chemotherapy question.

Treatment Planning

Brainstem gliomas and anaplastic astrocytomas are treated much like their supratentorial counterpart. Medulloblastoma and sometimes ependymoma are treated with CSI. This is discussed in the section on "Leukemia." However, it is not necessary to include the optic nerve, but the cribriform plate, which is a well-recognized site of recurrence (118), must be covered. The posterior fossa must be boosted, with the anterior border covering the posterior clinoids and the superior border including 1 cm above halfway between the foramen magnum and the vertex (superior extent to tentorium cerebelli). The use of MRI fusion on these cases is highly recommended. Inferiorly, the field should cover the foramen magnum. Conformal boosts are likely to become the standard of care in time, but at present they should be used only on protocol and the protocol guidelines should be followed. Newer studies, such as COG study ACNS0121 for ependymoma, have specific study goals based on conformal radiation technology and radiation dosimetry and are based on large data sets, where conformal radiation therapy at single institutions was felt to be safe, effective, and part of a formula with good surgery that allowed decreased late effects (119).

RETINOBLASTOMA

Clinical Overview

Retinoblastoma (RB) is 60% to 70% unilateral and is nearly always detected in the first 3 years of life. Although only ~10% of all patients (nearly all with bilateral disease) have a positive family history, it is estimated that ~30% are familial.

Patients are usually cured, and enucleation is recommended for eyes that have little potential for useful vision, that is, most unilateral disease and frequently the worse (blind) eye in bilateral retinoblastoma.

At present, there is a shift in the overall management paradigm for retinoblastoma as arterial chemotherapy has shown enormous promise in trials out of Japan and more recently Memorial Sloan Kettering. COG is actively initiating research on this technique. At issue is the ability for interventional radiologist to produce drug delivery in a reproducible fashion. In time, it is possible that radiation will be used only in rare instances for RB patients. The presentation here is meant to serve as a reference in this context.

For small tumors (2- to 3-disc diameter), cryotherapy or photocoagulation can be used. Radioactive plaques may also be employed (cobalt 60, iodine 125, iridium 192, palladium 109). Recommended doses are 50 Gy to the apex and 150 Gy to the base (120).

External-beam RT is employed for larger (>3-disc diameter) tumors in which there is hope of vision. Smaller tumors close to the optic nerve or macula may also be treated. Formerly, doses of 3 Gy three times weekly were used, but with effective anesthesia patients are now routinely treated 5 days a week. Larger (10-disc diameter) tumors or tumors with vitreous seeding may be treated to 50 Gy. Smaller tumors usually respond well to 40 to 45 Gy. On study, it may remain viable to use external-beam treatment for salvage of chemotherapy failures.

Blindness follows RT in ~70% of patients with larger tumors. Cataract formation is frequent unless only the posterior globe is treated by a lateral portal. Of most concern is the development of a second malignancy, although retinoblastoma itself, particularly bilateral disease, is also a predisposition. It has been estimated that the latent period for development of the second tumor in unirradiated patients is 5 years longer than that of irradiated children (121). Protons are often used on RB patients so as to minimize RT integral dose, as they are superior in this regard to photons and electrons. In these patients, one must think of integral dose during the entire treatment process.

Treatment Planning

The standard historical treatment for retinoblastoma is a single ipsilateral beam. The field is angled slightly to minimize the dose to the lens. Alternatively, if there is anterior involvement particularly, an anterior 9- to 12-MeV electron beam with a lens block can effectively treat the entire retina (122). Accurate treatment planning for the latter technique requires the use of a pencil-beam algorithm that correctly incorporates the inhomogeneities of the human eye and its surrounding anatomy. The eye is treated with a circular field of diameter sufficient to include the entire globe of the eye. Photons can also be used (123). Because many authors think the disease is multifocal, in many centers the combined anterior and lateral approach is used. The ratio of dose from lateral to anterior is ~2.5 to 1. Radiation is still a primary agent in advanced RB and those patients are currently eligible for ARET0321 (for stage II–IV disease, including trilaterals).

ACKNOWLEDGMENTS

The authors acknowledge the help and support of Drs. Patrick Thomas and Moody Wharam.

REFERENCES

1. Rutz HP, Lomax AJ. Donut-shaped high-dose configuration for proton beam radiation therapy. *Strahlenther Onkol* 2005;181(1):49–53.
2. Merchant TE. Proton beam therapy in pediatric oncology. *Cancer J* 2009;15(4):298–305.
3. Kozak KR, Adams J, Krejcarek SJ, et al. A dosimetric comparison of proton and intensity-modulated photon radiotherapy for pediatric parameningeal rhabdomyosarcomas. *Int J Radiat Oncol Biol Phys* 2009;74(1):179–186.
4. Taddei PJ, Mirkovic D, Fontenot JD, et al. Stray radiation dose and second cancer risk for a pediatric patient receiving craniospinal irradiation with proton beams. *Phys Med Biol* 2009;54(8):2259–2275.
5. Lee EK, Fox T, Crocker I. Simultaneous beam geometry and intensity map optimization in intensity-modulated radiation therapy. *Int J Radiat Oncol Biol Phys* 2006;64(1):301–320.
6. Huang E, Teh BS, Strother DR, et al. Intensity-modulated radiation therapy for pediatric medulloblastoma: early report on the reduction of ototoxicity. *Int J Radiat Oncol Biol Phys* 2002;52(3):599–605.
7. Rembielak A, Woo TC. Intensity-modulated radiation therapy for the treatment of pediatric cancer patients. *Nat Clin Pract Oncol* 2005;2(4):211–217.
8. Merchant TE, Boop FA, Kun LE, et al. A retrospective study of surgery and reirradiation for recurrent ependymoma. *Int J Radiat Oncol Biol Phys* 2008;71(1):87–97.
9. Wara WM, Wallner KE, Levin VA, et al. Retreatment of pediatric brain tumors with radiation and misonidazole. Results of a CCSG/RTOG phase I/II study. *Cancer* 1986;58(8):1636–1640.
10. Fortney JT, Halperin EC, Hertz CM, et al. Anesthesia for pediatric external beam radiation therapy. *Int J Radiat Oncol Biol Phys* 1999;44(3):587–591.
11. Goske MJ, Applegate KE, Boylan J, et al. Image Gently(SM): a national education and communication campaign in radiology using the science of social marketing. *J Am Coll Radiol* 2008;5(12):1200–1205.
12. Goske MJ, Frush DP, Schauer DA. Image Gently campaign promotes radiation protection for children. *Radiat Prot Dosimetry* 2009;135(4):276.
13. Song WY, Kamath S, Ozawa S, et al. A dose comparison study between XVI and OBI CBCT systems. *Med Phys* 2008;35(2):480–486.
14. Murphy MJ, Balter J, Balter S, et al. The management of imaging dose during image-guided radiotherapy: report of the AAPM Task Group 75. *Med Phys* 2007;34(10):4041–4063.
15. United Nations Scientific Committee on the Effects of Atomic Radiation (UNSCEAR) annual report for 1993. The report is freely available at: http://www.unscear.org/unscear/en/publications/1993.html.
16. Mettler FA Jr, Wiest PW, Locken JA, et al. CT scanning: patterns of use and dose. *J Radiol Prot* 2000;20(4):353–359.
17. Huda W, Scalzetti EM, Roskopf M. Effective doses to patients undergoing thoracic computed tomography examinations. *Med Phys* 2000;27(5):838–844.
18. Ware DE, Huda W, Mergo PJ, et al. Radiation effective doses to patients undergoing abdominal CT examinations. *Radiology* 1999;210(3):645–650.
19. Jin DH, Lamberton GR, Broome DR, et al. Effect of reduced radiation CT protocols on the detection of renal calculi. *Radiology* 2010;255(1):100–107.
20. Dion AM, Berger F, Helie O, et al. Dose reduction at abdominal CT imaging: reduced tension (kV) or reduced intensity (mAs)? *J Radiol* 2004;85(4 Pt 1):375–380.
21. Brandberg J, Lonn L, Bergelin E, et al. Accurate tissue area measurements with considerably reduced radiation dose achieved by patient-specific CT scan parameters. *Br J Radiol* 2008;81(970):801–808.
22. Aur RJ, Simone JV, Hustu HO, et al. A comparative study of central nervous system irradiation and intensive chemotherapy early in remission of childhood acute lymphocytic leukemia. *Cancer* 1972;29(2):381–391.
23. Nathan PC, Maze R, Spiegler B, et al. CNS-directed therapy in young children with T-lineage acute lymphoblastic leukemia: high-dose methotrexate versus cranial irradiation. *Pediatr Blood Cancer* 2004;42(1):24–29.
24. Melin AE, Adan L, Leverger G, et al. Growth hormone secretion, puberty and adult height after cranial irradiation with 18 Gy for leukaemia. *Eur J Pediatr* 1998;157(9):703–707.
25. Bongers ME, Francken AB, Rouwe C, et al. Reduction of adult height in childhood acute lymphoblastic leukemia survivors after prophylactic cranial irradiation. *Pediatr Blood Cancer* 2005;45(2):139–143.
26. Winick NJ, Smith SD, Shuster J, et al. Treatment of CNS relapse in children with acute lymphoblastic leukemia: a Pediatric Oncology Group study. *J Clin Oncol* 1993;11(2):271–278.
27. Unal S, Yetgin S, Cetin M, et al. The prognosis and survival of childhood acute lymphoblastic leukemia with central nervous system relapse. *Pediatr Hematol Oncol* 2004;21(3):279–289.
28. Gold DG, Neglia JP, Dusenbery KE. Second neoplasms after megavoltage radiation for pediatric tumors. *Cancer* 2003;97(10):2588–2596.
29. Broniscer A, Ke W, Fuller CE, et al. Second neoplasms in pediatric patients with primary central nervous system tumors: the St. Jude Children's Research Hospital experience. *Cancer* 2004;100(10):2246–2252.
30. Sohn JW, Schell MC, Dass KK, et al. Uniform irradiation of the craniospinal axis with a penumbra modifier and an asymmetric collimator. *Int J Radiat Oncol Biol Phys* 1994;29(1):187–190.
31. Bentel GC, Halperin EC. High-dose areas are unintentionally created as a result of gap shifts when the prescribed dose in the two adjacent areas are different. *Med Dosim* 1990;15(4):179–183.
32. Li C, Muller-Runkel R, Vijayakumar S, et al. Craniospinal axis irradiation: an improved electron technique for irradiation of the spinal axis. *Br J Radiol* 1994;67(794):186–193.

33. Endicott TJ, Fisher BJ, Wong E, et al. Pulmonary sequelae after electron spinal irradiation. *Radiother Oncol* 2001;60(3):267–272.

34. Hood C, Kron T, Hamilton C, et al. Correlation of 3D-planned and measured dosimetry of photon and electron craniospinal radiation in a pediatric an-thropomorphic phantom. *Radiother Oncol* 2005;77(1):111–116.

35. Lee CT, Bilton SD, Famiglietti RM, et al. Treatment planning with protons for pediatric retinoblastoma, medulloblastoma, and pelvic sarcoma: how do protons compare with other conformal techniques? *Int J Radiat Oncol Biol Phys* 2005;63(2):362–372.

36. Yuh GE, Loredo LN, Yonemoto LT, et al. Reducing toxicity from craniospinal irradiation: using proton beams to treat medulloblastoma in young children. *Cancer J* 2004;10(6):386–390.

37. Van Dyk J, et al. The physical aspects of total and half body irradiation. AAPM Report 17, New York, 1986.

38. Galvin J, Curran W, D'Angio G. Practical aspects of total body irradiation. Radiation oncology physics. New York: AAPM physics monograph, 1987.

39. Hui SK, Kapatoes J, Fowler J, et al. Feasibility study of helical tomotherapy for total body or total marrow irradiation. *Med Phys* 2005;32(10):3214–3224.

40. Abraham D, Colussi V, Shina D, et al. TBI treatment planning using the ADAC pinnacle treatment planning system. *Med Dosim* 2000;25(4):219–224.

41. Hughes DB, Smith AR, Hoppe R, et al. Treatment planning for Hodgkin's disease: a patterns of care study. *Int J Radiat Oncol Biol Phys* 1995;33(2):519–524.

42. Gustavsson A, Osterman B, Cavallin-Stahl E. A systematic overview of radiation therapy effects in Hodgkin's lymphoma. *Acta Oncol* 2003;42(5–6):589–604.

43. Meyer RM, Ambinder RF, Stroobants S. Hodgkin's lymphoma: evolving concepts with implications for practice. *Hematol Am Soc Hematol Educ Program* 2004:184–202.

44. Yahalom J. Transformation in the use of radiation therapy of Hodgkin lymphoma: new concepts and indications lead to modern field design and are assisted by PET imaging and intensity modulated radiation therapy (IMRT). *Eur J Haematol* 2005;75(Suppl. 66):90–97.

45. Hakvoort-Cammel FG, Buitendijk S, van den Heuvel-Eibrink M, et al. Treatment of pediatric Hodgkin disease avoiding radiotherapy: excellent outcome with the Rotterdam-HD-84-protocol. *Pediatr Blood Cancer* 2004;43(1):8–16.

46. Hudson MM. Achieving cure for early stage pediatric Hodgkin disease with minimal morbidity: are we there yet? *Pediatr Blood Cancer* 2006;46(2):122–126.

47. Wollner N, Burchenal JH, Lieberman PH, et al. Non-Hodgkin's lymphoma in children. A comparative study of two modalities of therapy. *Cancer* 1976;37(1):123–134.

48. Anderson JR, Wilson JF, Jenkin DT, et al. Childhood non-Hodgkin's lymphoma. The results of a randomized therapeutic trial comparing a 4-drug regimen (COMP) with a 10-drug regimen (LSA2-L2). *N Engl J Med* 1983;308(10):559–565.

49. Link MP, Donaldson SS, Berard CW, et al. Results of treatment of childhood localized non-Hodgkin's lymphoma with combination chemotherapy with or without radiotherapy. *N Engl J Med* 1990;322(17):1169–1174.

50. Donaldson SS. Role of radiation therapy in non-Hodgkin's lymphoma in the child. In: Cassady JR, ed. *Radiation therapy in pediatric oncology*. Berlin: Springer-Verlag, 1994:123–131.

51. Mandell LR, Wollner N, Fuks Z. Is cranial radiation necessary for CNS prophylaxis in pediatric NHL? *Int J Radiat Oncol Biol Phys* 1987;13(3):359–363.

52. D'Angio GJ, Breslow N, Beckwith JB, et al. Treatment of Wilms' tumor. Results of the Third National Wilms' Tumor Study. *Cancer* 1989;64(2):349–360.

53. D'Angio GJ, Evans A, Breslow N, et al. The treatment of Wilms' tumor: results of the Second National Wilms' Tumor Study. *Cancer* 1981;47(9):2302–2311.

54. D'Angio GJ, Evans AE, Breslow N, et al. The treatment of Wilms' tumor: results of the national Wilms' tumor study. *Cancer* 1976;38(2):633–646.

55. Thomas PR, Tefft M, Compaan PJ, et al. Results of two radiation therapy randomizations in the third National Wilms' Tumor Study. *Cancer* 1991;68(8):1703–1707.

56. Thomas PR, Tefft M, Farewell VT, et al. Abdominal relapses in irradiated second National Wilms' Tumor Study patients. *J Clin Oncol* 1984;2(10):1098–1101.

57. D'Angio GJ, Tefft M, Breslow N, et al. Radiation therapy of Wilms' tumor: results according to dose, field, postoperative timing and histology. *Int J Radiat Oncol Biol Phys* 1978;4(9–10):769–780.

58. Castleberry RP, Kun LE, Shuster JJ, et al. Radiotherapy improves the outlook for patients older than 1 year with Pediatric Oncology Group stage C neuroblastoma. *J Clin Oncol* 1991;9(5):789–795.

59. Paulino AC, Mayr NA, Simon JH, et al. Locoregional control in infants with neuroblastoma: role of radiation therapy and late toxicity. *Int J Radiat Oncol Biol Phys* 2002;52(4):1025–1031.

60. Haas-Kogan DA, Swift PS, Selch M, et al. Impact of radiotherapy for high-risk neuroblastoma: a Children's Cancer Group study. *Int J Radiat Oncol Biol Phys* 2003;56(1):28–39.

61. Kushner BH, Wolden S, LaQuaglia MP, et al. Hyperfractionated low-dose radiotherapy for high-risk neuroblastoma after intensive chemotherapy and surgery. *J Clin Oncol* 2001;19(11):2821–2828.

62. Kuroda T, Saeki M, Honna T, et al. Clinical significance of intensive surgery with intraoperative radiation for advanced neuroblastoma: does it really make sense? *J Pediatr Surg* 2003;38(12):1735–1738.

63. Haas-Kogan DA, Fisch BM, Wara WM, et al. Intraoperative radiation therapy for high-risk pediatric neuroblastoma. *Int J Radiat Oncol Biol Phys* 2000;47(4):985–992.

64. Paulino AC, Ferenci MS, Chiang KY, et al. Comparison of conventional to intensity modulated radiation therapy for abdominal neuroblastoma. *Pediatr Blood Cancer* 2006;46(7):739–744.

65. Hug EB, Nevinny-Stickel M, Fuss M, et al. Conformal proton radiation treatment for retroperitoneal neuroblastoma: introduction of a novel technique. *Med Pediatr Oncol* 2001;37(1):36–41.

66. Schwabe D, Sahm S, Gerein V, et al. 131-Metaiodobenzylguanedine therapy of neuroblastoma in childhood. One year of therapeutic experience. *Eur J Pediatr* 1987;146(3):246–250.

67. Klingebiel T, Berthold F, Treuner J, et al. Metaiodobenzylguanidine (mIBG) in treatment of 47 patients with neuroblastoma: results of the German Neuroblastoma Trial. *Med Pediatr Oncol* 1991;19(2):84–88.

68. Peschel RE, Chen M, Seashore J. The treatment of massive hepatomegaly in stage IV-S neuroblastoma. *Int J Radiat Oncol Biol Phys* 1981;7(4):549–553.

69. Maurer HM, Gehan EA, Beltangady M, et al. The Intergroup Rhabdomyosarcoma Study-II. *Cancer* 1993;71(5):1904–1922.

70. Crist W, Gehan EA, Ragab AH, et al. The third Intergroup Rhabdomyosarcoma Study. *J Clin Oncol* 1995;13(3):610–630.

71. Michalski JM, Sur RK, Harms WB, et al. Three dimensional conformal radiation therapy in pediatric parameningeal rhabdomyosarcomas. *Int J Radiat Oncol Biol Phys* 1995;33(5):985–991.

72. Wharam MD, Meza J, Anderson J, et al. Failure pattern and factors predictive of local failure in rhabdomyosarcoma: a report of group III patients on the third Intergroup Rhabdomyosarcoma Study. *J Clin Oncol* 2004;22(10):1902–1908.

73. Michalski JM, Meza J, Breneman JC, et al. Influence of radiation therapy parameters on outcome in children treated with radiation therapy for localized parameningeal rhabdomyosarcoma in Intergroup Rhabdomyosarcoma Study Group trials II through IV. *Int J Radiat Oncol Biol Phys* 2004;59(4):1027–1038.

74. Schuck A, Mattke AC, Schmidt B, et al. Group II rhabdomyosarcoma and rhabdomyosarcomalike tumors: is radiotherapy necessary? *J Clin Oncol* 2004;22(1):143–149.

75. Leung S. Treatment of pediatric genitourinary malignancy with interstitial brachytherapy: Peter MacCallum Cancer Institute experience with four cases. *Int J Radiat Oncol Biol Phys* 1995;31(2):393–398.

76. Healey EA, Shamberger RC, Grier HE, et al. A 10-year experience of pediatric brachytherapy. *Int J Radiat Oncol Biol Phys* 1995;32(2):451–455.

77. Merchant TE, Parsh N, del Valle PL, et al. Brachytherapy for pediatric soft-tissue sarcoma. *Int J Radiat Oncol Biol Phys* 2000;46(2):427–432.

78. Grier HE. Improved outcome in non-metastatic Ewings' sarcoma and PNET of bone with the addition of ifosfamide and etoposide to vincristine, Adriamycin, cyclophosphamide and actinomycin. *Proc Am Soc Clin Oncol* 1994;13:4–21.

79. Donaldson SS. Ewing sarcoma: radiation dose and target volume. *Pediatr Blood Cancer* 2004;42(5):471–476.

80. Krasin MJ, Davidoff AM, Rodriguez-Galindo C, et al. Definitive surgery and multiagent systemic therapy for patients with localized Ewing sarcoma family of tumors: local outcome and prognostic factors. *Cancer* 2005;104(2):367–373.

81. Zogopoulos G, Teskey L, Sung L, et al. Ewing sarcoma: favourable results with combined modality therapy and conservative use of radiotherapy. *Pediatr Blood Cancer* 2004;43(1):35–39.

82. Schuck A, Ahrens S, Paulussen M, et al. Local therapy in localized Ewing tumors: results of 1058 patients treated in the CESS 81, CESS 86, and EICESS 92 trials. *Int J Radiat Oncol Biol Phys* 2003;55(1):168–177.

83. Dunst J, Schuck A. Role of radiotherapy in Ewing tumors. *Pediatr Blood Cancer* 2004;42(5):465–470.

84. Paulussen M, Ahrens S, Lehnert M, et al. Second malignancies after Ewing tumor treatment in 690 patients from a cooperative German/Austrian/Dutch study. *Ann Oncol* 2001;12(11):1619–1630.

85. Rodriguez-Galindo C, Billups CA, Kun LE, et al. Survival after recurrence of Ewing tumors: the St Jude Children's Research Hospital experience, 1979–1999. *Cancer* 2002;94(2):561–569.

86. Paulussen M, Ahrens S, Dunst J, et al. Localized Ewing tumor of bone: final results of the cooperative Ewing's Sarcoma Study CESS 86. *J Clin Oncol* 2001;19(6):1818–1829.

87. Marcus RB Jr, Cantor A, Heare TC, et al. Local control and function after twice-a-day radiotherapy for Ewing's sarcoma of bone. *Int J Radiat Oncol Biol Phys* 1991;21(6):1509–1515.

88. Perez CA, Tefft M, Nesbit M, et al. The role of radiation therapy in the management of non-metastatic Ewing's sarcoma of bone. Report of the Intergroup Ewing's Sarcoma Study. *Int J Radiat Oncol Biol Phys* 1981;7(2):141–149.

89. Donaldson SS, Shuster J, Andreozzi CM. The Pediatric Oncology Group (POG) experience in Ewing's sarcoma of bone. *Med Pediatr Oncol* 1989;17:283.

90. Hayes FA, Thompson EI, Meyer WH, et al. Therapy for localized Ewing's sarcoma of bone. *J Clin Oncol* 1989;7(2):208–213.

91. Sposto R, Ertel IJ, Jenkin RD, et al. The effectiveness of chemotherapy for treatment of high grade astrocytoma in children: results of a randomized trial. A report from the Childrens Cancer Study Group. *J Neurooncol* 1989;7(2):165–177.

92. Finlay JL, August C, Packer R, et al. High-dose multiagent chemotherapy followed by bone marrow 'rescue' for malignant astrocytomas of childhood and adolescence. *J Neurooncol* 1990;9(3):239–248.

93. Albright AL, Wisoff JH, Zeltzer P, et al. Prognostic factors in children with supratentorial (nonpineal) primitive neuroectodermal tumors. A neurosurgical perspective from the Children's Cancer Group. *Pediatr Neurosurg* 1995;22(1):1–7.

94. Jakacki RI, Zeltzer PM, Boyett JM, et al. Survival and prognostic factors following radiation and/or chemotherapy for primitive neuroectodermal tumors of the pineal region in infants and children: a report of the Childrens Cancer Group. *J Clin Oncol* 1995;13(6):1377–1383.

95. Linstadt D, Wara WM, Edwards MS, et al. Radiotherapy of primary intracranial germinomas: the case against routine craniospinal irradiation. *Int J Radiat Oncol Biol Phys* 1988;15(2):291–297.

96. Allen JC, Kim JH, Packer RJ. Neoadjuvant chemotherapy for newly diagnosed germ-cell tumors of the central nervous system. *J Neurosurg* 1987;67(1):65–70.

97. Sebag-Montefiore DJ, Douek E, Kingston JE, et al. Intracranial germ cell tumours: I. Experience with platinum based chemotherapy and implications for curative chemoradiotherapy. *Clin Oncol (R Coll Radiol)* 1992;4(6):345–350.

98. Dunbar SF, Tarbell NJ, Kooy HM, et al. Stereotactic radiotherapy for pediatric and adult brain tumors:

preliminary report. *Int J Radiat Oncol Biol Phys* 1994; 30(3):531–539.

99. Sarkaria JN, Mehta MP, Loeffler JS, et al. Radiosurgery in the initial management of malignant gliomas: survival comparison with the RTOG recursive partitioning analysis. Radiation Therapy Oncology Group. *Int J Radiat Oncol Biol Phys* 1995;32(4):931–941.

100. Gannett D, Stea B, Lulu B, et al. Stereotactic radiosurgery as an adjunct to surgery and external beam radiotherapy in the treatment of patients with malignant gliomas. *Int J Radiat Oncol Biol Phys* 1995;33(2):461–468.

101. Hug EB, Muenter MW, Archambeau JO, et al. Conformal proton radiation therapy for pediatric low-grade astrocytomas. *Strahlenther Onkol* 2002;178(1):10–17.

102. Gajjar A, Sanford RA, Heideman R, et al. Low-grade astrocytoma: a decade of experience at St. Jude Children's Research Hospital. *J Clin Oncol* 1997;15(8):2792–2799.

103. Freeman CR, Krischer JP, Sanford RA, et al. Final results of a study of escalating doses of hyperfractionated radiotherapy in brain stem tumors in children: a Pediatric Oncology Group study. *Int J Radiat Oncol Biol Phys* 1993;27(2):197–206.

104. Tait DM, Thornton-Jones H, Bloom HJ, et al. Adjuvant chemotherapy for medulloblastoma: the first multi-centre control trial of the International Society of Paediatric Oncology (SIOP I). *Eur J Cancer* 1990;26(4): 464–469.

105. Evans AE, Jenkin RD, Sposto R, et al. The treatment of medulloblastoma. Results of a prospective randomized trial of radiation therapy with and without CCNU, vincristine, and prednisone. *J Neurosurg* 1990;72(4): 572–582.

106. Gajjar A, Mulhern RK, Heideman RL, et al. Medulloblastoma in very young children: outcome of definitive craniospinal irradiation following incomplete response to chemotherapy. *J Clin Oncol* 1994;12(6):1212–1216.

107. Walter AW, Mulhern RK, Gajjar A, et al. Survival and neurodevelopmental outcome of young children with medulloblastoma at St Jude Children's Research Hospital. *J Clin Oncol* 1999;17(12):3720–3728.

108. Thomas PR, Deutsch M, Kepner JL, et al. Low-stage medulloblastoma: final analysis of trial comparing standard-dose with reduced-dose neuraxis irradiation. *J Clin Oncol* 2000;18(16):3004–3011.

109. Mulhern RK, Palmer SL, Merchant TE, et al. Neurocognitive consequences of risk-adapted therapy for childhood medulloblastoma. *J Clin Oncol* 2005;23(24): 5511–5519.

110. St Clair WH, Adams JA, Bues M, et al. Advantage of protons compared to conventional X-ray or IMRT in the treatment of a pediatric patient with medulloblastoma. *Int J Radiat Oncol Biol Phys* 2004;58(3):727–734.

111. Phillips C, Willis D, Cramb J, et al. A modified technique for craniospinal irradiation in children designed to reduce acute and late radiation toxicity. *Australas Radiol* 2004;48(2):188–194.

112. Merchant TE, Kiehna EN, Thompson SJ, et al. Pediatric low-grade and ependymal spinal cord tumors. *Pediatr Neurosurg* 2000;32(1):30–36.

113. Merchant TE, Haida T, Wang MH, et al. Anaplastic ependymoma: treatment of pediatric patients with or without craniospinal radiation therapy. *J Neurosurg* 1997;86(6):943–949.

114. Merchant TE. Current management of childhood ependymoma. *Oncology (Williston Park)* 2002;16(5): 629–642, 644; discussion 645–626, 648.

115. Merchant TE, Fouladi M. Ependymoma: new therapeutic approaches including radiation and chemotherapy. *J Neurooncol* 2005;75(3):287–299.

116. Merchant TE, Mulhern RK, Krasin MJ, et al. Preliminary results from a phase II trial of conformal radiation therapy and evaluation of radiation-related CNS effects for pediatric patients with localized ependymoma. *J Clin Oncol* 2004;22(15):3156–3162.

117. Merchant TE, Kiehna EN, Li C, et al. Radiation dosimetry predicts IQ after conformal radiation therapy in pediatric patients with localized ependymoma. *Int J Radiat Oncol Biol Phys* 2005;63(5):1546–1554.

118. Jereb B, Krishnaswami S, Reid A, et al. Radiation for medulloblastoma adjusted to prevent recurrence to the cribriform plate region. *Cancer* 1984;54(3):602–604.

119. Merchant TE, Zhu Y, Thompson SJ, et al. Preliminary results from a Phase II trail of conformal radiation therapy for pediatric patients with localised low-grade astrocytoma and ependymoma. *Int J Radiat Oncol Biol Phys* 2002;52(2):325–332.

120. Hernandez JC, Brady LW, Shields JA. Radiotherapy of ocular tumors. In: Tobias IS, Thomas PR, eds. *Current radiation oncology.* London: Arnold Publishing, 1994: 101–125.

121. Abramson DH, Ellsworth RM, Kitchin FD, et al. Second nonocular tumors in retinoblastoma survivors: are they radiation-induced? *Ophthalmology* 1988;91:1351–1355.

122. Kirsner SM, Hogstrom KR, Kurup RG, et al. Dosimetric evaluation in heterogeneous tissue of anterior electron beam irradiation for treatment of retinoblastoma. *Med Phys* 1987;14(5):772–779.

123. Weiss DR, Cassady JR, Petersen R. Retinoblastoma: a modification in radiation therapy technique. *Radiology* 1975;114(3):705–708.

124. Palm A, Nilsson E, Herrnsdorf L. Absorbed dose and dose rate using the Varian OBI 1.3 and 1.4 CBCT system. *J Appl Clin Med Phys* 2010;11(1):3085.

Feng-Ming (Spring) Kong ■ Jian-Yue Jin ■ Jeffrey D. Bradley ■ Mary K. Martel

INTRODUCTION

Thoracic tumors include lung cancer, thymomas, mesothelioma, esophageal cancer, and other less common tumors, such as lymphoma, germ cell tumor, and sarcoma. This chapter will cover only lung cancer, thymomas, and mesothelioma since the others are covered elsewhere in this book. Lung cancer is the most commonly diagnosed cancer worldwide (1.3 millions in 2002, 1.6 millions in 2008) (1,2). In 2009, there were an estimated 219,440 new cases and 159,390 deaths from lung cancer in the United States (3). Thymic tumors (4) and mesothelioma, on the other hand, are relatively uncommon (5). Radiation therapy (RT) plays a significant role in the management of thoracic tumors. The majority of these tumors require radiation therapy (RT) as a local measure for (i) definitive treatment of medical inoperable or surgically unresectable diseases; (ii) part of a multimodality regimen for locally advanced disease; (iii) adjuvant intent, needed prior to (neoadjuvant) or after surgery (adjuvant); or (iv) palliation of symptoms in patients with stage IV disease. This chapter reviews RT planning procedures, including steps before RT decision is made, such as diagnosis and staging workup, defining the role of RT; and steps after RT decision is made, such as defining dose and fractionation, simulation, defining target, dosimetric treatment planning, and RT techniques, for tumors of lung, thymus, and mesothelial cells. This chapter will focus on lung cancer, including both non-small-cell lung cancer (NSCLC) and small cell lung cancer (SCLC), and cover thymomas and mesothelioma, with each of the disease site divided into two subsections: procedures before and after the RT decision is made.

LUNG CANCER

Lung cancer is the leading cause of cancer deaths in the United States—among both men and women. It claims more lives than colon, prostate, and breast cancer combined. Treatment for lung cancer is based on the type (NSCLC vs. SCLC), stage of tumor, and the patient's general medical condition. Options include surgery, chemotherapy, and most frequently, a combined modality therapy. It is estimated that >60% of lung cancer cases

require RT at least once, with about 45% receiving it as part of their initial treatment (6).

Diagnosis and Staging Workup

Correct diagnosis and staging is essential for determining treatment and providing prognostic information. The tumor, node, and metastasis (TNM) system (AJCC 2010) (Table 33.1) should be used for staging. For SCLC, the tumor is further grouped as limited and extensive stage. Limited-stage SCLC (LS-SCLC) defines tumors that are encompassed within a reasonable radiation port, which often requires that the tumors be confined to the hemithorax without malignancy pleural effusion. Staging workup should be sequential and logical in order to avoid unnecessary, expensive or invasive tests, and extensive staging is unnecessary for a clearly palliative treatment. The end points are to (i) establish a histology diagnosis; (ii) obtain precise anatomical, and if possible, pathological, staging of the patient; and (iii) assess resectability and operability or direct radiation treatment planning. The workup should follow three steps: (i) clinical history and physical examination, (ii) clinical image staging, and (iii) pathologic diagnosis and staging.

Clinical History and Physical

All patients with newly diagnosed lung cancer should undergo a clinical history and physical examination. Particular note should be made of the overall performance status of the patient and of any weight loss. These two factors have significant predictive value for survival (7,8). The physical examination should be directed toward signs and symptoms of primary and distant metastatic disease, including bone pain, adenopathy, hepatomegaly, neurological changes consistent with brain metastasis, and subcutaneous nodules. Any pleural effusion should undergo cytological evaluation. Blood tests, including hemoglobin, alkaline phosphatase, transaminases, and lactate dehydrogenase (LDH) should be performed to look for evidence of distant metastases, particularly for SCLC, where the LDH test is prognostic and should be included in the lab request (9).

Clinical Image Staging

Virtually all patients should undergo a computerized tomography (CT) scan of the chest and upper abdomen,

TABLE 33.1	American Joint Cancer Committee Staging System for Lung Cancer

Lung

Primary tumor (T)

TX   Primary tumor cannot be assessed, or tumor proven by the presence of malignant cells in sputum or bronchial washings but not visualized by imaging or bronchoscopy

T0   No evidence of primary tumor.

Tis   Carcinoma *in situ*

T1   Tumor 3 cm or less in greatest dimension, surrounded by lung or visceral pleura, without bronchoscopic evidence of invasion more proximal than the lobar bronchus (i.e., not in the main bronchus)[a]
    T1a   Tumor 2 cm or less in greatest dimension
    T1b   Tumor >2 cm but 3 cm or less in greatest dimension

T2   Tumor >3 cm but 7 cm or less with any of the following features (T2 tumors with these features are classified T2a if 5 cm or less):
    Involves main bronchus, 2 cm or more distal to the carina
    Invades the visceral pleura PL1 or PL2; Associated with atelectasis or obstructive pneumonitis that extends to the hilar region but does not involve the entire lung
    T2a   Tumor >3 cm but 5 cm or less in greatest dimension
    T2b   Tumor >5 but 7 cm or less in greatest dimension

T3   Tumor >7 cm or one that directly invades any of the following: parietal (PL3), chest wall (including superior sulcus tumors), diaphragm, phrenic nerve, mediastinal pleura, parietal pericardium; or tumor in the main bronchus (<2 cm distal to the carina[a] but without involvement of the carina; or associated atelectasis or obstructive pneumonitis of the entire lung or separate tumor nodule(s) in the same lobe

T4   Tumor of any size that invades any of the following: mediastinum, heart, great vessels, trachea, recurrent laryngeal nerve, esophagus, vertebral body, carina, separate tumor nodules in a different ipsilateral lobe

Regional lymph nodes (N)

NX   Regional lymph nodes cannot be assessed

N0   No regional lymph nodes metastasis

N1   Metastasis to ipsilateral peribronchial and/or ipsilateral hilar lymph nodes, and intrapulmonary nodes including involvement by direct extension

N2   Metastasis to ipsilateral mediastinal and/or subcarinal lymph node(s)

N3   Metastasis in contralateral mediastinal, contralateral hilar, ipsilateral or contralateral scalene, or supraclavicular lymph node(s)

Distant metastasis (M)

M0   No distant metastasis

M1   Distant metastasis
    M1a   Separate tumor nodule(s) in a contralateral lobe tumor with pleural nodules or malignant pleural (or pericardial) effusion[b]
    M1b   Distant metastasis

Stage Grouping

Sixth edition	Seventh edition	N0	N1	N2	N3
T/M descriptor	T/M				
T1 (≤2 cm)	T1a	IA	IIA	IIIA	IIIB
T1 (>2–3 cm)	T1b	IA	IIA	IIIA	IIIB
T2 (≤5 cm)	T2a	IB	**IIA**	IIIA	IIIB
T2 (>5–7 cm)	T2b	**IIA**	IIB	IIIA	IIIB
T2 (>7 cm)	T3	**IIB**	**IIIA**	IIIA	IIIB
T3 invasion		IIB	IIIA	IIIA	IIIB
T4 (same lobe nodules)		**IIB**	**IIIA**	**IIIA**	IIIB
T4 (extension)	T4	**IIIA**	**IIIA**	IIIB	IIIB
M1 (ipsilateral lung)		**IIIA**	**IIIA**	**IIIB**	**IIIB**

(continued)

| TABLE 33.1 | American Joint Cancer Committee Staging System for Lung Cancer (*Continued*) |

Lung

Stage Grouping

Sixth edition	Seventh edition	N0	N1	N2	N3
T4 (pleural effusion)	M1a	**IV**	**IV**	**IV**	**IV**
M1 (contralateral lung)		IV	IV	IV	IV
M1 (distant)	M1b	IV	IV	IV	IV

Source: Edge SB, ed. AJCC Cancer staging manual, 7th ed. New York, NY: Springer, 2010.

[a]The uncommon superficial spreading tumor of any size with its invasive component limited to the bronchial wall, which may extend proximally to the main bronchus, is also classified as T1a.

[b]Most pleural (and pericardial effusions with lung cancer are due to tumor. In a few patients, however, multiple cytopathologic examinations of pleural (pericardial) fluid are negative for tumor, and the fluid is nonbloody and is not an exudate. Where these elements and clinical judgment dictate that the effusion is not related to the tumor, the effusion should be excluded as a staging element, and the patient should be classified as M0.

Cells in bold indicate a change from the sixth edition for a particular TNM category.

which should include the liver, upper abdomen, and adrenal glands (10). Intravenous contrast should be administrated unless the patient has renal insufficiency or known allergic reaction to the contrast material. The CT scan provides excellent anatomical detail, which allows the T-stage to be established, including the relationship to fissures, mediastinal structures, or the pleura and chest wall. CT may provide signs for the resectability of masses contiguous with the mediastinum; criteria for probable resectability of masses include: (i) a contact length of <3 cm with the mediastinum; (ii) <90 degrees contact with the aorta; and (iii) preserved mediastinal fat layer between the mass and mediastinal structures (11). CT is less reliable with regard to signs of unresectability (11). Modern contrast-enhanced CT is highly accurate in detecting lymph node (LN) enlargement, but the clinical applicability of LN enlargement for staging the mediastinum is poor, because small nodes may contain metastasis and large nodes may be benign (e.g., in the case of post-obstructive pneumonia). Current practice uses >10 mm of the short-axis diameter as the criterion for nodal metastasis. A pooled data set yielded a sensitivity of 57%, a specificity of 82%, a positive predictive value (PPV) of 56%, and a negative predictive value (NPV) of 83%, with marked heterogeneity across individual studies for CT (Table 33.2) (12,13). CT can assist in selecting the best procedure for sampling suspected LN regions.

Positron emission tomography (PET) with 18 F-fluoro-2-deoxy-D-glucose (FDG-PET) is a standard component of current staging in patients with nonmetastatic NSCLC and SCLC. For NSCLC, PET is superior to CT in estimating T, N, and M disease. Although CT with its better spatial resolution remains the standard assessment of T-stage, FDG-PET may better characterize the primary tumor by differentiating tumor from the collapsed lung and add information in case of pleural involvement, where 89% sensitivity, 94% specificity, and 91% accuracy have been reported (14). Data on nodal staging with PET have been addressed in several meta-analyses (12,15,16) (Table 33.2),

and convincingly demonstrate that PET is superior to CT in staging mediastinal LN. In general, PET has an excellent NPV for nodal disease, which may allow omission of invasive staging in the case of an absence of FDG-uptake in the mediastinum in patients with low risk factors. However, a number of granulomatous or other inflammatory diseases also exhibit increased FDG-uptake. Positive findings on PET should be pathologically verified when possible, particularly when the disease is relatively confined to limited areas. PET-CT is better than FDG-PET alone. FDG-PET is also more accurate than other imaging modalities for detecting extrathoracic metastatic disease (17). In at least two studies, FDG-PET revealed unsuspected distant metastases in 10% to 30% of cases (17,18). Figure 33.1 shows examples of PET in assessing the extent of the primary tumor and detecting early nodal disease.

The ability of PET in better defining tumor extent has a significant impact on target delineation in the treatment planning of NSCLC, which will be discussed in section on "PET Scan on Target Definition." PET is also superior to CT in restaging patients with NSCLC, which could be performed after induction therapy before surgery, after completion of a definitive nonsurgical intervention, or at recurrence after surgical resection (19,20).

Interpretation of PET images could be improved by visual correlation with CT, due to better localization of PET abnormalities using the anatomical detail of CT. Fusion PET-CT scanners, obtaining the coregistration of functional-molecular and morphological-anatomical data, can further improve T, N, and M staging accuracy (19,21,22). FDG-PET-CT is also more accurate than other imaging studies for detecting extrathoracic metastatic disease (17).

Magnetic resonance imaging (MRI) is of limited value in staging lung cancer except in the case of intolerance to intravenous ionic contrast media, and in some special circumstances, such as assessment of the relationship of the tumor with large blood vessels, soft tissues, or vertebral body for patients with superior sulcus tumors (23).

TABLE 33.2	**Predictive Accuracy of Mediastinal Nodal Staging (12,13)**

A. Imaging staging studies

Study	No. of patients	Sensitivity	Specificity	Positive predictive value	Negative predictive value
CT	3,438	0.57	0.82	0.56	0.83
PET	1,045	0.84	0.89	0.79	0.93

B. Pathologic staging procedures[a]

Procedure	No. of patients	Sensitivity	Specificity[a]	Positive predictive value	Negative predictive value[a]
Transbronchial needle aspiration biopsy	910	0.76	0.96	1.00	0.71
Transthoracic needle aspiration biopsy	215	0.91	1.0	1.0	0.83
Esophageal ultrasound needle aspiration biopsy	215	0.88	0.91	0.98	0.77
Mediastinoscopy	5,687	0.81	1.0	1.0	0.91
Chamberlain procedure	84	0.74	1.0	1.0	0.94
Extended cervical mediastinoscopy	206	0.73	1.0	1.0	0.34

[a]All of the specificity and negative predictive values were limited by the accessibility of that specific procedure. For example, Chamberlain procedure can only access levels 5–6.
CT, computed tomography; PET, positron emission tomography.

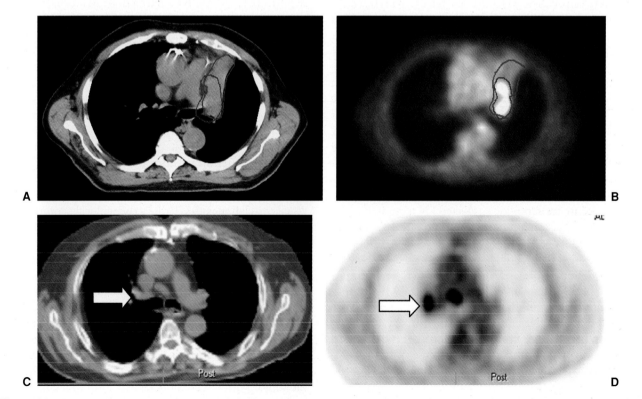

Figure 33.1. FDG-PET improves staging accuracy for non-small cell lung cancer. FDG-PET differentiates tumor from collapsed lung (**A** and **B**), and detects CT undetected node (*arrow* in **C** and **D**). Blue, CT lesion; red, PET tumor.

Ultrasound of the liver, and brain CT or MRI are recommended for evaluation of distant diseases for high-risk patients (such as stage III), or patients with stage I/II with symptoms from the bone, liver, or brain, and in high-risk patients with nonspecific features of metastasis. These include unexplained anemia, unexplained weight loss of >5% of normal body weight in the previous 6 months, abnormal alkaline phosphatase or transaminase levels, and clinical suspicion of metastatic disease (24). For patients who have already had a PET scan, a bone scan is of less value, as PET is also reported to be more accurate in detecting bone metastasis. Based on a retrospective review of 257 cases, the accuracy of the PET and bone scan were 94% and 85% ($p < 0.05$), sensitivity values were 91% and 75%, and the specificity values were 96% and 95%, respectively (25).

Pathologic Diagnosis and Staging

Histological diagnosis is mandatory and may be obtained using bronchoscopy, mediastinoscopy, and ultrasound-guided biopsy—bronchoscopy with biopsy is useful for T and N staging. Direct visualization and biopsy of the main bronchus and carina provide a 100% PPV for T4 disease. The same is true for transbronchial needle aspiration for mediastinal LN diseases. Endobronchial ultrasonography (EBUS) can visualize mediastinal LNs in the anterior, posterior, and inferior mediastinum at levels 2, 3, 4, and 7, as well as level 10 and 11 LNs. Esophageal ultrasonography (EUS) particularly visualizes LNs in the posterior part of levels 4 L, 3, 5, and 7, and in the inferior mediastinum at levels 8 and 9. The technique also complements mediastinoscopy and EBUS, for which cannot reach posterior subcarinal nodes or lower mediastinal nodes. Endoscopic ultrasonography may also help to exclude or confirm T4 disease in specific cases.

Mediastinoscopy remains the standard tool for invasive staging in patients without bulky mediastinal involvement. It has a good NPV and a 100% PPV (except for pathology misinterpretations) for nodal staging. Visual inspection at mediastinoscopy also distinguishes intra- from extra-nodal LN disease, and resectable from unresectable disease in difficult cases. Cervical mediastinoscopy—the most commonly used procedure—gives access to the pre-tracheal, right and left para-tracheal, and anterior subcarinal LN levels (levels 1, 2R, 4R, 2L, 4L, and 7), can be performed as an outpatient procedure and is reported to have very low mortality and morbidity in experienced hands (13). Patients with left upper lobe primary tumors may require additional evaluation of the subaortic area by left anterior mediastinotomy. Contraindications for mediastinoscopy are intolerance of general anesthesia, extreme kyphosis, and cutaneous tracheostomy. In some patients with central tumors, mediastinoscopy may also improve certainty of the T-stage, as it can prove unresectability due to the invasion of mediastinal central vascular structures. The sensitivity of cervical mediastinoscopy is reported as between 72% and 89%—on average 81% in a recent review with a pooled NPV of 91% (12). The results of the suboptimal sensitivity are partly explained by the fact that some LN stations (5, 6, 7 posterior, 8, 9) are not accessible

by cervical mediastinoscopy. The recently implemented video-assisted procedure may further improve the accuracy. Left anterior mediastinotomy—the Chamberlain procedure—through the left para-sternal second intercostal space gives extrapleural access to level 5 and 6 LNs and assessment of resectability by palpating the tumor. Extended mediastinoscopy has been described as a technique to allow exploration of level 5 and 6 nodes via the cervical approach, by inserting the mediastinoscope through the cervical incision above the aortic arch. These techniques are more challenging, thus should be performed in left upper lobe tumors with suspicion of LN metastases in levels 5 and 6 based on CT and/or PET.

Video-assisted thoracic surgery (VATS) is also an important staging tool, which can allow biopsy of lesions in the contralateral lung or pleura. Similarly, LNs beyond the reach of conventional mediastinoscopy such as the inferior mediastinal LNs (levels 8 and 9) can be biopsied. LN stations 5 and 6 can be explored at left thoracoscopy, as an alternative to left anterior mediastinotomy. VATS is also an approach used in patients with advanced primary lesions in order to identify suitable patients for induction chemoradiation (ChemRT). As imaging studies do not always allow one to distinguish resectable T3 disease from unresectable T4 disease, an exploratory thoracotomy may still have to be performed.

Table 33.3 summarizes American Association of Clinical Oncology (ASCO) staging guidelines between 2003 and 1997. The staging workup recommendation has not been changed remarkably from 2003. Workup should be stopped at any point if distant metastasis is confirmed. For those with localized disease and medically fit for definitive treatment, additional tests are often needed to assess operability or pretreatment conditions. These include pulmonary function tests and quantitative ventilation perfusion tests. Pulmonary function tests are always required for surgery or radiation-based management. Quantitative ventilation/perfusion SPECT is sometimes indicated to help planning of surgical resection or RT in patients with marginal pulmonary functional reserve (26) Cardiac or other medical evaluations should also be performed as indicated. Unfortunately, there is no consensus even in the surgical world regarding surgical contraindications, and many patients still receive substandard surgical care (27). In general, patients with FEV1 >60% are considered to be operable without need of further testing. For those with FEV1 ranged 40% to 60%, maximum oxygen consumption should be >15 mL/kg. One should be advised that determination of operabilities or resectability is not based on certain numbers, rather it should be a decision of board-certified thoracic surgeons who perform lung cancer surgery as a predominant part of their practice.

The Role of RT in NSCLC

The choice of treatment for NSCLC is highly dependent on (i) stage and resectability of the tumor, and (ii) medical operability of the patient. The therapeutic modality with

TABLE 33.3	Staging Workup Guidelines from the American Association of Clinical Oncology for Patients with Advanced Non-small-Cell Lung Cancer (24)	
Specific guidelines	**1997 Recommendations**	**2003 Recommendations**[a]
	Staging locoregional disease	
General	A chest x-ray and CT scan of chest and upper abdomen with IV contrast.	A chest x-ray and CT scan of chest and upper abdomen with IV contrast. FDG-PET if CT shows no evidence of distant metastasis
Clinically operable NSCLC	Biopsy for mediastinal lymph nodes ≥ 1.0 cm in shortest transverse axis.	Biopsy for mediastinal lymph nodes ≥1.0 cm in shortest transverse axis, or positive on FDG-PET scanning.
	Staging distant disease	
General		FDG-PET is required in patients with no distant metastasis on CT
Bone	A bone scan in patients with (a) bone pain, (b) chest pain, or (c) an elevated serum alkaline phosphatase level.	A bone scan is optional in patients with evidence of bone metastases on FDG-PET, unless there are suspicious symptoms in regions not imaged by FDG-PET. In patients with a surgically respectable primary lung lesion, bone lesions discovered on bone scan or FDG-PET require histologic confirmation, or corroboration by additional radiologic testing (x-ray, CT, and/or MRI).
Brain	Head CT or MRI brain with and without IV contrast only in patients who have signs or symptoms of CNS disease.	Head CT or MRI brain with and without IV contrast material only in patients who have signs or symptoms of CNS disease, and asymptomatic patients with stage III disease who are being considered for aggressive local therapy (chest surgery or radiation).
Adrenal and liver (If the patient is otherwise considered to be potentially resectable)	An isolated mass on ultrasonographic or CT scan requires biopsy to rule out metastatic disease	An isolated mass on ultrasonography, CT scan, or FDG-PET scan requires biopsy to rule out metastatic disease

[a]There has not been remarkable update in staging workup since 2003.
CT, computed tomography; FDG–PET, positron emission tomography with ^{18}F-fluoro-2-deoxy-D-glucose; NSCLC, non-small-cell lung cancer; MRI, magnetic resonance imaging; CNS, central nervous system.

the highest cure rates is surgical therapy by lobectomy or pneumonectomy (28–30). However, because of factors such as advanced stage, medical comorbidities, patient refusal, age, or other factors surgery may not be possible. It is estimated that only about 20% of patients initially presenting with lung cancer are eligible for definitive surgery (31,32).

A flow chart with recommended therapeutic management for NSCLC is presented in Figure 33.2. RT plays following important roles: definitive RT for resectable NSCLC patients with medically inoperable or who refuse surgical treatment (stages I and II), adjuvant or neoadjuvant RT for resectable or potentially resectable patients (limited stage IIIA), ChemRT for unresectable diseases

(stage III), and palliative RT for metastasis diseases (stage IV). Some patients with stage IV NSCLC could be treated aggressively when the distant disease burden is limited (such as solitary brain metastasis).

RT in Resectable NSCLC

Lobectomy is the treatment of choice for resectable NSCLC in patients who are medically fit for the procedure, with a 5-year survival rate after complete resection of 53%, 47%, 43%, 35%, and 26%, based on results of 68,463 patients of 20 countries treated from 1990 to 2000 from the IASLC database, for clinical stage T1a, T1b, T2a, T2b, and T3 disease, respectively (33). One must note that such procedure is associated with a significant morbidity

Cancers of the Thorax ■ **683**

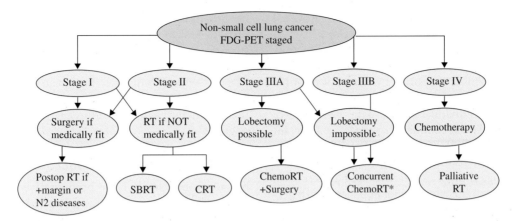

Figure 33.2. Schema of the therapeutic approach for newly diagnosed non-small cell lung cancer. RT, radiation therapy; ChemoRT, concurrent chemoradiation; 3DCRT, 3D conformal RT. * For patients with good performance status. Sequential chemoRT is recommended for patients with poor performance status. SBRT, stereotactic body radiation therapy; CRT, conformal radiation therapy. ChemoRT, chemoradiation.

and mortality. A surgical pattern of care analysis reported a perioperative mortality rate of 5.2%, which ranged from 4.0% in patients who did not require a transfusion, to 12.7% in patients who underwent a transfusion (27). This mortality reflects the considerable comorbidity typically found in elderly patients.

Definitive RT is the recommended treatment for patients with early stage NSCLC who are unfit for surgery and those who refuse surgical treatment. Radiation therapy improves survival in this group of patients (34). A median survival time of >30 months and a 5-year survival rate ±30% has been reported with fractionated RT alone (35,36). Local recurrence and distant metastasis are the main causes of failure, whereas regional nodal failure is uncommon (0%–7%) (7,37). A few selected studies from the use of conformal high dose RT reported 3-year sur-

vival rates around 20% to 30% (35,38–42). Stereotactic body radiotherapy (SBRT) is an emerging new technique and becomes the standard of care for T1 and T2 (<5 cm) N0, peripherally located NSCLC, with promising early results and limited acute toxicities (43–55). A meta-analysis of 30 studies (11 on 3DCRT, 11 on SBRT, 5 on proton, 3 on carbon ion) that reported 5-year overall survival rate in stage I inoperable NSCLC SBRT (42%) was significantly better than that for CRT (20%), similar to that of proton therapy (40%) and carbon-ion therapy (42%) (56). Tumor control outcome and results on radiation pneumonitis are shown in Table 33.4. RTOG 236, a recently published phase II trial from North America of 55 evaluable (44 patients with T1 tumors and 11 patients with T2 tumors) patients, reported an estimated 3-year primary tumor control rate of 97.6%—the 3-year primary tumor and

TABLE 33.4	Treatment Outcomes of SBRT and CRT (56)						
RT modality	No. of patients	No. of study	Dose (Gy)/ No. of fraction	RT duration (days)	% 2 years OS/DFS[a] (95%CI)	% 5 years OS/DFS (95%CI)	Grade ¾ Pneumonitis (%)[a]
CRT	1,326	11	20–90/20–58	14–70	53 (46–60)/ 67 (59–76)	19 (15–24)/ 43 (31–56)	0.23 (0.03–0.8)
SBRT	895	11	22–84/1–14	1–19	70 (63–77)/ 83 (75–92)	42 (34–50)/ 63 (50–75)	2.0 (1.1–3.2)
Proton	180	5	50–94/7–41	14–77	61 (47–75)/ 74 (61–87)	40 (24–55)/ 52 (32–72)	0.8 (0.02–4)
Carbon-Ion	210	3	53–95/4–18	1–42	74 (61–86)/ 82 (70–93)	42 (32–52)/ 64 (48–80)	1.4 (0.3–4)

[a]Not all studies reported this outcome.
RT, radiation therapy; CRT, conventionally fractionated RT; SBRT; stereotactic body RT; OS, overall survival; DFS, disease-free survival

involved lobe (local) control rate was 90.6% and overall survival of 55.8% (54).

After surgical resection, cisplatin-based chemotherapy is recommended in patients with completely resected stage IB to III NSCLC. This is supported by results of multiple randomized trials. A recent meta-analysis based on collected and pooled individual patient data from the five largest randomized trials conducted by the Lung Adjuvant Cisplatin Evaluation (LACE) demonstrated that cisplatin-based adjuvant chemotherapy improved survival in patients with stage II or III cancer after surgical resection (57). Chemotherapy effect was higher in patients with better performance status (58). Another meta-analysis of 12 trials plus an individual patient meta-analysis (7,334 patients) demonstrated significant differences in favor of chemotherapy for overall survival in all seven subpopulation, with a relative benefit of 7% to 12% and an absolute benefit ranging from 2.5% to 4.1% (59). A very recent two meta-analysis (surgery plus chemotherapy vs. surgery alone, surgery plus RT, and chemotherapy vs. surgery plus RT) reported that the addition of adjuvant chemotherapy after surgery for patients with operable NSCLC improves survival, irrespective of whether chemotherapy was adjuvant to surgery alone or adjuvant to surgery plus radiotherapy (60).

Radiation therapy may increase local control and potentially improve survival in patients who have had resection for lung cancer. Postoperative radiation to the primary tumor bed should be given to patients with positive or suspicious margins, as the rate of local recurrence for this condition is over 50% (61,62). For nodal disease, the role of radiation remains to be controversial (63–66). An earlier meta-analysis of postoperative radiation therapy (PORT) concluded that adjuvant RT was detrimental for survival, especially for stage N0/N1 NSCLC (2000)(67). However, these conclusions have been widely debated, with critics focusing on the inadequate staging of patients, inclusion of early-stage patients, outdated radiation equipment and techniques, and inappropriate radiation dose-fractionation schemes (36). For patients with N2 disease, however, postoperative radiation reduced local relapses in the Lung Cancer Study Group (68) and both local and distant failure in the MRC trial (69). Recent studies using modern RT have failed to detect the detrimental effects (70,71), and a retrospective analysis by Sawyer et al. even suggested a survival benefit from PORT in N2 disease (72). Within the Surveillance, Epidemiology, and End Results (SEER) database of 7,456 patients treated with lobectomy or pneumonectomy, PORT was associated with a survival benefit in patients with N2 nodal disease (hazard ratio [HR] = 0.855; 95% CI, 0.762–0.959; $p = 0.0077$), though it was detrimental in N0/N1 disease (73). A recent subgroup analysis of Adjuvant Navelbine International Trialist Association (ANITA) suggested a positive effect of PORT in pN2 disease and a negative effect on pN1 disease when patients treated with or without adjuvant chemotherapy (64). In summary, adjuvant RT should

be discouraged in patients with complete resected N0–1 NSCLC, and should be given in patients with positive or surpicious margins. Postoperative radiation with chemotherapy (after or concurrently) should be considered in patients with N2 disease. European Organization for Research and Treatment of Cancer (EORTC) trial to further evaluate the role of adjuvant RT in N2 disease is ongoing.

RT in Potentially Resectable NSCLC

Neoadjuvant ChemRT, or preoperative ChemRT, was reported to improve survival and decrease local recurrence rates in Pancoast tumors, which are tumors originating from the superior sulcus of the lung that invade the chest wall and adjacent structures, such as the brachial plexus (74,75). It improves 2-year survival rates from 50% to 55%, to around 70%, if a complete surgical resection can subsequently be performed (76,77). The historical survival rate was around 20% in patients receiving preoperative RT alone (74). The median survivals were only 11 months after surgery in T4 tumors invading mediastinum (78,79). Neoadjuvant chemoRT has also been evaluated in the treatment of resectable stage III NSCLC. The Intergroup 0139 trial demonstrated superior progression-free survival, but not overall survival after induction ChemRT and surgery, as opposed to ChemRT alone (80). The lack of survival benefit was due to the increased perioperative mortality in patients who underwent a pneumonectomy, especially a right pneumonectomy. At 5-year follow-up, 27% of patients who received ChemRT followed by surgery were alive compared to 20% patients who had ChemRT alone. An exploratory analysis showed improved survival with a trimodality approach in patients who had a lobectomy, but not pneumonectomy. These results suggest that preoperative ChemRT could be considered as an option for patients with resectable stage IIIA NSCLC if pneumonectomy can be avoided. However, even in patients with potentially resectable T1–3N2 NSCLC, non-surgical therapy can be justified as a standard treatment on the basis of the INT 0139 study (80).

RT in Unresectable NSCLC

The standard of care for stage III unresectable NSCLC disease is combined ChemRT. The results of RT alone for stage III tumors or those invading vital structures that are deemed unresectable or marginally resectable are poor, with 5-year survival ranging from 5% to 7% (81–83). RT alone is only used to treat patients who cannot tolerate chemotherapy. Addition of neoadjuvant chemotherapy resulted in 2 to 4 months' extension in median survival and 8% to 20% improvement in 2- to 3-year overall survival (84,85), ascertained by at least three randomized trials: the Cancer and Leukemia Group B (CALGB) 9433 (82), RTOG8808/ECOG4588 (83), and a French study (86). The French study also reported a significant reduction in distant recurrences.

While the standard care for unresectable NSCLC is chemotherapy and radiation, yet the optional combination of these two treatment modalities has yet to be defined.

Sequential Versus Concurrent ChemRT

Several prospective randomized trials examining the treatment of stage III unresectable NSCLC disease have demonstrated superior results from concurrent ChemRT compared to sequential ChemRT, with an additional 2 to 3 months' extension in median survival and 7% to 10% improvement in 3- to 5-year survival (87–89). A recent meta-analysis of six trials in 1,205 patients confirmed the benefit of concurrent ChemRT on overall survival (HR, 0.84; 95% CI, 0.74–0.95; $p = 0.004$), with an absolute improvement of 5.7% (from 18.1% to 23.8%) in 3 years and 4.5% in 5 years (90). Concurrent ChemRT had a borderline effect on locoregional progression (HR, 0.77; 95% CI, 0.62–0.95; $p = 0.01$) without a significant effect on distant progression (HR, 1.04; 95% CI, 0.86–1.25; $p = 0.69$). Concurrent chemoRT increased acute esophageal toxicity (grades 3 to 4) from 4% to 18% with a relative risk of 4.9 (95% CI, 3.1–7.8; $p < 0.001$) without a significant difference regarding acute pulmonary toxicity (Fig. 33.3). In patients with locally advanced NSCLC who are medically

fit, concurrent ChemRT should be considered as standard therapy.

Adjuvant or Induction Chemotherapy with Concurrent ChemRT

Although there is general agreement on the principle of using combined modality therapy with a concurrent regimen for stage III unresectable NSCLC in those medically fit, there is controversy over the optimal combined modality approach and sequence in this population. A number of phase II and III trials have established the use of both induction and consolidation chemotherapy (91–96). Researchers from the University of North Carolina reported a median survival of 24 months in patients treated with induction paclitaxel/carboplatin (CP) followed by concurrent ChemoRT. However, CALGB 39801, a phase III study comparing current ChemRT alone versus induction CP followed by concurrent ChemRT failed to show a significant survival difference between the two arms (97) The median survival was 14 months in the induction arm versus 11.4 months in the concurrent alone arm ($p = 0.154$). Although a median survival of 26 months was reported from SWOG 9504 using Taxotere adjuvant chemotherapy in unresectable stage III NSCLC (94), the HOG lung 01–24 study showed no

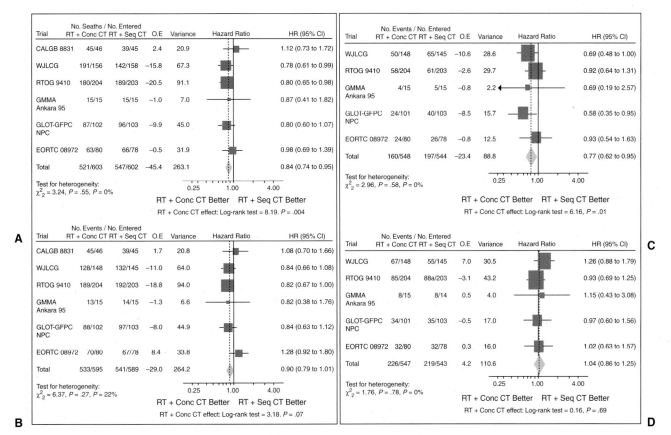

Figure 33.3. The role of concurrent chemoradiation in non-small cell lung cancer. This is a summary result from a recent meta-analysis, showing hazard ratio (HR) plots for (**A**) survival, (**B**) progression-free survival, (**C**) local progression, and (**D**) distant progression (90). Comparing to sequential treatment, concurrent chemoradiation has significantly better overall survival, locoregional progression without significant changes of distant progression.

significant benefit of adjuvant Taxotere after concurrent cis-platin and etoposide (98). The role of adjuvant CP after con-current CP has not been evaluated by a phase III study. The median overall survival result from the phase II study of locally advanced multiple modality protocol (LAMP) was 13, 12.7, and 16.3 months for sequential CP-RT, concurrent CP-RT with induction CP, and with adjuvant CP, respec-tively (95). Although the LAMP was not powered to answer the differences among modalities, it suggested that concur-rent CP-RT followed by adjuvant CP appeared to produce the best median survival. Neoadjuvant CP had the worst overall. CALGB 39801, a phase III study intended to evaluate role of neoadjuvant CP, demonstrated the same result show-ing no significant benefit of induction CP (99). Large phase III trials are still warranted to answer the definitive recom-mendations concerning the optimal combination of chemo-therapy and radiotherapy, and the role of adjuvant chemotherapy. Therefore, reasonable recommendations for unresectable stage III is RT with concurrent EP, with or with-out adjuvant EP, or concurrent CP followed by adjuvant CP.

Prophylactic Cranial Irradiation in Stage III NSCLC

Following potentially curative treatment for NSCLC, over-all central nervous system relapse rates range from 21% to 54%, and the central nervous system is the first site of relapse in 15% to 30% of cases (100,101). Brain metastases are more common in patients with adenocarcinoma (ADC) or large cell carcinoma, and in patients with locally advanced disease (102). Several randomized trials have demonstrated that prophylactic cranial irradiation (PCI) can significantly reduce the incidence of brain metastases to less than 10% to 15% (103,104). The fact that no sur-vival advantage has been demonstrated thus far could be attributed to the relatively poor local and systemic treat-ment results (82,83). PCI is not a standard practice in NSCLC, due to the lack of studies showing a survival ben-efit, and to concerns about the potential neurotoxicity of whole brain radiation. RTOG 0214 aimed to assess the effects of PCI on overall survival and toxicity in patients with stage III NSCLC who are treated with more modern and effective multimodality regimens, and who have no extracranial disease progression 4 months after comple-tion of their initial treatment. Unfortunately, the study closed prematurely due to slow accrual. Only 356 patients accrued of the targeted 1,058. Result of 340 evaluable patients demonstrated no significant difference in 1-year overall survival. Obviously, it is not powered to answer the primary endpoints on survival. The 1-year rates of brain relapse were significantly decreased after PCI (*p* <0.004; 7.7% vs. 18.0% for PCI vs. observation). Patients in the observation arm were 2.52 times more likely to develop BM than those in the PCI arm (unadjusted odds ratio, 2.52; 95% CI, 1.32–4.80) (105). There were no significant differences in global cognitive function or QOL after PCI, but there was a significant decline in memory assessed by Hopkins Verbal Learning Test at 1 year (106). The role of PCI in NSCLC will continue to be debatable.

RT in Metastatic NSCLC

Palliative Radiation for Extracranial Diseases

Palliative RT is often needed in the management of local thoracic symptoms from stage IV NSCLC. Such symptoms include, but are not limited to, hemoptysis, shortness of breath, obstructive pneumonia/atelectasis, superior venous cava syndrome, and chest wall invasion-induced pain (107–109). Approximately 60% of patients have objective or subjective improvement in these symptoms after a palliative course of treatment. RT remains the most effective palliative treatment for painful bone metastases (110), providing partial pain relief in about 60% patients, and complete pain control in over 30% with either single or multiple fractionated regimens (111).

Palliative Radiation for Brain Metastasis

Brain metastases are common in NSCLC. Solitary brain metastases can be treated by surgical resection or stereo-tactic radiosurgery in addition to whole brain radiation (112–114). RTOG 9508, a phase III trial comparing whole brain radiation versus brain with stereotactic surgery, has demonstrated that the addition of stereotactic radiosur-gery resulted in improved survival for patients with recur-sive partitioning analysis class 1 or favorable histology (113). Stereotactic radiosurgery group had a better sur-vival for patients with a single brain radiation metastasis (median survival time 6.5 months vs. 4.9 months, *p* = 0.0393). Thus, whole brain with either resection or stereo-tactic radiosurgery should be standard treatment for patients with a single brain metastasis and be considered for patients with two or three brain metastases. The role of stereotactic radiosurgery in patients with more than one brain metastasis is controversial (114). Whole brain radia-tion is the standard of care in patients with multiple brain metastases, though there are concerns about whole brain irradiation due to neurocognitive effects (115–119). One should note that the major cause of neurocognitive decline is brain relapse and whole brain radiation decreases the risk of brain relapses (116).

The Role of RT In SCLC

SCLCs make up approximately 15% to 20% of all newly diagnosed cases of lung cancer. There is a propensity for early metastasis and chemotherapy is the cornerstone of therapy. Up to 30% of patients can present with disease confined to one hemithorax with or without the regional lymph nodes, and these are classified as LS-SCLC. The standard of care for LS-SCLC involves the use of chemo-therapy, thoracic RT, and PCI for those who achieve a complete response.

Thoracic RT in LS-SCLC

Although chemotherapy is the primary modality for patients with LS-SCLC, those with disease confined to the chest, no pleural infusion, and encompassable with reasonable radiation fields should be considered for thoracic RT. The addition of thoracic RT has a small but clear survival advantage in this population. At least two large meta-analyses have confirmed the value of thoracic irradiation to decrease thoracic recurrence and to improve survival (120,121). Pignon et al. (120) found that the relative risk of death in the combined therapy group, as compared with the chemotherapy alone group, was 0.86, corresponding to a 14% reduction in the mortality rate. The benefit in terms of overall survival at 3 years was 5.4%. The meta-analysis by Warde and Payne was based on 11 randomized trials, and demonstrated that RT improved 2-year survival by 5.4% (120,121).

Thoracic RT in LS-SCLC should be delivered early and concurrently with chemotherapy rather than late in the course of chemotherapy or after (122). The National Cancer Institute of Canada performed a phase III prospective randomized trial to compare the outcomes of early versus late administration of RT (122). Patients were randomized to initiate RT in the second cycle of chemotherapy (week 3), or during the last cycle of chemotherapy (week 15). The median progression-free survival was 15.4 months in the early RT group versus 11.8 months in the late RT group ($p = 0.036$); the median overall survival was 21.2 months versus 16 months, respectively ($p = 0.008$). The Lung Cancer Study Group of the Japan Clinical Oncology Group conducted another phase III study in which patients were randomized to sequential ChemRT or concurrent ChemRT (123). RT was initiated after the fourth cycle of chemotherapy on the sequential arm and on day 2 on the concurrent arm. The median survival time was 19.7 months in the sequential arm versus 27.2 months in the concurrent arm ($p = 0.097$). The 5-year survival rate for patients who received sequential RT was 18.3%, as compared to 23.7% for the patients who received concurrent RT ($p = 0.097$). This study also suggests that chemotherapy and concurrent RT is more effective than the sequential regimen. Thus, early concurrent ChemRT is the recommended treatment for LS-SCLC.

Prophylactic Cranial RT in SCLC

Brain metastasis is commonly seen in patients with SCLC. Quite a few trials have been conducted to assess the role of PCI in SCLC treatment. Arriagada et al. (124) reported a prospective randomized study that the brain metastasis rate was significantly reduced by PCI, with a 2-year brain metastasis rate of 40% versus 67% for who did not receive PCI ($p = 0.0000$). The 2-year cumulative rate of brain metastasis as an isolated first site of relapse was 45% in the control group and 19% in the treatment group ($p < 10^{-6}$). The 2-year overall survival rate was 29% in the PCI group and 21.5% in the control group ($p = 0.14$). There were no significant differences between the two groups in terms of neuropsychological function or abnormalities indicated by CT brain scans. A multicenter randomized study reported by Gregor et al. (125) showed similar results, with a significant decrease in brain metastasis. In 1999,

Auperin et al. reported a meta-analysis on 987 patients with SCLC (847 patients with limited disease and 140 patients with extensive disease) who were in complete remission from seven trials that compared the use of PCI versus no PCI (125). PCI was associated with an absolute decrease of 25.3% in the cumulative incidence of brain metastasis in 3 years—from 58.6% in the control group to 33.3% in the PCI group. The relative risk of death in the treatment group as compared with the control group was 0.84 (95% confidence interval, 0.73 to 0.97; $p = 0.01$), which corresponded to an absolute increase in overall survival of 5.4% at 3 years—from 15.3% in the control group to 20.7% in the treatment group ($p = 0.01$). PCI has become a standard practice for patients with SCLC who have complete remission after ChemRT of the primary thoracic tumor.

RT in Extensive Stage SCLC

For extensive stage SCLC, the mainstay treatment is chemotherapy. Although many attempts have been made to develop new drugs, cisplatin-based combination chemotherapy remains the management mainstay (127).

PCI decreases brain relapse rate, improves overall survival, and is considered to be a standard of care for patients with responses to chemotherapy (Slotman). Radiation therapy to the thorax may be considered in those patients with excellent radiographical responses to chemotherapy, and may also be used as a palliative approach in some situations such as superior vena cava obstruction, obstructive pneumonia, or hemoptysis. Palliative radiation is often needed for (126) bone metastasis.

Dose and Fractionation in NSCLC

Conventional Dose and Fractionation

For conventionally fractionated RT, Table 33.5 summarizes the recommended dose/fractionation for different treatment types. A dose of 45 to 50 Gy in 1.8 to 2 Gy daily fractions is recommended for preoperative radiation. When postoperative RT is indicated, the mediastinum is commonly treated to 50 Gy in 25 fractions, and regions of extracapsular extension (ECE) and/or bulky nodal disease boosted by an additional 10 Gy. Areas of gross residual disease may be treated to 66 to 70 Gy, if the volume to the normal structure is limited. When T3N0 chest tumors with chest wall invasion are given postoperative RT, the regional nodal area does not require postoperative RT if it was adequately staged during surgery. However, the chest wall should receive up to 60 Gy postoperatively.

A regimen of 30 Gy in 10 daily fractions is usually used for palliative treatment (107–109). While using this dose regimen does initially relieve symptoms, it may not have a sustained effect. Another short course of radiation may be considered after a 2-week break. If the patients show improvement in their symptoms, and show continuing good performance status, an additional 20 Gy in four

TABLE 33.5	Common Radiation Dose Prescriptions for NSCLC	

Indications	Total dose/fractions (fx)
Medical inoperable early stage disease	
Definitive conventional radiation	±70 Gy in 30–35 fx
Stereotactic body radiotherapy	48–60 Gy in 3–5 fx
Postoperative radiation	
Positive or suspicious surgical margins	60 Gy in 30 fx
Mediastinal lymph nodes (N2 and above disease)	50–54 Gy in 25 fx
Chest wall invasion (T3 and T4)	50–60 Gy in 25–30 fx
Preoperative radiation combined with chemotherapy	45–50 Gy in 20–25 fx
Marginally operable patients (stage IIIa or Ib)	60 Gy in 30–33 fx
Unresectable patients	
Chemotherapy + concurrent chemoradiation	60–70 Gy in 30–35 fx
Concurrent chemoradiation + chemotherapy	60–70 Gy in 30–35 fx
Concurrent chemoradiation alone	60–70 Gy in 30–35 fx
Palliative radiotherapy	
External beam radiation	16–17 Gy in 2 fx, 48 Gy in 12 fx, 30–45 Gy in 10–15 fx, 50 Gy in 20 fx
Intraluminal brachytherapy	10–16 Gy in 2 fx

fractions to 30 Gy in 10 fractions may be given to these patients for a sustained palliative benefit. Other employed palliative regimens include 10 Gy × 1, 4 Gy daily × 5, 8.5 Gy weekly × 2, 3 Gy daily × 13 or 15, 2.5 Gy daily × 20, or even 2 Gy daily × 30, based on a recent survey performed among ASTRO members. Selection of regimen should be based on comprehensive consideration of age, performance status, tumor burden, and symptoms of each individual patient. Patients with poor performance status and with large distant tumor burden regardless of their performance status should be treated by a short course of relatively low dose radiotherapy. A definitive dose of radiation with combined chemotherapy may also be acceptable for patients with good performance and limited distant disease (such as solitary brain metastasis). There is limited evidence showing that higher dose thoracic radiation is associated with extension of survival in patients with good performance status (107).

Dose Escalation for Conventionally Fractionated RT

Historically, the tumor dose of 60 Gy was established as the standard of care in RTOG 73–01 randomized trial (81,128). However, long-term tumor control and survival are generally poor for such prescription dose. Evaluation by means of bronchoscopy and biopsy at 1 year after treatment completion revealed local control rates of only 15% to 17% (86), with 5-year overall survival reported to be <10% (82,83). Retrospective studies reported that stage I NSCLC patients received a dose of ≥70 Gy had better local tumor control compared to those had <70 Gy (39,129),

and ≥64 Gy was associated with superior survival in patients with stage III NSCLC disease (130). Using 3D-CT-based conformal RT techniques, several radiation dose escalation studies have shown much higher than 60 to 70 Gy to be feasible (71,131–133) (35,36,39,40,42,134), and higher doses appear to be associated with better local tumor control and survival in medically inoperable or unresectable NSCLC (7,130). In the settings of radiation alone or sequential ChemRT, the RTOG 9311 trial escalated the dose to 83.8 Gy for patients with V20 (the lung volume received >20 Gy) <37.5%, using daily fractions of 2.15 Gy (135). Investigators from Memorial Sloan-Kettering Cancer Center safely escalated to a dose of 84 Gy for NTCP of <25% (133). Using a lung volume-based escalation scheme, researchers from the University of Michigan have demonstrated that doses of 92.4 and 102.9 Gy in 2.1 Gy daily fractions can be delivered safely with minimal toxicity if the mean lung dose (MLD) is sufficiently small (42,132). For patients with newly diagnosed or recurrent stage I–III disease, multivariate analysis of this dose escalation trial found the radiation dose to be the only significant factor for local tumor control and overall survival (7), and demonstrated a positive relationship between dose and local/regional control, as well as overall survival in the dose range of 63 to 103 Gy. An increase of 1 Gy was associated with a >1% improvement in the 5-year tumor control, and a 3% decrease in the risk of death. Higher radiation doses may therefore be beneficial to patients with inoperable/unresectable NSCLC (Fig. 33.4). A recent secondary analysis from RTOG trials has demonstrated a

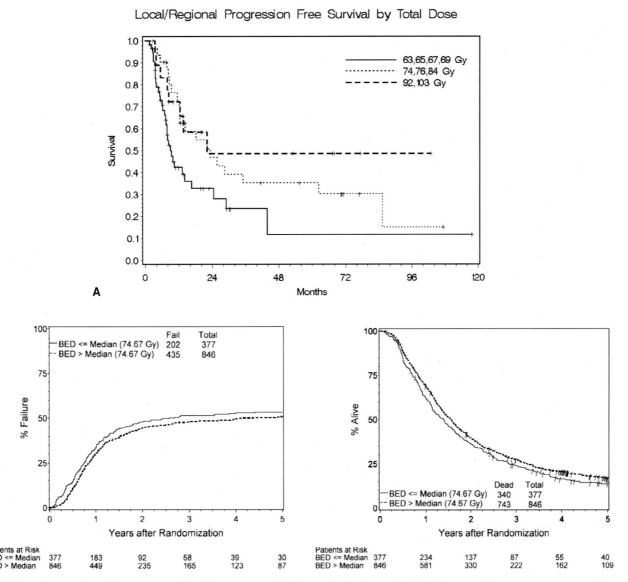

Figure 33.4. Radiation dose effect in non-small cell lung cancer. High dose radiation is associated with improved long-term tumor control in patients treated with radiation therapy alone or with sequential chemoradiation (**A**) (208), and concurrent chemoradiation (**B**) (136).

2% reduction of risk from death with each increase of 1 Gy biological equivalent dose (136). Bogart et al. used >2.25 Gy daily fraction to a total nominal dose up to 84 Gy (range: 60–84) and reported a promising overall tumor response rate of 88% (35% complete response and 53% partial response), actuarial median survival of 38 months, and 3-year overall survival of 60% in early stage medical inoperable NSCLC (36).

In the setting of concurrent ChemRT, the group from the University of North Carolina reported safe dose escalation up to 90 Gy with 2 Gy daily fractions, and with concurrent CP chemotherapy (137). However, RTOG 0117 demonstrated the maximum safe dose of 74 Gy with concurrent and adjuvant CP treatments (138). RTOG 0617 is ongoing phase III trial to compare the survival benefit between 74 Gy and 60 Gy. RTOG 1106 will escalate the radiation dose and shorten the treatment duration by

using isotoxicity and individualized adaptive dose prescription.

In summary, the dose of radiation should be individualized based on normal tissue tolerance particularly normal lung, and the use of chemotherapy. A dose of >70 Gy may be given with RT, or sequential ChemRT, and when the lung volume is limited (see later section for lung dose tolerance; Table 33.8). For large tumors when normal lung irradiation is extensive, or concurrent chemotherapy is given, the majority of the patients are unable to tolerate higher radiation doses due to severe toxicity; the most common prescription dose may still be around 60 to 70 Gy, depending on the results of RTOG 0617.

Hyperfractionated Accelerated RT

Dose escalation in conventional fractionation leads to extension of treatment duration, which may allow tumor re-population and decrease the probability of local tumor control and survival. Although hypofractionation may reduce treatment duration, it is usually not a choice because lung tissue has smaller alpha/beta than the tumor. Hyperfractionated accelerated RT (HART) or continuous hyperfractionated accelerated RT (CHART), which delivers multiple smaller fractions each day, was proposed to reduce the treatment duration and prevent excessive late tissue toxicities. Several trials showed benefit of reducing the treatment duration using CHART or HART. A phase III trial reported that 2-year survival was superior in the CHART arm (54 Gy delivered over 12 consecutive days) than the standard RT arm (60 Gy in 2 Gy fractions, Monday through Friday in 6 weeks) (139). The ECOG 2597 trial compared 64 Gy/32 fx/6.5 weeks with HART (57.6 Gy/ 36 fx/3 weeks) after induction chemotherapy in locally advanced stage III NSCLC, and reported a trend of improved survival with the HART arm (95).

With regard to hyperfractionated radiation therapy, RTOG 8311 was a phase I/II trial tested multiple RT regimens with different total tumor doses (60, 64.8, 69.6, 74.5, and 79.2 Gy). The study showed superior results with 69.6 Gy in 1.2 Gy twice daily fractions, compared to 60 Gy in 2 Gy daily fractions with a similar BED and treatment duration (140). The 69.6 Gy regimen also had better survival, than other regimens with higher doses, which often had extended treatment duration and delays due to acute esophagitis. Survival was significantly better in patients who completed treatment in the planned time, as compared with those who had treatment interruptions (140). However, randomized clinical trials have not shown an advantage for hyperfractionated RT (87,140,141). In the setting of neoadjuvant chemotherapy, RTOG 8808 did not show a significant advantage of using hyperfractionated radiation. Using concurrent ChemRT, RTOG 9410 showed that the hyperfractionated arm was associated with an increased incidence of esophagitis and inferior survival compared to the daily fractionated concurrent arm (88). In summary, hyperfractionated schemes are not recommended due to the lack of significant survival benefit in phase III trials, increased acute esophagitis, especially with concurrent chemotherapy, and the burden to the patients and radiation departments. Although HART may be an option for radiation alone, the "safe" fractionation prescription is still 1.8 to 2.0 Gy conventional fractionations, particularly when concurrent chemotherapy is given.

Nevertheless, prolonged treatment time is significantly associated with poorer survival. In a recent secondary analysis of three RTOG trials in patients with stage III NSCLC who were treated with immediate concurrent ChemRT, it was concluded that prolonged treatment time translated into a 2% increase in the risk of death for each day of prolongation in therapy (142). It was estimated that the tumor control probability of NSCLC decreases 1.6% per day after a 6-week duration of RT (143). Thus, every

effort should be made to limit treatment duration and avoid treatment delays. Currently, there are investigative efforts to increase daily fraction size to escalate total radiation dose without extending the treatment duration. One approach involves dose escalation using 2.25 Gy daily fractions (once or twice daily) but limiting treatment duration to 6 weeks (40). This approach was used to escalate radiation doses to 87.8 Gy in patients with limited lung volume. Another approach is to use higher fraction dose every day while limiting the treatment duration to 5 weeks (144). A dose of 86 Gy can be delivered within 6 weeks with daily fraction size ranging from 2.2 to 3.8 Gy (Kong ASTRO 2010). RTOG 1106 may validate this regimen in a multicenter setting.

Hypofractionated SBRT

Hypofractionated SBRT is an emerging new technique for T1 and T2 (<5 cm) N0, peripherally located NSCLC, to escalate tumor dose while shorten the treatment duration. There are wide variations in fractionation regimens. Quite a few studies reported that a higher BED is associated with better disease control. Researchers from Japan (44) reported a 3-year overall survival rate of 88.4% for medically operable diseases, when using a BED ≥ 100 Gy, compared to 69.4% for < 100 Gy ($p < 0.05$). Results of 241 patients from 13 Japanese Institutions reported the local recurrence rate of 20% when the BED <100 Gy, and 6.5% when the BED >100 Gy (144). Data from Germany reported that the dose to the CTV based on 4D dose calculation was closely correlated with local control: local control rates were 89% and 62% at 36 months for >100 Gy and <100 Gy BED ($p = 0.0001$), respectively (146). In the United States, researchers from Indiana University escalated safely to 60 Gy in three fractions and reported that fraction size of 18 Gy and above appeared to have less failure (46); in 47 patients with stage I disease, 10 patients had experienced local failure, of which nine occurred at doses <54 Gy in three fractions, with only one failure noted at higher doses (147). Experience from North America suggests that dose tumor control plateaus at about 18 to 20 Gy per fraction for three fractions (148,149). With this regimen, recent results from RTOG236 had only one primary tumor failure; the estimated 3-year primary tumor control rate was 97.6% (95% CI, 84.3–99.7%) in patients with medically inoperable stage I disease (<5 cm) (54).

A wide variety of fractionation schemes have been used in the management of NSCLC. One would ask if there is a particular condition under which a corresponding fractionation scheme would be preferable. In the context of lung normal tissue complication probability (NTCP), and the linear-quadratic models, a simulation study showed that the therapeutical ratio increases with increasing dose per fraction in the cases of higher prescription dose and small target volume, while it increases with decreasing dose per fraction in the cases of lower prescription dose and large target volume (150). As of current practice of tumor <5 cm, commonly employed SBRT schemes include (not limited by) 54 to 60 Gy delivered in three fractions over 8 to 14 days, 48 Gy in four fractions over 5 to 10 days, and 50 to 55 Gy in five fractions within 10 to 14 days—all with acceptable tumor control and normal tissue toxicity.

Dose and Fractionation in SCLC

Thoracic Irradiation

Thoracic radiation for LS-SCLC should be delivered early and concurrently with cisplatin-based chemotherapy, with 45 Gy in 1.5 Gy twice-daily fractions. If hyperfractionation is not possible, a dose of at least 54 to 60 Gy in 2 Gy daily fractions should be given. If the chemotherapy has been given prior to the thoracic RT, 50 to 54 Gy in 1.8 to 2.0 Gy should be given to the complete responders and 60 Gy to partial responders.

Accelerated hyperfractionated RT (45 Gy in 1.5 Gy twice-daily fractions) should be recommended whenever possible. This is supported by a randomized phase III clinical trial, INT 0096 (151) comparing once daily (45 Gy in 1.8 Gy daily fractions) versus twice daily RT (45 Gy given in twice daily 1.5 Gy fractions) in combination with concurrent cisplatin and etoposide therapy. An improved median survival time and a 5-year survival rate were observed in the accelerated arm compared with the once daily group, 23 months versus 19 months and 26% versus 16% respectively ($p = 0.04$). One must note that the accelerated hyperfractionated RT was associated with increased toxicity. A dose of 45 Gy in 1.8 Gy daily fractions is not biologically equivalent to 45 Gy in 1.5 Gy twice daily. Treatment duration may also impact the outcome of SCLC treatment. Using a similar regimen of hyperfractionated RT with a treatment break of 2.5 weeks, the North Central Cancer Treatment Group (NCCTG) failed to show a benefit of using hyperfractionated RT as compared to conventional RT (152,153). Nevertheless, 45 Gy in 30 fractions over 3 weeks concurrent with etoposide and cisplatin therapy generated superior results to other published reports and is the recommended regimen for the treatment of LS-SCLC. When twice daily radiation is impossible, daily fractionation with higher dose (60–70 Gy in 2 Gy fractions) is an acceptable alternative. CALGB39810/RTOG539 is ongoing to compare results of 45 Gy in 105 Gy BID with 70 Gy using standard fractionation (such as CALGB) and 61.2 Gy using concomitant boost.

Prophylactic Cranial Irradiation

The standard dose prescription for cranial irradiation for LS-SCLC is 25 to 30 Gy in 2 to 2.5 Gy daily fractions over 12 to 14 days for patients in complete remission (151,154). However, a review including 42 PCI trials with 4,749 patients revealed the optimal total RT dose to be 30 to 35 Gy given as 2 Gy fractions (155). A dose of 24 Gy in

3 Gy fractions also appeared safe based on data from a large randomized study. According to a comparison of four dose regimens: 8 Gy, 24 to 25 Gy, 30 Gy, and 36 to 40 Gy, higher doses of radiation appeared to be correlated with incremental decreases in the risk of brain metastasis (p for trend = 0.02), without significant impact on survival (126). Meanwhile, high-dose radiation may be associated with impaired neurocognitive function. Thus, more efficacious and less toxic treatment regimens were sought. This was directly addressed in a multinational phase III trial, in which 720 patients with limited-stage (LS)-SCLC and a complete response to their initial treatment were randomly assigned to PCI at a dose of either 25 Gy in 10 fractions or 36 Gy (administered either as 18 fractions of 2 Gy each or 24 fractions of 1.5 Gy given twice-daily)(156). Among the patients randomized to the 36 Gy treatment arm, 78% received once daily therapy. The 2-year incidence rates of brain metastases were 23% for the higher radiation dose and 29% with the lower dose, which was not statistically different ($p > 0.05$). However, the higher dose was associated with a significantly lower 2-year survival rate (37 vs. 42 %, HR 1.20, 95% CI, 1.00–1.44). There was no obvious explanation for the increased mortality in the group treated with higher doses of PCI. Nevertheless, the standard dose of PCI should be 25 Gy in 10 fractions within 2 weeks (Table 33.6).

Patient Simulation

Patient Immobilization

Immobilization is an important part in patient simulation to achieve reproducible positioning between simulation and treatment delivery and stable positioning during simulation and treatment delivery (157–159). Simple thorax board, Wing Board, T-bar devices, Alpha cradle, Vac-Lock, or Vacuum mattress (Fig. 33.5) can be used as the immobilization device for thoracic patients. Patients are usually positioned with both arms above the head to allow a greater choice of beam arrangement. However, for prolonged treatment preparation and delivery procedures, such as breath-holding, respiration-gated radiotherapy, and stereotactic radiotherapy, the patients may have difficulty tolerating this arms-above-head position. Devices providing stable arm support are preferred (157). With increasing use of imaging guidance systems, the role of the immobilization device is mainly to achieve patient comfortability and stability. Devices such as head and knee cushions are frequently used to ensure maximum comfortable level and minimize setup errors. Although it improves reproducibility of daily setup and reduces the main cause of setup errors, immobilization devices do not eliminate the errors. Conventional 3DCRT without using any immobilization devices may be acceptable in some centers when an adequate margin is added to cover the setup error (160).

TABLE 33.6	**EORTC Guidelines for Conformal Radiation Therapy (317)**

Summary of recommendations for high-precision radiotherapy in lung cancer

Patient positioning
1. Reproducible patient set-up can be achieved with the use of T-bar devices, and use of customized immobilization devices is not mandatory
2. Devices providing stable arm support are preferred for prolonged immobilization, e.g., when multiple CT scans are performed, and for breath-hold or gated treatment delivery

Planning CT scan
1. Spiral CT scans are superior to single-slice CT scans for target volume definition
2. The treatment isocenter should preferably be located in the tumor mass, and it should be defined at the time of CT scanning to minimize simulator set-up errors
3. Use of intravenous contrast may not be mandatory for radiotherapy planning when a recent contrast-enhanced diagnostic CT scan is available, and if CT slice thickness of <5 mm is used. Intravenous contrast use can improve the contouring of centrally located tumors
4. Thin CT slices (2–3 mm) enable the generation of high-resolution DRRs, which remove the need for a separate simulation step, and allows for use of smaller CTV–PTV margins

Accounting for tumor mobility
1. Fluoroscopy should not be relied upon for characterizing tumor mobility for 3D radiotherapy planning
2. The application of "standard" margins to GTVs derived from a single rapid CT scan is inappropriate
3. "Slow" CT scans capture more reproducible target volumes for peripheral lung cancers
4. A margin of at least 5 mm should be added to any contoured mediastinal node to account for nodal mobility
5. Margins between 10 and 15 mm are used to derive a PTV from the GTV, but a 10-mm margin is only justified if a representative GTV has been generated for radiotherapy planning, and when a set-up correction protocol is applied at the treatment unit

Investigational procedures:
6. Respiration-gated radiotherapy and/or breath-holding maneuvers can decrease the impact of tumor mobility, but the latter is often not well tolerated by patients with lung cancer
7. Reliable respiration-gated CT scanners are not routinely available
8. External breathing signals may not reflect the actual 3D tumor movement, and breath-holding or respiration-gated techniques should be used in conjunction with the actual monitoring of tumor position

Generating target volumes
1. The optimal CT window settings for contouring tumors in lung parenchyma or mediastinum should ideally be present at the planning workstations
2. The Naruke scheme for nodal stations should be referred to in radiotherapy planning, and nodes with a short-axis diameter of ≥1 cm should be included in the GTV
3. There is insufficient evidence to support the use of elective nodal irradiation for any patient with localized NSCLC (stages I–III), irrespective of whether chemotherapy is (or has been) administered
4. FDG-PET scans are superior to CT scans for staging mediastinal nodes, and incorporating FDG-PET findings into CT-based planning scan results in changes to radiotherapy plans in a significant proportion of patients

Treatment planning
1. Three-dimensional radiotherapy planning is essential for ensuring both optimal target coverage and the optimal sparing of normal tissues. If the random and systematic set-up errors in treatment planning and delivery are known, 3D margins for the PTV can be generated, which are based upon need to achieve a specified tumor coverage probability

Tumor:
2. The margins required for microscopic tumor extension in radiotherapy planning of NSCLC are approximately 5–6 mm

Lungs:
3. The risk of radiation pneumonitis can be estimated from the $V20$ (volume of both lungs minus the PTV, which receives a dose of 20 Gy), and by the mean lung dose

(continued)

TABLE 33.6	EORTC Guidelines for Conformal Radiation Therapy (*Continued*)

Esophagus:
4. The length of esophagus that is irradiated should be limited to reduce the incidence of high-grade toxicity during concurrent chemoradiotherapy or altered fractionation schemes
5. The volume receiving doses in excess of 50–55 Gy, and the portion of the organ circumference receiving a dose of 80 Gy or more, correlate with high-grade toxicity

CT, computed tomography; DRR, digital reconstructed radiographies; CTV, clinical target volume; PTV, planning target volume; GTV, gross tumor volume; NSCLC, non-small-cell lung cancer; FDG–PET, positron emission tomography with ^{18}F-fluoro-2-deoxy-D-glucose.
Please also see ACR-ASTRO guideline for external beam conformal plan on http://www.acr.org/SecondaryMainMenuCategories/quality_safety/guidelines/ro/3 d_external_beam.aspx. The authors are also recommended to review EORTC guideline on stereotactic body radiation therapy (318).

Conventional CT Simulation

Three-dimensional CT simulation is typically performed for 3DCRT. Simulation CT is normally performed from middle neck (the level of the cricoid cartilage) to middle abdomen (L2–3), so that the whole lung is included for dosimetric estimation. Intravenous contrast is recommended, if possible. This is helpful for differentiating centrally located tumor and enlarged lymph nodes in the hilum and mediastinum from adjacent organs (161,162). The use of intravenous contrast may be waived if a recent contrast-enhanced diagnostic CT scan or PET-CT simulation is available (163,164) or for a peripherally located tumor located. Study of a small series indicated that the impact of contrast on dose estimation is less than 2% to 3% of the prescription dose (165). CT scans with a slice thickness of 2 to 3 mm are recommended (166).

A treatment isocenter, which is preferably located within the tumor mass, is usually defined in the CT images immediately after CT scanning. The coordinator of the isocenter is then determined. Multiple laser setup points are aligned to the isocenter point according to the given coordinator. Tattoos or external markers are then marked on the patient's skin or the surface of the immobilization device for patient setup during treatment delivery. Digital reconstructed radiographies (DRRs) are computed from the CT images for the defined isocenter for setup verification. The DRRs from the CT simulation are similar to simulator films in 2D simulation (166).

4D-CT Simulation

Four-dimensional CT (4D-CT) is one of the important technological innovations impacting the radiation treatment of lung cancers. Internal target volume (ITV), which accounts for the uncertainty induced by the internal respiratory motion, can be determined through 4D-CT (167). 4D-CT images of different phases are reconstructed by first correlating the timing of imaging data with a respiratory motion signal, and retrospectively sorting the imaging data

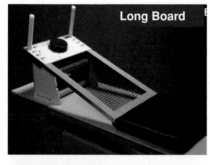
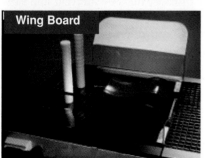
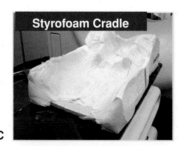
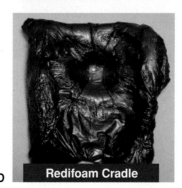
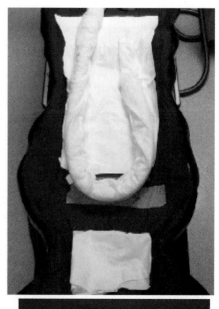

Figure 33.5. Immobilization devices for conventional radiation therapy in lung cancer (selected examples).

according to the phase and/or amplitude (168). The respiratory signal is usually obtained by detecting external motion of a patient (such as the surface of the stomach) by either an infrared-based respiratory position monitor (RPM) device or a belt wrapping around the stomach (169). Ten phases of 4D-CT images are usually reconstructed from a 4D-CT simulation. It can also be set to reconstruct a smaller number of phases (e.g., four phases at 25, 50, 75, and 100%) to reduce the burden of storing a large number of images (170,171). A maximum intensity projection (MIP) CT image set is then reconstructed from all phases of 4D-CT image (172). A composite gross tumor volume (GTVC) or internal gross tumor volume (IGTV) can be relatively conveniently contoured in the MIP image set. One should note that GTVC tends to be larger than true GTVs due to motion effect of normal tissues such as vessels. A motion display of each phase of images can then be used to verify if the GTVC encompass the tumor of each phase. An additional regular CT scan is often performed in many institutions for RT plan and dose calculation, particularly when the range of 4D-CT does not cover the whole spectrum of the OARs. 4D-CT can be set to just cover the tumor for motion assessment to reduce the imaging dose to the normal tissue, or a wider coverage of whole region of interest. When the 4D-CT has adequately covered the regions of interest for RT plan, an average CT image set can be reconstructed for dose calculation in treatment planning (173). 4D-CT should be performed for motion assessment for each definitive case whenever possible.

Treatment Target Definition

Traditional 2D radiation portals included regional lymphatic stations, and were defined according to anatomic landmarks visible in the radiography. The portals varied based on the primary tumor location. For upper-lobe tumors, bilateral upper mediastinum, supraclavicular regions, and subcarinal area (to 5 to 6 cm or two vertebral bodies below the carina) were encompassed. For middle or lower-lobe primaries without gross mediastinal lymph node involvement, the entire mediastinum (from the thoracic inlet to 8–9 cm below the carina) was encompassed without inclusion of the supraclavicular fossa. When gross mediastinal lymph node involvement is present, the supraclavicular areas were included along with the entire mediastinum. With wide availability of CT simulation and 3DCRT, 2D has become an uncommon practice, and is not a recommended radiation technique any more.

The modern 3DCRT requires precise definition of the treatment target and organs at risk (OARs). According to the guideline of International Commission of Radiation Units and Measurements (ICRU), the target planning target volume should consider the concept of gross tumor volume (GTV), clinical target volume (CTV), and (PTV). Figure 33.6 is a schematic display of the above volumes. The uses of 4D-CT and PET-CT have significantly improved the accuracy of target definition.

Determination of GTV

GTV includes the primary tumor (GTVT), and the nodal gross tumor (GTVN) that can usually be clearly identified in the imaging modalities. GTVN includes any abnormally enlarged regional lymph node (hilar and/or mediastinal), as well as mediastinal and/or supraclavicular nodes enlarged 1 cm or more in the short axis (166), unless metastases have been excluded by other means such as mediastinoscopy. GTVN should also include lymph nodes that are not enlarged but have been documented by mediastinoscopy/EUS/EBUS as being pathologically involved or have higher FDG activity than mediastinal blood pool. The measured diameter of tumors in lung parenchyma or mediastinum is highly dependent on the window width and level chosen during the delineating process (174). Lung primary tumors should be contoured using standard lung window/level settings, while the nodal disease and centrally located tumors are better contoured under mediastinum window/levels. The specific window widths and levels may vary with the CT scanner, software used, and the technique, with lung settings at $W = 400$ to $1,600$, $L = -400$ to -600, and mediastinum settings ranges $W = 400$ to $1,000$, $L = 0$ to 50 (166,174,175). One study found that the best concordance between measured and actual diameters and volumes was obtained with the following settings: $W = 1,600$ and $L = -600$ for parenchyma, and $W = 400$ and $L = 20$ for mediastinum (175). It is preferable that such parameters be specified in each center with the help of radiologist, and be preset in treatment planning workstations, in order to improve consistency in contouring.

Determination of CTV

CTV usually includes the GTV and a CTV margin around the GTV accounting for potential microscopic disease extension. It sometimes also includes regional lymph node areas that were not documented to have adenopathy or is proved by mediastinoscopy to be involved (176). The margins for CTV are controversial. It is challenging to estimate the extent of microscopic disease around the GTV. Giraud et al. examined NSCLC surgical specimens with ADC and squamous cell carcinoma (SCC) histology (175). The mean value of microscopic extension was 2.69 mm for ADC and 1.48 mm for SCC. A 5-mm margin covers 80% of the microscopic disease extension for ADC and 91% for SCC. To have 95% confidence that all tumor is included in the CTV, a margin of 8 mm and 6 mm must be chosen for ADC and SCC, respectively. The concept of nodal CTV includes CTV around the GTVN and the microscopic disease within clinically normal nodes. For CTV margins around GTVN, the nodal ECE was reported in 41.6% of patients (101/243) and 33.4% of lymph nodes (214/640) in one study (177). The extent of ECE was 0.7 mm in mean (range: 0–12.0 mm) and ≤3 mm in 95% of the nodes. Generally, extent of the CTV margin added to the GTVT to account for microscopic extent has been

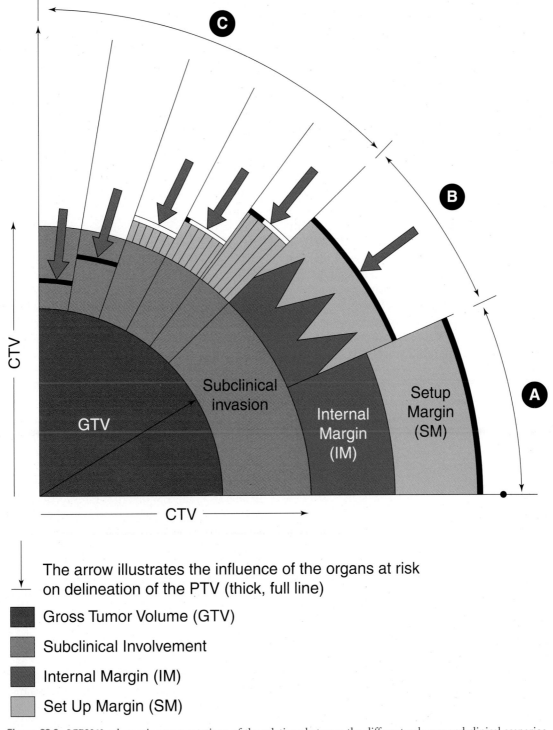

The arrow illustrates the influence of the organs at risk on delineation of the PTV (thick, full line)

Gross Tumor Volume (GTV)

Subclinical Involvement

Internal Margin (IM)

Set Up Margin (SM)

Figure 33.6. ICRU62 schematic representations of the relations between the different volumes and clinical scenarios. Gross tumor volume (GTV) is defined on CT scans. Clinical target volume (CTV) = GTV+ CTV margin. Internal target volume (ITV) = CTV+ IM (internal margin). Planning target volume (PTV) = CTV+IM+ SM (setup margin). PRV, planning organ at risk volume. **A:** PTV and CTV margins are added uniformly around GTV. **B:** The PTV margins (IM and SM) are compromised in some instances to decrease the dose to the adjacent structures. **C:** Both PTV and CTV margins are decreased in some regions due to presence of PRV. In some cases, the presence of organs at risk dramatically reduces the width of the acceptable safety margin (e.g., presence of the spinal cord and optical nerve). In other situations, larger safety margins may be accepted.

somewhat arbitrary, ranging from 5 to 8 mm, and GTVN ranging 3 to 5 mm.

The inclusion of the clinically uninvolved nodal regions into CTV has been a topic of debate and has been evolving over last several years. During the era of 1980s, this volume routinely included the mediastinum, bilateral hilum, and supraclavicular areas. Emami et al. (178) reported that inclusion of the contralateral hilum, the mediastinum, and supraclavicular lymph nodes in the field did not affect local control or survival. In 1990s, most centers have eliminated elective radiation of the contralateral hilum and/or the supraclavicular areas. However, whether or not the ipsilateral hilum lymph node group was included per protocol did appear to affect the local control and survival (179). Recent results with 3D conformal techniques without intentionally including these elective nodal regions have shown a low incidence (0–7%) of isolated nodal failure (7,37,42,134). There is no evidence to suggest that elective nodal irradiation is indicated in any patient group receiving curative or radical doses of RT for NSCLC.

Although most of the published results from the cooperative group used the elective radiation to most of the mediastinum regions, current practice in NSCLC and ongoing multicenter trials have a tendency to omit such radiation. If the treating physician believes that an elective nodal area (primarily of the mediastinum or ipsilateral hilum) should be indicated, it should be contoured and identified on CT scans (180). The definition of nodal stations are shown in Figure 33.7A. The University of Michigan has depicted an atlas of nodal regions on CT scan (Fig. 33.7B).

Determination of PTV

PTV includes the CTV and a margin around the CTV to compensate for errors in treatment setup and internal target motion during treatment. Traditionally, a uniform 7- to 10-mm margin was used to extend the CTV in all directions to form the PTV. However, because the internal target motion varies with direction (Table 33.7) (167,181), tumor location, size as well as patient condition such a practice is not ideal. It tends to include more normal lung than necessary and may lead to marginal miss (182). ICRU62 proposed to separate the PTV margin into two components: a setup margin (SM) and an internal margin (IM). The CTV plus the IM is defined as ITV. The PTV is thus the ITV plus the SM. The IM takes specifically the internal target motion into account and is patient-dependent. ITV may be reliably determined using 4D-CT and will be discussed in detail in section on "Determination of ITV." For clinics without 4D-CT, patient-specific IM may be used according to fluoroscopy data or data estimated from Table 33.7.

The SM takes into account all the variations/uncertainties in patients and beam positioning. It depends on the immobilization, simulation, and treatment techniques used at each individual institution. Therefore, it is more institution-dependent than patient-dependent. Setup errors include random and systematic variations; examples of random errors include unintentional movement of the patient's position while systematic errors may be from the offsets of the lasers used between the simulation and treatment room, and/or inaccurate marking on the setup points. If the random and systematic errors in treatment planning and delivery at an institution have been established for any particular tumor site, 3D margins for the SM can be calculated based upon the requirement for a certain coverage probability. For example, the SM margin can be expressed as $SM = 2.5\,\Sigma + 0.7^*\sigma$, where Σ and σ are the standard deviations of the systematic and random errors, respectively, considering a large part of the ITV (>95%) should receive >90% of the prescribed dose (183,184).

This relation can also be used for calculating the PTV margin applied to CTV. For example, one study (185) measured the overall setup errors in the chest were 1.3 ± 7.1 mm right–left, 3.3 ± 6.7 mm anterior–posterior, and 2.1 ± 8.3 mm superior–inferior. This study would indicate that a population-based standard PTV margin = $2.5^*1.3 + 0.7^*7.1 = 8.2$ mm in lateral, and 12.9 mm in AP, and 11.1 mm in SI directions. Such a margin would be too large for most patients and would unnecessarily encompass too much normal tissue, but may be too small for the outliers, leading to geographic miss of the PTV. If 4D-CT is used to determine the ITV, the SM from setup errors based on bony structure matching can be used to determine the PTV from the ITV. The setup error with bony structures is relatively small using the image guidance system. It was reported that the setup errors using a 2D x-ray image guidance system were 0.2 ± 1.0, 0.1 ± 0.9, and 0.2 ± 1.2 mm in lateral, AP, and SI directions, respectively, based on the match of bony structures such as vertebral column (186). Consequently, the SM can be <2 mm in each direction. However, there is uncertainty in defining the ITV, mainly due to the instability of respiratory motion of the patients. The SM should also include the uncertainty (or residual errors) of defining the ITV. Commonly, a margin of 3 to 5 mm may be added to the ITV if image guidance is used, and 5 to 7 mm if regular portal film is used.

Determination of ITV

ITV is the combination of CTV and margins for internal target motion (Fig. 33.6). It can be generated from the IGTV with addition of a CTV margin for microscopic diseases. IGTV can be determined by GTVs from 4D-CT images at different phases (170). Researchers from MD Anderson compared the IGTV from the following four approaches (187): (A) combining the GTVs from 10 respiratory phases; (B) combining the GTVs from two extreme respiratory phases (0% and 50%); (C) defining the GTV using the MIP images; and (D) defining the GTV using the MIP with modification based on visual verification of contours in individual respiratory phase. It was found that the IGTVs from the approaches B and C were statistically smaller than that from A, while the IGTV from D is similar to A. Increasing the number of phases in approach B

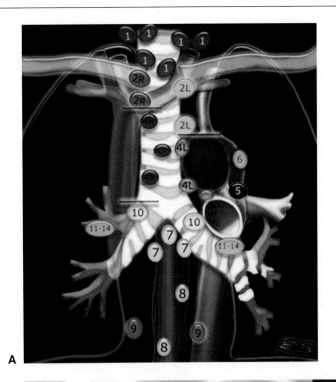

Figure 33.7. Considerations of mediastinal nodal clinical target volume (CTV). **A:** Nodal station definition. **Supraclavicular nodes 1. 1.** *Low cervical, supraclavicular, and sternal notch nodes.* From the lower margin of the cricoid to the clavicles and the upper border of the manubrium. The midline of the trachea serves as border between 1R and 1L. **Superior mediastinal nodes 2–4. 2R.** *Upper paratracheal.* 2R nodes extend to the left lateral border of the trachea. From upper border of manubrium to the intersection of caudal margin of innominate (left brachiocephalic) vein with the trachea. **2L.** *Upper paratracheal.* From the upper border of manubrium to the superior border of aortic arch. 2L nodes are located to the left of the left lateral border of the trachea. **3A.** *Pre-vascular.* These nodes are not adjacent to the trachea like the nodes in station 2, but they are anterior to the vessels. **3P.** *Prevertebral.* Nodes not adjacent to the trachea like the nodes in station 2, but behind the esophagus, which is prevertebral. **4R.** *Lower paratracheal.* From the intersection of the caudal margin of innominate (left brachiocephalic) vein with the trachea to the lower border of the azygos vein. 4R nodes extend from the right to the left lateral border of the trachea. **4L.** *Lower paratracheal.* From the upper margin of the aortic arch to the upper rim of the left main pulmonary artery. **Aortic nodes 5–6. 5.** *Subaortic.* These nodes are located in the AP window lateral to the ligamentum arteriosum. These nodes are not located between the aorta and the pulmonary trunk but lateral to these vessels. **6.** *Para-aortic.* These are ascending aorta or phrenic nodes lying anterior and lateral to the ascending aorta and the aortic arch. **Inferior mediastinal nodes 7–9. 7.** *Subcarinal.* **8.** *Paraesophageal.* Nodes below carina. **9.** *Pulmonary ligament.* Nodes lying within the pulmonary ligaments. **Hilar, lobar and (sub)segmental nodes 10–14.** These are all N1-nodes. **10.** *Hilar nodes.* These include nodes adjacent to the main stem bronchus and hilar vessels. On the right, they extend from the lower rim of the azygos vein to the interlobar region. On the left from the upper rim of the pulmonary artery to the interlobar region. **B:** Level 2, 3A, 3P, 4R, 4L, 5, 6, 7, and 8 on CT (180). *(continued)*

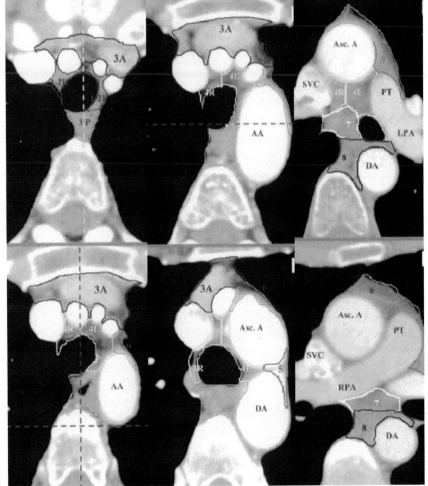

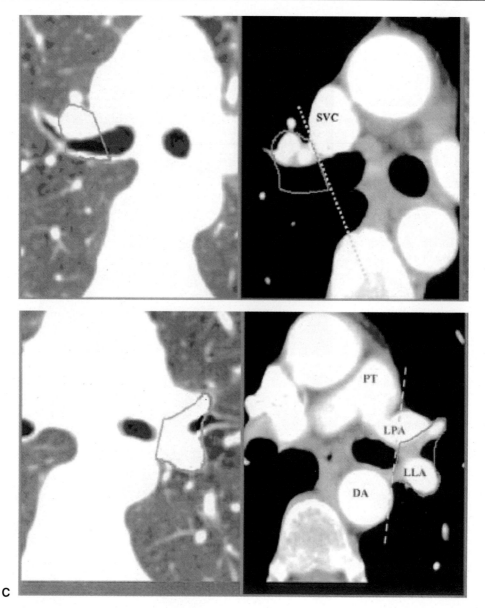

Figure 33.7. (*Continued*) **C:** Level 10 right (*top panel*) and left (*bottom panel*) under lung and mediastinal window-settings (180).

will increase the accuracy of defining the IGTV. Approach A is the most accurate, but has the heavy burden for the treatment planning computer to handle the large amount of data and for the radiation oncologists to delineate/check the target in each image set. Approach D may provide quick estimation but has a tendency to include vessels into the IGTV, particularly for the centrally located tumors. However, although statistically significant, the difference of IGTVs between B and C from that of A was small. Approach C may be still acceptable, especially when a large CTV margin and SM are applied to the IGTV to form the PTV—small misses will be ultimately included in the PTV. The extension of target motion and tumor size may also affect the requirement of the number of phases to define the IGTV. Using a motion phantom with various size/shape objects as virtual tumors, researchers from

Henry Ford Hospital in Detroit demonstrated that two gated CT scans at two extreme respiratory phases would be sufficient to determine the IGTV for tumor motion <1 cm and tumor volume >1 CC, and more phases would be required for tumors with 2-cm motion, especially for small tumors (170). An accurate and relatively easy method is to (i) generate the IGTV first based on 0% and 50% CTs, and (ii) expand this IGTV as indicated by scrolling through all phases, and double check the IGTV using the MIP scan.

ITV can also be determined without 4D-CT scanner. Methods such as three-phase breath-holding CT scans (188), multiple "slow" CT images (189), and a combination of one fast scan on shallow breathing with two breath-holding scans and a slow spiral CT scan (190) can be used to generate the IGTV. It should be noted that the

TABLE 33.7	Range of CTV Movements (236)			
Locations	**Mobility (mm)**			
	X direction	Y direction	Z direction	3D vector
Apical / 6 cm	3.8 ± 2.2	5.0 ± 3.3	4.2 ± 1.4	8.0 ± 3.1
Other	3.9 ± 2.5	6.6 ± 3.2	6.5 ± 2.7	10.7 ± 3.2
Supradiaphragmatic / 3 cm	6.2 ± 2.1	10.3 ± 4.6	6.2 ± 3.2	14.4 ± 2.4

tumor disposition during breath holding may be significantly larger from that during free breathing (such as that of 0% and 50% CT from 4D-CTs), as the patient often exaggerates the depth of their breathing. Residual uncertainty of defining the ITV exists for all the methods, including approach A and D using the 4D-CT images. Reproducibility of breathing pattern and amplitude is the major source of this residual uncertainty. Quality assurance of breathing reproducibility needs to be implemented to provide confident baseline estimations (181). Specifically, the patient should be coached appropriately that a deep breath should not be taken. Video assistant breathing coaching has also been developed to improve the breathing reproducibility.

PET Scan on Target Definition

FDG-PET has a significant impact on the delineation of the GTV for lung cancer because it images metabolically active tumor cells, and is superior to CT in estimating the disease extent, as described under Clinical Image Staging section (191–198). PET has the several advantages over CT: (i) it may distinguish tumor from collapsed lung or mediastinal structures (Figs. 33.1A and 33.8A); (ii) it detects mediastinal nodal involvement more accurately (Fig. 33.1B); (iii) it may estimate ITV as PET images are usually acquired over an extended period (196) (Fig. 33.8B); and (iv) it is reported to decrease interobserver and intra-observer variations in target delineation, particularly for tumors nearby hilum and mediastinum (200–201).

Using PET to delineate target delineation, however, is not straightforward for determining the edges of the tumor in the metabolically active area. Most of the studies mentioned above used an arbitrary threshold value of the maximum intensity (30%–50%) in the PET-avid area or a standardized uptake value (SUV) (range: 2–5). This threshold, however, was generated from phantom study of limited target size (202) and is not correct for the majority of patients with NSCLC (203). Figure 33.8C illustrates the problems with this method in underestimating GTV in a larger tumor. Researchers from Beaumont Hospital (203–204) performed a series of sphere phantom studies to determine an accurate and a uniformly applicable method for defining a GTV with FDG-PET. They found a strong linear relationship between the threshold SUV and the mean target SUV. Studies from University of Michigan further suggested that the threshold for the best match of CT GTV averaged 20% to 25% (range: 10%–50%), ITV 15% to 20% (range: 10%–50%), depending on the tumor size, activity, and location (205) Free-breathing PET can be used for determination of IGTV, ITV, or as a second QA for 4D-CT-based IGTV.

Another challenging issue of using PET for treatment planning is to register the PET image accurately when a PET-CT simulator or hybrid PET-CT is not available. An ideal registration method, which uses the entire volume of image data (i.e., intensities of the image voxels) for matching of "mutual information" and displays the two modalities simultaneously, would significantly improve the accuracy of PET in target delineation.

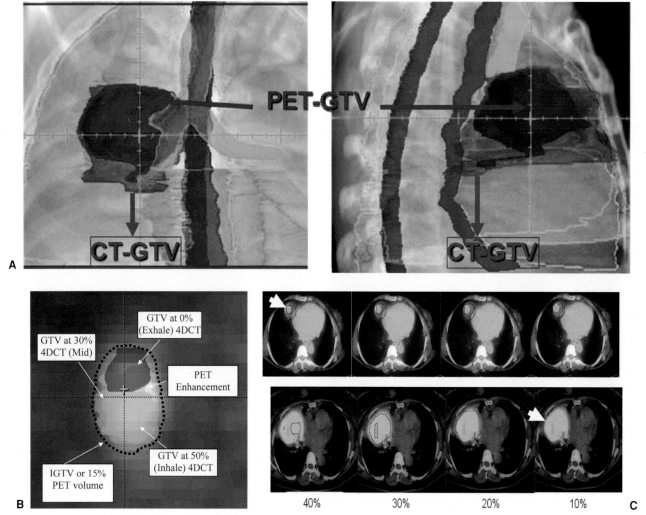

Figure 33.8. PET in target delineation and radiation treatment planning. **A:** PET differentiating active tumor from collapsed lung. This figure shows the difference of GTVs between PET and CT. The CT-GTV is larger than PET as it includes some collapsed lung. **B:** PET target volume and tumor motion: This picture depicts exhale CT-GTV (*red*), inhale CT-GTV (*green*), a middle-phase CT-GTV (*yellow*), the enhanced PET lesion (*in white*), and 15% threshold PET volume in the coronal plane from a non-small cell lung cancer of the left lower lobe. In this case, internal gross tumor volume (IGTV), a composite volume of all CT-GTVs matches with 15% +-PET threshold volume, indicating inclusion of motion effect in the PET volume. **C:** PET volume and CT gross tumor volume (GTV): PET target can be generated by using standard uptake value of 2.5, certain tumor back ground ratio, and maximum threshold method. The threshold generating best volumetric match between PET and CT depends on the size of the tumor. Figure 33.6C shows PET targets by thresholding an 10%, 20%, 30%, and 40%, respectively. A 40% threshold PET volume matches closely with CT GTV for a 2 cm tumor (the *top panel*), but largely underestimate the larger tumor (*bottom panel*). The best CT-PET match is around 10%–20% for the larger tumors.

Dosimetric Treatment Planning

After target definition, the next step is for dosimetrists to perform treatment planning in a treatment planning system (TPS). The TPS generally provides various functionalities for treatment simulation and planning, including setting radiation fields, calculating dose distribution, performing dosimetrical analysis such as dose-volume histogram (DVH) for the target and OARs, and so on. The dosimetric treatment planning process is an optimization process to achieve maximum dose coverage for the target and minimum dose to the OARs. In this section, we will discuss normal tissue dose constrains, beam arrangements (setting radiation fields), dose calculation and

evaluation, and inhomogeneity correction in dose calculation.

Normal Tissue Dose Constraints

In addition to accurate target definition, the critical structures or OARs should also be defined and delineated. The OARs for radiation of lung cancer are lung, esophagus, spinal cord, and heart. A set of criteria for tolerances of these normal tissues should be established from published studies and adapted for local clinical use (206,207). Table 33.8 shows some recommended dose/volume/outcome data for the lung, esophagus, spinal cord, and heart adapted from the recently published QUANTEC recommendation. For the lung, V20 ≤30% or a MLD of 20 Gy is

TABLE 33.8	Normal Tissue Dose Constraints Used for Conventionally Fractionated Radiotherapy			
Critical structure	DVH parameters	Limits	Toxicity rate	Toxicity endpoint
Spinal cord	Max dose	50 Gy	0.2%	Myelopathy
Spinal cord	Max dose	60 Gy	6%	Myelopathy
Spinal cord	Max dose	69 Gy	50%	Myelopathy
Lung	V20	≤30%	<20%	Symptomatic pneumonitis
Lung	Mean dose	7 Gy	5%	Symptomatic pneumonitis
Lung	Mean dose	13 Gy	10%	Symptomatic pneumonitis
Lung	Mean dose	20 Gy	20%	Symptomatic pneumonitis
Lung	Mean dose	24 Gy	30%	Symptomatic pneumonitis
Lung	Mean dose	27 Gy	40%	Symptomatic pneumonitis
Esophagus	Mean dose	<34 Gy	5%–20%	Grade 3+ esophagitis
Esophagus	V35	<50%	<30%	Grade 2+ esophagitis
Esophagus	V50	<40%	<30%	Grade 2+ esophagitis
Esophagus	V70	<20%	<30%	Grade 2+ esophagitis
Heart (pericardium)	Mean dose	<26 Gy	<15%	Pericarditis
Heart (pericardium)	V30	<46%	<15%	Pericarditis
Heart	V25	<10%	<1%	Long-term cardiac mortality

^{a}Vx = volume receiving ≥x Gy.
DVH, dose-volume histogram.
Source: Modified from QUANTEC Paper (207).

considered to correspond to 20% rate of symptomatic pneumonitis, which is considered as clinically acceptable to achieve best therapeutical ratio. For the esophagus, a mean dose <34 Gy corresponds to 5% to 20% rate of grade ≥ 3 acute esophagitis, while V35 = 50%, V50 = 40%, and V70 = 20% correspond to 30% rate of grade ≥2 acute esophagitis. For the spinal cord, a maximum dose of 50 Gy corresponds to 0.2% of myelopathy. For the heart, a mean dose of 26 Gy, or V30 of 46% of the pericardium corresponds to 15% of pericarditis. However, these data were based on limited clinical data and were "guesstimated" from clinical experience and consensus of the panel.

While either V20 or MLD is considered as a DVH parameter for lung toxicity in the QUANTEC recommendation, other parameters, such as V25, V30, V13, and V5, have been reported to be associated with the incidence of pneumonitis in multiple series (7). These parameters also highly correlate to each other. The problem with these point dosimetric factors is their high dependency on the shape of the DVH, which vary with the beam arranging pattern of each individual practicing physician. MLD seems to better represent the overall behavior of the DVH (7). Radiation pneumonitis increases remarkably after MLD reaching 15 to 20 Gy, and the curve is in agreement with the traditional sigmoid-shaped dose–response

relationship, with increasing steepness in the slope after passing a threshold dose. Using a cut-off of 20 Gy for MLD, the probability of freedom from pneumonitis in patients treated with radiation alone or sequential ChemRT (208), and concurrent ChemRT seems acceptable (209).

However, the MLD does not reflect the potential threshold characteristics of lung tissue dose–response. Lung effective volume (V_{eff}) and effective dose (D_{eff}), which are converted from lung DVH using more complicated functions, have also been used to model the lung NTCP (210). Because the lung is considered as a parallel organ, V_{eff} seems to better reflect the mechanism of the lung toxicity. The function to convert the lung DVH into V_{eff} can be considered as the dose–response curve for a single lung function unit receiving a uniform dose. The V_d model is a special case of V_{eff}, where the conversion function is a step function. In such a step function, a dose larger than a reference dose (d) completely damages the function unit, while a dose less than d has zero effect. A logistic function with two variables has been proposed to convert the DVH into V_{eff} (210). However, it has not showed significant superiority in predicting either moderate pneumonitis or clinical fibrosis (208). Recently, conversion functions combining V_d and MLD models, or V_d and logistic models, and with only one variable were proposed. In these functions, a dose larger than the reference dose (*d*) also completely damages the function unit, while a dose less than *d* has either linear effect or sigmoid curve effect (150). However, this model has not been tested with clinical data.

Esophagitis and resultant dysphagia and odynophagia are often the dose-limiting side effects of combined chemotherapy and radiotherapy to the chest (93,211–222). In practice, severe esophagitis ranges from 5% to 37%. Bradley et al. correlated the rate of ≥ grade 2 acute esophagitis to radiation dose–volume parameters for patients treated with or without concurrent chemotherapy (216). The data suggests that the use of concurrent chemotherapy effectively doubles the risk of clinically significant esophagitis. Hyperfractionation and concurrent chemotherapy also significantly increase the esophageal toxicity.

The heart does not, except under rare circumstances, contribute to the acute toxicity. However, cardiac toxicity in the form of pericardial disease or pericardial effusions and later myocardial and coronary artery disease has been reported in long-term survivors, making it desirable to reduce the dose to the entire heart as much as possible. However, one must note that radiation heart toxicity in general is poorly studied in patients with lung cancer.

The University of Michigan current ongoing trial set constraints for dose to normal tissue for patients receiving concurrent ChemRT as the following: the maximum dose to the spinal cord is a dose biologically equivalent to 50 Gy in 2 Gy fractions. The V_{eff} computed for the esophagus with a normalization dose biologically equivalent to 72 Gy in 2 Gy fractions must be less than one-third. The V_{eff} for the heart with a normalization dose of 40 Gy and 65 Gy must be less than 100% and 33%, respectively. The V_{eff} computed for both lungs minus the composite volume of inhale and exhale GTVs for the prescription dose must be generating <15% of NTCP, approximating a MLD of 20 Gy.

While limiting doses to critical structure, it is critical to define the normal tissues consistently. Figure 33.9 shows a recent atlas for OARs generated by a group of investigators from RTOG, SWOG, and EORTC (223).

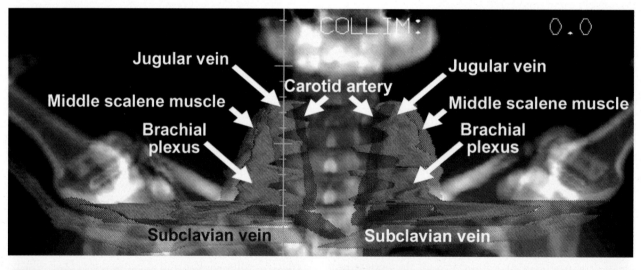

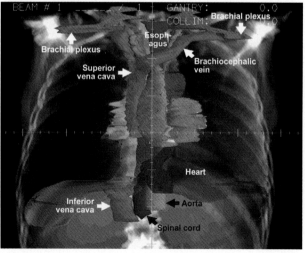

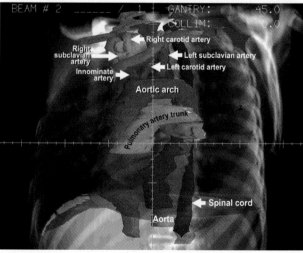

Figure 33.9. Atlas for organs at risk. **A:** Structures of digital reconstructed radiography. **B:** Example structures on CT axial cuts.

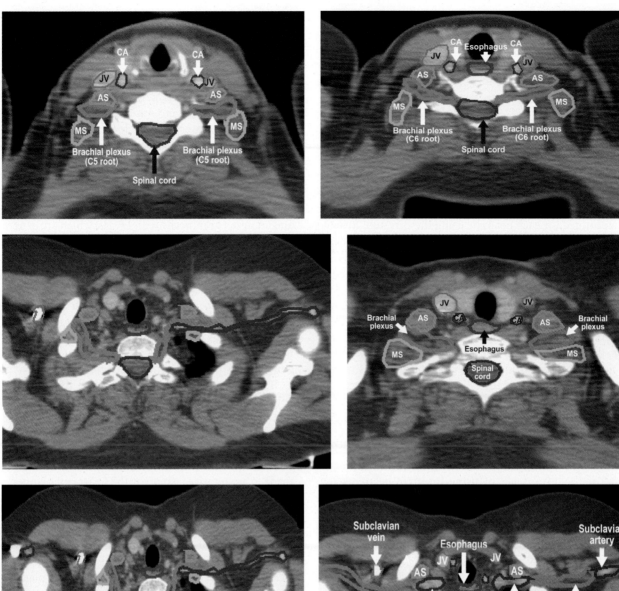

Figure 33.9. (*Continued*)

Beam Arrangements in 3DCRT

The basic principle of beam arrangement is to achieve maximum dose coverage for the target and minimum dose to the OARs. The design of radiation beam field or aperture depends on the treatment types and volume. In conventional 2D planning, corresponding lymph node stations are usually included as the radiation target. The beam selections are limited by the extensive volume of target, and consequently the tolerance of the critical organs

such as the lung, esophagus, and the spinal cord. Two parallel-opposed large fields from the anterior and posterior (AP/PA) directions of the patient are often used to minimize the dose to the lung. However, the AP/PA beam arrangement is limited by the tolerance dose of the cord; thus, one or more "off-cord" fields are always needed for definitive case when a dose of 60 Gy or higher is needed. In modern 3DCRT with selective ENI or without ENI, the target volume may be significantly reduced. Multiple coplanar or noncoplanar 3D conformal fields shaped to the target may be used to achieve more conformal dose to the target. However, the arrangement of AP/PA fields with off-cord oblique is still commonly used under 3DCRT, because the treatment target of lung cancer is often large so that lateral beam arrangement may increase the lung doses.

In conventional 2D-RT, the radiation fields are usually in a rectangular shape defined by the collimator jaws. The angles of the off-cord oblique fields can be selected by the use of the beam's eye view (BEV) tool in the TPS to avoid the cord. In modern 3DCRT, the beam shape is modified by designing a block or a block substitute called a multi-leaf collimator (MLC) shaper. Again, optimal angle can be determined for each beam by using the BEV tool to avoid direct irradiation of the OARs. The shape of each beam can also be formed by conforming the target in BEV. To cover the entire PTV with the prescription dose, an additional block (or MLC) margin should be added to each aperture to compensate the penumbra. Usually 5 to 10 mm block margin is needed for adequate coverage of PTV. It should be kept in mind that the block margin depends on the beam arrangement. For example, in a multiple-coplanar-beams setting, smaller lateral margin is needed for each beam because the radiation delivered outside the target along its pathway of one beam may compensate for the penumbra for the other beams, while relatively larger superior–inferior margins are needed because there is no beam coming from the superior–inferior direction. Reducing blocking margin with adequate PTV coverage is one of the advantages of using multiple-beam setting; however, this setting usually only benefits for cases with relatively smaller target volumes.

Selecting radiation beam energy is an important part of the beam arrangement. A photon energy of 6 MV is usually preferred to provide better PTV coverage in the boundary of the high density tumor and low density lung tissue. The imbalance of secondary electron flow between the high density and low density structures induces dose loss in the boundary region—the higher the photon energy, the greater the effect. This effect is usually not well demonstrated by most of the TPSs , even with sophisticated inhomogeneity corrections, except for those with Monte Carlo calculation algorithm. However, higher energy photons (15–18 MV) may be used in beams reaching targets without air gaps and/or to decrease the MU and provide better dose homogeneity for AP/PA mediastinal beams for large patients. Beam aids such as wedge or compensating filters are another part of the beam arrangement. In the case of a large sloping contour, they can be used to improve the dose distribution.

Dose Calculation and Evaluation

Once beam arrangement is set, dose calculation is performed according to the prescription dose and the patient geometry is defined by the 3D-CT images. Dose distributions are displayed with concentric curves for chosen dose levels (isodoses), which are displayed as overlays on ana-

tomic structures (Fig. 33.10). These curves are normalized to a reference dose, either at isocenter (ICRU point) or to the lowest isodose curve that encompasses the PTV.

The treatment plan can be evaluated as to whether it meets the objectives of PTV coverage and normal tissue avoidance. The idealized, perfect plan would be 100% coverage of a tumor target with a minimal amount of dose heterogeneity or overdose to achieve that 100% minimum dose coverage. This is very often an impossible goal. In practice, a 95% PTV coverage is acceptable for 3DRT. A set of criteria for normal tissue tolerances (discussed in the next section) must be given to guide the treatment planning. Dose distributions for 3D volumes can be displayed and analyzed graphically with DVHs, which are generated for each structure. The cumulative form of the DVH is a plot of the volume of a given structure receiving a certain dose or higher as a function of dose. Example DVHs for the target and critical structures are displayed in Figure 33.11. The DVH for normal lung is the addition of the dose distributions of both lungs but minus the dose distribution in the GTV. The GTV is selected instead of the PTV, since the PTV contains normal lung receiving a high dose, which influences the normal tissue toxicity rate.

If the treatment plan does not meet the given dose–volume objectives, beam arrangements or other parameters are adjusted. This can include a change of beam energy, beam angle, or adjustment of the beam intensity. For conventional conformal therapy, beam arrangements and adjustments are carried out manually, with changes made in an iterative fashion by the treatment planner. The inverse planning intensity-modulated radiation therapy (IMRT) technique will be discussed in detail in a separate section. Once the final beams are designed, x-ray images in the form of DRRs are generated from the treatment planning CT to compare to portal images taken before treatment for verification of radiation beam placement. Example DRRs are shown in Figure 33.12.

Tissue Heterogeneity Correction in Dose Calculation

A problem with dose calculation for lung cancer radiotherapy is that lung density is much smaller than that of tumor and other structures. Consequently, conventional dose calculation algorithms are often not accurate. Tissue heterogeneity correction is available in most TPSs; there are variations for different correction algorithms from different planning systems (224). An RTOG survey performed in 2004 showed that the majority of institutions had not taken the effects of lung density into account when prescribing dose to the PTV. Researchers at M.D. Anderson replanned 30 cases of early lung diseases with heterogeneity correction, using a commercial TPS with a convolution-superposition algorithm (225). They found that 14 of 30 original plans had <90% of PTV coverage if heterogeneity correction was turned on. To achieve equivalent PTV coverage (95% PTV coverage) as the original plan without correction, 8/30 cases required <2% increase of monitor units, while 13/30 cases required >5% monitor unit

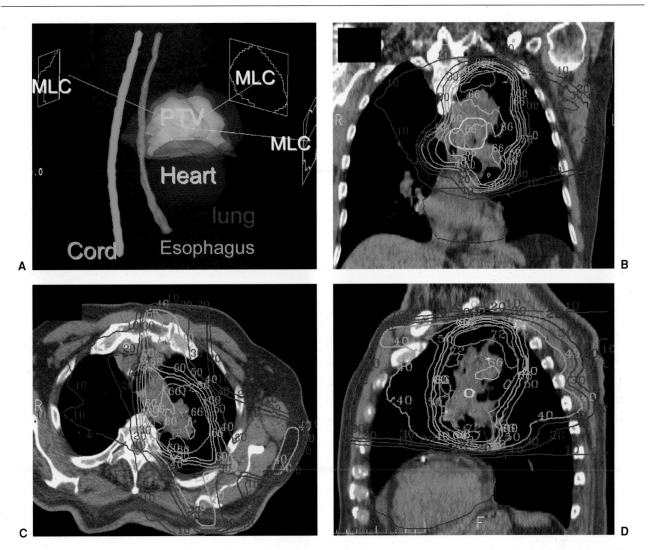

Figure 33.10. Example of 3D conformal radiotherapy planning. **A** shows 3D visualization of the MLC-shaped fields, PTV, and the surrounding normal structures. **B–D** show dose distributions at coronal, axial, and sagittal planes. MLC, multileaf collimator. The number shown in the figure is dose in Gy.

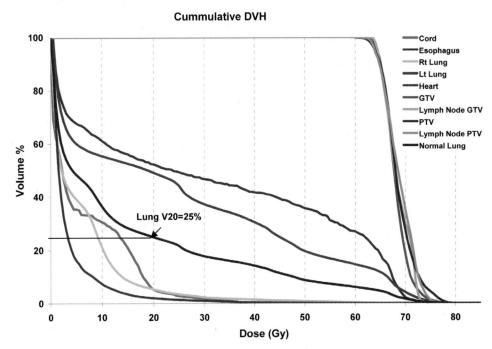

Figure 33.11. Dose-volume histogram (DVH) example of a typical 3D plan. The plot depicts accumulative DVHs of planning target volume (PTV) and organs at risk such as cord, esophagus, heart, and lung for the patient of Figure 33.10. Normal lung here represents the total lung volume with subtracting the overlapping gross tumor volume (GTV).

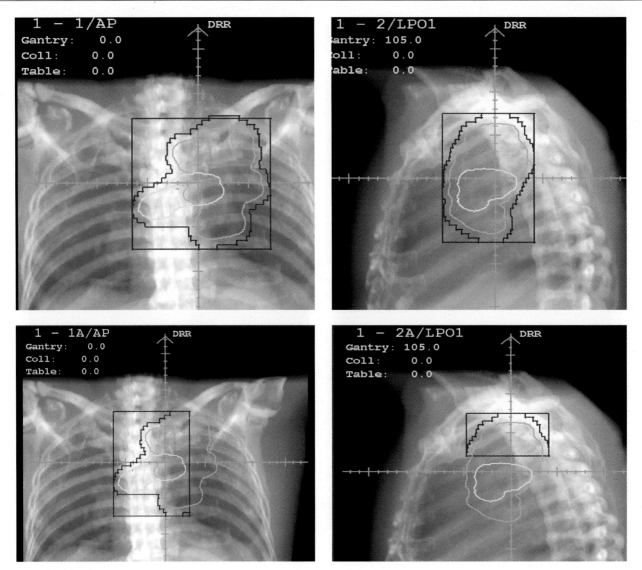

Figure 33.12. Examples of digital reconstructed radiography (DRR). These are two out of three fields used for the patient shown on Figures 33.10 and 33.11. To improve dose homogeneity, wedge or segmented fields (*bottom panel*) are often used. Red, collimator and multileaf shaped field borders; yellow, nodal planning target volume (PTV); purple, primary tumor PTV.

increase, with a maximum increase of 25%. Figure 33.13A shows examples of isodose distribution. The picture on the left was an original plan after correction is turned on; unfortunately, it had a rather large volume of CTV miss on the tumor peripheral zone, at a region adjacent to lung. The picture on the right shows a heterogeneity corrected plan, with nice, adequate target coverage. With the advancement of calculation software and supportive data from the phantom and patient, it is now the consensus of RTOG and AAPM that tissue heterogeneity needs to be corrected for treatment planning of lung cancer.

There are several density-correction algorithms available commercially, such as the equivalent-pathlength (EPL), equivalent-tissue-air ratio (ETAR), generalized Batho, and convolution-superposition (CS) methods. The EPL, Batho, and ETAR algorithms ignore lateral electron scatter in the tissue, thus are less accurate. The CS method

employs an empirical model to estimate the lateral electron transport in the calculation. Monte Carlo (MC) method is the only method that calculates explicitly the photon and electron transports within a material and is therefore likely to provide more accurate results at material interfaces and within lower density material (226). Studies demonstrated that the MC method provides the best match to the results of phantom measurement, and is considered to be the "gold standard" (227). For lung cancer cases, CS and MC recalculated dose distributions were characterized by reduced penetration and increased penumbra due to larger secondary electron range in the low-density media comparing to the pencil beam EPL method (226,228,229). Consequently, target dose was overestimated (though <10%), and the dose of adjacent lung was underestimated in the plans calculated by the EPL method. This effect is more prominent around the tumor–lung

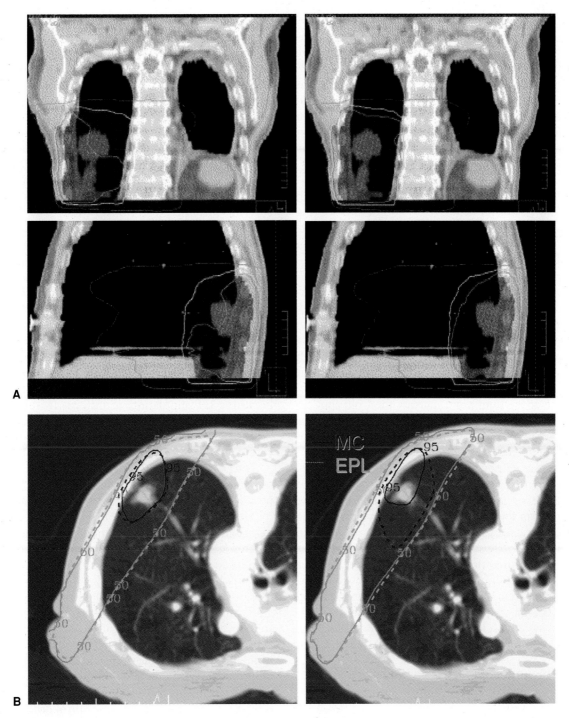

Figure 33.13. Tissue heterogeneity correction in lung cancer planning. **A.** Impact of heterogeneity correction on planning target volume (PTV) coverage in a patient with a tumor in the right lower lobe. This figure shows a remarkable underdosage of PTV in a plan generated by the traditional homogeneous prescription method with heterogeneity corrections (*right panel*) and the current heterogeneity-corrected prescription method (*left panel*) in the (a) sagittal and (b) coronal planes. Isodose lines are color-coded as follows: red, 76.Gy; orange, 66 Gy (prescribed dose); yellow, 60 Gy; green, 20 Gy. **B.** Impact of calculation algorithm on isodose distribution a lung treatment plan (two fields, 15-MV photons show isodose lines calculated with Monte Carlo (MC, *solid line*) and an equivalent path-length based algorithm (EPL, *dashed line*). Figure 33.11A shows that MC and EPL have almost same isodose distribution when heterogeneity correction is not turned on (i.e., the lung tissue is treated homogenously), while Figure 33.11B depicts remarkable overestimation of 95% isodose surface of the EPL-based dose computation comparing to that of MC calculation. (Courtesy of Indrin Chetty, Henry Ford Hospital, Detroit, Michigan.)

boundary, less at the PTV-mediastinal boundary. The MLD as determined by the CS and EPL algorithms differed on average by 17%, and the V20 differed on average by 12% (229). Figure 33.13B shows such an example recalculated by MC method. On the left panel, the dose was calculated without taking the tissue heterogeneity into account, and the isodose distributions are similar between the EPL and MC methods. On the right panel, a significant difference is seen in target coverage and normal lung doses.

In general, tissue heterogeneity effects depend on (i) the lung density; (ii) the lung length traversed; (iii) beam energy; and (iv) beam field size. In addition to altering PTV coverage, heterogeneity correction changes the ICRU prescription dose. Correction factors for a 6 MV photon AP/PA beams in lung range from 1.05 to 1.13, which varies with dose calculation algorithms. The CS and MC methods provide very close estimation. When dose was measured in a benchmark test phantom to a point in between two lungs, there was increased dose ranging from 5% to 14% relative to a phantom of unit density. The effect decreases as the photon energy increases. The use of high energy beams may minimize "hot spots" in lung treatment planning. However, higher energy beams tend to "spare" the surface of the tumor and increase the "cold spot" in this region due to increased range of secondary electrons in lung tissue (230). When a clinically relevant phantom study was performed (231), the dose delivered to the PTV with 6 MV was within 5% of prediction, but low by 11% with the use of 18 MV. Monte Carlo calculations showed that all target coverage indicators were significantly worse for 15 MV than for 6 MV, particularly the portion of the PTV receiving at least 95% of the prescription dose (232).

It is now generally accepted that density correction is better than no correction, and the CS method is better than the Batho, EPL, and TAR methods. Although it provides the most accurate estimation, the MC method is still in the process of validation, and only commercially available in few systems. A low energy photon beam should be used, especially for tumors imbedded in lung parenchyma.

Special Techniques in RT of Lung Cancers

Techniques for Tumor Motion Control

Tumor motion could be rather substantial and heterogeneous, ranging from a few millimeters to 25 mm based on tumor location, size, as well as patient's condition (233–235). The following techniques have been used to incorporate target motion into treatment planning, or control the tumor motion during treatment delivery (169): (i) Use a population-based internal margin (IM); (ii) use a patient-specific IM by estimating the amplitude of tumor motion in fluoroscopy; (iii) use ITV or IGTV by special simulation techniques such as 4D-CT; (iv) abdominal compression; (v) breath hold; (vi) gating; and (vii) Tracking tumor motion. Techniques (i)–(iii) only involve procedures during patient simulation and treatment planning,

while techniques (iv)–(vii) intend to control the motion, which not only involve procedures in simulation and planning, but also in treatment delivery.

The technique using a population based uniform PTV margin (or IM) of 10 to 15 mm had been a general approach before the 4D-CT era. The fluoroscopy technique with individual motion estimation can substantially reduce the PTV for patients with small motion, while provide adequate tumor coverage for patients with large motion (236,237). It was reported that with quiet respiration, the maximum movement in the craniocaudal direction was 12 mm, and the medio-lateral and anterior–posterior directions 5 mm (236). In another report, the movement ranged from 0 to 12.8 mm in the superior–inferior direction, 0 to 3.2 mm in the lateral direction, and 0 to 4.4 mm in the anterior–posterior direction (237). However, the fluoroscopy technique is limited by the facts including: (i) some tumors can be difficult to visualize with fluoroscopy x-rays; (ii) diaphragm motion may not correlate with tumor movement; and (iii) the shape change of the tumor cannot be measured clearly. In addition, because the tumor can be scanned in an extreme motion position (such as at the end of exhale) rather than its central motion position during the free-breathing CT simulation, a uniform IM expansion in both superior and inferior directions would include unnecessary normal tissue in one side, but not adequate coverage of the target in the other side.

The ITV technique using 4D-CT simulation overcomes the drawbacks of the fluoroscopy method. It is the state-of-art technique to assess the motion effect and integrate it into the treatment plan. The details of this technique are discussed in previous section under simulation.

The abdominal compression method reduces the amplitude of respiratory motion during CT simulation and treatment delivery (238). The breath-hold technique uses an active breathing control (ABC) device (239) to guide and control the patient's breathing holding pattern so that radiation treatment can be delivered in the controlled breathing holding phase. The tumor does not move in this fixed phase. However, many lung patients cannot hold their breath long and constantly. The gating technique uses an external motion signal (such as using an infrared device monitoring chest or abdominal surface movement) to control the linear accelerator so that radiation is only delivered in the specific defined phase window (169). The patient breathes freely during gating treatment. One problem with the breath hold and gating techniques is that radiation is only delivered in a selected phase window so that the treatment time extends. The tracking technique has been proposed to increase the efficiency by tracking the target motion with the moving MLC or treatment couch (240,241). However, all these techniques require repeatable breathing patterns and amplitudes during patient simulation and treatment. Some of the techniques may discomfort patients, require patient cooperation, and increase the time of the treatment procedure.

These factors could potentially increase the nonrespiratory motion during treatment. In addition, the external motion signal may significantly differ from the tumor motion. The external motion signals at different surface positions may also have different phase shifts (242). There are potential time delays in the control loop of acquiring motion signal, radiation delivery, moving MLC or couch (243). These may induce significant residual motion errors, and more importantly, if not handled properly, may cause severe adverse effect. Therefore, these techniques are still considered experimental procedures. Extensive clinical evaluation is required before they can be used widely in the clinic.

Another practical technique worth to mention is to utilize target motion to irradiate the CTV so that the CTV margin can be reduced or eliminated (244) (Fig. 33.14). This is based on the assumption that the tumor cell density (or tumor burden) in the microscopic extension is significantly less than that in the GTV. Consequently, the radiation dose required to control the tumor cells in this region is less than the full dose delivered to the GTV. With IGTV to encompass the GTV motion, a PTV margin is

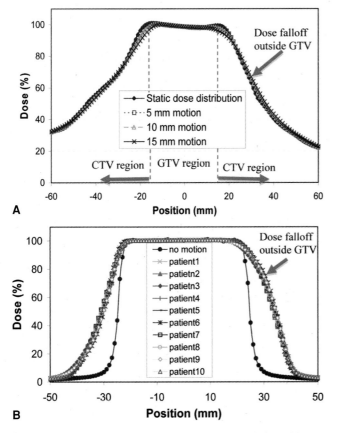

Figure 33.14. The effects of respiratory motion and clinical target volume (CTV) doses. **A.** In the axial (AP or lateral) direction, the natural dose falloff may cover the CTV; the respiratory motion has minimal effect on the dose coverage in this region. **B.** In the superior–inferior direction, the dose falloff without motion (*blue*) is very sharp, amplitude of 15 mm may generate enough gradual dose falloff to cover the CTV, based on measurements of 10 patients of different motion patterns (244). GTV, gross tumor volume.

added to the IGTV to account for the setup uncertainty. In such a setting, the GTV will receive full dose, while the CTV will receive partial of the prescription dose because respiratory motion shifts the CTV in and out of the field in different time.

Inverse Planning and Intensity-Modulated Radiation Therapy

IMRT is a treatment planning and delivery technique to achieve maximum dose coverage for the target and minimum dose to the critical structures. While the radiation intensity is uniform across the beam/field for conventional 3DCRT, it is highly varied or modulated for IMRT. The simplest modification of the intensity is a wedge-filter or a physical compensator placed in the machine head to achieve dose uniformity in the target. The MLC in a modern treatment machine can achieve the same goal by moving each pair of leaves during radiation delivery. The MLC can also achieve much more complicated form of intensity modulation, such as a checkerboard pattern. In a treatment plan, intensity modulation usually provides minimum intensity of radiation in the regions where critical structures appear in the BEV, while gives high intensity of radiation in the regions of "cold spots" due to the intensity modulation in other beams. An inverse planning process with a special computing algorithm is used to determine the intensity modulation pattern for each of the beams. A set of treatment planning goals, such as the dose coverage for the target and dose limitations for the OARs, usually represented by doses points in the corresponding DVH, and their relative weights, are first input into the IMRT inverse planning system. The beam arrangement, including the number of beams and their gantry angles, is also determined by the treatment planner. The computer then determines the corresponding intensity profiles to achieve the desired goal. Finally the computer will convert the intensity profiles into MLC leaf move sequences.

There has been several theoretical treatment planning studies published, with findings that higher levels of tumor dose can be achieved while maintaining the same normal lung dose–volume indices (245–248). Compared to 3DCRT, IMRT reduced the percentage of lung volume that received ≥20 Gy and the MLD, with a median reduction of 8% and 2 Gy, respectively (249). Treatment planning with IMRT under deep breath-hold results in lower V20 and lower modeled pneumonitis rates (250), allowing delivery higher dose to the target. IMRT is of significant value (compared to 3DCRT) in node-positive cases with target volumes close to the esophagus (220,248). Allowing nonuniform radiation to the target, Figure 33.15 shows an example IMRT plan delivering high equivalent uniform dose to the target, while sparing the esophagus (251). For such cases, IMRT can deliver RT doses 125% to 130% greater than an optimized 3DCRT plan and 130% to 140% greater than a plan including ENI (248). IMRT is of limited additional value (compared to 3DCRT) in node-negative cases (248) and may be associated with increased

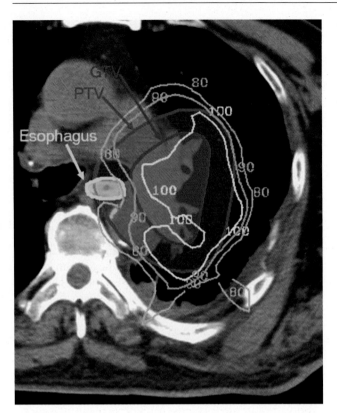

Figure 33.15. Plan of intensity-modulated radiation therapy (IMRT). The picture depicts an example isodose distribution of an optimized IMRT plan, showing sparing of esophagus from high dose region (<80%). Numbers on the figure show percentage of the dose referring to isocenter (180). GTV, gross tumor volume; PTV, planning target volume.

lung volume exposing to low doses (<10 Gy), for which the clinical impact on lung toxicity is not yet clear.

The major concern of using IMRT for lung cancer is the motion interplay effect (252,253). IMRT delivery is usually achieved by irradiating the target through multiple small segments. The sequence of the delivery of these multiple small fields induces an effect of moving the small fields within the entire large field. If the motion of these small fields synchronizes with target motion, radiation will be delivered to only one spot of the target instead of throughout the target. This motion interplay effect may induce significant errors for special circumstances. However, phantom and simulation studies have shown that the interplay effect may not be significant (252,253). To reduce the interplay effect, a proper collimator angle should be selected to avoid parallel motions between the MLC leave and the tumor. Retrospective studies from MD Anderson suggested that IMRT may improve treatment outcome while decrease treatment toxicity (254,255).

Stereotactic Body Radiation Therapy

Stereotactic body radiation therapy (SBRT) is an emerging new technique to treat medically inoperable early stage nodal negative NSCLC patients. As discussed above,

it delivers a very high dose in one or few fractions in a highly conformal fashion. The RTOG protocols such as RTOG618 (http://www.rtog.org/members/protocols/0618/0618.pdf) or RTOG813 (http://www.rtog.org/members/protocols/0813/0813.pdf) have a comprehensive and detailed method for this technique. Readers are strongly recommended to read the radiation technique section of RTOG protocols. Specifically, the conformal index (CI), defined as the ratio of the volume of the prescription isodose to the volume of the PTV, should be limited to <1.2; the gradient index (GI), defined as the ratio of the volume of the 50% prescription dose volume to the volume of the PTV, should be <4. The dose limits to normal structures as given in Table 33.9, should be respected.

The term "stereotactic" came from intracranial "stereotactic radiosurgery (SRS)." It can be defined as precisely directing radiation beams in 3D space toward a point target using an external 3D frame of reference usually based on the Cartesian coordinate system. The differences of SBRT from the conventional radiation treatment are mainly in three aspects: (i) "Targeting" or positioning; (ii) Delivery of radiation beams; and (iii) The dose and fractionation scheme.

The definition of "stereotactic" requires "targeting" to be conducted with the use of a well-defined 3D coordinate system. In brain stereotactic technique, a fiducial box attached to a head frame based immobilization system can well define the coordinate system, and associate it with the tumor position through CT and/or MR imaging in a reproducible and secure fashion. This is possible for brain, as the human skull is a relatively rigid structure, "stereotactic targeting" or patient positioning can be achieved by adjusting the head frame, which is rigidly attached to the patient skull, to a specific coordinate position according to the relative position of the tumor in the 3D coordinate system as determined in the process of treatment planning. A similar body frame was developed in the early stage of SBRT for "stereotactic targeting." However, because the body is not a rigid structure, and the tumor could move between simulation and treatment, the accuracy of such "stereotactic targeting" was suboptimal. The development of online image guidance systems enables the use of the implanted radioopaque markers, the neighboring bony anatomic landmarks, or the tumor itself as fiducials for "stereotactic targeting." Online image-guided positioning is currently the state-of-art technique, replacing the body frame based "stereotactic targeting" for more reliable and accurate positioning. Several points should be noted regarding the use of the online imaging guidance systems. First, the image guidance system cannot solve the tumor motion problem. Reliable motion control techniques such as abdominal compression may be used to reduce the motion amplitude. The ITV technique should be used to minimize the motion effect. Secondly, if a moving object, such as the tumor is used as the fiducial,

TABLE 33.9 Suggested Normal Tissue Dose Constraints for Lung SBRT.

Critical structure	Volume (cc)[a]	One fraction	3 fractions	5 fractions	Toxicity end point
Spinal cord	Point	14/14	7.3/21.9	6/30	Myelopathy
	<0.35	10/10	6/18	4.6/23	
	<1.2	7/7	4.1/12.3	2.9/14.5	
Lung	<1,500	7/7	3.5/10.5[a]	2.5/12.5	Basic lung function
Lung	<1,000	7.4/7.4	3.8/11.4[a]	2.7/13.5	Pneumonitis
Esophagus	Point	15.4/15.4	8.4/25.2	7/35	Stenosis/fistula
	<5	11.9/11.9	5.9/17.7	3.9/19.5	
Heart/pericardium	Point	22/22	10/30	7.6/38	Pericarditis
	<15	16/16	8/24	6.4/32	
Brachial plexus	Point	17.5/17.5	8/24	6.1/30.5	Neuropathy
	<3	14/14	6.8/20.4	5.4/27	
Rib	Point	30/30	12.3/36.9	8.6/43	Pain or fracture
	<1	22/22	9.6/28.8	7/35	
	<30 CC		10/30[a]		
Skin	Point	26/26	11/33	7.9/39.5	Ulceration
	<10	23/23	10/30	7.3/36.5	
Great vessel	Point	37/37	15/45	10.6/53	Aneurysm
	<10	31/31	13/39	9.4/47	
Trachea and large bronchus	Point	20.2/20.2	10/30	8/40	Stenosis/fistula
	<4	10.5/10.5	5/15	3.3/16.5	

Source: Adapted from American Association of Physicists in Medicine. Stereotactic body radiation therapy: The report of the AAPM Task Group 101. *Med Phys.* 2010;37:4078-4101, except for the data of lung in three fractions, which was adapted from Timmerman RD, Park C, Kavanagh BD. The North American experience with stereotactic body radiation therapy in non-small cell lung cancer. 2007; *J Thorac Oncol* 2(7 Suppl 3):S101–S112.

the online image must be synchronized with the simulation image. That is, both online and simulation images should be acquired in the same phase using a gating technique. Otherwise, the image of the tumor may be acquired in different extreme positions. Large setup error would be induced due to phase difference between simulation and online setup images. Therefore, matching of neighboring anatomic landmarks is recommended for volumetric image guidance systems, and the tumor in the online images should appear within the envelope of the PTV in the simulation image. Furthermore, reproducibility of immobilization systems should be utilized. The basic principle of using an immobilization device is that "the best immobilization method is the method that the patient feels most comfortable with," because the treatment process is long.

The second important component of SBRT is the "stereotactic directing" or delivery of radiation treatment. A large number of beams (201 beams in gamma knife or multiple arcs in linac-based SRS) from different directions in the 3D space are focused at the target for the cranial SRS. The result of such "stereotactic directing" is that it forms relatively isotropic dose falloff around the target. The advantage of such isotropic falloff of dose distribu-

tion is that the central region of the target, which usually has high tumor burden, receives relatively higher dose, while the peripheral and marginal regions, which usually have relatively low tumor burden, receive relatively lower dose. The gradually decreasing dose outside the target may also cover potential microscopic extension. Such dose distribution may also have the tendency to resist small setup errors, because a small shift in any direction causes small drop of the minimum target dose. However, in SBRT, many noncoplanar directions in the 3D space are prohibited due to gantry collision and geometric limitations (some treatment units with small and flexible gantry head may have more directions). Generally, for linacs with a regular large gantry head, 7 to 14 coplanar or noncoplanar beams are used in SBRT to form a dose distribution with relatively isotropic dose falloff in the axial plane (Fig. 33.16). The dose falloff in the superior–inferior direction is usually much sharper because the noncoplanar beams approximating this direction cause gantry collision. Such limited "stereotactic directing" seems to be not a bad choice in lung SBRT, possibility due to the following factors: (i) Lung SBRT uses relatively much larger PTV margin than the cranial SRS, especially in the inferior–superior direction; (ii) The respiratory motion in

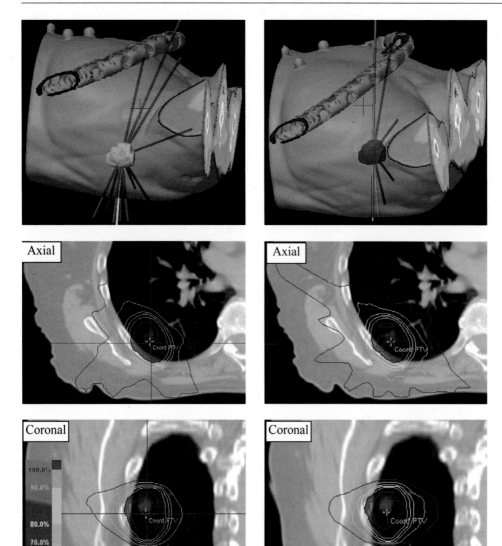

Axial

Axial

Coronal

100.0%

90.0%

80.0%

70.0%

50.0%

Coronal

| 14-beam non-coplanar, CI=1.17, GI=3.39 | 7-beam coplanar, CI=1.17, GI=3.62 |

Figure 33.16. Illustration of stereotactic body radiotherapy (SBRT) Plan. This figure shows 3D beam arrangement, isodose distributions in axial and coronal cuts for 14-beam noncoplanar (*left*), and 7-beam coplanar (*right*) SBRT plans. The conformal indexes (CI) are the same for two plans, the gradient index (GI) are 3.39 and 3.62, respectively.

inferior-superior direction has the effect to reduce the sharpness of the dose falloff in this direction to be similar to other directions; and (iii) Multiple coplanar beams significantly increase the amount of lung volume receiving low dose radiation.

The other important component of SBRT is high dose per fraction. This will enhance the BED of the tumor as well as the normal lung tissue. However, as the falloff of BED is normally rather sharp with such a technique, dose to normal tissue is much less than the tumor. That is, if the α/β ratio is same for the tumor and normal tissues, and the dose distribution has isotropic falloff, increasing dose per fraction can significantly improve the therapeutical ratio under very conformal plan. However, the lung tissue usually has much smaller α/β than the tumor, caution should be paid that such a fractionation regimen may not improve the ratio. Considering all factors together, it is estimated that hypofractionation higher dose prescription

may only benefit tumor control for tumors of small volume (150).

Brachytherapy

Brachytherapy may be an additional option both for palliation of NSCLC and, combined with external beam radiotherapy, for definitive treatment of NSCLC (256,257). The relief of symptoms has been reported to be better than 60%, and brachytherapy may be considered for patients who have endoscopically visible tumors that are not bulky and who could achieve an adequate dosimetric coverage of their tumor with brachytherapy delivery. Typical brachytherapy doses using high-dose rate (HDR) applicators are 6 Gy per fraction two or three times calculated at 1 cm from the center of the source. Brachytherapy catheters are placed bronchoscopically and should treat only the areas of visible disease (Fig. 33.17) (258).

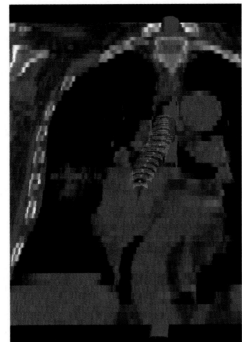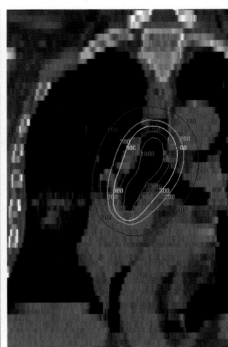

Figure 33.17. Example of brachytherapy for a patient with NSCLC of the right main bronchus and distal trachea. Spinal cord (*blue*), dummy seeds (*white dots*) in the bronchial on a coronal cut of CT scan (**A**) and isodose curves (**B**) are shown (258). (Courtesy of Suresh Senan, VU University Medical Center, Amsterdam, The Netherlands.)

TUMORS OF MEDIASTINUM-THYMOMA

Tumors of the mediastinum represent a wide diversity of disease states. The location and composition of a mass is critical to narrowing the differential diagnosis. The most common causes of an anterior mediastinal mass include the following: thymoma, teratoma, thyroid disease, and lymphoma. Masses of the middle mediastinum are typically congenital cysts, including foregut and pericardial cysts, while those that arise in the posterior mediastinum are often neurogenic tumors.

Rarer mediastinal tumors include germ cell tumors (seminomatous and nonseminomatous)—primary tracheal tumors. Primary mediastinal seminomas may be treated with radiotherapy alone or resection and postoperative radiotherapy—more currently chemotherapy. Chemotherapy is used for mediastinal nonseminomatous germ cell tumors and relapsed mediastinal seminomas. Surgical resection may also be appropriate for residual mass after chemotherapy or removal of bulky disease. Primary tracheal tumors, which are also rare, cause cough, dyspnea, and hemoptysis with primarily adenoid cystic or squamous cell histologies. Tracheal tumors are best treated with surgical resection and postoperative radiotherapy. For unresectable diseases, a multimodality regimen similar to that of NSCLC may be used for treatment.

Thymomas are the most common neoplasm of the anterior mediastinum, and will be the topic of this chapter.

Staging and the Role of Radiation

Thymomas are epithelial tumors of the thymus, which may or may not be extensively infiltrated by nonneoplastic lymphocytes. The term "thymoma" is customarily used to describe neoplasms that show no overt atypia of the epithelial component, while malignant thymoma refers to those thymomas invading through the capsule. Thymomas have a wide spectrum of histological diversity and are classified based on cell type predominance of lymphocytic, epithelial, or spindle cell variants. The classification has historically been controversial, but a system (Table 33.10) put forth by the World Health Organization (WHO) in 2004 has been generally accepted as a reproducible and clinically relevant classification. A thymic epithelial tumor that exhibits clear-cut cytological atypia and histological features no longer specific to the thymus is known as a thymic carcinoma (type c) will not be covered in this chapter.

The overall incidence of malignant thymoma in the United States was 0.15 per 100,000 person-years

TABLE 33.10	WHO Histologic Types of Thymomas

Type A thymoma (epithelial, spindle cell, medullary)
Type B thymoma, B1 (lymphocyte-rich, lymphocytic, predominantly cortical, organoid), B2 (cortical), B3 (epithelial, atypical, squamoid, well-differentiated thymic carcinoma)
Type AB thymoma (mixed A and B)
Type C thymic carcinoma, epidermoid keratinizing (squamous cell) carcinoma epidermoid nonkeratinizing carcinoma/lymphoepithelioma-like carcinoma, sarcomatoid carcinoma, carcinosarcoma, clear cell carcinoma, basaloid carcinoma, mucoepidermoid carcinoma, papillary carcinoma, undifferentiated carcinoma

(849 cases) in 2003. Thymoma incidence increased into the eighth decade of age and then decreased. Incidence was higher in males than females ($p = 0.007$) and was highest among Asians/Pacific Islanders (0.49 per 100,000 person-years) (259). Although rare in children, thymomas represent 20% of anterior mediastinal neoplasms in adults.

Thymomas should be staged surgically, while CT scan is important for evaluating surgical resectability. Thoracic CT scans also appear to be useful to differentiate B tumors from A and AB type (CT imaging revealed that type A and AB tumors tend to be round and have the smooth surface while type B1, B2, and B3 tumors are often flat and have irregular surface) (260). The vast majority (90–95%) of these tumors are localized (261,262), and resectable. The most commonly used staging system is the Masaoka system (Table 33.11). The most important determinants of long-term survival in thymoma are completeness of resection, Masaoka stage, and WHO classification (262–264). Radiotherapy plays an important adjuvant role in malignant (invasive) thymoma (i.e., stage II and above disease). Preoperative chemotherapy appears to be indicated for marginally resectable patients and metastatic disease.

Stage I thymomas are encapsulated and noninvasive, and can often be resected completely. Treatment results from surgical resection are excellent; 5- to 10-year survival rates are 95% to 100% and the local recurrence rate is <5% (265–267). Late recurrences that are limited to the mediastinum can often be treated by repeated re-excision (268). Thus, the use of RT is not justified in this subset of patients.

Adjuvant RT in completely resected stage II thymoma may be considered. Postoperative RT is often recommended to this group as total resection alone results in an unacceptably high local failure rate (up to 30%) with poor salvage therapy results (268–270). It is worth noting that there are retrospective studies that demonstrate only a minimal benefit of adjuvant RT in stage II disease with microscopic transcapsular invasion or macroscopic invasion into surrounding fatty tissue (266,267,271). The largest retrospective series, with inclusion of 1,320 patients, found no differences in recurrence rates between the adjuvant RT and the non-RT groups: 5 of 122 (4.1%) patients without additional RT and 4/86 (4.7%) patients with additional RT had recurrence (266). This study cannot disapprove the value of the adjuvant RT as those received RT were often those with higher risk factors and referred to radiation oncologists. On the other hand, one can argue that equivalent control rates of these two groups suggest the effectiveness of adjuvant RT. For Masaoka stage II disease with gross fibrous adhesion to pleura or histology-proven microscopic pleural invasion, local recurrence has been reported to be high and postoperative RT is often recommended (272).

For stage III thymic tumors, the benefit of adjuvant RT seems more apparent (269,273–275). The traditional rec-

TABLE 33.11	Masaoka Staging System for Thymomas
Masaoka stage	**Diagnostic criteria**
Stage I	Macroscopically and microscopically completely encapsulated
Stage II	Microscopic transcapsular invasion Macroscopic invasion into surrounding fatty tissue or grossly adherent to but not through mediastinal pleura or pericardium
Stage III	Macroscopic invasion into neighboring organs (i.e., pericardium, great vessels, lung) Without invasion of great vessels With invasion of great vessels
Stage IV	Pleural or pericardial dissemination Lymphogenous or hematogenous metastasis

AJCC/UICCTNM staging system for Thymoma

Primary tumor (T)
TX	Primary tumor cannot be assessed
T0	No evidence of primary tumor
T1	Tumor completely encapsulated
T2	Tumor invades pericapsular connective tissue
T3	Tumor invades into neighboring structures such as pericardium, mediastinal pleura, thoracic wall, great vessels and lung
T4	Tumor with pleural or pericardial dissemination

Regional lymph nodes (N)
NX	Regional nodes cannot be assessed
N0	No regional lymph node metastasis
N1	Metastasis in anterior mediastinal lymph nodes
N2	Metastasis in other intrathoracic lymph nodes excluding anterior mediastinal lymph nodes
N3	Metastasis in scalene and/or supraclavicular lymph nodes

Distant metastasis (M)
MX	Distant metastasis cannot be assessed
M0	No distant metastasis
M1	Distant metastasis

ommendation has been to offer adjuvant RT. This practice, however, has also been challenged by several retrospective reports that have shown no significant difference between those who received adjuvant RT and those who did not (276) Kondo et al. (277) found that for patients with stage III thymomas, 8/31 (26%) patients without additional RT and 8/78 (23%) patients with additional RT had a recurrence. The lack of demonstrated benefit from adjuvant RT may be due to the advancement to surgery, inclusion of a small number of cases, and the nature of retrospective analysis. In addition, the majority of these reports were not powered to perform such analysis as RT was normally recommended for this group of patients, and those who did not receive it may have had more favorable disease. It is obvious, for some special situations, that adjuvant RT provides a more consistent benefit (264,278). In a retrospective analysis of 228 resected cases, adjuvant chemotherapy did not appear to influence outcome, but adjuvant RT given to patients with completely resected type B2 and B3 thymomas prevented tumor recurrence in all patients treated, compared with a 33% local recurrence rate in those with stage III that did not receive adjuvant RT (264). Adjuvant RT may be recommended selectively in completely resected stage III thymomas.

For incompletely resected patients, adjuvant RT can improve local control and overall survival (264,269, 273,279). Strobel et al. reported on 75 patients with B2 and B3 thymomas with incomplete resection or tumor stage III or higher. The recurrence rate was 34% (*n* = 23) after 0.5 to 17 years (median: 5 years) in patients receiving adjuvant ChemRT, compared to 78% (7/9 patients) in patients without adjuvant ChemRT (264). As the data are consistent regarding the significantly poorer outcome in patients with incompletely resected disease, studies using preoperative measures, such as neoadjuvant chemotherapy and/or RT, to improve surgical resectability and local control, may be recommended in patients presenting with borderline resectable lesions (280,281). More aggressive adjuvant therapy such as combined ChemRT may also be beneficial to improve the long-term outcome.

For unresectable thymomas, a combined multimodality approach should be considered, although a few retrospective studies using RT alone have also shown modest disease control (279,281). A phase II Intergroup study was recently performed using four cycles of cisplatin–doxorubicin–cyclophosphamide chemotherapy and 54 Gy RT to the primary and nodal regions (282). The results in 23 patients demonstrated a high response rate of 69.6%. The progression-free and overall survival rates at 5 years were 54% and 52%, respectively. Recently, Kim et al. (283) at the M.D. Anderson Cancer Center conducted a prospective phase II study to assess the effect of a more aggressive treatment for unresectable malignant thymomas. Twenty-two patients with unresectable disease were treated with induction chemotherapy followed by surgical resection and then RT and consolidated chemotherapy. The long-term survival was promising, with a 5-year survival rate of 95% and a 7-year survival rate of 79%. Another study from Italy also showed promising results with the use of such an approach (284). Combined chemotherapy and RT treatment could increase the complete resection rate and improve the overall survival of these patients. With newly developed chemotherapeutic drugs and advanced radiation techniques, neoadjuvant ChemRT may significantly increase the rate of complete resection and improve the outcomes of locally advanced thymomas.

Radiation Treatment Planning

The dose and fractionation schemes depend on the indication. In the preoperative setting, a dose of 40 to 45 Gy is typically administered in 1.8 to 2.0 Gy daily dose fractions. The radiation dose currently used for postoperative radiation consists of 45 to 50 Gy for clear/close resection margins, 54 Gy for microscopically positive resection margins, and 60 Gy for grossly positive margins, with treatment administered in 1.8 to 2.0 Gy of daily dose fractions over a period of 5.0 to 6.6 weeks. While there is no clear evidence of a dose–response relationship due to the rarity of thymomas and the lack of prospective randomized trials, a dose of >60 Gy may be required to improve local control in unresectable cases (270). Also due to the paucity of cases and lack of prospective trials, there is limited evidence on dose–response relationship. For patients with gross residual or unresectable diseases, researchers from MD Anderson noted 50% in field local failure rate for those receiving <60 Gy. A total dose of 60 to 70 Gy may be prescribed to such cases if the normal tissue dose constraints are met.

Traditionally, the entire mediastinum (sometimes supraclavicular nodal regions) was encompassed within the ports in the postoperative treatment with 1- to 2-cm margins around any structures that were invaded. Doses of 40 to 50 Gy for thymomas are typically used, so off-cord obliques are usually not necessary. If spinal cord doses are excessive, however, posterior oblique beams may be used. The use of PA spinal cord blocks should be discouraged, as they result in an underdose to the mediastinum.

Currently, CT simulation and 3D conformal radiation therapy has become the standard care for adequate planning. GTV should include any grossly visible tumor—surgical clip if postoperatively. The CTV extension from the gross tumor is less clear. For cases of postoperative radiation, the CTV determination should be based on histology, preoperative radiographic extent, surgical findings, areas of suspicious subclinical disease, and adjacent regional lymphatics. Extensive elective nodal radiation (entire mediastinum and bilateral supraclavicular nodal regions) is not recommended, as such treatment is often rather morbid and there is no evidence on pattern of failure to support such practice. With better definition of target by CT simulation, inclusion of large elective nodal region is not a common practice any more. Consideration of PTV margin is similar to that of lung, though the tumor motion is yet to be studied. At least 10 to 15 mm margin should be added for motion and setup errors.

Radiation beam arrangements may include two apposed anterior–posterior ports (weighting more anteriorly), wedge pair technique, or multiple conformal fields, or IMRT (Fig. 33.18). Traditional wedge fields may generate

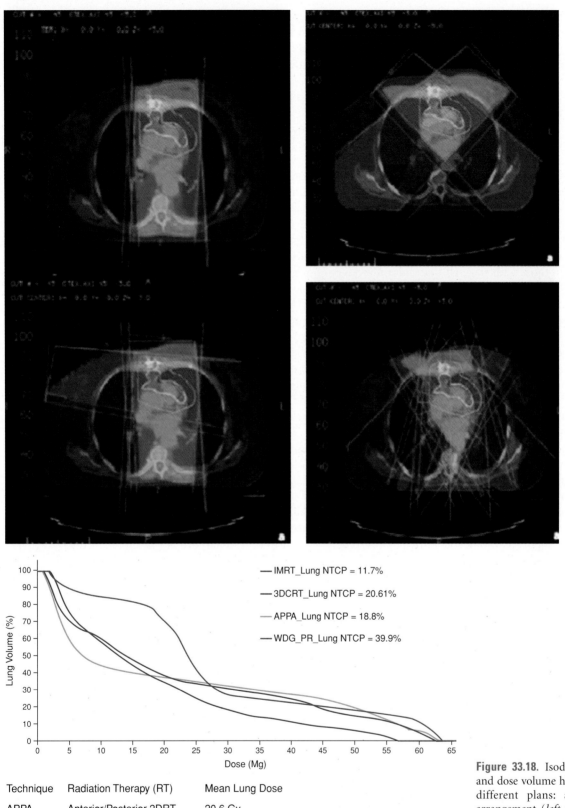

Technique	Radiation Therapy (RT)	Mean Lung Dose
APPA	Anterior/Posterior 2DRT	20.6 Gy
WDG	Wedge Paired 2DRT	27.8 Gy
IMRT	Intensity Modulated RT	17.2 Gy
3DCRT	3-D Conformal RT	21.4 Gy

Figure 33.18. Isodose distributions and dose volume histograms of four different plans: an AP/PA field arrangement (*left upper*), a wedge-paired field arrangement (*right upper*), 3D conformal radiation therapy (*left lower*), and IMRT (*right lower*) in postoperative case (prescription dose = 54 Gy to the ICRU reference point).

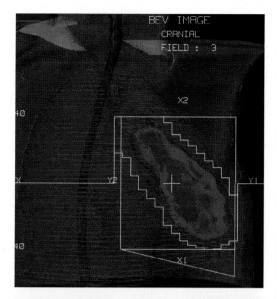
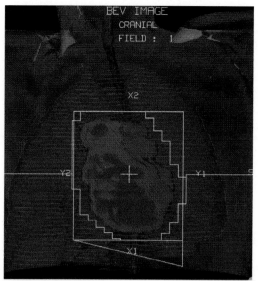
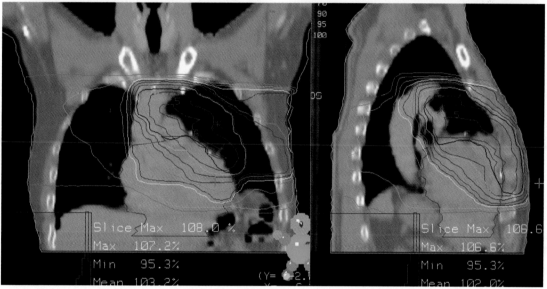

Figure 33.19. 3D conformal radiation for postoperative radiotherapy in a completely resected WHO type B3 thymoma. *Top panel:* Beam's eye view of two of three treatment portals used. *Bottom panel:* Isodose distribution for a three-field plan. Surgical clips are routinely placed in all patients undergoing thymic surgery in order to assist target delineation. (Courtesy of Suresh Senan, VU University Medical Center, Amsterdam, The Netherlands.)

excessive dose to normal lungs for large target; IMRT plan may provide some benefit of normal tissue sparing. While using 3D plan, selection of beam angles should be dictated by the shape of PTV aiming to confine the prescribed high dose to the target and minimize dose to adjacent critical structures. Figure 33.19 shows an example of 3D conformal plan, showing isodose curves along with BEV of a representative patient.

PLEURAL MESOTHELIAL CELLS—MALIGNANT PLEURAL MESOTHELIOMA

Malignant mesothelioma is uncommon, but its incidence is increasing over last 20 years, currently ranges from about 7 to 40 per 1,000,000 in industrialized Western nations, depending on the amount of asbestos exposure of the populations during the past several decades (285). It has been estimated that incidence may have peaked at 15 per 1,000,000 in the United States in 2004, with an incidence of over 3,000 new cases per year. For 2008, it was estimated as ~2,400 cases, with asbestos being likely the cause in 58% (286,287). They arise primarily from the surface serosal cells of the pleural, peritoneal, and pericardial cavities. About 85% of mesotheliomas arise in the pleura, the remaining from the peritoneum, and the pericardium or tunica vaginalis testis. Thus, the not otherwise specified mesotheliomas commonly refer to malignant pleural mesotheliomas (MPM). Most are associated with asbestos, although some have arisen in ports of prior radiation, and a reported association with simian virus 40 remains controversial. The histology of about half of mesotheliomas is epithelial (tubular papillary), with the remainder sarcomatous or mixed. Histologically, malignant mesotheliomas can show an epithelial morphology (malignant mesothelioma epithelial type), a fibrous morphology (malignant mesothelioma fibrous type, also called sarcomatoid type), or a combination of both. Most malignant mesotheliomas (50–60%) are of the epithelial type, ~10% are sarcomatoid, and the rest are biphasic malignant mesotheliomas. Histological diagnosis can be established by thoracentesis and closed pleural biopsy, biopsy under thoracoscopy, and in rare occasion opened pleural biopsy.

Staging and the Role of Radiation

The updated AJCC staging system should be used to stage MPM (Table 33.12). This was adopted from that of the International Mesothelioma Interest Group in 1995 and has been validated in a number of surgically based trials (288). Staging workup includes history and disease-related physical examination, blood test, imaging studies, and pathologic evaluations. Modern staging workups include CT, thoracoscopy with multiple pleural biopsies and talc pleurodesis, EBUS/EUS and one-stage transcervical extended mediastinal lymphadenectomy, and laparoscopy/peritoneal lavage and cytology of the fluid (289–290). MPM can have varying radiographic appearances, and many of the early changes are associated with a previous exposure to asbestos, including pleural plaques or parenchymal pulmonary fibrosis. The most common features on chest x-ray radiography include pleural effusion, diffuse pleural thickening, and nodularity. CT scan often shows asbestos-induced parenchymal changes such as subpleural lines and parenchymal bands, prominent pulmonary arcades, subpleural dependent densities, reticulation, and parenchymal honey comb patterns. Pleural changes on chest tomography will include pleural plaques, diffuse thickening, and effusion. Chest wall invasion include distortion of the intercostal spaces, infiltration of extrapleural soft tissue and ribs, and undefined densities infiltrating the chest wall musculature. A clear fat plane between the inferior diaphragmatic surface and the adjacent abdominal organs, as well as a smooth inferior diaphragmatic contour, might imply resectability. CT might reveal a hemidiaphragm encased by a mass or poor definition between the liver, stomach, and inferior diaphragmatic surface. CT can provide fairly good estimation of T and N stage. MRI is appealing because of its differential signal intensity, depending on the sequence used, and its ability to image in the coronal, sagittal, and transverse planes. Comparing to CT, MRI may provide more accurate estimation on diaphragm invasion and invasion of endothoracic fascia or a single chest wall focus, and differentiating fluid from solid tumor. MRI with gadolinium contrast enhancement MRI has implied a further improvement in defining tumor extent and detecting new lesions.

FDG-PET might be superior to CT for staging mediastinal lymph node involvement (291–294). PET can also detect additional extrathoracic, otherwise occult disease in 10% to 11% in newly diagnosed patients and 45% in patients who are followed after therapy with a PET scan. Data also suggest (295), SUV of the tumor before resection was significant in discriminating longer from shorter survival times. In a multivariable analysis of 65 patients, high SUV tumors were associated with a 3.3 times greater risk of death than low SUV tumors ($p = 0.03$). Median survivals were 14 and 24 months for the high and low SUV groups, respectively.

Pathologic staging should be performed if possible. Strategy for T and N staging is similar to that of NSCLC. Extended surgical staging procedures generally include a combination of laparoscopy, peritoneal lavage, and mediastinoscopy to more precisely stage patients with MPM, though emphasis should be placed on pleural evaluation in this disease (296).

The treatment recommendation depends on the resectability of the disease. The standard care of patients with unresectable diseases should be pemetrexed and cisplatin chemotherapy if the patient is medically fit. This regimen provides 3 to 4 months of survival benefit over single drug (297). Radiation might be used as a measure to palliate chest pain, dyspnea, and symptoms related with distant disease. For patients with resectable disease, the treatment recommendation apparently varies with culture. In the United Kingdom, only about half of the physician will refer patients for curative resection. In France, the focus has been on early detection and intrapleural treatment; surgery is performed after this therapy only to improve local control for stage I disease. In the United States, current standard of care involves a multimodality approach. The evolution of the use of surgery in MPM with or without intraoperative and/or postoperative innovative adjuvant therapies is being defined by some major cancer centers, within clinical trials. In general, surgical resection is the treatment of choice for patients with resectable diseases. Radiation alone has limited role in treating mesothelioma. Postoperative radiation therapy is often recommended for stage II or III diseases.

Adjuvant radiation therapy to the surgical bed may significantly decrease the incidence of local recurrence. Single modality with surgical resection such as pleurectomy/decortication, or extrapleural pneumonectomy has generated poor results on local tumor control and survival (298–301). The local recurrence rate after surgical resection, either alone or in combination with low-dose postoperative RT, ranges from 35% to 78%. When there is limited or no resection of disease, delivery of high-dose RT to the entire hemithorax in the setting of an intact lung has not been shown to be associated with any survival benefit, and the toxicity is clearly significant (302). After extrapleural pneumonectomy, however, higher dose adjuvant RT significantly reduced the local recurrence rate. For the 62 patients undergoing extrapleural pneumonectomy

TABLE 33.12	International Staging System for Malignant Pleural Mesothelioma

Primary tumor (T)
- T1
  - T1a
    - Tumor limited to the ipsilateral parietal ± mediastinal ± diaphragmatic pleura
    - No involvement of the visceral pleura
  - T1b
    - Tumor involving the ipsilateral parietal ± mediastinal ± diaphragmatic pleura
    - Tumor also involving the visceral pleura
- T2
  - Tumor involving each of the ipsilateral pleural surfaces (parietal, mediastinal, diaphragmatic, and visceral pleura) with at least one of the following features:
    - Involvement of diaphragmatic muscle
    - Extension of tumor from visceral pleura into the underlying pulmonary parenchyma
- T3
  - Describes locally advanced but potentially resectable tumor
  - Tumor involving all of the ipsilateral pleural surfaces (parietal, mediastinal, diaphragmatic, and visceral pleura) with at least one of the following features:
    - Involvement of the endothoracic fascia
    - Extension into the mediastinal fat
    - Solitary, completely resectable focus of tumor extending into the soft tissues of the chest wall
    - Nontransmural involvement of the pericardium
- T4
  - Describes locally advanced technically unresectable tumor
  - Tumor involving all the ipsilateral pleural surfaces surfaces (parietal, mediastinal, diaphragmatic, and visceral pleura) with at least one of the following features:
    - Diffuse extension or multifocal masses of tumor in the chest wall, with or without associated rib destruction
    - Direct transdiaphragmatic extension of tumor to the peritoneum
    - Direct extension of tumor to the contralateral pleura
    - Direct extension of tumor to the mediastinal organs
    - Direct extension of tumor into the spine
    - Tumor extending through to the internal surface of the pericardium with or without a pericardial effusion; or tumor involving the myocardium.

Regional lymph nodes (N)
NX: Regional lymph nodes cannot be assessed
N0: No regional lymph node metastases
N1: Metastases in the ipsilateral bronchopulmonary or hilar lymph nodes
N2: Metastases in the subcarinal or the ipsilateral mediastinal lymph nodes including the ipsilateral internal mammary and peridiaphragmatic nodes
N3: Metastases in the contralateral mediastinal, contralateral internal mammary, ipsilateral or contralateral supraclavicular lymph nodes

M: Metastasis, as same as lung cancer
Stage I: IA-T1aN0M0, IB-T1bN0M0
Stage II: T2N0M0
Stage III: Any T3, Any N1, Any N2, M0
Stage IV: Any T4, Any N3, Any M1

and adjuvant radiation, the sites of recurrence were locoregional in 2, locoregional and distant in 5, and distant only in 30. A retrospective review of 123 patients treated at the Memorial Sloan-Kettering Cancer Center revealed that the dose of adjuvant radiation appeared to significantly influence overall results (303). Those who received doses higher than 40 Gy might survive longer than those who receive doses <40 Gy ($p = 0.001$). A dose of 54 Gy to the entire hemithorax, the thoracotomy incision, and sites of chest drains was well tolerated; the adjuvant radiation dramatically reduced local recurrence and was associated with prolonged survival for early-stage tumors (304).

In summary, radiation plays adjuvant and palliative roles in the management of mesothelioma. The recommended treatment of MPM should be multimodality—median overall survival following aggressive multimodality ranges from 10.5 to 18 months (303,305).

Radiation Treatment Planning

Definitive postoperative RT: A total dose of 50 to 54 Gy in 1.8 to 2.0 Gy should be prescribed to surgical bed for microscopic diseases (304,305). A dose ≥60 Gy should be delivered to macroscopic residual tumors, if the doses to adjacent normal structures are limited. In addition to cover the surgical bed within the thorax, the volume of postoperative radiation should also include the surgical scars and biopsy tracks in the chest wall, as malignant seeding along tracts of cytology and biopsy needles, chest tubes, and surgical incisions have been reported in 19% to 40% of patients (306–308). The recurrent subcutaneous nodules are painful and often refractory to RT or respond only transiently to this treatment (307). Although a single dose of 10 Gy treatment with 9-MeV electrons appeared ineffective (309), adequate prophylactic radiation to these

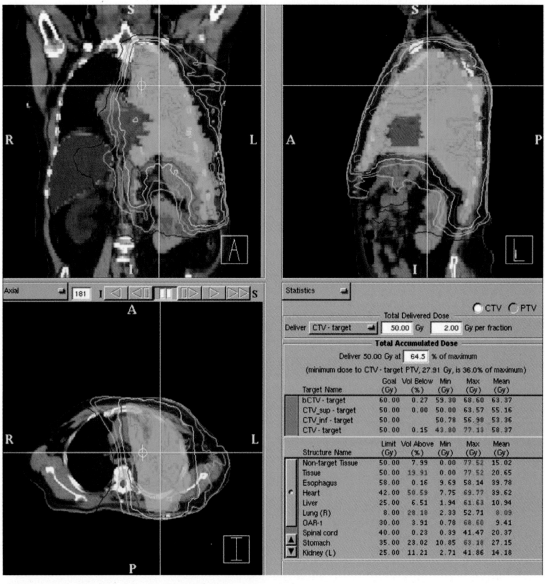

Figure 33.20. Intensity-modulated radiation therapy in a patient with malignant mesothelioma after left extrapleural pneumonectomy. Green, 50 Gy; Blue, 30 Gy. (Courtesy from C. Stevens, Moffitt Cancer Center, Tampa, Florida.)

sites may significantly reduce the scar recurrence. Using 21 Gy in three fractions using 12.5- to 15.0-MeV electron, Boutin et al. (306) reported that none of the 20 (0%) patients treated electively post surgical procedures developed entry tract metastasis, versus 8/20 (40%) patients not receiving prophylactic irradiation. For patients with residual tumors, some investigators have used brachytherapy or intraoperative external beam radiation in combination with surgery. Permanent ^{125}I brachytherapy implants, temporary ^{192}Ir implants, and a solution of ^{32}P might be used by experienced physicians.

IMRT: IMRT is a new and promising treatment technique that allows a more conformal high dose RT to the hemithorax, while protecting the surrounding normal tissue accurately (310,311). Researchers at the M.D. Anderson Cancer Center treated 28 patients with IMRT after extrapleural pneumonectomy (312,313). The hemithorax was treated with doses of 45 to 50 Gy. Some regions of the hemithorax were boosted to a total dose of 60 Gy. Radiation dose homogeneity to the entire hemithorax was excellent. Adverse effects included nausea, vomiting, dyspnea, and esophagitis. The median follow-up was 9 months and the local control rate was 100%. One-year survival was 65%. Treatment planning could be generated by using many commercially available systems, such Corvus, Eclipse, and Pinnacle (314). To deliver a dose of 50 Gy to the target, the monitor units used were 2786, 1451, and 1813; while the number of segments were 1050, 267, 173 for Corvus, Pinnacle, and Eclipse, respectively. Doses to spinal cord, lung, heart, liver, and contralateral kidney were acceptable for all planning systems. It is unclear, however, regarding the dose limit to the remaining side of lung. Safe dosimetric constraints for patients treated for lung cancer, such as MLD of 20 Gy, cannot be applied to the patients with mesothelioma who has had pneumonectomy. In such case, MLD should be limited within 9.5 Gy based on preliminary experience from MD Anderson Cancer Center, and Massachusetts General Hospital (personal communication from Craig Stevens). Figure 33.20 shows isodose distributions on coronal, sagittal, and axial cuts, along with a prescription page.

Palliative radiation: Radiation is an effective palliative treatment for relief of chest pain associated with mesothelioma. After local irradiation, 50% to 68% of patients experience symptom relief (307,315); however, almost all patients experience a recurrence of their symptoms several months after such radiation (315). Daily doses of 4 Gy appear to be more efficacious than fractions of <4 Gy in providing symptom relief (307,316), but the optimal daily and total dose of RT for palliative purposes remains unclear.

SUMMARY

In summary, many technological advances have become available in treatment and radiation therapy of thoracic tumors. In particular, 3D conformal therapy has put forward the first step in improving the targeting of dose to the tumor while sparing dose to normal tissue, and has facilitated radiation dose escalation to the tumor. Preliminary data from recent dose escalation trial has also shown that higher dose radiation may improve local control and survival. 4D technique provides us in-depth understanding of organ motion and thus improves the accuracy of targeting the tumor and sparing the critical structures, to decrease the geographical misses due to tumor motion from respiration. PET scan has a potential to significantly improve target definition. Improved construction of the PTV is an important first step in improving the treatment planning process. Algorithms to account for the effects of lower lung density have become available and will facilitate the accurate and realistic calculation of dose to the PTV and the normal structure. With the implementation of SBRT, treatment of thoracic cancer, particularly early stage NSCLC, has reached a new level of success. Further improvements in RT can be gained by even more sophisticated beam arrangement planning, intensity modulation with intelligent choice of clinically relevant normal tissue tolerance criteria, individualized radiation therapy, and combined multimodality therapy.

Acknowledgments

We are indebted to Suresh Senan, MD, PhD of VU University Medical Center of the Netherlands for his critical comments and significant contribution to the previous version. We are grateful to Daniel Tatro, CMD, from University of Michigan, for helping with the pictures.

REFERENCES

1. Parkin DM, Bray F, Ferlay J, et al. Global cancer statistics, 2002. *CA Cancer J Clin* 2005;55(2):74–108.
2. Ferlay J, Shin HR, Bray F, et al. GLOBOCAN 2008. Cancer Incidence and Mortality Worldwide: IARC Cancer Base, International Agency for Research on Cancer; 2010 No. 10 [Internet] (Lyon, France). Available from: http://globocan.iarc.fr
3. Jemal A, Siegel R, Ward E, et al. Cancer statistics, 2009. *CA Cancer J Clin* 2009;59(4):225–249.
4. Strollo DC, Rosado de Christenson ML, Jett JR. Primary mediastinal tumors. Part 1: tumors of the anterior mediastinum. *Chest* 1997;112(2):511–522.
5. Leigh J, Davidson P, Hendrie L, et al. Malignant mesothelioma in Australia, 1945–2000. *Am J Ind Med* 2002;41(3):188–201.
6. Tyldesley S, Boyd C, Schulze K, et al. Estimating the need for radiotherapy for lung cancer: an evidence-based, epidemiologic approach. *Int J Radiat Oncol Biol Phys* 2001;49(4):973–985.
7. Kong FM, Ten Haken R, Eisbruch A, et al. Non-small cell lung cancer therapy-related pulmonary toxicity: an update on radiation pneumonitis and fibrosis. *Semin Oncol* 2005;32(2 Suppl 3):S42–S54.

8. Maione P, Perrone F, Gallo C, et al. Pretreatment quality of life and functional status assessment significantly predict survival of elderly patients with advanced non-small-cell lung cancer receiving chemotherapy: a prognostic analysis of the multicenter Italian lung cancer in the elderly study. *J Clin Oncol* 2005;23(28):6865–6872.

9. Watine J, Friedberg B. Laboratory variables and stratification of metastatic colorectal cancer patients: recommendations for therapeutic trials and for clinical practice guidelines. *Clin Chim Acta* 2004;345(1–2):1–15.

10. Munden RF, Swisher SS, Stevens CW, et al. Imaging of the patient with non-small cell lung cancer. *Radiology* 2005;237(3):803–818.

11. Izbicki JR, Thetter O, Karg O, et al. Accuracy of computed tomographic scan and surgical assessment for staging of bronchial carcinoma. A prospective study. *J Thorac Cardiovasc Surg* 1992;104(2):413–420.

12. Toloza EM, Harpole L, McCrory DC, et al. Noninvasive staging of non-small cell lung cancer: a review of the current evidence. *Chest* 2003;123(Suppl 1):137S–146S.

13. Pass HI. Mediastinal staging 2005: pictures, scopes, and scalpels. *Semin Oncol* 2005;32(3):269–278.

14. Gupta NC, Rogers JS, Graeber GM, et al. Clinical role of F-18 fluorodeoxyglucose positron emission tomography imaging in patients with lung cancer and suspected malignant pleural effusion. *Chest* 2002;122(6):1918–1924.

15. Gould MK, Kuschner WG, Rydzak CE, et al. Test performance of positron emission tomography and computed tomography for mediastinal staging in patients with non-small-cell lung cancer: a meta-analysis. *Ann Intern Med* 2003;139(11):879–892.

16. Birim O, Kappetein AP, Stijnen T, et al. Meta-analysis of positron emission tomographic and computed tomographic imaging in detecting mediastinal lymph node metastases in nonsmall cell lung cancer. *Ann Thorac Surg* 2005;79(1):375–382.

17. Eschmann SM, Friedel G, Paulsen F, et al. Is standardised (18)F-FDG uptake value an outcome predictor in patients with stage III non-small cell lung cancer? *Eur J Nucl Med Mol Imaging* 2005;33(3):263–269.

18. Pieterman RM, van Putten JW, Meuzelaar JJ, et al. Preoperative staging of non-small-cell lung cancer with positron-emission tomography. *N Engl J Med* 2000;343(4):254–261.

19. Cerfolio RJ, Ojha B, Bryant AS, et al. The accuracy of integrated PET-CT compared with dedicated PET alone for the staging of patients with nonsmall cell lung cancer. *Ann Thorac Surg* 2004;78(3):1017–1023; discussion 1017–1023.

20. Roberts KB, Manus MP, Hicks RJ, et al. PET imaging for suspected residual tumour or thoracic recurrence of non-small cell lung cancer after pneumonectomy. *Lung Cancer* 2005;47(1):49–57.

21. Fritscher-Ravens A, Bohuslavizki KH, Brandt L, et al. Mediastinal lymph node involvement in potentially resectable lung cancer: comparison of CT, positron emission tomography, and endoscopic ultrasonography with and without fine-needle aspiration. *Chest* 2003;123(2):442–451.

22. Lardinois D, Weder W, Hany TF, et al. Staging of non-small-cell lung cancer with integrated positron-emission tomography and computed tomography. *N Engl J Med* 2003;348(25):2500–2507.

23. Vansteenkiste JF, Stroobants SG. The role of positron emission tomography with 18 F-fluoro-2-deoxy-D-glucose in respiratory oncology. *Eur Respir J* 2001;17(4):802–820.

24. Pfister DG, Johnson DH, Azzoli CG, et al. American Society of Clinical Oncology treatment of unresectable non-small-cell lung cancer guideline: update 2003. *J Clin Oncol* 2004;22(2):330–353.

25. Cheran SK, Herndon JE 2nd, Patz EF Jr. Comparison of whole-body FDG-PET to bone scan for detection of bone metastases in patients with a new diagnosis of lung cancer. *Lung Cancer* 2004;44(3):317–325.

26. Munley MT, Marks LB, Scarfone C, et al. Multimodality nuclear medicine imaging in three-dimensional radiation treatment planning for lung cancer: challenges and prospects. *Lung Cancer* 1999;23(2):105–114.

27. Little AG, Rusch VW, Bonner JA, et al. Patterns of surgical care of lung cancer patients. *Ann Thorac Surg* 2005;80(6):2051–2056; discussion 2056.

28. Martini N, Bains MS, Burt ME, et al. Incidence of local recurrence and second primary tumors in resected stage I lung cancer. *J Thorac Cardiovasc Surg* 1995;109(1):120–129.

29. Mountain CF. Staging classification of lung cancer. A critical evaluation. *Clin Chest Med* 2002;23(1):103–121.

30. Mountain CF, Hermes KE. Surgical treatment of lung cancer. Past and present. *Methods Mol Med* 2003;75:453–487.

31. Bach PB, Cramer LD, Warren JL, et al. Racial differences in the treatment of early-stage lung cancer. *N Engl J Med* 1999;341(16):1198–1205.

32. Potosky AL, Saxman S, Wallace RB, et al. Population variations in the initial treatment of non-small-cell lung cancer. *J Clin Oncol* 2004;22(16):3261–3268.

33. Rami-Porta R, Crowley JJ, Goldstraw P. The revised TNM staging system for lung cancer. *Ann Thorac Cardiovasc Surg* 2009;15(1):4–9.

34. Wisnivesky JP, Bonomi M, Henschke C, et al. Radiation therapy for the treatment of unresected stage I-II non-small cell lung cancer. *Chest* 2005;128(3):1461–1467.

35. Maguire PD, Marks LB, Sibley GS, et al. 73.6 Gy and beyond: hyperfractionated, accelerated radiotherapy for non-small-cell lung cancer. *J Clin Oncol* 2001;19(3):705–711.

36. Bogart JA, Aronowitz JN. Localized non-small cell lung cancer: adjuvant radiotherapy in the era of effective systemic therapy. *Clin Cancer Res* 2005;11(13 Pt 2):5004S–5010S.

37. Bradley JD, Wahab S, Lockett MA, et al. Elective nodal failures are uncommon in medically inoperable patients with Stage I non-small-cell lung carcinoma treated with limited radiotherapy fields. *Int J Radiat Oncol Biol Phys* 2003;56(2):342–347.

38. Rosenzweig KE, Dladla N, Schindelheim R, et al. Three-dimensional conformal radiation therapy (3D-CRT) for early-stage non-small-cell lung cancer. *Clin Lung Cancer* 3(2):141–144.

39. Bradley JD, Ieumwananonthachai N, Purdy JA, et al. Gross tumor volume, critical prognostic factor in patients treated with three-dimensional conformal

radiation therapy for non-small-cell lung carcinoma. *Int J Radiat Oncol Biol Phys* 2002;52(1):49–57.

40. Belderbos JS, De Jaeger K, Heemsbergen WD, et al. First results of a phase I/II dose escalation trial in non-small cell lung cancer using three-dimensional conformal radiotherapy. *Radiother Oncol* 2003;66(2): 119–126.

41. Bogart JA, Alpert TE, Kilpatrick MC, et al. Dose-intensive thoracic radiation therapy for patients at high risk with early-stage non-small-cell lung cancer. *Clin Lung Cancer* 2005;6(6):350–354.

42. Chen M, Hayman JA, Ten Haken RK, et al. Long-term results of high-dose conformal radiotherapy for patients with medically inoperable T1–3N0 non-small-cell lung cancer: Is low incidence of regional failure due to incidental nodal irradiation? *Int J Radiat Oncol Biol Phys* 2006;64(1):120–126.

43. Uematsu M, Shioda A, Suda A, et al. Computed tomography-guided frameless stereotactic radiotherapy for stage I non-small cell lung cancer: a 5-year experience. *Int J Radiat Oncol Biol Phys* 2001;51(3):666–670.

44. Onishi H, Araki T, Shirato H, et al. Stereotactic hypofractionated high-dose irradiation for stage I nonsmall cell lung carcinoma: clinical outcomes in 245 subjects in a Japanese multi-institutional study. *Cancer* 2004;101(7):1623–1631.

45. Wulf J, Haedinger U, Oppitz U, et al. Stereotactic radiotherapy for primary lung cancer and pulmonary metastases: a noninvasive treatment approach in medically inoperable patients. *Int J Radiat Oncol Biol Phys* 2004;60(1):186–196.

46. Timmerman R, Papiez L, McGarry R, et al. Initial report of a prospective phase II trial of stereotactic body radiation therapy for patients with medically inoperable stage I non-small cell lung cancer. *Int J Radiat Oncol Biol Phys* 2005;63(Suppl 1):S99.

47. Xia T, Li H, Sun Q, et al. Promising clinical outcome of stereotactic body radiation therapy for patients with inoperable Stage I/II non-small-cell lung cancer. *Int J Radiat Oncol Biol Phys* 2006;66(1):117–125.

48. Chang JY, Roth JA. Stereotactic body radiation therapy for stage I non-small cell lung cancer. *Thorac Surg Clin* 2007;17(2):251–259.

49. Hiraoka M, Ishikura S. A Japan clinical oncology group trial for stereotactic body radiation therapy of non-small cell lung cancer. *J Thorac Oncol* 2007;2(7 Suppl 3):S115–S117.

50. Bradley JD, El Naqa I, Drzymala RE, et al. Stereotactic body radiation therapy for early-stage non-small-cell lung cancer: the pattern of failure is distant. *Int J Radiat Oncol Biol Phys* 2010;77(4):1146–1150.

51. Crabtree TD, Denlinger CE, Meyers BF, et al. Stereotactic body radiation therapy versus surgical resection for stage I non-small cell lung cancer. *J Thorac Cardiovasc Surg* 2010;140(2):377–386.

52. Hiraoka M, Matsuo Y, Takayama K. Stereotactic body radiation therapy for lung cancer: achievements and perspectives. *Jpn J Clin Oncol* 2010;40(9):846–854.

53. Ricardi U, Filippi AR, Guarneri A, et al. Stereotactic body radiation therapy for early stage non-small cell lung cancer: results of a prospective trial. *Lung Cancer* 2010;68(1):72–77.

54. Timmerman R, Paulus R, Galvin J, et al. Stereotactic body radiation therapy for inoperable early stage lung cancer. *JAMA* 2010;303(11):1070–1076.

55. Zimmermann F, Wulf J, Lax I, et al. Stereotactic body radiation therapy for early non-small cell lung cancer. *Front Radiat Ther Oncol* 2010;42:94–114.

56. Grutters JP, Kessels AG, Pijls-Johannesma M, et al. Comparison of the effectiveness of radiotherapy with photons, protons and carbon-ions for non-small cell lung cancer: a meta-analysis. *Radiother Oncol* 2010;95(1):32–40.

57. Pignon JP, Tribodet H, Scagliotti GV, et al. Lung adjuvant cisplatin evaluation: a pooled analysis by the LACE Collaborative Group. *J Clin Oncol* 2008;26(21):3552–3559.

58. Suehisa H, Toyooka S. Adjuvant chemotherapy for completely resected non-small-cell lung cancer. *Acta Med Okayama* 2009;63(5):223–230.

59. Bria E, Gralla RJ, Raftopoulos H, et al. Magnitude of benefit of adjuvant chemotherapy for non-small cell lung cancer: meta-analysis of randomized clinical trials. *Lung Cancer* 2009;63(1):50–57.

60. Arriagada R, Auperin A, Burdett S, et al. Adjuvant chemotherapy, with or without postoperative radiotherapy, in operable non-small-cell lung cancer: two meta-analyses of individual patient data. *Lancet* 2010;375(9722):1267–1277.

61. Sawabata N. Malignant status at surgical margin of limited-resected non-small cell lung cancer: a crucial finding for predicting local relapse. *J Thorac Cardiovasc Surg* 2003;126(2):610–611; author reply 611.

62. Sawabata N, Takeda SI, Inoue M, et al. Spread of malignant cells in the surgical margin with stapled excision of lung cancer: comparison of aggressive clump and less traumatic jaw closure type staplers. *Thorac Cardiovasc Surg* 2006;54(6):418–424.

63. Decker RH, Wilson LD. Postoperative radiation therapy for non-small cell lung cancer. *Semin Thorac Cardiovasc Surg* 2008;20(3):184–187.

64. Douillard JY, Rosell R, De Lena M, et al. Impact of postoperative radiation therapy on survival in patients with complete resection and stage I, II, or IIIA non-small-cell lung cancer treated with adjuvant chemotherapy: the adjuvant Navelbine International Trialist Association (ANITA) Randomized Trial. *Int J Radiat Oncol Biol Phys* 2008;72(3):695–701.

65. Kelsey CR, Marks LB, Wilson LD. Postoperative radiation therapy for lung cancer: where do we stand? *Oncology (Williston Park)* 2008;22(3):301–310; discussion 310, 314–305, 319.

66. Saynak M, Higginson DS, Morris DE, et al. Current status of postoperative radiation for non-small-cell lung cancer. *Semin Radiat Oncol* 2010;20(3):192–200.

67. PORT Meta-analysis Trialists Group. Postoperative radiotherapy for non-small cell lung cancer. *Cochrane Database Syst Rev* 2000;(2):CD002142.

68. The Lung Cancer Study Group. Effects of postoperative mediastinal radiation on completely resected stage II and stage III epidermoid cancer of the lung. *N Engl J Med* 1986;315(22):1377–1381.

69. Stephens RJ, Girling DJ, Bleehen NM, et al. The role of post-operative radiotherapy in non-small-cell lung cancer: a multicentre randomised trial in patients with

pathologically staged T1–2, N1–2, M0 disease. Medical Research Council Lung Cancer Working Party. *Br J Cancer* 1996;74(4):632–639.

70. Machtay M, Lee JH, Shrager JB, et al. Risk of death from intercurrent disease is not excessively increased by modern postoperative radiotherapy for high-risk resected non-small-cell lung carcinoma. *J Clin Oncol* 2001;19(19):3912–3917.

71. Bradley JD, Paulus R, Graham MV, et al. Phase II trial of postoperative adjuvant paclitaxel/carboplatin and thoracic radiotherapy in resected stage II and IIIA non-small-cell lung cancer: promising long-term results of the Radiation Therapy Oncology Group–RTOG 9705. *J Clin Oncol* 2005;23(15):3480–3487.

72. Sawyer TE, Bonner JA, Gould PM, et al. Effectiveness of postoperative irradiation in stage IIIA non-small cell lung cancer according to regression tree analyses of recurrence risks. *Ann Thorac Surg* 1997;64(5):1402–1407; discussion 1407–1408.

73. Lally BE, Zelterman D, Colasanto JM, et al. Postoperative radiotherapy for stage II or III non-small-cell lung cancer using the surveillance, epidemiology, and end results database. *J Clin Oncol* 2006;24(19):2998–3006.

74. Attar S, Krasna MJ, Sonett JR, et al. Superior sulcus (Pancoast) tumor: experience with 105 patients. *Ann Thorac Surg* 1998;66(1):193–198.

75. Wright CD, Menard MT, Wain JC, et al. Induction chemoradiation compared with induction radiation for lung cancer involving the superior sulcus. *Ann Thorac Surg* 2002;73(5):1541–1544.

76. Rusch VW, Giroux DJ, Kraut MJ, et al. Induction chemoradiation and surgical resection for non-small cell lung carcinomas of the superior sulcus: Initial results of Southwest Oncology Group Trial 9416 (Intergroup Trial 0160). *J Thorac Cardiovasc Surg* 121(3):472–483.

77. Barnes JB, Johnson SB, Dahiya RS, et al. Concomitant weekly cisplatin and thoracic radiotherapy for Pancoast tumors of the lung: pilot experience of the San Antonio Cancer Institute. *Am J Clin Oncol* 2002;25(1):90–92.

78. Doddoli C, Rollet G, Thomas P, et al. Is lung cancer surgery justified in patients with direct mediastinal invasion? *Eur J Cardiothorac Surg* 2001;20(2):339–343.

79. Grunenwald DH. Resection of lung carcinomas invading the mediastinum, including the superior vena cava. *Thorac Surg Clin* 2004;14(2):255–263, vii.

80. Albain KS, Swann RS, Rusch VW, et al. Radiotherapy plus chemotherapy with or without surgical resection for stage III non-small-cell lung cancer: a phase III randomised controlled trial. *Lancet* 2009;374(9687):379–386.

81. Perez CA, Pajak TF, Rubin P, et al. Long-term observations of the patterns of failure in patients with unresectable non-oat cell carcinoma of the lung treated with definitive radiotherapy. Report by the Radiation Therapy Oncology Group. *Cancer* 1987;59(11):1874–1881.

82. Dillman RO, Herndon J, Seagren SL, et al. Improved survival in stage III non-small-cell lung cancer: seven-year follow-up of cancer and leukemia group B (CALGB) 8433 trial. *J Natl Cancer Inst* 1996;88(17):1210–1215.

83. Sause W, Kolesar P, Taylor S IV, et al. Final results of phase III trial in regionally advanced unresectable non-small cell lung cancer: Radiation Therapy Oncology Group, Eastern Cooperative Oncology Group, and Southwest Oncology Group. *Chest* 2000;117(2):358–364.

84. Marino P, Preatoni A, Cantoni A. Randomized trials of radiotherapy alone versus combined chemotherapy and radiotherapy in stages IIIa and IIIb nonsmall cell lung cancer. A meta-analysis. *Cancer* 1995;76(4):593–601.

85. Pritchard RS, Anthony SP. Chemotherapy plus radiotherapy compared with radiotherapy alone in the treatment of locally advanced, unresectable, non-small-cell lung cancer. A meta-analysis. *Ann Intern Med* 1996;125(9):723–729.

86. Le Chevalier T, Arriagada R, Quoix E, et al. Radiotherapy alone versus combined chemotherapy and radiotherapy in unresectable non-small cell lung carcinoma. *Lung Cancer* 1994;10(Suppl 1):S239–S244.

87. Furuse K, Fukuoka M, Kawahara M, et al. Phase III study of concurrent versus sequential thoracic radiotherapy in combination with mitomycin, vindesine, and cisplatin in unresectable stage III non-small-cell lung cancer. *J Clin Oncol* 1999;17(9):2692–2699.

88. Curran WJ, Scott CB, Langer CJ, et al. Long-term benefit is observed in a phase III comparison of sequential vs. concurrent chemo-radiation for patients with unresected stage III NSCLC: RTOG 9410 [abstract]. *Proc Am Soc Clin Oncol* 2003;22:621.

89. Zatloukal P, Petruzelka L, Zemanova M, et al. Concurrent versus sequential chemoradiotherapy with cisplatin and vinorelbine in locally advanced non-small cell lung cancer: a randomized study. *Lung Cancer* 2004;46(1):87–98.

90. Auperin A, Le Pechoux C, Rolland E, et al. Meta-analysis of concomitant versus sequential radiochemotherapy in locally advanced non-small-cell lung cancer. *J Clin Oncol* 2010;28(13):2181–2190.

91. Vokes EE. Induction chemotherapy followed by concomitant chemoradiotherapy for non-small cell lung cancer. *Oncologist* 2001;6(Suppl 1):25–27.

92. Albain KS, Crowley JJ, Turrisi AT 3rd, et al. Concurrent cisplatin, etoposide, and chest radiotherapy in pathologic stage IIIB non-small-cell lung cancer: a Southwest Oncology Group phase II study, SWOG 9019. *J Clin Oncol* 2002;20(16):3454–3460.

93. Rosenman JG, Halle JS, Socinski MA, et al. High-dose conformal radiotherapy for treatment of stage IIIA/IIIB non-small-cell lung cancer: technical issues and results of a phase I/II trial. *Int J Radiat Oncol Biol Phys* 2002;54(2):348–356.

94. Gandara DR, Chansky K, Albain KS, et al. Consolidation docetaxel after concurrent chemoradiotherapy in stage IIIB non-small-cell lung cancer: phase II Southwest Oncology Group Study S9504. *J Clin Oncol* 2003;21(10):2004–2010.

95. Belani CP, Choy H, Bonomi P, et al. Combined chemoradiotherapy regimens of paclitaxel and carboplatin for locally advanced non-small-cell lung cancer: a randomized phase II locally advanced multi-modality protocol. *J Clin Oncol* 2005;23(25):5883–5891.

96. Vokes EE. Optimal therapy for unresectable stage III non-small-cell lung cancer. *J Clin Oncol* 2005;23(25):5853–5855.

97. Vokes E, Herndon JE, Kelley MJ, et al. Induction chemotherapy followed by concomitant chemoradiotherapy versus chemoradiotherapy alone for regionally advanced unresectable non-small cell lung cancer: initial analysis of a randomized phase III trial. *J Clin Oncol* 2004;22(14 S):Suppl; abstr 7005.

98. Hanna N, Neubauer M, Yiannoutsos C, et al. Phase III study of cisplatin, etoposide, and concurrent chest radiation with or without consolidation docetaxel in patients with inoperable stage III non-small-cell lung cancer: the Hoosier Oncology Group and U.S. Oncology. *J Clin Oncol* 2008;26(35):5755–5760.

99. Stinchcombe TE, Hodgson L, Herndon JE 2nd, et al. Treatment outcomes of different prognostic groups of patients on cancer and leukemia group B trial 39801: induction chemotherapy followed by chemoradiotherapy compared with chemoradiotherapy alone for unresectable stage III non-small cell lung cancer. *J Thorac Oncol* 2009;4(9):1117–1125.

100. Stuschke M, Eberhardt W, Pöttgen C, et al. Prophylactic cranial irradiation in locally advanced non-small-cell lung cancer after multimodality treatment: long-term follow-up and investigations of late neuropsychologic effects. *J Clin Oncol* 1999;17(9):2700–2709.

101. Andre F, Grunenwald D, Pujol JL, et al. Patterns of relapse of N2 nonsmall-cell lung carcinoma patients treated with preoperative chemotherapy: should prophylactic cranial irradiation be reconsidered? *Cancer* 2001;91(12):2394–2400.

102. Figlin RA, Piantadosi S, Feld R. Intracranial recurrence of carcinoma after complete surgical resection of stage I, II, and III non-small-cell lung cancer. *N Engl J Med* 1988;318(20):1300–1305.

103. Arriagada R, Le Pechoux C, Baeza MR. Prophylactic cranial irradiation in high-risk non-small cell lung cancer patients. *Lung Cancer* 2003;42(Suppl 2):S41–S45.

104. Lester JF, MacBeth FR, Coles B. Prophylactic cranial irradiation for preventing brain metastases in patients undergoing radical treatment for non-small-cell lung cancer: a Cochrane Review. *Int J Radiat Oncol Biol Phys* 2005;63(3):690–694.

105. Gore EM, Bae K, Wong SJ, et al. Phase III comparison of prophylactic cranial irradiation versus observation in patients with locally advanced non–small-cell lung cancer: Primary Analysis of Radiation Therapy Oncology Group Study RTOG 0214. *J Clin Oncol* 2011;29(3):272–278.

106. Sun A, Bae K, Gore EM, et al. Phase III trial of prophylactic cranial irradiation compared with observation in patients with locally advanced non–small-cell lung cancer: neurocognitive and quality-of-life analysis. *J Clin Oncol* 2011;29(3):279–286.

107. Budach W, Belka C. Palliative percutaneous radiotherapy in non-small-cell lung cancer. *Lung Cancer* 2004;45(Suppl 2):S239–S245.

108. Macbeth FR, Bolger JJ, Hopwood P, et al. Randomized trial of palliative two-fraction versus more intensive 13-fraction radiotherapy for patients with inoperable non-small cell lung cancer and good performance status. Medical Research Council Lung Cancer Working Party. *Clin Oncol (R Coll Radiol)* 1996;8(3):167–175.

109. Cross CK, Berman S, Buswell L, et al. Prospective study of palliative hypofractionated radiotherapy (8.5 Gy × 2) for patients with symptomatic non-small-cell lung cancer. *Int J Radiat Oncol Biol Phys* 2004;58(4):1098–1105.

110. Wu JS, Wong R, Johnston M, et al. Meta-analysis of dose-fractionation radiotherapy trials for the palliation of painful bone metastases. *Int J Radiat Oncol Biol Phys* 2003;55(3):594–605.

111. Sze WM, Shelley MD, Held I, et al. Palliation of metastatic bone pain: single fraction versus multifraction radiotherapy–a systematic review of randomised trials. *Clin Oncol (R Coll Radiol)* 2003;15(6):345–352.

112. Patchell RA, Tibbs PA, Walsh JW, et al. A randomized trial of surgery in the treatment of single metastases to the brain. *N Engl J Med* 1990;322(8):494–500.

113. Mintz AH, Kestle J, Rathbone MP, et al. A randomized trial to assess the efficacy of surgery in addition to radiotherapy in patients with a single cerebral metastasis. *Cancer* 1996;78(7):1470–1476.

114. Andrews DW, Scott CB, Sperduto PW, et al. Whole brain radiation therapy with or without stereotactic radiosurgery boost for patients with one to three brain metastases: phase III results of the RTOG 9508 randomised trial. *Lancet* 2004;363(9422):1665–1672.

115. Petrovich Z, Yu C, Gainnotta SL, et al. Survival and pattern of failure in brain metastasis treated with stereotactic gamma knife radiosurgery. *J Neurosurg* 2002;97(Suppl 5):499–506.

116. Aoyama H, Tago M, Kato N, et al. Neurocognitive function of patients with brain metastasis who received either whole brain radiotherapy plus stereotactic radiosurgery or radiosurgery alone. *Int J Radiat Oncol Biol Phys* 2007;68(5):1388–1395.

117. Mintz A, Perry J, Spithoff K, et al. Management of single brain metastasis: a practice guideline. *Curr Oncol* 2007;14(4):131–143.

118. Nieder C, Astner ST, Grosu AL, et al. The role of postoperative radiotherapy after resection of a single brain metastasis. Combined analysis of 643 patients. *Strahlenther Onkol* 2007;183(10):576–580.

119. Andrews DW. Should surgery followed by whole-brain radiation therapy be the standard treatment for single brain metastasis? *Nat Clin Pract Oncol* 2008;5(10):572–573.

120. Pignon JP, Arriagada R, Ihde DC, et al. A meta-analysis of thoracic radiotherapy for small-cell lung cancer. *N Engl J Med* 1992;327(23):1618–1624.

121. Warde P, Payne D. Does thoracic irradiation improve survival and local control in limited-stage small-cell carcinoma of the lung? A meta-analysis. *J Clin Oncol* 1992;10(6):890–895.

122. Murray N, Coy P, Pater JL, et al. Importance of timing for thoracic irradiation in the combined modality treatment of limited-stage small-cell lung cancer. The National Cancer Institute of Canada Clinical Trials Group. *J Clin Oncol* 1993;11(2):336–344.

123. Takada M, Fukuoka M, Kawahara M, et al. Phase III study of concurrent versus sequential thoracic radiotherapy in combination with cisplatin and etoposide for limited-stage small-cell lung cancer: results of the Japan Clinical Oncology Group Study 9104. *J Clin Oncol* 2002;20(14):3054–3060.

124. Arriagada R, Le Chevalier T, Borie F, et al. Prophylactic cranial irradiation for patients with small-cell lung cancer in complete remission. *J Natl Cancer Inst* 1995;87(3):183–190.

125. Gregor A, Cull A, Stephens RJ, et al. Prophylactic cranial irradiation is indicated following complete response to induction therapy in small cell lung cancer: results of a multicentre randomised trial. United Kingdom Coordinating Committee for Cancer Research (UKCCR) and the European Organization for Research and Treatment of Cancer (EORTC). *Eur J Cancer* 1997;33(11):1752–1758.

126. Auperin A, Arriagada R, Pignon JP, et al. Prophylactic cranial irradiation for patients with small-cell lung cancer in complete remission. Prophylactic Cranial Irradiation Overview Collaborative Group. *N Engl J Med* 1999;341(7):476–484.

127. Spira A, Ettinger DS. Extensive-stage small-cell lung cancer. *Semin Surg Oncol* 2003;21(3):164–175.

128. Perez CA, Stanley K, Rubin P, et al. A prospective randomized study of various irradiation doses and fractionation schedules in the treatment of inoperable non-oat-cell carcinoma of the lung. Preliminary report by the Radiation Therapy Oncology Group. *Cancer* 1980;45(11):2744–2753.

129. Sibley GS, Mundt AJ, Shapiro C, et al. The treatment of stage III nonsmall cell lung cancer using high dose conformal radiotherapy. *Int J Radiat Oncol Biol Phys* 1995;33(5):1001–1007.

130. Rengan R, Rosenzweig KE, Venkatraman E, et al. Improved local control with higher doses of radiation in large-volume stage III non-small-cell lung cancer. *Int J Radiat Oncol Biol Phys* 2004;60(3):741–747.

131. Hayman JA, Martel MK, Ten Haken RK, et al. Dose escalation in non-small-cell lung cancer using three-dimensional conformal radiation therapy: update of a phase I trial. *J Clin Oncol* 2001;19(1):127–136.

132. Narayan S, Henning GT, Ten Haken RK, et al. Results following treatment to doses of 92.4 or 102.9 Gy on a phase I dose escalation study for non-small cell lung cancer. *Lung Cancer* 2004;44(1):79–88.

133. Rosenzweig KE, Fox JL, Yorke E, et al. Results of a phase I dose-escalation study using three-dimensional conformal radiotherapy in the treatment of inoperable nonsmall cell lung carcinoma. *Cancer* 2005;103(10):2118–2127.

134. Rosenzweig KE, Sim SE, Mychalczak B, et al. Elective nodal irradiation in the treatment of non-small-cell lung cancer with three-dimensional conformal radiation therapy. *Int J Radiat Oncol Biol Phys* 2001;50(3):681–685.

135. Bradley J, Graham MV, Winter K, et al. Toxicity and outcome results of RTOG 9311: a phase I-II dose-escalation study using three-dimensional conformal radiotherapy in patients with inoperable non-small-cell lung carcinoma. *Int J Radiat Oncol Biol Phys* 2005;61(2):318–328.

136. Machtay M, Bae K, Movsas B, et al. Higher biologically effective dose of radiotherapy is associated with improved outcomes for locally advanced non-small cell lung carcinoma treated with chemoradiation: An analysis of the Radiation Therapy Oncology Group. *Int J Radiat Oncol Biol Phys* 2010.

137. Socinski MA, Morris DE, Halle JS, et al. Induction and concurrent chemotherapy with high-dose thoracic conformal radiation therapy in unresectable stage IIIA and IIIB non-small-cell lung cancer: a dose-escalation phase I trial. *J Clin Oncol* 2004;22(21):4341–4350.

138. Bradley JD, Moughan J, Graham MV, et al. A phase I/II radiation dose escalation study with concurrent chemotherapy for patients with inoperable stages I to III non-small-cell lung cancer: phase I results of RTOG 0117. *Int J Radiat Oncol Biol Phys* 2010;77(2):367–372.

139. Saunders M, Dische S, Barrett A, et al. Continuous, hyperfractionated, accelerated radiotherapy (CHART) versus conventional radiotherapy in non-small cell lung cancer: mature data from the randomised multicentre trial. CHART Steering committee. *Radiother Oncol* 1999;52(2):137–148.

140. Cox JD, Azarnia N, Byhardt RW, et al. A randomized phase I/II trial of hyperfractionated radiation therapy with total doses of 60.0 Gy to 79.2 Gy: possible survival benefit with greater than or equal to 69.6 Gy in favorable patients with Radiation Therapy Oncology Group stage III non-small-cell lung carcinoma: report of Radiation Therapy Oncology Group 83–11. *J Clin Oncol* 1990;8(9):1543–1555.

141. Sause WT, Scott C, Taylor S, et al. Radiation Therapy Oncology Group (RTOG) 88–08 and Eastern Cooperative Oncology Group (ECOG) 4588: preliminary results of a phase III trial in regionally advanced, unresectable non-small-cell lung cancer. *J Natl Cancer Inst* 1995;87(3):198–205.

142. Machtay M, Hsu C, Komaki R, et al. Effect of overall treatment time on outcomes after concurrent chemoradiation for locally advanced non-small-cell lung carcinoma: analysis of the Radiation Therapy Oncology Group (RTOG) experience. *Int J Radiat Oncol Biol Phys* 2005;63(3):667–671.

143. Fowler JF, Chappell R. Non-small cell lung tumors repopulate rapidly during radiation therapy. *Int J Radiat Oncol Biol Phys* 2000;46(2):516–517.

144. Mehta M, Scrimger R, Mackie R, et al. A new approach to dose escalation in non-small-cell lung cancer. *Int J Radiat Oncol Biol Phys* 2001;49(1):23–33.

145. Hiraoka M, Matsuo Y, Nagata Y. Stereotactic body radiation therapy (SBRT) for early-stage lung cancer. *Cancer Radiother* 2007;11(1–2):32–35.

146. Guckenberger M, Wulf J, Mueller G, et al. Dose-response relationship for image-guided stereotactic body radiotherapy of pulmonary tumors: relevance of 4D dose calculation. *Int J Radiat Oncol Biol Phys* 2009;74(1):47–54.

147. McGarry RC, Papiez L, Williams M, et al. Stereotactic body radiation therapy of early-stage non-small-cell lung carcinoma: phase I study. *Int J Radiat Oncol Biol Phys* 2005;63(4):1010–1015.

148. Timmerman R, Bastasch M, Saha D, et al. Optimizing dose and fractionation for stereotactic body radiation therapy. Normal tissue and tumor control effects with large dose per fraction. *Front Radiat Ther Oncol* 2007;40:352–365.

149. Timmerman RD, Park C, Kavanagh BD. The North American experience with stereotactic body radiation therapy in non-small cell lung cancer. 2007;*J Thorac Oncol* 2(7 Suppl 3):S101–S112.

150. Jin JY, Kong FM, Chetty IJ, et al. Impact of fraction size on lung radiation toxicity: hypofractionation may be beneficial in dose escalation of radiotherapy for lung cancers. *Int J Radiat Oncol Biol Phys* 2010;76(3):782–788.

151. Turrisi AT 3rd, Kim K, Blum R, et al. Twice-daily compared with once-daily thoracic radiotherapy in limited small-cell lung cancer treated concurrently with cisplatin and etoposide. *N Engl J Med* 1999;340(4):265–271.

152. Bonner JA, Sloan JA, Shanahan TG, et al. Phase III comparison of twice-daily split-course irradiation versus once-daily irradiation for patients with limited stage small-cell lung carcinoma. *J Clin Oncol* 1999; 17(9):2681–2691.

153. Schild SE, Bonner JA, Shanahan TG, et al. Long-term results of a phase III trial comparing once-daily radiotherapy with twice-daily radiotherapy in limited-stage small-cell lung cancer. *Int J Radiat Oncol Biol Phys* 2004;59(4):943–951.

154. Komaki R, Byhardt RW, Anderson T, et al. What is the lowest effective biologic dose for prophylactic cranial irradiation? *Am J Clin Oncol* 1985;8(6):523–527.

155. Sorensen JB. The role of prophylactic brain irradiation in small cell lung cancer treatment. *Monaldi Arch Chest Dis* 2003;59(2):128–133.

156. Le Pechoux, C., et al., Standard-dose versus higher-dose prophylactic cranial irradiation (PCI) in patients with limited-stage small-cell lung cancer in complete remission after chemotherapy and thoracic radiotherapy (PCI 99-01, EORTC 22003-08004, RTOG 0212, and IFCT 99-01): a randomised clinical trial. *Lancet Oncol* 2009;10(5): 467–474.

157. Halperin R, Roa W, Field M, et al. Setup reproducibility in radiation therapy for lung cancer: a comparison between T-bar and expanded foam immobilization devices. *Int J Radiat Oncol Biol Phys* 1999;43(1):211–216.

158. Samson MJ, van Sornsen de Koste JR, de Boer HC, et al. An analysis of anatomic landmark mobility and setup deviations in radiotherapy for lung cancer. *Int J Radiat Oncol Biol Phys* 1999;43(4):827–832.

159. de Boer HC, van Sornsen de Koste JR, Senan S, et al. Analysis and reduction of 3D systematic and random setup errors during the simulation and treatment of lung cancer patients with CT-based external beam radiotherapy dose planning. *Int J Radiat Oncol Biol Phys* 2001;49(3):857–868.

160. Mirimanoff RO, Franzetti-Pellanda A. Immobilization devices in conformal radiotherapy for non-small cell lung cancer. *Cancer Radiother* 2000;4(4):279–284.

161. Senan S, van Sornsen de Koste J, Samson M, et al. Evaluation of a target contouring protocol for 3D conformal radiotherapy in non-small cell lung cancer. *Radiother Oncol* 1999;53(3):247–255.

162. Feng F, Kong F-M, Quint LE, et al. Target delineation in radiation therapy of non-small cell lung cancer: a correlation study with local tumor failure. *Int J Radiat Oncol Biol Phys* 2005;63(Suppl 1):S415–S416.

163. Cascade PN, Gross BH, Kazerooni EA, et al. Variability in the detection of enlarged mediastinal lymph nodes in staging lung cancer: a comparison of contrast-enhanced and unenhanced CT. *AJR Am J Roentgenol* 1998;170(4):927–931.

164. Patz EF Jr, Erasmus JJ, McAdams HP, et al. Lung cancer staging and management: comparison of contrast-enhanced and nonenhanced helical CT of the thorax. *Radiology* 1999;212(1):56–60.

165. Lees J, Holloway L, Fuller M, et al. Effect of intravenous contrast on treatment planning system dose calculations in the lung. *Australas Phys Eng Sci Med* 2005; 28(3):190–195.

166. de Koste JR, Lagerwaard FJ, de Boer HC, et al. Are multiple CT scans required for planning curative radiotherapy in lung tumors of the lower lobe? *Int J Radiat Oncol Biol Phys* 2003;55(5):1394–1399.

167. Underberg RW, Lagerwaard FJ, Cuijpers JP, et al. Four-dimensional CT scans for treatment planning in stereotactic radiotherapy for stage I lung cancer. *Int J Radiat Oncol Biol Phys* 2004;60(4):1283–1290.

168. Vedam S. Home birth versus hospital birth: questioning the quality of the evidence on safety. *Birth* 2003; 30(1):57–63.

169. Keall PJ, Mageras GS, Balter JM, et al. The management of respiratory motion in radiation oncology report of AAPM Task Group 76. *Med Phys* 2006;33(10):3874–3900.

170. Jin JY, Ajlouni M, Chen Q, et al. A technique of using gated-CT images to determine internal target volume (ITV) for fractionated stereotactic lung radiotherapy. *Radiother Oncol* 2005;78(2):177–178.

171. Rosu M, Balter JM, Chetty IJ, et al. How extensive of a 4D dataset is needed to estimate cumulative dose distribution plan evaluation metrics in conformal lung therapy? *Med Phys* 2007;34(1):233–245.

172. Underberg RW, Lagerwaard FJ, Slotman BJ, et al. Use of maximum intensity projections (MIP) for target volume generation in 4DCT scans for lung cancer. *Int J Radiat Oncol Biol Phys* 2005;63(1):253–260.

173. Glide-Hurst CK, Hugo GD, Liang J, et al. A simplified method of four-dimensional dose accumulation using the mean patient density representation. *Med Phys* 2008; 35(12):5269–5277.

174. Harris KM, Adams H, Lloyd DC, et al. The effect on apparent size of simulated pulmonary nodules of using three standard CT window settings. *Clin Radiol* 1993;47(4):241–244.

175. Giraud P, Antoine M, Larrouy A, et al. Evaluation of microscopic tumor extension in non-small-cell lung cancer for three-dimensional conformal radiotherapy planning. *Int J Radiat Oncol Biol Phys* 2000;48(4):1015–1024.

176. ICRU. Prescribing, recording and reporting photon beam therapy (Report 50) 1993.

177. Yuan S, Meng X, Yu J, et al. Determining optimal clinical target volume margins on the basis of microscopic extracapsular extension of metastatic nodes in patients with non-small-cell lung cancer. *Int J Radiat Oncol Biol Phys* 2007;67(3):727–734.

178. Emami B. Management of hilar and mediastinal lymph nodes with radiation therapy in the treatment of lung cancer. *Front Radiat Ther Oncol* 1994;28:102–120.

179. Emami B, Mirkovic N, Scott C, et al. The impact of regional nodal radiotherapy (dose/volume) on regional progression and survival in unresectable non-small cell lung cancer: an analysis of RTOG data. *Lung Cancer* 2003;41(2):207–214.

180. Chapet O, Kong FM, Quint LE, et al. CT-based definition of thoracic lymph node stations: an atlas from the University of Michigan. *Int J Radiat Oncol Biol Phys* 2005;63(1):170–178.

181. van Sornsen de Koste JR, Lagerwaard FJ, Nijssen-Visser MR, et al. Tumor location cannot predict the mobility of lung tumors: a 3D analysis of data generated from multiple CT scans. *Int J Radiat Oncol Biol Phys* 2003; 56(2):348–354.

182. Allen AM, Siracuse KM, Hayman JA, et al. Evaluation of the influence of breathing on the movement and modeling of lung tumors. *Int J Radiat Oncol Biol Phys* 2004;58(4):1251–1257.

183. Stroom JC, de Boer HC, Huizenga H, et al. Inclusion of geometrical uncertainties in radiotherapy treatment planning by means of coverage probability. *Int J Radiat Oncol Biol Phys* 1999;43(4):905–919.

184. van Herk M, Remeijer P, Rasch C, et al. The probability of correct target dosage: dose-population histograms for deriving treatment margins in radiotherapy. *Int J Radiat Oncol Biol Phys* 2000;47(4):1121–1135.

185. Schewe JE, Balter JM, Lam KL, et al. Measurement of patient setup errors using port films and a computer-aided graphical alignment tool. *Med Dosim* 1996; 21(2):97–104.

186. Jin JY, Ryu S, Rock J, et al. Evaluation of residual patient position variation for spinal radiosurgery using the Novalis image guided system. *Med Phys* 2008;35(3):1087–1093.

187. Ezhil M, Vedam S, Balter P, et al. Determination of patient-specific internal gross tumor volumes for lung cancer using four-dimensional computed tomography. *Radiat Oncol* 2009;4:4.

188. Balter JM, Ten Haken RK, Lawrence TS, et al. Uncertainties in CT-based radiation therapy treatment planning associated with patient breathing. *Int J Radiat Oncol Biol Phys* 1996;36(1):167–174.

189. Lagerwaard FJ, Van Sornsen de Koste JR, Nijssen-Visser MR, et al. Multiple "slow" CT scans for incorporating lung tumor mobility in radiotherapy planning. *Int J Radiat Oncol Biol Phys* 2001;51(4):932–937.

190. Shih HA, Jiang SB, Aljarrah KM, et al. Internal target volume determined with expansion margins beyond composite gross tumor volume in three-dimensional conformal radiotherapy for lung cancer. *Int J Radiat Oncol Biol Phys* 2004;60(2):613–622.

191. Nestle U, Walter K, Schmidt S, et al. 18 F-deoxyglucose positron emission tomography (FDG-PET) for the planning of radiotherapy in lung cancer: high impact in patients with atelectasis. *Int J Radiat Oncol Biol Phys* 1999;44(3):593–597.

192. Vanuytsel LJ, Vansteenkiste JF, Stroobants SG, et al. The impact of (18)F-fluoro-2-deoxy-D-glucose positron emission tomography (FDG-PET) lymph node staging on the radiation treatment volumes in patients with non-small cell lung cancer. *Radiother Oncol* 2000;55(3):317–324.

193. Erdi YE, Rosenzweig K, Erdi AK, et al. Radiotherapy treatment planning for patients with non-small cell lung cancer using positron emission tomography (PET). *Radiother Oncol* 2002;62(1):51–60.

194. Mah K, Caldwell CB, Ung YC, et al. The impact of (18) FDG-PET on target and critical organs in CT-based treatment planning of patients with poorly defined non-small-cell lung carcinoma: a prospective study. *Int J Radiat Oncol Biol Phys* 2002;52(2):339–350.

195. Bradley J, Thorstad WL, Mutic S, et al. Impact of FDG-PET on radiation therapy volume delineation in non-small-cell lung cancer. *Int J Radiat Oncol Biol Phys* 2004; 59(1):78–86.

196. De Ruysscher D, Wanders S, Minken A, et al. Effects of radiotherapy planning with a dedicated combined PET-CT-simulator of patients with non-small cell lung cancer on dose limiting normal tissues and radiation dose-escalation: a planning study. *Radiother Oncol* 2005; 77(1):5–10.

197. Fox JL, Rengan R, O'Meara W, et al. Does registration of PET and planning CT images decrease interobserver and intraobserver variation in delineating tumor volumes for non-small-cell lung cancer? *Int J Radiat Oncol Biol Phys* 2005;62(1):70–75.

198. Messa C, Ceresoli GL, Rizzo G, et al. Feasibility of [18 F] FDG-PET and coregistered CT on clinical target volume definition of advanced non-small cell lung cancer. *Quart J Nucl Med Mol Imaging* 2005;49(3):259–266.

199. Caldwell CB, Mah K, Skinner M, et al. Can PET provide the 3D extent of tumor motion for individualized internal target volumes? A phantom study of the limitations of CT and the promise of PET. *Int J Radiat Oncol Biol Phys* 2003;55(5):1381–1393.

200. Ashamalla H, Rafla S, Parikh K, et al. The contribution of integrated PET/CT to the evolving definition of treatment volumes in radiation treatment planning in lung cancer. *Int J Radiat Oncol Biol Phys* 2005;63(4):1016–1023.

201. Van Der Wel A, Nijsten S, Hochstenbag M, et al. Increased therapeutic ratio by 18FDG-PET CT planning in patients with clinical CT stage N2-N3M0 non-small-cell lung cancer: a modeling study. *Int J Radiat Oncol Biol Phys* 2005;61(3):649–655.

202. Erdi YE, Mawlawi O, Larson SM, et al. Segmentation of lung lesion volume by adaptive positron emission tomography image thresholding. *Cancer* 1997;80(Suppl 12):2505–2509.

203. Biehl K, Kong FM, Dehdashti, F., et al. 18F-FDG PET definition of gross tumor volume for radiotherapy of non-small cell lung cancer: is a single standardized uptake value threshold approach appropriate? *J Nucl Med* 2006;47(11):1808–1812.

204. Black QC, Grills IS, Kestin LL, et al. Defining a radiotherapy target with positron emission tomography. *Int J Radiat Oncol Biol Phys* 2004;60(4):1272–1282.

205. Fernando S, Kong F-M, Kessler M, et al. *Int J Radiat Oncol Biol Phy* 2005;63:s400–s401.

206. Emami B, Lyman J, Brown A, et al. Tolerance of normal tissue to therapeutic irradiation. *Int J Radiat Oncol Biol Phys* 1991;21(1):109–122.

207. Marks LB, Yorke ED, Jackson A, et al. Use of normal tissue complication probability models in the clinic. *Int J Radiat Oncol Biol Phys* 2010;76(Suppl 3):S10–S19.

208. Kong FM, et al., Final toxicity results of a radiation-dose escalation study in patients with non-small-cell lung cancer (NSCLC): predictors for radiation pneumonitis and fibrosis. *Int J Radiat Oncol Biol Phys* 2006; 65(4):1075–1086.

209. Liao Z, Wang SL, Wei X, et al. Analysis of clinical and dosimetric factors associated with radiation pneumonitis (RP) in patients with non-small cell lung cancer (NSCLC) treated with concurrent chemotherapy (ConChT) and three dimensional conformal radiotherapy (3D-CRT). *Int J Radiat Oncol Biol Phys* 2005;63(Suppl 1):S41.

210. Seppenwoolde Y, Lebesque JV, de Jaeger K, et al. Comparing different NTCP models that predict the incidence of radiation pneumonitis. Normal tissue complication probability. *Int J Radiat Oncol Biol Phys* 2003;55(3): 724–735.

211. Maguire PD, Sibley GS, Zhou SM, et al. Clinical and dosimetric predictors of radiation-induced esophageal toxicity. *Int J Radiat Oncol Biol Phys* 1999;45(1): 97–103.

212. Werner-Wasik M, Pequignot E, Leeper D, et al. Predictors of severe esophagitis include use of concurrent chemotherapy, but not the length of irradiated esophagus: a multivariate analysis of patients with lung cancer treated with nonoperative therapy. *Int J Radiat Oncol Biol Phys* 2000;48(3):689–696.

213. Hirota S, Tsujino K, Endo M, et al. Dosimetric predictors of radiation esophagitis in patients treated for non-small-cell lung cancer with carboplatin/paclitaxel/radiotherapy. *Int J Radiat Oncol Biol Phys* 2001; 51(2):291–295.

214. Komaki R, Seiferheld W, Ettinger D, et al. Randomized phase II chemotherapy and radiotherapy trial for patients with locally advanced inoperable non-small-cell lung cancer: long-term follow-up of RTOG 92–04. *Int J Radiat Oncol Biol Phys* 2002;53(3):548–557.

215. Singh AK, Lockett MA, Bradley JD. Predictors of radiation-induced esophageal toxicity in patients with non-small-cell lung cancer treated with three-dimensional conformal radiotherapy. *Int J Radiat Oncol Biol Phys* 2003;55(2):337–341.

216. Bradley JD, Dehdashti F, Mintun MA, et al. Positron emission tomography in limited-stage small-cell lung cancer: a prospective study. *J Clin Oncol* 2004;22(16): 3248–3254.

217. Patel AB, Edelman MJ, Kwok Y, et al. Predictors of acute esophagitis in patients with non-small-cell lung carcinoma treated with concurrent chemotherapy and hyperfractionated radiotherapy followed by surgery. *Int J Radiat Oncol Biol Phys* 2004;60(4):1106–1112.

218. Ahn SJ, Kahn D, Zhou S, et al. Dosimetric and clinical predictors for radiation-induced esophageal injury. *Int J Radiat Oncol Biol Phys* 2005;61(2):335–347.

219. Belderbos J, Heemsbergen W, Hoogeman M, et al. Acute esophageal toxicity in non-small cell lung cancer patients after high dose conformal radiotherapy. *Radiother Oncol* 2005;75(2):157–164.

220. Chapet O, Kong FM, Lee JS, et al. Normal tissue complication probability modeling for acute esophagitis in patients treated with conformal radiation therapy for non-small cell lung cancer. *Radiother Oncol* 2005; 77(2):176–181.

221. Kahn D, Zhou S, Ahn SJ, et al. "Anatomically-correct" dosimetric parameters may be better predictors for esophageal toxicity than are traditional CT-based metrics. *Int J Radiat Oncol Biol Phys* 2005;62(3):645–651.

222. Takeda K, Nemoto K, Saito H, et al. Dosimetric correlations of acute esophagitis in lung cancer patients treated with radiotherapy. *Int J Radiat Oncol Biol Phys* 2005;62(3):626–629.

223. Kong FM, Ritter T, Quint DJ, et al. Consideration of dose limits for organs at risk of thoracic radiotherapy: atlas for lung, proximal bronchial tree, esophagus, spinal cord, ribs, and brachial plexus. *Int J Radiat Oncol Biol Phys* 2010.

224. Orton CG, Chungbin S, Klein EE, et al. Study of lung density corrections in a clinical trial (RTOG 88–08). Radiation Therapy Oncology Group. *Int J Radiat Oncol Biol Phys* 1998;41(4):787–794.

225. Frank SJ, Forster KM, Stevens CW, et al. Treatment planning for lung cancer: traditional homogeneous point-dose prescription compared with heterogeneity-corrected dose-volume prescription. *Int J Radiat Oncol Biol Phys* 2003;56(5):1308–1318.

226. Chetty IJ, Charland PM, Tyagi N, et al. Photon beam relative dose validation of the DPM Monte Carlo code in lung-equivalent media. *Med Phys* 2003;30(4):563–573.

227. Chetty IJ, Curran B, Cygler JE, et al. Report of the AAPM Task Group No. 105: Issues associated with clinical implementation of Monte Carlo-based photon and electron external beam treatment planning. *Med Phys* 2007;34(12):4818–4853.

228. Wang L, Yorke E, Chui CS. Monte Carlo evaluation of 6 MV intensity modulated radiotherapy plans for head and neck and lung treatments. *Med Phys* 2002; 29(11):2705–2717.

229. De Jaeger K, Hoogeman MS, Engelsman M, et al. Incorporating an improved dose-calculation algorithm in conformal radiotherapy of lung cancer: re-evaluation of dose in normal lung tissue. *Radiother Oncol* 2003; 69(1):1–10.

230. Ekstrand KE, Barnes WH. Pitfalls in the use of high energy X rays to treat tumors in the lung. *Int J Radiat Oncol Biol Phys* 1990;18(1):249–252.

231. Klein EE, Morrison A, Purdy JA, et al. A volumetric study of measurements and calculations of lung density corrections for 6 and 18 MV photons. *Int J Radiat Oncol Biol Phys* 1997;37(5):1163–1170.

232. Wang JY, Chen KY, Wang JT, et al. Outcome and prognostic factors for patients with non-small-cell lung cancer and severe radiation pneumonitis. *Int J Radiat Oncol Biol Phys* 2002;54(3):735–741.

233. Seppenwoolde Y, Shirato H, Kitamura K, et al. Precise and real-time measurement of 3D tumor motion in lung due to breathing and heartbeat, measured during radiotherapy. *Int J Radiat Oncol Biol Phys* 2002;53(4):822–834.

234. Mageras GS, Pevsner A, Yorke ED, et al. Measurement of lung tumor motion using respiration-correlated CT. *Int J Radiat Oncol Biol Phys* 2004;60(3):933–941.

235. Shirato H, Seppenwoolde Y, Kitamura K, et al. Intrafractional tumor motion: lung and liver. *Semin Radiat Oncol* 2004;14(1):10–18.

236. Ekberg L, Holmberg O, Wittgren L, et al. What margins should be added to the clinical target volume in radiotherapy treatment planning for lung cancer? *Radiother Oncol* 1998;48(1):71–77.

237. Sixel KE, Ruschin M, Tirona R, et al. Digital fluoroscopy to quantify lung tumor motion: potential for patient-

specific planning target volumes. *Int J Radiat Oncol Biol Phys* 2003;57(3):717–723.

238. Negoro Y, Nagata Y, Aoki T, et al. The effectiveness of an immobilization device in conformal radiotherapy for lung tumor: reduction of respiratory tumor movement and evaluation of the daily setup accuracy. *Int J Radiat Oncol Biol Phys* 2001;50(4):889–898.

239. Wong JW, Sharpe MB, Jaffray DA, et al. The use of active breathing control (ABC) to reduce margin for breathing motion. *Int J Radiat Oncol Biol Phys* 1999;44(4):911–919.

240. D'Souza WD, Naqvi SA, Yu CX. Real-time intra-fraction-motion tracking using the treatment couch: a feasibility study. *Phys Med Biol* 2005;50(17):4021–4033.

241. Keall PJ, Joshi S, Vedam SS, et al. Four-dimensional radiotherapy planning for DMLC-based respiratory motion tracking. *Med Phys* 2005;32(4):942–951.

242. Jin JY, Ajlouni M, Ryu S, et al. A technique of quantitatively monitoring both respiratory and nonrespiratory motion in patients using external body markers. *Med Phys* 2007;34(7):2875–2881.

243. Jin JY, Yin FF. Time delay measurement for linac based treatment delivery in synchronized respiratory gating radiotherapy. *Med Phys* 2005;32(5):1293–1296.

244. Jin JY, Ajlouni M, Kong FM, et al. Utilize target motion to cover clinical target volume (CTV)—a novel and practical treatment planning approach to manage respiratory motion. *Radiother Oncol* 2008;89(3):292–303.

245. Derycke S, De Gersem WR, Van Duyse BB, et al. Conformal radiotherapy of Stage III non-small cell lung cancer: a class solution involving non-coplanar intensity-modulated beams. *Int J Radiat Oncol Biol Phys* 1998; 41(4):771–777.

246. van Sornsen de Koste J, Voet P, Dirkx M, et al. An evaluation of two techniques for beam intensity modulation in patients irradiated for stage III non-small cell lung cancer. *Lung Cancer* 2001;32(2):145–153.

247. Marnitz S, Stuschke M, Bohsung J, et al. Intraindividual comparison of conventional three-dimensional radiotherapy and intensity modulated radiotherapy in the therapy of locally advanced non-small cell lung cancer a planning study. *Strahlenther Onkol* 2002;178(11):651–658.

248. Grills IS, Yan D, Martinez AA, et al. Potential for reduced toxicity and dose escalation in the treatment of inoperable non-small-cell lung cancer: a comparison of intensity-modulated radiation therapy (IMRT), 3D conformal radiation, and elective nodal irradiation. *Int J Radiat Oncol Biol Phys* 2003;57(3):875–890.

249. Liu HH, Wang X, Dong L, et al. Feasibility of sparing lung and other thoracic structures with intensity-modulated radiotherapy for non-small-cell lung cancer. *Int J Radiat Oncol Biol Phys* 2004;58(4):1268–1279.

250. Manon RR, Jaradat H, Patel R, et al. Potential for radiation therapy technology innovations to permit dose escalation for non-small-cell lung cancer. *Clin Lung Cancer* 2005;7(2):107–113.

251. Chapet O, Thomas E, Kessler ML, et al. Esophagus sparing with IMRT in lung tumor irradiation: an EUD-based optimization technique. *Int J Radiat Oncol Biol Phys* 2005;63(1):179–187.

252. Chui CS, Yorke E, Hong L. The effects of intra-fraction organ motion on the delivery of intensity-modulated field with a multileaf collimator. *Med Phys* 2003;30(7): 1736–1746.

253. Li HS, Chetty IJ, Solberg TD, et al. Quantifying the interplay effect in prostate IMRT delivery using a convolution-based method. *Med Phys* 2008;35(5):1703–1710.

254. Yom SS, Liao Z, Lui HH, et al. Initial evaluation of treatment-related pneumonitis in advanced-stage non-small-cell lung cancer patients treated with concurrent chemotherapy and intensity-modulated radiotherapy. *Int J Radiat Oncol Biol Phys* 2007;68(1):94–102.

255. Sura S, Gupta V, Yorke E, et al. Intensity-modulated radiation therapy (IMRT) for inoperable non-small cell lung cancer: the Memorial Sloan-Kettering Cancer Center (MSKCC) experience. *Radiother Oncol* 2008; 87(1):17–23.

256. Gejerman G, Mullokandov EA, Bagiella E, et al. Endobronchial brachytherapy and external-beam radiotherapy in patients with endobronchial obstruction and extrabronchial extension. *Brachytherapy* 2002; 1(4):204–210.

257. Santos RS, Raftopoulos Y, Keenan RJ, et al. Bronchoscopic palliation of primary lung cancer: single or multimodality therapy? *Surg Endosc* 2004;18(6):931–936.

258. Senan S, Lagerwaard FJ, de Pan C, et al. A CT-assisted method of dosimetry in brachytherapy of lung cancer. Rotterdam Oncological Thoracic Study Group. *Radiother Oncol* 2000;55(1):75–80.

259. Engels EA, Pfeiffer RM. Malignant thymoma in the United States: demographic patterns in incidence and associations with subsequent malignancies. *Int J Cancer* 2003;105(4):546–551.

260. Tomiyama N, Muller NL, Ellis SJ, et al. Invasive and noninvasive thymoma: distinctive CT features. *J Comput Assist Tomogr* 2001;25(3):388–393.

261. Regnard JF, Magdeleinat P, Dromer C, et al. Prognostic factors and long-term results after thymoma resection: a series of 307 patients. *J Thorac Cardiovasc Surg* 1996;112(2):376–384.

262. Zhu G, He S, Fu X, et al. Radiotherapy and prognostic factors for thymoma: a retrospective study of 175 patients. *Int J Radiat Oncol Biol Phys* 2004;60(4):1113–1119.

263. Okumura M, Ohta M, Tateyama H, et al. The World Health Organization histologic classification system reflects the oncologic behavior of thymoma: a clinical study of 273 patients. *Cancer* 2002;94(3):624–632.

264. Strobel P, Bauer A, Puppe B, et al. Tumor recurrence and survival in patients treated for thymomas and thymic squamous cell carcinomas: a retrospective analysis. *J Clin Oncol* 2004;22(8):1501–1509.

265. Mangi AA, Wright CD, Allan JS, et al. Adjuvant radiation therapy for stage II thymoma. *Ann Thorac Surg* 2002;74(4):1033–1037.

266. Kondo K, Monden Y. Therapy for thymic epithelial tumors: a clinical study of 1,320 patients from Japan. *Ann Thorac Surg* 2003;76(3):878–884; discussion 884–875.

267. Singhal S, Shrager JB, Rosenthal DL, et al. Comparison of stages I-II thymoma treated by complete resection with or without adjuvant radiation. *Ann Thorac Surg* 2003;76(5):1635–1641; discussion 1641–1632.

268. Blumberg D, Port JL, Weksler B, et al. Thymoma: a multivariate analysis of factors predicting survival. *Ann Thorac Surg* 1995;60(4):908–913; discussion 914.

269. Curran WJ Jr, Kornstein MJ, Brooks JJ, et al. Invasive thymoma: the role of mediastinal irradiation following complete or incomplete surgical resection. *J Clin Oncol* 1988;6(11):1722–1727.

270. Pollack A, Komaki R, Cox JD, et al. Thymoma: treatment and prognosis. *Int J Radiat Oncol Biol Phys* 1992;23(5): 1037–1043.

271. Ruffini E, Mancuso M, Oliaro A, et al. Recurrence of thymoma: analysis of clinicopathologic features, treatment, and outcome. *J Thorac Cardiovasc Surg* 1997; 113(1):55–63.

272. Haniuda M, Miyazawa M, Yoshida K, et al. Is postoperative radiotherapy for thymoma effective? *Ann Surg* 1996;224(2):219–224.

273. Urgesi A, Monetti U, Rossi G, et al. Role of radiation therapy in locally advanced thymoma. *Radiother Oncol* 1990;19(3):273–280.

274. Gripp S, Hilgers K, Wurm R, et al. Thymoma: prognostic factors and treatment outcomes. *Cancer* 1998; 83(8):1495–1503.

275. Myojin M, Choi NC, Wright CD, et al. Stage III thymoma: pattern of failure after surgery and postoperative radiotherapy and its implication for future study. *Int J Radiat Oncol Biol Phys* 2000;46(4):927–933.

276. Mangi AA, Wain JC, Donahue DM, et al. Adjuvant radiation of stage III thymoma: is it necessary? *Ann Thorac Surg* 2005;79(6):1834–1839.

277. Kondo K, Monden Y. Therapy for thymic epithelial tumors: a clinical study of 1,320 patients from Japan. *Ann Thorac Surg* 2003;76(3):878–884; discussion 884-5.

278. Ogawa K, Uno T, Toita T, et al. Postoperative radiotherapy for patients with completely resected thymoma: a multi-institutional, retrospective review of 103 patients. *Cancer* 2002;94(5):1405–1413.

279. Ciernik IF, Meier U, Lütolf UM. Prognostic factors and outcome of incompletely resected invasive thymoma following radiation therapy. *J Clin Oncol* 1994;12(7): 1484–1490.

280. Fornasiero A, Daniele O, Ghiotto C, et al. Chemotherapy of invasive thymoma. *J Clin Oncol* 1990;8(8):1419–1423.

281. Akaogi E, Ohara K, Mitsui K, et al. Preoperative radiotherapy and surgery for advanced thymoma with invasion to the great vessels. *J Surg Oncol* 1996;63(1):17–22.

282. Loehrer PJ SR, Chen M, Kim K, et al. Cisplatin, doxorubicin, and cyclophosphamide plus thoracic radiation therapy for limited-stage unresectable thymoma: an intergroup trial. *J Clin Oncol* 1997;15(9):3093–3099.

283. Kim ES, et al., Phase II study of a multidisciplinary approach with induction chemotherapy, followed by surgical resection, radiation therapy, and consolidation chemotherapy for unresectable malignant thymomas: final report. *Lung Cancer* 2004;44(3):369–379.

284. Bretti S, Berruti A, Loddo C, et al. Multimodal management of stages III-IVa malignant thymoma. *Lung Cancer* 2004;44(1):69–77.

285. Robinson BW, Lake RA. Advances in malignant mesothelioma. *N Engl J Med* 2005;353(15):1591–1603.

286. Teta MJ, Mink PJ, Lau E, et al. US mesothelioma patterns 1973–2002: indicators of change and insights into background rates. *Eur J Cancer Prev* 2008;17(6):525–534.

287. Price B, Ware A. Time trend of mesothelioma incidence in the United States and projection of future cases: an update based on SEER data for 1973 through 2005. *Crit Rev Toxicol* 2009;39(7):576–588.

288. Pass HI, Lott D, Lonardo F et al. Asbestos exposure, pleural mesothelioma, and serum osteopontin levels. *N Engl J Med* 2005;353(15):1564–1573.

289. Richards WG, Godleski JJ, Yeap BY, et al. Proposed adjustments to pathologic staging of epithelial malignant pleural mesothelioma based on analysis of 354 cases. *Cancer* 116(6):1510–1517.

290. Zielinski M, Hauer J, Hauer L, et al. Staging algorithm for diffuse malignant pleural mesothelioma. *Interact Cardiovasc Thorac Surg* 2010;10(2):185–189.

291. Benard F, Sterman D, Smith RJ, et al. Metabolic imaging of malignant pleural mesothelioma with fluorodeoxyglucose positron emission tomography. *Chest* 1998;114(3):713–722.

292. Schneider DB, Clary-Macy C, Challa S, et al. Positron emission tomography with f18-fluorodeoxyglucose in the staging and preoperative evaluation of malignant pleural mesothelioma. *J Thorac Cardiovasc Surg* 2000;120(1):128–133.

293. Gerbaudo VH, Sugarbaker DJ, Britz-Cunningham S, et al. Assessment of malignant pleural mesothelioma with (18)F-FDG dual-head gamma-camera coincidence imaging: comparison with histopathology. *J Nucl Med* 2002;43(9):1144–1149.

294. Flores RM, Akhurst T, Gonen M, et al. Positron emission tomography defines metastatic disease but not locoregional disease in patients with malignant pleural mesothelioma. *J Thorac Cardiovasc Surg* 2003;126(1):11–16.

295. Flores RM. The role of PET in the surgical management of malignant pleural mesothelioma. *Lung Cancer* 2005;49 (Suppl 1): S27–S32.

296. Alvarez JM, Ha T, Musk W, et al. Importance of mediastinoscopy, bilateral thoracoscopy, and laparoscopy in correct staging of malignant mesothelioma before extrapleural pneumonectomy. *J Thorac Cardiovasc Surg* 2005;130(3):905–906.

297. Vogelzang NJ, Rusthoven JJ, Symanowski J, et al. Phase III study of pemetrexed in combination with cisplatin versus cisplatin alone in patients with malignant pleural mesothelioma. *J Clin Oncol* 2003;21(14):2636–2644.

298. Aisner J. Current approach to malignant mesothelioma of the pleura. *Chest* 1995;107(Suppl 6):332S–344S.

299. Baldini EH, Recht A, Strauss GM, et al. Patterns of failure after trimodality therapy for malignant pleural mesothelioma. *Ann Thorac Surg* 1997;63(2):334–338.

300. Pass HI, Kranda K, Temeck BK, et al. Surgically debulked malignant pleural mesothelioma: results and prognostic factors. *Ann Surg Oncol* 1997;4(3):215–222.

301. Hughes RS. Malignant pleural mesothelioma. *Am J Med Sci* 2005;329(1):29–44.

302. Baldini EH. External beam radiation therapy for the treatment of pleural mesothelioma. *Thorac Surg Clin* 2004;14(4):543–548.

303. Gupta V, Mychalczak B, Krug L, et al. Hemithoracic radiation therapy after pleurectomy/decortication for malignant pleural mesothelioma. *Int J Radiat Oncol Biol Phys* 2005;63(4):1045–1052.

304. Rusch VW, Rosenzweig K, Venkatraman E, et al. A phase II trial of surgical resection and adjuvant high-dose hemithoracic radiation for malignant pleural mesothelioma. *J Thorac Cardiovasc Surg* 2001;122(4): 788–795.

305. Ceresoli GL, Locati LD, Ferreri AJ, et al. Therapeutic outcome according to histologic subtype in 121 patients with malignant pleural mesothelioma. *Lung Cancer* 2001;34(2):279–287.

306. Boutin C, Rey F, Viallat JR. Prevention of malignant seeding after invasive diagnostic procedures in patients with pleural mesothelioma. A randomized trial of local radiotherapy. *Chest* 1995;108(3):754–758.

307. de Graaf-Strukowska L, van der Zee J, van Putten W, et al. Factors influencing the outcome of radiotherapy in malignant mesothelioma of the pleura–a single-institution experience with 189 patients. *Int J Radiat Oncol Biol Phys* 1999;43(3):511–516.

308. de Bree E, van Ruth S, Baas P, et al. Cytoreductive surgery and intraoperative hyperthermic intrathoracic chemotherapy in patients with malignant pleural mesothelioma or pleural metastases of thymoma. *Chest* 2002;121(2):480–487.

309. Bydder S, Phillips M, Joseph DJ, et al. A randomised trial of single-dose radiotherapy to prevent procedure tract metastasis by malignant mesothelioma. *Br J Cancer* 2004;91(1):9–10.

310. Munter MW, Thieke C, Nikoghosyan A, et al. Inverse planned stereotactic intensity modulated radiotherapy (IMRT) in the palliative treatment of malignant mesothelioma of the pleura: the Heidelberg experience. *Lung Cancer* 2005;49(Suppl 1):S83–S86.

311. Stevens CW, Wong PF, Rice D, et al. Treatment planning system evaluation for mesothelioma IMRT. *Lung Cancer* 2005;49(Suppl 1):S75–S81.

312. Ahamad A, Stevens CW, Smythe WR, et al. Intensity-modulated radiation therapy: a novel approach to the management of malignant pleural mesothelioma. *Int J Radiat Oncol Biol Phys* 2003;55(3):768–775.

313. Forster KM, Smythe WR, Starkschall G, et al. Intensity-modulated radiotherapy following extrapleural pneumonectomy for the treatment of malignant mesothelioma: clinical implementation. *Int J Radiat Oncol Biol Phys* 2003;55(3):606–616.

314. Stevens CW, Forster K, Zhu X, et al. Excellent local control and survival after extrapleural pneumonectomy and IMRT for mesothelioma. *Int J Radiat Oncol Biol Phys* 2005;63(Suppl 1):S103–S104.

315. Bissett D, Macbeth FR, Cram I. The role of palliative radiotherapy in malignant mesothelioma. *Clin Oncol (R Coll Radiol)* 1991;3(6):315–317.

316. Ball DL, Cruickshank DG. The treatment of malignant mesothelioma of the pleura: review of a 5-year experience, with special reference to radiotherapy. *Am J Clin Oncol* 1990;13(1):4–9.

317. Senan S, De Ruysscher D, Giraud P, et al. Literature-based recommendations for treatment planning and execution in high-dose radiotherapy for lung cancer. *Radiother Oncol* 2004;71(2):139–146.

318. De Ruysscher D, Faivre-Finn C, Nestle U, et al. European organisation for research and treatment of cancer recommendations for planning and delivery of high-dose, high-precision radiotherapy for lung cancer. *J Clin Oncol* 2010;28(36):5301–5310.

CHAPTER 34

Extremity Soft-Tissue Sarcomas

Michael T. Selch

INTRODUCTION

Soft-tissue sarcomas arise from extraskeletal connective tissue. These neoplasms are unusual despite the fact that soft tissues comprise over 40% of adult body weight. It is estimated that 10,600 new soft-tissue sarcomas occurred in 2009, accounting for 1% of all nonskin malignancies (1). These tumors can affect any portion of the body, including the rare visceral sarcomas. Excluding visceral tumors, soft-tissue sarcomas arise in the following locations: 40% to 50% lower extremity; 30% trunk (retroperitoneum, mediastinum, chest wall, abdominal wall, and breast); 10% to 15% upper extremity; 10% head and neck (2,3). Approximately 75% of all extremity soft-tissue lesions arise proximal to the elbow or knee joints.

The incidence of soft-tissue sarcomas demonstrates a bimodal age distribution. The median age varies from 52 to 62 years but soft-tissue sarcomas also represent 7% of all pediatric cancers (4,5). Adult sarcomas predominantly affect the limbs while pediatric tumors arise primarily in the pelvis or head and neck. There is a slight male predilection for soft-tissue sarcomas but no apparent racial difference. Soft-tissue sarcomas have been reported in association with chronic lymphedema, various genetic anomalies (Li-Fraumeni, von Recklinghausen's), environmental exposures (phenoxyacetic acid herbicides), and ionizing radiation but their etiology remains obscure.

Soft-tissue sarcomas were traditionally considered resistant to radiation therapy and their management largely depended upon surgical ablation. Local control following primary resection of an extremity soft-tissue sarcoma is related to the extent of surgery and the resulting margin obtained. Enneking and associates have defined four types of surgical margins for sarcoma surgery and the procedures required to achieve these margins (6). Intralesional excision is followed by local relapse in over 90% of cases (7,8). Marginal and wide excisions are accompanied by local recurrence in ~70% and 40%, respectively (9,10). Surgical therapy is successful only when a radical margin is obtained. This specific margin is achieved when the tumor and surrounding normal tissues are removed by dissection through at least one uninvolved tissue plane in both the longitudinal and transversal dimensions. Satisfying these surgical constraints has resulted in local relapse rates as low as 2% to 18% (11,12). Achieving a radical margin, however, historically required amputation in nearly one-half of patients. Those patients radically resected, but not amputated, also suffered significant cosmetic and functional tissue loss affecting quality of life.

Current management of extremity soft-tissue sarcomas typically involves function-preserving surgery plus adjunctive radiation therapy (limb salvage therapy). Following a relatively conservative wide excision of an extremity sarcoma, radiotherapy will be required to eliminate likely microscopic residual tumor cells. It is known from the pioneering studies of Gilbert Fletcher on epithelial cancers that minimal amounts of neoplastic clonogens can be more effectively controlled by radiotherapy than large bulky deposits (13). Cells comprising soft-tissue sarcomas, furthermore, are no longer considered inherently "radioresistant." In an *in vitro* model, the surviving fraction of fibrosarcoma cells after a 2-Gy exposure (SF_{2Gy}) is equivalent to adenocarcinomas of the breast (14). Since the initial experience with limb-sparing therapy, randomized and nonrandomized trials have demonstrated local control rates for sarcomas at least equivalent to those reported for radical surgery (5,15–22). A randomized trial performed by the National Cancer Institute demonstrated adjunctive radiotherapy is necessary in the setting of limb-sparing resection (23). The investigators randomized 91 patients with high-grade extremity sarcomas and 50 with low-grade tumors to limb-sparing surgery with or without postoperative external beam radiotherapy. After a median 10-year follow-up, the local control rate among patients with high-grade tumors was 100%, following postoperative radiotherapy compared to 78% after limb-sparing surgery alone ($p = 0.003$). For those with low-grade neoplasms, the respective local control rates were 95% and 70% ($p = 0.016$). Although the patients entered on these salvage protocols are not necessarily comparable to those previously undergoing radical surgeries, these data imply that limb-sparing approaches offer a viable alternative to local management of extremity sarcomas in selected situations. The best candidates for this procedure are those in whom a gross total excision can be performed with preservation of a reasonably functional extremity. The purpose of this chapter is to describe the radiation therapy techniques that ensure successful multimodal management of extremity soft-tissue sarcomas in adults.

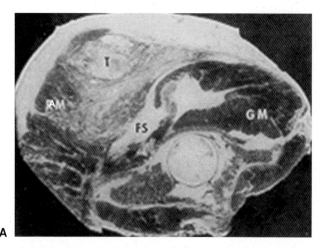 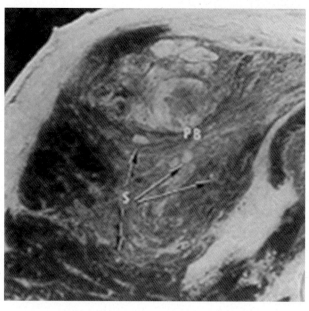

Figure 34.1. A: Gross morphology of a high-grade malignant fibrous histiocytoma. Tumor (T) expansion has resulted in surrounding atrophic reactive muscle (RM) compared to normal gluteus medius (GM) separated by the intermuscular fascial septa (FS). **B:** Compressed atrophic muscle results in a pushing border (PB). Satellite tumor deposits (S) are scattered throughout the border. *Source:* From Enneking WF, et al. The effect of the anatomic setting on the results of surgical procedures for soft parts sarcoma of the thigh. *Cancer* 1981;47:1005–1012.

NATURAL HISTORY

An extremity soft-tissue sarcoma typically presents as a painless mass situated deep within limb musculature. Symptoms occasionally encountered include pain, paresthesia, and edema. The rarity of these tumors and the resulting lack of clinical suspicion result in a diagnostic delay varying from 4 to 28 months (2).

Soft-tissue sarcomas demonstrate slow centrifugal expansion. This radial growth produces a peripheral pushing border composed of atrophic normal cells and edematous reactive tissue. The resulting compressed tissue mimics tumor encapsulation on gross inspection. It has become abundantly clear that the compressive zone is not an effective barrier to microscopic tumor extension (Fig. 34.1). The compressive zone is more properly a "pseudocapsule" commonly penetrated by sarcoma cells (6).

The normal extremity is composed of various muscle groups. Muscles with similar function are separated from other muscles by fascial barriers called major intermuscular septae. Although not strictly correct, these muscle groups and their accompanying neurovascular structures can be thought of as forming individual muscle compartments within an extremity (6). Muscles lying within a specific compartment are separated from each other by minor intermuscular septae. The growth of extremity soft-tissue sarcomas generally respects certain fascial barriers such as major intermuscular septae, interosseous membranes (tibia-fibula; ulna-radius), periosteum, perineurium and adventitia. Soft-tissue sarcomas arising within an extremity extend longitudinally, rather than radially, along the major fascial planes within the compartment of origin. As a consequence, undisturbed soft-tissue sarcomas generally

do not extend transversally into the neighboring compartments until quite late in their course. Extremity sarcomas can, however, extensively permeate minor septae and infiltrate intracompartmental muscle bundles for a considerable distance from the primary lesion (Fig. 34.2). As a consequence of the natural growth pattern of sarcomas, removal of the tumor plus pseudocapsule very likely leaves microscopic residual neoplasm within the remaining intracompartmental structures for an uncertain distance from the resection bed. Extremity soft-tissue sarcomas arising in an extracompartmental location, such as the popliteal fossa, inguinal area, or axilla, encounter fewer

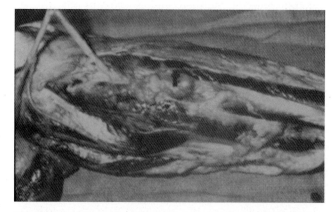

Figure 34.2. Gross inspection fibrosarcoma of the lower leg. Tumor (T) extends longitudinally within the structures of the lateral compartment to the fascia overlying the anterior compartment muscles, which are uninvolved by tumor. The common peroneal nerve is seen crossing the fibular head. *Source:* From Simon MA, et al. The management of soft-tissue sarcomas of the extremities. *J Bone Joint Surg* 1976; 58:317–327.

fascial restrictions and their pattern of spread is even less predictable. The subcutaneous tissue is also considered an extracompartmental location. Soft-tissue sarcomas arising in this area, however, usually display a less aggressive course than those lesions arising deep within the extremity.

Soft-tissue sarcomas of the extremity rarely involve regional lymphatics. Mazeron reviewed 2,500 literature cases and reported a 4% incidence of lymph node involvement over the entire course of the disease (24). Elective lymph node dissection reveals unsuspected sarcomatous adenopathy in 6% to 13% of patients (2,25,26). Lymphatic involvement appears higher for certain histotypes (rhabdomyosarcoma, epithelioid sarcoma, and angiosarcoma), although this observation may be more related to other histopathologic features than a real biologic difference. Lymph nodes are rarely an isolated site of sarcoma relapse following local tumor management.

Extremity soft-tissue sarcomas frequently recur within the pulmonary parenchyma. At the time of primary diagnosis, however, pulmonary metastases can be documented in only 4% to 11% of patients (5,27).

PATHOLOGY AND STAGING

Soft-tissue sarcomas are traditionally classified according to their presumed cell of origin. This histogenic classification scheme, proposed by Stout, defines the common following subtypes of tumors: fibrosarcoma, malignant fibrous histiocytoma, liposarcoma, leiomyosarcoma, rhabdomyosarcoma, angiosarcoma, lymphangiosarcoma, synovial cell sarcoma, and neurofibrosarcoma. All are of mesenchymal derivation except the latter which is of ectodermal origin. Tumors of uncertain histogenesis include alveolar soft part sarcoma, epithelioid sarcoma, clear cell sarcoma, and extraskeletal Ewing's sarcoma. The histogenic grouping is not an accurate predictor of the metastatic potential of soft-tissue sarcomas. The most consistent predictor of biologic behavior is sarcoma grade (28–30). Virtually, all histotypes of sarcoma display a spectrum of histologic grade. Occasionally, this grade spectrum can be noted within an individual tumor. Certain histotypes present more commonly as a particular grade. For instance, the liposarcoma is generally low grade while the angiosarcoma is usually high grade.

Grading schemes in use today are based on analysis of mitotic rate, necrosis, cellular pleomorphism, differentiation, and cellularity. Sarcomas are divided into low-, intermediate-, and high-grade tiers. Grade is the prime determinant of tumor stage according to the American Joint Commission on Cancer (Tables 34.1 and 34.2) (31). Grade is also a predictor of lymphatic involvement and pulmonary metastases at diagnosis (24). The radiation oncologist must also remember other determinants of local relapse: tumor size, tumor location, surgical margin status, and skin involvement by a deep tumor (32,33). These factors may not have prognostic impact indepen-

TABLE 34.1	American Joint Committee on Cancer Staging Classification for Soft-Tissue Sarcomas

TNM classification

T (primary tumor)

TX	Primary tumor cannot be assessed
T1	Tumor 5 cm or less in greatest diameter
T1a	Superficial tumor
T1b	Deep tumor
T2	Tumor more than 5 cm in greatest diameter
T2a	Superficial tumor
T2b	Deep tumor

N (regional lymph nodes)

NX	Regional lymph nodes cannot be assessed
N1	No regional lymph node metastasis
N2	Regional lymph node metastasis

M (distant metastasis)

MX	Presence of distant metastasis cannot be assessed
M0	No distant metastasis
M1	Distant metastasis

G (tumor grade)

G1	Well differentiated
G2	Moderately differentiated
G3	Poorly differentiated
G4	Poorly differentiated or undifferentiated (four tiered systems only)

dent of tumor grade but will influence treatment planning in the individual patient.

Recent attention has focused on molecular biology determinants of prognosis. The presence of a $t(x - 18)$ translocation is a significant predictor of metastasis-free survival for patients with synovial cell sarcoma (34). The impact of this translocation on local control, however, has

TABLE 34.2	American Joint Committee on Cancer Staging Classification for Soft-Tissue Sarcomas

Stage groupings

Stage IA	T1a,T1b, N0, M0 G1
Stage IB	T2a, T2b, N0, M0, G1
Stage IIA	T1a, T1b, N0, M0, G2–3
Stage IIB	T2a, T2b, N0, M0, G2
Stage III	T2a, T2b, N0, M0, G3 AnyT, N1, M0, Any G
Stage IV	Any T, Any N, M1, Any G

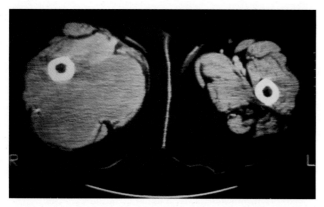

Figure 34.3. Axial CT scan of a patient with an angiosarcoma of the right thigh. The neoplasm involves all three thigh compartments.

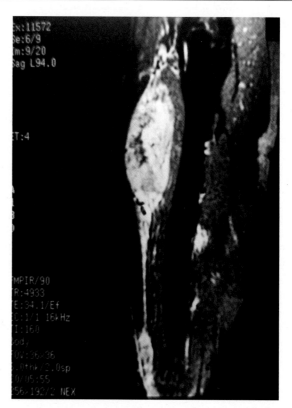

Figure 34.4. Coronal contrast-enhanced MRI demonstrating multifocal epithelioid sarcoma of the thigh (*arrows*).

not been analyzed. Overexpression of human telomerase is significantly more frequent in a group of locally recurrent soft-tissue sarcomas compared to those that are controlled (35). The influence of telomerase expression on local control has not been investigated prospectively. Finally, overexpression of aberrant p53 is a significant predictor of local recurrence for osseous chondrosarcoma (36). The influence of mutated p53 on the local relapse rate of soft-tissue sarcomas has not been studied. It is hoped that advances in molecular biology of soft-tissue sarcomas may lead to delineation of a subgroup of patients who are at extremely low risk of local recurrence and may, therefore, avoid adjunctive radiotherapy in the setting of limb-sparing surgery.

Although the prognostic significance of tumor histogenesis remains unreliable, the radiation oncologist should be cognizant of the peculiar growth patterns of specific extremity soft-tissue sarcomas. The angiosarcoma and lymphangiosarcoma typically arise in more than one compartment, suggesting a neoplastic process affecting an entire embryonic limb bud (Fig. 34.3). These cases are rarely amenable to nonamputative therapy or limited volume irradiation. The epithelioid sarcoma commonly arises on the hand or foot and is notorious for discontinuous spread ("skip metastases"), implying the requirement for wide-field irradiation regardless of tumor size (Fig. 34.4).

DIAGNOSIS AND EVALUATION

Definitive diagnosis of an extremity soft-tissue sarcoma requires tissue obtained by biopsy. Proper radiotherapy planning depends upon the knowledge of the type of biopsy procedure utilized. Excisional biopsy ("shelling out") is appropriate only for lesions <4 cm in diameter and located superficially. Such lesions are generally benign or low-grade sarcomas with an indolent course such as the subcutaneous malignant fibrous histiocytoma. Rarely, an aggressive soft-tissue lesion such as the angiosarcoma will present superficially in the limb. Aggressive superficial sar-

comas are more common in the trunk or head and neck. The majority of extremity soft-tissue sarcomas arise deep in the limb and are >5 cm in diameter. Incisional biopsy is the most appropriate procedure in this setting. Attempts at excisional biopsy of large, deep tumors are to be condemned (4). Excisional biopsy of this type of lesion may be associated with extensive postoperative eccymoses (Fig. 34.5). Areas of discoloration must be considered contaminated by sarcoma cells, thus vastly increasing the definitive surgical bed and radiotherapy field. Inappropriate biopsy also renders some limbs unsalvageable (37). Correct placement of the biopsy is also critical to the radiotherapy planning. The incision must be placed in the long axis of the limb and directly over the tumor (Fig. 34.6). A transversal approach, or one requiring extensive tunneling, may violate compartments not initially seeded with tumor. The transversal approach necessarily enlarges both the definitive surgical procedure and any radiotherapy field (Fig. 34.7). The entire biopsy site must be included in any patient undergoing preoperative radiotherapy and must be removed *in toto* during definitive resection. Image-guided core needle biopsy may supplant open procedures, provided the pathologist is skilled at the interpretation of small volume specimens (Fig. 34.8) (38). Positron emission tomography (PET) fused with computed tomography (CT) or magnetic resonance imaging (MRI) may assist in directing biopsy to the region of a heterogeneous tumor likely to harbor the highest grade elements (Fig. 34.9).

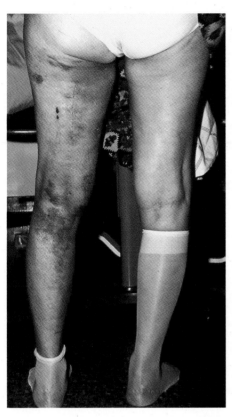

Figure 34.5. Extensive subcutaneous ecchymoses following excisional biopsy of a deep 8-cm sarcoma of the posterior thigh.

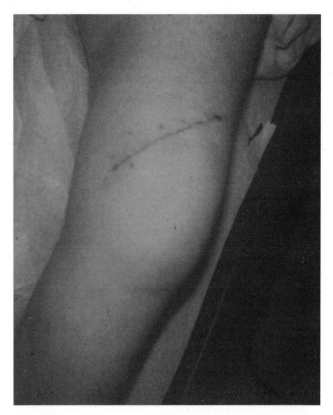

Figure 34.7. Oblique incision used for biopsy of a medial thigh mass. The incision extends into the adjacent anterior compartment.

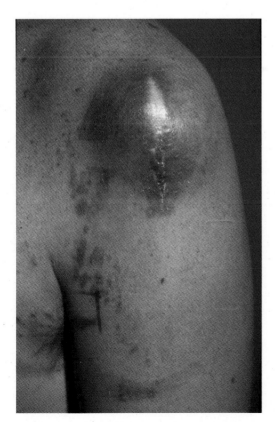

Figure 34.6. Appropriate placement of incisional biopsy for an extremity tumor.

Radiotherapy planning requires accurate assessment of tumor extent within the extremity. Plane radiographs, isotope bone scans, and angiography provide minimal clues to the topographic extent of extremity soft-tissue sarcomas (Fig. 34.10). Bone scans may reveal uptake near a sarcoma. Since skeletal invasion by a soft-tissue sarcoma is extremely unusual, this activity is misleading (5). Increased uptake is due to periosteal inflammatory response to an adjacent sarcoma and is not an absolute indication for amputation (Figs. 34.11 and 34.12). Pretreatment evaluation of extremity sarcomas demands modern imaging. Magnetic resonance (MR) scanning is superior to CT (39–42). MR yields better spatial resolution of tumor extent than CT and displays this in the three standard planes of reference (Fig. 34.13). MR yields superior definition of normal tissue planes, neurovascular bundles, and normal tissue–tumor interfaces. Prior biopsy procedures may exacerbate peritumoral edema resulting in an overestimation of tumor extent (43). Gadolinium administration may increase MR specificity in this situation. CT remains superior to MR only for detection of true bone invasion. It is a general rule that a sarcoma with both osseous and soft-tissue components represents a primary bone tumor with soft-tissue extension rather than a primary soft-tissue tumor with bone invasion. Neither MR nor CT accurately predicts tumor histogenesis or grade. These modern imaging studies must be available to the radiation oncologist in the simulator room and planning computer to expedite

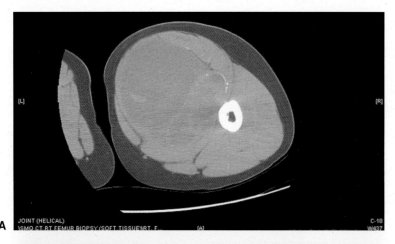

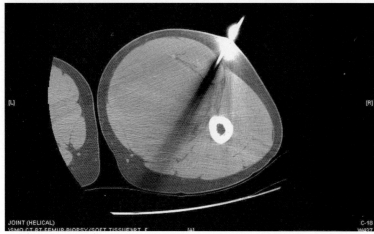

Figure 34.8. A: Axial CT demonstrating heterogeneous soft-tissue mass in the right thigh. **B:** Axial CT demonstrating core needle biopsy directed at the solid tumor component.

coverage of tissues at risk for tumor invasion with simultaneous exclusion of uninvolved normal tissue. PET is useful for the diagnosis of sarcoma and evaluation of tumor response to neoadjuvant therapies. The value of PET for radiotherapeutic treatment planning has not yet been established. Canadian investigators compared FDG-PET target volumes with T1-contrast enhanced MRI volumes in a series of 17 extremity soft-tissue sarcomas. For the purposes of target delineation on the PET study, threshold values of 2- to 10-times background and the 40% of maximum

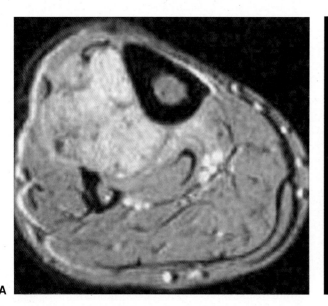

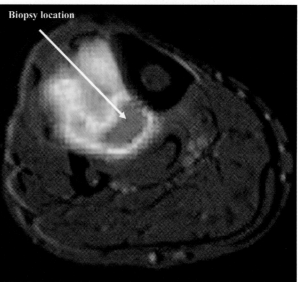

Figure 34.9. A: Axial MR demonstrating soft-tissue neoplasm of the lower leg. **B:** PET-MRI fusion image demonstrating soft-tissue neoplasm with regions of varying metabolic activity. Image-guided biopsy directed to region of highest activity (*red*).

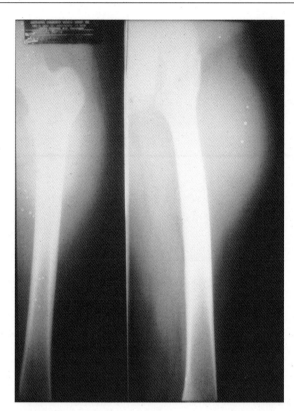

Figure 34.10. Plain extremity radiograph of a high-grade liposarcoma. Films reveal ill-defined soft-tissue density probably arising from the vastus lateralis.

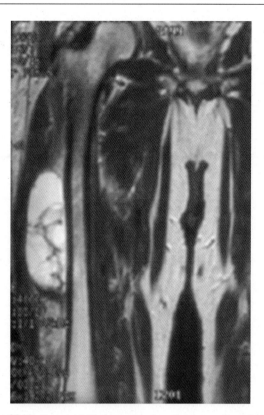

Figure 34.11. Coronal MR demonstrating abutment of a soft-tissue sarcoma to the periosteum of the femur.

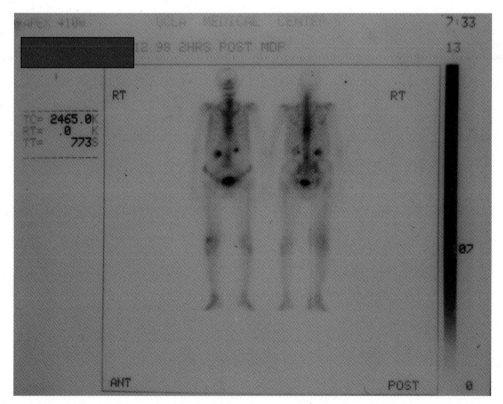

Figure 34.12. Isotope bone scan of a high-grade sarcoma of the distal right thigh. Study demonstrates increased tracer uptake due to periosteal reaction to overlying neoplasm.

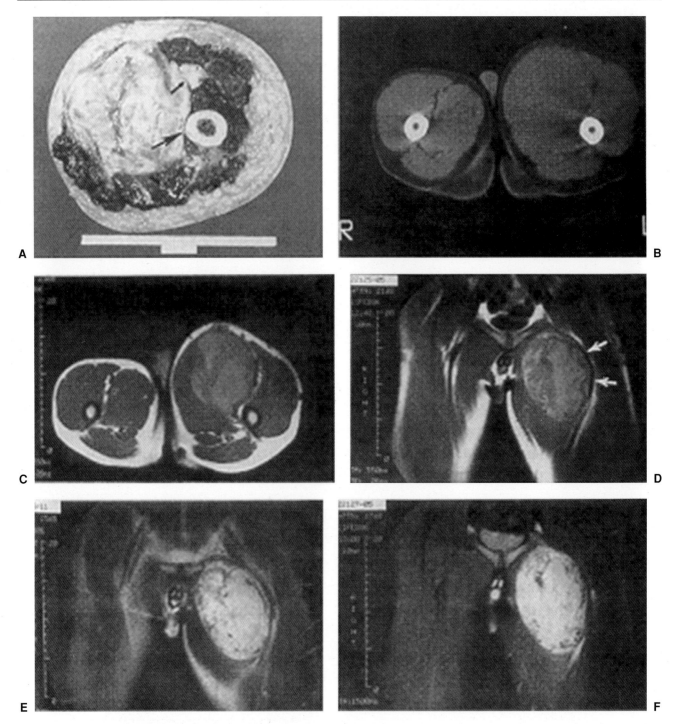

Figure 34.13. High-grade synovial sarcoma of the left proximal thigh requiring hemipelvectomy. **A:** Cross section through the tumor revealing abutment to femur (*large arrow*) and neurovascular bundle (*small arrow*). **B:** CT of thigh shows asymmetry but no demarcation between tumor and normal muscle. **C:** T1-weighted sagittal MR demonstrates distinct tumor/muscle interface and tumor/fat contrast. **D:** T1-weighted coronel MR demonstrate displacement of femoral vessels (*white arrows*) and visualization of craniocaudad tumor extent. **E:** T2-weighted coronal MR demonstrates increased tumor/muscle contrast and decreased tumor/fat contrast compared to T1 image. **F:** The IR pulse sequence demonstrates superior tumor/muscle and equivalent tumor/fat contrast compared with T1 images. *Source:* From Chang AE, et al. Magnetic resonance imaging versus computed tomography in the evaluation of soft-tissue tumors of the extremities. *Ann Surg* 1987;205:340–348.

uptake threshold were used. The authors found poor correlation between the PET-defined and MRI-defined volumes regardless of the threshold employed (44). Mean ratio of the GTV_{PET}/GTV_{MRI} ranged from 1.16 using a threshold value of 2 to 0.22 using a threshold of 10.

FIELD LENGTH

Radiotherapy should be directed to those tissues at risk for residual neoplastic cells. Theoretically, the entire compartment is implicated, but there is no proof that routinely

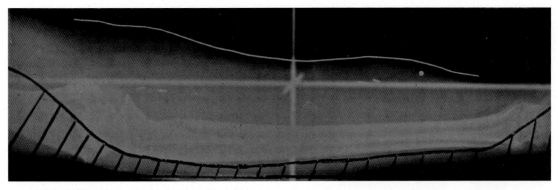

Figure 34.14. Simulation radiograph following resection of a high-grade neurofibrosarcoma of the volar right forearm. Lead tape depicts surgical scar. Radiodense vascular clips represent intraoperative extent of *en bloc* dissection of tumor plus normal tissue margin. Determination of postoperative radiotherapy volume based solely upon placement of clips would underestimate volume of tissue actually manipulated by the surgeon.

irradiating "origin to insertion" yields significantly better local control rates than a judiciously designed field encompassing the tumor or its resection bed plus a longitudinal margin of uninvolved tissue. The volume at risk for the radiation oncologist certainly includes all tissue manipulated by the surgeon, including drain sites. This volume will likely be larger when patients are treated postoperatively as opposed to preoperatively. Tepper has stressed that the length of the risk volume is not always equivalent to the length of the definitive incision in a postoperative setting (45). A better indication of the field length required for postoperative radiotherapy can be determined from radiodense vascular clips placed by the surgeon at the margins of resection. In practicality, these clips are not always utilized for outline of the resection site. In lieu of formal tumor bed clipping, the postoperative field traditionally extends 5- to 8-cm cephalocaudal to the surgical scar for low-grade tumors and ≥10 cm for intermediate-/high-grade tumors. Mundt et al. have recently challenged these recommendations in a review of postoperatively irradiated patients (46). Those with <5-cm initial, longitudinal margins around the tumor bed and scar had a 5-year local control rate of 30% compared to 93% for those with ≥5 cm ($p = 0.0003$). There was no significant local control difference, however, between those with initial margins of 5 to 9.9 versus ≥10 cm. This impact of field size applied only to intermediate- and high-grade tumors. No low-grade tumor recurred locally regardless of margins. The local control rate for intermediate grade tumors was 0% with an initial margin <5 cm compared to 92% with larger margins. Local control rates for high-grade tumors were 47% and 92%, respectively. There was no benefit to margins ≥10 cm for either intermediate or high-grade sarcomas compared to 5 to 9.9 cm. Margins of 5 to 9 cm, therefore, appear appropriate for intermediate-grade sarcomas. Five centimeters are sufficient for low-grade sarcoma, although routine adjuvant radiotherapy may not be necessary for a small low-grade tumor affecting a single muscle bundle and amenable to wide myomectomy. There is no need to electively irradiate the draining lymph nodal regions although satisfying field length requirements may unavoidably include these areas. Every attempt should be made to exclude major joint spaces from the radiotherapy beam, especially the weight-bearing hip and knee, while still fulfilling the above field length stipulations. Such protection may not be reasonable and, in some cases, the appropriate field length may be *longer* than the compartment in question due to the length of the scar (Fig. 34.14).

Extended treatment distances are often required to encompass these long fields. Modern rotational linear accelerators are capable of treating both anterior and posterior fields without turning patients and are strongly recommended for irradiating extremities (Fig. 34.15). If this

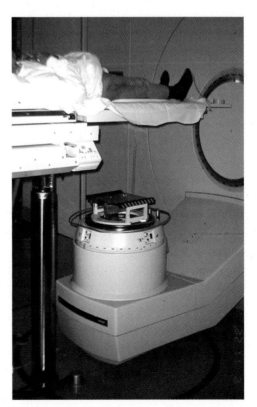

Figure 34.15. Linear accelerator couch at extreme elevation to provide the extended distance necessary to irradiate entire thigh with an isocentric anterior–posterior technique and a single field.

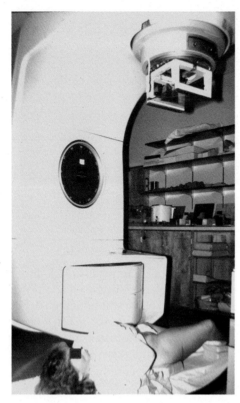

Figure 34.16. Patient receiving extended anterior distance treatment while supine on the floor. Extended distance posterior treatment will require prone reposition and a separate simulation.

equipment is not available, irradiation may be delivered on the treatment room floor with the necessity for turning the patient and individual simulations for each field (Fig. 34.16). Another solution would involve the use of matched fields with an appropriate skin gap calculation. This alternative would leave some superficial tissue, including the incision, undertreated unless the gap is moved periodically.

WIDTH

Although routine irradiation of the entire longitudinal extent of a compartment is not necessary, the entire transversal cross section of a compartment is at risk for tumor involvement (15,18,45). The radiation oncologist must have an in-depth knowledge of compartment boundaries in the axial plane in addition to the more available description of origin and insertion. The full circumference of the affected extremity must not be irradiated beyond the tolerance of the draining lymphatic channels or chronic lymphedema may result (47). In truth, distal edema due to circumferential extremity scarring has been reported when extraordinarily large total doses were delivered under tourniquet-induced hypoxia by hypofractionated techniques (48). From various animal experiments and inferential human experiences, peripheral lymphatics appear to tolerate 50 Gy in conventional fractionation (49–51). Any circumferential tissue sparing possible dur-

ing design of field width will improve outcome, but at least several centimeters are commonly advocated. The amount of circumferential sparing required to prevent the lymphedema has never been subjected to analysis by randomized trial. In a series of 41 patients, investigators at the University of Rochester postoperatively irradiated the entire cross-section extent of the relevant compartment to total doses of 55 to 64.8 Gy (52). A small strip of tissue was excluded from the high-dose volume and received <40 Gy. The percentage of limb circumference spared varied from 1% to 78% (mean 30%). Absolute volume of the limb spared ranged from 26 to 6,990 cm^3 (median 900 cm^3). The authors reported that the volume spared, either as a percentage of limb circumference or as an absolute volume, did not significantly correlate with the onset of the delayed lymphedema. Volumes as low as 26 cm^3 and percentages as low as 1 were not associated with poor outcome.

The neurovascular structures within the femoral triangle can be considered the medial border of the anterior compartment of the thigh. Failure to encompass the contents of the compartment may result in local relapse (Fig. 34.17). Slight obliquity of the incident beam during irradiation of the anterior thigh compartment allows both medial tissue sparing and inclusion of the depth of the target compartment (Fig. 34.18). The landmark for the lateral extent of the medial thigh compartment (e.g., adductor) is the femur. Sarcomas arising in the medial compartment can usually be irradiated with anterior–posterior fields with the lateral border at the femur (Fig. 34.19). Tumors of the distal posterior compartment can be treated with the patient in the ipsilateral decubitus position (Fig. 34.20). The affected limb is placed straight on the treatment couch. The contralateral limb is maximally flexed at the hip, placed beyond the portal, and supported by a cushion. The lateral position permits sparing tissue in both the anterior and the medial thigh compartments. The gluteal fold may require taping to remain out of the field for proximal tumors. The lateral position is also advised for tumors of the popliteal fossa. Another alternative, specifically for distal lesions of the thigh, involves placing the patient supine and elevating the affected limb off the treatment couch by way of hip flexion and irradiating via lateral fields. Tumors arising within the proximal portion of the posterior compartment lend themselves to irradiation via anterior–posterior fields. Attempts to utilize the lateral decubitus orientation are frustrated by proximity of the tumor or the cephalad field margin to the radiosensitive perineum and anorectal tissue.

The lower leg and forearm are each composed of only two compartments. These are separated by a thick interosseous membrane. By placing the affected limb on the simulator couch and externally rotating either the hand or foot, the membrane is placed parallel to the beam axis. A simulator radiograph or CT in this position will show near superimposition of the radius-ulna or tibia-fibula

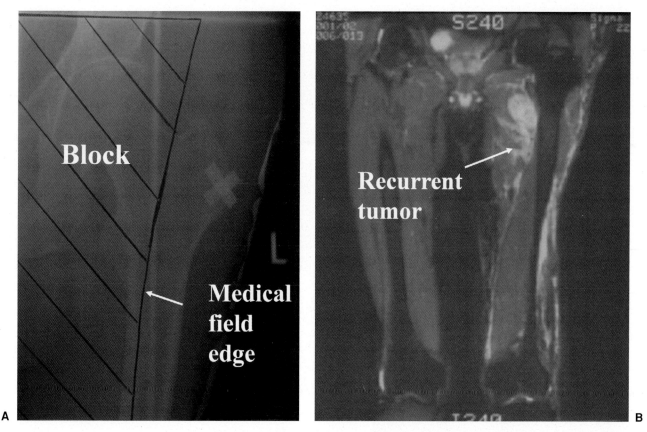

Figure 34.17. A: Analog simulator radiograph demonstrating field edge for postoperative treatment of a high-grade sarcoma arising in the anterior compartment musculature. **B:** Coronal MRI demonstrating local tumor recurrence near the medial field edge.

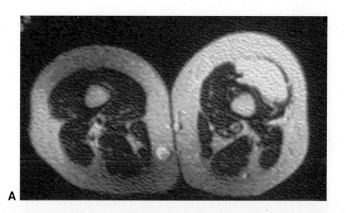

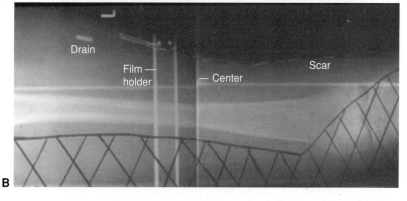

Figure 34.18. A: Magnetic resonance imaging (MRI) of a high-grade liposarcoma of the anterior compartment musculature. Note the relationship of the tumor to the underlying femur. **B:** Forty-five degree field arrangement to irradiate the affected region with sufficient margin while sparing medial thigh tissue. Note relation of medial field margin to the adjacent femur.

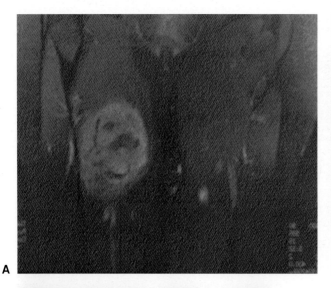

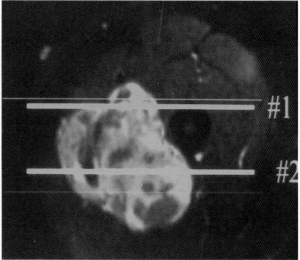

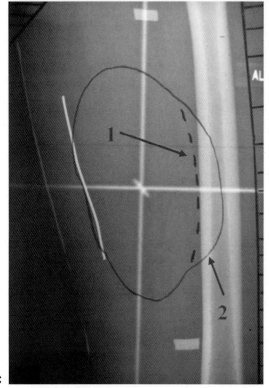

Figure 34.19. (A) Coronal and (B) axial MRI of a biphasic synovial cell sarcoma of the medial compartment. Coronal image corresponds to level 1 on the axial scan. Note location of the lateral tumor margin, apparently adjacent to the femur. Axial image level 2, however, demonstrates that the tumor extends posterior to the femur. (C) Tumor area transposed to anterior analog simulation radiograph using MRI depiction of tumor volume. *Dashed line* represents lateral tumor margin according to information from coronal image and axial level 1. *Solid line* represents lateral margin determined from axial level 2 image. Marginal relapse might have resulted from field design based only on coronal MRI. Long wire marks skin edge; short wire marks biopsy scar; lead tape for off-axis calculations.

(Figs. 34.21 and 34.22). Placing the field border adjacent to these osseous landmarks effectively separates the contents of the two compartments and permits transversal sparing with confidence.

Field-size recommendations have not been subjected to randomized trials. Those authors advocating routine radiotherapy of the full compartment (32,53–55) do not report local control rates superior to those employing more restricted fields (5,15–17,46). Investigators at Washington University retrospectively analyzed local control using various postoperative field sizes (18). Local relapse was reported in 6 of 31 receiving radiotherapy to the entire compartment. Relapse occurred in only 1 of 10 receiving treatment to the full compartmental width but field length restricted to 5 cm beyond the resection bed. Four of nine recurred locally if neither the full length nor width were irradiated.

IMMOBILIZATION

Reproducibility of fields required for extremity radiotherapy is problematic, particularly if couch pressure causes discomfort. Patients in a neutral position may require only simple tape or sandbag reinforcement. Angled or rotated limbs may require rigid fixation devices, the Alpha Cradle (Moldmaker Inc., Smithers Medical Products, Hudson, Ohio) being the most popular. Attention must be given to

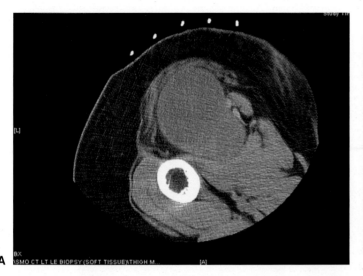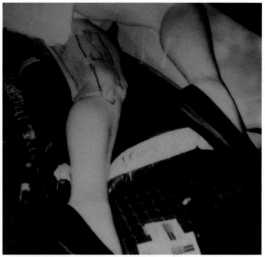

Figure 34.20. **A:** Prone CT done for image-guided core needle biopsy of a posterior thigh mass. **B:** Left lateral patient position for irradiation of a left posterior compartment ("hamstrings") thigh sarcoma. The right lower extremity has been positioned out of the field and the knee supported. The tumor site can be irradiated with anterior–posterior fields.

preventing loss of skin sparing due to extensive limb coverage by the fixation device (Fig. 34.23). Immobilization material should be placed at the proximal and distal ends of the limb in regions not included within the radiotherapy field. This approach allows reproducibility, skin sparing, and physician access to the tumor site (Fig. 34.24). The upper arm may be treated with the patient seated next to the couch with the arm abducted and resting on the transmission tray. Alternatively, the patient can assume a supine position with the upper arm supported by an arm rest typically used for breast irradiation (Fig. 34.25). A third method involves the prone position with the ipsilateral arm raised above the head. In this position, however,

the entire length of the target volume is often not perpendicular to the beam, resulting in variability in depth of the isocenter along the field. Proper elbow elevation will eliminate this slope (Fig. 34.26). The forearm can be treated with the patient prone or seated. Thigh abduction will prevent unnecessary dose buildup during treatment of medial compartment tumors. Therapy couches are frequently too narrow to permit maximal, yet stable, abduction unless both legs are placed in a centered alpha cradle. Reproducibility can be documented by periodic portal films or, in difficult cases, real-time megavoltage imaging (MVI).

FIELD SHAPING

Simple square or rectangular fields are rarely appropriate for extremity radiotherapy. Shielding of the Achilles tendon, pretibial skin, olecranon, patella, groin, joints, and a portion of the full extremity circumference are to be strived for in order to decrease late effects. Sparing one-half the diameter of any long bone within the field will decrease the risk of fracture. Methods to shape the field include custom design using Cerrobend, prefabricated hand blocks, or a multileaf collimator (Fig. 34.27). The latter method proves less time and labor intensive for most departments compared to block construction methods. External scatter to the testes can be reduced with a testicular shield (clam shell).

DOSIMETRY

Beam energies <10 MV are appropriate for extremity treatment. These energies will not underdose superficial tissue, including the incision, if postoperative therapy is delivered. If appropriate energies are not available, the

Figure 34.21. Reproducible position for irradiation of the forearm. Pronation to a "thumb up" position superimposes ulna and radius, effectively separating the two forearm compartments. Extensor or flexor compartment can be irradiated with anterior–posterior field arrangement.

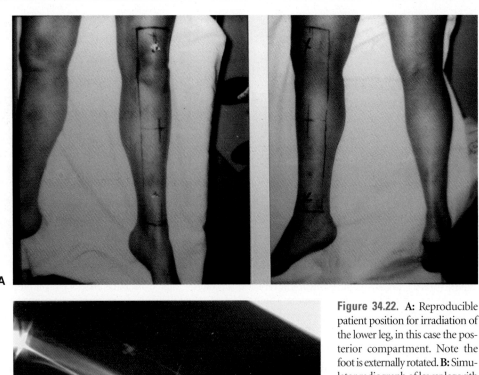

Figure 34.22. A: Reproducible patient position for irradiation of the lower leg, in this case the posterior compartment. Note the foot is externally rotated. **B:** Simulator radiograph of lower leg with appropriate external rotation. Superimposition of the tibia-fibula serves as a landmark for the interosseous membrane separating the two compartments of the lower leg. Radiotherapy fields can now be designed to include the tissue affected while sparing much uninvolved leg.

incision dose should be monitored by thermal luminescent dosimetry (TLD). Bolus can be applied if the incision is underdosed. Bolus will not be necessary if the scar is tangential to the beam. Using megavoltage photons and the treatment distances necessary for thigh tumors, the authors have noted inhomogeneity less than ±10% for most cases. Inhomogeneity may be greater for other extremity locations that do not require extended distance. Mixing available photon energies serves to reduce dose inhomogeneity. CT-based conformal treatment planning is particularly advantageous in three situations: noncoplanar beam arrangements, tangential irradiation of buttock

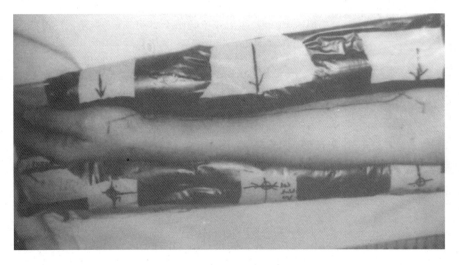

Figure 34.23. Patient immobilized in an Alpha Cradle for irradiation of a forearm sarcoma. Note that the immobilization device may eliminate posterior field skin sparing.

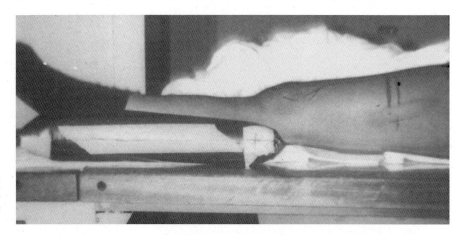

Figure 34.24. Patient immobilized for irradiation of a thigh sarcoma. Note that all immobilization materials are restricted to the lower leg.

tumors, and anterior–posterior irradiation of a volume that varies greatly in thickness (Fig. 34.28). The radiation oncologist must remember to request that treatment planning scans be performed with the patient on a flat table mimicking the accelerator couch. CT planning provides the radiation oncologist with dosimetry in all three standard planes of view, an advantage compared to conventional analog simulation (Fig. 34.29).

The clinical impact of IMRT has not been established for extremity soft-tissue sarcomas. There are no large retrospective reviews or prospective clinical trials for this innovation comparable to the experience with head and neck or prostate cancers. Dosimetry studies document an advantage for IMRT compared to conformal planning techniques (56,57). Hong et al. reported a dosimetric comparison of IMRT and 3D-CRT approaches in a feasibility study of 10 patients with sarcomas of thigh approaching, but not involving, the femur (57). For the purposes of the study, a radial CTV margin of 1.5 cm was used unless this margin extended beyond the bone–soft-tissue interface. In

that situation, the CTV margin was restricted to the bone interface only. An additional 0.5-cm margin of adjacent tissue was added for the PTV. Thus, at most 0.5 cm of the adjacent bone was included within the PTV (Fig. 34.30). Cranio-caudal margins followed traditional guidelines. The authors advised that the PTV was extended to the skin surface at the region of any surgical scar. There was no significant difference in PTV coverage between IMRT and CRT. Homogeneity and conformality were significantly improved with IMRT planning and this was particularly true for tumors with large variation in contour. Dose to the adjacent bone was also significantly reduced with IMRT planning. The respective $V_{100\%}$ values were 18.6% compared to 44.7% ($p < 0.01$) and the respective mean bone doses were 38.5 Gy compared to 40.9 Gy ($p = 0.06$). Femur dose reduction was most pronounced for a GTV that encompassed <50% of the femur circumference. The femur dose advantage with IMRT planning is a consequence of greater capacity for achieving a concave isodose distribution. IMRT planning also resulted in significant reduction to surrounding normal soft tissue and skin surface.

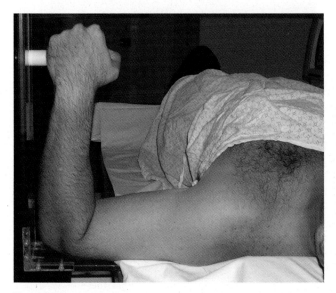

Figure 34.25. Arm board immobilization for irradiation of a patient with a sarcoma of the biceps muscle.

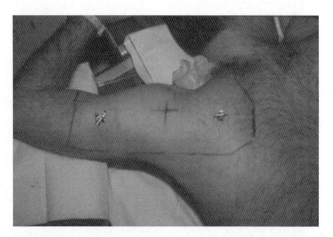

Figure 34.26. Patient with a proximal arm sarcoma placed in the prone position with the affected arm abducted above the head. The ipsilateral elbow is supported by pads so that the target volume is level with the treatment couch.

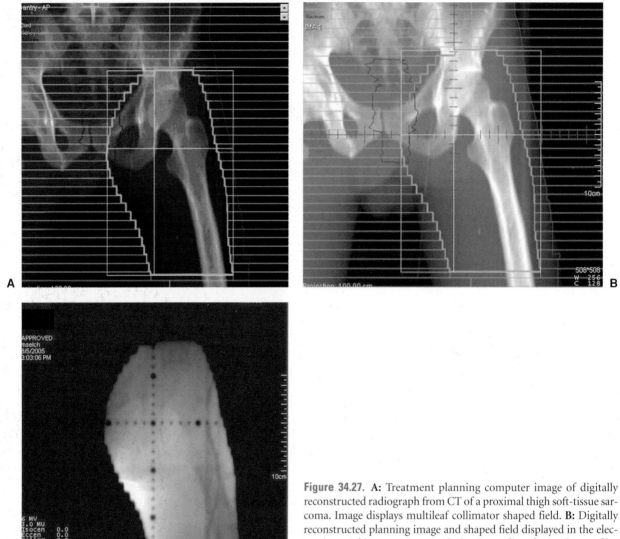

Figure 34.27. **A:** Treatment planning computer image of digitally reconstructed radiograph from CT of a proximal thigh soft-tissue sarcoma. Image displays multileaf collimator shaped field. **B:** Digitally reconstructed planning image and shaped field displayed in the electronic portal image computer. **C:** Corresponding electronic port film of field design shown in (**A**).

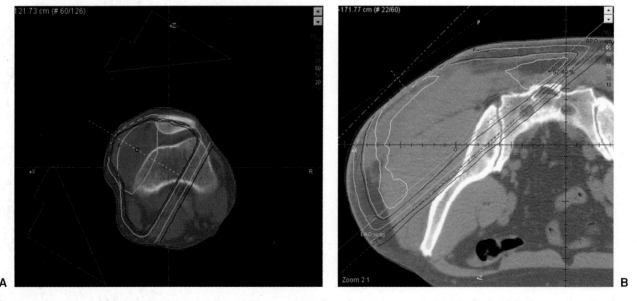

Figure 34.28. **A:** Isodose distribution for noncoplanar field arrangement for soft-tissue sarcoma arising in the distal thigh. **B:** Isodose distribution for tangential irradiation of a buttock sarcoma.

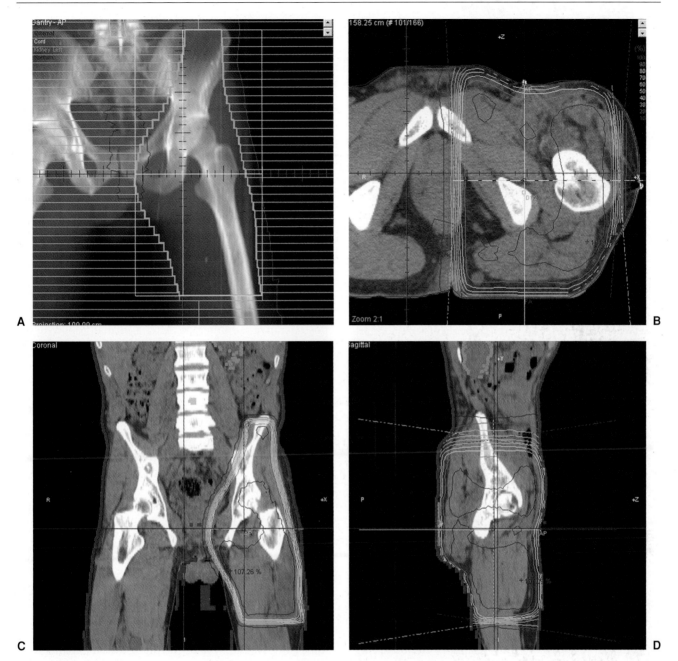

Figure 34.29. **A:** Treatment planning computer image of digitally reconstructed radiograph from CT of a proximal thigh soft-tissue sarcoma. Image displays multileaf collimator shaped field. **B:** Axial plane through field center with isodose distribution. **C:** Coronal plane through field center with isodose distribution. **D:** Sagittal plane through field center with isodose distribution.

Griffen et al. confirmed dose reduction to the skin with IMRT planning for extremity soft-tissue sarcomas (58). The authors retrospectively compared dose distribution to "virtual" skin flaps in patients receiving preoperative radiotherapy planned with conventional AP–PA technique, 3D-CRT or IMRT. Mean dose to the potential skin flaps needed for planned wound closure with the conventional technique was 42.6 Gy compared to 40.1 Gy for 3D-CRT and 27.6 Gy for IMRT ($p = 0.0008$). The respective $V_{\geq 30\%}$ values were 86.4%, 83.4%, and 34% ($p = 0.0001$). The respective conformality indices were 2.34, 1.76, and 1.27 ($p = 0.0001$).

It is hypothesized that IMRT techniques should result in a reduction in serious acute/late effects compared to more traditional methods of dose delivery. Alektiar and colleagues reported morbidity in a series of 31 extremity soft-tissue sarcomas patients receiving pre- or postoperative radiotherapy employing the IMRT approach published by Hong et al. (57,59). The incidence of grade 3 acute skin reaction was 10% and wound complications 23% (infectious 13%, noninfectious 10%). After a median follow-up of 23 months, delayed pathologic fracture was reported in 6% and limb edema 30%.

There is concern that the increase in conformality inherent in IMRT may compromise local control, particularly for soft-tissue sarcomas which have a propensity for occult extension along fascial planes. Alektiar et al. have

Anterior

MAO   MAO2   LAO

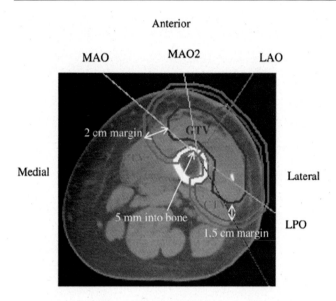

Medial   Lateral

LPO

Figure 34.30. Illustration of gross tumor volume (GTV), planning target volume (PTV), and beam arrangement guidelines. The medial-anterior oblique (MAO) beam is chosen as the most medial-anterior beam to avoid the uninvolved leg and the genital organs; beam MAO2 was midway between MAO and LAO; the lateral-posterior oblique (LPO) beam was chosen as the most lateral-posterior beam to avoid the uninvolved leg and genital organs; beam LPO2, if desirable, was about 30 degrees more medially from the LPO. Beam MAO and beam LPO were most likely the beams used in conventional plans, which are nearly opposed. Beam LAO or MAO2 was sometimes used as a third beam in conventional plans. *Source:* From Hong L, et al. Intensity-modulated radiotherapy for soft-tissue sarcoma of the thigh. *Int J Radiat Oncol Biol Phys* 2004;59:752–759.

documented no significant decrement in local control rate associated with IMRT delivery compared to historic values associated with conventional techniques. The authors irradiated pre- or postoperatively 41 patients with high risk extremity sarcomas: 90% deep, 68% ≥10 cm, 22% requiring periosteal stripping, 12% positive margins. The IMRT technique followed the guidelines of Hong et al. After a 35 month follow-up, the 3- and 5-year actuarial local control rates were 94%. Two local relapses were judged in-field and not marginal (60). There was no impact of margin status or periosteal stripping on local control. The results imply the definition of the radial margin used for IMRT planning and the resulting concave isodose distribution is not associated with an undue risk of local relapse in the setting of extremity soft-tissue sarcomas.

The hand and foot are locations traditionally excluded from limb salvage due to presumed poor tolerance of these end-vascular structures to radiotherapy and difficulty achieving gross tumor removal. These areas are amenable to adjuvant irradiation if patients are stringently selected and properly informed (61–65). Candidates include nonsmokers free of hypertension, diabetes mellitus, and peripheral vascular disease. Patients with a sarcoma near the heel or a digit are very poor candidates. Patients with tumors on the hand or dorsum of the foot are good candidates, while those with involvement of the

sole are intermediate. Thin structures like the foot and hand require treatment aids to ensure homogeneity. Both sites are ideally irradiated in a water bath (Figs. 34.31 and 34.32). Dose buildup for hand tumors can also be provided by the use of bolus and a single appositional beam (Fig. 34.33). These techniques, while ensuring homogeneity, serve to abrogate the skin sparing effects of high-energy photons.

DOSE–TIME PARAMETERS

The initial experience with adjuvant irradiation in the setting of limb preservation concerned postoperative treatment. Limb salvage using postoperative radiotherapy has been shown equivalent to amputation in a randomized trial performed by Rosenberg et al. at the NCI (5). The authors assigned 43 eligible patients to amputation or function-preserving wide resection plus 60- to 70-Gy postoperative radiotherapy. After a median follow-up of 52 months, 4 of 27 limb salvage patients had locally recurred compared to none of the 16 amputated patients ($p = 0.06$). The actuarial 5-year survival rates were 88% and 83%, respectively. A subsequent analysis of all 211 extremity soft-tissue sarcomas treated at the NCI, whether randomized or not, revealed local relapse in 12 of 128 (9%) limb salvage patients compared to none of the 83 amputated patients ($p = 0.004$) (66). Again, the difference in local control rates did not result in a significant difference in survival rates.

Theoretic advantages to preoperative radiotherapy include: enhanced tumor resectability, destruction of microscopic tumor foci that may lie outside the surgical site, delivery of radiotherapy to a well-oxygenated tumor, and decrease potential tumor seeding during resection. Enneking and colleagues reported a prospective, nonrandomized trial of preoperative radiotherapy for 38 patients with soft-tissue sarcomas (67). Local failure occurred in 5% of the irradiated patients with wide or marginal resections compared to 37% of the unirradiated patients with similar margins. Surgery alone was able to achieve local control rates equivalent to the preoperative radiotherapy group only if amputations or compartmental resections were performed.

Numerous centers have reported their results with each form of adjuvant irradiation (Tables 34.3 and 34.4). No significant overall difference in local control rates can be detected using these disparate forms of radiotherapy. Comparison of pre- and postoperative treatment within a single institution demonstrates a potential superiority of preoperative therapy for large, high-grade tumors (Table 34.5) (33). These data have led to a gradual trend toward preoperative therapy in many centers for all but the simplest of extremity tumors. The actual approach to be employed depends upon the philosophy and expertise of the responsible oncology team members. Definitive surgical resection should be delayed 2 to 4 weeks after

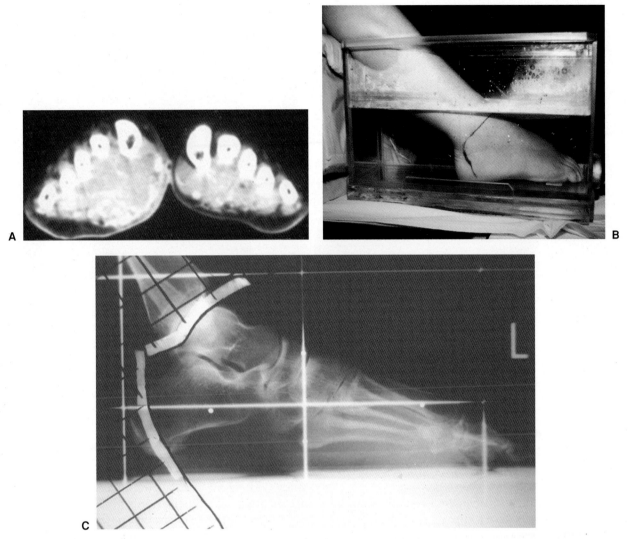

Figure 34.31. **A:** MR of a high-grade synovial sarcoma of the plantar aspect of the foot. **B:** Simulator radiograph of preoperative radiotherapy field. Note exclusion of calcaneous and metatarsal-phalangeal joints. **C:** Affected extremity placed in water bath for treatment. Note field outline on patient's skin.

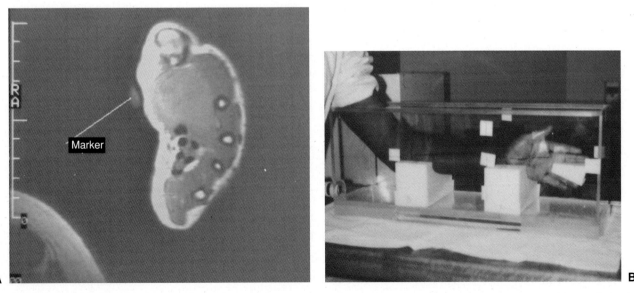

Figure 34.32. **A:** MRI demonstrating low-grade soft-tissue sarcoma of the thenar eminence. **B:** Treatment setup for postoperative irradiation in a water bath.

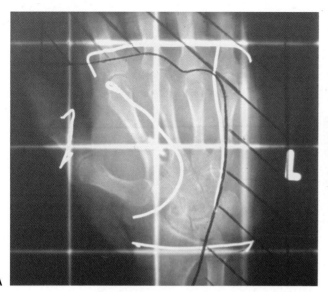
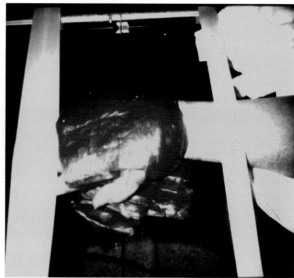

A   B

Figure 34.33. **A:** Simulator radiograph of postoperative radiotherapy field for patient with soft-tissue sarcoma of the thenar eminence. Note exclusion of hypothenar tissue and metacarpal-phalangeal joints. **B:** Use of moldable plastic bolus material. The patient was treated with an anterior field.

preoperative radiotherapy. Postoperative radiotherapy should be delayed until the surgical wound is healed, generally by weeks 3 to 6. Ballo et al. reported a statistically nonsignificant decrease in 10-year local control rate in patients with a >30-day delay between surgery and the initiation of irradiation compared to <30 days. (68). A delay of >4 months resulted in a significant reduction in local control compared to shorter delays in a retrospective review by Schwarz and associates (69).

Investigators at the Canadian NCI recently reported results of a randomized trial comparing preoperative versus postoperative radiotherapy in the management of extremity soft-tissue sarcomas (72). The trial randomized 190 patients to either 50 Gy preoperatively or 66 to 70 Gy postoperatively. Approximately one-third of patients in each arm had tumors >10 cm in size. After a median

follow-up of 3 years, the local control rates were 90% in each arm. Local control according to tumor size and extremity site was not reported for the respective treatment groups. The trial was stopped early due to significant differences in acute morbidity (*vide infra*).

A distinct advantage to preoperative radiotherapy may be the smaller required field size. Neilsen et al. compared potential postoperative and preoperative fields in a unique study (73). Twenty-six patients underwent simulation of actual preoperative fields. After resection, the patients were resimulated to determine potential postoperative field size. In both settings, the longitudinal margins around the target volume were 5 cm for low- or intermediate-grade tumors and 7 cm for high-grade lesions. The target volume in the preoperative setting was the tumor volume determined by imaging. The target volume for

TABLE 34.3	Results of Postoperative Radiotherapy for Extremity Soft-Tissue Sarcomas			
Series	**# Patients**	**Dose (Gy)**	**Local control (%)**	**Survival (%)**
Karakousis (15), RPMI	60	65	94	60
Leibel (16), UCSF	29	50–75	90	68
Lindberg (167, MDAH	223	60–75	78	61
Rosenberg (5), NCI	27	60–70	85	71
Pao (18), Mallinckrodt	50	45–68	78	52
Suit (33), MGH	131	60–68	85	73
Mundt (46), Chicago	50	60–68	88	—
Fein (70), Fox Chase	67	40–70	87	—

PRMI, Roswell Park Memorial Institute; UCSF, University of California at San NCI, National Cancer Institute; MGH, Massachusetts General Hospital Francisco; MDAH, Marion D. Anderson Hospital.

TABLE 34.4	Results of Preoperative Radiotherapy for Extremity Soft-Tissue Sarcomas			
Series	**No. of patients**	**Dose (Gy)**	**Local control (%)**	**Survival (%)**
Barkley (21), MDAH	110	50–60	90	61
Brant (20), Florida	58	50	90	—
Nielson (73), Canada	26	50	100	92
Suit (33), MGH	989	50–56	90	65
Eilber (71), UCLA	402	17.5–35	86	—

MDAH, Marion D. Anderson Hospital; MGH, Massachusetts General Hospital; UCLA, University of California at Los Angeles.

postoperative treatment was the length of the incision. The authors found that both the field size and the number of irradiated joints were significantly less with preoperative radiotherapy. Field size for patients randomized to preoperative radiotherapy was also significantly smaller than for those in the postoperative group according to the recent Canadian NCI trial.

The dose–response of soft-tissue sarcomas in the setting of limb preservation has not been established. When patients with gross residual tumor are excluded from analysis, there is little evidence for a dose–response relationship for local control using postoperative therapy over the range of 50 to 75 Gy (66). Investigators at the University of Chicago recently demonstrated no significant local control rate difference between patients receiving 60 to 63.9 Gy versus 64 to 66 Gy postoperative radiotherapy following gross total removal of intermediate-/high-grade sarcomas (46). Investigators at Fox Chase, however, have reported contradictory findings (70). The 5-year local control rate for patients receiving ≤62.5 Gy was 78% compared to 95% for those receiving >62.5 Gy ($p = 0.04$). Interestingly, the group receiving the higher radiotherapy dose had larger tumors, higher grade tumors, and more

frequent positive surgical margins. The MDAH group retrospectively reviewed 775 patients, including 573 extremity tumors (74). Total postoperative dose varied nonrandomly from 40 to 75 Gy. After a median follow-up of 12 years, the 15-year actuarial local control rate was 82% in patients receiving ≤64 Gy compared to 76% in those receiving >64 ($p = 0.034$). Higher radiotherapy dose, however, was not beneficial in all settings. In addition to dose, factors significant for local control on multivariate analysis included margin status (positive/uncertain versus negative), presentation (primary versus recurrent), primary site (extremity/superficial trunk versus deep trunk), and histology (malignant fibrous histiocytoma/nerve sheath/epitheliod versus all others). The authors recommended 60 Gy postoperatively for uncomplicated, low-risk patients; 64 Gy for those with any risk factor other than positive/uncertain margins; 68 Gy for those with positive margins. In the UCLA experience with preoperative chemoradiotherapy, a necrosis score of <95% and primitive neuroectodermal histology were independent predictors of local relapse by multivariate analysis (75).

The impact of positive margins on the control of extremity soft-tissue sarcomas remains controversial. At

TABLE 34.5	Results of Preoperative and Postoperative Radiotherapy for Extremity Soft-Tissue Sarcomas				
	Preoperative		**Postoperative**		
Stage	**No. of patients**	**Local control (%)**	**No. of patients**	**Local control (%)**	
IA	3	100	12	100	
IB	8	70	17	100	
IIA	7	100	25	83	
IIB	28	100	25	74	
IIIA	6	83	25	95	
IIIB	35	83	26	68	

Source: Suit HD, et al. Treatment of the patient with M0 soft tissue sarcoma. *J Clin Oncol* 1988;6:854–862.

Fox Chase, margin status significantly influenced local control in a multivariate analysis. Local control was obtained in 98% with negative or close margins compared to 72% with positive margins ($p = 0.007$). In that analysis, tumor grade and size did not influence local control. Others have reported no independent impact of margin status on success of limb salvage but radiotherapy dose is tailored to the amount of residual disease (16,66). A total dose of 64 Gy is necessary for those with minimal amounts of residual tumor. Those with gross residual disease, as well as those with the rare unresectable sarcoma undergoing primary radiotherapy, require doses. Investigators at the Massachusetts General Hospital reported the results of radiotherapy for 112 patients with gross soft-tissue sarcoma (76). The overall 5-year local control rate in those receiving <63 Gy was 22% compared to 60% among those receiving higher doses. For those patients with ≤5-cm tumors, the local control rate was 22% with <63 Gy compared to72% with higher doses. For those with gross tumor >5 and ≤10 cm, the respective local control rates were 49% and 42%. For those with >10-cm lesions, the respective control rates were 0% and 25%. These local control rates demonstrate the clinical advantage of gross tumor removal for the effective management of soft-tissue sarcoma.

Preoperative radiotherapy is generally limited to 45 to 50 Gy. Histologic response to preoperative treatment is related to sarcoma grade and size. Willet and associates have demonstrated enhanced histologic response following hyperfractionated preoperative irradiation (77).

An unresolved issue is the necessity for boost irradiation following preoperative radiotherapy. Investigators at Massachusetts General Hospital have routinely used a boost, either by intraoperative technique, brachytherapy, or delayed external beam (33). Recent experiences at other centers demonstrate no diminution of local control without resort to routine boost (20,21). Reserving boost therapy for those patients with residual disease after preoperative irradiation is appropriate. If the tumor removal is known to be incomplete in the operating theater, the patient may undergo brachytherapy or further external beam treatment. Those with a finding of positive margins only after complete histologic analysis of the resected specimen receive further external beam treatment. Boost external beam necessarily involves prolonged delay from the conclusion of preoperative radiotherapy until the surgical wound is healed. Overall duration of radiotherapy did not significantly influence local control in the Fox Chase experience, suggesting that sarcoma cells do not exhibit significant repopulation. Patients in that center, however, were treated in a continuous course and did not have a long delay to boost therapy.

The technique of interstitial implantation of afterloading catheters for boost therapy of extremity sarcomas has

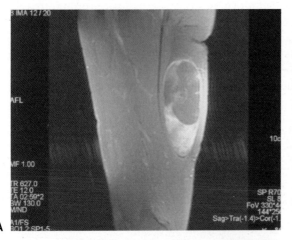

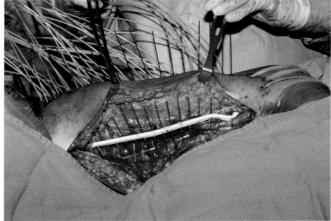

Figure 34.34. A: Sagittal magnetic resonance (MR) image of a high-grade sarcoma of the posterior compartment of the thigh. **B:** Transverse parallel needle placement used for three plane interstitial implantation of the surgical bed following tumor excision. **C:** Nylon afterloading tubes for high dose rate brachytherapy have replaced needles in the surgical bed and the wound has been closed with metallic staples. (Courtesy of D. Jeffrey Demanes, M.D.)

been reviewed elsewhere (77,78), but several important details must be stressed. The catheters should be placed perpendicular to the surgical wound (Fig. 34.34). The implant volume should encompass the resection bed plus a small amount of normal tissue. Schray et al. advocate a 2-cm margin (79). Gemer and colleagues have demonstrated that the implant volume must exceed the tumor volume whether or not the implant is supplemented by external beam radiotherapy (80). The radiation oncologist must ensure uniform implant geometry both during the direct placement of silastic catheters and when the wound is closed. Iridium-192 is the isotope of choice and the implant should deliver ~20 Gy. Afterloading should be delayed until at least postoperative day 3 to 5 to decrease the chance of major wound morbidity (79,81). The skin dose should be monitored by TLD and should be less than 20 Gy (79). Although brachytherapy to a dose of 45 Gy has been employed as sole adjuvant therapy for *de novo* soft-tissue sarcomas, this approach cannot be advised.

COMPLICATIONS

Serious acute complications of adjuvant irradiation are unlikely in the setting of limb salvage therapy. Dry desquamation and skin erythema are frequent but manageable with standard topical measures. In the Canadian NCI trial, grade ≥ 2 skin toxicity was recorded in 36% in the preoperative group and 68% in the postoperative group ($p < 0.0001$). Severe moist desquamation requiring an interruption of radiotherapy occurs in <5% of cases (72). Gastrointestinal/genitourinary reactions are possible if the superior border of the field extends into the pelvis for sarcomas of the groin or proximal thigh musculature. Delayed wound healing occurs to some degree in 20% to 34% following resection alone (20–22,32,82,83). Severe disturbance of wound healing occurs in 6% to 10% following surgery alone. The incidence of severe wound healing complications does not appear to be increased by postoperative radiotherapy. Mundt and colleagues reported a 3% rate of RTOG grades 3 to 4 wound healing complications with the postoperative therapy (40). Wound complications following preoperative irradiation are greater than after surgery alone or postoperative treatment, a fact confirmed by the Canadian NCI randomized trial. The rate of wound complications was 35% in the preoperative group compared to 17% in the postoperative patients ($p = 0.01$). A second operation was required due to wound complications in 16% of the preoperative group compared to 12% in the postoperative group. The risk of wound complications according to treatment group was associated with tumor location ($p = 0.026$). The rate of wound complications in patients with sarcomas of the upper leg was 45% in the preoperative group compared to 28% in the postoperative patients. The respective rates among those with lower leg sarcomas were 38% and 5%. Wound complications were unusual in patients with sar-

comas affecting the upper extremity, regardless of radiotherapy schedule. Of 37 total patients with upper extremity tumors, a single wound complication occurred in a preoperatively irradiated patient. Long-term morbidity has not been reported from this trial. There is no apparent impact of neoadjuvant chemotherapy on the incidence of wound morbidity in patients receiving either preoperative or postoperative radiotherapy (84).

Serious late effects are uncommon following either preoperative or postoperative irradiation according to the experience at MD Anderson Hospital (85). In patients presenting with gross tumor, the 10-year actuarial risk of late tissue injury was 9% in those receiving postoperative treatment compared to 5% among those undergoing preoperative radiotherapy ($p = 0.03$). For those patients undergoing re-excision following gross tumor removal elsewhere, the respective risks were 8% and 3% ($p = 0.08$) Late effects are directly related to radiotherapy dose. Mundt and associates demonstrated a statistically significant difference in complication rate between those patients receiving <63 Gy and those receiving ≥ 63 Gy (46). The lower dose group had significantly lower rates of both overall and severe complications than the higher dose group. Soft-tissue fibrosis was related to the volume of irradiation by investigators at the University of Rochester (52). In a group of patients receiving a mean postoperative dose of 59 Gy, significant univariate predictors of fibrosis included peak dose, $V_{50-54Gy}$ and $V_{55-59Gy}$. Investigators at the NCI reported that the incidence of serious late effects was associated with inclusion of >75% of an extremity cross section in the field, field length greater than 35 cm, irradiation across joints, and total dose in excess of 63 Gy (86). Eilber et al. demonstrated a direct relationship between tumor size and late complications (22). This observation is due to the larger resections and radiotherapy field sizes required for bulkier tumors. Late pathologic fracture of a long bone is related both to the use of radiotherapy and removal of the periosteum during definitive tumor resection. Investigators at the Memorial-Sloan Kettering Cancer Center reported an 8.6% 5-year actuarial rate of femur fracture in a group of 205 patients with thigh sarcomas undergoing limb-sparing surgery and radiotherapy (87). Periosteal stripping was the strongest predictor of fracture. All patients with a femur fracture had periosteal stripping. The risk of fracture was 29% among those 54 patients requiring stripping compared to 0% in the group of 151 not requiring this surgical procedure ($p < 0.0001$). There was no significant difference in radiotherapy dose between those with and without fracture. No pathologic fractures were noted in patients undergoing postoperative radiotherapy without antecedent periosteal stripping. In a review of 691 lower extremity soft-tissue sarcomas, Dickie and colleagues documented 31 pathologic fractures (88). Three-dimensional volumetric bone dosimetry was available for 21 of the fracture patients. Maximum bone dose, mean bone dose, and V_{40Gy} were significantly greater among the fracture patients compared to matched controls. The authors suggested that fracture risk could be minimized if radiation dose was kept below the following thresholds: bone maximum dose 59 Gy, mean bone dose 37 Gy, V_{40Gy} 64%.

The use of brachytherapy has been associated with wound complication rates greater than after surgery alone or adjunctive external beam radiotherapy (79). This disturbing finding is related to implant technique. With attention to several details, the rate of serious complications following brachytherapy should be no higher than after teletherapy (79,81). Complications can be reduced by the use of supplemental, external beam therapy and limitation of the implant dose to no more than 20 Gy. The skin overlying the implant should receive <20 Gy and there should be sufficient postoperative delay to loading radioactive sources. Finally, proper wound closure with vascularized tissue flaps is advised.

Despite these late effects, more than 80% of patients receiving pre- or postoperative radiotherapy retain a useful limb. Physical therapy has been shown to enhance long-term functional outcome (89). Although a majority of patients undergoing limb-preserving therapy maintain a functional extremity, quality of life assessments are not always superior to amputated patients (90). Longitudinal studies are required since some specific measurements of quality in salvaged patients show a decrement over time (91).

REFERENCES

1. Jemal A, Siegel R, Ward E, et al. Cancer statistics, 2009. *CA Cancer J Clin* 2010;59:225–249.
2. Lawrence W, Donegan WL, Nataranjan N, et al. Adult soft tissue sarcomas. A pattern of care survey of the American College of Surgeons. *Ann Surg* 1987;205: 349–359.
3. Collin C, Godbold J, Hajdu S, et al. Localized extremity soft tissue sarcomas: an analysis of factors affecting survival. *J Clin Oncol* 1987;5:601–612.
4. Eilber FR. Soft tissue sarcomas of the extremity. *Curr Probl Cancer* 1984;8:1–41.
5. Rosenberg SA, Tepper J, Glatstein E, et al. The treatment of soft-tissue sarcomas of the extremities. Prospective randomized evaluations for (1) limb sparing surgery plus radiation therapy compared with amputation and (2) the role of adjuvant chemotherapy. *Ann Surg* 1982;196: 305–315.
6. Enneking WF, Spanier SS, Lalawer MM, et al. The effect of anatomic setting on the results of surgical procedures for soft parts sarcoma of the thigh. *Cancer* 1981;47:1005–1012.
7. Cantin J, McNeer GP, Chu FC, et al. The problem of local recurrence after treatment of soft tissue sarcoma. *Ann Surg* 1968;168:47–53.
8. Brennhoud IO. The treatment of soft tissue sarcomas—a plea for a more urgent and aggressive approach. *Acta Chir Scand* 1966;131:438–442.
9. Gerner RE, Moore GE, Pickren JW. Soft tissue sarcomas. *Ann Surg* 1975;181:803–808.
10. Yang JC, Rosenberg SA. Surgery for adult patients with soft tissue sarcomas. *Semin Oncol* 1989;16:289–296.
11. Simon MA, Enneking WF. The management of soft-tissue sarcomas of the extremities. *J Bone Joint Surg* 1976; 58:317–327.
12. Shiu MM, Castro EB, Hajdu SI, et al. Surgical treatment of 297 soft tissue sarcomas of the lower extremity. *Ann Surg* 1975;182:597–602.
13. Fletcher, GH. Subclinical disease. *Cancer* 1984;53:1274–1284.
14. Ruka W, Taghian A, Grocoso D, et al. Comparison between the in vitro intrinsic radiation sensitivity of human soft tissue sarcoma and breast cancer. *J Surg Oncol* 1996;61:290–294.
15. Karakousis CP, Emrich LJ, Vesper DS. Feasibility of limb salvage and survival in soft tissue sarcomas. *Cancer* 1988;57:484–491.
16. Leibel SA, Tranbaugh RF, Wara WM. Soft tissue sarcomas of the extremities. Survival and patterns of failure with conservative surgery and postoperative irradiation compared to surgery alone. *Cancer* 1982;50:1076–1083.
17. Lindberg RD, Martin RG, Romsdahl MM. Conservative surgery and postoperative radiotherapy in 300 adults with soft-tissue sarcomas. *Cancer* 1981;47:2391–2397.
18. Pao WJ, Pilepich MV. Postoperative radiotherapy in the treatment of extremity soft tissue sarcomas. *Int J Radiat Oncol Biol Phys* 1990;19:907–911.
19. Suit, HD, Russell WO, Martin RG. Management of patients with sarcoma of soft tissue in an extremity. *Cancer* 1973;31:1247–1255.
20. Brant TA, Parsons JT, Marcus RB, et al. Preoperative irradiation for soft tissue sarcomas of the trunk and extremities. *Int J Radiat Oncol Biol Phys* 1990;19:899–906.
21. Barkley HT, Martin RG, Romsdahl MM, et al. Treatment of soft tissue sarcomas by preoperative irradiation and conservative surgical resection. *Int J Radiat Oncol Biol Phys* 1988;14:693–699.
22. Eilber FR, Giuliano AE, Huth J, et al. Limb salvage for high grade soft tissue sarcomas of the extremity: experience at the University of California, Los Angeles. *Cancer Treat Symp* 1985;3:49–57.
23. Yang JC, Chang AE, Baker AR, et al. Randomized prospective study of the benefit of adjuvant radiation therapy in the treatment of soft tissue sarcomas of the extremity. *J Clin Oncol* 1998;16:197–203.
24. Mazeron JJ, Suit HD. Lymph nodes as sites of metastases from sarcomas of soft tissue. *Cancer* 1987;60:1800–1808.
25. Collin CF, Griedrich C, Godbold J, et al. Prognostic factors for local recurrence and survival in patients with localized extremity soft-tissue sarcoma. *Semin Surg Oncol* 1988; 4:30–37.
26. Ariel IM. Incidence of metastasis to lymph nodes from soft tissue sarcomas. *Semin Surg Oncol* 1988;4:27–34.
27. Shieber W, Graham P. An experience with sarcomas of the sot tissues in adults. *Surgery* 1962;52:295–298.
28. Levyraz S, Costa J. Histological diagnosis and grading of sot tissue sarcomas. *Semin Surg Oncol* 1988;4:3–6.
29. Costa J, Wesley RA, Glatstein E, et al. The grading of soft tissue sarcomas. Results of a clinicopathologic correlation in a series of 163 cases. *Cancer* 1984;53:530–541.
30. Trojani M, Contesso G, Coindre JM, et al. Soft tissue sarcomas of adults: study of pathological prognostic

variables and definition of a histopathological grading system. *Int J Cancer* 1984;33:37–42.

31. Edge SB, Byrd DR, Compton CC, et al. eds. *American Joint Commission on Cancer, manual for staging cancer*, 7th ed. New York, NY: Springer, 2010:291–298.

32. Robinson E, Neugut AI, Wylie P. Clinical aspects of postirradiation sarcoma. *J Natl Cancer Inst* 1988;80:233–240.

33. Suit HD, Mankin HJ, Wood WC, et al. Treatment of the patient with stage M_0 soft tissue sarcoma. *J Clin Oncol* 1988;6:854–862.

34. Kawai A, Woodruff J, Healy JH, et al. SYT-SYX gene fusion as a determinant of morphology and prognosis in synovial sarcoma. *N Engl J Med* 1998;338:153–160.

35. Tomoda R, Seto M, Tsumuki H, et al. Telomerase activity and human telomerase reverse transcriptase mRNA expression are correlated with clinical aggressiveness in soft tissue sarcomas. *Cancer* 2002;95:1127–1133.

36. Oshino Y, Chatyedu U, Haydern D, et al. Altered p53 is associated with aggressive behavior of chondrosarcoma. A long term follow-up study. *Cancer* 1998;83:2324–2334.

37. Mankin JH, Lange TA, Spanier SS, et al. The hazards of biopsy in patients with malignant primary bone and soft-tissue tumors. *J Bone Joint Surg* 1982;64(A):1121–1127.

38. Hau A, Kim I, Kattapuran S, et al. Accuracy of CT-guided biopsies in 359 patients with musculoskeletal lesions. *Skeletal Radiol* 2002;31:349–353.

39. Bland KI, McCoy DM, Kenard RE, et al. Application of magnetic resonance imaging and computerized tomography as an adjunct to the surgical management of soft tissue sarcomas. *Ann Surg* 1987;205:473–481.

40. Chang AE, Maroty YL, Duyer AJ, et al. Magnetic resonance imaging versus computed tomography in the evaluation of soft tissue tumors of the extremities. *Ann Surg* 1987;205:340–348.

41. Demas BE, Heelan RT, Lane J, et al. Soft tissue tumors of the extremity: comparison of MR and CT in determination of extent of disease. *AJR* 1988;150:615–620.

42. Pestanick JP, Turener DA, Charters JR, et al. Soft tissue masses of the locomotor system: comparison of MR imaging with CT. *Radiology* 1986;160:125–133.

43. Manaster BJ: Musculoskeletal oncologic imaging. *Int J Radiat Oncol Biol Phys* 1991;21:1643–1651.

44. Karam I, Devic S, Hickeson M, et al. PET/CT for radiotherapy treatment planning in patients with soft tissue sarcomas. *Int J Radiat Oncol Biol Phys* 2009;75:817–821.

45. Tepper J, Rosenberg SA, Glatstein E. Radiation therapy techniques in soft tissue sarcomas of the extremity-policies for treatment at the National Cancer Institute. *Int J Radiat Oncol Biol Phys* 1982;8:263–273.

46. Mundt AJ, Awan A, Sibley GS, et al. Conservative surgery and adjuvant radiation therapy in the management of adult soft tissue sarcoma of the extremities: clinical and radiobiological results. *Int J Radiat Oncol Biol Phys* 1995;32:977–985.

47. Suit HD, Russell WO. Radiation therapy of soft tissue sarcomas. *Cancer* 1975;36:759–764.

48. Wylie JP, O'Sullivan B, Catton C, et al. Contemporary radiotherapy for soft tissue sarcoma. *Semin Surg Oncol* 1999;17:33–46.

49. Jovanovic D. The influence of radiation on blood vessels and circulation. *Current Top Radiat Res Q* 1974;10: 85–97.

50. Leeds SE. The pulmonary lymph flow after irradiation of the lung of dogs. *Chest* 1971;9:203–207.

51. Ariel IM, et al. The effects of irradiation (external and internal) on lymphatic dynamics. *Am J Roentgenol Radium Ther Nucl Med* 1967;99:404–414.

52. Karasek K, Constine LS, Rosier R. Sarcoma therapy: functional outcome and relationship to treatment parameters. *Int J Radiat Oncol Biol Phys* 1992;24:651–656.

53. Coe MA, Madden FJ, Mould RF. The role of radiotherapy in the treatment of soft tissue sarcoma: a retrospective study 1958–73. *Clin Radiol* 1981;32:47–51.

54. Mantravadi RV, Trippon MJ, Patel MK, et al. Limb salvage in extremity soft tissue sarcomas: combined modality therapy. *Radiology* 1984;152:523–526.

55. Weisenburger TH, Eilber FR, Grant TT, et al. Multi-disciplinary "limb salvage" treatment of soft tissue and skeletal sarcomas. *Int J Radiat Oncol Biol Phys* 1981;7: 1495–1499.

56. Chan MF, Chui CS, Schupak K, et al. The treatment of large extraskeletal chondrosarcoma of the leg: comparison of IMRT and conformal radiotherapy techniques. *J Appl Clin Med Phys* 2001;2:3–8.

57. Hong L, Alektiar KM, Hunt M, et al. Intensity-modulated radiotherapy for soft tissue sarcoma of the thigh. *Int J Radiat Oncol Biol Phys* 2004;59:752–759.

58. Griffen AM, Euler CI, Sharpe MB, et al. Radiation planning comparison for superficial tissue avoidance in radiotherapy for soft tissue sarcoma of the lower extremity. *Int J Radiat Oncol Biol Phys* 2007;67:847–856.

59. Alektiar KM, Hong L, Brennan MF, et al. Intensity modulated radiation therapy for primary soft tissue sarcoma of the extremity: preliminary results. *Int J Radiat Oncol Biol Phys* 2007;68:458–464.

60. Alektiar KM, Brennan MF, Healy JH, et al. Impact of intensity modulated radiation therapy on local control in primary soft-tissue sarcoma of the extremity. *J Clin Oncol* 2008;20:3440–3444.

61. Kinsella TJ, Loeffler JS, Frasco BA, et al. Extremity preservation by combined modality therapy in sarcomas of the hand and foot: an analysis of local control, disease free survival and functional result. *Int J Radiat Oncol Biol Phys* 1983;9:1115–1119.

62. OKunieff P, Suit HD, Proppe KH. Extremity preservation by combined modality treatment of sarcomas of the hand and wrist. *Int J Radiat Oncol Biol Phys* 1986; 12:1223–1229.

63. Selch MT, Kopald KH, Ferriero GA, et al. Limb salvage therapy for soft tissue sarcomas of the foot. *Int J Radiat Oncol Biol Phys* 1990;19:41–48.

64. Talbert ML, Zagars GK, Sherman NE, et al. Conservative surgery and radiation therapy for soft tissue sarcoma of wrist, hand, ankle and foot. *Cancer* 1990;66:2482–2491.

65. Wexler AM, Eilber FR, Miller TA, et al. Therapeutic and functional results of limb salvage to treat sarcomas of the forearm and hand. *J Hand Surg* 1988;13A:292–296.

66. Potter DA, Kinsella T, Glatstein E, et al. High-grade soft tissue sarcomas of the extremities. *Cancer* 1986;58: 190–205.

67. Enneking WF, McAuliffe JA. Adjunctive preoperative radiation therapy in treatment of soft tissue sarcomas: a preliminary report. *Cancer Treat Symp* 1985;3:37–42.

68. Ballo MT, zagars GK, Cormier JN, et al. Interval between surgery and radiotherapy: effect on local control of soft tissue sarcoma. *Int J Radiat Oncol Biol Phys* 2004;58:1461–1467.

69. Schwarz DL, Einch J, Hunt K, et al. The effect of delayed postoperative irradiation on local control of soft tissue sarcomas of the extremity and torso. *Int J Radiat Oncol Biol Phys* 2002;52:1352–1359.

70. Fein DA, Lee WR, Lanciano RM, et al. Management of extremity soft tissue sarcomas with limb-sparing surgery and postoperative irradiation: do total dose, overall treatment time and the surgery-interval impact on local control? *Int J Radiat Oncol Biol Phys* 1995;32:969.

71. Eilber FR, Eckardt J, Rosen G, et al. Preoperative therapy for soft tissue sarcoma. *Hematol Oncol Clin North Am* 1995;9:817–823.

72. O'Sullivan B, Davis AM, Turcotte R, et al. Preoperative versus postoperative radiotherapy in soft tissue sarcoma of the limbs: a randomized trial. *Lancet* 2002;359:2235–2241.

73. Nielson OS, Cummings B, O'Sullivan B, et al. Preoperative and postoperative irradiation of soft tissue sarcomas: effect on radiation field size. *Int J Radiat Oncol Biol Phys* 1991;21:1595–1599.

74. Zagars GK, Ballo MT. Significance of dose in postoperative radiotherapy of soft tissue sarcomas. *Int J Radiat Oncol Biol Phys* 2003;56:473–481.

75. Eilber FC, Rosen G, Eckardt J, et al. Treatment-induced pathologic necrosis: a predictor of local recurrence and survival in patients receiving neoadjuvant therapy for high-grade extremity soft tissue sarcoams. *J Clin Oncol* 2001;19:3203–3209.

76. Kepka L, DeLaney TF, Suit HD, et al. Results of radiation therapy for unresected soft-tissue sarcomas. *Int J Radiat Oncol Biol Phys* 2005;63:852–859.

77. Willet CG, Schiller AL, Suit HD, et al. The histologic response of soft tissue sarcoma to radiation therapy. *Cancer* 1987;60:1500–1504.

78. Shiu MH, Hilaris BS, Harrison LB, et al. Brachytherapy and function-saving resection of soft tissue sarcoma arising in the limb. *Int J Radiat Oncol Biol Phys* 1991;21:1485–1492.

79. Schray, MF, Gunderson LL, Sim FH, et al. Soft tissue sarcoma. Integration of brachytherapy, resection and external irradiation. *Cancer* 1990;66:451–456.

80. Gemer LS, Trowbridge DR, Neff J, et al. Local recurrence of soft tissue sarcoma following brachytherapy. *Int J Radiat Oncol Biol Phys* 1991;20:587–592.

81. Ormsby MV, Hilaris B, Nori D. Wound complications of adjuvant radiation therapy in patients with soft tissue sarcomas. *Ann Surg* 1989;210:93–99.

82. Arbeit JM, Hilaris B, Brevusom MF. Wound complications in the multimodality treatment of extremity and superficial truncal sarcomas. *J Clin Oncol* 1987;5:480–488.

83. Skibber JM, Lotze MT, Seipp CA, et al. Limb-sparing surgery for soft tissue sarcoma: wound related morbidity in patients undergoing wide local excision. *Surgery* 102:447, 1987.

84. Meric F, Milas M, Hunt KK, et al. Impact of neoadjuvant chemotherapy on postoperative morbidity in soft tissue sarcomas. *J Clin Oncol* 2000;18:3378–3383.

85. Zagars GK, Ballo MT, Pisters PWT, et al. Preoperative vs. postoperative radiation therapy for soft tissue sarcoma: a retrospective comparative evaluation of disease outcome. *Int J Radiat Oncol Biol Phys* 2003;56:482–488.

86. Stinson SF, DeLaney TF, Greenberg J, et al. Acute and long-term effects on limb function of combined modality limb sparing therapy for extremity soft-tissue sarcoma. *Int J Radiat Oncol Biol Phys* 1991;21:1493–1499.

87. Lin PP, Schupak KD, Bolovel PJ, et al. Pathologic femoral fracture after periosteal excision and radiation for treatment of soft tissue sarcoma. *Cancer* 1998;82:2356–2365.

88. Dickie CL, Parent AL, Griffin AM, et al. Bone fracture following external beam radiotherapy and limb-preservation surgery for lower extremity soft tissue sarcoma: relationship to irradiated bone length, volume, tumor location and dose. *Int J Radiat Oncol Biol Phys* 2009;75:1119–1124.

89. Lampert MH, Gerber LH, Glatstein E, et al. Soft tissue sarcoma; functional outcome of wide local excision and radiation therapy. *Arch Phys Med Rehabil* 1984;65:47–50.

90. Weddington WW, Saegraves KB. Psychological outcome of extremity sarcoma survivors undergoing amputation or limb salvage. *J Clin Oncol* 1985;3:1393–1399.

91. Chang AE, Steinberg SM, Culnane M, et al. Functional and psychosocial effects of multimodality limb-sparing therapy in patients with soft tissue sarcoma. *J Clin Oncol* 1984;7:1217–1228.

INDEX

Note: Page numbers followed by f indicate figures; those followed by t indicate tables.

17 MeV electron isodose curves, effect of compact bone on, 373f

A

A Practical Manual of Brachytherapy, 326
AAPM. *See* American Association of Physicists in Medicine (AAPM)
AAPM Radiation Therapy Committee Task Group 53 report, 184
AAPM Reports 50, 389
AAPM Reports 74, 389
AAPM Task Group 102, 160
AAPM Task Group 121, 218
AAPM TG40, 59
AAPM TG-43, 520
AAPM TG-51, 389
AAPM TG-72, 389
Abdomen, 554
   radiation-induced toxicity of, 429
ABS. *See* American Brachytherapy Society (ABS)
ABS Cervical Cancer Brachytherapy Task Group, 302
ABS Guidelines Definitive Radiation Therapy
   for cervical cancer HDR intracavitary brachytherapy, 488t
   for cervical cancer LDR intracavitary brachytherapy, 488t
Absolute dosimetry
   in scanned proton fields, 401
   in scattered proton fields, 399–400
Accelerated fractionation, 411
Accelerated hyperfractionation, 411
Accelerator-mounted imaging systems, 10–11
Acceptance testing
   for IMRT, 154
   process proposed IAEA, 154
   in quality assurance, 90–91, 149, 152–154
Acoustic neuroma, isocenters for, 272f
ACR. *See* American College of Radiology (ACR)
Acrylic phantom, contaminated electron ionization, 98f
Active breathing control (ABC) system, 46
   components of, 46f
Acute esophagitis, 428–429
Acute leukemia, 638
Acute lymphoblastic leukemia (ALL), 653–657
   central nervous system irradiation in, 654–655
   clinical overview, 653–654
   indications for irradiation in, 653t
   local recurrence of, 656
   testicular irradiation, 655–656
   total body irradiation, 656–657
   treatment planning, 654–657
Adaptive histogram equalization (AHE), 173
Adjuvant radiation therapy, for prostate cancer, 517
ADT. *See* Androgen deprivation therapy (ADT)

AJCC staging system
   for breast cancer, 609t–610t
   for prostate cancer, 503t
   for thorax cancers, 678t–679t
AJCC TNM staging system
   for bladder cancer, 530t
   for soft tissue sarcomas, 735t
   for testicular cancer, 539t
Algorithms, for treatment planning, 144
   brachytherapy, 110–123
   calculation, 147
   clinical application of, 149
   computer programs for, 147, 147t
   development and implementation, 146–149
   IAEA TRS-430 questionnaire, 148t
   model-based photon dose calculations, 93–108
   radiation database for, 147–149
   radiation therapy process and, 145f
American Association of Physicists in Medicine (AAPM), 13, 115, 144
American Brachytherapy Society (ABS), 487
   selection criteria for partial breast irradiation, 620t
American College of Radiology (ACR), 11
American Society for Radiation Oncology (ASTRO), 144
American Society of Breast Surgeons (ASBS), 620t
Anal cancer, 449–453
   chemotherapy for, 453
   diagnostic evaluation of, 449
   prognosis in, 453
   radiotherapy target for, 450
   treatment options in, 449
   treatment planning of, 449–453
      boost planning, 453
      normal tissue tolerances, 450
      radiotherapy dose in, 450–451
      radiotherapy fields and techniques in, 451–453
      simulation in, 449–450
Androgen deprivation therapy (ADT), 504
Angiography, in cranial radiosurgery, 362–263
Anisotropy function
   Amersham CDCS-M type ^{137}Cs source, 314t
   for Amersham model 6711 ^{125}I seed, 313t
   for Amersham model 200 ^{103}Pd seed, 314t
   for ^{192}Ir source with stainless steel encapsulation, 313t
APBI, 619–620
Applicators
   for cervical cancer intracavitary insertions, 359f
   in HDR brachytherapy, 337
Arm board immobilization, for irradiation of biceps muscle sarcoma, 747f
Arm board support, 68f
Assorted foam wedges, 63f

ASTRO. *See* American Society for Radiation Oncology (ASTRO)
^{198}Au radionuclide, 306–307
Automated image segmentation, of multiple repeat CT data set, 243f
Axial computed tomography image
   from IMRT plan, 516f
   of seminal vesicles, 513f
   of thorax, 172f
Axillary region, 554
Axis percentage depth-dose curves, electron central, 366f

B

Base of tongue cancer, 575, 575f
Beacon transponders, 54–55
Beam coordinate system, in positioning, 51
Beam determination, in 3-DCRT, 179–184
Beam's eye views (BEV), 28, 87f
   display anterior lung field, 179f
   dose distribution, 182f
   of tangential breast, 28f
BED model. *See* Biologically effective dose (BED) model
Belly board, for positioning, 71, 71f
BEV. *See* Beam's eye views (BEV)
Biochemical relapse-free survival (bRFS), 518
Biological equivalent dose (BED)
   basic fallacies of, 422
   caution of, 422
   dose/fractionation, 422
   in high dose-rate brachytherapy, 340–341
Biologically effective dose (BED) model, 412–415
Biophysical indices, in 3-DCRT, 189–190
Bite blocks, 74, 74f
   in head and neck cancer, 563
Bladder, radiation-induced toxicity of, 429–430
Bladder cancer
   bladder-sparing approaches, 531–532. *See also* Prostate cancer
   diagnosis of, 529–531
   dosage in, 535
   fractionation in, 535
   non-bladder sparing treatment approaches for, 531
   overview, 529
   prognosis of, 535
   risk straification in, 529
   RTOG protocols for invasive, 532t
   staging in, 529–531, 530t
   survival rate after radical cystectomy for, 531t
   treatment options for, 531–532
   treatment planning for, 532–535
      pelvic fields in, 533–534
      simulation and, 533
      target volume, 532–533
      Tumor Boost, 534
      whole bladder field in, 534
   treatment technique for, 534–535